Red Bo

2021–2024 Report of the Committee on Infectious Diseases
32ND Edition

Author:

Committee on Infectious Diseases,
American Academy of Pediatrics

David W. Kimberlin, MD, FAAP, Editor

Elizabeth D. Barnett, MD, FAAP, Associate Editor
Ruth Lynfield, MD, FAAP, Associate Editor
Mark H. Sawyer, MD, FAAP, Associate Editor

American Academy of Pediatrics
345 Park Blvd
Itasca, IL 60143

Suggested citation: American Academy of Pediatrics. [Chapter title.] In: Kimberlin DW, Barnett ED, Lynfield R, Sawyer MH, eds. *Red Book: 2021 Report of the Committee on Infectious Diseases*. Itasca, IL: American Academy of Pediatrics: 2021 [page numbers]

32nd Edition
1st Edition – 1938
2nd Edition – 1939
3rd Edition – 1940
4th Edition – 1942
5th Edition – 1943
6th Edition – 1944
7th Edition – 1945
8th Edition – 1947
9th Edition – 1951
10th Edition – 1952
11th Edition – 1955
12th Edition – 1957
13th Edition – 1961
14th Edition – 1964
15th Edition – 1966
16th Edition – 1970
16th Edition Revised – 1971
17th Edition – 1974
18th Edition – 1977
19th Edition – 1982
20th Edition – 1986
21st Edition – 1988
22nd Edition – 1991
23rd Edition – 1994
24th Edition – 1997
25th Edition – 2000
26th Edition – 2003
27th Edition – 2006
28th Edition – 2009
29th Edition – 2012
30th Edition – 2015
31st Edition – 2018

ISSN No. 1080-0131
ISBN No. 978-1-61002-521-8
eBook: 978-1-61002-522-5
MA1024

Quantity prices on request. Address all inquiries to:
American Academy of Pediatrics
345 Park Blvd
Itasca, IL 60143

or Phone:
1-888-227-1770 Publications

The recommendations in this publication do not indicate an exclusive course of treatment or serve as a standard of medical care. Variations, taking into account individual circumstances, may be appropriate.

Publications from the American Academy of Pediatrics benefit from expertise and resources of liaisons and internal (AAP) and external reviewers. However, publications from the American Academy of Pediatrics may not reflect the views of the liaisons of the organizations or government agencies that they represent.

The American Academy of Pediatrics has neither solicited nor accepted any commercial involvement in the development of the content of this publication.

3-358/0421   1 2 3 4 5 6 7 8 9 10

Committee on Infectious Diseases
2018-2021

Yvonne A. Maldonado, MD, FAAP,
    Chairperson
Sean T. O'Leary, MD, MPH, FAAP, Vice
    Chairperson
Ritu Banerjee, MD, PhD, FAAP
Elizabeth D. Barnett, MD, FAAP, *Red Book*
    Associate Editor
James D. Campbell, MD, MS, FAAP
Mary T. Caserta, MD, FAAP
Jeffrey S. Gerber, MD, PhD, FAAP
Athena P. Kourtis, MD, PhD, MPH, FAAP
Ruth Lynfield, MD, FAAP, *Red Book*
    Associate Editor

Flor M. Munoz, MD, MSc, FAAP
Dawn Nolt, MD, MPH, FAAP
Ann-Christine Nyquist, MD, MSPH, FAAP
Adam J. Ratner, MD, MPH
Mark H. Sawyer, MD, FAAP, *Red Book*
    Associate Editor
Samir S. Shah, MD, MSCE, FAAP
William J. Steinbach, MD, FAAP
Ken Zangwill, MD, FAAP
Theoklis E. Zaoutis, MD, MSCE, FAAP

Ex Officio

David W. Kimberlin, MD, FAAP, *Red Book* Editor
Henry H. Bernstein, DO, MHCM, FAAP, *Red Book* Online Associate Editor
H. Cody Meissner, MD, FAAP, Visual *Red Book* Associate Editor

Liaisons

Amanda C. Cohn, MD, FAAP	Centers for Disease Control and Prevention
Karen M. Farizo, MD	US Food and Drug Administration
Marc Fischer, MD, FAAP	Centers for Disease Control and Prevention
Natasha B. Halasa, MD, MPH, FAAP	Pediatric Infectious Disease Society
David Kim, MD	Office of Infectious Disease and HIV/AIDS Policy (OIDP), Office of the Assistant Secretary for Health, US Department of Health and Human Services
Nicole Le Saux, MD, FRCP(C)	Canadian Paediatric Society
Eduardo López Medina, MD, MSc	Sociedad Latinoamericana de Infectología Pediátrica (SLIPE)
Scot B. Moore, MD, FAAP	AAP Committee on Practice and Ambulatory Medicine
Neil S. Silverman, MD	American College of Obstetricians and Gynecologists
Jeffrey R. Starke, MD, FAAP	American Thoracic Society
James J. Stevermer, MD, MSPH, FAAFP	American Academy of Family Physicians
Kay M. Tomashek, MD, MPH, DTM	National Institutes of Health

Staff
Jennifer M. Frantz, MPH

Collaborators

Francisca Abanyie, MD, MPH, Centers for Disease Control and Prevention, Atlanta, GA

Mark J. Abzug, MD, University of Colorado School of Medicine and Children's Hospital Colorado, Aurora, CO

Anna M. Acosta, MD, Centers for Disease Control and Prevention, Atlanta, GA

Edward P. Acosta, PharmD, University of Alabama at Birmingham, Birmingham, AL

Paula Ehrlich Agger, MD, MPH, Food and Drug Administration, Silver Spring, MD

Ibne Karim Ali, PhD, Centers for Disease Control and Prevention, Atlanta, GA

Maria C. Allende, MD, Food and Drug Administration, Silver Spring, MD

Evan J. Anderson, MD, Emory University School of Medicine, Atlanta, GA

Jon Kim Andrus, MD, University of Colorado, Denver, CO, and George Washington University, Washington, DC

Kristina M. Angelo, DO, MPH&TM, Centers for Disease Control and Prevention, Atlanta, GA

Grace Dufie Appiah, MD, Centers for Disease Control and Prevention, Atlanta, GA

Paige A. Armstrong, MD, MHS, Centers for Disease Control and Prevention, Atlanta, GA

Stephen S. Arnon, MD, MPH, California Department of Public Health, Richmond, CA

Naomi E. Aronson, MD, Uniformed Services University of the Health Sciences, Bethesda, MD

David M. Asher, MD, Food and Drug Administration, Silver Spring, MD

Negar Ashouri, MD, CHOC Children's Hospital, Orange, CA

T. Prescott Atkinson, MD, PhD, University of Alabama at Birmingham, Birmingham, AL

Rachael D. Aubert, PhD, Centers for Disease Control and Prevention, Atlanta, GA

Laura Bachmann, MD, MPH, Centers for Disease Control and Prevention, Atlanta, GA

Lorraine Backer, PhD, MPH, Centers for Disease Control and Prevention, Chamblee, GA

John W. Baddley, MD, MSPH, University of Maryland, Baltimore, MD

Bethany Baer, MD, Food and Drug Administration, Silver Spring, MD

Gerri Baer, MD, Food and Drug Administration, Silver Spring, MD

Carol J. Baker, MD, University of Texas Health Science Center, McGovern Medical School, Houston, TX

Robert S. Baltimore, MD, Yale School of Medicine, New Haven, CT

Ana Cecilia Bardossy, MD, Centers for Disease Control and Prevention, Atlanta, GA

Margaret Bash, MD, MPH, Food and Drug Administration, Silver Spring, MD

Melisse S. Baylor, MD, Food and Drug Administration, Silver Spring, MD

Judy A. Beeler, MD, Food and Drug Administration, Silver Spring, MD

Karlyn D. Beer, MS, PhD, Centers for Disease Control and Prevention, Atlanta, GA

Ermias Belay, MD, Centers for Disease Control and Prevention, Atlanta, GA

Yodit Belew, MD, Food and Drug Administration, Silver Spring, MD

Melissa Bell, MSc, Centers for Disease Control and Prevention, Atlanta, GA

Tanvir Bell, MD, FACP, FIDSA, Food and Drug Administration, Gaithersburg, MD

Roy Benaroch, MD, Emory University, Dunwoody, GA

Ivan Benavides, MD, Universidad del Valle, Cali, Valle, Columbia

Kaitlin Benedict, MPH, Centers for Disease Control and Prevention, Atlanta, GA
William E. Benitz, MD, Stanford University School of Medicine, Palo Alto, CA
Stephanie R. Bialek, MD, MPH, Centers for Disease Control and Prevention, Atlanta, GA
Holly Biggs, MD, MPH, Centers for Disease Control and Prevention, Atlanta, GA
Jessica Biggs, PharmD, BCPPS, University of Maryland Medical Center, Baltimore, MD
Alison M. Binder, MS, Centers for Disease Control and Prevention, Atlanta, GA
Danae Bixler, MD, MPD, Centers for Disease Control and Prevention, Brookhaven, GA
David D. Blaney, MD, MPH, Centers for Disease Control and Prevention, Atlanta, GA
Karen C. Bloch, MD, MPH, Vanderbilt University Medical Center, Nashville, TN
Juri Boguniewicz, MD, University of Colorado School of Medicine, Aurora, CO
Michael A. Bolaris, MD, Harbor-UCLA Medical Center, Torrance, CA
Suresh B. Boppana, MD, University of Alabama at Birmingham, Birmingham, AL
Anna Bowen, MD, MPH, Centers for Disease Control and Prevention, Atlanta, GA
William Alfred Bower, MD, Centers for Disease Control and Prevention, Atlanta, GA
Thomas G. Boyce, MD, MPH, Levine Children's Hospital, Charlotte, NC
John S. Bradley, MD, University of California San Diego/Rady Children's Hospital San Diego, San Diego, CA
Joseph S. Bresee, MD, Centers for Disease Control and Prevention, Atlanta, GA
Karen R. Broder, MD, Centers for Disease Control and Prevention, Atlanta, GA
Samantha Anne Brokenshire, PharmD, Monroe Carell Jr. Children's Hospital at Vanderbilt, Nashville, TN
Patricia C. Brown, MD, Food and Drug Administration, Silver Spring, MD
Kevin E. Brown, MD, MRCP FRCPath, Public Health England, London, England
Sarah K. Browne, MD, Food and Drug Administration, Silver Spring, MD
Beau B. Bruce, MD, PhD, Centers for Disease Control and Prevention, Atlanta, GA
Gale R. Burstein, MD, MPH, Erie County Department of Health, Buffalo, NY
Diego H. Caceres, BSc, MSc, Centers for Disease Control and Prevention, Atlanta, GA
Susan B. Cali, MSN, RN, MHA, Centers for Disease Control and Prevention, Conyers, GA
Angela J. P. Campbell, MD, MPH, Centers for Disease Control and Prevention, Atlanta, GA
Doug Campos-Outcalt, MD, MPA, University of Arizona, College of Public Health, Phoeniz, AZ
Maria Cano, MD, MPH, Centers for Disease Control and Prevention, Atlanta, GA
Paul T. Cantey, MD, MPH, Centers for Disease Control and Prevention, Atlanta, GA
Joseph B. Cantey, MD, MPH, University of Texas Health San Antonio, San Antonio, TX
Michael Cappello, MD, Yale School of Medicine, New Haven, CT
Cristina V. Cardemil, MD, MPH, Centers for Disease Control and Prevention, Atlanta, GA
Jessica R. Cataldi, MD, MSCS, University of Colorado School of Medicine, Denver, CO
Robert M. Centor, MD, University of Alabama at Birmingham, Birmingham, AL
Ellen Gould Chadwick, MD, Northwestern University Feinberg School of Medicine, Ann & Robert H. Lurie Children's Hospital of Chicago, Chicago, IL
Rana Chakraborty, MD, MSc, FRCPCH, DPhil (Oxon), Mayo Clinic Alix School of Medicine, Rochester, MN

Kirk M. Chan-Tack, MD, Food and Drug Administration, Silver Spring, MD
Kevin Chatham-Stephens, MD, MPH, Centers for Disease Control and Prevention, Chamblee, GA
Rana Chattopadhyay, PhD, Food and Drug Administration, Silver Spring, MD
Sofia Chaudhry, MD, Food and Drug Administration, Silver Spring, MD
Michelle Chen, BA, Cohen Children's Medical Center of New York, New Hyde Park, NY
Cara Cherry, DVM, MPH, Centers for Disease Control and Prevention, Atlanta, GA
Dena Cherry-Brown, MPH, Centers for Disease Control and Prevention, Decatur, GA
Preeti Chhabra, PhD, Centers for Disease Control and Prevention, Atlanta, GA
Mary Choi, MD, MPH, Centers for Disease Control and Prevention, Atlanta, GA
Nancy A. Chow, PhD, Centers for Disease Control and Prevention, Atlanta, GA
John C. Christenson, MD, Indiana University School of Medicine, Indianapolis, IN
Paul R. Cieslak, MD, Oregon Health Authority, Portland, OR
Kevin L. Clark, MD, Food and Drug Administration, Silver Spring, MD
Susan E. Coffin, MD, MPH, Children's Hospital of Philadelphia, Philadelphia, PA
Mark L. Cohen, MD, Case Western Reserve University, Cleveland, OH
Jennifer P. Collins, MD, MSc, Centers for Disease Control and Prevention, Decatur, GA
Joseph Wayne Conlan, BSc, PhD, National Research Council, Ottawa, Ontario, Canada
Roxanne Connelly, PhD, Centers for Disease Control and Prevention, Fort Collins, CO
Despina G. Contopoulos-Ioannidis, MD, Stanford University School of Medicine, Stanford, CA
Laura A. Cooley, MD, MPHTM, Centers for Disease Control and Prevention, Atlanta, GA
Jennifer Rittenhouse Cope, MD, MPH, Centers for Disease Control and Prevention, Atlanta, GA
Margaret M. Cortese, MD, Centers for Disease Control and Prevention, Atlanta, GA
Lisa A. Cosgrove, MD, FAAP, Jacksonville, FL
Tamera Coyne-Beasley, MD, MPH, University of Alabama Birmingham, Children's of Alabama, Birmingham, AL
Sue E. Crawford, PhD, Baylor College of Medicine, Houston, TX
Matthew Brian Crist, MD, MPH, Centers for Disease Control and Prevention, Atlanta, GA
Richard N. Danila, PhD, MPH, Minnesota Department of Health, St. Paul, MN
Toni A. Darville, MD, University of North Carolina School of Medicine, Chapel Hill, NC
Shom Dasgupta-Tsinikas, MD, Harbor-UCLA Medical Center & Los Angeles County TB Control Program, Torrance, CA
Alma C. Davidson, MD, Food and Drug Administration, Silver Spring, MD
Roberta Lynn DeBiasi, MD, MS, Children's National Health System/The George Washington University School of Medicine and Health Sciences, Washington, DC
Mark R. Denison, MD, Vanderbilt University Medical Center, Nashville, TN
Sheila Dollard, PhD, Centers for Disease Control and Prevention, Atlanta, GA
Kenneth Dominguez, MD, MPH, Centers for Disease Control and Prevention, Atlanta, GA
Dorothy E. Dow, MD, MSc, Duke University Medical Center, Durham, NC
Naomi A. Drexler, MPH, Centers for Disease Control and Prevention, Atlanta, GA

Christine L. Dubray, MD, MSc, Centers for Disease Control and Prevention, Atlanta, GA

Jeffrey S. Duchin, MD, Public Health - Seattle & King County and the University of Washington, Seattle, WA

Jonathan Duffy, MD, MPH, Centers for Disease Control and Prevention, Atlanta, GA

Diana Dunnigan, MD, Native Health, Phoenix, AZ

Judith K. Eckerle, MD, University of Minnesota, Minneapolis, MN

Morven S. Edwards, MD, Baylor College of Medicine, Houston, TX

Samer El-Kamary, MD, MPH, Food and Drug Administration, Baltimore, MD

Sean P. Elliott, MD, University of Arizona College of Medicine, Tucson, AZ

Mindy G. Elrod, Centers for Disease Control and Prevention, Atlanta, GA

Delia A. Enría, MD, MPH, Scientific Advisor, Pergamino, Argentina

Roselyn E. Epps, MD, Food and Drug Administration, Silver Spring, MD

Guliz Erdem, MD, Nationwide Children's Hospital and the Ohio State University, Columbus, OH

Darcie Lyn Everett, MD, MPH, Food and Drug Administration, Silver Spring, MD

Julia C. Feinstein, BA, Cohen Children's Medical Center of New York, New Hyde Park, NY

Meghan Ferris, MD, MPH, Food and Drug Administration, Silver Spring, MD

Amy Parker Fiebelkorn, MSN, MPH, Centers for Disease Control and Prevention, Atlanta, GA

Doran L. Fink, MD, PhD, Food and Drug Administration, Silver Spring, MD

Theresa Finn, Food and Drug Administration, Silver Spring, MD

Anthony Fiore, MD, MPH, Centers for Disease Control and Prevention, Atlanta, GA

Katherine E. Fleming-Dutra, MD, Centers for Disease Control and Prevention, Atlanta, GA

Gary W. Floyd, MD, FAAP, Keller, TX

Patricia Michelle Flynn, MD, MS, St. Jude Children's Research Hospital, Memphis, TN

Kaitlin Forsberg, MPH, Centers for Disease Control and Prevention, Atlanta, GA

Monique A. Foster, MD, MPH, Centers for Disease Control and Prevention, Atlanta, GA

Sheila Fallon Friedlander, MD, University of California San Diego School of Medicine, San Diego, CA

Cindy R. Friedman, MD, Centers for Disease Control and Prevention, Atlanta, GA

Yasuko Fukuda, MD, FAAP, Pacific Pediatrics, San Francisco, CA

Sara Gagneten, PhD, Food and Drug Administration, Silver Spring, MD

Renee Galloway, Centers for Disease Control and Prevention, Atlanta, GA

Pooja D. Gandhi, MPH, CHES, Centers for Disease Control and Prevention, Atlanta, GA

Amanda G. Garcia-Williams, PhD, MPH, Centers for Disease Control and Prevention, Atlanta, GA

Jay Edward Gee, PhD, Centers for Disease Control and Prevention, Atlanta, GA

Susan Gerber, MD, Centers for Disease Control and Prevention, Atlanta, GA

Anne A. Gershon, MD, Columbia University College of Physicians and Surgeons, New York, NY

Mayurika Ghosh, MD, FACP, FIDSA, Food and Drug Administration, Silver Spring, MD

Francis Gigliotti, MD, University of Rochester School of Medicine and Dentistry, Rochester, NY

Janet R. Gilsdorf, MD, University of Michigan Medical Center, Ann Arbor, MI

Dominique G. Godfrey, BS, MPH, Centers for Disease Control and Prevention, Atlanta, GA

Brittany E. Goldberg, MD, MS, Food and Drug Administration, Gleneg, MD

Ellie J.C. Goldstein, MD, R M Alden Research Laboratory, Santa Monica, CA

Gerardo A. Gomez, BS, BA, Centers for Disease Control and Prevention, Atlanta, GA

Carolyn Virginia Gould, MD, MSCR, Centers for Disease Control and Prevention, Fort Collins, CO

Elizabeth B. Gray, MPH, Centers for Disease Control and Prevention, Atlanta, GA

Christopher Gregory, MD, MPH, Centers for Disease Control and Prevention, Fort Collins, CO

Patricia M. Griffin, MD, Centers for Disease Control and Prevention, Atlanta, GA

Daniel Griffin, MD, PhD CTropMed CTH, Columbia University, New York, NY

Lisa A. Grohskopf, MD, MPH, Centers for Disease Control and Prevention, Atlanta, GA

Alice Y. Guh, MD, MPH, Centers for Disease Control and Prevention, Atlanta, GA

Kriti Gupta, MD, Cohen Children's Medical Center of New York, New Hyde Park, NY

Julie Gutman, MD, MSc, Centers for Disease Control and Prevention, Atlanta, GA

Penina Haber, MPH, Centers for Disease Control and Prevention, Atlanta, GA

Jesse Hackell, MD, Pomona Pediatrics, A Division of Boston Children's Health Physicians, Pomona, NY

Aron J. Hall, DVM, MSPH, Centers for Disease Control and Prevention, Atlanta, GA

Scott A. Halperin, MD, Dalhousie University, IWK Health Centre, Halifax, Nova Scotia, Canada

Davidson H. Hamer, MD, University of Vermont College of Medicine, Boston, MA

Susan Hariri, PhD, Centers for Disease Control and Prevention, Atlanta, GA

Kathleen H. Harriman, PhD, MPH, RN, California Department of Public Health, Richmond, CA

Theresa Harrington, MD, MPH&TM, Centers for Disease Control and Prevention, Atlanta, GA

Aaron M. Harris, MD, MPH, Centers for Disease Control and Prevention, Atlanta, GA

Jason B. Harris, MD, MPH, Massachusetts General Hospital, Boston, MA

Elizabeth S. Hart, MD, Food and Drug Administration, Washington, DC

Joshua D. Hartzell, MD, MS-HPEd, Walter Reed National Military Medical Center, Bethesda, MD

Fiona P. Havers, MD, MHS, Centers for Disease Control and Prevention, Atlanta, GA

Andrew Haynes, MD, Children's Hospital Colorado, Aurora, CO

Jessica M. Healy, PhD, Centers for Disease Control and Prevention, Atlanta, GA

Yosefa Hefter, MD, Food and Drug Administration, Silver Spring, MD

Kristen Nichols Heitman, MPH, Centers for Disease Control and Prevention, Atlanta, GA

Tobin Hellyer, Food and Drug Administration, Silver Spring, MD

Katherine Ann Hendricks, MD, MPH&TM, Centers for Disease Control and Prevention, Atlanta, GA

Adam L. Hersh, MD, PhD, University of Utah, Salt Lake City, UT

Barbara L. Herwaldt, MD, MPH, Centers for Disease Control and Prevention, Atlanta, GA

Maureen Hess, MPH, RD, Food and Drug Administration, Silver Spring, MD

Beth Hibbs, MPH, RN, Centers for Disease Control and Prevention, Decatur, GA
Sheila M. Hickey, MD, University of New Mexico, Albuquerque, NM
Carole J. Hickman, PhD, Centers for Disease Control and Prevention, Atlanta, GA
Susan L. Hills, MBBS, MTH, Centers for Disease Control and Prevention, Fort Collins, CO
Alison F. Hinckley, PhD, Centers for Disease Control and Prevention, Fort Collins, CO
Hiwot Hiruy, MD, PhD, Food and Drug Administration, Silver Spring, MD
Michele C. Hlavsa, RN, MPH, Centers for Disease Control and Prevention, Atlanta, GA
Aimee C. Hodowanec, MD, Food and Drug Administration, Silver Spring, MD
Megan Hofmeister, MD, MS, MPH, Centers for Disease Control and Prevention, Atlanta, GA
Katherine K. Hsu, MD, MPH, Massachusetts Department of Public Health, Boston University Medical Center, Jamaica Plain, MA
Christine M. Hughes, MPH, Centers for Disease Control and Prevention, Atlanta, GA
Joseph P. Icenogle, PhD, Centers for Disease Control and Prevention, Atlanta, GA
Ilan Irony, MD, Food and Drug Administration, Silver Spring, MD
Brendan R. Jackson, MD, MPH, Centers for Disease Control and Prevention, Atlanta, GA
Ruth A. Jajosky, DMD, MPH, Centers for Disease Control and Prevention, Atlanta, GA
Denise Jamieson, MD, MPH, Emory University, Atlanta, GA
Emily N. Jenkins, MPH, Centers for Disease Control and Prevention, Atlanta, GA
Emily S. Jentes, PhD, MPH, Centers for Disease Control and Prevention, Atlanta, GA
John Jereb, MD, Centers for Disease Control and Prevention, Atlanta, GA
Ravi Jhaveri, MD, Ann & Robert H. Lurie Children's Hospital of Chicago/Northwestern University Feinberg School of Medicine, Chicago, IL
Caroline J. Jjingo, MD, MPH, Food and Drug Administration, Silver Spring, MD
Chandy C. John, MD, Indiana University School of Medicine, Riley Hospital for Children at IU Health, Indianapolis, IN
Jefferson M. Jones, MD, MPH, Centers for Disease Control and Prevention, Atlanta, GA
Nicola L. Jones, MD, FRCPC, PhD, Division of Gastroenterology, SickKids, Toronto, Canada
S. Patrick Kachur, MD, MPH, Columbia University Irving Medical Center, New York, NY
Laura H. Kahn, MD, MPH, MPP, Woodrow Wilson School of Public and International Affairs, Princeton University, Princeton, NJ
Alexander Kallen, MD, MPH, Centers for Disease Control and Prevention, Atlanta, GA
Mary L. Kamb, MD, MPH, Centers for Disease Control and Prevention, Atlanta, GA
Saleem S.M. Kamili, PhD, Centers for Disease Control and Prevention, Atlanta, GA
Sheldon L. Kaplan, MD, Baylor College of Medicine, Houston, TX
Ben Z. Katz, MD, Northwestern University Feinberg School of Medicine, Ann & Robert H. Lurie Children's Hospital of Chicago, Chicago, IL
Carol A. Kauffman, MD, VA Ann Arbor Healthcare System, University of Michigan Medical School, Ann Arbor, MI
Susana Williams Keeshin, MD, University of Utah, Salt Lake City, UT
Gilbert J. Kersh, PhD, Centers for Disease Control and Prevention, Atlanta, GA
David L. Kettl, MD, Food and Drug Administration, Silver Spring, MD
Grishma Kharod, Centers for Disease Control and Prevention, Atlanta, GA

Peter W. Kim, MD, MS, Food and Drug Administration, Silver Spring, MD
Charles H. King, MD, MS, Case Western Reserve University, Cleveland, OH
Miwako Kobayashi, Centers for Disease Control and Prevention, Atlanta, GA
Philip R. Krause, MD, Food and Drug Administration, Silver Spring, MD
Kristen Kreisel, PhD, Centers for Disease Control and Prevention, Atlanta, GA
Andrew T. Kroger, MD, MPH, Centers for Disease Control and Prevention, Atlanta, GA
David Kuhar, MD, Centers for Disease Control and Prevention, Atlanta, GA
Adam J. Langer, DVM, MPH, Centers for Disease Control and Prevention, Atlanta, GA
Gayle Langley, MD, MPH, Centers for Disease Control and Prevention, Atlanta, GA
Paul M. Lantos, MD, MS, Duke University, Greensboro, NC
Tatiana M. Lanzieri, MD, MPH, Centers for Disease Control and Prevention, Atlanta,
    GA
Brent Lasker, PhD, Centers for Disease Control and Prevention, Atlanta, GA
Ana Lauer, BS, PhD, Centers for Disease Control and Prevention, Lilburn, GA
Mark E. Laughlin, DVM, MPH-VPH, DACVPM, Centers for Disease Control and
    Prevention, Atlanta, GA
Ralph Eli LeBlanc, MD, MPH, DTMH, PhD, Food and Drug Administration, Baltimore,
    MD
Joohee Lee, MD, Food and Drug Administration, Silver Spring, MD
Lucia H. Lee, MD, Food and Drug Administration, Silver Spring, MD
Myron M. Levine, MD, DTPH, Center for Vaccine Development and Global Health,
    University of Maryland School of Medicine, Baltimore, MD
Stephen Lindstrom, PhD, Centers for Disease Control and Prevention, Atlanta, GA
John J. LiPuma, MD, University of Michigan, Ann Arbor, MI
Lindy Liu, MPH, Centers for Disease Control and Prevention, Atlanta, GA
Eloisa Llata, MD, MPH, Centers for Disease Control and Prevention, Atlanta, GA
Shawn R. Lockhart, PhD, Centers for Disease Control and Prevention, Atlanta, GA
Benjamin D. Lorenz, MD, Food and Drug Administration, Silver Spring, MD
Xiaoyan Lu, Centers for Disease Control and Prevention, Atlanta, GA
Carolina Lúquez, PhD, Centers for Disease Control and Prevention, Atlanta, GA
Anna Mandra, DVM, MPH, Centers for Disease Control and Prevention, Atlanta, GA
Mona Marin, MD, Centers for Disease Control and Prevention, Atlanta, GA
Lauri E. Markowitz, MD, Centers for Disease Control and Prevention, Atlanta, GA
Mariel Marlow, Centers for Disease Control and Prevention, Atlanta, GA
Zachary A. Marsh, MPH, Centers for Disease Control and Prevention, Atlanta, GA
Gary S. Marshall, MD, University of Louisville School of Medicine, Louisville, KY
Barbara J. Marston, MD, Centers for Disease Control and Prevention, Atlanta, GA
Emily Toth Martin, PhD, MPH, University of Michigan School of Public Health, Ann
    Arbor, MI
Grace E. Marx, MD, MPH, Centers for Disease Control and Prevention, Fort Collins,
    CO
Sarah R. Maxwell, MD, MPH, University of Colorado, Children's Hospital of Colorado,
    Aurora, CO
Sarah Mbaeyi, MD, MPH, Centers for Disease Control and Prevention, Atlanta, GA
Orion McCotter, MPH, Centers for Disease Control and Prevention, Atlanta, GA
Anita K. McElroy, MD, PhD, University of Pittsburgh, Pittsburgh, PA

Olivia Lauren McGovern, PhD, MS, Centers for Disease Control and Prevention, Atlanta, GA

Susan L.F. McLellan, MD, MPH, University of Texas Medical Branch, Galveston, TX

Lucy A. McNamara, PhD, MS, Centers for Disease Control and Prevention, Atlanta, GA

Michael M. McNeil, MD, MPH, Centers for Disease Control and Prevention, Atlanta, GA

John McQuiston, PhD, Centers for Disease Control and Prevention, Atlanta, GA

Elissa Meites, MD, MPH, Centers for Disease Control and Prevention, Atlanta, GA

Asuncion Mejias, MD, PhD, MsCS, Nationwide Children's Hospital and The Ohio State University, Columbus, OH

Ian C. Michelow, MD, DTM&H, Warren Alpert Medical School of Brown University, Providence, RI

Claire M. Midgley, PhD, Centers for Disease Control and Prevention, Atlanta, GA

Elaine R. Miller, BSN, MPH, Centers for Disease Control and Prevention, Atlanta, GA

Eric Mintz, MD, MPH, Centers for Disease Control and Prevention, Atlanta, GA

John F. Modlin, MD, Bill and Melinda Gates Foundation, Seattle, WA

Tina Khoie Mongeau, MD, MPH, Food and Drug Administration, Silver Spring, MD

Martha P. Montgomery, MD, MHS, Centers for Disease Control and Prevention, Atlanta, GA

José G. Montoya, MD, Stanford University and Palo Alto Medical Foundation Toxoplasma Serology Laboratory, Stanford, CA

Anne C. Moorman, MPH, Centers for Disease Control and Prevention, Atlanta, GA

Pedro L. Moro, MD, MPH, Centers for Disease Control and Prevention, Atlanta, GA

William Moss, MD, MPH, Johns Hopkins Bloomberg School of Public Health, Baltimore, MD

Charu Mullick, MD, Food and Drug Administration, Silver Spring, MD

Barbara E. Murray, MD, University of Texas Health Science Center at Houston, Houston, TX

Oidda Ikumboka Museru, MSN, MPH, Centers for Disease Control and Prevention, Atlanta, GA

Christina A. Muzny, MD, MSPH, Centers for Disease Control and Prevention, Birmingham, AL

Sumathi Nambiar, MD, MPH, Food and Drug Administration, Germantown, MD

Srinivas Acharya Nanduri, MBBS, MD, MPH, Centers for Disease Control and Prevention, Atlanta, GA

Theodore E. Nash, MD, National Institue of Health (Retired), Asheville, NC

James Nataro, MD, PhD, MBA, University of Virginia, Charlottesville, VA

Mark S. Needles, MD, Food and Drug Administration, Silver Spring, MD

Christina Nelson, MD, MPH, Centers for Disease Control and Prevention, Fort Collins, CO

Noele P. Nelson, MD, PhD, MPH, Centers for Disease Control and Prevention, Atlanta, GA

Steven R. Nesheim, MD, Centers for Disease Control and Prevention, Atlanta, GA

Jason G. Newland, MD, MEd, Washington University School of Medicine, St. Louis, MO

Megin Nichols, DVM, MPH, Centers for Disease Control and Prevention, Atlanta, GA

William L. Nicholson, BSc, MSc, PhD, Centers for Disease Control and Prevention, Atlanta, GA

William Allan Nix, Centers for Disease Control and Prevention, Atlanta, GA
Thomas B. Nutman, MD, National Institutes of Health, Bethesda, MD
Steve Oberste, PhD, Centers for Disease Control and Prevention, Atlanta, GA
Tina S. Objio, MSN, MHA, Centers for Disease Control and Prevention, Atlanta, GA
Andrew O'Carroll, DVM, Food and Drug Administration, Silver Spring, MD
Theresa Jean Ochoa, MD, Universidad Peruana Cayetano Heredia, Lima, Peru
Titilope Oduyebo, MD, MPH, Centers for Disease Control and Prevention, Atlanta, GA
Sara E. Oliver, MD, MSPH, Centers for Disease Control and Prevention, Atlanta, GA
Christina M. Osborne, MD, University of Colorado School of Medicine, Aurora, CO
Elizabeth O'Shaughnessy, MB, BCh, Food and Drug Administration, Silver Spring, MD
Gary D. Overturf, MD, University of New Mexico, Albuquerque, NM
Sherry Michele Owen, PhD, Centers for Disease Control and Prevention, Atlanta, GA
Christopher D. Paddock, MD, MPHTM, Centers for Disease Control and Prevention, Atlanta, GA
Mark A. Pallansch, PhD, Centers for Disease Control and Prevention, Atlanta, GA
Lakshmi Panagiotakopoulos, MD, MPH, Centers for Disease Control and Prevention, Atlanta, GA
Pia S. Pannaraj, MD, MPH, Children's Hospital Los Angeles/University of Southern California, Los Angeles, CA
Ina U. Park, MD, MS, Centers for Disease Control and Prevention, Berkeley, CA
Manisha Patel, MD, MS, Centers for Disease Control and Prevention, Atlanta, GA
Sheral Patel, MD, FAAP, FASTMH, FIDSA, Food and Drug Administration, Silver Spring, MD
Nehali Patel, MD, St. Jude Children's Research Hospital, Memphis, TN
Thomas F. Patterson, MD, FACP, FIDSA, UT Health San Antonio and South Texas Veterans Health Care System, San Antonio, TX
Stephen I. Pelton, MD, Boston University Schools of Medicine and Public Health, Boston Medical Center, Boston, MA
Teresa C.T. Peret, PhD, Centers for Disease Control and Prevention, Atlanta, GA
John R. Perfect, MD, Duke University Medical Center, Durham, NC
Kiran M. Perkins, MD, MPH, Centers for Disease Control and Prevention, Brookhaven, GA
Joseph F. Perz, DrPH, MA, Centers for Disease Control and Prevention, Decatur, GA
Brett W. Petersen, MD, MPH, Centers for Disease Control and Prevention, Atlanta, GA
Amy E. Peterson, DVM, PhD, Centers for Disease Control and Prevention, Atlanta, GA
Andreas Pikis, MD, Food and Drug Administration, Silver Spring, MD
Tamara Pilishvili, PhD, MPH, Centers for Disease Control and Prevention, Atlanta, GA
Ana Yecê das Neves Pinto, MD, Evandro Chagas Institute, Ananindeua City, Pará, Brazil
Paul Joseph Planet, MD, PhD, University of Pennsylvania, Children's Hospital of Philadelphia, Philadelphia, PA
Ian D. Plumb, MBBS, MSc, Centers for Disease Control and Prevention, Atlanta, GA
Nicole M. Poole, MD, MPH, University of Colorado, Aurora, CO
Drew L. Posey, MD, MPH, Centers for Disease Control and Prevention, Atlanta, GA
Ann M. Powers, PhD, Centers for Disease Control and Prevention, Fort Collins, CO
R. Douglas Pratt, MD, MPH, Food and Drug Administration, Silver Spring, MD
Christopher Prestel, MD, Centers for Disease Control and Prevention, Atlanta, GA

Nathan Price, MD, University of Arizona, Tucson, AZ

Gary W. Procop, MD, MS, Cleveland Clinic, Cleveland, OH

Karen M. Puopolo, MD, PhD, Children's Hospital of Philadelphia, Philadelphia, PA

Laura A. S. Quilter, MD, MPH, Centers for Disease Control and Prevention, Atlanta, GA

Shawn L. Ralston, MD, MA, MS, Johns Hopkins Children's Center, Baltimore, MD

Octavio Ramilo, MD, Nationwide Children's Hospital and The Ohio State University, Columbus, OH

Agam Kumari Rao, MD, Centers for Disease Control and Prevention, Atlanta, GA

Anuja Rastogi, MD, MHS, Food and Drug Administration, Silver Spring, MD

Mobeen Hasan Rathore, MD, University of Florida Center for AIDS/HIV, Research, Education and Service, Jacksonville, FL

Logan C. Ray, MPH, Centers for Disease Control and Prevention, Atlanta, GA

Sujan C. Reddy, Centers for Disease Control and Prevention, Atlanta, GA

Susan Reef, MD, Centers for Disease Control and Prevention, Atlanta, GA

Rebecca Reindel, MD, Food and Drug Administration, Silver Spring, MD

Hilary E. Reno, MD, PhD, Centers for Disease Control and Prevention, Saint Louis, MO

Melissa Reyes, MD, MPH, DTMH, Food and Drug Administration, Silver Spring, MD

Brian Rha, MD, MSPH, Centers for Disease Control and Prevention, Atlanta, GA

Frank Richards, Jr., MD, The Carter Center, Atlanta, GA

Nicholas Rister, MD, Food and Drug Administration, Fort Worth, TX

Virginia A. Roberts, MSPH, Centers for Disease Control and Prevention, Atlanta, GA

Jeff Roberts, MD, Food and Drug Administration, Silver Spring, MD

Candice L. Robinson, MD, MPH, Centers for Disease Control and Prevention, Atlanta, GA

Joan L. Robinson, MD, FRCPC, University of Alberta, Edmonton, Alberta, Canada

Martin Rodriguez, MD, University of Alabama at Birmingham, Birmingham, AL

Dawn M. Roellig, MS, PhD, Centers for Disease Control and Prevention, Atlanta, GA

José R. Romero, MD, University of Arkansas for Medical Sciences and Arkansas Children's Hospital, Little Rock, AR

Shannon Ross, MD, MSPH, The University of Alabama at Birmingham, Birmingham, AL

John Alden Rossow, DVM, MPH, Centers for Disease Control and Prevention, Decatur, GA

Janell A. Routh, MD, MHS, Centers for Disease Control and Prevention, Atlanta, GA

Anne H. Rowley, MD, Northwestern University Feinberg School of Medicine, Ann & Robert H. Lurie Children's Hospital of Chicago, Chicago, IL

Sharon L. Roy, MD, MPH, Centers for Disease Control and Prevention, Atlanta, GA

Lorry G. Rubin, MD, Steven and Alexandra Cohen Children's Medical Center of New York, New Hyde Park, NY

A. Blythe Ryerson, PhD, MPH, Centers for Disease Control and Prevention, Atlanta, GA

Hari Cheryl Sachs, MD, Food and Drug Administration, Silver Spring, MD

Johanna S. Salzer, DVM, PhD, Centers for Disease Control and Prevention, Atlanta, GA

Hugh A. Sampson, BA, MD, Icahn School of Medicine at Mount Sinai, New York, NY

Sara R. Saporta-Keating, MD, MS, Children's Hospital Colorado, Aurora, CO

Kim Sapsford-Medintz, PhD, Food and Drug Administration, Silver Spring, MD

Jason B. Sauberan, PharmD, Neonatal Research Institute, Sharp Mary Birch Hospital for Women and Newborns, San Diego, CA

Christian J. Sauder, PhD, Food and Drug Administration, Silver Spring, MD

Ilana J. Schafer, DVM, MSPH, Centers for Disease Control and Prevention, Atlanta, GA

Sarah Schillie, MD, MPH, MBA, Centers for Disease Control and Prevention, Atlanta, GA

Julia Ann Schillinger, MD, MSc, Centers for Disease Control and Prevention, New York, NY

D. Scott Schmid, PhD, Centers for Disease Control and Prevention, Atlanta, GA

Eileen Schneider, MD, MPH, Centers for Disease Control and Prevention, Stone Mountain, GA

Stacey Schultz-Cherry, PhD, St. Jude Children's Research Hospital, Memphis, TN

Gordon E. Schutze, MD, Baylor College of Medicine, Houston, TX

Ann T. Schwartz, MD, Food and Drug Administration, Gaithersburg, MD

Justin B. Searns, MD, University of Colorado School of Medicine, Aurora, CO

W. Evan Secor, PhD, Centers for Disease Control and Prevention, Atlanta, GA

Isaac See, MD, Centers for Disease Control and Prevention, Atlanta, GA

Andi L. Shane, MD, MPH, MSc, Emory University School of Medicine and Children's Healthcare of Atlanta, Atlanta, GA

Virginia M.W. Sheikh, MD, MHS, Food and Drug Administration, Silver Spring, MD

Margaret Sherin, BA, Cohen Children's Medical Center of New York, New Hyde Park, NY

Tom T. Shimabukuro, MD, MPH, MBA, Centers for Disease Control and Prevention, Atlanta, GA

Azadeh Shoaibi, PhD, MHS, Food and Drug Administration, Silver Spring, MD

Trevor R. Shoemaker, PhD, MPH, Centers for Disease Control and Prevention, Atlanta, GA

Timothy R. Shope, MD, MPH, Children's Hospital of Pittsburgh of UPMC, Pittsburgh, PA

Stanford T. Shulman, MD, Ann & Robert H. Lurie Children's Hospital of Chicago, Chicago, IL

Scott H. Sicherer, MD, Icahn School of Medicine at Mount Sinai, New York, NY

Benjamin Silk, PhD, Centers for Disease Control and Prevention, Atlanta, GA

Rosalyn J. Singleton, MD, MPH, Alaska Native Tribal Health Consortium, Anchorage, AK

Anders Sjöstedt, MD, PhD, Umeå University, Umeå, Sweden

Tami H. Skoff, MS, Centers for Disease Control and Prevention, Atlanta, GA

Thomas Smith, MD, Food and Drug Administration, Silver Spring, MD

Heidi L. Smith, MD, PhD, Food and Drug Administration, Silver Spring, MD

Thomas D. Smith, MD, Food and Drug Administration, Silver Spring, MD

P. Brian Smith, MD, MPH, MHS, Duke University Medical Center, Durham, NC

Kirk Smith, DVM, MS, PhD, Minnesota Department of Health, St Paul, MN

Sunil Kumar Sood, MD, Cohen Children's & Southside Hospitals, Northwell Health, Bay Shore, NY

Paul W. Spearman, MD, Cincinnati Children's Hospital, Cincinnati, OH

Stanley M. Spinola, MD, Indiana University School of Medicine, Indianapolis, IN
Philip R. Spradling, MD, Centers for Disease Control and Prevention, Atlanta, GA
Sancta B. St. Cyr, MD, MPH, Centers for Disease Control and Prevention, Atlanta, GA
Mary Allen Staat, MD, MPH, Cincinnati Children's Hospital Medical Center, Cincinnati,
    OH
J. Erin Staples, MD, PhD, Centers for Disease Control and Prevention, Fort Collins, CO
William M. Stauffer, MD, MSPH, University of Minnesota, Lake Elmo, MN
Irving Steinberg, PharmD, University of Southern California, Schools of Pharmacy and
    Medicine, Los Angeles, CA
David S. Stephens, MD, Emory University School of Medicine, Atlanta, GA
Shannon Stokley, DrPH, MPH, Centers for Disease Control and Prevention, Atlanta, GA
Anne M. Straily, DVM, MPH, Centers for Disease Control and Prevention, Atlanta, GA
Tara W. Strine, MPH, PhD, Centers for Disease Control and Prevention, Atlanta, GA
Nancy A. Strockbine, PhD, Centers for Disease Control and Prevention, Atlanta, GA
John R. Su, MD, PhD, MPH, Centers for Disease Control and Prevention, Atlanta, GA
Maria E. Negron Sureda, DVM, PhD, MS, Centers for Disease Control and Prevention,
    Atlanta, GA
Adam M. Szewc, BS, SM(ASCP), MB, QLS, Centers for Disease Control and Prevention,
    Atlanta, GA
Peter G. Szilagyi, MD, UCLA School of Medicine, Los Angeles, CA
Danielle M. Tack, DVM, MPVM, Centers for Disease Control and Prevention, Atlanta,
    GA
Pranita D. Tamma, MD, MHS, Johns Hopkins University School of Medicine, Ellicott
    City, MD
Kathrine R. Tan, MD, MPH, Centers for Disease Control and Prevention, Atlanta, GA
Gillian Taormina, DO, MS, Food and Drug Administration, Silver Spring, MD
Cheryl Tarr, Centers for Disease Control and Prevention, Atlanta, GA
Edna Termilus, MD, MPH, Food and Drug Administration, Washington, DC
Eyasu Habtu Teshale, MD, Centers for Disease Control and Prevention, Atlanta, GA
Brenda L. Tesini, MD, University of Rochester, Rochester, NY
Alan T.N. Tita, MD, PhD, University of Alabama at Birmingham, Birmingham, AL
Tejpratap S.P. Tiwari, MD, Centers for Disease Control and Prevention, Atlanta, GA
Melissa Tobin-D'Angelo, MD, MPH, Georgia Department of Public Health, Atlanta, GA
Mitsuru Toda, PhD, Centers for Disease Control and Prevention, Atlanta, GA
Rita M. Traxler, MHS, Centers for Disease Control and Prevention, Atlanta, GA
Sean R. Trimble, MPH, Centers for Disease Control and Prevention, Atlanta, GA
Stephanie Troy, MD, Food and Drug Administration, Silver Spring, MD
Richard W. Truman, PhD, LSU School of Veterinary Medicine, Baton Rouge, LA
Ronald B. Turner, MD, University of Virginia School of Medicine, Charlottesville, VA
Elizabeth R. Unger, PhD, MD, Centers for Disease Control and Prevention, Atlanta, GA
Chris A. Van Beneden, MD, MPH, Centers for Disease Control and Prevention, Altanta,
    GA
John A. Vanchiere, MD, PhD, Louisiana State University, Health Sciences Center,
    Shreveport, LA
Antonio Vieira, DVM, MPH, PhD, Centers for Disease Control and Prevention, Atlanta,
    GA

Joseph M. Vinetz, MD, Yale University School of Medicine, New Haven, CT

Jan Vinje, PhD, Centers for Disease Control and Prevention, Atlanta, GA

Prabha Viswanathan, MD, Food and Drug Administration, Silver Spring, MD

Duc J. Vugia, MD, MPH, California Department of Public Health, Richmond, CA

Timothy J. Wade, MD, United States Environmental Protection Agency, Research Triangle Park, NC

Emmanuel B. Walter, MD, MPH, Duke University School of Medicine, Durham, NC

Robin Warner, MD, Union Pediatrics, PSC, Union, KY

Richard L. Wasserman, MD, PhD, Medical City Children's Hospital, Dallas, TX

Stephen H. Waterman, MD, MPH, Centers for Disease Control and Prevention, San Juan, PR

Louise K. Francois Watkins, MD, MPH, Centers for Disease Control and Prevention, Atlanta, GA

John T. Watson, MD, MSc, Centers for Disease Control and Prevention, Atlanta, GA

Michelle Weinberg, MD, MPH, Centers for Disease Control and Prevention, Atlanta, GA

Eric Weintraub, MPH, Centers for Disease Control and Prevention, Atlanta, GA

Mark K. Weng, MD, MSc, FAAP, Centers for Disease Control and Prevention, Atlanta, GA

J. Gary Wheeler, MD, Arkansas Department of Health, Little Rock, AR

A. Clinton White, Jr., MD, University of Texas Medical Branch, Galveston, TX

Hilary K. Whitham, PhD, MPH, Centers for Disease Control and Prevention, Atlanta, GA

Richard James Whitley, MD, University of Alabama at Birmingham, Birmingham, AL

Rodney E. Willoughby, Jr., MD, Medical College of Wisconsin, Milwaukee, WI

Kelly Wilt, MD, Children's Hospital Colorado, Denver, CO

Alison Winstead, MD, Centers for Disease Control and Prevention, Atlanta, GA

Carla Winston, PhD, MA, Centers for Disease Control and Prevention, Atlanta, GA

A. Patricia Wodi, MD, Centers for Disease Control and Prevention, Atlanta, GA

Joellen Wolicki, BSN, Centers for Disease Control and Prevention, Atlanta, GA

Susan K. Wollersheim, MD, Food and Drug Administration, Silver Spring, MD

Karen K. Wong, MD, MPH, Centers for Disease Control and Prevention, Atlanta, GA

Emily Jane Woo, MD, MPH, Food and Drug Administration, Silver Spring, MD

Meklit Workneh, MD, MPH, Food and Drug Administration, Silver Spring, MD

Kimberly Workowski, MD, FACP, FIDSA, Centers for Disease Control and Prevention, Atlanta, GA

Alexandra S. Worobec, MD, Food and Drug Administration, Silver Spring, MD

Mary A. Worthington, PharmD, BCPS, BCPPS, Samford University McWhorter School of Pharmacy, Birmingham, AL

Pablo Yagupsky, MD, Soroka University Medical Center, Ben-Gurion University of the Negev, Herzliya, Israel

Albert C. Yan, MD, Children's Hospital of Philadelphia - Perelman School of Medicine at the University of Pennsylvania, Philadelphia, PA

Carolyn L. Yancey, MD, Food and Drug Administration, Silver Spring, MD

April H. Yarbrough, PharmD, BCPS, Children's of Alabama, Birmingham, AL

Alexandra B. Yonts, MD, Food and Drug Administration, Silver Spring, MD

Jonathan Zenilman, MD, Johns Hopkins University, Baltimore, MD

Rachel Zhang, MD, Food and Drug Administration, Silver Spring, MD

AAP Committee on Bioethics
AAP Committee on Coding and Nomenclature
AAP Committee on Continuing Medical Education
AAP Committee on Drugs
AAP Committee on Fetus and Newborn
AAP Committee on Hospital Care
AAP Committee on Medical Liability and Risk Management
AAP Committee on Native American Child Health
AAP Committee on Pediatric AIDS
AAP Committee on Pediatric Emergency Medicine
AAP Committee on Practice and Ambulatory Medicine
AAP Committee on Substance Use and Prevention
AAP Council on Child Abuse and Neglect
AAP Council on Children and Disasters
AAP Council on Children With Disabilities
AAP Council on Clinical Information Technology
AAP Council on Early Childhood
AAP Council on Environmental Health
AAP Council on Foster Care, Adoption, and Kinship Care
AAP Council on School Health
AAP FamilY Partnerships Network
AAP Payer Advocacy Advisory Committee
AAP Section on Administration and Practice Management
AAP Section on Allergy and Immunology
AAP Section on Breastfeeding
AAP Section on Cardiology and Cardiac Surgery
AAP Section on Critical Care
AAP Section on Dermatology
AAP Section on Emergency Medicine
AAP Section on Epidemiology, Public Health, and Evidence
AAP Section on Gastroenterology, Hepatology, and Nutrition
AAP Section on Hematology/Oncology
AAP Section on Home Care
AAP Section on Hospital Medicine
AAP Section on Infectious Diseases
AAP Section on Lesbian, Gay, Bisexual, and Transgender Health and Wellness
AAP Section on Minority Health, Equity, and Inclusion
AAP Section on Nephrology
AAP Section on Neurology
AAP Section on Ophthalmology
AAP Section on Oral Health
AAP Section on Otolaryngology - Head and Neck Surgery
AAP Section on Pediatric Pulmonology and Sleep Medicine
AAP Section on Rheumatology
AAP Section on Surgery
AAP Section on Uniformed Services
AAP Section on Urology

Committee on Infectious Diseases, 2018-2021

TOP ROW, LEFT TO RIGHT: Ritu Banerjee, Elizabeth D. Barnett, Henry H. Bernstein, James D. Campbell, Mary T. Caserta, Amanda C. Cohn, Karen M. Farizo, Jennifer M. Frantz

SECOND ROW, LEFT TO RIGHT: Jeffrey S. Gerber, Natasha B. Halasa, David Kim, David W. Kimberlin, Athena P. Kourtis, Nicole Le Saux, Eduardo López Medina, Ruth Lynfield

THIRD ROW, LEFT TO RIGHT: Yvonne A. Maldonado, H. Cody Meissner, Scot B. Moore, Flor M. Munoz, Dawn Nolt, Ann-Christine Nyquist, Sean T. O'Leary, Adam Ratner

FOURTH ROW, LEFT TO RIGHT: Mark H. Sawyer, Samir S. Shah, Neil S. Silverman, Jeffrey R. Starke, William J. Steinbach, James J. Stevermer, Kenneth M. Zangwill, Kay M. Tomashek

NOT PICTURED: Theoklis E. Zaoutis, Marc Fischer

2021 *Red Book* Dedication for Louis Z. Cooper, MD, FAAP

Unprecedented. As we continue to move through the coronavirus pandemic that started at the end of 2019 and accelerated throughout 2020, use of this word has skyrocketed not only as it applies to medicine but also in business, politics, the media, and countless other aspects of our everyday lives. Truth increasingly is called into question, and basic facts are disputed to the point where it is challenging to find common language to try to chart our path forward. We truly are living in unsettled and unsettling times, and it can sometimes feel overwhelming and, yes, unprecedented.

But rarely is a given circumstance completely novel. Almost always, we can reach back to an earlier time, with earlier leaders, to learn how challenges were met and ultimately overcome. There is precedent even in the unprecedented. The 2021 *Red Book* is dedicated to such a visionary leader from an earlier era. A man who stared down an earlier pandemic—rubella—and helped lead the world through it in the 1960s. A man who went on to lead the American Academy of Pediatrics (AAP) at the turn of the new millennium, as the world was being forever changed following the September 11, 2001, terrorist attacks. Across all of these decades, Louis Z. Cooper, MD, FAAP, exhibited both the compassion and the determination that we can learn from as we face our current global crisis today. It is for all of these reasons that the 2021 *Red Book* is dedicated to him.

During his residency in Boston, Lou studied penicillin-resistant *Staphylococcus aureus*. After serving in the United States Air Force, he completed a public health service fellowship, during which he worked with Saul Krugman, MD, on development of a rubella vaccine. During this time, the world was immersed in the rubella pandemic of 1964–65. In the United States alone, an estimated 12.5 million people were infected with rubella, 11 000 pregnant women lost their babies, 2100 newborn infants died, and 20 000 infants were born with congenital rubella syndrome (CRS). Literally moving from the bench to the bedside, Lou isolated rubella virus and measured antibody responses in the laboratory while also evaluating hundreds of mothers and infants with CRS. Through these efforts, Lou established the clinical definition, features, and health impacts of CRS.

Realizing that defining the disease and diagnosing the infection were only a part of what was needed, in 1965 Lou founded the Rubella Project with initial funding from a March of Dimes grant and public health department support. The clinic delivered medical and psychosocial care to 300 patients with CRS in the first year alone. The project eventually evolved into a multidisciplinary medical, educational, and social service organization, and laws passed in New York with the strong backing of the Rubella Project later served as examples for a federal special education law.

In addition to service to patients and their families, Lou served the Academy across many years. He was District II Chair, New York Chapter 3 Chair, and a member of the AAP Committee on Child Health Financing and Task Force on Pediatric AIDS. In 2001–02, he was the AAP President, helping to guide our field during another most challenging period following the September 11 terrorist attacks in New York, Washington, DC, and Pennsylvania. In later years, he resumed his work on rubella as a senior adviser of the Measles & Rubella Initiative, a global eradication project supported by the Academy.

Lou died on October 3, 2019, of pancreatic cancer at the age of 87. He did not see this current pandemic, but I believe that we can glean from his lifetime of accomplishments what his advice to us would be. He would tell us to roll up our sleeves, find a way to help, and run the race that is ours to complete. He would tell us to always put our patients at the center of all that we do. He would tell us that, together, all of us can make a difference and change the outcome of this current crisis. After all, when Lou entered Saul Krugman's laboratory, the rubella pandemic had not yet flared, but he was in the right place at the right time, and this, coupled with his passions and energies, changed the course of that pandemic. I believe that Lou would say that nothing is unprecedented—we just need to know where to look to find the guidance from the past to lead us through the challenges of the present.

PREVIOUS *RED BOOK* DEDICATION RECIPIENTS:
2018 Larry K. Pickering, MD, FAAP, and Carol J. Baker, MD, FAAP
2015 Stanley Plotkin, MD, FAAP
2012 Samuel L. Katz, MD, FAAP
2009 Ralph Feigin, MD, FAAP
2006 Caroline Breese Hall, MD, FAAP
2003 Georges Peter, MD, FAAP
2000 Edgar O. Ledbetter, MD, FAAP
1997 Georges Peter, MD, FAAP
1988 Jean D. Lockhart, MD, FAAP

Preface

The *Red Book*, now in its 32nd edition, has been a unique and valuable source of information on infectious diseases and immunizations for pediatric practitioners since 1938. In the 21st century, with the practice of pediatric infectious diseases changing rapidly and the limited time available to the practitioner, the *Red Book* remains an essential resource to quickly obtain current, accurate, and easily accessible information about vaccines and vaccine recommendations, emerging infectious diseases, diagnostic modalities, and treatment recommendations. The Committee on Infectious Diseases of the American Academy of Pediatrics (AAP), the editors of the *Red Book*, and the 500 *Red Book* contributors are dedicated to providing the most current and accurate information available in the concise, practical format for which the *Red Book* is known.

As with the 2018 edition, the print version of the *Red Book* will be provided to every AAP member as part of their member benefit. This commitment reflects the Academy's strong interest in its members' needs. In addition, AAP members also will continue to have access to *Red Book* content on *Red Book* Online (**www.aapredbook.org**). AAP policy statements, clinical reports, and technical reports and recommendations endorsed by the AAP are posted on *Red Book* Online as they become available during the 3 years between *Red Book* editions, and online chapters are modified as needed to reflect these changes. The Outbreaks section of *Red Book* Online is a new resource that concisely summarizes current infectious disease outbreaks that affect the pediatric population and that have been identified in multiple US states; other outbreak types may be covered occasionally as situations warrant. *Red Book* users also are encouraged to sign up for e-mail alerts on **www.aapredbook.org** to receive new information and policy updates between editions.

Another important resource is the visual library of *Red Book* Online, which is continually updated and expanded to include more images of infectious diseases, examples of classic radiologic and other findings, and recent information on epidemiology of infectious diseases. The Committee on Infectious Diseases relies on information and advice from many experts, as evidenced by the lengthy list of contributors to the *Red Book*. We especially are indebted to the many contributors from other AAP committees, sections, and councils; the American Academy of Family Physicians; the American College of Obstetricians and Gynecologists; the American Thoracic Society; the Canadian Paediatric Society; the Centers for Disease Control and Prevention; the US Food and Drug Administration; the National Institutes of Health; the National Vaccine Program Office; the Pediatric Infectious Diseases Society; la Sociedad Latinoamericana de Infectología Pediátrica; the World Health Organization; and many other organizations and individuals who have made this edition possible. In addition, suggestions made by individual AAP members to improve the presentation of information on specific issues and on topic selection have been incorporated whenever possible.

Most important to the success of this edition is the dedication and work of the editors, whose commitment to excellence is unparalleled. This new edition was made possible under the able leadership of David W. Kimberlin, MD, Editor, along with Associate

Editors Elizabeth D. Barnett, MD, Ruth Lynfield, MD, and Mark H. Sawyer, MD. We also are indebted to H. Cody Meissner, MD, for his untiring efforts to gather and organize the slide materials that make up the visual library of *Red Book* Online and are part of the electronic versions of the *Red Book,* and to Henry H. Bernstein, DO, MHCM, for his continuous efforts to maintain up-to-date content as Editor of *Red Book* Online.

As noted in previous editions of the *Red Book,* some omissions and errors are inevitable in a book of this type. We ask that AAP members continue to assist the committee actively by suggesting specific ways to improve the quality of future editions. The committee membership and editorial staff hope that the 2021 *Red Book* will enhance your practice and benefit the children you serve.

Yvonne A. Maldonado, MD, FAAP
Chairperson, Committee on Infectious Diseases

Introduction

The Committee on Infectious Diseases (COID) of the American Academy of Pediatrics (AAP) is responsible for developing and revising guidance from the AAP for management and control of infectious diseases in infants, children, and adolescents. Every 3 years, the COID issues the *Red Book: Report of the Committee on Infectious Diseases*, which contains a composite summary of current recommendations representing the policy of the AAP on various aspects of infectious diseases, including updated vaccine recommendations for the most recent US Food and Drug Administration (FDA)-licensed vaccines for infants, children, and adolescents. These recommendations represent a consensus of opinions based on consideration of the best available evidence by members of the COID, in conjunction with liaison representatives from the Centers for Disease Control and Prevention (CDC), the FDA, the National Institutes of Health, the National Vaccine Program Office, the Canadian Paediatric Society, the American Thoracic Society, the Pediatric Infectious Diseases Society, the American Academy of Family Physicians, the American College of Obstetricians and Gynecologists, *Red Book* consultants, and scores of collaborators. This edition of the *Red Book* is based on information available as of February 2021. The *Red Book* is your own personal infectious disease consultant, on your bookshelf and ready for you 24 hours a day, 7 days a week. Arguably, it is most valuable in those circumstances in which definitive data from randomized controlled trials are lacking. It is in those situations that guidance from experts in the field is most critical, and the COID has literally hundreds of years of cumulative expertise to bring to bear on such recommendations.

Preparation of the *Red Book* is a team effort in the truest sense of the term. Within weeks following the publication of each *Red Book* edition, all *Red Book* chapters are sent for updates to primary reviewers who are leading national and international experts in their specific areas. For the 2021 *Red Book*, one third of primary reviewers were new to this process, ensuring that the most up-to-date information has been included in this new edition. Following review by the primary reviewer, each chapter is returned to the assigned Associate Editor for incorporation of the reviewer's edits. The chapter then is disseminated to content experts at the CDC and FDA and to members of all AAP Sections, Committees, and Councils that agree to review specific chapters for their additional edits as needed, after which it again is returned to the assigned Associate Editor for harmonization and incorporation of edits as appropriate. Two designated COID reviewers then complete a final review of the chapter, and it is returned to the assigned Associate Editor for inclusion of any needed additional modifications. Chapters requiring consideration by the full committee then are debated at the "Marathon Meeting," where the chapters are finalized. Copyediting by the Editor and Senior Medical Copy Editor, Jennifer Shaw, follows, and the book then is reviewed by the *Red Book* reviewers appointed by the AAP Board of Directors. In all, 1000 hands have touched the 2021 *Red Book* prior to its publication! That so many contributors dedicate so much time and expertise to this product is a testament to the role the *Red Book* plays in the care of children.

As with literally everything in the world in 2020, the SARS-CoV-2 pandemic necessitated on-the-fly modifications to the production process. The Marathon Meeting typically is held in person in March of the year prior to publication. With the rolling restrictions on travel during the spring of 2020, the Marathon Meeting initially was pushed to April and then finally changed to a virtual meeting in June 2020. This put us 3 months behind in the production cycle, at a time when pediatricians more than ever needed timely guidance with the management of infectious diseases and when the pediatric infectious diseases experts who are the members of COID were being stretched more thinly than ever before. The responses of the committee members were simply amazing, and quite honestly I have never been more proud to be in the field of pediatric infectious diseases. As a direct consequence of their commitment and that of the AAP Board of Directors reviewers, and the tireless effort of Senior Medical Copy Editor Jennifer Shaw, we were able to make up 3 months of delay to bring this edition to you on time in the midst of a once-in-a-century pandemic.

Through the deliberative and inclusive process that defines the production of the *Red Book*, the COID endeavors to provide current, relevant, evidence-based recommendations for the prevention and management of infectious diseases in infants, children, and adolescents. Seemingly unanswerable scientific questions, the complexity of medical practice, ongoing innovative technology, continuous new information, and inevitable differences of opinion among experts all are addressed during production of the *Red Book*. In some cases, other committees and experts may differ in their interpretation of data and resulting recommendations, and occasionally no single recommendation can be made because several options for management are equally acceptable. In such circumstances, the language incorporated in the chapter acknowledges these differing acceptable management options by use of the phrases "most experts recommend..." and "some experts recommend..." Both phrases indicate valid recommendations, but the first phrase signifies more agreement and support among the experts. Inevitably in clinical practice, questions arise that cannot be answered easily on the basis of currently available data. When this happens, the COID still provides guidance and information that, coupled with clinical judgment, will facilitate well-reasoned, clinically relevant decisions. Through this process of lifelong learning, the committee seeks to provide a practical guide for physicians and other health care professionals in their care of infants, children, and adolescents.

To aid physicians and other health care professionals in assimilating current changes in recommendations in the *Red Book*, a list of major changes between the 2018 and 2021 editions has been compiled (see Summary of Major Changes, p xxxv). However, this list only begins to cover the many in-depth changes that have occurred in each chapter and section. Throughout the *Red Book*, internet addresses enable rapid access to new information. In addition, new information between editions from the COID, in the form of Policy Statements, Clinical Reports, and Technical Reports, are posted on *Red Book* Online (**www.aapredbook.org),** and online chapters are modified as needed with clear indications of where changes have been made. These completed work products are a result of the continuous reassessment by the COID of its current positions across the spectrum of pediatric infectious diseases and demonstrate the dynamic process by which the committee's deliberations always are inclusive of new data and perspectives.

Information on use of antimicrobial agents is included in the package inserts (product labels) prepared by manufacturers, including contraindications and adverse events. The *Red Book* does not attempt to provide this information comprehensively, because it is available readily in the Physicians' Desk Reference (**www.pdr.net**) and in package inserts.

As in previous editions of the *Red Book*, recommended dosage schedules for antimicrobial agents are provided (see Section 4, Antimicrobial Agents and Related Therapy) and may differ from those of the manufacturer as provided in the package insert. Antimicrobial agents recommended for specific infections in the *Red Book* may or may not have an FDA indication for treatment of that infection. Physicians also can reference additional information in the package inserts of vaccines licensed by the FDA (which also may differ from COID and ACIP/CDC recommendations for use) and of immune globulins, as well as recommendations of other committees (see Sources of Vaccine Information, p 0), many of which are included in the *Red Book*.

Likewise, we strive to utilize the accurate terminology for licensure, approval, or clearance of drugs and devices by the FDA. The correct term used depends on the classification of the product (eg, drug, biological product, or device) and, for devices, whether a "premarket notification" or a "premarket application" has been submitted. Drugs are approved by the FDA, biologic products (eg, vaccines, immunoglobulin preparations) are licensed by the FDA, and vaccines are approved for use in certain populations and age groups. The FDA "clears" devices after reviewing premarket notifications, but "approves" devices after reviewing a premarket application. Whether a premarket notification or premarket application needs to be filed depends on the classification of the medical device. "Cleared" devices (also called "510 (k)" or "premarket notification" devices) can be searched at **www.fda.gov/medical-devices/device-approvals-denials-and-clearances/510k-clearances.** Devices@FDA (**www.fda.gov/medical-devices**) is more comprehensive and includes both "cleared" and "approved" tests and other devices. Where we fail in the *Red Book* to select the appropriate term for a given product, we apologize for any (additional) confusion this adds to this regulatory structure.

This book could not have been prepared without the dedicated professional competence of many people. The AAP staff has been outstanding in its committed work and contributions, particularly Jennifer Shaw, Senior Medical Copy Editor; Linda Rutt, Project Specialist; Jennifer Frantz, Senior Manager, who serves as the administrative director for the COID and coordinated preparation of the *Red Book;* Theresa Wiener, Manager of Publishing and Production Services; and all of the directors and staff of the AAP publishing and marketing groups who make the full *Red Book* product line possible.

Marc Fischer, MD, of the CDC, and Karen M. Farizo, MD, of the FDA, devoted time and effort in providing significant input from their organizations. Lisa Cosgrove, MD, Gary Floyd, MD, and Yasuko Fukuda, MD, served as *Red Book* reviewers appointed by the AAP Board of Directors, spending scores of hours reviewing the final chapters for consistency and accuracy. I am especially indebted to the Associate Editors Elizabeth D. Barnett, MD, Ruth Lynfield, MD, and Mark H. Sawyer, MD, for their expertise, tireless work, good humor, and immense contributions in their editorial and committee work. Members of the COID contributed countless hours and deserve appropriate recognition for their patience, dedication, revisions, and reviews. The COID appreciates the guidance and dedication of Yvonne A. Maldonado, MD, COID Chairperson, whose knowledge, dedication, insight, and leadership are reflected in the quality and productivity of the committee's work. I thank my wife, Kim, for always being there and for her patience, understanding, and never-ending support as this edition of the *Red Book* came to fruition.

I also would like to personally thank Mark Del Monte, JD, Chief Executive Officer/Executive Vice President of the Academy, for his calm demeanor and exceptional support throughout what likely is the most stressful year that any of us have ever experienced. His steady hand on the rudder of the AAP directly results in the productivity that we have been able to achieve during these extraordinary times. All pediatricians across the country, and the patients they serve, owe him a debt of gratitude.

There are many other contributors whose professional work and commitment have been essential in the committee's preparation of the *Red Book*. Please forgive any omissions I have made in expressing my gratitude. As stated in the African proverb, if you want to go fast, go alone; if you want to go far, go together. This edition of the *Red Book*, produced in the most unusual and difficult of times, shows just how far we can go, together.

David W. Kimberlin, MD, FAAP, Editor

Table of Contents

SECTION 2
RECOMMENDATIONS FOR CARE OF CHILDREN IN SPECIAL CIRCUMSTANCES

SECTION 3
SUMMARIES OF INFECTIOUS DISEASES

SECTION 4
ANTIMICROBIAL AGENTS AND RELATED THERAPY

SECTION 5
ANTIMICROBIAL PROPHYLAXIS

APPENDICES

Summary of Major Changes in the 2021 *Red Book*

MAJOR CHANGES: GENERAL

1. All chapters in the last edition of the *Red Book* were assessed for relevance in the dynamic environment that is the practice of pediatric medicine today. The School Health chapter was noted to have significant overlap with the Children in Out-of-Home Child Care chapter, so they were merged in the 2021 edition into a single chapter titled **Children in Group Child Care and Schools**. In addition, the Vaccine Injury Table appendix was deleted. Two chapters have been added to the 2021 edition: ***Pseudomonas aeruginosa* Infections** and a new **Systems-based Treatment Table** that is designed to aid in initial antibiotic selections by clinical condition, before the specific pathogen is known.

2. The 2018 *Red Book* had 9% fewer chapters compared with the 2015 edition, and yet the total book was 60 pages longer. As we started work on the 2021 *Red Book*, we therefore identified the 31 chapters that were 10 pages or longer in the 2018 edition, and made a targeted effort to trim them so that all relevant information could more easily and quickly be located. Although some of these 31 chapters (eg, the antibiotic or antiparasitic tables) could not be truncated, we overall achieved our goal by decreasing the 2021 *Red Book* by 41 pages compared with the 2018 edition.

3. Every chapter in the 2021 *Red Book* has been modified since the last edition. The listing below outlines the more major changes throughout the 2021 edition.

4. To ensure that the information presented in the *Red Book* is based on the most accurate and up-to-date scientific data, the primary reviewers of each *Red Book* chapter were selected for their specific academic expertise in each particular area. In this edition of the *Red Book*, 32% of the primary reviewers were new for their assigned chapters. This ensures that the *Red Book* content is viewed with fresh eyes with each publication cycle.

5. Throughout the *Red Book*, the number of websites where additional current and future information can be obtained has been updated. All websites are in bold type for ease of reference, and all have been verified for accuracy and accessibility.

6. Reference to evidence-based policy recommendations from the American Academy of Pediatrics (AAP), the Advisory Committee on Immunization Practices (ACIP) of the Centers for Disease Control and Prevention (CDC), and other select professional organizations have been updated throughout the *Red Book*.

7. Standardized approaches to disease prevention through immunizations, antimicrobial prophylaxis, and infection-control practices have been updated throughout the *Red Book*.

8. Policy updates released after publication of this edition of the *Red Book* will be posted on *Red Book* Online.

9. Appropriate chapters throughout the *Red Book* have been updated to be consistent with 2021 AAP and CDC vaccine recommendations, CDC recommendations for immunization of health care personnel, and drug recommendations from *2021 Nelson's Pediatric Antimicrobial Therapy*.[1]

10. Several tables and figures have been added for ease of information retrieval.

SECTION 1. ACTIVE AND PASSIVE IMMUNIZATION

1. Internet resources for vaccine information have been updated in **Sources of Information About Immunization.**

2. The CDC's new "Vaccinate with Confidence" program, launched in 2019, has been added to the **Discussing Vaccines With Patients and Parents** chapter.

3. The table on "Vaccines Approved for Immunization and Distributed in the United States and Their Routes of Administration" in the **Active Immunization** chapter has been updated to include the newly approved dengue vaccine.

4. The **Vaccine Ingredients** chapter has been restructured to more clearly delineate the excipients that may be present in vaccines.

5. Information on vaccine transport has been expanded in **Vaccine Handling and Storage.**

6. In the **Vaccine Administration** chapter, information on needle length and site of injection for intramuscularly administered vaccines is provided by age group.

7. Sequence and interval between PCV13 and PPSV23 has been added to the section on administration of multiple vaccines in the **Timing of Vaccines and the Immunization Schedule** chapter.

8. A link to the CDC's General Best Practice Guidelines for Immunization document has been added to **Minimum Ages and Minimum Intervals Between Vaccine Doses.**

9. In the **Interchangeability of Vaccine Products** chapter, clarification has been added that if different brands of a particular vaccine require a different number of doses for series completion and a provider mixes brands in the primary series, then the higher number of doses is recommended for series completion.

10. Data have been updated on the small increased risk of febrile seizure when IIV and PCV13 are administered simultaneously in the chapter on **Simultaneous Administration of Multiple Vaccines.**

11. The new hexavalent vaccine to prevent diphtheria, tetanus, pertussis, poliomyelitis, hepatitis B, and invasive disease due to *Haemophilus influenzae* type b, Vaxelis, has been added to the table in the **Combination Vaccines** chapter.

12. A link to the recommended intervals between vaccine doses has been added to enhance discussion of **Lapsed Immunizations.**

13. In the **Unknown or Uncertain Immunization Status** chapter, a statement has been added that serologic testing may not satisfy some school immunization requirements.

---

[1] Bradley JS, Nelson JD, Barnett ED, et al, eds. *2021 Nelson's Pediatric Antimicrobial Therapy.* 27th ed. Elk Grove Village, IL: American Academy of Pediatrics; 2021

14. Table 1.11 (Recommended Intervals Between Receipt of Blood Products and Administration of MMR, Varicella, or MMRV Vaccines) has been significantly revised in the chapter on **Active Immunization of People Who Recently Received Immune Globulin and Other Blood Products.**

15. The listing of the National Academy of Medicine's causality conclusions regarding evidence for a causal relationship between the specific vaccines and other adverse event has been expanded in the **National Academy of Medicine Reviews of Adverse Events After Immunization** chapter.

16. The **Vaccine Adverse Event Reporting System** chapter has updated information on reporting of adverse events.

17. The description of the FDA's active postmarket surveillance system, the Biologics Effectiveness and Safety (BEST) Initiative, has been updated in the chapter **FDA CBER Sentinel Program.**

18. Information about funding and award distribution of the Vaccine Injury Compensation Program has been added to the **Vaccine Injury Compensation** chapter.

19. **Immune Globulin Intramuscular** recommendations for hepatitis A prophylaxis have been updated.

20. In the **Immune Globulin Intravenous** chapter, high-titer polyclonal RSV IGIV preparation has been added, the impact on IGIV on ESR has been added, and availability of an anti-IgA assay has been updated.

21. Utility of **Immune Globulin Subcutaneous** for immunomodulation in autoimmune neurologic conditions has been added.

22. Administration of rotavirus vaccine to patients while still in the NICU has been added to **Immunization in Special Clinical Circumstances.**

23. Discussion of live vaccines and pregnancy, including cholera vaccine, has been expanded in the **Immunization in Pregnancy** chapter.

24. In the chapter on **Immunization and Other Considerations in Immunocompromised Children**, the timing of immunization following resolution of severe immunization has been added. Meningococcal booster dose information for some immunocompromising conditions has been added. Use of penicillin or amoxicillin prophylaxis "can be considered" for duration of eculizumab treatment and until immune competence has returned. And MenQuadfi (meningococcal groups A, C, Y, W conjugate vaccine [Sanofi Pasteur Inc]) has been added.

25. The small increased risk of febrile seizure when IIV and PCV13 or when IIV and DTaP are administered simultaneously has been added to the **Immunization in Children With a Personal or Family History of Seizures** chapter.

26. The CDC link with guidance on vaccinating people with increased bleeding risk has been added to the **Immunization in Children With Chronic Diseases** chapter.

27. The new PRP-OMP containing hexavalent combination vaccine (DTaP-IPV-Hib-HepB) has been added to the chapter on **Immunization in American Indian/ Alaska Native Children and Adolescents.**

28. In **Immunization in Health Care Personnel,** Heplisav-B has been added, and a distinction has been made between numbers of doses for it versus Engerix-B or Recombivax HB.

29. The new dengue vaccine is mentioned in the **International Travel** chapter. Catch-up HepA administration has been added. The option of Heplisav-B for adults is included. Information on yellow fever vaccine has been expanded in the text. And MenQuadfi (meningococcal groups A, C, Y, W conjugate vaccine [Sanofi Pasteur Inc]) has been added.

SECTION 2. RECOMMENDATIONS FOR CARE OF CHILDREN IN SPECIAL CLINICAL CIRCUMSTANCES

1. The human milk chapter has been retitled as **Breastfeeding and Human Milk**. Specific infections during which breastfeeding is not advised have been added. Information on Ebola and breastfeeding has been added. Information on cholera vaccine and breastfeeding has been added.

2. The **School Health** chapter and the **Children in Out-of-Home Child Care** chapter have been merged into the new **Children in Group Child Care and Schools** chapter. Content has been harmonized with the American Academy of Pediatrics' "Purple Book" (*Managing Infectious Diseases in Child Care and Schools: A Quick Reference Guide*, 5th ed. Aronson SS, Shope TR, eds. Itasca, IL: American Academy of Pediatrics; 2019).

3. Respiratory hygiene and cough etiquette have been added to the Standard Precautions section of the **Infection Control and Prevention for Hospitalized Children** chapter, and the chapter has been shortened.

4. CDC guidance on the appropriate use of serologic testing for assessing immunity has been added to the **Infection Control and Prevention in Ambulatory Settings** chapter.

5. The chapter on **Sexually Transmitted Infections in Adolescents and Children** has been restructured and shortened. It also has been harmonized with the CDC 2021 Sexually Transmitted Infections Treatment Guidelines.

6. Hepatitis C testing and malaria screening recommendations for international adoptees have been updated in the **Medical Evaluation for Infectious Diseases for Internationally Adopted, Refugee, and Immigrant Children** chapter.

7. Data on infection risks from discarded needles have been updated in the **Injuries From Discarded Needles in the Community** chapter.

8. Factors increasing risk for penetrating trauma to the cranium have been added to the **Bite Wounds** chapter.

9. Discussion of dengue prevention has been expanded in the **Prevention of Mosquitoborne and Tickborne Infections** chapter, and recommendations for use of insect repellents have been updated.

10. In **Prevention of Illnesses Associated With Recreational Water Use**, incidence data on infections associated with recreational water use have been updated. Information on cyanobacteria has been added. Recommendations on when not to swim in lakes, rivers, and oceans has been added.

SECTION 3. SUMMARIES OF INFECTIOUS DISEASES

1. **Actinomycosis** disease in people receiving biologic response modifiers has been added. The list of alternative antibiotics that can be used has been narrowed.

2. Treatment options for **Adenovirus Infections** are discussed in greater detail.

3. Molecular diagnostics for intestinal **Amebiasis** have been expanded. *Dientamoeba fragilis* epidemiology, diagnosis, and treatment has been added to the chapter.

4. The sequence of diagnostic testing for **Amebic Meningoencephalitis and Keratitis** is provided in greater detail. Miltefosine availability has been updated. *Sappinia* has been removed from the discussion.

5. The clinical manifestations of **Anthrax** have been expanded.

6. Heartland virus has been added to the **Arboviruses** chapter, and Toscana virus has been removed. Dengue and yellow fever vaccine availabilities have been updated. Dosing in adults and booster dose in children for Japanese encephalitis vaccine has been added.

7. Treatment options for ***Arcanobacterium haemolyticum* Infections** are discussed in greater detail.

8. Test of cure assessments of stool following treatment of ***Ascaris lumbricoides* Infections** are presented in greater detail.

9. Discussion of intrinsic and acquired antifungal resistance for **Aspergillosis** has been expanded, including empiric treatment options for areas with high levels of azole resistance.

10. Viral shedding prior to onset of symptoms from **Astrovirus Infections** has been added.

11. The **Babesiosis** chapter has been aligned with the IDSA babesiosis guidelines released in 2020. Diagnostic options and treatment recommendations have been updated.

12. The listing of foods implicated in ***Bacillus cereus*** outbreaks has been expanded.

13. The role of *Gardnerella vaginalis* in **Bacterial Vaginosis** has been updated. Diagnostic options have been expanded.

14. Treatment options for ***Bacteroides, Prevotella,* and Other Anaerobic Gram-Negative Bacilli Infections** have been expanded.

15. Treatment options for ***Balantidium coli* Infections** have been updated.

16. Clinical manifestations of ***Bartonella henselae*** are provided in greater detail. Challenges with some diagnostic tests are discussed.

17. Clinical manifestations of ***Baylisascaris* Infections** are provided in greater detail.

18. Etiologic information on ***Blastocystis hominis*** has been updated.

19. The diagnostic section of the **Blastomycosis** chapter has been updated.

20. Interpretation of diagnostic test results for **Bocavirus** has been expanded.

21. Transmission and serologic detection of ***Borrelia* Infections Other Than Lyme Disease** are provided in greater detail.

22. Serologic testing information for **Brucellosis** has been expanded.

23. Treatment options for ***Burkholderia* Infections** have been updated.

24. Molecular and antigenic testing for ***Campylobacter* Infections** has been updated.

25. Treatment recommendations for **Candidiasis** have been modified.

26. The diagnostic section of the **Chancroid and Cutaneous Ulcers** chapter has been updated, and the chapter has been harmonized with the CDC 2021 Sexually Transmitted Infections Treatment Guidelines.

27. Risk factors for long-term sequelae following **Chikungunya** have been added. Epidemiologic data have been updated.

28. Isolation precautions for *Chlamydia pneumoniae* infections have been updated.

29. Control measures for *Chlamydia psittaci* infections have been expanded.

30. Epidemiologic data for *Chlamydia trachomatis* have been updated. Diagnostic options have been expanded based upon newer tests. Possible need for retreatment of neonatal infection has been added. Timing of test-of-cure in pregnant women has been modified. The chapter has been harmonized with the CDC 2021 Sexually Transmitted Infections Treatment Guidelines.

31. Diagnostic assessment for foodborne **Botulism** has been added.

32. Discussion of when testing is appropriate for *Clostridioides difficile* has been expanded. Fidaxomicin is now approved for use in the pediatric population (6 months of age and older). Bezlotoxumab is approved in adults to reduce recurrence.

33. A recommended sequential approach to diagnostic evaluation of **Coccidioidomycosis** has been added.

34. The **Coronavirus** chapter has been updated to include the worst global pandemic in 100 years, with specific information on SARS-CoV-2.

35. Information on antifungal resistance has been added to the **Cryptococcus neoformans and Cryptococcus gattii Infections** chapter. Timing of antiretroviral therapy after starting induction therapy for HIV-infected children with cryptococcal meningitis, in order to avoid immune reconstitution inflammatory syndrome, has been added.

36. Sources of **Cryptosporidiosis** infection have been updated to incorporate outbreaks in recent years.

37. Treatment options for **Cutaneous Larva Migrans** have been expanded.

38. Sources of **Cyclosporiasis** infection have been updated to incorporate outbreaks in recent years. Treatment options have been expanded.

39. Diagnostic tests for **Cystoisosporiasis** have been updated.

40. Role of race, ethnicity, and nonprimary infections in the incidence of congenital **Cytomegalovirus** infections has been added. The role of human milk in CMV transmission in preterm infants, and its prevention, has been expanded. Specific recommendations from *Bright Futures* for audiologic follow-up in congenital CMV have been added.

41. WHO classification of **Dengue** presentation has been added. Vertical transmission risks have been added. Dengue incidence rates in US states and territories have been updated. Chimeric yellow fever dengue-tetravalent dengue vaccine (Dengvaxia), approved on May 1, 2019, has been added to the chapter, along with detailed discussion of the complexity of determining whether and when to use it.

42. Changes in national reporting implemented in 2019 have been added to the **Diphtheria** chapter.

43. A taxonomy table has been added to the **Ehrlichia, Anaplasma, and Related Infections** chapter. Discussions of *Anaplasma* and *Ehrlichia* have been separated throughout chapter for ease of distinguishing between them.

44. Treatment of carbapenemase-producing gram negative organisms has been expanded in the **Serious Bacterial Infections Caused By *Enterobacteriaceae*** chapter. Discussion of pseudomonal infections has been removed and placed in a new *Pseudomonas* Infections chapter.

45. Discussion of acute flaccid myelitis (AFM) has been expanded in the **Enterovirus (Nonpoliovirus) Infections** chapter. Therapeutic options have been updated.

46. Genetic mutations that impede control of **Epstein-Bar Virus Infections** have been expanded. Rituximab treatment for post-transplant lymphoproliferative disorder (PTLD) has been added.

47. Discussion of atypical EPEC strains has been added to the ***Escherichia coli* Diarrhea** chapter. Challenges interpreting culture-independent diagnostic methods that detect EAEC, EPEC, and ETEC on multiplex panels are discussed.

48. Otogenic and nonotogenic clinical manifestations of infection have been expanded in the ***Fusobacterium* Infections** chapter.

49. Descriptions of clinical manifestations of ***Giardia intestinalis*** have been extensively rewritten. Treatment of recurrent *Giardia* infections has been expanded.

50. The **Gonococcal Infections** chapter has been extensively revised, shortening by approximately one third. Specific dosages of antibiotics largely have been removed from the chapter, with cross-refencing of the STI Treatment Table 4.4 in Section 4. Use of gentamicin in neonates receiving intravenous calcium (in whom ceftriaxone is contraindicated) for prevention of neonatal ophthalmia has been added. The chapter has been harmonized with the CDC 2021 Sexually Transmitted Infections Treatment Guidelines.

51. The evolving epidemiology of Hia has been updated in the ***Haemophilus influenzae* Infections** chapter. The new PRP-OMP containing hexavalent combination vaccine (DTaP-IPV-Hib-HepB) has been added to the chapter.

52. Data on the geographic distribution of **Hantavirus Pulmonary Syndrome** has been added. A diagnostic criteria screening tool has been added.

53. Tables with treatment options for first-line treatment and rescue therapies for children with ***Helicobacter pylori* Infections** have been added to the chapter. The risks for peptic ulcer disease and gastric cancer have been added.

54. The number of viruses mentioned in the **Hemorrhagic Fevers Caused by Arenaviruses** chapter has been expanded.

55. The list of countries with recent outbreaks of **Hemorrhagic Fevers Caused by Bunyaviruses** has been expanded.

56. Discussion of in utero transmission has been expanded in the **Hemorrhagic Fevers Caused by Filoviruses: Ebola and Marburg** chapter. The recent licensure of the first Ebola vaccine, for use in adults, has been added to the chapter.

57. HIV and homelessness have been added as risk groups for **Hepatitis A** infection. The recommendation of catchup immunization with HepA vaccine in people 2 to 18 years of age has been added. Use of HepA vaccine in 6- through 11-month-olds traveling internationally (in whom MMR also is being administered) has been added.

58. The **Hepatitis B** chapter extensively revised, shortening by approximately one quarter. A figure has been added for administration of the birth dose of hepatitis B vaccine by maternal HBsAg status. The new hexavalent vaccine, Vaxelis, has been added to Table 3.21: Recommended Dosages of Hepatitis B Vaccines.

59. Testing recommendations for **Hepatitis C** have been aligned with recommendations from the US Preventive Services Task Force. IDSA and AASLD recommendations for universal testing of pregnant women have been added. Antiviral therapies for HCV infection are now approved and recommended for people 3 years and older.

60. Specific examples of when **Hepatitis D** testing should be conducted have been added.

61. A recommendation has been added to discourage breastfeeding among confirmed **Hepatitis E** virus-infected mothers until further data are available.

62. Clarification has been added that suppressive therapy is not indicated following preemptive antiviral treatment to prevent **Herpes Simplex Virus** exposure at delivery from developing into neonatal HSV disease.

63. Using both urine and blood antigen testing to increase sensitivity of **Histoplasmosis** testing has been added to chapter.

64. Diagnostic methods to increase sensitivity for **Hookworm Infections** have been added.

65. Diagnostic approaches to distinguish chromosomally integrated HHV-6 DNA versus acute HHV-6 infection have been added to the **Human Herpesvirus 6 (Including Roseola) and 7** chapter.

66. Clinical manifestations of **Human Herpesvirus 8** in young children have been added.

67. The **Human Immunodeficiency Virus Infection** chapter has been extensively revised, shortening by approximately one third. The diagnostic approach following perinatal exposure has been summarized in 2 new figures.

68. The **Influenza** chapter has been shortened by approximately one third and harmonized with the most recent AAP and CDC recommendations as well as IDSA antiviral treatment guidelines.

69. Differences in aspirin dosing in the United States versus Japan and Western Europe have been added to the **Kawasaki Disease** chapter.

70. Discussion of antibiotics to use in ***Kingella kingae* Infections** has been expanded.

71. Sources of transmission of ***Legionella pneumophila*** have been expanded, as have prevention strategies.

72. Discussion of post-kala-azar dermal **Leishmaniasis** has been expanded. Worldwide geographic distribution has been updated.

73. Discussion of the varied presentations of the skin lesions of **Leprosy** is provided. Treatment recommendations now reference contact of the National Hansen's Disease Program.

74. Recommendations for convalescent serologic testing for **Leptospirosis** have been broadened.

75. Risks during pregnancy for acquiring ***Listeria monocytogenes* Infections** have been updated.

76. The **Lyme Disease** chapter has been harmonized with 2020 IDSA Lyme Guidelines. Management of partial therapeutic response of Lyme arthritis has been expanded. Options for second tier diagnostic testing have been expanded.

77. Hematologic manifestations of **Malaria** have been expanded. Impact of premature discontinuation of malaria prophylaxis on timing of disease presentation has been added. Quinidine has been removed as a treatment option because it has been removed from the US market. Tafenoquine has been added as a prophylaxis option.

78. **Measles** inclusion body encephalitis has been added. Newer estimates of incidence of SSPE have been added. Immunologic amnesia following measles infection has been added. A new table summarizing postexposure prophylaxis recommendations has been created.

79. Booster dosing for MenB vaccines has been added to the **Meningococcal Infections** chapter. The newly approved MenQuadfi has been added to the chapter.

80. Cross-reference to the AAP clinical practice guideline on bronchiolitis has been added to the management section of the **Human Metapneumovirus** chapter.

81. Treatment options for **Microsporidia Infections** have been expanded.

82. A preferential ranking of treatment options for **Molluscum Contagiosum** has been added.

83. Epidemiologic data on **Mumps** outbreaks among college-aged young adults and people previously receiving 2 doses of MMR vaccine have been updated.

84. *Mycoplasma genitalium* has been added to the ***Mycoplasma pneumoniae* and Other *Mycoplasma* Species Infections** chapter, including diagnosis and treatment.

85. Diagnostic methods for **Nocardiosis** have been updated.

86. Discussion of coinfection with other gastrointestinal tract pathogens has been added to the **Norovirus and Sapovirus Infections** chapter.

87. Moxidectin has been added to the treatment section for **Onchocerciasis (River Blindness)**.

88. Discussion of screening programs for **Human Papillomavirus**-associated cancers has been expanded. Age ranges for use of HPV vaccines have been standardized.

89. Treatment options for **Paracoccidioidomycosis** have been updated.

90. Extrapulmonary manifestations of **Paragonimiasis** in children have been added. Access to triclabendazole has been updated in the chapter.

91. Diagnostic approaches for **Parainfluenza Viral Infections** have been updated.

92. The table of **Parasitic Diseases** has been updated with diagnostic testing and clinical manifestations.

93. The propensity for neurologic sequelae following **Parechovirus Infections** has been emphasized.

94. Management of **Parvovirus B19** in the immunocompromised host has been expanded.

95. The need to assess for rabies prophylaxis when diagnosing ***Pasteurella* Infections** has been added to chapter.

96. The table "Pediculicides for the Treatment of Head Lice" has been updated in the **Pediculosis Capitis** chapter, including the newly approved abametapir by prescription and the availability of ivermectin lotion over the counter.

97. Follow-up assessments and possible retreatment have been added to the **Pediculosis Pubis** chapter.

98. The **Pelvic Inflammatory Disease** chapter has been harmonized with the CDC 2021 Sexually Transmitted Infections Treatment Guidelines. The polymicrobial

nature of PID has been emphasized. Treatment tables have been moved from this chapter and merged into Table 4.4.

99. In the **Pertussis (Whooping Cough)** chapter, allowance has been added for using either Tdap or Td in situations where previously only Td would have been permitted.

100. Treatment of refractory or recurrent **Pinworm Infections** has been addressed.

101. Diagnostic approaches for **Pityriasis Versicolor** have been expanded.

102. Recommendations for management of **Plague** have been harmonized with 2020 CDC guidance. These include recommendations for combination therapy. Treatment of neonates whose mothers have plague also has been added.

103. The epidemiology of **Pneumococcal Infections** in the PCV13 era has been updated.

104. Discussion of prophylaxis for ***Pneumocystis jirovecii* Infections** in solid organ transplant recipients has been expanded.

105. Global eradication efforts for **Poliovirus Infections** have been updated, including the vaccines being used.

106. Members of the family *Polyomaviridae* have been expanded in the **Polyomaviruses** chapter.

107. The mechanism by which abnormal protein folding occurs in **Prion Diseases** is explained in greater detail.

108. ***Pseudomonas aeruginosa* Infections** is an entirely new chapter.

109. Association of anticardiolipin antibodies with severe complications of **Q Fever** has been added. Situations that increase aerosolization risks have been added.

110. KEDRAB Rabies Immune Globulin has been added to the **Rabies** chapter.

111. The diagnostic section of **Rat-Bite Fever** has been updated to include 16S ribosomal RNA gene sequencing and matrix-assisted laser desorption/ionization time-of-flight (MALDI-TOF) mass spectrometry.

112. Discussion of isolation precautions in **Respiratory Syncytial Virus** infections have been expanded. The chapter has been harmonized with the forthcoming technical report. Although the overall recommendations for palivizumab have not changed, the basis for maintaining those recommendations now includes recent publications.

113. The role of **Rhinovirus Infections** as a major viral cause of exacerbations of asthma, cystic fibrosis, and chronic obstructive pulmonary disease has been expanded.

114. *Rickettsia akari* has been added to the **Rickettsial Infections** chapter, and a CDC website is provided for information on spotted fevers occurring outside of the United States.

115. Duration of doxycycline therapy for **Rickettsialpox** has been made more precise.

116. The proportion of **Rocky Mountain Spotted Fever** cases not reporting tick bites (approximately half) has been added. Serologic testing has been updated to indicate IgM being relatively less specific.

117. Administration of rotavirus vaccine to patients while still in the NICU has been added to the **Rotavirus Infections** chapter. Rotavirus vaccine use in HIV-infected people has been added. Vaccination of infants who have had rotavirus gastroenteritis has been addressed.

118. Isolation guidance for **Rubella** in the hospital and school settings has been updated to include PCR testing.
119. Global resistance rates for ***Salmonella* Infections** have been updated, with a subsequent impact on empiric antibiotic recommendations. A new conjugate typhoid vaccine available outside of the United States has been added.
120. Information about environmental disinfection for crusted **Scabies** has been added.
121. Use of repeat dosing of praziquantel in chronic **Schistosomiasis** has been clarified.
122. Increasing fluoroquinolone and azithromycin resistance patterns for ***Shigella* Infections** have been added, along with CDC's request for treatment failure information.
123. Tecovirimat (TPOXX or ST-246) has been licensed by the FDA for the treatment of **Smallpox.** A third-generation vaccine (JYNNEOS) that is an attenuated, live, replication-deficient vaccinia virus has been approved.
124. Situations in which serologic testing for **Sporotrichosis** may be beneficial have been added.
125. Mention of commercially available tests for enterotoxin in **Staphylococcal Food Poisoning** has been added.
126. Management of secondary MRSA pneumonias following influenza infections has been expanded in the ***Staphylococcus aureus*** chapter. Discussion of second- and third-tier MRSA therapeutics has been expanded. Preoperative antibacterial prophylaxis in MRSA colonized people has been modified.
127. Discussion of second-tier therapeutics for **Coagulase-Negative Staphylococcal Infections** has been expanded.
128. Complications of **Group A Streptococcal Infections**, and management thereof, have been updated and expanded.
129. The **Group B Streptococcal Infections** chapter has been harmonized with the 2019 AAP clinical report and the 2019 statement from the American College of Obstetricians and Gynecologists on GBS.
130. The treatment section of the **Non-Group A or B Streptococcal and Enterococcal Infections** chapter has been updated, and antibiotic options are more thoroughly explained.
131. People at risk for *Strongyloides* hyperinfection syndrome are more thoroughly described. The diagnostic section has been updated in the **Strongyloidiasis** chapter.
132. The **Syphilis** chapter has been harmonized with the CDC 2021 Sexually Transmitted Infections Treatment Guidelines. The chapter has been decreased in length by greater than 10%. Epidemiologic data have been updated, including the increase in incidence of congenital syphilis. Therapeutic options for patients with severe penicillin allergy have been provided.
133. The diagnostic section of the **Tapeworm Diseases** chapter has been updated.
134. Therapeutic options and when test of cure is indicated have been updated across the pathogens described in the **Other Tapeworm Infections** chapter.
135. Recommendations for how to respond to inadvertent Tdap doses have been added to the **Tetanus** chapter. Risk factors in the United States for tetanus have been added.
136. Treatment options for **Tinea Capitis** have been updated.

137. The table on "Products for Topical Treatment of Tinea Corporis, Cruris, and Pedis" has been updated in the **Tinea Corporis** chapter.
138. Oral options for **Tinea Cruris** infections recalcitrant to topical management have been added.
139. A differential diagnosis listing has been added to the **Tinea Pedis and Tinea Unguium** chapter.
140. Clinical manifestations of **Toxocariasis** are presented in greater detail.
141. The chapter on ***Toxoplasma gondii* Infections** has been decreased in length by one third. Treatment recommendations are presented in table form for ease of access.
142. The ***Trichomonas vaginalis* Infections** chapter has been harmonized with the CDC 2021 Sexually Transmitted Infections Treatment Guidelines. The diagnostic section has been updated.
143. The diagnostic section of the **Trichuriasis** chapter has been updated.
144. Clinical manifestations of **African Trypanosomiasis (African Sleeping Sickness)** are presented in greater detail. Interim WHO treatment guidelines are referenced.
145. CDC algorithms for evaluation of pregnant women and infants with **American Trypanosomiasis (Chagas Disease)** have been added. American Heart Association guidance on management of Chagas cardiomyopathy is referenced.
146. The terminology in the **Tuberculosis** chapter has changed to tuberculosis infection (TBI, formerly LTBI) and tuberculosis disease (TBD). The chapter has been harmonized with new AAP clinical report titled "Tuberculosis Infection in Children: Testing and Treatment," including new treatment options for multidrug-resistant tuberculosis and a new table for treatment dosing for TBI.
147. Treatment recommendations for **Nontuberculous Mycobacteria** have been harmonized with the upcoming IDSA/ATS guidelines for NTM treatment.
148. Geographic areas in the United States where **Tularemia** is found have been updated.
149. Clinical manifestations of **Murine Typhus** are presented in greater detail.
150. Clinical manifestations of **Louseborne Typhus** are presented in greater detail.
151. Sepsis with hyperammonemia in lung transplant recipients has been added ***Ureaplasma urealyticum* and *Ureaplasma parvum* Infections** chapter. The treatment section has been updated.
152. Isolation precautions in **Varicella-Zoster Virus Infections** have been separated by patient (eg, mother, neonate) in the Control Measures section of the chapter.
153. Discussion of vaccines for prevention of **Cholera** has been updated.
154. The diagnostic section of the **Other *Vibrio* Infections** chapter has been updated.
155. Epidemiologic data for **West Nile Virus** have been updated.
156. Incidence data for ***Yersinia enterocolitica* and *Yersinia pseudotuberculosis* Infections** have been updated.
157. The time interval for avoiding sex or using condoms following return from an area with **Zika** has been changed from 6 months to 3 months.

SECTION 4. ANTIMICROBIAL AGENTS AND RELATED THERAPY

1. Warnings concerning fluoroquinolones have been strengthened in **Antimicrobial Agents and Related Therapy**. A table has been added presenting cephalosporin cross-reactivity with other beta lactam antibiotics.
2. The antimicrobial stewardship portion of the **Antimicrobial Resistance and Antimicrobial Stewardship: Appropriate and Judicious Use of Antimicrobial Agents** chapter has been aligned with the new AAP policy statement on antimicrobial stewardship.
3. The **Tables of Antimicrobial Drug Dosages** have been updated with new antibiotics and with new dosages based on recent publications.
4. The **Sexually Transmitted Infections** tables have been harmonized with the CDC 2021 Sexually Transmitted Infections Treatment Guidelines.
5. Activity and age indications for the newer azoles have been updated in the **Antifungal Drugs for Systemic Fungal Infections** chapter.
6. Newer pediatric dosages have been added to the **Recommended Doses of Parenteral and Oral Antifungal Drugs** table.
7. Newer **Topical Drugs for Superficial Fungal Infections** have been added, and ones that are no longer available have been deleted.
8. New antivirals, including many HCV antivirals, have been added to the **Non-HIV Antiviral Drugs** table.
9. Updated dosing recommendations based on new guidance have been incorporated throughout the **Drugs for Parasitic Infections** table.
10. The **Systems-based Treatment Table** is a completely new table, and the first time the *Red Book* has grouped recommendations by body system.

SECTION 5. ANTIMICROBIAL PROPHYLAXIS

1. Recommendations based on new studies for prophylaxis for UTIs have been added to the **Antimicrobial Prophylaxis** chapter.
2. Delabeling of antibiotic allergies has been added to the **Antimicrobial Prophylaxis in Pediatric Surgical Patients** chapter.
3. Approaches to erythromycin shortages have been added to the **Prevention of Neonatal Ophthalmia** chapter. Recommendations have been added for gonococcal prophylaxis following exposure at birth in a newborn infant who cannot receive ceftriaxone (eg, receiving continuous intravenous calcium, as in parenteral nutrition).

APPENDICES

1. Telephone and website addresses for organizations listed in the **Directory of Resources** have been updated.
2. **Codes for Commonly Administered Pediatric Vaccines/Toxoids and Immune Globulins** have been updated.
3. The diseases listed in the **Nationally Notifiable Infectious Diseases in the United States** table are those required for 2020 and include coronavirus disease 2019 (COVID-19).

4. The table in **Guide to Contraindications and Precautions to Immunizations** has been deleted, and the link to the CDC General Recommendations table is provided.

5. The **Prevention of Disease From Contaminated Food Products** appendix has been updated to take into account recent outbreaks. Raw dough has been added.

6. The **Clinical Syndromes Associated With Foodborne Diseases** table has been updated with recent information from foodborne outbreaks.

7. The **Diseases Transmitted by Animals (Zoonoses)** table has been updated with the 2019 DHHS Zoonotic Diseases Report.

Active and Passive Immunization

PROLOGUE

The ultimate goal of immunization is control of infection transmission, elimination of disease, and ideally, eradication of the pathogen that causes the infection and disease; the immediate goal is prevention of disease in people or groups. To accomplish these goals, physicians must make timely immunization a high priority in the care of infants, children, adolescents, and adults. The global eradication of smallpox in 1977, elimination of poliomyelitis disease from the Americas in 1991, elimination of endemic measles transmission in the United States in 2000 and in the Americas in 2002, elimination of rubella and congenital rubella syndrome from the United States in 2004 and from the Americas in 2015, and global eradication of type 2 wild poliovirus in 2015 and type 3 wild poliovirus in 2019 serve as models for fulfilling the promise of disease control through immunization. These accomplishments were achieved by combining a comprehensive immunization program providing consistent, high levels of vaccine coverage with intensive surveillance and effective public health disease-control measures. The resurgence of measles and mumps in the United States, however, illustrates how precarious the substantial gains to date can be without vigilant commitment by physicians, public health officials, and members of the public. Worldwide eradication of polio, measles, and rubella remains possible through implementation of proven prevention strategies, and in the case of polio is tantalizingly close, but diligence must prevail until eradication is achieved, or success itself is imperiled. The complexity of completing guiding eradication programs to fruition is even more challenging given alarming declines in immunizations globally during the initial months of the coronavirus pandemic that began in late 2019.

High immunization rates, in general, have reduced dramatically the incidence of all vaccine-preventable diseases (see Table 1.1) in the United States. Yet, because pathogens that cause vaccine-preventable diseases persist in the United States and elsewhere around the world, ongoing immunization efforts must be not only maintained but also strengthened. All vaccine-preventable diseases are, at most, 18 hours away by air travel from any part of the world.

Discoveries in immunology, molecular biology, and medical genetics have resulted in groundbreaking advances in vaccine research. Licensing of new, improved, and safer vaccines; establishment of an adolescent immunization platform; development of vaccines against cancer (eg, human papillomavirus and hepatitis B vaccines); and application of novel vaccine-delivery systems promise to continue the advances in preventive medicine achieved during the latter half of the 20th century. The extremely rapid pace of development of a vaccine against severe acute respiratory syndrome-coronavirus 2 (SARS-CoV-2) beginning in early 2020 is a testament to the scientific investments in vaccinology over 70 years. The advent of population-based postlicensure studies of vaccines facilitates detection of rare adverse events temporally associated with immunization that were undetected during large prelicensure clinical trials as well as detection of changes over time in vaccine effectiveness that directly inform recommendations on use of specific vaccines.

Table 1.1. Comparison of Prevaccine Era Estimated Average Annual Morbidity With Current Estimates

Disease	Prevaccine Era Annual Case Estimate[a]	2017 Reported Cases[b]	Percent Decrease
Diphtheria	21 053	0	100
Haemophilus influenzae type b (Hib) <5 y of age	20 000	33	>99
Hepatitis A	117 333	3 366	98
Hepatitis B (acute)	66 232	2 866	96
Measles	530 217	122	>99
Mumps	162 344	5 629	97
Pertussis	200 752	15 808	92
Polio (paralytic)	16 316	0	100
Pneumococcus (invasive)			
All ages	63 067	16 251	74
<5 y	16 069	971	94
Rubella	47 745	9	>99
Congenital rubella syndrome	152	2	99
Smallpox	29 005	0	100
Tetanus	580	31	95
Varicella	4 085 120	7 059	>99

[a] Roush SW, Murphy TV, Vaccine-Preventable Disease Table Working Group. Historical comparisons of morbidity and mortality for vaccine-preventable diseases in the United States. *JAMA*. 2007;298(18):2155-2163
[b] Centers for Disease Control and Prevention. NNDSS Notifiable Diseases and Mortality Tables. Available at: **www.cdc. gov/mmwr/mmwr_nd/nd_data_tables.html.**

Each edition of the *Red Book* provides recommendations for immunization of infants, children, adolescents, and young adults. These recommendations, which are harmonized among the American Academy of Pediatrics (AAP), the Advisory Committee on Immunization Practices (ACIP) of the Centers for Disease Control and Prevention (CDC), and the American Academy of Family Physicians (AAFP), are based on careful analysis of disease epidemiology, benefits, and risks of immunization; feasibility of implementation; and cost-benefit analysis. ACIP recommendations utilize Grading of Recommendations Assessment, Development and Evaluation (GRADE), when feasible, in evaluating the evidence of benefits and risks for a given vaccine, further ensuring that the recommendations are evidence based and objectively assessed.

Use of trade names and commercial sources in the *Red Book* is for identification purposes only and does not imply endorsement by the AAP. Internet sites referenced in the *Red Book* are provided as a service to readers and may change without notice; citation of websites does not constitute AAP endorsement.

SOURCES OF INFORMATION ABOUT IMMUNIZATION

In addition to the latest print edition of the *Red Book*, the following sources can assist providers in remaining up-to-date with information pertaining to vaccines and immunization recommendations and finding answers to questions that arise in practice. For many of these resources, providers can sign up for e-mail alerts to receive new information as soon as it is available.

- **American Academy of Pediatrics (AAP)**—*Red Book Online* includes the print edition content plus updates and is available on the Internet (**http://redbook.solutions.aap.org/Redbook.aspx**) and as a mobile app for iOS and Google Play to AAP members and subscribers. The website has links to the latest implementation guidance, immunization schedules, and the Vaccine Status Table, which provides information on recently submitted, approved, and recommended vaccines and biologics. New recommendations are summarized in *AAP News* (**www.aappublications.org/news**), the official newsmagazine of the AAP, and are published in *Pediatrics* (**http://pediatrics.aappublications.org**), the official journal of the Academy. The AAP also maintains a website (**www.aap.org/en-us/advocacy-and-policy/aap-health-initiatives/immunizations/Pages/Immunizations-home.aspx**) that contains useful links to immunization resources for providers as well as a website with information geared toward parents (**https://healthychildren.org**).

- **Centers for Disease Control and Prevention (CDC)**—The CDC immunization website (**www.cdc.gov/vaccines/**) contains a wealth of information, including annually updated immunization schedules; vaccine safety information; recommendations from the Advisory Committee on Immunization Practices (ACIP); vaccine supply updates; vaccine coverage and disease surveillance data; recommendations for specific patient populations; information about storage, handling, and administration of vaccines; legal requirements; and education and training. ACIP recommendations become "official" when they are published in the *Morbidity and Mortality Weekly Report (MMWR)*, but the CDC may post provisional recommendations that can assist providers in making decisions on use of new vaccines prior to the publication of final recommendations. Noteworthy CDC Internet resources are listed in Table 1.2. CDC experts also are available to answer immunization-related questions by email at **nipinfo@cdc.gov.**

- **Food and Drug Administration (FDA)**—The FDA maintains a website that includes information on its evaluation of safety and effectiveness of FDA-licensed vaccines and a repository of current FDA-approved prescribing information (**www.fda.gov/vaccines-blood-biologics/vaccines/vaccines-licensed-use-united-states**). The FDA-approved prescribing information (also referred to as the "label" or "package insert") contains detailed information for health care providers to ensure safe and effective use. The approved indications in the package insert are supported by substantial evidence of effectiveness based on data evaluated by the FDA. The FDA does not issue guidelines or recommendations for vaccine use, and in some instances recommendations of the AAP and ACIP may differ from FDA-approved prescribing information.

Table 1.2. CDC Immunization Web Page Quick Reference

Content	URL
Glossary, acronyms, abbreviations, foreign language terms	**www.cdc.gov/vaccines/terms/**
Information for parents	**www.cdc.gov/vaccines/parents/index.html**
Provider resources for vaccine conversations with parents	**www.cdc.gov/vaccines/hcp/conversations/ conv-materials.html**
ACIP recommendations	**www.cdc.gov/vaccines/hcp/acip-recs/ index.html**
General best practice guidelines for immunization	**www.cdc.gov/vaccines/hcp/acip-recs/ general-recs/index.html**
Schedules	**www.cdc.gov/vaccines/schedules/hcp/ index.html**
Child Vaccine Assessment Tool	**www2a.cdc.gov/vaccines/childquiz/**
Vaccine Information Statements	**www.cdc.gov/vaccines/hcp/vis/index.html**
Vaccines for Children Program	**www.cdc.gov/vaccines/programs/vfc/ index.html**
Travel	**wwwnc.cdc.gov/travel/destinations/list**
CDC Health Information for International Travel (also known as the Yellow Book)	**wwwnc.cdc.gov/travel/page/yellowbook- home**
Epidemiology and Prevention of Vaccine- Preventable Diseases (also known as the Pink Book)	**www.cdc.gov/vaccines/pubs/pinkbook/ index.html**
Manual for the Surveillance of Vaccine- Preventable Diseases	**www.cdc.gov/vaccines/pubs/surv-manual/ index.html**
Morbidity and Mortality Weekly Report (MMWR)	**www.cdc.gov/mmwr/index.html**

- **Immunization Action Coalition (IAC)**—Working in partnership with the CDC, the IAC maintains a website (**www.immunize.org**) replete with copyright-free information about virtually every aspect of vaccine practice. Unique content includes Vaccine Information Statement (VIS) translations in more than 50 languages; *Ask the Experts*, a repository of answers to challenging immunization questions; handouts for patients and staff; *Unprotected People Reports*, containing personal accounts of encounters with vaccine-preventable diseases; updated information about state mandates and exemptions; expansive image and video libraries; and screening tools for contraindications and precautions. The IAC also maintains websites for the public (**www.vaccineinformation.org**) and for immunization coalitions (**www.immunizationcoalitions.org**). The IAC's weekly e-mail newsletter, *IAC Express*, is available free of charge.

- **Vaccine Manufacturers—Vaccine manufacturers maintain websites with** current information concerning new products, contact information for medical questions, and updated package inserts. Contact information for manufacturers is available online (**www.cdc.gov/vaccines/hcp/admin/storage/downloads/manufact-dist-contact.pdf**).
- **Other Resources**—Table 1.3 lists major national and international organizations that are involved in immunization policy, education, implementation, and advocacy, along with their respective websites. The Directory of Resources in Appendix I (p 1027) also is a source of contact information for these and other organizations.

Table 1.3. Internet Resources for Vaccine Information for Health Care Professionals and Parents

Resource	URL
Government	
Centers for Disease Control and Prevention: Vaccines & Immunization	**www.cdc.gov/vaccines/**
Clinical Immunization Safety Assessment (CISA) Project	**www.cdc.gov/vaccinesafety/ ensuringsafety/monitoring/cisa**
National Institute of Allergy and Infectious Diseases	**www.niaid.nih.gov**
US Food and Drug Administration: Vaccines, Blood & Biologics	**www.fda.gov/vaccines-blood-biologics/vaccines**
National Vaccine Injury Compensation Program	**www.hrsa.gov/vaccine-compensation/index.html**
Vaccine Adverse Event Reporting System	**www.vaers.hhs.gov/index**
Office of Infectious Diseases and HIV/AIDS Policy	**www.hhs.gov/vaccines**
National Vaccine Advisory Committee	**www.hhs.gov/nvpo/nvac**
International	
Pan American Health Organization	**www.paho.org/hq**
World Health Organization	**www.who.int/en**
Professional Associations	
American Academy of Pediatrics	**www.aap.org/en-us**
American Academy of Family Physicians	**www.aafp.org**
American Medical Association	**www.ama-assn.org**
American College Health Association	**www.acha.org**
American College of Nurse Midwives	**www.midwife.org**
American College of Physicians	**www.acponline.org**
American College of Obstetricians and Gynecologists	**www.acog.org**

Table 1.3. Internet Resources for Vaccine Information for Health Care Professionals and Parents, continued

Resource	URL
American Immunization Registry Association	www.immregistries.org
American Nurses Association	www.nursingworld.org
American Osteopathic Association	www.osteopathic.org
American Pharmacists Association	www.pharmacist.com
American Public Health Association	www.apha.org
Association for Prevention Teaching and Research	www.aptrweb.org
Association of State and Territorial Health Officials	www.astho.org
Association of Immunization Managers	www.immunizationmanagers.org
Council of State and Territorial Epidemiologists	www.cste.org
Infectious Diseases Society of America	www.idsociety.org
National Association of County and City Health Officials	www.naccho.org
National Association of Pediatric Nurse Practitioners	www.napnap.org
National Foundation of Infectious Diseases	www.nfid.org
National Medical Association	www.nmanet.org
Pediatric Infectious Diseases Society	www.pids.org
Society for Adolescent Health and Medicine	www.adolescenthealth.org
Society for Healthcare Epidemiology of America	www.shea-online.org
Society of Teachers of Family Medicine	www.stfm.org

Advocacy and Implementation

Resource	URL
Children's Hospital of Philadelphia Vaccine Education Center	www.chop.edu/centers-programs/vaccine-education-center
Families Fighting Flu	www.familiesfightingflu.org
Global Alliance for Vaccines and Immunization	www.gavi.org
Immunization Action Coalition	www.immunize.org
Immunization for Women (American College of Obstetricians and Gynecologists)	www.immunizationforwomen.org
National Foundation for Infectious Diseases	www.nfid.org
National Meningitis Association	www.nmaus.org
Parents of Kids With Infectious Diseases	www.pkids.org
Texas Children's Hospital Center for Vaccine Awareness and Research	www.texaschildrens.org/departments/center-vaccine-awareness-and-research-cvar
Vaccinate Your Family (the next generation of Every Child by Two)	www.vaccinateyourfamily.org
Voices for Vaccines	www.voicesforvaccines.org

DISCUSSING VACCINES WITH PATIENTS AND PARENTS

Patients and their families should be informed about both the benefits and risks of vaccines.[1] The importance of confident and strong support by health care professionals for all recommended vaccines cannot be overemphasized. The single most important factor in parents' acceptance of vaccines is the recommendation of a well-informed, caring, and concerned clinician. Questions should be encouraged, and adequate time should be allowed so that the information provided is understood (**www.cdc.gov/ vaccines/hcp/conversations/index.html**). Parents should receive a clear and confident message that vaccines are safe and effective and that serious disease can occur when children are not immunized.

Addressing Parents' Questions About Vaccine Safety and Effectiveness

Although parents receive information about vaccines from multiple sources, they consider health care professionals—their primary care physician as well as all members of the health care team in clinical practice settings—to be their most trusted source of health information. Several factors contribute to parental concerns about vaccines, including: (1) lack of information about the vaccine being administered and about immunizations in general; (2) lack of understanding of the severity and communicability of vaccine-preventable diseases; (3) varied information and misinformation from other sources (eg, alternative medicine practitioners, social media, and the Internet); (4) perceived risk of serious vaccine adverse effects; (5) mistrust of the source of information regarding vaccines (eg, vaccine manufacturer, schools, the government); and (6) sometimes a less-than-enthusiastic recommendation from health care professionals. Some caregivers view the risk involved with immunization as disproportionately greater than the risk of disease, in part because of the relative infrequency of vaccine-preventable diseases in the United States, which of course is a direct result of the success of the immunization program. Others may focus on sociopolitical issues, such as mandatory immunization, informed consent, and the argument for the primacy of individual rights over that of societal benefit. Acknowledging parents' concerns, listening respectfully, and providing accurate information about both benefits and risks of vaccines helps forge a trusting relationship. Identifying the specific uncertainties or apprehensions that parents may have about particular vaccines will help to focus the discussion and avoid making assumptions about caregivers' concerns.

Common Misconceptions About Immunizations

Misconceptions and misinformation regarding vaccines should be addressed clearly and specifically. Table 1.4 includes facts that refute common misconceptions and myths about immunizations. The National Academy of Medicine (NAM), formerly

---

[1] Edwards KM, Hackell JM; American Academy of Pediatrics, Committee on Infectious Diseases, Committee on Practice and Ambulatory Medicine. Countering vaccine hesitancy. *Pediatrics*. 2016;138(3):e20162146

Table 1.4. Common Misconceptions/Myths About Immunizations[a,b]

Claims	Facts
Natural methods of enhancing immunity are better than vaccinations.	The only "natural way" to be immune is to have the disease. Immunity from a preventive vaccine provides protection against disease when a person is exposed to it in the future. That immunity is usually similar to what is acquired from natural infection, although several doses of a vaccine may have to be administered for a child to develop an adequate immune response.
Giving multiple vaccines at the same time causes an "overload" of the immune system.	Vaccination does not overburden a child's immune system; the recommended vaccines use only a small portion of the immune system's "memory." Although the number of unique vaccines administered has risen over recent decades, the number of antigens administered has decreased because of advances in science and manufacturing. The National Academy of Medicine (NAM) has concluded that there is no evidence that the immunization schedule is unsafe (see text).
Vaccines are ineffective.	Vaccines have spared millions of people the effects of devastating diseases.
Prior to the use of vaccinations, these diseases had begun to decline because of improved nutrition and hygiene.	In the 19th and 20th centuries, some infectious diseases began to be better controlled because of improvements in sanitation, clean water, pasteurized milk, and pest control. However, vaccine-preventable diseases decreased dramatically after the vaccines for those diseases were approved and were administered to large numbers of children.
Vaccines cause poorly understood illnesses or disorders, such as autism, sudden infant death syndrome (SIDS), immune dysfunction, diabetes, neurologic disorders, allergic rhinitis, eczema, and asthma.	These claims are false. Multiple, high-quality scientific studies have failed to substantiate any link between vaccines and these health conditions. See NAM reports.
Vaccines weaken the immune system.	Vaccines actually strengthen the immune system. Vaccinated children have decreased risk of infections. Importantly, natural infections like influenza, measles, and chickenpox can weaken the immune system, increasing the risk of other infections.

Table 1.4. Common Misconceptions/Myths About Immunizations,[a,b] continued

Claims	Facts
Giving many vaccines at the same time is untested.	New vaccines are tested in concomitant use studies with existing vaccines that are administered on the same or overlapping schedule. These studies are performed to ensure that new vaccines do not affect the safety or effectiveness of existing vaccines administered at the same time and that existing vaccines administered at the same time do not affect the safety or effectiveness of new vaccines.
Vaccines can be delayed, separated, and spaced out without consequences.	Many vaccine-preventable diseases occur in early infancy. Optimal vaccine-induced immunity may require a series of vaccines over time. Any delay in receiving age-appropriate immunization increases the risk of diseases that vaccines are administered to prevent. Spacing out vaccine may also have psychological consequences, because many more office visits will be associated with injections.

Adapted from: Myers MG, Pineda D. *Do Vaccines Cause That? A Guide for Evaluating Vaccine Safety Concerns.* Galveston, TX: Immunizations for Public Health; 2008:79.
[a] See National Academy of Medicine Reviews of Adverse Events After Immunization (p 43).
[b] Other common misconceptions are detailed online (**www.cdc.gov/vaccines/parents/tools/parents-guide/index.html**).

the Institute of Medicine (IOM), reviewed evidence on the safety of 8 individual vaccines in 2011 (**www.nap.edu/catalog/13164/adverse-effects-of-vaccines-evidence-and-causality**) and, in 2013, the safety of the immunization schedule (**www.nap.edu/catalog/13563/the-childhood-immunization-schedule-and-safety-stakeholder-concerns-scientific-evidence**). The NAM concluded that health problems caused by individual vaccines are quite rare and that there is no evidence that the immunization schedule is unsafe. The NAM also found no links between the immunization schedule and autoimmune diseases, asthma, hypersensitivity, seizures, child developmental disorders, learning or developmental disorders, autism spectrum disorders, or attention deficit or disruptive disorders. In addition to reaffirming the safety of the recommended immunization schedule, the NAM noted that the use of nonstandard schedules is potentially harmful, because it extends the period of risk of susceptibility to acquiring vaccine-preventable diseases and increases the risk of incomplete immunization. (Also see National Academy of Medicine Reviews of Adverse Events after Immunization, p 43.)

Parents may have encountered sources, including the media, social media, or websites, that may suggest there is controversy regarding routine vaccines. Information from such sources may be presented incompletely or inaccurately. When a parent initiates discussion about an alleged vaccine controversy, the health care professional is encouraged to listen carefully to the parent's concerns, acknowledge how frightening these sound, and then confidently and patiently discuss these specific concerns using factual information, personal experiences, and nonjudgmental language appropriate for parents and other care providers.

Safety information should be presented in a nonconfrontational dialogue with the parents while listening to and acknowledging their concerns. Providing specific examples and anecdotes about the diseases prevented by immunization and sharing personal choices and experiences surrounding vaccination can provide a compelling message about the confidence of the provider in the safety and efficacy of vaccines.

Resources for Optimizing Communications With Parents About Vaccines

Information that can help health care professionals respond to questions and misconceptions about vaccines and vaccine-preventable diseases is readily available (see Table 1.2 and Table 1.3). Helpful and credible information sources to which parents may be directed include the "Parent's Guide to Childhood Immunization" (**www.cdc.gov/vaccines/parents/tools/parents-guide/index.html**), the Food and Drug Administration (FDA) "Vaccines for Children - A Guide for Parents and Caregivers" (**www.fda.gov/vaccines-blood-biologics/consumers-biologics/vaccines-children-guide-parents-and-caregivers**), and the Centers for Disease Control and Prevention (CDC) Internet hotline service (**www.cdc.gov/info**). Additionally, in 2019 the CDC launched the new "Vaccinate with Confidence" program designed to strengthen public trust in vaccines (**www.cdc.gov/vaccines/partners/vaccinate-with-confidence.html**). This will be achieved by leveraging data from the Vaccines for Children program and the Immunization Information Systems to identify and respond to community pockets of low vaccination coverage, empowering parents to choose to vaccinate, engaging with state policy makers, and working with social media companies to promote trustworthy vaccine information. Further key resources include the American Academy of Pediatrics (AAP) Immunization Initiative (**www2.aap.org/immunization/**), the Immunization Action Coalition (**www.immunize.org**), and the Vaccine Education Center at Children's Hospital of Philadelphia (**www.chop.edu/centers-programs/vaccine-education-center**).

The CDC, the AAP, and the American Academy of Family Physicians have developed "Provider Resources for Vaccine Conversations with Parents" (**www.cdc.gov/vaccines/hcp/conversations/index.html**). These educational materials build on the latest research in both vaccine and communication science and are designed to help health care professionals remain current on vaccine topics and strengthen communication and trust with parents. Health care providers can download these materials and enroll to receive email updates when new resources are posted. The materials include the following:

- Strategies on Talking with Parents about Vaccines for Infants.
- Current vaccine safety topics, such as Understanding MMR and Vaccine Safety; Understanding Thimerosal, Mercury, and Vaccine Safety; Ensuring the Safety of US Vaccines; The Childhood Immunization Schedule; and more.
- Basic and in-depth fact sheets on 14 vaccine-preventable diseases for parents. Fact sheets are available in English and Spanish for a variety of reading levels, and many

include stories of families whose children have experienced a vaccine-preventable disease.

- "If You Choose Not to Vaccinate Your Child, Understand the Risks and Responsibilities," which helps parents appreciate the risks if they choose to delay or decline a vaccine.
- Interactive, online childhood immunization scheduler and waiting room videos, such as Get the Picture: Childhood Immunization Video.

Parental Refusal of Immunizations

Administration of all vaccines should adhere to age ranges for vaccine administration provided in the "Recommended Immunization Schedule for Children and Adolescents Aged 18 Years or Younger" (**http://redbook.solutions.aap.org/ SS/Immunization_Schedules.aspx**). Many parents have concerns related to specific vaccines, as opposed to vaccines in general. Pediatricians and other health care providers should discuss the benefits and risks of each vaccine, because a parent who is reluctant to accept administration of one vaccine may be willing to accept others. Parents who have concerns about administering multiple injections to a child in a single visit may have their concerns addressed by using methods to reduce the pain of injection (see Managing Injection Pain, p 30) or by using combination vaccines. Concerns about the number of antigens administered at one time may be addressed by discussing the ability of the immune system to respond to many antigens at once as well as the advances in science and manufacturing so that it is easier than in the past to be sure that vaccines are both highly safe and effective.

Parents or caregivers who decline one or more vaccines for their child should be advised that all states have laws prohibiting unimmunized children from attending school during outbreaks of vaccine-preventable diseases. Parents should be encouraged to be familiar with the applicable laws in their state. Information on state-specific laws regarding religious, philosophical, and other nonmedical exemptions from immunization requirements is available online (**www.immunize.org/laws** and **www.ncsl. org/research/health/school-immunization-exemption-state-laws.aspx**). Discussions about delaying or declining vaccines should be documented in the patient's health record. If one or more scheduled vaccines is declined, a signed *informed refusal* document should note that the parent was informed about why the immunization was recommended, the benefits and risks of immunization, and the possible consequences of not being immunized. Parents or caregivers must understand that they have an obligation to inform health care professionals when children who are not fully immunized are seeking care for an acute illness so that vaccine-preventable diseases be considered in the evaluation and differential diagnosis of the child's illness and so that the ill child may be isolated from other vulnerable children who might also be in the health care facility. A sample Refusal to Vaccinate form can be found on the AAP website (**www. aap.org/en-us/Documents/immunization_refusaltovaccinate.pdf**).

When parents or caregivers refuse vaccines for their child, clinicians should revisit the immunization discussion on subsequent visits. Continued refusal after adequate discussion should be documented in the heath record. If failure to vaccinate puts the child at significant risk of immediate harm (eg, during an epidemic), the pediatrician should determine whether this constitutes medical neglect and act accordingly. When significant differences in philosophy of care exist or where poor communication persists, a substantial level of distrust may develop in the pediatrician's relationship with the family. When this occurs, the individual pediatrician may consider dismissal of families who refuse vaccination as an acceptable option. The physician must provide medical care for a period of time until a new physician can be secured, in accordance with local and state regulations.

Immunization Documentation

The National Childhood Vaccine Injury Act (NCVIA) of 1986 established the Vaccine Injury Compensation Program (VICP) and included requirements for notifying *all* patients and parents about vaccine benefits and risks. Whether vaccines are purchased with private or public funds, this legislation mandates that a current vaccine information statement (VIS) be provided *each* time a vaccine covered under the VICP is administered (see Table 1.5). The VIS must be provided at the time of the immunization and for take-away, if desired. Copies of current VISs in English, Spanish, and other languages are available online from the CDC (**www.cdc.gov/vaccines/hcp/vis/ index.html**). In addition, the Immunization Action Coalition (**www.immunize. org**) provides VIS documents with translations into more than 40 languages available. If the translated VIS version is older than the current VIS, it is acceptable to give the translated VIS even though it is not the most current edition. Online availability of the VIS on the physician's website provides the opportunity for the parent or guardian to review the information before the routine immunization visit, which can allow for a more productive discussion at the time of the visit. The NCVIA requires that personnel administering VICP-covered vaccines record in the patient's health record the information shown in Table 1.6, as well as confirmation that the relevant VIS was provided to the patient or guardian at the time of each immunization. Parents' or patients' signatures are not required by the federal NCVIA statute but may be required by state law to indicate that they have read and understood material in the VIS.

Table 1.5. Guidance in Using Vaccine Information Statements (VISs)[a]

Distribution:
Must be provided each time a VICP-covered vaccine is administered.[b]
Must be provided to and discussed with the patient (nonminor), parent, and/or legal representative.[b,c]
Must be the current version.[d]
Providers can add (not substitute) other written materials or audiovisual aids in addition to VISs.[e]

VICP indicates Vaccine Injury Compensation Program.
[a]VISs are available on the Centers for Disease Control and Prevention (CDC) website (**www.cdc.gov/vaccines/hcp/ vis/index.html**).
[b]Required under the National Childhood Vaccine Injury Act.
[c]Definition of a consenting adolescent may vary by state.
[d]Required by CDC regulations for vaccines purchased through CDC contract. See the VIS website for current versions.
[e]An electronic version of the VIS can be transmitted to the patient's electronic device.

Table 1.6. Documentation Requirements Under the National Childhood Vaccine Injury Act

Document in the Patient's Health Record

Vaccine manufacturer, lot number, and date of administration[a]

Name, title, and business address of the health care professional administering the vaccine and date that the VIS is provided (and VIS publication date)[a]

Site (eg, deltoid area) and route (eg, intramuscular) of administration and expiration date of the vaccine[b]

[a]Required under the National Childhood Vaccine Injury Act.
[b]Recommended by the American Academy of Pediatrics and the Centers for Disease Control and Prevention (CDC).

The vast majority of parents or caregivers who express concerns about vaccines simply have questions about this critically important part of their child's health care. As caregivers' most trusted source of health care information, it is important for the clinician to address these concerns and questions confidently and with sensitivity and understanding, because this is the most effective way to achieve full vaccine uptake for the benefit of all children.

ACTIVE IMMUNIZATION

Active immunization involves administration of all or part of a microorganism or a modified product of a microorganism (eg, a toxoid, a purified antigen, or an antigen produced by genetic engineering) to evoke an immunologic response and clinical protection that mimics that of natural infection but usually presents little or no risk to the recipient. Immunization can result in antitoxin, anti-adherence, anti-invasive, or neutralizing activity or other types of protective humoral or cellular responses in the recipient. Some vaccines provide nearly complete and lifelong protection against disease, some provide protection against the more severe manifestations and/or consequences of the infection if exposed, and some must be readministered periodically to maintain protection. The immunologic response to vaccination is dependent on the type and dose of antigen, the effect of adjuvants, and host factors related to age, preexisting antibody, nutrition, concurrent disease, or genetics of the host. The effectiveness of a vaccine is assessed by evidence of protection against the natural disease. For some infectious diseases, induction of antibodies following vaccination is an indirect measure that predicts protection (eg, antitoxin against *Clostridium tetani* or neutralizing antibody against measles virus), but for others, serum antibody concentration does not always predict protection.

Vaccines are categorized as live (viral or bacterial, which almost always are attenuated) or inactivated. The term "inactivated vaccines," for simplicity, includes antigens that are toxoids or other purified proteins, purified polysaccharides, protein-polysaccharide or oligosaccharide conjugates, inactivated whole or partially purified viruses, recombinant proteins, and proteins assembled into virus-like participles. Recommendations for vaccines routinely advised for immunocompetent and immunocompromised children and adolescents are updated annually in the harmonized schedule developed by the AAP, Centers for Disease Control and Prevention (CDC), the American Academy of Family Physicians (AAFP), the American College of Obstetricians and Gynecologists (ACOG), and the American College of Nurse Midwives (ACNM) (**http://redbook.solutions.aap.org/SS/Immunization_ Schedules.aspx**), and for simplicity are referred to as being "on the annual immunization schedule." Vaccines approved for use in the United States are listed in Table 1.7. The US Food and Drug Administration (FDA) maintains and updates a website listing vaccines approved for immunization and distribution in the United States with supporting documents (**www.fda.gov/vaccines-blood-biologics/vaccines/ vaccines-licensed-use-united-states**). Appendix II provides information on the billing codes for commonly administered pediatric vaccines and toxoids used for vaccine administration. A regularly updated listing of *Current Procedural Terminology* (CPT) product codes for commonly administered pediatric vaccines can be found at **www. aap.org/en-us/Documents/coding_vaccine_coding_table.pdf.**

Among currently approved vaccines in the United States, there are 3 live attenuated bacterial vaccines (oral typhoid, oral cholera, and bacille Calmette-Guérin vaccines) and several live attenuated viral vaccines. Although active bacterial or viral replication ensues after administration of these vaccines, because the pathogen has been attenuated, few or no symptoms of illness occur. Sufficient antigenic characteristics of the virus or bacteria are retained during attenuation so that a protective immune response develops in the vaccine recipient.

Vaccines for some viruses (eg, hepatitis A, hepatitis B, human papillomavirus) and most bacteria are inactivated, component, subunit (purified components) preparations or inactivated toxins. Some vaccines contain purified bacterial polysaccharides conjugated chemically to immunobiologically active proteins (eg, tetanus toxoid, diphtheria toxoid, nontoxic variant of mutant diphtheria toxin, meningococcal outer membrane protein complex). Viruses and bacteria in inactivated, subunit, and conjugate vaccine preparations are not capable of replicating in the host; therefore, these vaccines must contain sufficient antigen content and possibly include an adjuvant to stimulate a desired response. In the case of conjugate polysaccharide vaccines, the linkage between the polysaccharide and the carrier protein enhances vaccine immunogenicity by converting the vaccine from a T-lymphocyte–independent antigen to a T-lymphocyte–dependent antigen. Maintenance of long-lasting immunity with inactivated viral or bacterial vaccines and toxoid vaccines may require periodic administration of booster doses. Although inactivated vaccines may not elicit the range of immunologic response provided by live attenuated agents, efficacy of approved inactivated vaccines in children is high. For example, an injected inactivated viral vaccine may evoke sufficient serum antibody or cell-mediated immunity but evoke only minimal mucosal antibody in the form of secretory immunoglobulin (Ig) A. Mucosal protection after administration of inactivated vaccines generally is inferior to mucosal immunity induced by live attenuated vaccines. Nonetheless, the demonstrated efficacy for such vaccines against invasive infection is high. Bacterial polysaccharide conjugate vaccines (eg, *Haemophilus influenzae* type b, pneumococcal, and meningococcal ACWY conjugate vaccines) reduce nasopharyngeal colonization through exudated IgG.

Viruses and bacteria in inactivated vaccines cannot replicate in or be excreted by the vaccine recipient as infectious agents and, thus, do not present the same safety

Table 1.7. Vaccines Approved for Immunization and Distributed in the United States and Their Routes of Administration[a]

Vaccine	Type	Route of Administration
Anthrax	Inactivated[b]	IM or SC
BCG	Live bacteria	Percutaneous using multiple puncture device
Cholera	Live attenuated bacteria	Oral
Dengue[c]	Live attenuated chimeric viruses	SC
Diphtheria-tetanus (DT, Td)	Toxoids	IM
DTaP	Toxoids and inactivated bacterial components	IM
DTaP, hepatitis B, and IPV	Toxoids and inactivated bacterial components, recombinant viral antigen, inactivated virus	IM
DTaP-IPV	Toxoids and inactivated bacterial components, inactivated virus	IM
DTaP, hepatitis B, Hib (*Haemophilus influenzae* type b), and IPV	Toxoids and inactivated bacterial components, recombinant viral antigen, polysaccharide-protein conjugate, inactivated virus	IM
Hepatitis A (HepA)	Inactivated virus	IM
Hepatitis B (HepB)	Recombinant viral antigen	IM
Hepatitis A-hepatitis B	Inactivated virus and recombinant viral antigens	IM
Hib (*Haemophilus influenzae* type b) conjugate (tetanus toxoid)[d]	Bacterial polysaccharide-protein conjugate	IM
Hib conjugate (meningococcal protein conjugate)	Bacterial polysaccharide-protein conjugate	IM
Human papillomavirus (9vHPV)	Recombinant viral antigens	IM
Influenza (IIV)	Inactivated viral components	IM
Influenza (IIV)	Inactivated viral components	ID[e]
Influenza (LAIV)	Live attenuated viruses	Intranasal
Japanese encephalitis	Inactivated virus	IM
Meningococcal ACWY conjugate (MCV4 or MenACWY)	Bacterial polysaccharide-protein conjugate	IM

Table 1.7. Vaccines Approved for Immunization and Distributed in the United States and Their Routes of Administration,[a] continued

Vaccine	Type	Route of Administration
Meningococcal serogroup B (MenB)	Bacterial recombinant protein	IM
MMR	Live attenuated viruses	SC
MMRV	Live attenuated viruses	SC
Pneumococcal polysaccharide (PPSV23)	Bacterial polysaccharide	IM or SC
Pneumococcal conjugate (PCV13)	Bacterial polysaccharide-protein conjugate	IM
Poliovirus (IPV)	Inactivated viruses	SC or IM
Rabies	Inactivated virus	IM
Rotavirus (RV1 and RV5)	Live attenuated virus	Oral
Tdap	Toxoids and inactivated bacterial components	IM
Tetanus	Toxoid	IM
Typhoid	Bacterial capsular polysaccharide	IM
Typhoid	Live attenuated bacteria	Oral
Varicella (VAR)	Live attenuated virus	SC
Yellow Fever	Live attenuated virus	SC
Zoster (HZ/su)	Recombinant viral antigens	IM

BCG indicates bacille Calmette-Guérin; ID, intradermal; SC, subcutaneous; DT, diphtheria and tetanus toxoids (for children younger than 7 years of age); Td, diphtheria and tetanus toxoids (for children 7 years of age or older and adults); IM, intramuscular; DTaP, diphtheria and tetanus toxoids and acellular pertussis, adsorbed; IPV, inactivated poliovirus; Hib, *Haemophilus influenzae* type b; PRP-T, polyribosylribitol phosphate-tetanus toxoid; HPV, human papillomavirus; MMR, live measles, mumps, rubella; MMRV, live measles, mumps, rubella, varicella (monovalent measles, mumps, and rubella components are not being produced in the United States); Tdap, tetanus toxoid, reduced diphtheria toxoid, and acellular pertussis.

[a] Other vaccines approved in the United States but not distributed include adenovirus (types 4, 7), anthrax, smallpox, H5N1 influenza vaccines, influenza A (H1N1) monovalent 2009 vaccine, JE-virus vaccine (JE-VAX), pneumococcal conjugate vaccine (PCV7), HepB-Hib (Comvax), and bivalent HPV vaccine (Cervarix). The FDA maintains a website listing currently approved vaccines in the United States (**www.fda.gov/vaccines-blood-biologics/vaccines/vaccines-licensed-use-united-states**). The AAP maintains a website (**http://aapredbook.aappublications.org/news/vaccstatus.dtl**) showing status of licensure and recommendations for newer vaccines.

[b] **https://pediatrics.aappublications.org/content/133/5/e1411.** Anthrax vaccine is not approved for use in children. Federal/state authorities would oversee emergency use under an investigational new drug application for children, should the need arise.

[c] Dengue vaccine is indicated only for individuals 9 through 16 years of age with laboratory confirmed prior dengue infection and living in areas with endemic infection.

[d] See Table 3.11, p 351.

[e] Intradermal influenza vaccine is recommended only for people 18 through 64 years of age.

concerns for immunosuppressed vaccine recipients or contacts of vaccine recipients as might live attenuated vaccines. For example, live rotavirus vaccines pose risk and are contraindicated in children with severe combined immunodeficiency disease. Furthermore, the AAP, the Advisory Committee on Immunization Practices (ACIP) of the Centers for Disease Control and Prevention, and the Healthcare Infection Control Practices Advisory Committee (HICPAC) recommend against administering live attenuated influenza vaccine to close contacts and caregivers of severely immunosuppressed people who require a protected environment.

Recommendations for dose, vaccine storage and handling (see Vaccine Handling and Storage, p 19), route and technique of administration (see Vaccine Administration, p 26), and immunization schedules should be followed for predictable, effective protection (also see disease-specific chapters in Section 3). Adherence to recommended guidance in terms of sequence, timing, route of administration, and dosage is critical to the success of immunization practices at both the individual and the societal levels.

Vaccine Ingredients

As part of the licensure process, the US Food and Drug Administration (FDA) reviews the laboratory and clinical data on vaccines and their components to ensure their safety and efficacy. In addition to one or more antigens, a vaccine may contain other ingredients, each of which serves a specific purpose, as listed on its package insert. A catalog of package inserts for vaccines currently licensed for use in the United States is available at **www.fda.gov/vaccines-blood-biologics/vaccines/vaccines-licensed-use-united-states.** A summary table of ingredients other than antigens that are used in vaccines can be accessed at **www.cdc.gov/vaccines/pubs/pink-book/downloads/appendices/B/excipient-table-2.pdf.**

Allergic reactions may occur if the vaccine recipient is sensitive to any ingredient in the vaccine. Therefore, a careful screening for allergy to a vaccine or a vaccine component is indicated. Standardized screening checklists are available to assist clinicians in screening for allergies and other potential contraindications to immunization. An example can be found at **www.immunize.org/catg.d/p4060.pdf.** The safety and effectiveness of vaccines and vaccine ingredients licensed for use in the United States are continuously monitored by the FDA and the Centers for Disease Control and Prevention (CDC).

ANTIGENS

Antigens in vaccines, sometimes referred to as immunogens, are toxoids, viruses, bacteria, or their components that result in active immunization, which is the process by which a person becomes protected from a disease. Some vaccines consist of a single antigen that is a highly defined constituent (eg, tetanus and diphtheria toxoids). Some vaccines consist of multiple antigens, which vary in chemical composition, structure, and number (eg, acellular components in pertussis vaccines; polysaccharide protein conjugates in 13-valent pneumococcal conjugate vaccine and serogroups A, C, W, and Y meningococcal conjugate vaccines; and recombinant proteins in 9-valent human papillomavirus vaccine). Other vaccines contain live attenuated viruses (eg, measles, mumps, and rubella vaccines), live reassorted viruses (eg, rotavirus vaccines), or killed whole cell viruses (eg, inactivated poliovirus vaccines and hepatitis A vaccines).

CONJUGATES

Conjugates are proteins that chemically combine with polysaccharide antigens to increase immunogenicity in children younger than 18 months who do not consistently respond to polysaccharide antigens and fail to induce immunologic memory and to boost antibody response to multiple doses of a vaccine. Some vaccines are chemically conjugated to protein carriers with proven immunologic potential (eg, diphtheria toxoid and meningococcal outer membrane protein complex) to improve the immune response (eg, *Haemophilus influenzae* type b and certain pneumococcal and meningococcal vaccines).

ADJUVANTS

Adjuvants are vaccine ingredients that are included to improve the immune response to antigens but do not themselves provide immunity. Adjuvants stimulate an immune response via cytokine release. Not all vaccines use adjuvants. For example, live vaccines such as measles, mumps, rubella, varicella, and rotavirus vaccines do not include adjuvants. Because the purpose of adjuvants is to generate stronger immune response, adjuvanted vaccines may cause local and systemic reactions more frequently compared with nonadjuvanted vaccines. Adjuvants have been ingredients in vaccines licensed for use in the United States for decades. Aluminum salts, a class of adjuvants that has been used safely in the United States since the 1930s and remains widely in use, are often in vaccines that contain subunit antigens of a cell (eg, hepatitis B vaccine) or toxoids (eg, diphtheria and tetanus toxoids). Newer adjuvants currently in use in the United States are generally limited to vaccines routinely recommended for adults. They include oil-in-water emulsions (used in adjuvanted influenza vaccine), deacylated monophosphoryl lipid A and saponin in a liposomal formulation (used in recombinant zoster vaccine), and cytosine-phosphate-guanine enriched oligodeoxynucleotide motifs (used in Heplisav-B). Adjuvants can also be "antigen sparing," in which a reduced amount of antigen can stimulate an equivalent immune response. Adjuvants also permit the production of multifold numbers of vaccine doses from limited antigen supply when large numbers of people need them, such as during an influenza pandemic.

STABILIZERS

Stabilizers are ingredients used in vaccines to help ensure that vaccine potency is not affected by adverse conditions such as heat and abnormal pH during the vaccine manufacturing process or during transport and storage. Stabilizers used in vaccines include sugars (eg, lactose or sucrose in *H influenzae* type b vaccines), amino acids (eg, glycine or monosodium salt of glutamic acid in live attenuated influenza vaccine), or proteins (eg, gelatin in varicella vaccine and some inactivated influenza vaccines).

PRESERVATIVES

Preservatives are included in multidose vials of vaccines as a safety measure to prevent the growth of microorganisms that may be introduced into the vaccine when the vial is penetrated repeatedly to withdraw doses of the vaccine. Examples of preservatives include thimerosal, formaldehyde, and phenol derivatives. Thimerosal is an ethyl mercury-containing organic compound that has been widely used as a preservative in many vaccines since the 1930s to help prevent contamination. Although there are minor side effects associated with vaccines containing thimerosal, such as redness and swelling at the injection site, the use of thimerosal in vaccines is safe. Regardless of the safe record of thimerosal in vaccines, all routinely recommended vaccines for infants and children in the United States are available thimerosal free. Inactivated influenza vaccines for pediatric use are available as thimerosal free or thimerosal containing (for multidose vials) formulations. Additional information on thimerosal in vaccines is available from the FDA at **www.fda.gov/vaccines-blood-biologics/safety-availability-biologics/thimerosal-and-vaccines.** Formaldehyde is used in vaccines to detoxify bacterial toxins (eg, diphtheria and tetanus toxoids) and inactivate viruses (eg, several inactivated influenza vaccines). Although almost all formaldehyde is removed during production of vaccines that use formaldehyde, very low amounts may remain. Formaldehyde exposure at such a residual level is far less than what occurs naturally in the environment. Phenols are used as a preservative in the 23-valent pneumococcal polysaccharide vaccine.

ANTIBIOTICS

As a class of preservatives, antibiotics are sometimes used during the vaccine manufacturing process to inhibit bacterial growth, and trace amounts can remain in the final product. During production, several inactivated influenza vaccines use antibiotics such as neomycin, gentamicin, and polymyxin B. Other vaccines that have trace amounts of antibiotics include the measles, mumps, and rubella vaccine and hepatitis A vaccines.

DILUENTS

Some vaccines are supplied as a lyophilized powder that must be reconstituted with their supplied liquid diluent prior to use. For some vaccines, the diluent is sterile water (eg, measles, mumps, rubella, and varicella combination vaccine). Other diluents contain vaccine antigens themselves (eg, serogroups A, C, W, and Y meningococcal conjugate vaccine) or the vaccine adjuvant component (eg, recombinant zoster vaccine). Diluents are specifically formulated for each vaccine. Therefore, only the specific diluent supplied for each vaccine should be used.

Vaccine Handling and Storage

For vaccines to be optimally effective, they must be stored properly from the time of manufacturing until they are administered. Immunization providers are responsible for proper storage and handling from the time the vaccine arrives at their facility until the vaccine is administered. All staff should be knowledgeable about the importance of proper storage and handling of vaccines and the implications of improper storage and handling. The administration of improperly stored and handled vaccines is a frequent error reported to the Vaccine Adverse Event Reporting System (VAERS) (see Vaccine Safety, p 42).

Recommendations for handling and storage of vaccines are summarized in the package insert for each product (**www.immunize.org/fda**) and should be reviewed. Additional information can be obtained directly from manufacturers. Contact information for manufacturers is available online (**www.cdc.gov/vaccines/hcp/admin/storage/downloads/manufact-dist-contact.pdf**). The Centers for Disease Control and Prevention (CDC) Vaccine Storage and Handling toolkit is a useful resource for quality-control systems for safe handling and storage of vaccines in an

office or clinic setting (**www.cdc.gov/vaccines/hcp/admin/storage/toolkit/
storage-handling-toolkit.pdf**).

A written vaccine-specific storage and handling plan should be available for reference by all staff members and kept on or near the unit used for storing vaccines. This plan should be updated annually. It should detail both routine management of vaccines and emergency measures for vaccine retrieval and storage and for standard operating procedures for documenting these activities.

Most vaccines are designated for optimal storage between +2°C and +8°C (+36°F and +46°F). Varicella vaccine has both refrigerated and frozen formulations. The refrigerated formulation should be stored between +2°C and +8°C (+36°F and +46°F), and the frozen formulation should be stored between −50°C and −15C° (−58°F and +5°F). The measles, mumps, and rubella (MMR) and measles, mumps, rubella, and varicella (MMRV) vaccines can be stored in either location with a safe temperature range between −50°C and +8°C (−58°F and +46°F).

It is imperative that great care be taken to avoid exposing refrigerated vaccines to freezing temperatures, even for brief periods. Such exposure can compromise the integrity of refrigerated vaccines even without generating ice crystals or other changes in physical appearance of the vaccine. Visual inspection cannot reliably detect a vaccine that has been compromised by freeze exposure; thus, only careful monitoring of the temperatures used to store these vaccines will allow identification of potentially altered vaccines. Refrigerator or freezer thermostats should be set at the factory-set or midpoint temperature, which will decrease the likelihood of temperature excursions.

Vaccines exposed to temperatures outside their approved storage ranges are generally considered ineffective, especially when no records exist about the temperature excursion or light exposure. They should be segregated in a bag or container, marked **"Do Not Use,"** and kept under the appropriate storing conditions (vaccine refrigerator or freezer). They should not be used until the specifics of the temperature excursion are reviewed. Protocols after the event vary depending on individual state or agency policies. Providers should contact their state immunization program, vaccine manufacturer, or both for guidance. Advice regarding disposition of improperly handled or stored vaccines should be documented. In general, manufacturers analyze information about the magnitude of the temperature excursion and the total amount of time that temperatures were out of range, as well as information about the vaccine in question, to determine whether a vaccine is likely to still be viable. Ideally, a temperature excursion should be immediately identified and immunization using affected vaccine halted until a vaccine viability determination can be made. If vaccine exposed to a temperature excursion is administered and subsequently determined not to be viable, the doses administered using the nonviable vaccine should be considered invalid. Providers should refer to state or agency policy on management of patients in receipt of invalid doses because of temperature excursion and vaccine administration errors. Manufacturers can be asked about possible replacement of nonviable vaccine.

Generally, all vaccines should be protected from light during long-term storage. Many vaccines, including human papillomavirus (HPV), MMR, MMRV, varicella, hepatitis B (HepB) (Recombivax), most influenza vaccines, meningococcal group B (Bexsero), inactivated poliovirus, and rotavirus vaccines, must be protected from light exposure of more than 30 minutes. Protection from light exposure can be accomplished by keeping each vial or syringe in its original carton while in recommended storage and until immediate use.

The diluent component of vaccines that need reconstitution may require storage at a different temperature than the antigen component and generally cannot be frozen. For appropriate storage of the diluent component, the recommendations in the package insert should be followed.

PERSONNEL

A primary staff vaccine coordinator and an alternate vaccine coordinator should be trained and responsible for vaccine storage and handling. In addition, a physician or manager with understanding of the importance of appropriate vaccine storage should be engaged with the responsible vaccine coordinating staff. The CDC offers online training on vaccine storage and handling, and information can be found at **www2a. cdc.gov/nip/isd/ycts/mod1/courses/sh/ce.asp.** Vaccine coordinators and all staff handling vaccines should have training and education on vaccine storage and handling as part of new employee orientation, annually (refresher training), when new vaccines are added to the inventory, and when recommendations for storage and handling of vaccines are updated (**www.cdc.gov/vaccines/ed/index.html**). The vaccine coordinator should be responsible for:

- Ordering vaccines.
- Overseeing proper receipt and storage of shipments.
- Documenting vaccine inventory information.
- Organizing vaccines in storage units.
- Setting up temperature-monitoring devices.
- Checking and recording storage unit temperatures on a log (at the start of each workday if using a device that displays minimum/maximum temperatures or the current temperature at the start and end of the workday if using a device that does not display minimum/maximum temperatures).
- Daily physical inspection of the storage unit.
- Rotating stock so that vaccines closest to expiration date are used first.
- Contacting the state Vaccines for Children (VFC) program vaccine coordinator if it appears that VFC vaccines will expire before they will be used in the practice.
- Monitoring expiration dates and ensuring expired vaccines are removed from the refrigerator/freezer.
- Responding to potential storage temperature excursions and calling the manufacturer, VFC program, or both to obtain guidance for temperature excursion events.
- Overseeing proper vaccine transport, either routine or in an emergency.
- Maintaining all appropriate vaccine storage and handling documentation, including temperature excursion responses.
- Maintaining storage equipment and records, including VFC program documentation.
- Informing all people who will be handling vaccines about specific storage requirements and stability limitations of the products they will encounter. The details of proper storage conditions should be posted on or near each refrigerator or freezer used for vaccine storage or should be readily available to staff. Receptionists, mail clerks, and other staff members who also may receive shipments should be educated in these matters as well.

EQUIPMENT

- Store vaccines in refrigerator and freezer units that can maintain the appropriate temperature range and are large enough to maintain the largest anticipated inventory without crowding. Use purpose-built or pharmaceutical-grade units designed to either refrigerate or freeze. These units can be compact, under-the-counter style, or large.
- Household-grade units can be an acceptable alternative to pharmaceutical-grade or purpose-built vaccine storage units in some situations. However, these units should be replaced with stand-alone units as soon as is practical. Household-grade units are primarily designed for home use. The freezer compartment is not recommended to store vaccines, and certain areas of the refrigerator should be avoided as well, including directly under cooling vents, in deli, fruit, or vegetable drawers, or in door shelves, because of instability of temperatures and air flow in these areas. A separate freezer unit is necessary if the facility provides frozen vaccines.
- Dormitory-style or bar-style combined refrigerator/freezer units are not acceptable for vaccine storage under any circumstances and are not allowed for vaccine storage of VFC program products. These units have a single exterior door and an evaporator plate/cooling coil, usually located in an icemaker/freezer compartment. These units pose a significant risk of freezing vaccine, even when used for temporary storage.
- Inspection of door seals, vacuuming coils, and other maintenance of refrigeration units should be performed at least annually.
- Use refrigerators with wire—not glass—shelving to improve air circulation in the unit, and do not place bins or boxes against rear or side walls of the refrigerator. The CDC recommends that each vaccine storage unit should be monitored by a digital data logger with accuracy of $+/- 0.5°C$ ($1°F$). The temperature-monitoring device should be capable of continuous frequent measurements (no less frequently than every 30 minutes and with a detachable probe that best reflects vaccine temperatures, such as those in a temperature buffer [eg, biosafe glycol, glass beads, sand, Teflon]), should display daily minimum and maximum temperatures, and should be readable without opening the unit door. The buffered probe(s) should be located in the center of the vaccines, away from the walls, vents, and floor of the vaccine storage unit. Temperature data should be displayed graphically and should be able to be stored for 3 years. The graphic data should be reviewed, and corrective efforts should be documented if daily minimum and maximum values are found to be outside of acceptable ranges.
- Use a temperature-monitoring device with a buffered probe and a Certificate of Calibration Testing (also known as Report of Calibration). Such temperature-monitoring devices have been individually tested for accuracy against a recognized reference standard by a laboratory with accreditation from an International Laboratory Accreditation Cooperation (ILAC) Mutual Recognition Arrangement (MRA) signatory body, or by a laboratory or manufacturer with documentation that calibration testing performed meets ISO/IEC 17025 international standards for calibration testing and traceability. These devices are sold with an individually numbered certificate documenting this testing. Providers who receive VFC vaccines or other vaccines purchased with public funds should consult their state's immunization program

regarding the required methods and timeframe for temperature-monitoring device calibration testing. The National Institute of Standards and Technology maintains a website devoted to vaccine storage education (**www.nist.gov/pml/div685/grp01/vaccines.cfm**). Calibration testing and traceability must be performed every 1 to 2 years from the last calibration testing date (date certificate issued) or suggested calibration timelines from the manufacturer of the device must be used. Temperature accuracy of temperature-monitoring devices can be checked using an ice melting point test (**www.nist.gov/pml/div685/grp01/upload/Ice-Melting-Point-Validation-Method-for-Data-Loggers.pdf**). Providers should check with their state VFC program for specific requirements related to calibration testing of temperature-monitoring devices. Do not drill through the refrigerator or freezer to route a temperature probe.

- Providers should use a remote alarm notification system that sends an alert if temperature is out of range. These alarms usually have the capability to send notifications via email, telephone, or text. Redundant, multiple alerts are recommended to ensure receipt. Provision should be made to ensure alerts are still sent if there is loss of power and/or internet.

PROCEDURES

- Maintain a vaccine inventory log, which should include vaccine name, number of doses, arrival condition of the vaccine, manufacturer and lot numbers, and expiration date.
- Formally accept vaccine on receipt of shipment:
  - Ensure that the expiration date of the delivered product has not passed and identify any soon-to-expire products.
  - Examine the merchandise and its shipping container for any evidence of damage during transport.
  - Determine whether the interval between shipment from the supplier and arrival of the product at its destination is within the allowable limit noted on the shipping insert or container, and whether the product has been exposed to excessive heat or cold that might alter its integrity. Review vaccine time and temperature indicators, both chemical and electronic, if included in the vaccine shipment.
  - Find and inspect any temperature excursion devices (electronic or temperature-tape) found in the shipment for evidence of temperature excursions. Do not accept the shipment if reasonable suspicion exists that the delivered product may have been damaged by environmental insult or improper handling during transport.
    - However, if you are a VFC provider, do not refuse vaccine shipments. In the case of vaccine shipment compromise or a problem with the temperature monitors, the VFC provider must contact the McKesson Specialty Contact Center and/or VFC program immediately using the telephone number dedicated to receiving provider calls about vaccine usability: 1-877-TEMP123.
  - Contact the vaccine supplier or manufacturer when unusual circumstances raise questions about the stability of a delivered vaccine. Store suspect vaccine under proper conditions and label it **"Do Not Use"** until the usability has been determined.

- Inspect the refrigerator and freezer:
  - If using a household-grade combination refrigerator-freezer, determine the placement of the cold air vents and do not put vaccines on the top shelf or near the vents. A minimum-maximum temperature-monitoring device in a thermal buffer is preferred to record extremes in temperature fluctuation and reset to baseline daily. Consider use of an alarm system capable of phone/text message/email notification if there is equipment failure, power outage, or temperature excursion. The refrigerator temperature should be maintained between +2°C and +8°C (+36°F and +46°F), and the freezer temperature should be maintained between −50°C and −15°C (−58°F and +5°F). A "**Do Not Unplug**" sign should be affixed directly next to the refrigerator electrical outlet and to the circuit breaker controlling that circuit.
- Train and designate staff to respond immediately to temperature recordings outside the recommended range and to document response and outcome.
  - Inspect the unit weekly for outdated vaccine and either dispose of or return expired products appropriately.
- Establish routine procedures:
  - Store vaccine where temperature remains constant.
  - Store vaccines according to temperatures specified in the package insert.
  - Rotate vaccine supplies so that the shortest-dated vaccines are in front to reduce wastage because of expiration.
  - Promptly remove expired (outdated) vaccines from the refrigerator or freezer and dispose of them appropriately or return to manufacturer to avoid accidental use.
  - Store both opened and unopened vials in the original packaging, which facilitates temperature stability, inventory management, and rotation of vaccine by expiration date and avoids light exposure. Mark the outside of boxes of opened vaccines with a large "X" to indicate that it has been opened.
  - Keep opened vials of vaccine in a tray so that they are readily identifiable.
  - Indicate on the label of each vaccine vial the date and time the vaccine was reconstituted or first opened.
  - Unless immediate use is planned, avoid reconstituting multiple doses of vaccine or drawing up multiple doses of vaccine in multiple syringes. Predrawing vaccine increases the possibility of medication errors and causes uncertainty of vaccine stability.
  - Because different vaccines can share similar components/names (eg, diphtheria and tetanus and acellular pertussis vaccines [DTaP and Tdap], or pneumococcal, meningococcal, and influenza products), care should be taken during storage to ensure that the different products are stored separately in a manner to avoid confusion and possible medication errors.
  - Each vaccine and diluent vial should be inspected carefully for damage or contamination prior to use. The expiration date printed on the vial or box should be checked. Vaccine can be used through the last day of the month indicated by the expiration date unless otherwise stated on the package labeling. The expiration date or time for some vaccines changes once the vaccine vial is opened or the vaccine is reconstituted. This information is available in the product package insert. Regardless of expiration date, vaccine and diluent should only be used as long as their appearance is as described in the product package insert and have

been stored and handled properly. Expired vaccine or diluent should never be used.

* All reconstituted vaccines should be administered as soon as possible after reconstitution and within the time interval specified in the package insert. All reconstituted vaccines should be refrigerated during the interval in which they may be used unless alternative temperatures are specified in the package insert.
* Always store vaccines in the refrigerator or freezer as indicated until immediately prior to administration. Do not open more than 1 vial of a specific vaccine at a time.
* Do not keep food or drink in refrigerators in which vaccine is stored. This is not a best practice for medication storage. This will reduce frequent opening of the unit that leads to thermal instability.
* Do not store radioactive materials in the same refrigerator in which vaccines are stored.
* Discuss with all clinic or office personnel any violation of protocol for handling vaccines or any accidental temperature excursion. Follow temperature excursion procedures until the vaccine manufacturers can be contacted to determine the disposition of the affected vaccine.

SUMMARY

Best equipment and practices for storage of refrigerated vaccines are as follows:
1. Purpose-built or pharmaceutical-grade refrigerator is recommended for vaccine storage.
2. Wire shelving and an interior circulating fan.
3. A digital data logger with a buffered probe should be placed in the center of the vaccines within each storage unit.
4. Displays with current temperature and resettable maximum and minimum temperatures visible on the outside of the unit.
5. Audible temperature alarm with capability for rapid user notification via phone/text message/email should temperature excursion be detected.
6. Extra space in a household-grade unit should be filled with water bottles to serve as a cold mass and to prolong safe storage in the event of refrigerator failure. Follow manufacturer's guidance for purpose-built and pharmaceutical-grade vaccine storage units, because this practice may not be necessary or recommended in those units.

VACCINE TRANSPORT

Transport of vaccines is not routinely recommended but may be necessary in emergency situations (eg, entire stock is being relocated for its protection) and may be appropriate for off-site clinics or when relocation of stock is required (eg, another site needs your excess supply). Vaccines should only be transported using appropriate packing materials that provide the maximum protections. Vaccines should never be moved, even over a short distance, without the use of an appropriate transport system. Portable vaccine refrigerator or freezer units are preferred, but qualified containers and packouts may also be used for either emergency or other necessary vaccine transport. The conditioned water bottle transport system may only be used for emergency transport. The manufacturer's original shipping container may only be used in an emergency as a last resort. Soft-sided food and beverage coolers should never be used; however, soft-sided containers engineered specifically for vaccine transport may be used. Phase change materials at +4°C to +5°C (+39°F to +41°F) can be purchased to maintain proper temperatures. Follow the manufacturer's instructions for use to reduce the risk of freezing vaccines during transport.

- Do not use frozen gel packs or coolant packs from original vaccine shipments to pack refrigerated vaccines. They can still freeze vaccines even if they are conditioned or appear to be "sweating." Do not use dry ice, even for temporary storage. Dry ice might expose the vaccines to temperatures colder than −50°C (−58°F).
- Use a continuous temperature-monitoring device, preferably a digital data logger with a probe that best reflects vaccine temperatures such as a buffered probe, for monitoring and recording temperatures while transporting vaccines. Place the buffered probe directly with the vaccines.
- Keep the temperature-monitoring device display on top of vaccines so the temperature can be seen easily.
- Ensure staff are trained on emergency procedures, and roles and responsibilities are clearly detailed in a written plan that is easily accessible to all staff.

EMERGENCY VACCINE STORAGE AND HANDLING

In addition to emergency transport instructions, practices should develop a written plan for emergency management of vaccine in the event of a catastrophic event or malfunction of the storage unit, train personnel, and make the plan easily accessible. Refrigerators vary and may maintain their +2°C to +8°C temperature for only 2 to 3 hours without power. This plan should include establishing an agreement with at least one alternate storage facility even if you have a generator or battery-powered back-up equipment. Ensure 24-hour access to alternate facilities as well as after-hours access to your own facility. Refer to emergency transport plans in the event you need to move vaccine to an alternate facility.

After a power outage or mechanical failure, it should not be assumed that vaccine exposed to temperature above the recommended range is unusable without first contacting the vaccine manufacturer (or, for VFC vaccines, the McKesson Specialty Contact Center at 1-877-TEMP123 and/or VFC program) for guidance before discarding vaccine. Guidance on vaccine transport is available from the AAP (**www.aap. org/en-us/advocacy-and-policy/aap-health-initiatives/immunization/ Pages/vaccine-storage-and-handling-guidance.aspx**) and CDC (**www.cdc. gov/vaccines/hcp/admin/storage/toolkit/index.html**).

Vaccine Administration

GENERAL CONSIDERATIONS

Proper vaccine administration is critical to ensure safe and effective delivery of the vaccine antigen to the recipient. In addition, health care personnel who administer vaccines should be trained in proper vaccine preparation, infection control practices, and care of patients before and after vaccine administration.

TRAINING AND EDUCATION. Competency-based training on vaccination should be integrated into existing staff education programs such as new staff orientation and annual continuing education requirements. Numerous in-person and online vaccination training opportunities are available, including the web-based education and training modules available at **www.aap.org/en-us/advocacy-and-policy/ aap-health-initiatives/immunizations/Practice-Management/Pages/ Vaccine-Administration.aspx** and **www.cdc.gov/vaccines/ed/index.html.** Additionally, demonstration videos and other resources can be found at **www.aap. org/en-us/advocacy-and-policy/aap-health-initiatives/immunizations/ Practice-Management/Pages/Practice-Management.aspx, www.cdc.gov/ vaccines/hcp/admin/resource-library.html,** and **immunize.org/clinic/ administering-vaccines.asp.**

INFECTION CONTROL. Health care personnel who administer vaccines should take appropriate precautions to protect themselves and minimize the risk of disease spread. Proper hand hygiene is required before preparing and administering vaccines and with each new patient contact. The use of gloves is not required when administering vaccines unless the health care provider has an open lesion on the hand or expects to come in contact with body fluids or when gloves are required because of isolation precautions for the patient. Proper hand hygiene should be practiced regardless of whether or not gloves are used, and gloves should be changed between patients. Syringes and needles must be sterile and not reused. Discard used syringes and needles promptly in a proper punctureproof, labeled container located in the room where the vaccine is administered. To prevent inadvertent needlesticks or reuse, needles should not be recapped after use.

VACCINE PREPARATION. Vaccines and diluents should be used only if they have been stored and handled properly. Vaccines should be prepared immediately before administration using aseptic technique. If the vaccine requires reconstitution, only the diluent supplied by the manufacturer should be used. Each vaccine and diluent should be carefully inspected for damages on the container or vial and evidence of contamination (eg, unusual coloration or sediments), and to ensure that the vaccine and diluent have not expired. For vaccine and diluent in a multidose vial that should be used within a certain timeframe after its content was first drawn ("beyond use date"), the beyond use date on the package insert should be identified and noted on the vial. Changing needles between drawing vaccine into a syringe and its injection is not necessary unless the needle has been damaged.

PATIENT CARE BEFORE, DURING, AND AFTER VACCINE ADMINISTRATION. A patient should be comfortably seated or lying down before an injection and, if necessary, adequately restrained (see Managing Injection Pain, p 30). Because of the rare possibility of a severe allergic reaction to a vaccine or its components, health care personnel who administer vaccines should be able to recognize and treat allergic reactions, including anaphylaxis (see Hypersensitivity Reactions After Immunization, p 51). Syncope can occur following vaccine administration, particularly in adolescents and young adults. Health care personnel should take appropriate measures to prevent injuries if weakness, dizziness, or loss of consciousness occurs. However, syncope can occur without presyncopal symptoms, so patients should be seated or lying down during vaccination. Consideration should be given to observing patients while *seated or lying down for 15 minutes* after vaccine administration to avoid the risk of fall if syncope occurs. Syncope following vaccination is not a contraindication to that or any other vaccine in the future.

SITES AND ROUTES OF VACCINE ADMINISTRATION

Vaccines are administered parenterally, orally, or intranasally. Parenteral routes include intramuscular (IM), subcutaneous (SC), and intradermal injections. Most vaccines are administered intramuscularly and some are administered subcutaneously, such as the measles, mumps, rubella, and varicella vaccines. Intradermal and intranasal influenza vaccines are available, and the inactivated poliovirus and pneumococcal polysaccharide vaccines can be administered intramuscularly or subcutaneously. Additional information is available at **www.aap.org/en-us/advocacy-and-policy/ aap-health-initiatives/immunizations/Practice-Management/Pages/ Vaccine-Administration.aspx** and **www.cdc.gov/vaccines/hcp/admin/ admin-protocols.html.**

PARENTERAL VACCINATION. Approved sites and routes of administration can be found in package inserts of vaccines and in Table 1.7 (p 16). When multiple parenteral vaccines are indicated, separate injection sites should be used. If the same limb must be used as the injection site for 2 or more vaccinations, separate injections by at least 1 inch so that local reactions can be differentiated if they develop. Multiple vaccines should not be mixed in a single syringe.

IM Administration. Vaccines administered intramuscularly should be injected at a site that minimizes risks for neural, vascular, or tissue injury. Most commonly used vaccines are administered intramuscularly. For IM injections, the site of choice between thigh and arm depends on the age of the vaccine recipient, degree of muscle development, and thickness of adipose tissue at the injection site. In children younger than 2 years, the anterolateral aspect of the upper thigh provides the largest muscle and is the preferred site. In older children, the deltoid muscle is usually large enough for IM injection. Decisions on needle length should be based on the size of the muscle and the thickness of adipose tissue at the injection site. Needles should be long enough to reach the muscle mass and prevent vaccine from seeping into subcutaneous tissue and causing local reactions but not so long as to reach underlying nerves, blood vessels, or bone. The use of a 22- to 25-gauge needle is generally recommended for IM injections. Suggested needle lengths are described in Table 1.8. Note that the upper, outer aspect of buttocks generally should not be used for vaccination, because the gluteal region is covered by a significant layer of subcutaneous fat. Because of diminished immunogenicity, hepatitis B and rabies vaccines should not be administered in the buttocks at any age. Localized swelling, redness, and pain can occur at the IM injection site, but serious complications are rare. Reported adverse events include infections, bleeding, nerve injury, and shoulder injury related to vaccine administration (SIRVA) from inadvertent injection into the joint space. In general, vaccines containing adjuvants (eg, aluminum) are recommended to be injected deep into the muscle mass. If administered subcutaneously or intradermally, these vaccines can cause local irritation, inflammation, granuloma formation, and tissue necrosis. For patients with a known bleeding disorder or receiving anticoagulant therapy, bleeding complications following IM injection can occur. Additional information on vaccinating patients with bleeding disorders and other special populations such as preterm infants and pregnant women are available at **www.cdc.gov/vaccines/hcp/acip-recs/general-recs/ special-situations.html.**

Table 1.8. Site and Needle Length by Age for Intramuscular Immunization[a]

Age Group	Needle Length, inches (mm)	Suggested Injection Site
Newborns (preterm and term) and infants <1 mo of age	⅝ (16 mm)[b]	Anterolateral thigh muscle
Infants, 1–12 mo of age	1 (25 mm)	Anterolateral thigh muscle
Toddlers, 1–2 years	1–1¼ (25–32 mm)	Anterolateral thigh muscle (preferred)
	⅝[b]–1 (16–25 mm)	Deltoid muscle of the arm
Children, 3–10 years	⅝[b]–1 (16–25 mm)	Deltoid muscle of arm (preferred)
	1–1¼ (25–32 mm)	Anterolateral thigh muscle
Children, 11–18 years	⅝[b]–1 (16–25 mm)	Deltoid muscle of arm (preferred)
	1–1½ (25–38 mm)	Anterolateral thigh muscle
Adults		
Female and male, weight <130 lb	1 (25 mm)[c]	Deltoid muscle of the arm
Female and male, weight 130–152 lb	1 (25 mm)	Deltoid muscle of the arm
Female, weight 153–200 lb	1–1½ (25–38 mm)	Deltoid muscle of the arm
Male, weight 153–260 lb	1–1½ (25–38 mm)	Deltoid muscle of the arm
Female, weight >200 lb	1½ (38 mm)	Deltoid muscle of the arm
Male, weight >260 lb	1½ (38 mm)	Deltoid muscle of the arm

[a] Adapted from General Best Practice Guidelines for Immunization: Best Practices Guidance of the Advisory Committee on Immunization Practices (ACIP), Vaccine Administration, Table 6-2, **www.cdc.gov/vaccines/hcp/acip-recs/general-recs/administration.html#t6_2**

[b] If the skin is stretched tightly and subcutaneous tissues are not bunched.

[c] Some experts recommend a ⅝-inch needle for men and women who weigh less than 130 lb. If used, skin must be stretched tightly (do not bunch subcutaneous tissue).

SC Administration. Several routinely recommended vaccines are administered subcutaneously, including measles, mumps, rubella; measles, mumps, rubella, varicella; and varicella vaccines. Inactivated poliovirus and pneumococcal conjugate vaccines can be administered subcutaneously or intramuscularly. SC injections place the vaccine in the tissue between the dermal and muscle layers. SC administration is made at the anterolateral aspect of the thigh or the upper outer triceps area by inserting the needle in a pinched-up fold of skin at a 45° angle. A 23- to 25-gauge needle of ⅝ inch length is generally recommended. Like other vaccines that are administered parenterally, localized swelling, redness, and pain can occur at the injection site, but serious complications are rare.

Intradermal Administration. No intradermal vaccine is approved for use in patients younger than age 18 years, because they may not have sufficient skin thickness. Intradermal inactivated influenza vaccine is available for patients 18 through 64 years of age.

ORAL VACCINATION. Only rotavirus vaccines and oral typhoid vaccine are approved for oral administration in children. For infants, oral vaccines should be administered slowly down one side of the inside of the cheek between the cheek and gum toward the back of the mouth, but not so far as to trigger the gag reflex. Do not squirt the vaccine directly into the throat. Detailed information on oral delivery of vaccines is included in package inserts. Breastfeeding does not appear to diminish response to rotavirus vaccines, and the infant can eat or drink immediately following oral vaccination. If a dose of rotavirus vaccine is regurgitated or spat or vomited out, do not readminister the vaccine. Currently, there are no data available on the benefits or risks of repeating the dose. The infant should receive the remaining recommended doses of rotavirus vaccine following the routine schedule.

INTRANASAL VACCINATION. Live attenuated influenza vaccine (LAIV) is the only vaccine currently approved for intranasal administration. LAIV is approved for use for healthy, nonpregnant people 2 years through 49 years of age. The vaccine is prepared inside a special sprayer device that divides the dose into equal parts for delivery into each nostril. The dose need not be repeated if the patient sneezes after vaccination. LAIV can be administered during minor illnesses, but if nasal congestion might impede delivery of the vaccine, administration of injectable influenza vaccine or deferral of the use of LAIV until the symptom resolves should be considered.

Managing Injection Pain

A planned approach to decreasing the child's anxiety before, during, and after immunization and to decreasing pain from the injection is helpful for children of any age. The Advisory Committee on Immunization Practices (ACIP),[1] the Canadian Medical Association,[2] and the World Health Organization[3] provide guidance on a variety of pain mitigation interventions during vaccination. Parents, children 3 years and older, and health care providers administering vaccine injections should be educated about evidence-based techniques for reducing injection pain or distress. Combination vaccines should be used when feasible to reduce the number of injections and their attendant pain.

PHYSICAL AND PSYCHOLOGICAL TECHNIQUES FOR MINIMIZING INJECTION PAIN AND ANXIETY

Strategies to reduce pain include tactile stimulation and holding the child, which is routinely recommended in children younger than 3 years. If multiple vaccines are to be given, they should be administered in order from least to most painful. The

---

[1]Ezeanolue E, Harriman K, Hunter P, Kroger A, Pellegrini C. General best practice guidelines for immunization. Best practice guidance of the advisory committee on immunization practices (ACIP). Available at: **www.cdc.gov/vaccines/hcp/acip-recs/general-recs/downloads/general-recs.pdf.** Accessed July 26, 2020

[2]Taddio A, McMurtry M, Shah V, et al. Reducing pain during vaccine injections: clinical practice guideline. *CMAJ.* 2015;187(13):975-982

[3]World Health Organization. Reducing pain at the time of vaccination: WHO position paper – September 2015. *Wkly Epidemiol Rec.* 2015;90(39):505-510

appropriately sized needle should be plunged rapidly through the skin without aspiration. Aspiration before injection is not necessary, because large blood vessels are not present at the recommended injection sites and pain may be increased with longer needle dwell time in the tissue. Breastfeeding, feeding sweet-tasting solutions, and applying topical anesthetics at the site of injection are other tools that have been used before vaccine administration to decrease pain. Distraction strategies, including pinwheels, deep breathing exercises, music, videos, and toys, have been used in older children to decrease anxiety and pain. Adolescents should be seated or lying down during vaccination to reduce the risk of injury should syncope develop. Consideration should be given to observing patients while *seated or lying down for 15 minutes* after vaccine administration to avoid the risk of fall if syncope occurs. Warming a vaccine by rubbing it between the hands is not recommended because of concern for altering vaccine effectiveness.

PHARMACOLOGIC TECHNIQUES FOR MINIMIZING INJECTION PAIN

If topical anesthesia is used, planning ahead is necessary so that the anesthetic is applied to allow the minimum 30 to 60 minutes required to provide effective anesthesia. Strategies can include applying the anesthetic en route to the office visit or immediately on arrival. Lidocaine 4% (LMX4) is approved by the US Food and Drug Administration (FDA) for children older than 2 years, is available over the counter, and takes effect 30 minutes after application. Lidocaine 2.5%/prilocaine 2.5% (EMLA), available by prescription, is approved by the FDA for neonates >37 weeks' estimated gestational age, infants, and children and takes effect 60 minutes after application. These products should be applied under occlusion. Topical application of ethyl chloride, a topical coolant sprayed onto a cotton ball that is then placed over the injection site for 15 seconds prior to administering the injection, has been shown to decrease injection pain in school-aged children. Administration of oral analgesics such as acetaminophen prior to vaccinations has not been shown to reduce pain and may have a detrimental effect on the immune response to the vaccine(s) being administered. Acetaminophen can be used after immunization to treat pain and to reduce the discomfort of fever.

Immunization Schedule and Timing of Vaccines

The purpose of a vaccine is to prompt the development of immunity against a disease in a person without the person developing the disease. The balance between timely protection and optimal immunologic response is the basis of the immunization schedule. The vaccination schedule—including dose, frequency, and timing, along with the age and health status of the person—should consider available clinical and epidemiologic data on vaccine safety and efficacy and programmatic considerations (eg, incorporating vaccinations into scheduled health maintenance visits).

RECOMMENDED IMMUNIZATION SCHEDULE

The "Recommended Child and Adolescent Immunization Schedule for Ages 18 Years or Younger, United States" represents a consensus of the Advisory Committee on Immunization Practices (ACIP), a federal advisory committee administered by the

Centers for Disease Control and Prevention (CDC), and the American Academy of Pediatrics (AAP) and the American Academy of Family Physicians (AAFP). The immunization schedule, available at **www.cdc.gov/vaccines/schedules/index.html** is reviewed annually and published in February each year.

AGE INDICATIONS FOR VACCINES

The age at which a vaccine is indicated depends on immunologic maturity or status of the patient, risk of exposure to the pathogen for which the vaccine is effective, vaccine safety, and optimal booster effect if the vaccine is a part of a series. In general, a vaccine is recommended for the youngest age of patients who are at risk for disease for which the vaccine is safe and provides protection. With a parenterally administered live vaccine for infants, the inhibitory effect of residual maternal antibody determines the optimal age at which the infant should receive the vaccine. For example, a measles-containing vaccine provides suboptimal seroconversion during the first year of life of an infant because of an interference by maternal antibody acquired through transplacental passage as well as the infant's own immature immune system.

MULTIPLE DOSES OF THE SAME VACCINE

Some vaccines are administered as a series of doses to provide optimal protection. For example, one dose of the measles, mumps, and rubella vaccine (MMR) is 93% effective against measles, 78% effective against mumps, and 97% effective against rubella. A small number of vaccine recipients may fail to respond to 1 dose of measles-containing vaccine; however, 97% respond to the second dose. In addition, a second dose of MMR is believed to be 88% effective against mumps. The protection provided by some vaccines wanes over time, and booster doses are periodically indicated. For example, tetanus and diphtheria toxoids require booster doses to maintain protective antibody concentrations. For a multidose primary vaccination series, administration at recommended intervals optimizes the immunologic response and minimizes possible adverse reactions (eg, increased local and systemic reactions to diphtheria and tetanus toxoids administration).

MULTIPLE VACCINES ADMINISTERED AT THE SAME TIME

In general, different vaccines administered at the same time are safe and effective and routinely recommended in the immunization schedule. Administration of multiple vaccines at the same time promotes adherence to completion of vaccination series (ie, reduced medical visits) and ensures optimal protection. In addition, simultaneous administration of vaccines is particularly important for scheduling immunizations for children with lapsed or missed immunizations, for children requiring early or rapid protection, and for people preparing for international travel (see Simultaneous Administration of Multiple Vaccines, p 36).

More than 1 live-virus vaccine (eg, MMR and varicella vaccines) may be administered at the same time. Immune responses may be impaired when 2 or more parenterally administered live-virus vaccines are not administered simultaneously but within 28 days of each other; therefore, live-virus vaccines not administered on the same day should be given at least 28 days (4 weeks) apart whenever possible (Table 1.9). This restriction does not apply to the nasally administered live attenuated influenza vaccine, which does not interfere with immune responses to MMR or varicella vaccination. In

Table 1.9. Guidelines for Spacing of Live and Inactivated Antigens

Antigen Combination	Recommended Minimum Interval Between Doses
2 or more inactivated[a]	May be administered simultaneously or at any interval between doses
Inactivated plus live	May be administered simultaneously or at any interval between doses
2 or more live[b]	28-day minimum interval if not administered simultaneously

[a] See text for exceptions.
[b] An exception is made for live oral vaccines, which can be administered simultaneously or at any interval before or after inactivated or live parenteral vaccines.

addition, live oral vaccines—Ty21a typhoid vaccine and rotavirus vaccine—may be administered simultaneously with or at any interval before or after inactivated or live injectable vaccine (Table 1.9).

No minimum interval is required between administration of different inactivated vaccines, with 3 exceptions: 1) when both 13-valent pneumococcal conjugate vaccine (PCV13) and 23-valent pneumococcal polysaccharide vaccine (PPSV23) are indicated, PCV13 should be administered first, followed by PPSV23 at least 8 weeks later (see *Streptococcus pneumoniae* (Pneumococcal) Infections, p 717); 2) when MenACWY-D (Menactra) is administered 30 days after diphtheria and tetanus toxoids and acellular pertussis (DTaP) vaccine, it interferes with the immune response for all 4 meningococcal serogroups, and therefore, MenACWY-D should be administered either before or at the same time as DTaP; and 3) for children for whom quadrivalent meningococcal conjugate vaccine is indicated, MenACWY-D (Menactra) should not be administered concomitantly OR within 4 weeks of administration of PCV13 immunization, to avoid potential interference with the immune response to PCV13. Because of their high risk for invasive pneumococcal disease, children with functional or anatomic asplenia should not be immunized with MenACWY-D (Menactra) before 2 years of age so that they can complete their PCV13 series; MenACWY-CRM (Menveo) can be used before 2 years of age, however, because it is licensed for use down to 2 months of age and has been shown to not interfere with the immune response to PCV13.

COMBINATION VACCINES

Combination vaccine products may be administered when they are age appropriate and any of the component vaccine is indicated and other components are not contraindicated. The use of a combination vaccine generally is preferred over separate injections of its equivalent component vaccines (see Combination Vaccines, page 37).

Web-based childhood immunization schedulers using the current vaccine recommendations are available for parents, caregivers, and health care professionals to facilitate making schedules for children 0 through 6 years of age (**www.cdc.gov/vaccines**). Most state and regional immunization information systems (also known as immunization registries) also will forecast immunizations that are due according to the immunization schedule.

Minimum Ages and Minimum Intervals Between Vaccine Doses

Immunizations generally are recommended for members of the youngest age group at risk of experiencing the disease for whom efficacy, effectiveness, immunogenicity, and safety of the vaccine have been demonstrated. Most vaccines in the childhood and adolescent immunization schedule require 2 or more doses for stimulation of an adequate and persisting immune response. The schedule is determined based on studies demonstrating safety and effectiveness of individual vaccines evaluated in the context of the existing childhood immunization schedule (**www.cdc.gov/vaccines/ schedules/index.html**).

Vaccines generally should not be administered at intervals less than the recommended minimum or at an age earlier than the recommended minimum (ie, accelerated schedules). Administering doses of a multidose vaccine at intervals shorter than those recommended in the childhood and adolescent immunization schedule might be necessary in circumstances in which an infant or child is behind schedule and needs to be brought up to date quickly or when international travel is anticipated. For example, during a measles outbreak or for international travel, measles vaccine may be administered as early as 6 months of age. However, if a measles-containing vaccine is administered before 12 months of age, the dose is not counted toward the 2-dose measles vaccine series, and the child should be reimmunized at 12 through 15 months of age with a measles-containing vaccine; a third dose of a measles-containing vaccine then is indicated at 4 through 6 years of age but can be administered as early as 4 weeks after the second dose (see Measles, p 503).

Certain circumstances, such as the need for an additional office visit or a patient or parent poorly adherent to scheduled visits, could lead to consideration of administering a vaccine up to 4 days before the minimum interval or age. In general, vaccine doses administered (intentionally or inadvertently) 4 days or fewer before the minimum interval or age can be counted as valid. Health care professionals should be aware that state and school guidelines may consider such doses invalid and require additional vaccinations. Doses administered 5 days or more before the minimum interval or age should not be counted as valid doses and should be repeated as age appropriate. The repeat dose should be spaced by the recommended minimum interval after the invalid dose. Because of the unique schedule for rabies vaccine, consideration of days of a shortened interval between doses must be individualized.

The latest recommendations can be found in the annual immunization schedule (**http://redbook.solutions.aap.org/SS/Immunization_Schedules.aspx**).

Additional information from CDC can be found on the CDC website (**www.cdc. gov/vaccines/hcp/acip-recs/general-recs/index.html**).

Interchangeability of Vaccine Products

Similar vaccines made by different manufacturers can vary in several ways: the type, number, and amount of antigenic components; the formulation of adjuvants and conjugating agents; and the choice of stabilizers and preservatives. These differences may lead to variation in the immune response elicited. When possible, effort should be made to complete a series with vaccine made by the same manufacturer. If different brands of a particular vaccine require a different number of doses for series completion (eg, *Haemophilus influenzae* type b [Hib] and rotavirus vaccines) and a provider mixes brands in the primary series, the higher number of doses is recommended for series completion. Although data documenting the effects of interchangeability are limited, available results are reassuring for adequate immune responses, and most experts have considered vaccines interchangeable when administered according to their recommended schedule and dosing regimen. Approved vaccines that may be used interchangeably during a vaccine series from different manufacturers, according to recommendations from the AAP or ACIP, include diphtheria and tetanus toxoids vaccines, hepatitis A vaccines, hepatitis B vaccines, and rabies vaccines.

An example of similar vaccines that are not recommended as interchangeable is the adult formulation of Recombivax HB (see Hepatitis B, p 381), which is approved for adolescents 11 through 15 years of age; adolescent patients who start their hepatitis B schedule with this vaccine are not candidates to complete their series with the adult formulation of Engerix-B. Likewise, because each of the 2 meningococcal B vaccines uses very different protein antigens and because there are no data on their interchangeability, the same vaccine must be used for all doses to complete the full meningococcal B series.

Approved rotavirus (RV) vaccines (RV5, RotaTeq; RV1, Rotarix) are considered interchangeable as long as recommendations concerning conversion from a 2-dose regimen (RV-1) to a 3-dose regimen (RV-5) are followed (see Rotavirus, p 644). Similarly, approved Hib conjugate vaccines are considered interchangeable as long as recommendations for a total of 3 doses in the first year of life are followed (ie, if 2 doses of Hib-OMP are not administered, 3 doses of a Hib-containing vaccine are required). When a vaccine with increased serotype content replaces a previously recommended product (eg, PCV13 for PCV7, or 9vHPV for 4vHPV), the vaccines are considered interchangeable, so the series can be completed with the broader serotype product.

Minimal data on safety and immunogenicity and no data on efficacy are available for interchangeability of DTaP vaccines from different manufacturers. When feasible, DTaP from the same manufacturer should be used for the primary series (see Pertussis, p 578). However, in circumstances in which the DTaP product received previously is not known or the previously administered product is not readily available, any of the DTaP vaccines may be used according to licensure for dose and age. Matching of booster doses of DTaP and adolescent Tdap by manufacturer is not necessary. Single-component vaccines from the same manufacturer of combination vaccines, including DTaP-IPV-Hib-HepB, DTaP-HepB-IPV, and DTaP-IPV/Hib are interchangeable (see Combination Vaccines, p 37).[1]

---

[1]Ezeanolue E, Harriman K, Hunter P, Kroger A, Pellegrini C. General best practice guidelines for immunization. Best practices guidance of the Advisory Committee on Immunization Practices (ACIP). Available at: **www.cdc.gov/vaccines/hcp/acip-recs/general-recs/downloads/general-recs.pdf.** Accessed July 26, 2020

Simultaneous Administration of Multiple Vaccines

Simultaneous administration of most vaccines according to the immunization schedule is safe, effective, and recommended. Infants and children have sufficient immunologic capacity to respond to multiple vaccines administered at the same time. There is no contraindication to simultaneous administration of multiple vaccines routinely recommended for infants and children, with 2 exceptions: (1) for children for whom quadrivalent meningococcal conjugate vaccine is indicated, MenACWY-D (Menactra) should not be administered concomitantly OR within 4 weeks of administration of PCV13 immunization, to avoid potential interference with the immune response to PCV13; MenACWY-CRM (Menveo) can be used before 2 years of age, however, because it has been shown to not interfere with the immune response to PCV13; and (2) when both 13-valent pneumococcal conjugate vaccine (PCV13) and 23-valent pneumococcal polysaccharide vaccine (PPSV23) are indicated, PCV13 should be administered first, followed by PPSV23 at least 8 weeks later.

The immune response to one vaccine generally does not interfere with responses to other vaccines. Simultaneous administration of IPV, MMR, varicella, or DTaP vaccines results in rates of seroconversion and of adverse events similar to those observed when vaccines are administered at separate visits. A slightly increased risk of febrile seizures is associated with the first dose of MMRV compared with MMR and monovalent varicella vaccine administered simultaneously at separate sites among children 12 through 23 months of age; after dose 1 of MMRV vaccine, 1 additional febrile seizure is expected to occur per approximately 2300 to 2600 young children immunized, compared with MMR and monovalent varicella. Evidence from several epidemiologic studies indicated that during the 2 influenza seasons spanning 2010–2012, there was an increased risk of febrile seizures in young children, mostly concentrated in children 6 through 23 months of age, when inactivated influenza vaccine (IIV) is administered simultaneously with PCV13 or DTaP-containing vaccines. This risk occurs on the day of vaccination to the day after; there did not appear to be an increased risk when IIV was administered without PCV13 or DTaP-containing vaccines. The risk was small with, at most, 1 additional febrile seizure per 3333 children vaccinated with any combination of simultaneous administration of these vaccines. More recently, a sentinel Center for Biologics Evaluation and Research (CBER)/Post-licensure Rapid Immunization Safety Monitoring (PRISM) surveillance report evaluating influenza vaccines and febrile seizures found no evidence of an elevated risk of febrile seizures in children 6 through 23 months of age following IIV administration during the 2013–2014 and 2014–2015 influenza seasons, noting that the risk of seizures after PCV13 or concomitant PCV13 and IIV was low compared with a child's lifetime risk of febrile seizures from other causes. Overall, simultaneous administration of IIV and PCV13 continues to be recommended when both vaccines are indicated because of the preponderance of benefit relative to the risk.

Because simultaneous administration of routinely recommended vaccines is not known to alter the effectiveness or safety of any of the recommended childhood vaccines, simultaneous administration of all vaccines that are appropriate for the age and immunization status of the recipient is recommended.[1] When vaccines are administered simultaneously,

---

[1] Ezeanolue E, Harriman K, Hunter P, Kroger A, Pellegrini C. General best practice guidelines for immunization. Best practices guidance of the Advisory Committee on Immunization Practices (ACIP). Available at: **www.cdc.gov/vaccines/hcp/acip-recs/general-recs/downloads/general-recs.pdf.** Accessed July 26, 2020

separate syringes and separate sites should be used, and injections into the same extremity should be separated by at least 1 inch so that any local reactions can be differentiated.

Individual vaccines should never be mixed in the same syringe unless they are specifically approved and labeled for administration in 1 syringe. If an inactivated vaccine and an Immune Globulin product are indicated concurrently (eg, hepatitis B vaccine and Hepatitis B Immune Globulin, rabies vaccine and Rabies Immune Globulin, tetanus-containing vaccine and Tetanus Immune Globulin), they should be administered at separate anatomic sites.

Combination Vaccines

Combination vaccines can decrease the number of injections during a single clinic visit and generally are preferred over separate injections of equivalent component vaccines. Table 1.10 lists combination vaccines approved for use and the age groups for which they are approved in the United States. Factors that could be considered by the provider, in consultation with the parent, include the routinely recommended schedule for vaccines based on age, health status, and other indications; vaccine safety and availability; cost; the number of injections needed; and whether the patient is likely to return for follow-up and complete vaccine series. Not all providers stock all vaccines that are routinely recommended. In addition, the use of combination vaccines involves complex economic and logistic considerations for providers.

Table 1.10. Combination Vaccines Approved by the US Food and Drug Administration (FDA)[a]

Vaccine[b]	Trade Name (Year Approved)	FDA Licensure Age Group	Use in Immunization Schedule
HepA-HepB	Twinrix (2001)	≥18 y	Three doses on a 0-, 1-, and 6-mo schedule
DTaP-HepB-IPV	Pediarix (2002)	6 wk through 6 y	Three-dose series at 2, 4, and 6 mo of age
MMRV[c]	ProQuad (2005)	12 mo through 12 y	Two doses usually at 12–15 mo and 4–6 y of age (see Varicella-Zoster Infections, p 831); separate by at least 1 mo between measles-containing vaccine and ProQuad and at least 3 mo between varicella-containing vaccine and ProQuad
DTaP-IPV	Kinrix (2008)	4 y through 6 y	Booster for fifth dose of DTaP and fourth dose of IPV in children who have received 3 doses of Pediarix or Infanrix and a fourth dose of Infanrix

Table 1.10. Combination Vaccines Approved by the US Food and Drug Administration (FDA),[a] continued

Vaccine[b]	FDA Licensure		
	Trade Name (Year Approved)	Age Group	Use in Immunization Schedule
DTaP-IPV/Hib	Pentacel (2008)	6 wk through 4 y	Four-dose series administered at 2, 4, 6, and 15 mo through 18 mo of age
DTaP-IPV	Quadracel (2015)	4 y through 6 y	Single dose approved for use in children 4 through 6 years of age as a fifth dose in DTaP series and as a fourth or fifth dose in IPV series, in children who have received 4 doses of Pentacel and/or Daptacel vaccine
DTaP-IPV-Hib-HepB	Vaxelis (2018)	6 wk through 4 y	Three dose series administered at 2, 4, and 6 months of age[d]

HepA indicates hepatitis A vaccine; HepB, hepatitis B vaccine; HepA-HepB, hepatitis A and hepatitis B combination vaccine; DTaP, diphtheria and tetanus toxoids and acellular pertussis vaccine; IPV, inactivated poliovirus vaccine; MMRV, measles, mumps, rubella, varicella vaccine; Hib, *Haemophilus influenzae* type b vaccine.

[a] Excludes measles, mumps, rubella vaccine (MMR); DTaP; tetanus and diphtheria toxoids and acellular pertussis vaccine (Tdap), and tetanus and diphtheria toxoids (Td), for which individual component vaccines are not available. IPV is not available as a single-antigen vaccine.

[b] Dash (-) indicates products in which the active components are supplied in their final (combined) form by the manufacturer; slash (/) indicates products in which active components must be mixed by the user.

[c] The American Academy of Pediatrics expresses no preference between MMR plus monovalent varicella vaccine or MMRV for toddlers receiving their first immunization of this kind. Parents should be counseled about the rare possibility of their child developing a febrile seizure 1 to 2 weeks after immunization with MMRV for the first immunizing dose.

[d] A fourth dose of acellular pertussis vaccine is needed to complete the pertussis primary series in infants who receive 3 doses of Vaxelis.

When patients have received the recommended series of immunizations for a particular antigen, administering an extra dose of this antigen as part of a combination vaccine is permissible and doing so will reduce the number of injections required, as long as the vaccines are age appropriate and there are no contraindications.

Confusing ambiguities in the names of vaccines and vaccine combinations benefit from development of electronic systems that automate bar code scanning, which reduce potential recording errors enhancing the convenience and accuracy of transferring vaccine-identifying information into health records and immunization information systems.

Lapsed Immunizations

A lapse in an immunization series does not require restarting the series or adding doses to the series. If a dose in a vaccine series is missed or delayed, it should be administered at the next opportunity, and the series should resume for completion as recommended from the time of the catch-up vaccination. A summary of recommended intervals between doses in vaccine series can be found at **www.cdc.gov/vaccines/hcp/acip-recs/general-recs/timing.html#t-01.**

Not all childhood vaccine series are required to be completed if there is an extended gap between doses or delay in series initiation. For rotavirus vaccination, the doses in the series are age limited, and catch-up vaccination may not be indicated (see Rotavirus Infections, p 644). The rotavirus vaccination series should not start at or after age 15 weeks, 0 days, and the final dose in the series should not be administered after age 8 months, 0 days.

Children 6 months through 8 years of age who are receiving influenza vaccine for the first time or have received only 1 dose before the current influenza season should receive 2 doses of influenza vaccine separated by at least 4 weeks. Detailed influenza vaccination recommendations can be found in the Influenza chapter (p 447) and the annual influenza policy statement of the American Academy of Pediatrics (**https:// redbook.solutions.aap.org/ss/influenza-resources.aspx**).

Health records of children for whom immunizations have been missed or delayed should be flagged as a reminder to resume their immunization series at the next opportunity and to implement reminder/recall communications to the family. An interactive app developed by the CDC is available for downloading and has up-to-date information on the childhood immunization schedule, including catch-up timing of missed vaccines (**www.cdc.gov/vaccines/schedules/hcp/schedule-app.html**).

Unknown or Uncertain Immunization Status

Many children, adolescents, and young adults do not have adequate documentation of their immunizations, which reinforces the need to include all vaccinations in state-based immunization information systems. Parent, guardian, or child recollection of immunization history may not be accurate. Only written/electronic, dated, authentic records should be accepted as evidence of immunization. In general, when in doubt, a person with unknown or uncertain immunization status should be considered disease susceptible, and recommended immunizations should be initiated without delay on a schedule appropriate for the person's current age. If the primary series has been started but not completed, the series should be completed, but there is no need to repeat doses or restart the full course.

Serologic testing is an alternative to vaccination for certain antigens (eg, measles, rubella, hepatitis A, and tetanus). However, commercial serologic testing takes time, can lead to a failed immunization opportunity, and may not always be sufficiently sensitive to indicate protection. Importantly, no evidence suggests that administration of vaccines to already immune recipients is harmful. In addition, serologic testing may not satisfy some school immunization requirements.

Vaccine Dose

Recommended vaccine doses are those that have been determined to be both safe and effective for their specified indication in prelicensure clinical trials; alternative doses or intervals for administration may not be safe or effective. Reducing or exceeding a recommended dose volume or collecting residual volumes to make up a dose is never recommended. Reducing or dividing doses of any vaccine, including vaccines administered to preterm or low birth weight infants, can result in inadequate immune responses. A previous immunization with a dose that was less than the standard dose or one administered by a nonstandard route should not be counted as valid, and the person should be reimmunized as recommended for age.

Active Immunization After Receipt of Immune Globulin or Other Blood Products

Donor-derived antibodies contained in polyclonal immune globulin (IG) preparations, including hyperimmune globulins like Hepatitis B Immune Globulin (HBIG), can inactivate certain live-virus vaccines and reduce their immunogenicity. As such, these vaccines should be deferred for varying periods of time when IG preparations have been administered. Other blood products, such as plasma or packed red blood cells, also may contain antibodies capable of inactivating live vaccines. However, because the concentration of antibodies in these blood products is generally low, the length of vaccine deferral is less.

In the United States, the issue of interference by passively administered antibodies is only relevant for measles, mumps, rubella vaccine (MMR); varicella vaccine (VAR); and the combination measles, mumps, rubella, and varicella vaccine (MMRV). Table 1.11 shows the suggested intervals between receipt of blood products, including IG, and vaccine administration. This varies depending on the product type, the calculated amount of immunoglobulin G (IgG) in the product, and the dose of the product. Blood products and inactivated vaccines may be administered at any time in relation to each other. When both IG and vaccine are indicated to provide short- and long-term protection, respectively (eg, HBIG and hepatitis B vaccine [HepB] for infants of mothers who have positive serology for hepatitis B surface antigen [HBsAg]), the products should be administered at different anatomic sites. For additional information, see chapters on specific diseases in Section 3. The respiratory syncytial virus monoclonal antibody, palivizumab, does not interfere with the immunogenicity of any vaccine.

Table 1.11. Recommended Intervals Between Receipt of Blood Products and Administration of MMR, Varicella, or MMRV Vaccines[a]

Indications or Blood Product	Route	Usual Dose	Interval, Mo[b]
Blood transfusion			
Washed RBCs	IV	10 mL/kg (negligible IgG/kg)[c]	0
RBCs, adenine-saline added	IV	10 mL/kg (10 mg IgG/kg)[c]	3
Packed RBCs	IV	10 mL/kg (60 mg IgG/kg)[c]	6
Whole blood	IV	10 mL/kg (80–100 mg IgG/kg)[c]	6
Plasma or platelet products	IV	10 mL/kg (160 mg IgG/kg)	7
Hyperimmune Globulin			
Botulinum Immune Globulin	IV	1 mL/kg (50 mg IgG/kg)	6
Cytomegalovirus Immune Globulin	IV	150 mg/kg (max)	6
Hepatitis B Immune Globulin	IM	0.06 mL/kg (10 mg IgG/kg)	3
Rabies Immune Globulin	IM	20 IU/kg (22 mg IgG/kg)	4
Tetanus Immune Globulin	IM	250 U (10 mg IgG/kg)	3
Varicella Immune Globulin	IM	125 U/10 kg (60–200 mg IgG/kg) (max 625 U)	5

Table 1.11. Recommended Intervals Between Receipt of Blood Products and Administration of MMR, Varicella, or MMRV Vaccines,[a] continued

Indications or Blood Product	Route	Usual Dose	Interval, Mo[b]
Immune Globulin			
Hepatitis A prophylaxis			
Contact prophylaxis	IM	0.1 mL/kg (3.3 mg IgG/kg)	6
International travel (short-term <1 month stay)	IM	0.1 mL/kg (3.3 mg IgG/kg)	6
International travel (long-term ≥1 month stay)	IM	0.2 mL/kg (10 mg IgG/kg)	6
Measles prophylaxis			
Not pregnant or immunocompromised[d]	IM	0.5 mL/kg (80 mg IgG/kg)	6
Pregnant or immunocompromised[e]	IV	400 mg/kg	8
Varicella prophylaxis	IV	400 mg/kg	8
Replacement for immunodeficiency	IV	300–400 mg/kg	8
Treatment of immune thrombocytopenic purpura	IV	400 mg/kg OR 1000 mg/kg	8 / 10
Treatment of Kawasaki disease	IV	2000 mg/kg	11

Adapted from General Best Practice Guidelines for Immunization: Best Practices Guidance of the Advisory Committee on Immunization Practices (ACIP), Vaccine Administration, Table 3–5, **www.cdc.gov/vaccines/hcp/acip-recs/general-recs/timing.html#t-05.**

IM indicates intramuscular; IV, intravenous; MMR, measles, mumps, rubella; MMRV, measles, mumps, rubella, varicella; RBCs, red blood cells.

[a] Live vaccines may be contraindicated in patients receiving certain blood products because of immunosuppression caused by their underlying disease.

[b] These intervals should provide sufficient time for decreases in passive antibodies that would allow for an adequate response to measles vaccine. Physicians should not assume that children are protected fully against measles during these intervals, and if measles virus is circulating in the community or if the child is traveling to an area where measles may be circulating, a measles containing vaccine should be administered, but not counted towards adequate immunization. Measles vaccine should be readministered after the appropriate interval has passed from the receipt of blood product (as per immunization schedule). If a blood product must be given within 14 days after administration of a measles- or varicella-containing vaccine, these vaccines should be administered again after the appropriate interval. One exception to this rule is when serologic testing is performed at an appropriate interval after IG administration documents seroconversion (although this is not expected to be performed routinely).

[c] For neonates, transfusion volume may be 15 mL/kg of washed, adenine-saline added, or packed RBCs. Above interval lengths are still applicable. Whole blood transfusions of >10 mL/kg may be used for cardiopulmonary surgery, exchange transfusions, or responding to trauma.

[d] This table is not intended for determining the correct indications and dosages for using antibody-containing products. Unvaccinated people might not be protected fully against measles during the entire recommended interval, and additional doses of IG or measles vaccine might be indicated after measles exposure. Concentrations of measles antibody in an IG preparation can vary by manufacturer's lot. Rates of antibody clearance after receipt of an IG preparation also might vary. Recommended intervals are extrapolated from an estimated half-life of 30 days for passively acquired antibody and an observed interference with the immune response to measles vaccine for 5 months after a dose of 80 mg IgG/kg.

[e] Immune Globulin Intravenous is recommended for pregnant women without evidence of measles immunity and for severely immunocompromised hosts regardless of immunologic or vaccination status, including patients with severe primary immunodeficiency; patients who have received a bone marrow transplant until at least 12 months after finishing all immunosuppressive treatment, or longer in patients who have developed graft-versus-host disease; patients on treatment for acute lymphocytic leukemia within and until at least 6 months after completion of immunosuppressive chemotherapy; individuals who have received a solid organ transplant; and people with HIV infection who have severe immunosuppression, defined as CD4+ T-lymphocyte percentage <15% (all ages) or CD4+ T-lymphocyte count <200 lymphocytes/mm³ (older than 5 years), and those who have not received MMR vaccine since receiving effective antiretroviral therapy.

Live intranasal (live attenuated influenza vaccine [LAIV]) and oral (rotavirus vaccine [RV] and Ty21A typhoid vaccine) vaccines do not need to be deferred, because parenterally administered antibodies are unlikely to achieve significant concentrations at mucosal surfaces. Also, donor blood in the United States is unlikely to have neutralizing antibodies to *Salmonella* Typhi and currently circulating strains of influenza. Likewise, yellow fever vaccine does not need to be deferred, because blood donors are unlikely to have experienced yellow fever virus infection or vaccination. No data are available on the use of live oral cholera vaccine after receipt of blood products.

Vaccine Safety

RISKS AND ADVERSE EVENTS

Prior to licensure, all vaccines in the United States undergo rigorous immunogenicity and safety testing, but adverse events can occur following the administration of any vaccine. Many adverse events following vaccination are coincidental events that occur in temporal association but are unrelated to vaccination. The mere occurrence of an adverse event following vaccination does not mean the vaccine caused the symptoms or signs. Mild and self-limited reactions (eg, local pain and tenderness at the injection site, fever) are common and clearly associated with vaccine administration. Serious causally related adverse events also can occur but are rare. Highly effective vaccines have dramatically reduced the threat of many infectious diseases, and because of this success, some people now are more concerned about potential vaccine adverse effects than about the illnesses vaccines prevent. As vaccinations successfully control their target diseases, health care providers need to communicate benefits and risks of vaccination to a population whose first-hand experience with vaccine-preventable diseases increasingly is rare.

As with all interventions in medicine, the benefits and risks from vaccines must be weighed, and vaccine recommendations are based on this assessment. Recommendations are made to maximize protection and minimize risk by providing specific advice on dose, route, and timing and by identifying precautions or contraindications to vaccination.

Common vaccine adverse reactions usually are mild to moderate in severity (eg, fever or injection site reactions, such as swelling, redness, and pain) and have no permanent sequelae. Examples include local inflammation after administration of either DTaP, Td, or Tdap vaccines, and fever and rash 1 to 2 weeks after administration of MMR or MMRV vaccines. Because many suspected adverse events are merely coincidental with administration of a vaccine, definitive assessment of causality often requires careful epidemiologic studies comparing the incidence of the event in vaccinated versus unvaccinated individuals or other comparison group(s) of similar age, or comparing the incidence of the adverse event in a specific time frame following immunization with the incidence in other timeframes. Although rare, a causal link with a live-virus vaccine may be established if the vaccine-strain virus can be identified in biologic specimens from an ill child with compatible symptoms (eg, rotavirus vaccine-associated diarrhea in a patient with severe combined immunodeficiency or varicella-vaccine strain from a vesicular lesion).

The Brighton Collaboration is a nonprofit international voluntary consortium formed to develop globally accepted and standardized case definitions for adverse events following immunization that can be used in vaccine safety surveillance and research. It provides guidelines for collecting, analyzing, and presenting vaccine safety data in a way that facilitates sharing and comparison of vaccine data among professionals working in the area of vaccine safety worldwide. Brighton Collaboration guidelines as well as case definitions for adverse events following immunization can be found online (**https://brightoncollaboration.org**).

The National Childhood Vaccine Injury Act of 1986 (**www.congress.gov/ bill/99th-congress/house-bill/5546**) requires health care providers and vaccine manufacturers to report any condition listed in the Vaccine Adverse Event Reporting System (VAERS) Table of Reportable Events Following Vaccination (**vaers.hhs. gov/docs/VAERS_Table_of_Reportable_Events_Following_Vaccination. pdf**) or listed in the product package insert as a contraindication to further doses. Providers are encouraged to report any clinically important adverse event following vaccination to VAERS (**vaers.hhs.gov/reportevent.html**) (see p 46) even if they are not sure it was caused by the vaccine. When analyzed in conjunction with other VAERS reports, this information can provide evidence of safety signals for unanticipated, potentially causally related vaccine adverse events. It is important to understand that VAERS is not designed to assess whether a vaccine caused an adverse event but rather as a system to generate hypotheses (to detect signals) to be tested subsequently through well-designed epidemiologic studies. Other vaccine safety monitoring systems, such as the Vaccine Safety Datalink (VSD) (**www.cdc.gov/vaccinesafety/ensuringsafety/monitoring/vsd/index.html**), which uses large linked databases to conduct epidemiologic studies, or the CDC's Clinical Immunization Safety Assessment (CISA) Project (**www.cdc.gov/vaccinesafety/ensuringsafety/monitoring/ cisa/index.html**), which conducts clinical research related to vaccine safety, provide mechanisms to scientifically evaluate vaccine safety concerns. A nationally notifiable vaccine-preventable disease (see Appendix III, p 1033) that occurs in a child or adolescent at any time, including after vaccination (vaccine failure), should be reported to the local or state health department. A National Academy of Medicine report published in January 2013 (**nationalacademies.org/hmd/reports/2013/the-childhood-immunization-schedule-and-safety.aspx**) reviewed and affirmed existing data sources and systems involved in vaccine safety surveillance and research regarding the childhood immunization schedule.

NATIONAL ACADEMY OF MEDICINE REVIEWS OF ADVERSE EVENTS AFTER IMMUNIZATION

Through a series of comprehensive reviews, the National Academy of Medicine (NAM), formerly called the Institute of Medicine (IOM), independently concluded that current childhood immunizations and the immunization schedule are safe and that following the complete childhood immunization schedule is strongly associated with a reduction in vaccine-preventable diseases. The committee members for these reviews included individuals with expertise in medicine, medical subspecialties, immunology, immunotoxicology, epidemiology, biostatistics, ethics, law, and other scientific disciplines.

IMMUNIZATION SAFETY REVIEW

During the years 2001-2004, the Immunization Safety Review Committee of the NAM evaluated 8 existing and emerging vaccine safety concerns. One of these reports, published in 2004, examined hypotheses about associations between vaccines and autism (**nationalacademies.org/hmd/reports/2004/immunization-safety-review-vaccines-and-autism.aspx**). The committee concluded that the evidence favors rejection of a causal relationship between the MMR vaccine and autism and between thimerosal-containing vaccines and autism.[1] In a subsequent review, the NAM convened a committee of experts to review the epidemiologic, clinical, and biological evidence regarding adverse health events associated with specific vaccines covered by the National Vaccine Injury Compensation Program (VICP). The 2011 NAM report titled "Adverse Effects of Vaccines: Evidence and Causality"[2] (**nationalacademies.org/HMD/ Reports/2011/Adverse-Effects-of-Vaccines-Evidence-and-Causality.aspx**) reviewed 8 different types of vaccines covered by the VICP: combination measles, mumps, rubella vaccine (MMR); varicella vaccine (VAR); influenza vaccine; hepatitis A vaccine (HepA); hepatitis B vaccine (HepB); human papillomavirus (HPV) vaccine; diphtheria toxoid-, tetanus toxoid-, and acellular pertussis-containing vaccines other than those containing whole-cell pertussis component; and meningococcal conjugate vaccines. The vaccines and adverse events associated with these vaccines were selected based on successful or unsuccessful claims made through the VICP. The review also covered the injection-related adverse events of complex regional pain syndrome, deltoid bursitis, and syncope. Two lines of evidence supported the committee's causality conclusions: epidemiologic evidence and mechanistic evidence. The benefit and effectiveness of vaccines were not assessed during this review. The NAM committee developed 158 specific vaccine-adverse event pairings and assigned each to 1 of 4 categories of causation. A summary of the NAM committee's causality conclusions regarding evidence for a causal relationship between the specific vaccines and other adverse event is as follows:

Category 1: Evidence convincingly supports a causal relationship:

- VAR and 5 specific adverse events:
  - disseminated vaccine-strain varicella-zoster virus (VZV) infection without other organ involvement
  - disseminated vaccine-strain VZV infection with other organ involvement, including pneumonia, meningitis, or hepatitis, in immunodeficient individuals
  - vaccine-strain viral reactivation without other organ involvement
  - vaccine-strain viral reactivation with subsequent infection resulting in meningitis or encephalitis
  - anaphylaxis
- MMR and 3 specific adverse events:
  - measles inclusion body encephalitis in immunodeficient individuals
  - febrile seizures
  - anaphylaxis

---

[1]Institute of Medicine. Immunization Safety Review: Vaccines and Autism. Washington, DC: National Academies Press; 2004

[2]Institute of Medicine. Adverse Effects of Vaccines: Evidence and Causality. Washington, DC: National Academies Press; 2011

- Influenza vaccines and 1 specific adverse event:
  - anaphylaxis
- HepB and 1 specific adverse event:
  - anaphylaxis
- Vaccines containing tetanus toxoid and 1 specific adverse event:
  - anaphylaxis
- Meningococcal conjugate vaccines and 1 specific adverse event:
  - anaphylaxis
- Injection-related (ie, injectable vaccines) events and 2 specific adverse events:
  - deltoid bursitis
  - syncope

Category 2: Evidence favors acceptance of a causal relationship (evidence is strong and generally suggestive but not firm enough to be described as convincing):
- Certain inactivated influenza vaccines previously used in Canada and oculo-respiratory syndrome
- MMR and transient arthralgia in women and children
- HPV vaccines and anaphylaxis

Category 3: Evidence favors rejection of a causal relationship:
- MMR and autism
- MMR and type 1 diabetes mellitus
- DT, TT, or acellular pertussis-containing vaccines and type 1 diabetes mellitus
- Inactivated influenza vaccines and Bell's palsy
- Inactivated influenza vaccines and exacerbation of asthma or reactive airways disease in children and adults

Category 4: Evidence is inadequate to accept or reject a causal relationship for the other 135 vaccine-adverse event pairs.

CHILDHOOD IMMUNIZATION SCHEDULE AND SAFETY

In response to a recommendation by the National Vaccine Advisory Committee, in 2013 the NAM issued a report, "The Childhood Immunization Schedule and Safety: Stakeholder Concerns, Scientific Evidence, and Future Studies"[1] (**nationalacademies. org/HMD/Reports/2013/The-Childhood-Immunization-Schedule-and-Safety.aspx**). The committee reviewed scientific findings and stakeholder concerns related to the safety of the recommended childhood immunization schedule. The committee also identified potential research approaches, methodologies, and study designs that could inform this question, upon consideration for strengths, weaknesses, and ethical and financial feasibility of each approach. The NAM committee concluded that the recommended childhood immunization schedule is safe. The committee based its conclusion on a "lack of conclusive evidence linking adverse events to multiple immunizations" and recommended continued research on the safety of the childhood immunization schedule. The committee also concluded that following the complete childhood immunization schedule is associated strongly with reductions in vaccine-preventable diseases.

---

[1]Institute of Medicine. The Childhood Immunization Schedule and Safety: Stakeholder Concerns, Scientific Evidence, and Future Studies. Washington, DC: National Academies Press; 2013

VACCINE ADVERSE EVENT REPORTING SYSTEM

The Vaccine Adverse Event Reporting System (VAERS) is a national passive surveillance system that monitors the safety of vaccines licensed for use in the United States (**www.cdc.gov/vaccinesafety/ensuringsafety/monitoring/vaers/index.html**). Jointly administered by the Centers for Disease Control and Prevention (CDC) and the US Food and Drug Administration (FDA), VAERS accepts reports of suspected adverse events occurring in temporal association following vaccine administration. The strengths of VAERS are that it is national in scope, can detect signals of possible safety problems, and can detect rare and unexpected adverse events. The purposes of VAERS are:

- Detect new, unusual, or rare vaccine adverse events;
- Monitor increases in known adverse events;
- Identify potential patient risk factors for particular types of adverse events;
- Assess the safety of newly licensed vaccines;
- Determine and address possible reporting clusters (eg, temporarily or geographically localized or product-/batch-/lot-specific adverse event reporting); and
- Recognize persistent safe-use problems and administration errors.

Like all passive surveillance systems, VAERS is subject to limitations, including reporting biases such as lack of denominator data, underreporting, stimulated reporting, inconsistent data quality and completeness, and absence of an unvaccinated comparison group. Because of these limitations, it is generally not possible to determine, through VAERS reports alone, whether a vaccine caused an adverse event. VAERS encourages the reporting of any medically important health event that occurs after vaccination, even if the reporter is not certain that a vaccine caused the event. A reported adverse event may be coincidental (not related to the vaccine) or causal (related to the vaccine).

The National Childhood Vaccine Injury Act of 1986 (**www.congress.gov/bill/99th-congress/house-bill/5546**) requires physicians and other health care professionals who administer vaccines covered under the National Vaccine Injury Compensation Program (**www.hrsa.gov/vaccine-compensation/index.html**) to maintain permanent vaccination records. Additionally, the Act requires health care providers and vaccine manufacturers to report to VAERS any condition listed in the VAERS Table of Reportable Events Following Vaccination or listed in the product package insert as a contraindication to further doses. Vaccines covered under this Act include all vaccines on the Recommended Child and Adolescent Immunization Schedule. Health care professionals are encouraged to report any medically important health event occurring after vaccination, regardless of whether or not it is listed on the VAERS Table of Reportable Events Following Vaccination. People other than health care professionals, including patients and parents, also may submit a report of a suspected adverse event to VAERS. Vaccine manufacturers are required to report any adverse event that comes to their attention.

Information in VAERS reports is evaluated and analyzed by the CDC and FDA to determine whether there are unusual or unexpected patterns of adverse event reporting (ie, safety signals). Approximately 40 000 VAERS reports are filed each year, 85% to 90% of which describe mild side effects such as fever, arm soreness, and crying or mild irritability. The remaining reports are classified as serious, which means that the reported adverse event resulted in permanent disability, hospitalization, life-threatening illness, congenital anomaly/birth defect, or death. Although these problems occur after vaccination, they are rarely caused by the vaccine. Medical records are requested for serious reports and other reports of special interest and are reviewed by FDA and CDC clinicians.

In addition to adverse events, vaccine failure, vaccine product problems, and vaccine administration errors can be reported to VAERS. VAERS reports may be submitted online or by uploading a writable PDF report. Instructions for reporting to VAERS are available at **vaers.hhs.gov/reportevent.html.** Additional assistance is available via e-mail at **info@vaers.org** or by phone at 1-800-822-7967. The Health Insurance Portability and Accountability Act (HIPAA) Privacy Rule permits reporting of protected health information to public health authorities. A patient's consent is not required to release medical records to VAERS. All patient-identifying information and reporter-identifying information is kept confidential.

After licensure of a vaccine for use in children, the FDA presents a summary of the first 18 months of safety data to an independent pediatric advisory committee. Vaccine safety data are presented routinely to the Advisory Committee on Immunization Practices (ACIP) of the CDC (**www.cdc.gov/vaccines/acip/ index.html**) to inform deliberations around vaccine recommendations. Periodically, reviews of vaccine and adverse event-specific surveillance summaries from VAERS data are published by CDC and FDA staff. These summary reports often provide reassurance of the safety of a vaccine. However, they also may describe findings of possible safety concerns that require further evaluation. Vaccine safety concerns identified in VAERS as sentinel events usually require further studies for confirmation using established systems, such as the Vaccine Safety Datalink (**www.cdc.gov/vaccine-safety/ensuringsafety/monitoring/vsd/index.html**) or other systems that use controlled epidemiologic methods.

VACCINE SAFETY DATALINK PROJECT

The Vaccine Safety Datalink (VSD) project is a collaborative partnership between the Centers for Disease Control and Prevention (CDC) and 8 large managed-care organizations. Established in 1990, the VSD project is an active surveillance system designed to monitor and evaluate vaccine safety (**www.cdc.gov/vaccinesafety/ ensuringsafety/monitoring/vsd/index.html**). The VSD project is one of the most important sources of scientific information about the safety of vaccines. As an active surveillance system, the VSD project complements the broader, passive Vaccine Adverse Event Reporting System (VAERS) administered by the CDC.

The VSD project provides access to comprehensive medical and immunization histories on more than 9 million people annually. The VSD project allows for retrospective and prospective observational vaccine safety studies as well as timely monitoring of newly approved vaccines. It has the ability to assess rates of potential adverse events following vaccinations compared with their background rates, rates in a historical cohort, or rates in unexposed populations in the VSD cohort.

From each participating site, the VSD collects electronic health data, including vaccines administered, dates of vaccines administered, and other vaccines administered on the same day. To contextualize the vaccination information, the VSD also collects information on medical illnesses that have been diagnosed during patient visits to physicians' offices, urgent care clinics, and emergency departments as well as hospitalizations. The VSD project conducts vaccine safety studies based on questions or concerns raised in the medical literature and from reports to the VAERS. When a new vaccine is recommended for use in the United States or when there is a change in vaccination recommendation, the VSD monitors it for safety.

The VSD project has supported many studies to address vaccine safety concerns, including a white paper on studying the safety of the childhood immunization schedule, safety of vaccines for children that contain additives or preservatives, intussusception and other adverse events after rotavirus vaccinations, risks of febrile seizures associated with childhood vaccines, and human papillomavirus vaccine safety. A list of publications based on VSD data are available at **www.cdc.gov/vaccinesafety/ ensuringsafety/monitoring/vsd/publications.html.**

FDA CBER SENTINEL PROGRAM

The 2007 Food and Drug Administration Amendments Act required the US Food and Drug Administration (FDA) to develop an active risk identification and analysis system to monitor and analyze postmarket performance of regulated medical products including drugs, vaccines, and other biologics. Since 2009, the FDA Center for Biologics Evaluation and Research (CBER) has evaluated vaccine safety, currently with the Biologics Effectiveness and Safety (BEST) Initiative, an active postmarket surveillance system that is a part of the FDA-wide Sentinel Initiative. The BEST Initiative, which replaced the Post-licensure Rapid Immunization Safety Monitoring (PRISM) program, monitors a large network of administrative claims and electronic health records data covering over 100 million people in the United States for safety and effectiveness of regulated biologic products including vaccines. The BEST Initiative generates safety signals that prompts the FDA to investigate possible associations between vaccines and detected adverse events, including events detected among women during pregnancy. Sources of potential vaccine safety signals include passive adverse events reports, randomized controlled clinical trials, reports in the literature, and reports from other countries. The BEST Initiative's large population base allows detection of rare adverse events associated with vaccines. The BEST Initiative complements other vaccine safety monitoring systems such as the Vaccine Safety Datalink (VSD), administered by the Centers for Disease Control and Prevention and 8 collaborating health care organizations (see Vaccine Safety Datalink Project, p 47). Postmarket vaccine surveillance systems are critical to enable continued monitoring and evaluation of vaccine safety and effectiveness and resulted in the detection of an increased risk of intestinal intussusception in infants after they receive a specific rotavirus vaccine and the conclusion that there is no increased risk of febrile seizures in children after they receive the influenza vaccine.

CLINICAL IMMUNIZATION SAFETY ASSESSMENT (CISA) PROJECT

The number of participants enrolled in prelicensure vaccine clinical trials may be insufficient to detect rare, clinically important adverse events following immunization, and health care providers may see them too infrequently to be able to provide standardized evaluation. In addition, high-quality studies are needed to identify risk factors for adverse events following immunization, especially in special populations, and to develop strategies to prevent or reduce the severity of adverse events following immunization. The Centers for Disease Control and Prevention (CDC) established the CISA Project to improve the understanding of adverse events following immunization at the patient level (**www.cdc.gov/vaccinesafety/ensuringsafety/monitoring/cisa/index.html**).

The CISA Project's goals are (1) to serve as a resource for vaccine safety information for US health care providers who have complex vaccine safety questions about a specific patient to assist with immunization decision-making; (2) to conduct clinical research to better understand vaccine safety and identify preventive strategies for adverse events following immunization; and (3) to assist the CDC and its partners in evaluating emerging vaccine safety issues. The CISA Project is a collaboration among the CDC, 7 medical research centers, and other federal partners. The medical research centers have expertise in vaccines and vaccine safety, epidemiology, biostatistics, clinical trials, and a wide range of specialty areas, such as allergy, immunology, neurology, infectious diseases, and obstetrics and gynecology.

The CISA Project facilitates the CDC's collaboration with vaccine safety experts at leading academic medical centers and strengthens national capacity for vaccine safety monitoring. CISA advises health care providers who have vaccine safety questions about specific patients in the United States involving US-licensed vaccines that are not readily available in Advisory Committee on Immunization Practices (ACIP) recommendations or professional medical society guidelines. For example, CISA may provide an opinion on whether a patient who has had an unusual adverse event following immunization after 1 dose of a vaccine should receive a future dose of the same vaccine. In a CISA evaluation, vaccine safety experts from the CDC's Immunization Safety Office and the CISA medical centers meet via scheduled teleconferences to review complex vaccine safety cases from US health care providers. The experts discuss the case, review the literature on the topic, and form a general assessment and recommended plan. This review is then shared with the health care provider. Advice from the CDC and CISA is meant to assist in decision making rather than to direct patient management, because patient-management decisions are the responsibility of the treating health care provider.

US health care providers who have a vaccine safety question about a specific patient residing in the United States can contact the CDC (email: **CISAeval@cdc.gov**) to request a CISA evaluation. Upon review by CDC medical officers, select inquiries are forwarded for CISA evaluation, and inquiring health care providers will be notified about the status of their request shortly after submission. If a case is accepted for a CISA consult, then the health care provider is requested to assist in obtaining medical records for review. The health care provider may attend the CISA case presentation and participate in the discussion. Patient confidentiality is protected during CISA case consultations. There is no cost to the health care provider for the CISA evaluation. Clinical vaccine safety questions that are not accepted for a CISA consultation will be addressed through other channels.

CISA has published and continues to develop research studies that address vaccine safety priorities, such as those identified in the US National Vaccine Plan (**www.hhs.gov/nvpo/national-vaccine-plan/index.html**). Current priority areas for CISA research (registered at **www.clinicaltrials.gov**) include influenza vaccine safety and vaccine safety in pregnant women and other special populations. CISA studies complement postlicensure vaccine safety surveillance systems and usually address clinical vaccine safety questions by prospectively enrolling up to hundreds of subjects receiving US-licensed vaccines. Whereas a large database system like the Vaccine Safety Datalink (VSD) managed by CISA (**www.cdc.gov/vaccinesafety/ensuring-safety/monitoring/vsd/index.html**) is best used to assess risk for rare, medically attended events in vaccinated populations, CISA's research is designed to study more common, nonmedically attended events (eg, fever or injection-site reactions) and to collect biological specimens after vaccination. CISA investigators also have access to special populations (eg, preterm infants) and links to specialists who care for these patients.

VACCINE INJURY COMPENSATION

Although vaccines are extremely safe products, rare, serious adverse events, such as allergic reactions, can result from vaccine administration. The Vaccine Injury Compensation Program (VICP) was established in 1988 as a means to stabilize the nation's vaccine supply by reducing excess liability that could lead vaccine manufacturers to exit the US market. It was developed as an alternative to civil litigation and to simplify the process of settling vaccine injury claims. The VICP is a no-fault system in which compensation may be sought if people are believed to have experienced an injury as a result of administration of a covered vaccine.

The VICP compensates for injuries that have occurred as a result of the administration of a vaccine routinely recommended for children from birth through 18 years of age, although the vaccine recipient and beneficiary can be of any age. Vaccines not routinely recommended for children, including zoster vaccines, pneumococcal polysaccharide vaccine (PPSV23), and travel vaccines are not covered by the VICP. Claims must be filed within 36 months after the first symptom appeared following immunization, and death claims must be filed within 3 years after the first symptom of the vaccine injury or within 2 years of a death and 4 years after the start of the first symptom of the vaccine injury that resulted in the death. People seeking compensation for alleged injuries from covered vaccines must first file claims with the VICP before pursuing civil litigation against manufacturers or vaccine providers. To ensure that legal expenses are not a barrier to entry into the program, the VICP may pay lawyer's fees and other legal costs related to a claim, regardless of the judgment, if certain minimal requirements are met and the claim is determined to have been filed on a reasonable basis and in good faith. If the claimant accepts the judgment of the VICP, neither vaccine providers nor manufacturers can be sued in civil litigation. If the claimant rejects the VICP judgment, he or she has the option of filing a claim against the vaccine company and the health care professional who administered the vaccine, although this seldom happens.

The VICP compensates for vaccine-related injuries that are included on the Vaccine Injury Table (**www.hrsa.gov/sites/default/files/hrsa/vaccine-compensation/vaccine-injury-table.pdf**). The table lists the vaccines covered by the VICP as well as injuries, disabilities, illnesses, and conditions for which compensation may be awarded. The Vaccine Injury Table defines the time during which the first symptoms or significant aggravation of an injury must appear after immunization. If an injury listed in the Vaccine Injury Table is shown to exist, claimants receive a legal presumption of causation, thus avoiding the need to prove causation. If the claim pertains to conditions not listed in the Vaccine Injury Table, claimants still may file a claim.

In 2009, a separate program, the Countermeasure Injury Compensation Program, was created to cover medical countermeasures developed and/or used in response to public health emergencies, such as in an influenza pandemic or a bioterrorism attack (eg, smallpox, anthrax, botulism). The 21st Century Cures Act, signed into law in December 2016, amended the legislation that created the VICP to include coverage for vaccines recommended for routine use in pregnant women, ensuring that both a woman who received a covered vaccine while pregnant and her child (in utero at the time) are covered by the program.

The VICP is funded by a $0.75 tax on every vaccine antigen administered (ie, $0.75 for a vaccine with a single antigen and $2.25 for a vaccine with 3 antigens). The average time from filing a claim to a judgement is under 3 years. Between 2006 and 2016, more than 3.1 billion doses of covered vaccines were distributed in the United States. During this same time period, 5564 petitions were considered by the Court and 3,773 were compensated. Thus, for every 1 million doses of vaccine that were distributed, approximately 1 individual was compensated for a vaccine-related injury. Approximately 70% of compensation awards resulted from a negotiated settlement between parties, with no conclusion reached that a vaccine caused the injury.

Information about the VICP and the Vaccine Injury Table can be obtained from the following: Parklawn Building, 5600 Fishers Lane, 8N146B Rockville, MD 20857; telephone: 800-338-2382; website: **www.hrsa.gov/vaccine-compensation/index.html.**

People wishing to file a claim for a vaccine injury should telephone or write to the following: United States Court of Federal Claims, 717 Madison Place, NW, Washington, DC 20439; telephone: 202-357-6400. Information on the VICP is available to parents or guardians through Vaccine Information Statements (**www.cdc.gov/vaccines/hcp/vis/index.html),** which are required to be provided before administering each dose of vaccines covered through the program.

HYPERSENSITIVITY REACTIONS AFTER IMMUNIZATION

Anaphylaxis to a vaccine generally is a contraindication to future vaccination (see Treatment of Anaphylactic Reactions, p 64). However, such reactions to constituents of vaccines are rare. Medications, equipment, and competent staff necessary to respond to these medical emergencies, to maintain patency of the airway, and to manage cardiovascular collapse should be available to treat anaphylaxis in all settings in which vaccines are administered. This recommendation includes administration of vaccines in schools, pharmacies, or other nontraditional vaccination settings.

In general, children who have experienced an immediate-type hypersensitivity reaction to a vaccine should be evaluated by an allergist before receiving subsequent doses of the suspect vaccine or other vaccines containing the offending ingredient. This evaluation and appropriate allergy testing may determine whether the child currently is allergic to a vaccine component, which vaccines pose a risk, and whether alternative vaccines (without the allergen) are available. Even when the child truly is allergic and no alternative vaccines are available, in almost all cases, the risk of remaining unimmunized exceeds the risk of careful, graded vaccine administration under observation where personnel, medications, and equipment are available to treat anaphylaxis, should it occur.

Hypersensitivity reactions related to vaccine constituents can be immediate or delayed and often are attributable to an excipient rather than the immunizing agent itself.

IMMEDIATE-TYPE ALLERGIC REACTIONS

Immediate allergic reactions may be caused by the vaccine antigen, residual animal protein, or other vaccine components. Almost all anaphylactic reactions to vaccines occur within minutes to 1 to 2 hours after vaccination.

ALLERGIC REACTIONS TO EGG PROTEIN (OVALBUMIN). Current measles and mumps vaccines (and some rabies vaccines) are derived from chicken embryo fibroblast tissue cultures and do not contain significant amounts of egg proteins. Studies indicate that children with egg allergy, even children with severe hypersensitivity, are at low risk of anaphylactic reactions to these vaccines, singly or in combination (eg, measles, mumps, and rubella [MMR] or measles, mumps, rubella, and varicella [MMRV]). Most immediate hypersensitivity reactions after measles or mumps immunization appear to be reactions to other vaccine components, such as gelatin. Therefore, children with egg allergy may receive MMR or MMRV vaccines without special precautions.

Although most inactivated influenza vaccines (IIVs) and the live attenuated influenza vaccine (LAIV) are produced in eggs, data have shown that these vaccines are well tolerated by essentially all recipients who have an egg allergy, including severely egg-allergic patients, likely because the volume of ovalbumin in these vaccines is well below the threshold required to induce an allergic reaction. All children with egg allergy of any severity can receive any influenza vaccine without any additional precautions beyond those recommended for all vaccines.[1]

Yellow fever vaccine may contain a larger amount of egg protein than influenza vaccines, and there are fewer reports on administering the vaccine to egg-allergic patients. A history of egg allergy should be sought prior to administration. The vaccine package insert describes a protocol involving skin testing the patient with the vaccine and if positive, giving the vaccine in graded doses. Such a procedure would best be performed by an allergist.

ALLERGIC REACTIONS TO GELATIN. Some vaccines, such as MMR, MMRV, varicella, yellow fever (YF-VAX), LAIV, and some rabies vaccines, contain gelatin of porcine or bovine origin as a stabilizer. The Vero cell culture-derived Japanese encephalitis (JE-VC) vaccine and the recombinant zoster vaccine do not contain gelatin stabilizers. People with a history of food allergy to gelatin may develop anaphylaxis after receipt of gelatin-containing vaccines. In addition, people without any apparent clinical allergy to oral ingestion of gelatin may experience an immediate hypersensitivity reaction following injection of a vaccine containing gelatin. Patients believed to be allergic to gelatin should be evaluated by an allergist with immediate-type allergy skin testing before receiving gelatin-containing vaccines. If gelatin is found to be the triggering allergen, the subsequent gelatin-containing vaccines should be administered in graded doses under observation, with competent personnel, medications, and equipment available to manage anaphylaxis.

[1]American Academy of Pediatrics, Committee on Infectious Diseases. Recommendations for prevention and control of influenza in children, 2020-2021. *Pediatrics*. 2020; 146(4):e2020024588

ALLERGIC REACTIONS TO YEAST. Hepatitis B and human papillomavirus vaccines are manufactured using recombinant technology in *Saccharomyces cerevisiae* (baker's or brewer's yeast). Allergy to yeast is rare; however, patients claiming such an allergy should be evaluated by an allergist before receiving yeast-containing vaccines to confirm the yeast allergy. If the history and testing suggest immediate hypersensitivity, the vaccine should be administered, in graded doses, under observation, with competent personnel, medications, and equipment available to manage anaphylaxis.

ALLERGIC REACTIONS TO LATEX. Dry natural rubber latex contains native proteins that may be responsible for allergic reactions. Some vaccine vial stoppers and syringe plungers contain latex, although allergic reactions to such vaccines in latex-allergic recipients are exceedingly rare. Other vaccine vials and syringes contain synthetic rubber, which does not pose risk to the latex-allergic child. Information about latex used in vaccine packaging is available in the manufacturer's package inserts or on the Centers for Disease Control and Prevention website (**www.cdc. gov/vaccines/pubs/pinkbook/downloads/appendices/B/latex-table. pdf**). Latex-allergic patients should receive vaccines with natural rubber latex in the packaging in the normal manner, but under observation, with competent personnel, medications, and equipment available to manage the rare allergic reaction, should it occur.

DELAYED-TYPE ALLERGIC REACTIONS

As with most cell-mediated, delayed-type allergic reactions, the allergens usually are small molecules. The molecules present in vaccines capable of producing such reactions include preservatives like thimerosal, adjuvants like aluminum, and antimicrobial agents.

ALLERGIC REACTIONS TO THIMEROSAL. Most patients with delayed-type hypersensitivity reactions to thimerosal tolerate injection of vaccines containing thimerosal uneventfully or with only a temporary nodule or swelling at the injection site. This is not a contraindication to receive a vaccine that contains thimerosal. Thimerosal was removed from childhood vaccines in 2001. Only multidose vials of influenza vaccines currently contain thimerosal, and many thimerosal-free influenza vaccines in prefilled syringes are available.

ALLERGIC REACTIONS TO ALUMINUM SALTS. Sterile abscesses or persistent nodules have occurred at the site of injection of certain adjuvanted vaccines. These abscesses may result from a delayed-type hypersensitivity response to the aluminum salts used as vaccine adjuvants such as aluminum hydroxide, aluminum phosphate, alum (potassium aluminum sulfate), or mixed aluminum salts. In some instances, these reactions may be caused by inadvertent subcutaneous inoculation of a vaccine intended for intramuscular use (Table 1.7, p 16). Aluminum-related abscesses recur frequently with subsequent dose(s) of vaccines containing aluminum. Only if such reactions were severe would they constitute a contraindication to further vaccination with aluminum-containing vaccines.

ALLERGIC REACTIONS TO ANTIMICROBIAL AGENTS. Many vaccines contain trace amounts of streptomycin, neomycin, or polymyxin B. Some people have delayed-type allergic reactions to these agents and may develop an injection site papule 48 to

96 hours after vaccine administration. This minor reaction is not a contraindication to future doses of vaccines containing these agents. The rare patients with a history of an anaphylactic reaction to one of these antimicrobial agents should be evaluated by an allergist before receiving vaccines containing them. No vaccine currently approved for use in the United States contains penicillin or its derivatives, cephalosporins, or fluoroquinolones.

OTHER VACCINE REACTIONS

People who have high serum concentrations of tetanus immunoglobulin (Ig) G antibody, usually as the result of frequent booster immunizations, may have an increased incidence of large injection site swelling after vaccine administration, presumed to be immune complex mediated (Arthus reaction). These reactions are self-limited and do not contraindicate future doses of vaccines at appropriate intervals. Such reactions had been believed to be common with tetanus-containing vaccines, but studies suggest that the reactions are uncommon, even with short intervals between immunizations. Therefore, when indicated, a tetanus-containing vaccine should be administered regardless of interval since the last tetanus-containing vaccine.

Reactions resembling serum sickness have been reported in approximately 6% of patients after a booster dose of human diploid rabies vaccine, probably resulting from sensitization to human albumin that had been altered chemically by the virus-inactivating agent. Such patients should be evaluated by an allergist but likely will be able to receive additional vaccine doses.

··

PASSIVE IMMUNIZATION

Passive immunization entails administration of preformed antibody to a recipient and, unlike active immunization, confers immediate protection but for only a short period of time. Passive immunization is indicated in the following general circumstances for prevention or amelioration of infectious diseases:

- As replacement, when people are deficient in synthesis of antibody as a result of congenital (eg, severe combined immunodeficiency) or acquired antibody production defects, alone or in combination with other immunodeficiencies (eg, immunosuppressive therapy or human immunodeficiency virus [HIV] infection).
- For prophylaxis when a person susceptible to a disease is exposed to or has a high likelihood of exposure to a specific infectious agent. This is especially important when that person has a high risk of complications from the disease or when time does not permit adequate protection by active immunization alone (eg, Rabies Immune Globulin, Varicella Zoster Immune Globulin, Hepatitis B Immune Globulin).
- Therapeutically, when a disease already is present, whereby administration of preformed antibodies (ie, passive immunization) may ameliorate or aid in suppressing the effects of a toxin (eg, foodborne, wound, or infant botulism; diphtheria; or tetanus), ameliorate or suppress clinical disease (eg, anthrax, vaccinia, post-transplantation hepatitis B, post-transplantation cytomegalovirus [CMV]), or suppress the inflammatory response (eg, Kawasaki disease).

Passive immunization can be accomplished with several types of products. The choice is dictated by the types of products available, the type of antibody desired, the route of administration, timing, and other considerations. These products include standard Immune Globulin Intramuscular (IGIM); standard Immune Globulin Intravenous (IGIV); hyperimmune globulins, some of which are for intramuscular use (eg, hepatitis B, rabies, tetanus, varicella) and some of which are for intravenous use (eg, botulism, CMV, vaccinia); antibodies of animal origin (eg, foodborne botulism, black widow spider, coral snake, rattlesnake, and scorpion antitoxins); and monoclonal antibodies (eg, respiratory syncytial virus [RSV]). Although the use of Immune Globulin Subcutaneous (IGSC) for replacement has become increasingly common, IGSC usually is not preferred for prophylactic or therapeutic use because of the slower absorption and diminished bioavailability compared with IGIV.

Indications for administration of IG preparations other than those relevant to infectious diseases or Kawasaki disease are not reviewed in the *Red Book*.

Immune Globulin Intramuscular (IGIM)

IGIM is derived from pooled plasma of adults by a cold ethanol fractionation procedure (Cohn fraction II). IGIM consists of at least 90% immunoglobulin (Ig) G with trace amounts of IgA and IgM. It is treated with solvent/detergent to inactivate lipid-enveloped viruses, is sterile, and is not known to transmit any virus or other infectious agent. IGIM is a concentrated protein solution (approximately 16.5% or 165 mg/mL) containing specific antibodies that reflect the infectious and immunization experience of the population from whose plasma the IGIM was prepared. Many donors (1000 to 60 000 donors per lot of final product) are used to include a broad spectrum of antibodies. Products sold in the United States are derived from plasma collected exclusively in US-licensed facilities.

IGIM is licensed and recommended for IM administration. Therefore, IGIM should be administered deep into a large muscle mass (see Sites and Routes of Immunization, p 28). Ordinarily, no more than 5 mL should be administered at one site in an adult, adolescent, or large child; a lesser volume per site (1–3 mL) should be given to small children and infants. Health care professionals should refer to the package insert for total maximal dose at one time. Peak serum concentrations usually are achieved 2 to 3 days after administration.

Standard human IGIM should not be administered intravenously. Intradermal use of IGIM is not recommended. For information on hyperimmune globulins for intramuscular use (eg, hepatitis B, rabies, tetanus, varicella), see chapters on specific diseases in Section 3.

INDICATIONS FOR THE USE OF IGIM

HEPATITIS A PROPHYLAXIS. IGIM is indicated for **postexposure prophylaxis (PEP)** to provide short-term protection against hepatitis A in previously unvaccinated patients. PEP with IGIM alone should be used for infants younger than 12 months and for people who have serious allergy to the hepatitis A vaccine (HepA) or its components. For patients older than 40 years, depending on the clinician's risk assessment (**https://stacks.cdc.gov/view/cdc/59777**), IGIM may be administered in addition to HepA. For patients 12 months through 40 years of age, HepA vaccine alone is preferred for PEP against hepatitis A.

For unvaccinated patients traveling to areas with high or intermediate hepatitis A endemicity, IGIM alone can be used for **preexposure prophylaxis (PrEP)** in infants younger than 6 months and people who have serious allergy to HepA or its components. For protection of infant travelers 6 through 11 months of age, preexposure HepA vaccine is preferred to IGIM. For healthy travelers 12 months through 40 years of age, HepA vaccine alone is recommended. For people older than 40 years, immunocompromised people of all ages, and people with chronic liver disease or other chronic medical condition, HepA vaccine should be administered and in addition IGIM can be considered (see Hepatitis A, p 373).

IGIM is not indicated for people with clinical manifestations of hepatitis A infection or for people exposed to hepatitis A more than 14 days earlier.

MEASLES PROPHYLAXIS. IGIM administered to exposed, measles-susceptible (not previously vaccinated or immunocompromised) people will prevent or attenuate infection if administered within 6 days of exposure (see Measles, p 503). The effectiveness of IGIM is titer dependent. Vaccine-eligible people 12 months or older exposed to measles should preferably receive measles, mumps, and rubella vaccine (MMR), if it can be administered within 72 hours of initial exposure. Measles vaccine and IGIM should not be administered at the same time. Subsequent vaccination with MMR is recommended in nonimmune people exposed to measles who received IG for PEP. The appropriate interval between IGIM administration and measles immunization varies with the dose of IGIM and the specific product (see Table 1.11, p 41).

RUBELLA PROPHYLAXIS. Administration of Immune Globulin to susceptible people experimentally exposed to rubella virus can prevent clinical rubella. However, there have also been many reports of the failure of Immune Globulin to prevent the anomalies of congenital rubella. For this reason, the routine use of IGIM for the prevention of rubella in an exposed pregnant patient is not recommended.

REPLACEMENT THERAPY IN ANTIBODY DEFICIENCY DISORDERS. Most experts no longer consider IGIM appropriate for replacement therapy in immunodeficiency because of the pain of administration and the inability to achieve therapeutic blood concentrations of IgG. If IGIM is used for this indication, the usual dose (limited by muscle mass and the volume that should be administered) is 100 mg/kg (equivalent to 0.66 mL/kg) every 3 weeks. Customary practice is to administer twice this dose initially and to adjust the interval between administration of the doses (2–4 weeks) on the basis of trough IgG concentrations and clinical response (absence of or decrease in infections).

ADVERSE REACTIONS TO IGIM

- Almost all recipients experience local discomfort and many experience pain at the site of IGIM administration that is related to the volume administered per injection site. Discomfort is lessened if the preparation is at room temperature at the time of injection. Less common reactions include nausea, flushing, chills, headache, and aseptic meningitis.
- Serious reactions are uncommon; these reactions can be anaphylactic or anaphylactoid in nature and manifest as chest pain or constriction, dyspnea, or hypotension and shock.
- Both IGIM and IGSC are associated with thrombosis, particularly for individuals at increased risk. To minimize thrombosis, recipients should be adequately hydrated before IGIM administration.

- An increased risk of systemic reactions, including renal dysfunction, hemolysis, and transfusion-related acute lung injury (TRALI), may result from inadvertent intravenous administration. Standard IGIM should not be administered intravenously.
- People requiring repeated doses of IGIM have been reported to experience systemic reactions, such as fever, chills, sweating, and shock.
- IGIM should not be administered to people with known selective IgA deficiency (serum IgA concentration <7 mg/dL; IgG and IgM concentrations normal). Because IGIM contains trace amounts of IgA, people who have selective IgA deficiency may develop anti-IgA antibodies on rare occasions and on a subsequent dose of IGIM may experience an anaphylactic reaction with systemic symptoms such as chills, fever, and shock. In rare cases in which reactions related to anti-IgA antibodies have occurred, subsequent use of a licensed IGIV preparation with the lowest IgA concentration may decrease the likelihood of further reactions. Because these reactions are rare, routine screening for IgA deficiency is not recommended.

PRECAUTIONS FOR THE USE OF IGIM

- Caution should be used when administering IGIM to a patient with a history of adverse reactions to IGIM. In this circumstance, some experts recommend administering a test dose (1%–10% of the intended dose) before the full dose.
- Although systemic reactions to IGIM are rare (see Adverse Reactions to IGIM, p 56), epinephrine and other means of treating serious, acute reactions (eg, saline for intravenous administration) should be immediately available. Health care professionals administering IGIM should have training in the management of anaphylaxis and shock.
- Unless the benefit will outweigh the risk, IGIM should not be used in patients with severe thrombocytopenia or any coagulation disorder that would preclude IM injection. In such cases, use of IGIV is recommended.

Immune Globulin Intravenous (IGIV)

IGIV is a highly purified preparation of IgG antibodies extracted from the pooled plasma of 1000 to 60 000 qualified adult donors using methods that vary by manufacturer. IGIV comprises more than 95% IgG, with trace amounts of IgA and IgM. IGIV is available as a lyophilized powder or as a formulated liquid solution, with final concentrations of IgG of 5% and 10% depending on the product. IGIV does not contain thimerosal or any other preservative. IGIV products vary in their sodium content, type of stabilizing excipients (eg, sugars, amino acids), osmolarity/osmolality, pH, IgA content, and recommended infusion rate. Each of these factors may contribute to tolerability and the risk of serious adverse events. All IGIV preparations must have a minimum concentration of antibodies to measles virus, *Corynebacterium diphtheriae* toxoid, poliovirus, and hepatitis B virus. Antibody concentrations against other pathogens, such as *Streptococcus pneumoniae*, cytomegalovirus, and respiratory syncytial virus (RSV), vary widely among products and even between lots from the same manufacturer. One product, Asceniv, is produced from donors with high anti-RSV titers and has a consistent amount of anti-RSV antibody; it is approved for treatment of primary immunodeficiency, but the clinical impact of the high anti-RSV titers on this or other patient populations is unknown.

Table 1.12. Uses of Immune Globulin Intravenous (IGIV) for Which There is Approval by the US Food and Drug Administration[a]

Primary immunodeficiency disorders such as common variable immunodeficiency, X-linked agammaglobulinemia, Wiskott-Aldrich syndrome

Kawasaki disease, for prevention of coronary aneurysms

Immune-mediated thrombocytopenia, to increase platelet count

Secondary immunodeficiency attributable to therapy for B-cell chronic lymphocytic leukemia or autoimmunity

Chronic inflammatory demyelinating polyneuropathy, to improve neuromuscular disability

Multifocal motor neuron neuropathy, to improve muscle strength

Reduction of serious bacterial infection in children with HIV infection

[a]Not all IGIV products are approved by the FDA for all indications and not all products are approved for children or for all ages of the pediatric population.

INDICATIONS FOR THE USE OF IGIV

IGIV preparations available in the United States currently are licensed by the US Food and Drug Administration (FDA) for use in 7 conditions (Table 1.12). IGIV products may be useful for other conditions, although demonstrated efficacy from controlled trials is not available for many of them. Blood sample(s) needed for diagnostic serologic tests for infectious diseases or to evaluate for immunologic disorders must be obtained before IGIV administration, because antibodies present in IGIV may confound test interpretation. Administration of IGIV can independently increase the erythrocyte sedimentation rate (ESR), so monitoring of C-reactive protein (CRP) after IGIV use may be more helpful in certain clinical scenarios.

All IGIV products are licensed to prevent serious infections in primary immunodeficiency, but not all licensed products are approved for the other indications listed in Table 1.12. Not all products are licensed for the entire pediatric age spectrum, and in some cases only a single product has certain indications. Therapeutic differences among IGIV products from different manufacturers may exist, but there are no comparative clinical trials of currently available products. Most experts believe that licensed IGIV and IGSC products are equally efficacious except for Kawasaki disease, which should be treated with IGIV. Hyperimmune globulins (eg, BabyBIG, Varicella-Zoster Immune Globulin) as well as animal-derived immune globulin products are not discussed in this chapter. Among the licensed IGIV products, but not necessarily for each product individually, indications for prevention or treatment of infectious diseases in children and adolescents include the following:

- **Replacement therapy in antibody-deficiency disorders.** The typical dose of IGIV in primary immune deficiency is 400 to 600 mg/kg but may be as high as 800 mg/kg or higher, administered by IV infusion approximately every 21 to 28 days. Because of the half-life of administered IgG, dosing intervals greater than 28 days are not recommended. Dose and frequency of infusions should be based on clinical effectiveness in an individual patient and in conjunction with an expert on primary immune deficiency disorders. When possible, the same brand of IGIV should be administered longitudinally, because changing products is associated with an increased risk of adverse reactions.

- **Kawasaki disease.** Administration of IGIV at a dose of 2 g/kg as a single dose within the first 10 days of onset of fever, when combined with salicylate therapy, decreases the frequency of coronary artery abnormalities and shortens the duration of symptoms. IGIV treatment for children with symptoms of Kawasaki disease for more than 10 days is recommended, although data on efficacy are not available (see Kawasaki Disease, p 457). Repeat doses of IGIV may be indicated for refractory Kawasaki disease.
- **Pediatric HIV infection.** In children with HIV infection and hypogamma-globulinemia, IGIV may be used to prevent serious bacterial infection.[1] IGIV also might be considered for HIV-infected children who have recurrent serious bacterial infection but is recommended only in unusual circumstances (see Human Immunodeficiency Virus Infection, p 427).
- **Immune thrombocytopenia (ITP).**[2] Several IGIV products are licensed for the treatment of ITP and are considered first line therapy by some experts. Studies have demonstrated a more rapid rise in platelet count with IGIV therapy compared to other treatments.

IGIV has been used for many other conditions, some of which are listed below.

- **Guillain-Barré syndrome (GBS), chronic inflammatory demyelinating polyneuropathy (CIDP), and multifocal motor neuropathy (MMN).** In GBS, IGIV treatment has been demonstrated to have efficacy equivalent to that of plasmapheresis and is easier to manage. Based on phase III trials, IGIV has been licensed for treatment of CIDP and MMN in adults. IGIV is equivalent to steroids and plasmapheresis in treatment of CIDP, although individual patients may respond better to one treatment than another. MMN, unlike GBS and CIDP, responds only to IGIV, not steroids or plasmapheresis.
- **Toxic shock syndrome.** IGIV has been administered to patients with severe staphylococcal or streptococcal toxic shock syndrome and necrotizing fasciitis. Therapy appears most likely to be beneficial when used early in the course of illness.
- **Low birth weight infants.** Results of most clinical trials have indicated that IGIV does not decrease the incidence or mortality rate of late-onset infections in infants who weigh less than 1500 g at birth. IGIV is not recommended for routine use in preterm infants to prevent early-onset or late-onset infection.
- **Other potential uses.** IGIV may be useful for sustained hypogammaglobulinemia secondary to anti-B cell therapy for autoimmunity or malignancy, severe anemia caused by parvovirus B19 infection, neonatal autoimmune thrombocytopenia that is unresponsive to other treatments, immune-mediated neutropenia, decompensation in myasthenia gravis, dermatomyositis, polymyositis, stiff person syndrome, transplant rejection, and severe thrombocytopenia that is unresponsive to other treatments.

---

[1] Panel on Opportunistic Infections in HIV-Exposed and HIV-Infected Children. Guidelines for the Prevention and Treatment of Opportunistic Infections in HIV-Exposed and HIV-Infected Children. Department of Health and Human Services. Available at **https://clinicalinfo.hiv.gov/sites/default/files/inline-files/oi_guidelines_pediatrics.pdf** Accessed July 27, 2020

[2] Neunert C, Terrell DR, Arnold DM, et al. American Society of Hematology 2019 guidelines for immune thrombocytopenia. *Blood Adv.* 2019;3(23):3829-3866

TRANSMISSION OF INFECTION BY IGIV

Following an outbreak of hepatitis C virus infection associated with IGIV in the United States in 1993, changes in the preparation of IGIV, including additional viral inactivation steps (such as solvent/detergent exposure, pH 4 incubation, trace enzyme exposure, nanofiltration, and heat treatment), have been instituted to prevent transmission of hepatitis C virus and other enveloped viruses, nonenveloped viruses, and prions via IG preparations. Most manufacturers use 3 or 4 different pathogen removal/inactivation procedures. All products currently available in the United States are believed to be free of known pathogens, and the risk of transmission of infection with IGIV administration is extremely low. Transmission of HIV by any IGIV product licensed in the United States has never been reported.

ADVERSE REACTIONS TO IGIV

INFUSION REACTIONS. Reactions such as fever, headache, myalgia, chills, nausea, and vomiting often are related to the rate of IGIV infusion and may occur in as many as 25% of patients. These systemic adverse events usually are mild to moderate and self-limited (Table 1.13). There have been numerous documented cutaneous reactions to IGIV, including urticaria, eczematous or lichenoid eruptions, petechiae, erythroderma, nonspecific macular or maculopapular rashes, and pruritus. The cause of most acute reactions is uncertain. Product-to-product variations in adverse effects occur among individual patients, but it is not possible at this time to predict the reactogenicity of one product relative to others.

Table 1.13. Managing IGIV Reactions[a]

Timing	Symptoms	Management
During infusion	Anaphylactic/anaphylactoid	Stop the infusion. Administer epinephrine and fluid support, diphenhydramine, and glucocorticoid.
	Headache, fever, chills, sinus tenderness, cough, mild hypotension	Slow the infusion until symptoms resolve. Administer diphenhydramine, NSAID; consider glucocorticoid. When symptoms resolve, the infusion rate may be increased. Pretreatment with NSAID, diphenhydramine, or glucocorticoid or a combination may lesson or prevent a reaction.
After infusion	Headache	Administer NSAID, triptan, glucocorticoid. Consider an alternative product or change to IGSC if there are repeated reactions.
	Myalgia/malaise	Administer NSAID, glucocorticoid. Consider an alternative product or change to IGSC if there are repeated reactions.

NSAID indicates nonsteroidal anti-inflammatory drug.

[a]There are no studies of the management of IGIV adverse effects, only expert opinion.

SERIOUS ADVERSE REACTIONS. Acute, severe reactions including hypersensitivity and anaphylactoid reactions occur infrequently and are marked by flushing, changes in blood pressure, tachycardia, and shock. Anaphylactic reactions induced by anti-IgA are very rare and only occur in some patients with selective IgA deficiency (ie, total absence of circulating IgA, IgA <7 mg/dL, with normal anti-protein antibody forming ability) who have been previously sensitized to IgA, rarely in patients with common variable immunodeficiency who develop IgE antibodies to IgA, and in a small number of patients with primary humoral immunodeficiency. Infusion of licensed IGIV products with a low concentration of IgA may reduce the likelihood of further reactions but rarely is needed. Because of the extreme rarity of these reactions, screening for IgA deficiency is not recommended.

Other potentially life-threatening adverse reactions include thrombosis, isoimmune hemolysis, renal insufficiency and failure, aseptic meningitis, noncardiogenic pulmonary edema, and transfusion-related acute lung injury. Products are screened for antibody to A and B blood group antigens (hemolysis risk) and coagulation factor 11 (FXIa) contamination (thrombosis risk). Although products now are tested for presence of thrombogenic substances, occasional events still may occur, particularly in patients with underlying thrombosis risk factors. Renal failure occurs mainly in patients with preexisting renal dysfunction and diabetes mellitus. Renal failure also may occur secondary to acute hemolysis mediated by isoagglutinins.

Hemolytic events are observed mainly in patients with A, B, or AB blood types receiving high doses of IGIV (approximately 80% of patients received ≥1.5 g/kg). Patients receiving high doses of IGIV should be monitored for hemolysis, which can be acute or can evolve over 5 to 10 days. Complications of severe hemolysis include need for transfusion, renal failure, and rarely, disseminated intravascular coagulation. If transfusion is needed, type O blood cells are recommended.

Aseptic meningitis syndrome beginning several hours to 2 days following IGIV treatment may be associated with severe headache, nuchal rigidity, fever, nausea, and vomiting. Pleocytosis frequently is present in the cerebrospinal fluid.

Risk factors for these adverse reactions include hypertension, diabetes mellitus, history of thrombosis, other thrombotic risk factors, prior renal compromise, and underlying hyperviscosity. The risk of some reactions can be mitigated by limiting the dose and infusion rate or by subcutaneous administration using IGSC (see Immune Globulin Subcutaneous, p 62). The rate and type of adverse events is one factor that should be considered when deciding on a mode of IG administration.

PRECAUTIONS FOR THE USE OF IGIV

- Patients receiving IGIV should be adequately hydrated to reduce the risk of renal dysfunction, which can occur in volume depleted patients.
- Caution should be used when administering IGIV to a patient with a history of adverse reactions to IG.
- Because acute anaphylactic or anaphylactoid reactions to IGIV can occur (see Adverse Reactions to IGIV, p 60), experienced personnel, medications, and equipment to manage anaphylaxis should be immediately available. If an anaphylactic or anaphylactoid reaction occurs, the risk versus benefit of further infusions should be evaluated. If IG therapy is continued, IGSC or enzyme-facilitated subcutaneous infusion (see Immune Globulin Subcutaneous, p 62) is recommended because of the decreased incidence of systemic adverse events compared with IGIV. Whichever

modality of administration is used, the product that elicited the reaction should not be used again.

- As practitioners have gained experience with IGSC (see Immune Globulin Subcutaneous), many experts recommend a change to subcutaneous administration instead of manipulating methods of IV infusion or administering premedications to patients who have had reactions to IGIV.
- Reducing either the rate of infusion or the IGIV dose often can alleviate mild to moderate infusion-related nonallergic adverse reactions (excluding life-threatening subacute adverse events). Patients sensitive to one product often tolerate alternative products. Although there are no studies to support the practice, most experts pretreat patients who have experienced significant reactions with a nonsteroidal anti-inflammatory agent such as ibuprofen or aspirin, acetaminophen, diphenhydramine, or a glucocorticoid to modify or relieve symptoms. Clinicians should balance the benefits of routine, long-term glucocorticoid premedication with the known accumulating risks of ongoing exposure. Significant adverse effects of IGIV administration should prompt consultation with an immunologist or other specialist experienced in managing this problem.
- Seriously ill patients with compromised cardiac function who are receiving large volumes of IGIV may be at increased risk of vasomotor or cardiac complications manifested as elevated blood pressure, cardiac failure, or both. In this setting, a low-sodium, high-IgG concentration product should be used if available. In hospitalized patients, these and other IGIV adverse event risks can be mitigated by using very slow infusion rates (approximately 30 mL/hour of a 10% IGIV product).

Immune Globulin Subcutaneous (IGSC)

Subcutaneous (SC) administration of IG using manual syringe push or mechanical or battery-driven pumps has been shown to be safe and effective in adults and children with primary immunodeficiencies. Because the SC delivery method does not require intravenous nor implanted venous access devices, most parents or patients can be taught to infuse IGSC at home. IGSC uses smaller doses administered more frequently (ie, daily to biweekly) providing a more consistent IgG concentration.

Both mild and severe systemic reactions are substantially less frequent with IGSC than with IGIV therapy, and no premedication is usually required for IGSC. The most common adverse effects of IGSC are infusion-site reactions, including local swelling, redness, itching, soreness, induration, and local heat. These most often occur during or soon after completion of infusion and generally resolve over 1 to 2 days. Such reactions occur more frequently during the first months of treatment. The most common systemic reaction is headaches. Systemic infusion reactions should be treated as discussed for IGIV (p 60). Infusing daily to several times a week decreases or eliminates systemic adverse effects in most patients.

Factors involved in selection of IGSC versus IGIV are listed in Table 1.14. Several products, ranging in concentration from 10% to 20%, are licensed in the United States for conventional SC use. There are reports that IGSC is well tolerated in patients with thrombocytopenia and those receiving anticoagulant therapy. High-dose IGSC has been shown to be effective for immunomodulation in autoimmune neurologic conditions, and a 20% SCIG product has been licensed for the treatment of chronic inflammatory demyelinated polyneuropathy. Because there are limited data on the efficacy of

Table 1.14. Comparison of Routes for IG Administration

Attribute	IGIV	Conventional IGSC	IGHY
Infusion frequency	Typically every 3–4 weeks	Most often daily to every 2 weeks	Every 2–4 weeks
Administration requirements	IV access, usually by a health care provider	No IV access, self-administered	No IV access, self-administered or by a health care provider
Sites/month	1	4–30	1–2
Systemic adverse events	Higher than with IGSC	Lower than with either IGIV or IGHY	Lower than IGIV
Local adverse events	Infrequent	Common	Similar to conventional IGSC

IGHY indicates recombinant human hyaluronidase.

IGSC for conditions requiring high-dose IG, only IGIV should be used for the treatment of Kawasaki disease.

Because the subcutaneous space limits infusion volume (typically to a maximum of 60 mL/site), multiple infusion sites and frequent infusions are needed to achieve an adequate IG dose using conventional IGSC. Pretreatment with recombinant human hyaluronidase (IGHY) (a spreading factor) permits the subcutaneous infusion of larger volumes (up to 600 mL) of IG at a single site, although many clinicians prefer to limit infusions to 300 mL/site. Products have been developed that include both the hyaluronidase for preinfusion and the IGSC and are known as IGHY. The efficacy of IGHY products is comparable with that of standard IGSC and of IGIV. The infusion frequency and number of needlesticks required for IGHY are similar to those for IGIV, and IGHY has less than half the frequency of systemic adverse events compared with IGIV. The peak serum IgG concentration achieved following IGHY administration occurs several days following infusion and is far lower than that of IGIV. Unlike the consistent steady-state serum concentration achieved following IGSC, trough concentrations associated with IGHY are comparable to those following administration of IGIV.

TRANSMISSION OF INFECTION BY IGSC

The transmission of infections by IGSC products is considered to be the same as with IGIV and is exceedingly low.

PRECAUTIONS FOR THE USE OF IGSC AND IGHY

- Caution should be used when administering IGSC to a patient with a history of adverse reactions to IGSC. In this circumstance, most experts recommend use of an alternate product. Some suggest administering a fraction (1/30) of the monthly dose daily.
- Although immediate, systemic reactions to IGSC are substantially less common and usually less severe than with IGIV (see Adverse Reactions to IGIV, p 60), epinephrine should be immediately available (ie, epinephrine autoinjector). Health care professionals administering IGSC should have training in the management of

emergencies (particularly anaphylactic shock). Parents and patients should be trained on the use of epinephrine autoinjector in case of anaphylaxis outside of a medical setting.

- Life-threatening, subacute systemic adverse reactions (thrombosis, hemolysis, renal injury) appear to be less common following IGSC than with IGIV but do occur (see Adverse Reactions to IGIV, p 60). Clinicians should be mindful of risk factors for adverse reactions (hypertension, diabetes mellitus, history of thrombosis, renal compromise, and hyperviscosity), because high-dose, intravenous route, and rapid rate of administration are additive risk factors.

Treatment of Anaphylactic Reactions

Health care professionals administering biologic products or serum must be able to recognize and treat systemic anaphylaxis. Medications, equipment, and competent staff necessary to maintain the patency of the airway and to manage cardiovascular collapse must be available.[1,2] In the event of a severe reaction requiring interventions beyond the capacity of the initial treatment team, emergency medical services should be requested to initiate additional emergency care prior to and during transport to a site for higher level of care.

The emergency treatment of systemic anaphylactic reactions is based on the type of reaction. In all instances, epinephrine is the primary drug. Delayed administration of epinephrine is believed to be the major contributor to fatalities. Mild manifestations, such as skin reactions alone (eg, pruritus, erythema, localized urticaria, or angioedema), may be the first signs of an anaphylactic reaction, but intrinsically and in isolation are not dangerous and can be treated with antihistamines. However, using clinical judgment, an injection of epinephrine may be administered, depending on the clinical situation (Table 1.15). Epinephrine should be injected promptly (eg, goal of <4 minutes) for anaphylaxis, which is likely (although not exclusively) occurring if the patient has 2 or more organ systems involved: (1) skin and mucosal involvement (generalized urticaria or angioedema, flush, swollen lips/tongue/uvula); (2) respiratory compromise (dyspnea, wheeze, bronchospasm, stridor, or hypoxemia); (3) low blood pressure; or (4) gastrointestinal tract involvement (eg, crampy abdominal pain or vomiting). If a patient is known to have had a previous severe allergic reaction to the biologic product/serum, onset of skin, cardiovascular, or respiratory symptoms alone may warrant treatment with epinephrine.[3] Epinephrine should be administered intramuscularly, because higher in vivo concentrations are achieved more rapidly compared with subcutaneous administration. Use of readily available commercial epinephrine autoinjectors (available in 3 dosages based on patient weight; 0.1, 0.15, and 0.3 mg/dose; see Table 1.15) are preferred and have been shown to reduce time to drug administration and dosing errors. Aqueous epinephrine (1:1000 dilution, 0.01 mg/kg; maximum dose,

---

[1]Hegenbarth MA; American Academy of Pediatrics, Committee on Drugs. Preparing for pediatric emergencies: drugs to consider. *Pediatrics.* 2008;121(2):433–443 (Reaffirmed February 2016)

[2]Sicherer SH; American Academy of Pediatrics, Section on Allergy and Immunology. Epinephrine for first-aid management of anaphylaxis. *Pediatrics.* 2017;139(3):e20164006

[3]Lieberman P, Nicklas RA, Randolph C, et al. Anaphylaxis–a practice parameter update 2015. *Ann Allergy Asthma Immunol.* 2015;115(5):341-384

Table 1.15. Epinephrine in the Treatment of Anaphylaxis[a]

Intramuscular (IM) administration

Epinephrine autoinjector (0.1 mg per dose for children 7.5–14 kg; 0.15 mg per dose for children 15–29 kg; or 0.3 mg per dose for children 30 kg or greater) IM (anterolateral thigh), repeated every 5–15 min up to 3 doses.

OR

Epinephrine 1:1000 (1 mg/mL) (aqueous): IM (anterolateral thigh), 0.01 mL/kg per dose, up to 0.5 mL, repeated every 5–15 min, up to 3 doses[b]

Intravenous (IV) administration

An initial bolus of IV epinephrine is given to patients not responding to IM epinephrine using a dilution of 1:10 000 (0.1 mg/mL) rather than a dilution of 1:1000. This dilution can be made using 1 mL of the 1:1000 dilution in 9 mL of physiologic saline solution. The dose is 0.01 mg/kg (0.1 mL/kg) of the 1:10 000 dilution.

A continuous infusion should be started if repeated doses are required. One milligram (1 mL) of 1:1000 dilution of epinephrine added to 250 mL of 5% dextrose in water, resulting in a concentration of 4 µg/mL, is infused initially at a rate of 0.1 µg/kg per minute and increased gradually to 1 µg/kg per minute to maintain blood pressure.

[a] In addition to epinephrine, maintenance of the airway and administration of oxygen are critical.
[b] If agent causing anaphylactic reaction was given by injection, epinephrine can be injected into the same site to slow absorption.

0.5 mg) or autoinjector can be administered intramuscularly every 5 to 15 minutes, as necessary, to control symptoms and maintain blood pressure. Repeat doses of epinephrine are required in up to 35% of cases of anaphylaxis. Injections can be given at shorter than 5-minute intervals if deemed necessary. Most patients being treated for anaphylaxis should be placed in a supine position. If a patient is having difficulty breathing, he or she may be asked to sit up. When the patient's condition improves and remains stable, oral antihistamines and possibly oral corticosteroids (1.5–2.0 mg/kg per day of prednisone; maximum, 60 mg/day) can be given for an additional 24 to 48 hours but is not always necessary.

Maintenance of the airway and administration of oxygen should be instituted promptly. Severe or potentially life-threatening systemic anaphylaxis involving severe bronchospasm, laryngeal edema, other airway compromise, shock, and cardiovascular collapse necessitates additional therapy. Rapid intravenous (IV) bolus infusion of isotonic fluids adequate to maintain blood pressure must be instituted to compensate for the loss of circulating intravascular volume.

Epinephrine is administered intramuscularly immediately while IV access is being established. IV epinephrine (note further dilution: 1:10 000 dilution) may be indicated for bolus infusion but should be used with caution (see Table 1.15). Administration of epinephrine intravenously can lead to lethal arrhythmia; cardiac monitoring is recommended. A slow, continuous, low-dose epinephrine infusion is preferable to repeated bolus administration, because the dose can be titrated to the desired effect, and accidental administration of large boluses of epinephrine can be avoided. Nebulized

Table 1.16. Dosages of Commonly Used Secondary Drugs in the Treatment of Anaphylaxis

Drug	Dose
H₁ receptor-blocking agents (antihistamines)	
Diphenhydramine	Oral, IM, IV: 1–2 mg/kg, every 4–6 h (40 mg, maximum single dose <12 y; 100 mg, maximum single dose for 12 y and older)
Hydroxyzine	Oral, IM: 0.5–1 mg/kg, every 4–6 h (100 mg, maximum single dose)
Cetirizine	Oral: 2.5 mg, 6–23 mo; 2.5–5 mg, 2–5 y; 5–10 mg, >5 y (single dose daily)
H₂ receptor-blocking agents (also antihistamines)	
Cimetidine	IV: 5 mg/kg, slowly over a 15-min period, every 6–8 h (300 mg, maximum single dose)
Ranitidine	IV: 1 mg/kg, slowly over a 15-min period, every 6–8 h (50 mg, maximum single dose)
Corticosteroids	
Methylprednisolone	IV: 1 mg/kg, every 4–6 h (125 mg, maximum single dose)
Prednisone	Oral: 1.5–2 mg/kg, single morning dose (60 mg, maximum single dose); use corticosteroids as long as needed
B₂-agonist	
Albuterol	Nebulizer solution: 0.5% (5 mg/mL), 0.05–0.15 mg/kg per dose in 2–3 mL isotonic sodium chloride solution, maximum 5 mg/dose every 20 min over a 1-h to 2-h period, or 0.5 mg/kg/h by continuous nebulization (15 mg/h, maximum dose)
Vasopressor	
Dopamine	5–20 µg/kg/min IV drip

IM indicates intramuscular; IV, intravenous.

albuterol is indicated for bronchospasm (see Table 1.16). In some cases, the use of other inotropic agents, such as dopamine (see Table 1.16), may be necessary for blood pressure support. The combination of histamine H_1 and H_2 receptor-blocking agents (see Table 1.16) may be synergistic in effect and could be used as adjunctive therapy. Corticosteroids have no role in the acute treatment of anaphylaxis but may also be used as an adjunctive therapy to decrease the likelihood of a biphasic or prolonged reaction, although the evidence for this practice is weak (see Table 1.16).

All patients showing signs and symptoms of systemic anaphylaxis, regardless of severity, should be observed for several hours in an appropriate facility, even after remission of immediate symptoms. Anaphylactic reactions can be uniphasic, biphasic, or protracted over 24 to 36 hours despite early and aggressive management. Although a specific period of observation has not been established, a reasonable period of observation would be 4 hours for a mild episode and as long as 24 hours for a severe episode.

Anaphylaxis occurring in people who are taking beta-adrenergic–blocking agents can be more profound and significantly less responsive to epinephrine and other beta-adrenergic agonist drugs. More aggressive therapy with epinephrine may override receptor blockade in some patients. For epinephrine-refractory anaphylaxis, some experts recommend use of IV glucagon (20–30 mg/kg in children; maximum 1 g, administered intravenously over 5 minutes, followed by an infusion at 5 to 15 mg/min titrated to clinical response). Inhaled atropine sometimes is used for management of bradycardia or bronchospasm in these patients. At the time of discharge, all patients should be provided with an epinephrine autoinjector, a written emergency plan to treat future reactions, and a referral to an allergist to identify the triggering allergen, if unknown. The patient and/or parent(s) should be trained on the use of the specific autoinjector pen provided.

IMMUNIZATION IN SPECIAL CLINICAL CIRCUMSTANCES

Immunization in Preterm and Low Birth Weight Infants

Infants born preterm (at less than 37 weeks of gestation) or of low birth weight (less than 2500 g) who are clinically stable should, with few exceptions, receive all routinely recommended childhood vaccines at the same chronologic age as term and normal birth weight infants. Although studies have shown decreased immune responses to several vaccines administered to neonates with very low birth weight (less than 1500 g) and neonates of very early gestational age (less than 29 weeks of gestation), most preterm infants, including infants who receive corticosteroids for chronic lung disease, produce sufficient vaccine-induced immunity to prevent disease. Vaccine dosages administered to term infants should not be reduced or divided when administered to preterm or low birth weight infants.

Preterm and low birth weight infants tolerate most childhood vaccines as well as do term infants. Some studies show that cardiorespiratory events may increase in extremely (less than 1000 g) and very (less than 1500 g) low birth weight infants who receive selected vaccines. Apnea within 24 hours prior to immunization, younger age, or weight less than 2000 g at the time of immunization and 12-hour Score for Neonatal Acute Physiology II[1] greater than 10 have been associated with development of postimmunization apnea, and it may be prudent to monitor infants with these characteristics for 48 hours after immunization if they are still in the hospital.

Medically stable preterm infants who remain in the hospital at 2 months of chronologic age should receive all inactivated vaccines recommended at that age (see Recommended Child and Adolescent Immunization Schedule for Ages 18 Years or Younger [**http://redbook.solutions.aap.org/SS/Immunization_Schedules. aspx**]). A medically stable infant is defined as one who does not require ongoing management for serious infection; metabolic disease; or acute renal, cardiovascular,

---

[1]Zupancic JAF, Richardson DK, Horbar JD, Carpenter JH, Lee SK, Escobar GJ. Vermont Oxford Network SNAP Pilot Project Participants. Revalidation of the Score for Neonatal Acute Physiology in the Vermont Oxford Network. *Pediatrics*. 2007;119(1):e156-e163

neurologic, or respiratory tract illness and who demonstrates a clinical course of sustained recovery and a pattern of steady growth. All immunizations required at 2 months of age can be administered simultaneously to preterm or low birth weight infants, with the possible exception of live oral rotavirus vaccine in hospitalized infants (see below and Rotavirus, 644). The number of vaccine injections at 2 months of age can be minimized by using combination vaccines. When limited injection sites preclude simultaneous administration, vaccines recommended at 2 months of age may be administered at different times with any interval between doses of different inactivated parenteral vaccines. The choice of needle lengths used for IM vaccine administration is determined by available muscle mass of the preterm or low birth weight infant (see Table 1.8, p 29).

Hepatitis B vaccine administered to preterm or low birth weight infants weighing 2000 g or more at birth produces an immune response comparable to that in term infants. Medically stable infants weighing less than 2000 g demonstrate a lower hepatitis B antibody response. Hepatitis B vaccine schedules for infants weighing <2000 g and infants weighing ≥2000 g born to mothers with positive, negative, and unknown hepatitis B surface antigen (HBsAg) status are provided in Hepatitis B, Special Considerations, including Table 3.21 (p 393). Only monovalent hepatitis B vaccine should be used for preterm or term infants younger than 6 weeks. Administration of a total of 4 doses of hepatitis B vaccine is permitted when a combination vaccine containing hepatitis B vaccine is administered after the birth dose.

Because all preterm infants are considered at increased risk of complications of influenza, 2 doses of inactivated influenza vaccine, administered 1 month apart, should be offered for all preterm infants beginning at 6 months of chronologic age (see Influenza, p 447). Influenza vaccine should be given to all pregnant women during pregnancy (may be administered at any time during pregnancy) to protect the mother and to provide passive protection of young infants. Because preterm infants younger than 6 months and infants of any age with chronic complications of preterm birth are extremely vulnerable to influenza virus infection, it is very important that household contacts, child care providers, and hospital nursery personnel caring for preterm infants receive influenza vaccine annually (see Influenza, p 447).

Preterm infants younger than 6 months, who are too young to have completed the primary immunization series, are at increased risk of pertussis infection and pertussis-related complications. Tetanus toxoid, reduced diphtheria toxoid, and acellular pertussis (Tdap) vaccine should be administered to all pregnant women (optimally, early in the interval between weeks 27 and 36 of gestation, to maximize passive antibody transfer to the infant) during every pregnancy. Tdap should be administered immediately postpartum for women who were not immunized during pregnancy and never have received a previous dose of Tdap. Health care personnel caring for pregnant women and infants, and household contacts and child care providers of all infants who have not previously received Tdap, also should be vaccinated (see Pertussis, p 578).

Preterm infants born before 29 weeks, 0 days of gestation; infants born with certain congenital heart defects; and certain infants with chronic lung disease of prematurity or hemodynamically significant heart disease may benefit from monthly immunoprophylaxis with palivizumab (respiratory syncytial virus monoclonal antibody) during respiratory syncytial virus season (see Respiratory Syncytial Virus, p 628). Routine childhood immunizations should be administered on schedule in infants receiving palivizumab.

Rotavirus vaccine virus is shed by some infants in the weeks after vaccination. There are limited published studies on the transmission of vaccine virus in hospital settings, including neonatal intensive care units that have not documented nosocomial transmission. Individual institutions may consider administering rotavirus vaccine at the recommended chronologic age to otherwise eligible infants during hospitalization, including in the neonatal intensive care unit. Otherwise, the first dose of rotavirus vaccine should be administered at the time of discharge to eligible infants.

Immunization in Pregnancy[1]

Immunization is an essential component of care in pregnancy. Several vaccine-preventable diseases, such as influenza, are associated with increased morbidity and mortality during pregnancy, and others, like pertussis, can affect newborn infants who are too young to begin active vaccination until months after delivery. The benefits of vaccinating the expectant mother and providing protection for the infant through maternally acquired antibodies have led to recommendations for select vaccinations during pregnancy.[2] Vaccines routinely recommended during pregnancy are safe for the mother and the fetus and infant. Obstetric care providers play a critical role in reviewing the expectant mother's vaccination history and ensuring that they receive recommended vaccines. Pediatricians are also frequently asked about vaccines during pregnancy by parents and play an important role in reinforcing the importance of vaccines. This chapter covers active immunization during pregnancy. Passive maternal-neonatal immunization topics related to breastfeeding are covered in the chapter Breastfeeding and Human Milk (p 107).

Two vaccines are specifically recommended for routine administration during pregnancy—tetanus and diphtheria toxoids and acellular pertussis vaccine (Tdap) and inactivated influenza vaccine (IIV).

- **Tdap With Each Pregnancy.** Tdap administered during the third trimester of pregnancy reduces pertussis infection in infants. The Centers for Disease Control and Prevention (CDC), the American Academy of Pediatrics (AAP), the American College of Obstetricians and Gynecologists (ACOG), and the American Academy of Family Physicians (AAFP) recommend administration of Tdap during every pregnancy to ensure that babies have high concentrations of pertussis-specific antibodies at the time of birth. The recommended timing for administration of Tdap is as early as possible during the interval between 27 and 36 weeks' gestation, to maximize the maternal antibody response and passive antibody transfer to the infant. Tdap may be safely administered at any time during pregnancy if needed for wound management, pertussis outbreaks, or other extenuating circumstances. For women never previously vaccinated with Tdap, if Tdap was not administered during the current pregnancy, Tdap should be administered immediately postpartum. If a Td booster is indicated for wound management during pregnancy, Tdap should be administered if it was not administered during the current pregnancy (see Pertussis, p 578). Tdap and inactivated influenza vaccine can be administered together safely, and Tdap can be safely administered after a recent dose of Td.

---

[1]See adult immunization schedule available at **www.cdc.gov/vaccines/schedules/hcp/adult.html.**
[2]**www.cdc.gov/vaccines/pregnancy/index.html**

- **Influenza Vaccine Each Influenza Season.** Pregnancy increases risks of influenza even among those who do not have underlying medical conditions. Influenza vaccination is recommended for everyone 6 months of age or older who does not have a contraindication, and pregnancy is a specific indication for vaccination with IIV. In addition to protecting the mother, IIV in pregnancy also protect infants younger than 6 months of age who are too young to be vaccinated. IIV may be administered at any time during pregnancy (see Influenza, p 447). Pregnancy is a contraindication for live attenuated influenza vaccine (LAIV).

LIVE ATTENUATED VACCINES

Pregnancy is generally a contraindication for live-virus vaccines, except when susceptibility and exposure are highly probable, the disease to be prevented poses a greater threat than the theoretical risk of the vaccine, and there is no other effective prevention option. The background rate of major and minor structural fetal malformations in otherwise uncomplicated pregnancies, commonly accepted as 3% to 5%, needs to be taken into account when discussing concerns regarding a birth defect diagnosed before or after birth that could be attributed inappropriately to a vaccine. This consideration is particularly important when vaccination with a live or live-attenuated vaccine has occurred after completion of embryogenesis in the first trimester. Inadvertent administration of live-virus vaccines in early pregnancy has not been shown to result in specific embryopathy and is not an indication to consider pregnancy termination. Pregnancy should be avoided for 4 weeks after receiving a live-virus vaccine.

- **Measles, Mumps, and Rubella Vaccine.** Measles, mumps, rubella, and varicella vaccines are contraindicated for pregnant women. Efforts should be made to immunize women without evidence of immunity against these viruses before they become pregnant or in the immediate postpartum period. Following receipt of measles, mumps, and rubella vaccine (MMR), women should avoid pregnancy for at least 4 weeks. No case of embryopathy caused by live rubella vaccine has been reported; however, a rare theoretical risk of embryopathy from inadvertent administration cannot be excluded. Because pregnancy might result in a higher risk for severe measles disease and complications, Immune Globulin Intravenous (IGIV) should be administered to pregnant women who do not have evidence of measles immunity and have been exposed to measles (see Measles, p 503). IGIV does not prevent rubella or mumps infection after exposure and is not recommended for that purpose.

- **Varicella Vaccine.** Like MMR, varicella-containing vaccines (varicella vaccine [VAR]; measles, mumps, rubella, and varicella vaccine [MMRV]) are live vaccines and are contraindicated in pregnancy. This contraindication is based on a theoretical risk for congenital varicella syndrome, although there is no association between inadvertent administration of VAR or MMRV and adverse pregnancy outcome based on available safety surveillance. A pregnant woman living in a household is not a contraindication for another household member to be vaccinated against varicella. Pregnant women who do not have evidence of immunity to varicella are at risk for severe disease and disease complications. Varicella-Zoster Immune Globulin is recommended for pregnant women without evidence of immunity who have been exposed and should ideally be administered within 96 hours of exposure for greatest effectiveness but can be administered up to 10 days after exposure (see Varicella-Zoster Virus Infections, p 831). The purpose of using Varicella-Zoster Immune

Globulin during pregnancy is to prevent complications in the mother and not to protect the fetus/infant, because maternal receipt of Varicella-Zoster Immune Globulin does not prevent fetal infection or neonatal disease. If Varicella-Zoster Immune Globulin is not available, some experts suggest use of IGIV. Published data on the benefit of acyclovir as postexposure prophylaxis among immunocompromised individuals are limited, although the use of acyclovir during pregnancy is not contraindicated if clinically indicated.

- **Live Attenuated Influenza Vaccine (LAIV).** Although influenza vaccination is recommended during pregnancy, LAIV, as a live vaccine, is contraindicated. Any licensed inactivated influenza vaccine (IIV) that is otherwise appropriate for age should be used instead.
- **Yellow Fever Vaccine.** Unlike most other live vaccines, the yellow fever vaccine is not contraindicated in pregnancy. It nevertheless poses a theoretical risk, and pregnancy is a precaution to yellow fever vaccine administration because of rare cases of transmission of the vaccine virus in utero, albeit without adverse effects in the infant. Whenever possible, pregnant women should defer travel to areas where yellow fever is endemic. If travel to an area with endemic disease is unavoidable and risks for yellow fever virus exposure are believed to outweigh the vaccination risks, a pregnant woman should be vaccinated. Breastfeeding also is a precaution for yellow fever vaccine administration (see Breastfeeding and Human Milk, p 107).
- **Typhoid Vaccine.** There are 2 types of typhoid vaccine currently available in the Unites States—a live attenuated vaccine for oral administration and a polysaccharide vaccine for parenteral administration. No information is available on the safety of either typhoid vaccine in pregnancy. Generally, live vaccines should be avoided in pregnancy.
- **Cholera Vaccine.** Pregnant women are at increased risk for poor outcomes from cholera infections. No information is available on the safety of live attenuated cholera vaccine in pregnancy. The vaccine is not absorbed from the recipient's gastrointestinal tract. Thus, administration of the vaccine to a pregnant woman is not expected to result in fetal vaccine virus exposure. When considering cholera vaccination during pregnancy, for travel to areas of cholera transmission, the benefit of protection offered by the vaccine should be weighed against the risk of possible adverse events.
- **Smallpox Vaccine.** The use of live smallpox virus (vaccinia) vaccine is limited to laboratory workers who work with the virus or other orthopoxviruses that infect humans, (eg, monkeypox). Smallpox causes more severe disease in pregnant than nonpregnant women. In the absence of a smallpox outbreak, however, use of vaccinia vaccine in pregnant women is not recommended.

INACTIVATED VACCINES

- **Pneumococcal Vaccines.** Pregnant women with underlying conditions that warrant pneumococcal immunization may be vaccinated when the benefit of the vaccination is considered to outweigh any potential risks.
- **Meningococcal Vaccines.** Although not extensively studied in pregnant women, serogroups A, C, W, and Y meningococcal conjugate vaccine (MenACWY) and serogroup B meningococcal vaccine (MenB) may be administered to pregnant women when there is increased risk of disease, as detailed in Table 3.38 in the Meningococcal Infections chapter (p 528).

- **Hepatitis A and Hepatitis B Vaccines.** Infection with hepatitis A virus or hepatitis B virus can result in severe disease in the mother and, in the case of hepatitis B, chronic infection in the infant. If not already vaccinated with hepatitis A vaccine (HepA) and hepatitis B vaccine (HepB), the vaccine(s) should be administered in pregnancy if there is an indication.
- **Inactivated Poliovirus Vaccine.** Although data on safety of inactivated poliovirus (IPV) vaccine for a pregnant woman or developing fetus are limited, no adverse effect has been found. IPV vaccine can be administered to pregnant women who never have received poliovirus vaccine, are immunized partially, or are immunized completely but require a booster dose (see Poliovirus Infections, p 601). Oral poliovirus (OPV) vaccine should not be administered to pregnant women.
- **Human Papillomavirus Vaccine.** The HPV vaccine is not recommended for use during pregnancy because of limited information about safety. The health care professional should inquire about pregnancy in patients who are known to be sexually active, but a pregnancy test is not required before starting the HPV vaccination series. If a vaccine recipient becomes pregnant, subsequent doses should be postponed until she is no longer pregnant. If a dose has been administered inadvertently during pregnancy, no intervention is needed. Data to date show no evidence of adverse effect of any HPV vaccine on outcomes of pregnancy. Health care professionals can report inadvertent administrations of 9vHPV to pregnant women by calling the vaccine manufacturer at 1-800-986-8999.
- **Rabies Vaccine.** The serious consequences of rabies dictate prompt postexposure prophylaxis and the rabies vaccine should be administered regardless of pregnancy status. Studies have shown that there is no association between rabies vaccination and increases in spontaneous abortions, premature births, or other adverse pregnancy outcomes. If the risk of exposure to rabies during pregnancy is substantial, preexposure prophylaxis also may be indicated.
- **Japanese Encephalitis Vaccine.** No studies in humans have assessed the safety of Japanese encephalitis virus vaccine for pregnant women. Women should be immunized before conception, if possible. Immunization during pregnancy may be considered if travel to an area with endemic infection is unavoidable and the risk of disease outweighs the risk of adverse events in pregnancy (see Arboviruses, p 202).
- **Anthrax Vaccine.** Anthrax vaccine is not licensed for use in pregnant women; however, in a postevent setting that poses a high risk of exposure to aerosolized *Bacillus anthracis* spores, pregnancy is neither a precaution nor a contraindication to its use in postexposure prophylaxis (see Anthrax, p 196).

Immunization and Other Considerations in Immunocompromised Children

The safety and effectiveness of vaccines in people with immunodeficiency depends on the nature and extent of their immunosuppression. Even though these individuals represent a heterogeneous population, their immunodeficiency can be classified into primary and secondary disorders. Primary disorders of the immune system generally are inherited and can involve any part of the immune defenses. Secondary disorders of the immune system are acquired, including conditions related to infection, malignancies, and chronic diseases and their treatments (see Table 1.17). The Infectious Diseases

Table 1.17. Immunization of Children and Adolescents With Primary and Secondary Immune Deficiencies

Category	Example of Specific Immunodeficiency	Vaccine Contraindications[a]	Comments
Primary			
B lymphocyte (humoral)	Severe antibody deficiencies (eg, X-linked agammaglobulinemia and common variable immunodeficiency)	OPV,[b] BCG, smallpox vaccine, LAIV, YF vaccine, and live-bacteria vaccines[c]; no data for rotavirus vaccines	Effectiveness of any vaccine is uncertain if dependent only on humoral response (eg, PPSV23). Replacement IG therapy interferes with response to live vaccines MMR and VAR. Annual IIV is the only vaccine administered routinely to patients receiving IG replacement therapy. All inactivated vaccines are safe to administer as part of immune response assessment prior to instituting IG therapy.
	Less severe antibody deficiencies (eg, selective IgA deficiency and IgG subclass deficiencies)	OPV,[a] BCG, YF vaccine	All inactivated and live-virus vaccines[d] on the standard annual schedule are safe, likely are effective (although responses may be attenuated), and should be administered.[e] PPSV23 should be administered beginning at 2 years of age.[f]
T lymphocyte (cell-mediated and humoral)	Complete defects (eg, severe combined immunodeficiency; complete DiGeorge syndrome)	All live-bacteria and live-virus vaccines (including rotavirus vaccine)[c,d,g]	All inactivated vaccines probably are ineffective. Annual IIV is the only vaccine administered routinely to patients receiving IG replacement therapy, if there is some residual antibody-producing capacity.
	Partial defects (eg, most patients with DiGeorge syndrome, hyperIgM syndrome, Wiskott-Aldrich syndrome, ataxia telangiectasia)	All live-bacteria and live-virus vaccines[c,d,g]	All inactivated vaccines on the standard annual schedule are safe, may be effective depending on the degree of the immune defect, and should be administered.[e] Those with ≥500 CD3+ T lymphocytes/mm^3, ≥200 CD8+ T lymphocytes/mm^3, and normal mitogen response could be considered to receive MMR and VAR vaccine (but not MMRV). PPSV23 should be administered beginning at 2 years of age.[f] Consider MenACWY-CRM series beginning in infancy[h]; and the MenB series beginning at 10 years of age depending on splenic dysfunction.

Table 1.17. Immunization of Children and Adolescents With Primary and Secondary Immune Deficiencies, continued

Category	Example of Specific Immunodeficiency	Vaccine Contraindications[a]	Comments
T lymphocyte (cell-mediated and humoral)	Interferon-alpha; interferon-gamma; interleukin 12 axis deficiencies; STAT1 deficiencies	All live-bacteria vaccines[e] and YF vaccine; other live-virus vaccines[d] if severely lymphopenic	All inactivated vaccines on the standard annual schedule are safe, likely are effective, and should be administered.[e] Based on experience in HIV-infected children with the measles vaccine, MMR and VAR (but not MMRV) probably are safe and may be preferable to the risk of disease. Inactivated typhoid vaccine (Typhoid Vi) should be used for people living in areas with endemic typhoid.
Complement	Persistent complement component, properdin, mannan-binding lectin, or factor B deficiency; secondary deficiency because receiving eculizumab	None	All inactivated and live-virus vaccines on the standard annual schedule are safe, likely are effective, and should be administered.[e] PPSV23 should be given beginning at 2 years of age[f]; MenACWY-CRM series beginning in infancy[h], and the MenB series beginning at 10 years of age. Meningococcal vaccination may be ineffective in patients receiving eculizumab; prophylactic antimicrobial therapy such as amoxicillin or penicillin can be considered for duration of treatment and until immune competence has returned.
Phagocytic function	Chronic granulomatous disease	Live-bacteria vaccines[e]	All inactivated and live-virus vaccines[d] on the standard annual schedule are safe, likely are effective and should be administered.[e,i]
	Phagocytic deficiencies that are ill-defined or accompanied by defects in T-lymphocyte and natural killer cell dysfunction (such as Chediak-Higashi syndrome, leukocyte adhesion defects, and myeloperoxidase deficiency)	All live-bacteria[e] and live-virus vaccines[d]	All inactivated vaccines on the standard annual schedule are safe, likely are effective, and should be given. PPSV23 should be administered beginning at 2 years of age.[f] Consider MenACWY-CRM series beginning in infancy[h] and the MenB series beginning at 10 years of age depending on splenic dysfunction.

Table 1.17. Immunization of Children and Adolescents With Primary and Secondary Immune Deficiencies, continued

Category	Example of Specific Immunodeficiency	Vaccine Contraindications[a]	Comments
Secondary			
	HIV/AIDS	OPV,[a] smallpox vaccine, BCG, LAIV, MMRV, MMR, VAR in highly immunocompromised children; YF vaccine may have a contraindication or precaution depending on indicators of immune function[j]	All inactivated vaccines on the standard annual schedule are safe, may be effective, and should be administered.[e] Rotavirus vaccine should be administered on the standard schedule. MMR and VAR are recommended for children with HIV infection who are asymptomatic or have only low-level immunocompromise.[k] PPSV23 should be administered beginning at 2 years of age.[f] MenACWY-CRM series should be administered beginning in infancy.[h] Hib is indicated for under- or unimmunized children ≥5 years of age.[l]
	Malignancy, transplantation, autoimmune disease, immunosuppressive or radiation therapy	All live-virus and live-bacteria vaccines, depending on immune status[c,d]	Refer to text for guidance. All inactivated vaccines on the standard annual schedule are safe and may be effective depending on degree of immunocompromise.[e] Annual IIV is recommended unless receiving intensive chemotherapy or anti-B cell antibodies. PPSV23 should be administered beginning at 2 years of age.[f] Hib vaccine is indicated in under- or unimmunized children <5 years of age only.[e]
	Asplenia (functional, congenital anatomic, surgical)	LAIV	All inactivated and live-virus vaccines on the standard annual schedule are safe, likely are effective, and should be administered.[e] PPSV23 should be administered beginning at 2 years of age.[f] MenACWY-CRM series beginning in infancy,[h] and the MenB series beginning at 10 years of age. Hib is indicated for under- or unimmunized children ≥5 years of age.[l]
	Chronic renal failure	None	All inactivated and live-virus vaccines, except LAIV, on the standard annual immunization schedule are safe, likely are effective, and should be administered.[e] PPSV23 should be administered beginning at 2 years of age.[f] HepB is indicated if not previously immunized.

Table 1.17. Immunization of Children and Adolescents With Primary and Secondary Immune Deficiencies, continued

Category	Example of Specific Immunodeficiency	Vaccine Contraindications[a]	Comments
CNS	CNS anatomic barrier defect (cochlear implant, congenital dysplasia of the inner ear, persistent CSF communication with naso-oropharynx)	LAIV	All inactivated and live-virus vaccines on the standard annual immunization schedule are safe and effective and should be administered.[e] PPSV23 should be administered beginning at 2 years of age.[f]

AIDS indicates acquired immune deficiency syndrome; BCG, bacille Calmette-Guérin; CNS, central nervous system; CSF, cerebrospinal fluid; HepB, hepatitis B vaccine; Hib, *Haemophilus influenzae* type b vaccine; HIV, human immunodeficiency virus; IG, Immune Globulin; IgA, immunoglobulin A; IgG, immunoglobulin G; IIV, inactivated influenza vaccine; LAIV, live attenuated influenza vaccine; MenACWY, serogroups A, C, W, and Y meningococcal conjugate vaccine; MenACWY-CRM, MenACWY (Menveo); MenB, serogroup B meningococcal conjugate vaccine; MMR, measles, mumps, and rubella vaccine; MMRV, measles, mumps, rubella, and varicella vaccine; OPV, oral poliovirus vaccine; PPSV23, 23-valent pneumococcal polysaccharide vaccine; STAT1, signal transducer and activator of transcription 1; VAR, varicella vaccine; YF, yellow fever.

[a] This table refers to contraindications for nonemergency vaccination as recommended by the Advisory Committee on Immunization Practices, Centers for Disease Control and Prevention.

[b] OPV vaccine not available in the United States.

[c] Live-bacteria vaccines: BCG, Ty21a *Salmonella* Typhi vaccine, cholera vaccine.

[d] Live-virus vaccines: MMR, VAR, MMRV, OPV, YF vaccine, vaccinia (smallpox vaccine), and rotavirus vaccine. Except for severe T-lymphocyte deficiency, data to contraindicate rotavirus vaccine are lacking; the immunocompromised state generally is considered a precaution for rotavirus vaccine. LAIV is not indicated for any person with a potentially immunocompromising condition.

[e] Children who are under- or unimmunized for age should receive routinely recommended vaccines, according to age and the catch-up schedule, with urgency to administer needed Hib and 13-valent pneumococcal conjugate vaccine (PCV13).

[f] PPSV23 is begun at ≥2 years of age for patients with complement deficiency other than those with a deficiency limited to terminal complement components. If PCV13 is required (ie, for children <6 years who have not received all required doses, and for those ≥26 years of age who never received PCV13), PCV13 dose(s) should be administered first, followed by PPSV23 at least 8 weeks later; a second dose of PPSV23 is given 5 years after the first (see *Streptococcus pneumoniae* (Pneumococcal) Infections, p 717).

[g] Regarding T-lymphocyte immunodeficiency as a contraindication to rotavirus vaccine, data only exist for severe combined immunodeficiency syndrome.

[h] Age and schedule of doses depend on the product; repeated doses are required (see Meningococcal Infections, p 519).

[i] Additional pneumococcal vaccine is not indicated for children with chronic granulomatous disease beyond age-based standard recommendations for PCV13, because these children are not at increased risk of pneumococcal disease.

[j] YF vaccine is contraindicated in children with HIV infection younger than 6 years who are highly immunosuppressed (see text). There is a precaution for use of YF vaccine in asymptomatic children with HIV infection younger than 6 years with total lymphocyte percentage of 15% to 24%, and older than 6 years with CD4+ T-lymphocyte counts of 200–499 cells/mm^3 (Centers for Disease Control and Prevention. Yellow fever vaccine: recommendations of the Advisory Committee on Immunization Practices [ACIP]. *MMWR Recomm Rep.* 2010;59[RR-07]:1-27).

[k] Live-virus vaccines (MMR and VAR) can be administered to asymptomatic children with HIV infection and adolescents without severe immunosuppression (ie, to children 1 year through 13 years of age with a CD4+ T-lymphocyte percentage ≥15%, and to adolescents ≥14 years of age with a CD4+ T-lymphocyte count ≥200 lymphocytes/mm^3). Severely immunocompromised infants, children, adolescents, and young adults with HIV infection (ie, children 1 year through 13 years of age with a CD4+ T-lymphocyte percentage <15%, and adolescents ≥14 years of age with a CD4+ T-lymphocyte count <200 lymphocytes/mm^3) should not receive measles virus–containing vaccine, because vaccine-related pneumonia has been reported. MMRV should not be administered to children with HIV infection, regardless of degree of immunosuppression, because of lack of safety data in this population.

[l] A single dose of Hib is indicated for unimmunized children and adolescents ≥5 years of age (children and adolescents who have not received a primary series and booster dose or at least 1 dose of Hib after 14 months of age are considered unimmunized) who have anatomic or functional asplenia (including sickle cell disease), who will undergo splenectomy, or who have HIV infection.

Society of America (IDSA), in collaboration with the Centers for Disease Control and Prevention (CDC), the American Academy of Pediatrics (AAP), and other professional societies and organizations, has developed immunization guidelines for children and adults with primary and secondary immune deficiencies.[1] Health care providers should consult these guidelines for vaccinating children and adults with specific health conditions (eg, hematopoietic stem cell or solid organ transplant recipients) and life circumstances (eg, international travel or providing care for people with immune deficiencies). This chapter includes general principles and specific recommendations when the primary care physician is more likely to deliver care without the patient's continuous management by a subspecialist. Subspecialists who care for immunocompromised patients share responsibility with the primary care physician for ensuring appropriate vaccinations for immunocompromised patients and members of their households and other close contacts.

GENERAL PRINCIPLES

Certain generalizations regarding degree of immune suppression in patients with a primary or secondary immunodeficiency are useful for the health care provider and were adopted in the IDSA guideline.

High-level immunosuppression includes patients who:

- Have combined B- and T-lymphocyte primary immunodeficiency (eg, severe combined immunodeficiency [SCID]).
- Receive cancer chemotherapy.
- Receive chemotherapeutic agents (eg, cyclophosphamide, methotrexate, mycophenolate) and combination immunosuppressive drugs for rheumatologic conditions.
- Have HIV infection and a CD4+ T-lymphocyte percentage <15% for children age 1 year through 13 years, or a CD4+ T-lymphocyte count <200 lymphocytes/mm^3 in adolescents age ≥14 years.
- Receive daily corticosteroid therapy at a dose ≥20 mg (or ≥2 mg/kg/day for patients weighing <10 kg) of prednisone or equivalent for ≥14 days.
- Receive certain biologic immune modulators (eg, tumor necrosis factor-alpha [TNF-α] antagonists, anti–B-lymphocyte monoclonal antibodies, anti-T-lymphocyte monoclonal antibodies, or checkpoint inhibitors).
- Are within 2 months of solid organ transplantation (SOT).
- Are within 2 to 3 months of receiving hematopoietic stem cell transplant (HSCT) at a minimum and frequently for a much longer period (HSCT recipients can have prolonged high degrees of immunosuppression depending on type of transplant [allogeneic > autologous], type of donor and stem cell source, and post-transplant complications [eg, graft versus host disease {GVHD}] and their treatments).

Low-level immunosuppression includes patients who:

- Have HIV infection without symptoms and with a CD4+ T-lymphocyte percentage ≥15% for children age 1 year through 13 years, or a CD4+ T-lymphocyte count ≥200 lymphocytes/mm^3 in adolescents age ≥14 years.

---

[1]Rubin LG, Levin MJ, Ljungman P, et al. 2013 IDSA clinical practice guideline for vaccination of the immunocompromised host. *Clin Infect Dis.* 2014;58(3):309-318. Available at: **www.idsociety.org/Templates/Content.aspx?id=32212256011**

- Receive a lower daily dose of systemic corticosteroid than for high-level immunosuppression for ≥14 days or receive alternate-day corticosteroid therapy.
- Receive methotrexate at a dosage of ≤0.4 mg/kg/week, azathioprine at a dosage of ≤3 mg/kg/day, or 6-mercaptopurine at a dosage of ≤1.5 mg/kg/day.

TIMING OF VACCINES. For patients in whom initiation of immunosuppressive medication is planned, vaccinations should be administered before immunosuppression, when feasible. Live vaccines should be administered as indicated no closer than 4 weeks before initiation of immunosuppression or transplantation. If administration is not possible within this time restriction, immunization should be deferred until after recovery and/or reduction of profound immunosuppression. Inactivated vaccines should be administered at least 2 weeks before immunosuppression or transplantation, if feasible.

Certain vaccines may be administered to children while they are modestly immunosuppressed, especially when the immunosuppressed state is likely to be lengthy or lifelong. Examples include some children with HIV infection and those having received solid organ transplants. Currently, there is no universally approved revaccination guidelines for nontransplanted childhood cancer survivors, and therefore, the exact timing of when to revaccinate and/or catch-up children with cancer remains unclear. IDSA recommends reimmunization at 3 months following cessation of chemotherapy, but other societies recommend waiting 6 months. Some inactivated vaccines have been given during maintenance chemotherapy for children with acute leukemia, including inactivated influenza vaccine (IIV). However, as described later in this chapter, live attenuated vaccines are generally contraindicated in immunocompromised people. Expert consultation is warranted if a live-virus vaccine is being considered for immunocompromised people, including certain children after SOT, with HIV infection, and after HSCT.

The interval between cessation of immunosuppressive therapy and immune reconstitution varies. Therefore, it is often not possible to make a definitive recommendation for an interval after cessation of immunosuppressive therapy when inactivated vaccines can be administered effectively or when or whether live-virus vaccines can be administered safely and effectively. Immunodeficiency that follows use of certain recombinant human proteins with anti-inflammatory properties, such as the anti-B-lymphocyte monoclonal antibody rituximab, is prolonged and patients who receive such treatment are unlikely to respond to vaccines for at least 6 months and often much longer (see Biologic Response-Modifying Drugs Used to Decrease Inflammation, p 82).

Vaccinations after reduction or cessation of immunosuppression following transplantation vary depending on the vaccine, underlying disorder, specific immunosuppressive therapy, and presence or absence of GVHD.[1] Timing for inactivated and live-virus vaccines could vary from as early as 3 months after cessation of chemotherapy for acute leukemia to 24 months or longer for measles, mumps, and rubella vaccine (MMR) or varicella vaccine (VAR) after HSCT in a patient without ongoing immunosuppression or GVHD. Timing also may be delayed for solid organ transplant recipients with graft rejection.

---

[1]Rubin LG, Levin MJ, Ljungman P, et al. 2013 IDSA clinical practice guideline for vaccination of the immunocompromised host. *Clin Infect Dis*. 2014;58(3):309-318. Available at: **www.idsociety.org/Templates/Content.aspx?id=32212256011**

LIVE VACCINES. In general, people who are severely immunocompromised or in whom immune function is uncertain should not receive live vaccines because of the risk of disease caused by the vaccine strains. However, there are particular immune deficiency disorders in which some live vaccines are safe and, for certain immunocompromised children and adolescents, the benefits may outweigh risks for use of particular live vaccines (see Table 1.17, p 73).

INACTIVATED VACCINES. Inactivated vaccines do not convey substantial increased risk to an immunocompromised child compared with an immunocompetent child and, therefore, the decision to administer an inactivated vaccine to children with immunodeficiency is based on an assessment of the likelihood of benefit. Inactivated vaccines administered during immunosuppressive therapies generally are not counted as valid in the recommended immunization schedule. Annual vaccination with inactivated influenza vaccine (IIV) is recommended for immunocompromised patients 6 months of age and older. Other than IIV, inactivated vaccines are generally not routinely administered to patients receiving immunoglobulin therapy for major antibody deficiency disorders or severe combined immunodeficiencies because of lack of added benefit.

Inactivated vaccines not administered universally or at specific ages sometimes may be specifically indicated for children with inherited and acquired immunodeficient conditions because of their high risk for infection. These might include pneumococcal vaccine (ie, 13-valent pneumococcal conjugate vaccine [PCV13] followed by 23-valent pneumococcal polysaccharide vaccine [PPSV23], PCV13 after the age of 6 years if not previously vaccinated with PCV13), serogroups A, C, W, and Y meningococcal conjugate vaccine (MenACWY) beginning in infancy, serogroup B meningococcal conjugate vaccine (MenB) beginning at 10 years of age, and *Haemophilus influenzae* type b vaccine (Hib) after the age of 5 years.

Table 1.17 (p 73) provides guidance for some immunocompromising conditions. Additional information can be found in the IDSA clinical practice guideline for vaccination of the immunocompromised person (**https://academic.oup.com/cid/article/59/1/144/405127**) and in the annually updated child and adolescent immunization schedule (**https://redbook.solutions.aap.org/SS/Immunization_Schedules.aspx**).

Because patients with congenital or acquired immunodeficiencies may not have an adequate response to vaccines, they may remain susceptible to infections despite having been immunized. Positive serologic test results are not always reliable markers of protection. Health care providers should generally assume susceptibility to infections when considering postexposure intervention strategies for these patients.

PRIMARY IMMUNODEFICIENCIES

Vaccine recommendations for primary immunodeficiency disorders depend on the specific immunologic abnormality and degree of impairment (Table 1.17, p 73). All live-virus and inactivated vaccines can be administered to children with isolated immunoglobulin (Ig) A deficiency. Inactivated vaccines other than IIV are not routinely administered to patients with major antibody deficiencies or SCID during IG therapy. For these patients, inactivated vaccines can be administered as part of immunologic assessment prior to Immune Globulin Intravenous (IGIV) therapy without safety concerns. For patients with common variable immunodeficiency, MenACWY should be administered beginning at 2 months of age because of their splenic dysfunction and lack of substantial meningococcal antibodies in IGIV.

Live-virus vaccines such as MMR and VAR should not be administered to patients with major antibody deficiencies, SCID, and T-lymphocyte immunodeficiencies, including any of the following conditions: DiGeorge syndrome with CD3+ T-lymphocyte count <500 cells/mm³, other combined immunodeficiencies with similar CD3+ T-lymphocyte counts, Wiskott-Aldrich syndrome, or X-linked lymphoproliferative disease or familial disorders that predispose to hemophagocytic lymphohistiocytosis.

Patients with primary complement deficiencies of early classic pathway, alternate pathway, or severe mannose-binding lectin deficiency should receive all routine inactivated and live vaccines on the immunization schedule. For patients with complement deficiencies other than isolated terminal component deficiencies, PPSV23 should be administered at 2 years of age (and ≥8 weeks after last dose of PCV13) and again 5 years after the initial dose. The MenACWY series should be initiated at age 2 months or older and the MenB series should be administered starting at age 10 years. MenACWY and MenB booster doses are indicated for those at chronic, increased risk for meningococcal disease (eg, functional [eg, sickle cell disease] and anatomical [eg, splenectomy] asplenia, HIV infection, persistent complement component deficiency) (see Meningococcal Infections, p 519). Both meningococcal vaccines are recommended for patients receiving eculizumab, which inhibits the complement cascade by binding to complement component 5 (C5).

Patients with phagocytic cell deficiencies (eg, chronic granulomatous disease [CGD], leukocyte adhesion deficiency [LAD], Chediak-Higashi syndrome, cyclic neutropenia) and patients with innate immune defects that result in defects of cytokine generation or response or cellular activation (eg, defects of interferon-gamma/interleukin [IL]-12 axis) should receive all inactivated vaccines on the annual immunization schedule. Live-virus vaccines (eg, MMR) should be administered to patients with CGD and cyclic neutropenia, but live-bacterial vaccines (eg, oral typhoid vaccine [Ty21a]) should not be administered to these patients. Live-bacterial and live-virus vaccines should not be administered to patients with LAD, Chediak-Higashi syndrome, or defects within the interferon-gamma or IL-12 pathway.

SECONDARY (ACQUIRED) IMMUNODEFICIENCIES

Several factors should be considered in immunization of children with secondary immunodeficiencies (Table 1.17, p 73), including the underlying disease, the specific immunosuppressive regimen (dose and schedule), and the patient's infectious disease and immunization history. Live-virus vaccines generally are contraindicated because of a proven or theoretical increased risk of vaccine virus disease. For example, in children with an immunocompromising condition or HIV infection and CD4+ T-lymphocyte percentage <15% or count <200/mm³, MMR and VAR are contraindicated. LAIV should not be administered to children with HIV infection. Rotavirus vaccine should be administered to HIV-exposed and HIV-infected infants irrespective of CD4+ T-lymphocyte percentage or count (see Human Immunodeficiency Virus Infection, p 427). Rotavirus vaccine may be indicated for infants with other acquired immunocompromising conditions if the potential benefit of protection outweighs the risk of adverse reaction.

HOUSEHOLD MEMBERS OF IMMUNOCOMPROMISED PATIENTS

Household contacts of immunocompromised patients should receive all age- and exposure-appropriate vaccines, with the exception of smallpox vaccine, to minimize the exposure of the immunocompromised patient to vaccine-preventable infections. LAIV may be administered to healthy household and other close contacts of people with altered immunocompetence. However, if the person with altered immunocompetence is in a protected environment, then LAIV recipients should avoid close contact with the immunocompromised person for 7 days.

Live vaccines, when indicated for travel (eg, yellow fever and oral typhoid vaccines), should also be administered to household contacts, with the exception of oral poliovirus vaccine (OPV), which still is available in many countries outside of the United States. Although the risk of transmission is low, immunocompromised patients should avoid contact with people who develop skin lesions after receipt of VAR until the lesions clear. When transmission of vaccine-strain varicella virus has occurred, the virus is expected to maintain its attenuated characteristics and susceptibility to acyclovir. Therefore, administration of Varicella-Zoster Immune Globulin or IGIV to an immunocompromised person after exposure to a person with skin lesions developed after varicella vaccination is not indicated. All members of the household should wash their hands after changing the diaper of an infant who received rotavirus vaccine to minimize rotavirus transmission, as shedding of the virus may occur up to 1 month after the last dose.

SPECIAL SITUATIONS/HOSTS

CORTICOSTEROIDS. Before starting corticosteroid therapy for inflammatory or auto-immune diseases, patients should be current in their vaccinations based on their age and other indications. Inactivated vaccines should be administered at least 2 weeks before, and live-virus vaccines should be administered at least 4 weeks before initiating corticosteroid therapy.

Guidance for Administration of Inactivated Vaccines During Corticosteroid Therapy. Inactivated vaccines can still be administered to patients while they are on steroid therapy long-term. Inactivated vaccine administration can be deferred temporarily until corticosteroids are discontinued if the hiatus is expected to be brief and adherence to return appointment is likely. Inactivated vaccines need not be avoided because of concern for exacerbation of an inflammatory or immune-mediated condition.

Guidance for Administration of Live-Virus Vaccines During Corticosteroid Therapy.
Recommendations depend on potency, route of administration, and duration of corticosteroid therapy:

- **High doses of systemic corticosteroids given daily for 14 days or more.** Children receiving ≥2 mg/kg per day of prednisone or its equivalent, or ≥20 mg/day if they weigh 10 kg or more, for 14 days or more should not receive live-virus vaccines until 4 weeks after discontinuation of treatment.
- **High doses of systemic corticosteroids given daily or on alternate days for fewer than 14 days.** Children receiving ≥2 mg/kg per day of prednisone or its equivalent, or ≥20 mg/day if they weigh 10 kg or more, can receive live-virus vaccines immediately after discontinuation of treatment. Some experts suggest delaying administration of live-virus vaccines until 2 weeks after discontinuation.

- **Low or moderate doses of systemic corticosteroids or locally administered corticosteroids in children who have a disease (eg, systemic lupus erythematosus) that itself is immunosuppressive, or who are receiving immunosuppressive medication other than corticosteroids,** should not receive live-virus vaccines during therapy, except in special circumstances during which the potential benefit of protection and the risk of adverse reaction are weighed.
- **Low or moderate doses of systemic corticosteroids given daily or on alternate days.** Children receiving <2 mg/kg per day of prednisone or its equivalent, or <20 mg/day if they weigh 10 kg or more, can receive live-virus vaccines during corticosteroid treatment.
- **Physiologic maintenance doses of corticosteroids.** Children who are receiving only maintenance physiologic doses of corticosteroids can receive live-virus vaccines.
- **Topical therapy, local injections, or aerosol use of corticosteroids.** Application of low-potency topical corticosteroids to localized areas on the skin; administration by aerosolization; application on conjunctiva; or intra-articular, bursal, or tendon injections of corticosteroids usually do not result in immunosuppression that limit the use of live-virus vaccines.

BIOLOGIC RESPONSE-MODIFYING DRUGS USED TO DECREASE INFLAMMATION. Biologic response modifiers (BRMs) are drugs used to treat immune-mediated conditions, including juvenile idiopathic arthritis, rheumatoid arthritis, and inflammatory bowel disease. Their immune-modulating effects can last for weeks to months after discontinuation. These BRMs are often used in combination with other immunosuppressive drugs, such as methotrexate or corticosteroids.

Vaccination status of patients who need BRMs should be assessed and recommended vaccines should be administered in advance (Table 1.18). Recommended vaccines include PPSV23 for patients 2 years or older (8 weeks or more after PCV13 doses on the routine schedule are completed) and PCV13 for patients 6 years or older who previously did not receive PCV13.

BRMs are considered highly immunosuppressive, and live-virus vaccines are contraindicated during therapy; inactivated vaccines, including IIV, should be administered as per the immunization schedule and should not be withheld because of concern for an exaggerated inflammatory response. The interval following therapy until live-virus vaccines can be administered safely has not been established and is likely to vary by agent.

Infants exposed in utero to maternally administered BRMs can have detectable drug concentrations for many months following delivery, resulting in concern for immunosuppression among infants in the 12 months after the last maternal dose during pregnancy. Data are sparse on the safety of rotavirus vaccines in infants who were exposed to maternally administered BRMs in utero. Considering that rotavirus disease is rarely life threatening in the United States, rotavirus vaccines should be avoided in infants for the first 12 months after the last in utero exposure to most BRMs. Exceptions include certolizumab, which is not transferred across the placenta because of its structure as a pegylated Fab fragment, and likely infliximab, although the data are more sparse for it; rotavirus vaccination of infants can be considered when

Table 1.18. Recommendations for Evaluation Prior to Initiation of Biologic Response-Modifying Drugs

- Perform tuberculin skin test (TST) or interferon-gamma release assay (IGRA) (see Tuberculosis, p 786)
- Consider chest radiograph on the basis of clinical and epidemiologic findings
- Document vaccination status and, if required, administer:
  - Inactivated vaccines (including annual IIV) a minimum of 2 weeks before initiation of biologic response-modifying drug
  - Live-virus vaccines a minimum 4 weeks before initiation of biologic response modifier therapy, unless contraindicated by condition or other therapies
- Counsel household members regarding risk of infection and ensure vaccination (see Household Members of Immunocompromised Patients, p 81)
- Consider serologic testing for *Histoplasma* species, *Toxoplasma* species, and other intracellular pathogens depending on risk of past exposure
- Perform serologic testing for hepatitis B virus and vaccinate/revaccinate if HBsAb is <10 mIU/mL
- Consider serologic testing for varicella-zoster virus and Epstein-Barr virus
- Counsel regarding:
  - Food safety (**www.cdc.gov/foodsafety**)
  - Maintenance of dental hygiene
  - Risks of exposure to garden soil, pets, and other animals
  - Avoiding high-risk activities (eg, excavation sites or spelunking because of risk of *Histoplasma capsulatum*)
  - Avoiding travel to areas with endemic pathogenic fungi (eg, certain areas of southwestern United States for risk of *Coccidioides* species) or to areas where tuberculosis is endemic

IIV indicates inactivated influenza vaccine; HBsAb, hepatitis B surface antibody.
Modified from Le Saux N; Canadian Paediatric Society, Infectious Diseases and Immunization Committee. *Paediatr Child Health.* 2012;17(3):147-150 and Davies HD; American Academy of Pediatrics, Committee on Infectious Diseases. Infectious complications with the use of biologic response modifiers in infants and children. *Pediatrics.* 2016;138(2):e20161209.

mothers received treatment during pregnancy with either of these BRMs. As more data become available for the other BRMs, recommendations are likely to change, so consultation with a pediatric infectious diseases physician is recommended. Because MMR, VAR, and measles, mumps, rubella, and varicella vaccine (MMRV) are recommended routinely at 12 months of age, previous receipt of BRMs during pregnancy does not preclude the infant from receiving these live vaccines at the recommended time. For measles prevention in infants younger than 12 months following exposure during outbreak settings or for travel, MMR or Immune Globulin Intramuscular should be used. The choice depends on several factors (eg, age, time elapsed since exposure, which BRM was administered during pregnancy). International travel for infants who were exposed to BRMs in utero (other than certolizumab) should be discouraged for the 12 months following the last maternal dose during pregnancy. These recommendations may not apply to management of infants born in other countries, where risks of wild-type infection may differ from the United States and where additional live vaccines may be administered in early infancy (eg, bacille Calmette-Guérin [BCG], OPV).

HEMATOPOIETIC STEM CELL TRANSPLANTATION. Patients for whom HSCT is planned should receive all routinely recommended inactivated vaccines (including IIV) at least 2 weeks before the start of the conditioning period, when possible. Routinely recommended live-virus vaccines should be administered if the patient is not already immunosuppressed and the interval to the start of the conditioning period is at least 4 weeks. By vaccinating the nonimmune patient before HSCT, some protection likely will persist in the months after transplant. The HSCT donor, if known and feasible, should be current with routinely recommended vaccines, but vaccination of the donor solely for benefit of the recipient is not recommended. Administration of MMR, MMRV, and VAR should be avoided within 4 weeks of hematopoietic stem cell harvest but may be contraindicated because of the reason for HSCT.

Household members of HSCT recipients should be fully immunized (see Household Members of Immunocompromised Patients, p 81). Timing of immune reconstitution of HSCT recipients varies greatly depending on type of transplantation, interval since transplantation, receipt of immunosuppressive medications, and presence or absence of GVHD and other complications. Routine and additional vaccinations needed for medical conditions are an important part of patient management in collaboration with the patient's specialty care providers. Revaccination for certain inactivated vaccines, such as pneumococcal vaccines and IIV, can be given starting 3 to 6 months after transplantation. Live vaccines can be given as early as 2 years following transplantation but may be delayed if HSCT recipients still have active GVHD and/or high degree of immunosuppression.

SOLID ORGAN TRANSPLANTATION. Children and adolescents with chronic heart, lung, liver, or kidney disease should receive all vaccinations as appropriate for age and health condition. Similarly, SOT candidates should be current with their vaccination status and if feasible should receive inactivated vaccines at least 2 weeks prior and live vaccines 4 week prior to SOT. SOT candidates who are 2 years or older should receive pneumococcal vaccination (PCV13, PPSV23) as described in the annual immunization schedule. SOT candidates who have negative hepatitis B surface antigen (HBsAg) and hepatitis B surface antibody (anti-HBsAb) test results should complete the hepatitis B vaccine (HepB) series, followed by serologic testing to confirm immunity. Additional doses of HepB may be indicated if serologic test results are negative. Patients 12 months or older who have not completed the hepatitis A vaccine (HepA) series or have negative hepatitis A serologic test results should complete the HepA series. MMR can be administered to infants 6 through 11 months of age who are SOT candidates and who are not immunocompromised. A second dose of MMR at ≥12 months is indicated if the infant is still awaiting a transplant that will not occur within 4 weeks of the second dose of MMR. Living SOT donors should be current on their vaccination status, with considerations for required vaccines the same as for HSCT donors (see Hematopoietic Stem Cell Transplantation). Donors should avoid receiving live-virus vaccines within 4 weeks before donation. Household members of SOT recipients should be current on their vaccination status.

HIV INFECTION (ALSO SEE HUMAN IMMUNODEFICIENCY VIRUS INFECTION, P 427). HIV-infected children and adolescents should receive all inactivated vaccines as indicated on the annual immunization schedule. PPSV23 should be administered to people 2 years of age or older, at least 8 weeks after the last required PCV13 dose. Meningococcal conjugate vaccine (MenACWY) should be administered beginning at 8 weeks of age. Depending on age of the patient and the vaccine manufacturer, the number of doses and the intervals between doses can vary. Booster does of MenACWY are recommended 3 to 5 years after the primary series, depending on age at vaccination (see Meningococcal Infections, p 519). Currently, MenB is not specifically recommended for people with HIV infection. Rotavirus vaccine should be administered to HIV-exposed and HIV-infected infants irrespective of CD4+ T-lymphocyte percentage or count. MMR and VAR should be administered to children 12 months or older who are stable clinically and who have CD4+ T-lymphocyte percentage $\geq15\%$ or count ≥200 cells/mm^3 (see General Principles, p 77). Children with HIV infection should not receive MMRV or LAIV.

In the United States, BCG is contraindicated for HIV-infected patients. In areas of the world with a high incidence of tuberculosis, the World Health Organization (WHO) recommends administering BCG vaccine to children with HIV infection who are asymptomatic.

ASPLENIA AND FUNCTIONAL ASPLENIA. The asplenic state can result from the following: (1) surgical removal of the spleen (eg, after trauma, for treatment of hemolytic conditions); (2) functional asplenia (eg, from sickle cell disease or thalassemia); or (3) congenital asplenia or polysplenia. Special recommendations for patients with asplenia apply to all 3 categories. All infants, children, adolescents, and adults with asplenia have an increased risk of fulminant septicemia, especially associated with encapsulated bacteria, which is associated with a high mortality rate. In comparison with immunocompetent children who have not undergone splenectomy, the incidence of and mortality rate from septicemia are increased in children who have had splenectomy after trauma and in children with sickle cell disease by as much as 350-fold, and the rate may be even higher in children who have had splenectomy for thalassemia. The risk of invasive bacterial infection is higher in younger children than in older children, and the risk may be greater during the years immediately after surgical splenectomy. Fulminant septicemia, however, has been reported in adults as long as 25 years after splenectomy.

Streptococcus pneumoniae is the most common pathogen causing septicemia in children with asplenia. Less common vaccine-preventable causes include *Haemophilus influenzae* type b and *Neisseria meningitidis.*

Pneumococcal vaccination is vital for children with asplenia (see *Streptococcus pneumoniae* [Pneumococcal] Infections, p 717). Following administration of an appropriate number of primary series or catch-up doses of PCV13, PPSV23 should be administered to children 24 months or older at least 8 weeks after the last PCV13 dose. A second dose of PPSV23 should be administered 5 years later (see *Streptococcus pneumoniae* [Pneumococcal] Infections, p 717). For children 2 through 18 years of age who have not received PCV13, even if they previously received PCV7 series or already received PPSV23 or both, 1 dose of PCV13 should be administered. When splenectomy is planned for a patient 2 years or older who is PPSV23 naïve, PPSV23 should be administered at least 8 weeks after indicated dose(s) of PCV13 and at least 2 weeks before surgery.

Previously unimmunized children with asplenia younger than 5 years should receive appropriate number of doses of and intervals for *Haemophilus influenzae* type b vaccine (Hib) according to the catch-up schedule as described in the annual immunization schedule. Unimmunized children 5 years or older should receive a single dose of Hib.

MenACWY should be administered to children with asplenia, as recommended for those with primary complement component deficiencies (see Primary Immunodeficiencies, p 79), with one important caveat. MenACWY-D (Menactra) should not be used before 2 years of age and sooner than 4 weeks after completion of the 4-dose series of PCV13 series because of interference with antibody response to some serotypes contained in PCV13 when the vaccines are administered concurrently. In this instance, MenACWY-CRM (Menveo) should be used as indicated by age, without concern for significant interference with PCV13. For patients with asplenia who are younger than 7 years, an additional dose of either MenACWY-D or MenACWY-CRM is recommended 3 years after the primary series and then every 5 years; for patients with asplenia who are 7 years and older, the initial booster dose following the primary series should be at 5 years instead of 3 years, and then every 5 years thereafter. Use of MenACWY vaccine (beginning in infancy) and MenB vaccine (beginning at 10 years of age) can be considered on a case-by-case basis for children with other primary or secondary splenic dysfunction.

When surgical splenectomy is planned, Hib, pneumococcal, and meningococcal vaccine history should be reviewed, and needed vaccines should be administered at least 2 weeks before surgery. If splenectomy is performed on an emergency basis or if needed vaccines were not administered before splenectomy, they should be administered as soon as possible when the patient's condition is stable.

In addition to immunization, antibiotic prophylaxis against pneumococcal infections is recommended for many children with asplenia (see *Streptococcus pneumoniae* [Pneumococcal] Infections, p 717).

CENTRAL NERVOUS SYSTEM ANATOMIC BARRIER DEFECTS. Patients of all ages scheduled to receive a cochlear implant as well as patients with congenital dysplasias of the inner ear or persistent cerebrospinal fluid (CSF) communication with the naso-oropharynx should receive vaccines recommended routinely on the annual immunization schedule. In addition, they should receive PCV13 as recommended for children with asplenia and at 24 months or older should receive PPSV23 (≥8 weeks after receipt of PCV13). Indicated doses of PCV13 and PPSV23 should be administered at least 2 weeks before cochlear implant surgery, when feasible.

There is no well-established evidence for use of antimicrobial prophylaxis for patients with CSF communication with the naso-oropharynx or middle ear. Risk of bacterial meningitis is highest in the first 7 to 10 days following acute traumatic breach. Some physicians recommend empiric parenteral antimicrobial therapy in the immediate post-traumatic period. Parenteral antimicrobial therapy also is given in the perioperative period for cochlear implantation and reparative neurosurgical procedures. Chronic antimicrobial prophylaxis is not indicated for persistent CSF communications or following cochlear implantation.

Immunization in Children With a Personal or Family History of Seizures

Studies have demonstrated a short-term increased risk of a febrile seizure (ie, generalized, brief, self-limited seizure) following receipt of several vaccines (eg, diphtheria and tetanus toxoids and whole-cell pertussis vaccine [DTwP]; measles, mumps, and rubella vaccine [MMR]; measles, mumps, rubella, and varicella vaccine [MMRV]; and 13-valent pneumococcal conjugate vaccine [PCV13] and influenza vaccine). Infants and children with a personal or family history of seizures of any etiology might be at greater risk of having a febrile seizure after receipt of these vaccines compared with children without such histories. No evidence indicates that febrile seizures cause permanent brain damage or epilepsy, aggravate neurologic disorders, or affect the prognosis for children with underlying disorders.

An increased incidence of seizures has not been found with the currently recommended DTaP vaccines that have replaced the whole-cell DTwP vaccines in the United States. In the case of pertussis immunization during infancy, vaccine administration could coincide with or hasten the recognition of a disorder associated with seizures, such as infantile spasms or severe myoclonic epilepsy of infancy, which could cause confusion about the role of pertussis immunization. Hence, pertussis immunization in infants with a history of recent seizures generally is deferred until the course of the neurologic disorder is clarified. DTaP should be administered to infants and children with a stable neurologic condition, including well-controlled seizures. Although reports of febrile seizures have been associated with other vaccines, with the exception of DTaP vaccine discussed previously, vaccination should not be deferred in children with a personal or family history of seizures. Postimmunization seizures in these children are uncommon, and if they occur, they usually are febrile in origin, have a benign outcome, and are not likely to be confused with manifestations of a previously unrecognized neurologic disorder.

Immunization in Children With Chronic Diseases

Chronic disease in children may be defined as having a medical condition that is currently not curable and that has been present for at least 3 months, will likely last longer than 3 months, or has occurred at least 3 times in the past year and likely will recur. Chronic diseases may increase children's susceptibility to infections and may increase the severity of infection-related manifestations and complications. Unless specifically contraindicated, immunizations recommended for healthy children should be administered to children with chronic diseases. The importance of annual influenza immunization should be particularly emphasized in this population and their household contacts. Children with hemophilia or other bleeding disorders should be immunized following the Centers for Disease Control and Prevention (CDC) guidelines for vaccinating persons with increased bleeding risk.[1] For children with chronic and immunocompromising conditions or therapies, see "Immunization and Other Considerations in Immunocompromised Children" (p 72) and "Recommended Child and Adolescent Immunization Schedule for Ages 18 Years or Younger, United States," which is

[1] **www.cdc.gov/vaccines/hcp/acip-recs/general-recs/special-situations.html#bleeding**

updated annually (**www.cdc.gov/vaccines/schedules/hcp/imz/child-ado-lescent.html** and **https://redbook.solutions.aap.org/SS/Immunization_Schedules.aspx**).

Children with certain chronic diseases such as allergic, respiratory, cardiovascular, hematologic, metabolic, and renal disorders are at increased risk of complications from pneumococcal infection and may need to receive pneumococcal vaccine(s) (13-valent pneumococcal conjugate vaccine [PCV13], 23-valent pneumococcal polysaccharide vaccine [PPSV23], or both), as recommended for age and condition (see *Streptococcus pneumoniae* [Pneumococcal] Infections, p 717). All children with chronic liver disease are at risk of severe clinical manifestations of acute hepatitis virus infections and should receive hepatitis A (HepA) and hepatitis B (HepB) vaccines if not previously vaccinated (see Hepatitis A, p 373, and Hepatitis B, p 381). Household members of children with chronic diseases should be current on recommended vaccines based on their age and health conditions. (**https://redbook.solutions.aap.org/SS/Immunization_Schedules.aspx**).

In 2012, the National Academy of Medicine (NAM) assessed whether vaccines (measles, mumps, and rubella; acellular pertusis-containing diphtheria and tetanus; tetanus toxoid; influenza; hepatitis A; hepatitis B; and human papillomavirus vaccines) were a potential trigger for a flare or the onset of chronic inflammatory diseases. The NAM review concluded that, although the evidence was inadequate to establish or refute a causal relationship between these vaccines and onset or exacerbation of multiple sclerosis, systemic lupus erythematosus, vasculitis, rheumatoid arthritis, or juvenile idiopathic arthritis,[1] overall, clinical evidence indicates that vaccines are not important triggers of these diseases or disease exacerbations and should not be withheld because of these concerns.

Immunization in American Indian/Alaska Native Children and Adolescents

Indigenous populations worldwide have high morbidity and mortality from infectious diseases, including vaccine-preventable infections (**wwwnc.cdc.gov/eid/article/7/7/pdfs/01-7732.pdf**). This chapter focuses on the US population of American Indian and Alaska Native (AI/AN) people and considerations for use of vaccines and biologic products that are special to these populations. For AI/AN people who live on or near reservation communities, geographic isolation and socioeconomic factors such as poverty, household crowding, substandard housing, poor indoor air quality, and lack of indoor plumbing are the major drivers of the persistence of elevated rates of infectious diseases. Currently, more than half of AI/AN people do not reside on reservation lands or in Alaska Native villages; the little data available indicate relative risk of vaccine-preventable and other infectious diseases for this subset of AI/AN people are lower compared with AI/AN living on reservations.

Historically, compared with children from other racial groups, AI/AN children living on reservation lands or in Alaska Native villages have higher rates of certain vaccine-preventable diseases, such as *Haemophilus influenzae* type b, *Streptococcus pneumoniae*, hepatitis A, and hepatitis B. Although the rate of mortality from pneumonia and influenza among AI/AN infants has steadily declined over recent decades, disparities persist.

---

[1]Stratton K, Andrew F, Rusch E, Clayton E. *Adverse Effects of Vaccines: Evidence and Causality.* Washington, DC: National Academies Press; 2012

During the past 2 decades, childhood immunizations for hepatitis A and hepatitis B in the United States have eliminated disease disparities for these pathogens in most populations of AI/AN children. Significant decreases have been documented in varicella hospitalizations and invasive disease caused by *H influenzae* type b and *S pneumoniae*. However, the historically high rates of infection and ongoing disparities highlight the importance of ensuring that recommendations for universal childhood immunization be implemented for all AI/AN children. Specific vulnerabilities are as follows.

- **Haemophilus influenzae type b.** There are important differences among the currently available *H influenzae* type b (Hib) vaccines that should be considered by clinicians caring for AI/AN children. Before availability and routine use of Hib conjugate vaccines, the incidence of invasive *H influenzae* type b disease was up to 10 times higher among young AI/AN children compared with non-AI/AN children. Because of the historically high risk of invasive *H influenzae* type b disease within the first 6 months of life in many AI/AN infant populations, the Indian Health Service (IHS) and the AAP recommend that the first dose of Hib conjugate vaccine be PedvaxHIB, which contains polyribosylribitol phosphate-meningococcal outer membrane protein (PRP-OMP). The administration of the PRP-OMP–containing PedvaxHIB vaccine leads to more rapid development of protective concentrations of antibody compared with other Hib vaccines, and failure to use vaccine containing PRP-OMP has been associated with excess cases of *H influenzae* type b disease in Alaska Native infants. Because of the lack of information on immunogenicity after the first dose of the new PRP-OMP-containing combination vaccine (DTaP-IPV-Hib-HepB) marketed as Vaxelis, this vaccine does not have a preferential recommendation for use in AI/AN infants at this time. If the first vaccination dose of PedvaxHIB is delayed by >1 month, the recommended catch-up schedule (available at **https://redbook.solutions.aap.org/SS/Immunization_Schedules. aspx**) should be followed. A booster dose (dose 3) in the PRP-OMP schedule or dose 4 in other Hib conjugate vaccine schedules is recommended at age 12 through 15 months; regardless of vaccine used in the primary series, there is no preferred vaccine formulation for the booster dose (ie, any approved Hib conjugate vaccine is acceptable **[www.cdc.gov/mmwr/preview/mmwrhtml/rr6301a1.htm]**). Availability of more than one Hib vaccine product in a clinic, however, has been shown to lead to errors in vaccine administration. To avoid confusion for health care professionals who serve AI/AN children predominantly, it may be prudent to use only PRP-OMP–containing Hib vaccines, if feasible.
- **Streptococcus pneumoniae.** Recommendations for 13-valent pneumococcal conjugate vaccine (PCV13) for AI/AN children are the same as for other US children. Before introduction of heptavalent pneumococcal conjugate vaccine (PCV7), the incidence of invasive pneumococcal disease (IPD) in certain AI/AN children (Alaska Native, Navajo, and White Mountain Apache) was 5 to 24 times higher than the incidence among other US children. Use of PCV7 in AI/AN infants resulted in near-elimination of disease caused by vaccine serotypes and decreased incidence of overall IPD. Use of PCV13 has further reduced the incidence of IPD in AI/ AN children. However, rates of IPD among some AI/AN children (Alaska Native, Navajo, and White Mountain Apache) remain more than fourfold higher than the rate among children in the general US population, largely attributable to serotypes

not targeted by the vaccine (**www.cdc.gov/mmwr/preview/mmwrhtml/rr5911a1.htm**).

- **Hepatitis viruses.** Before the introduction of hepatitis vaccines, rates of hepatitis A and hepatitis B in the AI/AN population exceeded those of the general US population. In 1970, Alaska Native people had an overall prevalence of hepatitis B surface antigen (HBsAg) of >6%, leading to high rates of hepatocellular carcinoma in Alaska Native people younger than 30 years. Universal infant immunization and population-wide screening and vaccination eliminated symptomatic hepatitis B infection and hepatocellular carcinoma in Alaska Native people younger than 20 years. Similarly, after initiation of universal childhood hepatitis A vaccination, hepatitis A infection rates among AI/AN people declined 20-fold during 1997-2001 to a rate similar to that of the general US population. Special efforts continue to be needed to ensure catch-up hepatitis A and hepatitis B immunization of previously unimmunized adolescents.

- **Influenza virus.** The disparity in influenza-related mortality rates in the AI/AN population compared with the general US population was confirmed during the 2009 H1N1 epidemic; the H1N1 death rate among AI/AN people in 12 states (representing 50% of the AI/AN population in the United States) was 4 times higher than the H1N1 death rate for all other racial and ethnic populations combined. For this reason, the AI/AN population is listed among the groups at risk of severe complications from influenza. When vaccine or antiviral medication supplies are limited or delayed, AI/AN people are considered a high-risk priority group. Studies also have documented the value of maternal immunization to protect both the mother and infants too young to be vaccinated. Given the elevated risk of influenza in the AI/AN population, maternal influenza immunization is an important strategy.

- **Respiratory syncytial virus (RSV).** The rates of hospitalization for RSV have been much higher for AI/AN infants in rural Alaska and southwest IHS regions than for other US infants. Hospitalization rates for AI/AN infants in these areas are similar to rates among medically high-risk and preterm infants in the overall US population. RSV hospitalization rates in Alaska Native children are related, in part, to household crowding and lack of plumbed water. Improvements in these risk factors and changes in RSV epidemiology contributed to a decline in the RSV hospitalization rate among Alaska Native children during 1994-2012; however, current RSV hospitalization rates in rural Alaska Native infants and Navajo/White Mountain Apache infants still are at least threefold higher than rates in other US children. Use of RSV-specific monoclonal antibody prophylaxis (palivizumab), as recommended by the AAP, should be optimized among high-risk AI/AN infants (see Respiratory Syncytial Virus, p 628). The RSV season may be different in northern latitudes, including Alaska, and RSV prophylaxis should reflect local seasonality and risk factors in this population.

- **Rotavirus.** In the 1990s, diarrhea-associated hospitalization rates in AI/AN infants were nearly twice those of the general US infant population. Following introduction of rotavirus vaccination, diarrhea-associated hospitalization rates in AI/AN children younger than 5 years during 2008, 2009, and 2010 were 24%, 37%, and 44%, respectively, lower than expected. These numbers suggest that rotavirus played a significant role in AI/AN infant hospitalizations and reinforces the importance of this vaccine for AI/AN infants.

Immunization in Adolescent and College Populations

Immunization recommendations for adolescents and college students have become routine and are reflected on the adolescent immunization schedule that is published annually (**www.cdc.gov/vaccines/schedules/index.html** and **www.vaccines.gov/who_and_when/college/index.html**). The adolescent population presents many immunization challenges, including less frequent visits for preventive care, scheduling conflicts because of age-appropriate activities, and providers missing opportunities to immunize. In addition, the ability of minors to consent to immunization varies by state. Providers should know and abide by the laws in their state governing minor consent for immunizations. The Society for Adolescent Health and Medicine has a position paper on adolescents consenting for vaccination and the potential impact on immunization rates (**www.adolescenthealth.org/SAHM_Main/media/Advocacy/Positions/Oct-13-Consent-Vaccination.pdf**). Updates on state laws are available from the Centers for Disease Control and Prevention (CDC).[1]

To ensure age-appropriate immunization, all youth should have an annual comprehensive preventive health visit, including routine visits at 11 through 12 years of age and 16 through 18 years of age for administration of appropriate vaccines.[2] During all adolescent visits, immunization status should be reviewed, and deficiencies should be corrected according to the recommended immunization schedule. The use of patient reminder-recall systems, provider reminders, and standing orders have been shown to increase immunization rates. Linking to statewide or regional immunization information systems will facilitate keeping adolescents appropriately immunized. Lapses in the immunization schedule do not necessitate reinitiation of a vaccine series or extra doses for any vaccine.

Tetanus toxoid, reduced diphtheria toxoid, and acellular pertussis vaccine (Tdap), serogroups A, C, W, and Y meningococcal vaccine (MenACWY), and human papillomavirus (HPV) vaccine should be administered at the 11- through 12-year-old visit. Only 2 doses of HPV vaccine are required for individuals whose first dose was given before their 15th birthday, and 3 doses are required for those starting HPV vaccination at 15 years or older (see Human Papillomavirus, p 440). If possible, making appointments for subsequent doses of HPV vaccine can enhance series completion. Providers can choose to begin HPV vaccine series as early as 9 years of age if they deem this the optimal age to attain acceptance and completion prior to the risk of acquisition of HPV. When HPV vaccine is begun at 9 or 10 years, other adolescent vaccines (eg, MenACWY and Tdap) still are recommended to be initiated at 11 to 12 years. A MenACWY booster dose is recommended at 16 years of age. Serogroup B meningococcal vaccine (MenB) is not a routine recommendation for adolescents in the absence of an outbreak or an underlying high-risk condition (eg, complement deficiency or asplenia) (see Meningococcal Infections, p 519).

---

[1] **www.cdc.gov/phlp/publications/topic/vaccinationlaws.html**

[2] American Academy of Pediatrics, Committee on Practice and Ambulatory Medicine and Bright Futures Periodicity Schedule Workgroup. 20120 recommendations for preventive pediatric health care. *Pediatrics.* 2020;145(3):e20200013

VACCINATION OF COLLEGE-AGED PEOPLE

A history should be obtained from all late adolescents to assess missing vaccines and risk factors that would require consideration for administration of additional vaccines, such as hepatitis A vaccine (HepA), MenB, *Haemophilus influenzae* type b vaccine (Hib), 13-valent pneumococcal conjugate vaccine (PCV13), and 23-valent pneumococcal polysaccharide vaccine (PPSV23). Specific indications for each of these vaccines are provided in the respective disease-specific chapters in Section 3.

Residential schools, colleges, and universities should establish a system to ensure that all students are protected against vaccine-preventable diseases and also to be able to identify unimmunized or underimmunized students in the event of an outbreak. Because outbreaks of vaccine-preventable diseases, including measles, mumps, and meningococcal disease, have occurred at colleges and universities, the American College Health Association encourages a comprehensive institutional prematricula-tion immunization policy consistent with recommendations from the CDC Advisory Committee on Immunization Practices (**www.acha.org/ACHA/Resources/ Topics/Vaccine.aspx**). Many colleges and universities are mandated by state law to require vaccination for specific vaccine, either for all matriculating students or only those living in campus housing. Information regarding state laws requiring prematricu-lation immunization is available (**www.immunize.org/laws**).

The suspected occurrence of illness attributable to a vaccine-preventable disease in a school or college should be reported promptly to local health officials for aid in man-agement, for assessment of public health implications, and to comply with state law (see Appendix III, p 1033).

Immunization in Health Care Personnel

People whose occupations place them in contact with patients with contagious diseases are at increased risk of contracting vaccine-preventable diseases and, if infected, trans-mitting them to their coworkers and patients. For the purposes of this section, health care personnel (HCP) are defined as those who have face-to-face contact with patients, or anyone who works in a building where patient care is delivered or is employed or contracted by a health care facility (eg, laboratory personnel). The definition of HCP includes trainees and volunteers. All HCP should protect themselves and susceptible patients by receiving appropriate immunizations. Physicians, health care facilities, and schools for health care professionals should play an active role in promoting policies to maximize immunization of HCP. Vaccine-preventable diseases of special concern to people involved in the health care of children are as follows (see the disease-specific chapters in Section 3 for further recommendations).

- **Pertussis.** Pertussis outbreaks involving adults occur in the community and the workplace. HCP frequently are exposed to *Bordetella pertussis*, have substantial risk of illness, and can be sources for spread of infection to patients, colleagues, families, and the community. HCP of all ages who work in hospitals or ambulatory-care set-tings should receive a dose of tetanus toxoid, reduced diphtheria toxoid, and acellu-lar pertussis vaccine (Tdap) as soon as is feasible if they previously have not received Tdap. Hospitals and ambulatory-care facilities should provide Tdap for HCP using approaches that maximize immunization rates.

Either Td or Tdap can be used regardless of prior receipt of Tdap for the routine decennial tetanus-diphtheria booster and for wound prophylaxis when indicated. In addition, if there is an increased risk of pertusssis in a health care setting, as evidenced by documented or suspected health care-associated transmission of pertussis, revaccination of HCP with Tdap vaccine may be considered. (**www.cdc.gov/vaccines/vpd/pertussis/tdap-revac-hcp.html**). In these cases, it is important to consider that vaccinating HCP with Tdap is not a substitute for infection prevention and control measures, including postexposure antimicrobial prophylaxis, and therefore, revaccinated HCP still should receive postexposure antimicrobial prophylaxis when applicable. If implemented, HCP who work with infants or pregnant women should be prioritized for revaccination.

- **Hepatitis B.** Hepatitis B vaccine (HepB) is recommended for all HCP whose work- and training-related activities involve reasonably anticipated risk of exposure to blood or other infectious body fluids. The Occupational Safety and Health Administration (OSHA) of the US Department of Labor issued a regulation requiring employers of personnel at risk of occupational exposure to hepatitis B to offer HepB immunization to personnel at the employer's expense. The employer shall ensure that employees who decline to accept HepB immunization offered by the employer sign a declination statement. To determine the need for revaccination and to guide postexposure prophylaxis, postvaccination serologic testing should be performed for all recently vaccinated HCP at risk of occupational percutaneous or mucosal exposure to blood or body fluids. Postvaccination serologic testing is performed 1 to 2 months after administration of the last dose of the vaccine series using a method that allows detection of the protective concentration of hepatitis B surface antibody (anti-HBs [$\geq$10 mIU/mL]). People determined to have anti-HBs concentrations of $\geq$10 mIU/mL, at any time after receipt of the primary vaccine series, are considered immune and the result should be documented. Future testing is not required.

  Although vaccine-induced anti-HBs wanes over time, protection persists for immunocompetent vaccine responders (eg, those with anti-HBs $\geq$10 mIU/mL at their postvaccination serologic testing). Therefore, testing HCP for anti-HBs years after vaccination (eg, when HepB vaccination was received as part of routine infant immunization) might not distinguish vaccine responders from nonresponders. Preexposure assessment of anti-HBs results at the time of hiring or matriculation, followed by one or more additional doses of HepB vaccine when needed helps to ensure that remotely vaccinated HCP will be protected. HCP who lack documentation of prior immunity to hepatitis B and who have anti-HBs <10 mIU/mL should be reimmunized with a single dose of vaccine and retested for anti-HBs within 1 to 2 months after that dose. HCP whose anti-HBs remains <10 mIU/mL should receive additional doses to complete the second vaccine series. For the 3-dose vaccine series using Engerix-B or Recombivax HB, this would require 2 additional doses of vaccine, and for the 2-dose series using Heplisav-B, this would require 1 additional dose. For very recently vaccinated HCP with anti-HBs <10 mIU/mL, in whom the low antibody concentration is more likely to reflect a failure to respond rather than waning antibody concentration, it may be more practical to revaccinate with an entire second series (3 doses of Engerix-B or Recombivax HB; 2 doses of Heplisav-B) followed by anti-HBs testing 1 to 2 months after the last dose. Heplisav-B may be used for revaccination following an initial HepB vaccine series that consisted of doses from a different manufacturer. [1,2]

People who do not respond to the second series and remain hepatitis B surface antigen (HBsAg) negative should be considered susceptible to hepatitis B virus infection and will need to receive Hepatitis B Immune Globulin (HBIG) prophylaxis after any known or probable exposure to blood or body fluids infected with hepatitis B virus.

- **Influenza.** Because HCP can transmit influenza to patients and because health care-associated outbreaks of influenza do occur, annual influenza immunization should be considered a patient safety responsibility and a requirement for employment in a health care facility unless an individual has a recognized medical contraindication to immunization.[3] HCP should be educated about the benefits of influenza immunization and the potential health consequences of influenza illness for themselves and their patients. Influenza vaccine should be offered at no cost, and efforts should be made to ensure that vaccine is readily available to HCP on all shifts, such as through use of mobile immunization carts. A signed declination form should be obtained from personnel who decline for reasons other than medical contraindications in any facility that does not have a formal mandatory vaccine policy. Mandatory education about the benefits of vaccination should be required for all people who decline influenza immunization. Any approved influenza vaccine product is appropriate if otherwise indicated with the exception of live attenuated vaccine, which should not be used for personnel who will have close contact with patients with altered immunocompetence who are in a protected environment; HCP receiving LAIV should avoid close contact with these immunocompromised people for 7 days following vaccination.

- **Measles.** Because measles in HCP has contributed to spread of this disease during outbreaks, evidence of immunity to measles should be required for HCP. Evidence of immunity is established by laboratory confirmation of infection, laboratory evidence of immunity (positive serologic test result for measles antibody), or documented receipt of 2 appropriately spaced doses of live virus-containing measles vaccine, the first of which was administered on or after the first birthday. People born before 1957 generally are considered immune to measles. However, because measles cases have occurred in HCP in this age group, health care facilities should consider offering 2 doses of measles-containing vaccine to HCP who lack proof of immunity to measles. In communities with documented measles outbreaks, 2 doses of MMR vaccine are recommended for unvaccinated HCP born before 1957 unless evidence of serologic immunity is demonstrated.

---

[1]Schillie S, Vellozzi C, Reingold A, et al. Prevention of hepatitis B virus infection in the United States: recommendations of the Advisory Committee on Immunization Practices. *MMWR Recomm Rep.* 2018;67(RR-1):1–31

[2]Schillie S, Harris A, Link-Gelles R, et al. Recommendations of the Advisory Committee on Immunization Practices for Use of a Hepatitis B Vaccine with a Novel Adjuvant. *MMWR Morb Mortal Wkly Rep.* 2018;67(15):455-458

[3]American Academy of Pediatrics, Committee on Infectious Diseases. Policy statement: Influenza immunization for all health care personnel: keep it mandatory. *Pediatrics.* 2015;136(4):809-818

- **Mumps.** Transmission of mumps in health care facilities can be disruptive and costly. All people who work in health care facilities should be immune to mumps. Evidence of immunity is established by laboratory confirmation of infection, laboratory evidence of immunity (positive serologic test result for mumps antibody), documented receipt of 2 appropriately spaced doses of live virus-containing mumps vaccine, the first of which was administered on or after the first birthday, or birth before 1957. During an outbreak, a second dose of MMR vaccine should be offered to HCP born during or after 1957 who have only received 1 dose of MMR vaccine. HCP born before 1957 without a history of MMR immunization should obtain a mumps antibody titer to document their immune status and, if negative, should receive 2 appropriately spaced doses of MMR vaccine.
- **Rubella.** Transmission of rubella from HCP to pregnant women has been reported. Although the disease is mild in adults, the risk to a fetus necessitates documentation of rubella immunity in HCP of both genders. People should be considered immune on the basis of a positive serologic test result for rubella antibody or documented proof of 1 dose of rubella-containing vaccine. A history of rubella disease is unreliable and should not be used in determining immune status. All susceptible HCP who may be exposed to patients with rubella or who take care of pregnant women, as well as people who work in educational institutions or provide child care, should be immunized with 1 dose of MMR to prevent infection for themselves and to prevent transmission of rubella to pregnant patients.
- **Varicella.** Evidence of varicella immunity is recommended for all HCP. Evidence of immunity to varicella in HCP includes any of the following: (1) documentation of 2 doses of varicella vaccine at least 28 days apart, the first of which was administered on or after the first birthday; (2) history of varicella diagnosed or verified by a physician (for a patient reporting a history of or presenting with an atypical case, a mild case, or both, the physician should seek either an epidemiologic link with a typical varicella case or evidence of laboratory confirmation, if it was performed at the time of acute disease); (3) history of herpes zoster diagnosed by a physician; or (4) laboratory evidence of immunity or laboratory confirmation of disease. Birth in the United States before 1980 should not be considered as evidence of immunity for HCP, pregnant women, or immunocompromised people (**www.cdc.gov/chickenpox/hcp/immunity.html**). The Centers for Disease Control and Prevention's Advisory Committee on Immunization Practices (ACIP) and Health Infection Control Practices Advisory Committee (HICPAC) do not recommend serologic testing of HCP for immunity to varicella after receiving varicella-zoster virus vaccine. Commercially available serologic assays may not be sufficiently sensitive to detect immunization-induced antibody.
- **Meningococcus.** Meningococcal vaccination is not recommended for HCP performing direct patient care. However, clinical microbiologists routinely exposed to isolates of *Neisseria meningitidis* are at increased risk of severe meningococcal disease if exposed to a clinical isolate and should be vaccinated with serogroup A, C, W, and Y meningococcal vaccine (MenACWY) and serogroup B meningococcal vaccine (MenB).

Children Who Received Immunizations Outside the United States or Whose Immunization Status is Unknown or Uncertain

IMMUNIZATIONS RECEIVED OUTSIDE THE UNITED STATES

People immunized in other countries, including international students, internationally adopted children, refugees, and other immigrants, should be immunized according to recommended schedules (including minimal ages and intervals) in the United States (**www.cdc.gov/vaccines/schedules/index.html**). The Immigration and Nationality Act (INA) of 1996 requires all people immigrating to the United States as legal permanent residents (ie, green card holders) to provide "proof of vaccination" with vaccines recommended by the Centers for Disease Control and Prevention (CDC) Advisory Committee on Immunization Practices (ACIP) before entry into the United States. Vaccines required for immigration must fulfill the following criteria: (1) must be an age-appropriate vaccine as recommended by the ACIP for the general US population; and (2) either must protect against a disease that has the potential to cause an outbreak or protect against a disease that has been eliminated or is in the process of being eliminated in the United States. For example, human papillomavirus (HPV) vaccine is not required. For vaccination instructions including the list of required vaccines, see the website: **www.cdc.gov/immigrantrefugeehealth/exams/ti/panel/vaccination-panel-technical-instructions.html.**

Internationally adopted children who are 10 years and younger may obtain a waiver of exemption from the INA regulations pertaining to immunization of immigrants before arrival in the United States (**www.cdc.gov/immigrantrefugeehealth/adoption/overseas-exam.html**). Children adopted from countries that are not part of the Hague Convention can receive waivers to have their immunizations delayed until arrival in the United States (**https://travel.state.gov/content/travel/en/Intercountry-Adoption/Adoption-Process/understanding-the-hague-convention.html**). When an exemption is granted, adoptive parents are required to sign a waiver indicating their intention to comply with ACIP-recommended immunizations within 30 days after the child arrives in the United States.

Refugees are not required to meet immunization requirements of the INA at the time of initial entry into the United States but must show proof of immunization when they apply for permanent residency, typically 1 year after arrival. Selected refugees bound for the United States are immunized in their country of departure before arrival in the United States. Clinicians may review the CDC Refugee Health Guidelines for the current overseas immunization schedule for US-bound refugees at **www.cdc.gov/immigrantrefugeehealth/guidelines/overseas/interventions/immunizations-schedules.html.** Guidance on evaluating and updating immunizations during the domestic medical examination for refugees after arrival in the United States is available at **www.cdc.gov/immigrantrefugeehealth/guidelines/domestic/immunizations-guidelines.html.**

An increasing number of vaccines are being incorporated into routine immunization schedules in countries outside the United States. In general, written documentation of immunizations can be accepted as evidence of previous immunization if the vaccines, dates of administration, number of doses, intervals between doses, and age of the child at the time of immunization are consistent internally and are comparable to current US or World Health Organization schedules (**www.who.int/immuniza-tion/policy/immunization_tables/en/**). Any vaccination documented on the official Department of State health immigration form (DS-3025) should be accepted. Inaccuracies, inconsistencies, and fraudulent data should be considered during review of records.

Record review also should include consideration of ACIP recommendations for poliovirus vaccination, which require protection against all 3 poliovirus types by age-appropriate vaccination with inactivated poliovirus (IPV) or trivalent oral poliovirus (tOPV) vaccines. Some countries may have provided monovalent or bivalent oral poliovirus (OPV) vaccine during polio vaccination campaigns after April 1, 2016. If OPV was administered before April 1, 2016, OPV can be counted as tOPV. If OPV was administered after April 1, 2016, it may not be counted as tOPV; in the absence of adequate written vaccination records documenting the doses as tOPV, vaccination or revaccination in accordance with the age-appropriate US IPV schedule is recommended (see Poliovirus Infections, p 601, for further recommendations).

Studies performed in internationally adopted children have demonstrated that the majority of children with documentation of immunizations have antibodies consistent with those immunizations. Limited country-specific data are available regarding serologic verification of immunization records for other categories of immigrant children. Evaluation of concentrations of antibody to vaccine-preventable diseases can be useful in some circumstances to ensure that vaccines were administered and were immunogenic, and to document immunity from past infection (see Serologic Testing to Document Immunization Status).

UNKNOWN OR UNCERTAIN IMMUNIZATION STATUS IN US CHILDREN

There are circumstances in which the immunization status for a child born in the United States is uncertain or unknown because of lack of documentation, an incomplete or inaccurate record, or a recording inconsistent with a recommended product or schedule. Serologic testing can be performed to determine whether antibody concentrations are present for some of the vaccine-preventable diseases (see Serologic Testing to Document Immunization Status). A combined strategy of serologic testing for antibodies to some vaccine antigens and immunization for others may be used.

SEROLOGIC TESTING TO DOCUMENT IMMUNIZATION STATUS

Usefulness, validity, and interpretation of serologic testing to guide management of vaccinations can be complex and varies by age. Cost of testing versus cost of administering a given immunization, as well as likelihood of adherence for completing the immunization series, also should be considered in these decisions.

When validity of immunization records is in doubt, or when documentation of response to vaccine is desired for other reasons in children 6 months or older, serologic testing to document antibodies to diphtheria and tetanus toxoids (ie, ≥ 0.1 IU/mL) or *Haemophilus influenzae* type b for a child younger than 60 months (ie, ≥ 1.0 µg/mL) may be considered to determine whether the child likely has received and responded to dose(s) of the vaccine in question. Even if the child has a "protective" level of antibodies, the immunization series should be completed as appropriate for that child's age. If a child does not have a protective level of antibodies, the series should be restarted, with the understanding that for some vaccine-preventable diseases, fewer doses of vaccine are needed to complete the series as a child ages. The immunization record, plus presence of antibody to diphtheria and tetanus toxoids, can be used as proxy for receipt of pertussis-containing vaccine dose(s).

Hepatitis A, measles, mumps, rubella, and varicella antibody concentrations could be measured in children 12 months or older to determine whether the child is immune; these antibody tests should not be performed in children younger than 12 months because of the potential presence of maternal antibody. Usefulness of measuring measles antibody alone is limited, because many foreign-born children will need mumps and rubella vaccines as these vaccines are administered less frequently in resource-limited countries and they are available in the Unites States only as MMR vaccine. Two doses of MMR vaccine should be administered for mumps coverage, even if measles antibodies are present. Rubella coverage is achieved following 1 dose of a rubella-containing vaccine. Documented receipt of 2 doses of varicella vaccine or positive varicella antibody is the best indication of immunity to varicella. *H influenzae* type b vaccine (Hib) is not indicated for immunocompetent children 5 years or older, even if none was administered previously; serologic testing should not be performed, because children in this age group frequently have antibody concentrations <1.0 µg/ mL yet are not susceptible to *H influenzae* type b infection. Age-appropriate pneumococcal vaccine dose(s) should be administered if a completed series is not documented; serologic testing should not be performed for validation or evidence of immunity. Serologic tests to assess immunity to poliovirus and rotavirus are not available.

Serologic testing for hepatitis B surface antigen (HBsAg) should be performed for all immigrant, refugee, and internationally adopted children to identify chronic hepatitis B virus infection (**www.cdc.gov/immigrantrefugeehealth/guidelines/ domestic/hepatitis-screening-guidelines.html**). When the HBsAg test result is negative, the result of the antibody to HBsAg (anti-HBs) test will determine whether the child is immune. Children who have documentation of an incomplete hepatitis B immunization series should complete the series even if the result of testing for anti-HBs is positive. Refugee children who are receiving vaccinations overseas as part of the Refugee Vaccination Program are tested for HBsAg before vaccination. The result of this test is documented on the Department of State official health immigration forms. Transient presence of HBsAg can occur following receipt of HepB vaccine, with HBsAg being detected as early as 24 hours after and up to 3 weeks following administration of the vaccine, so prevaccination assessment is important. Some immigrant or refugee children may have had previous hepatitis A infection, and the presence of immunoglobulin (Ig) G-specific antibody to hepatitis A virus would preclude need for hepatitis A vaccine.

If serologic testing is not available or is too costly or if a positive result would not mitigate need for further immunization, the prudent course is to repeat or administer the immunizations in question. Some state laws stipulate that only certain serologic tests are accepted for school attendance; testing may not be worthwhile in this circumstance as vaccine will still need to be administered.

International Travel

Children are at risk for illness when traveling internationally, and some may require medical care or hospitalization. US-born children of immigrants are especially likely to travel at young ages to visit relatives. Consultation with a health care provider who is knowledgeable or specializes in travel medicine can mitigate this risk but requires advance planning to allow time to complete necessary pretravel vaccinations and obtain necessary medications. Parents should be made aware that there is increased risk of exposure to vaccine-preventable diseases when traveling outside the United States, even in countries perceived to be without substantial risk of infectious diseases. Routine immunizations should be up-to-date before international travel, and some may be administered early or on an accelerated schedule to optimize protection. Vaccines to prevent influenza, typhoid fever, yellow fever, meningococcal disease, rabies, Japanese encephalitis, and cholera may be indicated depending on the age of the child, destination, season of travel, duration of the trip, and activities during travel (see disease-specific chapters in Section 3). Families should arrange travel consultation about 4 to 6 weeks before planned departure, because travel vaccines may not be available at all sites and some vaccines, such as Japanese encephalitis and rabies vaccine, require multiple doses before departure.

Travelers also may be at risk for exposure to malaria, dengue, chikungunya, Zika, diarrheal and respiratory illnesses, tickborne infections, and skin diseases for which vaccines are not available. A dengue vaccine was licensed in 2019 by the Food and Drug Administration (FDA) for use in individuals 9 through 16 years of age who reside in areas with endemic dengue and who have laboratory confirmation of a previous dengue infection, which does not include travelers. Antimalarial chemoprophylaxis is recommended for travelers to areas with endemic malaria, and insect bite prevention should be addressed for all travelers at risk of vector-borne diseases. Attending to hand hygiene, choosing safer foods, and limiting exposure to contaminated sand, soil, and water may reduce travelers' risk of acquiring other communicable diseases.

Up-to-date information, including alerts about current disease outbreaks that may affect international travelers, is available on the CDC Travelers' Health website (**wwwnc.cdc.gov/travel/**) or the WHO website (**www.who.int/health-topics/travel-and-health#tab=tab_1**). *Health Information for International Travel* (the "Yellow Book," **wwwnc.cdc.gov/travel/page/yellowbook-home**) is revised every 2 years by the CDC and is available to travelers and health professionals. Local and state health departments and travel clinics[1] also can provide updated information. Many colleges have clinics where pretravel counseling and immunizations can be obtained. Information about cruise ship sanitation inspection scores and reports can be found on the CDC website (**www.cdc.gov/nceh/vsp/default.htm**).

RECOMMENDED IMMUNIZATIONS

Infants and children traveling internationally should be up-to-date with immunizations recommended for their age. Some vaccines may be administered before the age of routine immunization (hepatitis A vaccine [HepA]; meningococcal conjugate vaccine;

---

[1]Sources for travel clinics: Center for Disease Control and Prevention (**wwwnc.cdc.gov/travel/page/find-clinic**), American Society of Tropical Medicine and Hygiene (**www.astmh.org/for-astmh-members/clinical-consultants-directory**), and International Society for Travel Medicine (**www.istm.org/AF_CstmClinicDirectory.asp**).

measles, mumps, and rubella vaccine [MMR]) or be administered on an accelerated schedule (MMR) to optimize immunity before departure.

HEPATITIS A. HepA is recommended routinely in a 2-dose series ≥6 months apart for all children at 12 through 23 months of age in the United States, with catch-up vaccination recommended through 18 years of age. HepA is recommended for all people >6 months of age who are unimmunized and traveling to areas with intermediate or high rates of hepatitis A infection (see Table 3.18, p 379). These include all areas of the world except Australia, Canada, Japan, New Zealand, and most of Western Europe. For children 6 through 11 months of age, this dose of HepA does not count toward the routine 2-dose series, which should be started at age 12 months. Immune Globulin Intramuscular (IGIM) is recommended for HepA preexposure prophylaxis prior to travel for infants <6 months of age. People with chronic liver disease as well as adults aged >40 years, immunocompromised people, and people with other chronic medical conditions planning to depart to an area with high or intermediate hepatitis A endemicity in <2 weeks should receive the initial dose of HepA vaccine and also simultaneously may receive IGIM at a separate anatomic injection site (**www.cdc.gov/ mmwr/volumes/67/wr/mm6743a5.htm**). The dose of IGIM administered for hepatitis A prevention may interfere with the immune response to varicella and MMR vaccines for several months (see Table 1.11, p 40, for details). A combination HepA-HepB (hepatitis B) vaccine (Twinrix) is available for people 18 years and older.

HEPATITIS B. HepB is recommended for all children in the United States and for people traveling to areas where the prevalence of chronic hepatitis B virus infection is 2% or greater (see Hepatitis B, p 381). Ideally, HepB vaccination should be administered ≥6 months before travel so that a 3-dose regimen can be completed. If fewer than 4 months are available before departure, the alternative 4-dose schedule of 0, 1, 2, and 12 months, licensed for the Engerix-B vaccine (see Table 3.20, p 388), might provide opportunity for more rapid development of protection. Individual health care providers may choose to use an accelerated schedule (eg, doses at days 0, 7, and 21–30, with a booster at 12 months) for travelers who will depart before an approved immunization schedule can be completed. People who receive immunization on an accelerated schedule that is not licensed by the FDA also should receive a dose at 12 months after initiation of the series to promote long-term immunity. For adults, the 2-dose regimen of Heplisav-B can be completed in one month and offers greater flexibility before travel.

MEASLES. Importation of measles remains an important source for measles cases in the United States. People traveling anywhere outside the United States should be immune to measles to provide personal protection and minimize importation. Immunity to measles is defined by laboratory confirmation of prior infection; laboratory evidence of immunity (positive serologic test result for measles antibody); documented receipt of 2 appropriately spaced doses of live virus-containing measles vaccine, the first of which was administered on or after the first birthday; or birth in the United States before 1957 (see Measles, p 503). Children who travel or live abroad should be vaccinated beginning at 6 months of age. Children 6 through 11 months of age should receive 1 dose of MMR vaccine at least 2 weeks before departure if possible, and then should receive a second dose of measles-containing vaccine at 12 through 15 months of age (at least 28 days after the initial measles immunization) and a third dose at 4 through 6 years of age. Children 12 months or older as well as adults who have received 1 dose and are traveling to areas where measles is endemic or epidemic should receive their second dose before departure, provided the interval between doses is 28 days or more. MMR should not be administered to pregnant women. Live-virus vaccines (MMR, varicella, yellow fever) generally should be administered either on the same day or separated by at least 4 weeks, and attention should be paid to the timing of immune globulin products administration if these are indicated (see Simultaneous Administration of Multiple Vaccines, p 36, and Table 1.11, p 40).

POLIOVIRUS. Significant efforts have been made to achieve global eradication of polio, but spread of disease continues in some areas. Travelers should be up to date with poliovirus immunization for age before travel. Travelers to countries with wild-type or vaccine-derived polio circulation (**http://polioeradication.org/polio-today/polio-now/public-health-emergency-status/**) within the past 12 months may require additional doses of vaccine according to current CDC guidance. Travelers 18 years or older visiting regions identified on the CDC Travelers' Health website (**wwwnc.cdc.gov/travel**) as being at risk for circulation of poliovirus should receive a booster dose of inactivated poliovirus vaccine (IPV). Current recommendations should be verified before departure (**wwwnc.cdc.gov/travel/yellowbook/2020/travel-related-infectious-diseases/poliomyelitis**).

TRAVEL-RELATED IMMUNIZATIONS

Other immunizations may be required or recommended for international travelers depending on factors such as destination, planned activities, and length of stay (see **wwwnc.cdc.gov/travel/** and disease-specific chapters in Section 3).

CHOLERA. An oral cholera vaccine (Vaxchora [CVD 103-HgR, PaxVax Bermuda Ltd, Redwood City, CA]) is approved in the United States for use in people 2 through 64 years of age. Vaccine is not recommended routinely for most travelers. Immunization would be most appropriate for those traveling to areas with active cholera transmission (**wwwnc.cdc.gov/travel/news-announcements/cholera-vaccine-for-travelers**). A pediatric study of this vaccine in children and adolescents 2 through 17 years of age is evaluating safety and immunogenicity in this age group.

JAPANESE ENCEPHALITIS.[1] Japanese encephalitis (JE) virus, a mosquitoborne Flavivirus, is the most common vaccine-preventable cause of encephalitis in Asia. Risk of JE is low for most travelers to Asia but varies on the basis of destination, duration, season, accommodations, and activities (**wwwnc.cdc.gov/travel/page/yellowbook-home**). Travelers to countries with endemic JE should be informed about the disease and should use personal protective measures to reduce the risk of mosquito bites during the night. JE vaccine can reduce the risk for infection further. JE vaccine is recommended for those taking up residence in a JE endemic country, longer-term travelers (eg, a month or longer), and frequent travelers to areas with endemic JE. JE vaccine also should be considered for shorter-term travelers if they plan to travel outside of an urban area and have an itinerary or activities that will increase their risk of mosquito exposure in an area with endemic infection. Information on the location of JE

---

[1] Hills SL, Walter EB, Atmar RL, Fischer M. Japanese encephalitis vaccine: recommendations of the Advisory Committee on Immunization Practices. *MMWR Recomm Rep.* 2019;68(RR-2):1–33

virus transmission and detailed information on vaccine recommendations and adverse events can be obtained from the CDC (**www.cdc.gov/vaccines/hcp/acip-recs/ vacc-specific/je.html**).

An inactivated Vero cell culture-derived JE virus vaccine (Ixiaro) is approved and available in the United States for use in adults and children 2 months and older. The primary vaccination series for children and adolescents aged <18 years is 2 doses administered 28 days apart. An interval of as short as 7 days may be used for travelers 18 to 65 years of age with imminent departures. A booster dose should be administered at 1 year or longer after the primary series if ongoing exposure or reexposure is expected.

INFLUENZA. Influenza immunization is recommended for travelers and may be needed outside the times when annual influenza immunization is recommended in the United States. Influenza season is different in the northern and southern hemispheres and epidemic strains may differ. Antigenic composition of influenza vaccines used in Northern and Southern hemispheres may be different, and timing of administration may vary (see Influenza, p 447).

MENINGOCOCCUS. Meningococcal conjugate vaccines against serogroups A, C, W, and Y (MenACWY) are recommended for use in people age ≥2 months traveling to areas where there is a high burden of meningococcal disease, such as sub-Saharan Africa or other areas with ongoing meningococcal outbreaks. Meningococcal conjugate vaccines vary in conjugating protein, ages of approved use, and dosing schedules. The following MenACWY vaccines are available for travelers: MenACWY-CRM · (Menveo; ages 2 months to 55 years of age), MenACWY-D (Menactra; ages 9 months to 55 years of age), and MenACWY-TT (MenQuadfi; ages 2 years and older). MenACWY-D (Menactra) should not be administered concomitantly OR within 4 weeks of administration of PCV13 immunization, to avoid potential interference with the immune response to PCV13. Completion of the entire series is preferred prior to travel. Booster doses are recommended for people who are at continuous or repeated increased risk of meningococcal infection, after 3 years for those who received their last dose at <7 years of age and after 5 years for those who received their last dose at ≥7 years of age, and every 5 years thereafter for people at continued risk. Immunization against serogroup B meningococcal disease is not recommended routinely for travel unless there are other indications to provide this vaccine or there is an outbreak at the travel destination. The Kingdom of Saudi Arabia requires an International Certificate of Vaccination or Prophylaxis (ICVP) documenting immunization against meningococcal serogroups A, C, W, and Y for pilgrims attending the Hajj or Umrah pilgrimages.

RABIES. The mainstay of prevention of rabies is education of families about avoidance of animals and the need for immediate medical care if a bite or other exposure occurs. Rabies preexposure prophylaxis should be considered for children who will be traveling to areas with endemic rabies where they may encounter wild or domestic animals (particularly dogs). Preexposure prophylaxis consists of a 3-dose series of rabies vaccine administered on days 0, 7, and 21 or 28 by intramuscular injection (see Rabies, p 619). Postexposure prophylaxis includes cleaning wounds thoroughly with soap and water and then receiving postexposure prophylaxis promptly (PEP; see Rabies, p 619). For individuals who have not received the 3 doses of vaccine for preexposure prophylaxis, PEP consists of Rabies Immune Globulin (RIG), 20 IU/kg infiltrated into the wound, plus 4 doses of rabies vaccine (days 0, 3, 7, and 14). For those who have received preexposure prophylaxis, 2 doses of rabies vaccine (days 0 and 3) constitute PEP. Travelers who have completed a 3-dose preexposure series or have received the full PEP series do not require routine boosters, except after a presumed rabies exposure. Testing for rabies virus-neutralizing antibody is not necessary for routine international travelers. The World Health Organization recently recommended use of intradermal rabies immunization as an alternative to intramuscular administration to reduce costs, but the FDA and the Centers for Disease Control and Prevention's (CDC's) Advisory Committee on Immunization Practices (ACIP) have not endorsed this recommendation. Travelers can be informed that the treatment they may be offered for an exposure outside the United States may differ from what they would receive in the United States.

TUBERCULOSIS. Risk of being infected with *Mycobacterium tuberculosis* during international travel depends on the activities of the traveler, duration of travel, and the epidemiology of tuberculosis at the destination. Risk of acquiring infection during usual tourist activities appears to be low, and pre- or post-travel testing is not recommended routinely. Risk may be higher for travelers living or working among the general population of a country with a high prevalence of tuberculosis. Children with a history of significant travel to countries with endemic tuberculosis infection who have substantial contact with the resident population should be tested with a tuberculin skin test (TST) or interferon-gamma release assay (IGRA). Some experts define significant travel as birth, travel, or residence in a country with an elevated tuberculosis rate for at least 1 month. If the child is well and has no history of exposure, the TST or IGRA should be delayed for 10 weeks after return. Pretravel administration of bacille Calmette-Guérin vaccine generally is not recommended.

TYPHOID. Typhoid vaccine is recommended for travelers who may be exposed to contaminated food or water. Two typhoid vaccines are available in the United States: an oral vaccine containing live attenuated *Salmonella enterica* serovar Typhi (Ty21a strain), approved for people 6 years and older (the capsules must be swallowed whole), and a parenteral Vi capsular polysaccharide (ViCPS) vaccine, approved for people 2 years and older. The Ty21a vaccine series consists of 1 enteric-coated capsule every other day for a total of 4 capsules and should be completed at least 1 week before anticipated exposure, whereas the ViCPS vaccine is administered as a single intramuscular injection that should be given at least 2 weeks before anticipated exposure. Typhoid immunization is not 100% effective; both vaccines protect 50% to 80% of recipients and do not provide adequate protection against paratyphoid fever. Revaccination is recommended 5 years after oral live-attenuated and 2 years after inactivated vaccine if continued or subsequent exposure to *Salmonella enterica* serovar Typhi is expected. Reimmunization includes completing the entire 4-dose series again for the Ty21a oral vaccine and receiving 1 intramuscular dose for the ViCPS parenteral vaccine. For specific recommendations, see *Salmonella* Infections (p 655). The oral live-attenuated vaccine capsules should be refrigerated and should not be administered during use of any antimicrobial agent other than the antimalarial agents mefloquine and chloroquine when used in prophylactic doses (**www.cdc.gov/mmwr/preview/mmwrhtml/mm6411a4.htm**). Typhoid immunization is not a substitute for careful selection of food and beverages.

YELLOW FEVER. Yellow fever (YF) occurs in parts of sub-Saharan Africa and tropical South America. YF continues to be reported rarely among unimmunized travelers but may be fatal. Prevention measures against YF should include protection against mosquito bites (see Prevention of Mosquitoborne and Tickborne Infections, p 175) and immunization. Current country requirements and recommendations for YF immunization change frequently and can be obtained from the CDC Travelers' Health website (**wwwnc.cdc.gov/travel/**). Travelers should verify entry requirements for their destination. YF vaccine should be administered at least 10 days before travel.

YF vaccine is recommended for people 9 months and older who are traveling to or living in areas of South America and Africa in which risk exists for YF virus transmission. Booster doses of yellow fever vaccine are no longer recommended for most travelers, because a single dose of YF vaccine provides long-lasting protection.[1] Additional doses of YF vaccine are recommended for women who were pregnant when they received their initial dose of vaccine, people who received a hematopoietic stem cell transplant after receiving a dose of YF vaccine, and people infected with HIV when they received their last dose of YF vaccine (**wwwnc.cdc.gov/travel/ yellowbook/2020/travel-related-infectious-diseases/yellow-fever**).

YF immunization should be limited to people at risk of exposure to YF or who require proof of vaccination for country entry, because of risk of rare but serious adverse events including vaccine-associated neurologic and viscerotropic (multiple-organ system failure) disease. As of 2020, the only yellow fever vaccine licensed in the United States (YF-VAX) is not available because of manufacturing issues. In the interim, the manufacturer of YF-VAX (Sanofi Pasteur) has worked with the FDA to import its yellow fever vaccine Stamaril under an investigational new drug (IND) application and distribute it in the United States in an Expanded Access Program. Stamaril is manufactured by Sanofi Pasteur in France and uses the 17D-204 strain of yellow fever virus, which is the same strain as in YF-VAX. More than 430 million doses have been distributed worldwide, and its safety and efficacy profile is comparable to YF-VAX vaccine. During this period of shortage of YF-VAX, health care providers of yellow fever vaccine can direct their patients to Stamaril vaccine sites (**wwwnc.cdc. gov/travel/page/search-for-stamaril-clinics**).

OTHER CONSIDERATIONS. Travelers outside the United States may be exposed to mosquitoborne diseases, such as malaria, which can be life threatening; dengue or chikungunya viruses; or Zika virus, which for pregnant women may pose risk of congenital transmission. Prevention strategies include mosquito-bite prevention (see Prevention of Mosquitoborne and Tickborne Infections, p 175) and, for malaria, use of antimalarial chemoprophylaxis. For recommendations on appropriate use of chemoprophylaxis, including recommendations for pregnant women, infants, and breastfeeding mothers see Malaria (p 493).

Travelers' diarrhea affects up to 60% of travelers but may be mitigated by attention to foods and beverages ingested (such as avoiding ice). Chemoprophylaxis generally is not recommended. Educating families about self-treatment, particularly oral

[1]Staples JE, Bocchini JA, Rubin L, Fischer M. Yellow fever vaccine booster doses: recommendations of the Advisory Committee on Immunization Practices, 2015. *MMWR Morb Mortal Wkly Rep.* 2015;64(23):647–650

rehydration, is critical. Packets of oral rehydration salts can be obtained before travel and are available in most pharmacies throughout the world, including in resource-limited countries, where diarrheal diseases are most common. During international travel, families may want to carry an antimicrobial agent (eg, azithromycin or a fluoro-quinolone, for up to 3 days). Taking antimicrobial agents increases risk of colonization with resistant bacteria, so treatment should be reserved for moderate to severe cases of travelers' diarrhea. Antimotility agents may be considered for older children and adolescents (see *Escherichia coli* Diarrhea, p 322) for mild to moderate diarrhea (and may be used along with an antimicrobial agent) but generally should be avoided in cases of bloody diarrhea or diarrhea associated with fever. Bismuth subsalicylate has been approved for treatment of diarrhea by the FDA for use in children ≥12 years of age and has been shown to reduce the severity of travelers' diarrhea (**wwwnc. cdc.gov/travel/page/travelers-diarrhea** and **wwwnc.cdc.gov/travel/ yellowbook/2020/preparing-international-travelers/travelers-diarrhea**).

Travelers should be aware of potential acquisition of respiratory tract viruses, including novel strains of coronavirus or influenza. They should be counseled on hand hygiene and avoidance of close contact with animals (dead or live). Swimming, water sports, and ecotourism involving exposure to fresh water carry risks of acquisition of infections from environmental contamination (notably schistosomiasis and leptospirosis from lakes, streams, or rivers). Pyogenic skin infections and cutaneous larva migrans may be acquired.

Recommendations for Care of Children in Special Circumstances

BREASTFEEDING AND HUMAN MILK

Breastfeeding provides numerous health benefits to infants, including protection against morbidity and mortality from infectious diseases of bacterial, viral, and parasitic origin. In addition to providing an optimal source of infant nutrition, human milk contains immune-modulating factors, including secretory antibodies, glycoconjugates, anti-inflammatory components, prebiotics, probiotics, and antimicrobial compounds such as lysozyme and lactoferrin, which contribute to the formation of a health-promoting microbiota and an optimally functioning immune system. Breastfed infants have high concentrations of protective bifidobacteria and lactobacilli in their gastro-intestinal tracts, which diminish the risk of colonization and infection with pathogenic organisms. Protection by human milk is established most clearly for pathogens causing gastrointestinal tract infection. In addition, human milk likely provides protection against otitis media and upper and lower respiratory tract infections. Breastfeeding decreases the severity of upper and lower respiratory tract respiratory infections, including bronchiolitis, resulting in more than a 70% reduction in hospitalizations. Evidence indicates that human milk may modulate the development of the immune system of infants. Maternal milk and pasteurized donor human milk are clearly superior to formula for preterm and very low birth weight infants, as they are associated with decreased rates of serious infections and necrotizing enterocolitis and better feeding tolerance, growth, and neurodevelopmental outcomes.[1-3]

AAP Recommendations on Breastfeeding

The American Academy of Pediatrics (AAP) recommends exclusive breastfeeding for the first 6 months of life, with introduction of complementary foods at about 6 months of age, while continuing breastfeeding up to 2 years of age.[2] The AAP publishes policy statements[2,3] and a manual on infant feeding[4] that provide additional information about the benefits of breastfeeding, recommended feeding practices, and potential

---

[1]World Health Organization. *Guidelines on Optimal Feeding of Low Birth-Weight Infants in Low- and Middle-Income Countries.* Geneva, Switzerland: World Health Organization; 2011. Available at: **www.who.int/ maternal_child_adolescent/documents/infant_feeding_low_bw/en/**

[2]American Academy of Pediatrics, Section on Breastfeeding. Breastfeeding and the use of human milk. *Pediatrics.* 2012;129(3):e827-e841

[3]American Academy of Pediatrics, Committee on Nutrition, Section on Breastfeeding, Committee on Fetus and Newborn. Donor human milk for the high-risk infant: preparation, safety, and usage options in the United States. *Pediatrics.* 2017;139(1):e20163440

[4]American Academy of Pediatrics. *Breastfeeding Handbook for Physicians.* 2nd ed. Schanler RJ, Krebs NF, Mass SB, eds. Elk Grove Village, IL: American Academy of Pediatrics; 2013

contaminants of human milk. In the *Pediatric Nutrition Handbook*[1] and in the AAP policy statements on human milk and pasteurized donor human milk, issues regarding immunization of lactating mothers and breastfeeding infants, transmission of infectious agents via human milk, and potential effects on breastfed infants of antimicrobial agents administered to lactating mothers are addressed.

Contraindications to Breastfeeding

Breastfeeding provides the most complete nutrition for infants, including preterm and ill newborn infants, and therefore, health care providers should carefully consider any decision not to start, to interrupt, or to stop breastfeeding. There are only a few instances when mothers should not breastfeed or feed expressed milk to their infants because of infectious diseases. These include: maternal infection with human immunodeficiency virus (HIV), human T-cell lymphotropic virus type I or type II, or Ebola virus. Temporary suspension of breastfeeding is suggested when mothers have active herpetic (herpes simplex virus) lesions on the breast (see p 111) or are infected with untreated brucellosis. Women with infections that require airborne precautions (tuberculosis, varicella, measles) should avoid contact with the infant, but the infant can be fed the mother's expressed milk.

Immunization of Mothers and Infants

EFFECT OF MATERNAL IMMUNIZATION

Women who have not received recommended immunizations before or during pregnancy may be immunized during the postpartum period, regardless of lactation status. With the exception of yellow fever vaccine,[2] no evidence exists to validate any clinical concern about the presence of other live vaccine viruses in maternal milk if the mother is immunized while lactating. Lactating women should be immunized as recommended for adults and adolescents (**www.cdc.gov/vaccines**). If previously unimmunized or if traveling to an area with endemic poliovirus circulation, a lactating mother may receive inactivated poliovirus vaccine (IPV). Mothers who are susceptible to any of the viruses contained in the measles, mumps, and rubella vaccine (MMR) should be immunized during the early postpartum period. In lactating women who receive live attenuated varicella vaccine, neither varicella DNA in human milk (by polymerase chain reaction assay) nor varicella antibody in the infant can be detected. If not administered during pregnancy, tetanus toxoid, reduced diphtheria toxoid, and acellular pertussis vaccine (Tdap) should be administered immediately postpartum. Nonimmunized breastfeeding women should receive influenza vaccine.[3,4] Inactivated

[1]American Academy of Pediatrics, Committee on Nutrition. *Pediatric Nutrition Handbook*. Kleinman RE, Greer FR, eds. 8th ed. Itasca, IL: American Academy of Pediatrics; 2019

[2]Centers for Disease Control and Prevention. Yellow fever vaccine: recommendations of the Advisory Committee on Immunization Practices (ACIP). *MMWR Recomm Rep*. 2010;59(RR-7):1-27

[3]Grohskopf LA, Alyanak E, Broder KR, Walter EB, Fry AM, Jernigan DB. Prevention and control of seasonal influenza with vaccines: recommendations of the Advisory Committee on Immunization Practices—United States, 2019–20 influenza season. *MMWR Recomm Rep*. 2019;68(RR-3):1–21. For annual updates, see **www.cdc.gov/vaccines**

[4]American Academy of Pediatrics, Committee on Infectious Diseases. Recommendations for prevention and control of influenza, 2019-2020. *Pediatrics*. 2019;144(4):e20192478. For updates, see **https://redbook. solutions.aap.org/ss/influenza-resources.aspx**

influenza vaccine (IIV) or live attenuated influenza vaccine (LAIV) may be administered during the postpartum period, if not otherwise contraindicated.

Breastfeeding is a precaution for yellow fever vaccine administration. Three cases of yellow fever vacine-associated neurologic disease have been reported in exclusively breastfed infants whose mothers received yellow fever vaccine while lactating. All 3 infants were younger than 1 month at the time of exposure and had a diagnosis of encephalitis. The risk of potential yellow fever vaccine virus exposure through breastfeeding is unknown. Pregnant and breastfeeding mothers should avoid travel to areas with yellow fever. If travel is unavoidable and the risks of vaccination are believed to outweigh the likelihood of yellow fever virus exposure, a pregnant or breastfeeding woman should be issued a medical waiver to fulfill health regulations. If the risk of yellow fever virus exposure outweighs the vaccination risks, a pregnant or breastfeeding woman should be vaccinated. Although there are no data, some experts recommend that breastfeeding women who receive yellow fever vaccine should temporarily suspend breastfeeding and pump and discard expressed milk for at least 2 weeks.

The world's first Ebola vaccine, ERVEBO, is a vesicular stomatitis platform-based live-virus (sVSV-ZEBOV) vaccine. No information is yet available on the safety of this vaccine during lactation. Similarly, no data are available on the live attenuated cholera vaccine in breastfeeding women. However, the live attenuated cholera vaccine is not absorbed from the gastrointestinal tract, so maternal exposure to the vaccine is not expected to result in exposure of the fetus. Pregnant women and their clinicians should consider the risks associated with traveling to areas of active cholera transmission.

EFFICACY AND SAFETY OF IMMUNIZATION IN BREASTFED INFANTS

Infants should be immunized according to the recommended childhood and adolescent immunization schedule (**https://redbook.solutions.aap.org/SS/Immunization_Schedules.aspx**), regardless of the mode of infant feeding. Theoretically, high concentrations of poliovirus antibody in human milk could interfere with the immunogenicity of oral poliovirus vaccine; this is not a concern with inactivated poliovirus vaccine (IPV), which is the only poliovirus vaccine used in the United States. There is in vitro evidence that human milk from women who live in areas with endemic rotavirus contains antibodies that can neutralize live rotavirus vaccine virus. However, in licensing trials, the effectiveness of rotavirus vaccine in breastfed infants was comparable to that in nonbreastfed infants. Postmarketing immunogenicity studies conducted outside the United States did not demonstrate improved antibody response following rotavirus vaccine when breastfeeding was temporarily withheld before and after vaccine administration. Furthermore, breastfeeding reduces the likelihood of rotavirus disease in infancy.

Transmission of Infectious Agents via Human Milk

BACTERIA

Postpartum mastitis occurs in one third of breastfeeding women in the United States and leads to breast abscesses in up to 10% of cases. Both mastitis and breast abscesses have been associated with the presence of bacterial pathogens in human milk. In cases of breast abscess or cellulitis, breastfeeding on the affected breast should continue, even if a drain is present, as long as the infant's mouth is not in direct contact with purulent drainage or infected tissue. In general, infectious mastitis resolves with continued lactation during appropriate antimicrobial therapy and does not pose a significant risk for the infant. Breastfeeding on the affected side in cases of mastitis generally is recommended; however, even when breastfeeding is interrupted on the affected breast, breastfeeding may continue on the unaffected breast.

Women with tuberculosis who have been treated appropriately for 2 or more weeks and who are not considered contagious (negative sputum) may breastfeed. Women with tuberculosis disease suspected of being contagious should refrain from breastfeeding and from other close contact with the infant because of potential spread of *Mycobacterium tuberculosis* through respiratory tract droplets or airborne transmission (see Tuberculosis, p 786). However, expressed human milk can be fed to the infant, as long as there is no evidence of tuberculosis mastitis, which is rare.

Expressed human milk can become contaminated with a variety of bacterial pathogens, including *Staphylococcus* species and gram-negative bacilli. Outbreaks of gram-negative bacterial infections in neonatal intensive care units occasionally have been attributed to contaminated human milk specimens that have been improperly collected or stored. Liquid human milk fortifiers are preferred, because receipt of powdered human milk fortifiers and powdered infant formula has been associated with invasive bacteremia and meningitis attributable to *Cronobacter* species (formerly *Enterobacter sakazakii*), resulting in death in approximately 40% of cases. Consequently, the AAP has advised against the use of powdered infant formulas/human milk fortifiers in preterm or immunocompromised infants. Routine culturing or heat treatment of a mother's milk fed to her infant has not been demonstrated to be necessary or cost-effective (see Human Milk Banks, p 114). Because of the immune-protective factors in human milk, there is a hierarchical preference for the mother's freshly expressed milk, followed by the mother's previously refrigerated or frozen milk, followed by pasteurized donor milk as the third best option for feeding of sick and/or preterm infants.[1]

VIRUSES

CYTOMEGALOVIRUS. Cytomegalovirus (CMV) may be shed intermittently in human milk. Although CMV has been found in human milk of women who delivered preterm infants, case reviews of preterm infants acquiring CMV postnatally have not demonstrated long-term clinical sequelae over several years of follow-up after infants were discharged from the neonatal intensive care unit (NICU). Very low birth weight preterm infants, however, are at greater potential risk of developing symptomatic disease shortly after postnatal acquisition of CMV, including through human milk. Decisions about breastfeeding of preterm infants by mothers known to be CMV seropositive should include consideration of the potential benefits of human milk and the risk of CMV transmission. Mothers who deliver infants at <32 weeks' gestation can be screened for CMV. When available, Holder pasteurization (62.5°C [144.5°F] for 30 minutes) and short-term pasteurization (72°C [161.6°F] for 5 seconds) of human milk appear to inactivate CMV; short-term pasteurization may be less harmful to the

---

[1] American Academy of Pediatrics, Committee on Nutrition, Section on Breastfeeding, Committee on Fetus and Newborn. Donor human milk for the high-risk infant: preparation, safety, and usage options in the United States. *Pediatrics*. 2017;139(1):e20163440

beneficial constituents of human milk. Freezing human milk at $-20°C$ ($-4°F$) for the sole purpose of reducing CMV infectivity is not advised, because although it may reduce the viral load of CMV, it does not change the risk of CMV sepsis-like syndrome, and freezing reduces the bioactivity of human milk.

EBOLA VIRUS. Ebola virus has been detected in human milk during and in the first month after infection. The duration of Ebola virus shedding in human milk is unknown. Genomic analysis in a case of fatal Ebola in a 9-month-old strongly suggested Ebola virus transmission through human milk. When safe alternatives to breastfeeding and infant care exist, a mother with confirmed or suspected Ebola virus infection should not have close contact with her infant (including breastfeeding) to reduce the risk of transmitting Ebola virus to her child. There is not enough evidence to provide guidance on precisely when it is safe to resume breastfeeding after recovery. Where available, testing of human milk for the presence of Ebola virus RNA can help to guide decisions about when breastfeeding can be safely resumed. Additional recommendations may be found at **www.cdc.gov/vhf/ebola/clinicians/evd/neonatal-care.html** and **www.cdc.gov/vhf/ebola/clinicians/evd/pregnant-women.html.**

HEPATITIS B VIRUS. Hepatitis B surface antigen (HBsAg) has been detected in milk from HBsAg-positive women. However, studies from Taiwan and England have indicated that breastfeeding by HBsAg-positive women does not significantly increase the risk of infection among their infants. In the United States, infants born to known HBsAg-positive women should receive the initial dose of hepatitis B vaccine within 12 hours of birth, and Hepatitis B Immune Globulin should be administered concurrently but at a different anatomic site. This combination effectively will eliminate any theoretical risk of transmission through breastfeeding (see Hepatitis B, p 381). There is no need to delay initiation of breastfeeding until after the infant is immunized.

HEPATITIS C VIRUS. Hepatitis C virus (HCV) RNA and antibody to HCV have been detected in milk from mothers infected with HCV, but transmission of HCV via breastfeeding has not been documented in mothers who have positive test results for anti-HCV antibody but negative test results for HIV antibody. According to current guidelines of the US Public Health Service, maternal HCV infection is not a contraindication to breastfeeding. The decision to breastfeed should be based on an informed discussion between a mother and her health care professional. Mothers infected with HCV should consider abstaining from breastfeeding from a breast with cracked or bleeding nipples.

HERPES SIMPLEX VIRUS TYPE 1. Women with herpetic lesions may transmit herpes simplex virus (HSV) to their infants by direct contact with the lesions. Transmission may be reduced with hand hygiene and covering of lesions with which the infant might come into contact. Women with herpetic lesions on a breast or nipple should refrain from breastfeeding an infant from the affected breast until lesions have resolved but may breastfeed from the unaffected breast when lesions on the affected breast are covered completely to avoid transmission. In addition, a woman with active herpes lesions on her breast can feed expressed milk from that breast to her infant, as there is no concern of herpes transmission through the milk. However, no part of the breast pump or expressed milk should come in contact with the lesions during expression, if the milk will be fed to the infant. If the pump does come in contact with the herpetic lesions, the mother should still express to maintain her milk supply and prevent mastitis, but the milk should be discarded.

HUMAN IMMUNODEFICIENCY VIRUS. All pregnant women in the United States should be screened for HIV infection as part of a prenatal testing panel (see Human Immunodeficiency Virus Infection, p 447). All women found to have HIV infection should receive appropriate antiretroviral therapy for their own health and for prevention of vertical transmission. All HIV-infected women should be counseled regarding breastfeeding.[1] HIV has been isolated from human milk and can be transmitted through breastfeeding. The risk of transmission is higher for women who acquire HIV infection during pregnancy and lactation (ie, postpartum) than for women with preexisting infection. In the absence of antiretroviral therapy, the transmission risk appears to be higher in the first few months of life and during weaning; however, transmission can occur throughout lactation. In resource-limited settings, replacement feeding and/ or short-course breastfeeding (4 to 6 months) has been associated with very high rates of infant morbidity and mortality. Multiple African studies have revealed that exclusive breastfeeding for the 4 to 6 months after birth lowers, but does not eliminate, the risk of HIV transmission through human milk compared with infants who received mixed feedings (breastfeeding and other foods or milks).

Randomized clinical trials have demonstrated that both maternal triple antiretroviral therapy and daily infant prophylaxis (nevirapine or nevirapine/zidovudine) during breastfeeding significantly decreases the risk of postnatal transmission via human milk. However, neither maternal nor infant postpartum antiretroviral therapy is sufficient to eliminate completely the risk of HIV transmission through breastfeeding.[2] Penetration of antiretroviral agents into human milk also raises potential concerns regarding infant toxicity as well as the selection of antiretroviral-resistant virus within human milk. Thus, decisions related to breastfeeding must balance the risks of HIV transmission against the risk of non-HIV morbidity and mortality. In settings like the United States, where the risk of infant morbidity and mortality from infectious diseases and malnutrition is low and alternative sources of feeding are available, HIV-infected women should be counseled to avoid breastfeeding and donating human milk. If HIV-infected women in the United States choose to breastfeed, consultation with a pediatric HIV expert is recommended so that HIV transmission risk is minimized.[2,3]

In resource-limited settings, the World Health Organization, UNICEF, and UNAIDS have recommended that countries adopt national or subnational infant feeding guidelines based socioeconomic and public health considerations including the availability and quality of health services available.[4] The most appropriate feeding

---

[1]Centers for Disease Control and Prevention. Revised recommendations for HIV testing of adults, adolescents, and pregnant women in health-care settings. *MMWR Recomm Rep.* 2006;55(RR-14):1–17

[2]Panel on Treatment of Pregnant Women with HIV Infection and Prevention of Perinatal Transmission. Recommendations for the use of antiretroviral drugs in pregnant women with HIV infection and interventions to reduce perinatal HIV transmission in the United States. Available at: **https://clinicalinfo.hiv. gov/en/guidelines/perinatal/whats-new-guidelines.** Accessed July 27, 2020

[3]American Academy of Pediatrics, Committee on Pediatric AIDS. Infant feeding and transmission of human immunodeficiency virus in the United States. *Pediatrics.* 2013;131(2):391-396 (Reaffirmed April 2016)

[4]World Health Organization, United Nations Children's Fund. *Guideline: Updates on HIV and Infant Feeding: The Duration of Breastfeeding, and Support from Health Services to Improve Feeding Practices Among Mothers Living with HIV.* Geneva, Switzerland: World Health Organization; 2016

option for an HIV-infected mother in a resource-limited setting needs to be based on her individual circumstances (eg, access to safe alternative replacement feeding, access to antiretroviral medications, and HIV viral load) and should consider the benefits of breastfeeding and the risk of transmission of HIV by breastfeeding. HIV-infected women who breastfeed should do so exclusively for the first 6 months, and breast-feeding should be extended through at least 12 months as complementary foods are introduced. Breastfeeding may continue for up to 24 months or longer while being supported for antiretroviral adherence. Weaning should occur gradually over a month. Antiretroviral prophylaxis (maternal triple antiretroviral therapy or extended infant prophylaxis) should be provided throughout the breastfeeding and weaning periods.

HUMAN T-LYMPHOTROPIC VIRUS TYPE 1. Human T-lymphotropic virus type 1 (HTLV-1), which is endemic in Japan, the Caribbean, and parts of South America, is associated with development of malignant neoplasms and neurologic disorders among adults. Epidemiologic and laboratory studies suggest that mother-to-infant transmission of human HTLV-1 occurs primarily through breastfeeding, although freezing/thawing of expressed human milk may decrease infectivity of human milk. Women in the United States who are HTLV-1 seropositive should be advised not to breastfeed and not to donate to human milk banks.

HUMAN T-LYMPHOTROPIC VIRUS TYPE 2. Human T-lymphotropic virus type 2 (HTLV-2) is a retrovirus that has been detected among American and European injection drug users and some American Indian/Alaska Native groups. Although apparent maternal-infant transmission has been reported, the rate and timing of transmission have not been established. Until additional data about possible transmission through breastfeeding become available, women in the United States who are HTLV-2 seropositive should be advised to not breastfeed and to not donate to human milk banks. Routine screening for both HTLV-1 or HTLV-2 during pregnancy is not recommended.

RUBELLA. Wild and vaccine strains of rubella virus have been isolated from human milk. However, the presence of rubella virus in human milk has not been associated with significant disease in infants, and transmission is more likely to occur via other routes. Women with rubella or women who have been immunized recently with a live attenuated rubella virus-containing vaccine may continue to breastfeed.

SARS-COV-2. Severe acute respiratory syndrome-coronavirus 2 (SARS-CoV-2) has been detected rarely in human milk, but there have been no documented cases of transmission to breastfeeding infants. Mothers shedding SARS-CoV-2 may express milk after appropriate breast and hand hygiene, and this milk may be fed to the infant by designated caregivers. Breast pumps and components should be thoroughly cleaned between pumping sessions using standard center policies that must include cleaning the pump with disinfectant wipes and washing pump attachments with hot, soapy water. Mothers who want to breastfeed directly should be encouraged to properly wash their hands with soap and water before handling the infant and advised to wear a mask while nursing. When not nursing, the infant can be cared for by a healthy caregiver, if available, and/or maintained in a separate room or at least 6 feet away from the mother. Additional information is available at **https://services.aap.org/en/pages/2019-novel-coronavirus-covid-19-infections/clinical-guidance/breastfeeding-guidance-post-hospital-discharge/**.

VARICELLA. Secretion of attenuated varicella vaccine virus in human milk has not been documented. Breastfeeding is not a contraindication to immunization (see Varicella-Zoster Infections, p 831). Expressed/pumped milk from a mother with varicella or zoster can be fed to the infant, provided no lesions are on the breast.

WEST NILE VIRUS. West Nile virus RNA has been detected in human milk collected from a woman with disease attributable to West Nile virus. Her breastfed infant developed West Nile virus immunoglobulin M antibodies but remained asymptomatic. Such transmission appears to be rare, and no adverse effects on infants have been described. Because the benefits of breastfeeding outweigh the risk of WNV disease in breastfeeding infants, mothers should be encouraged to breastfeed even in areas with ongoing WNV transmission.

ZIKA VIRUS. Although Zika virus has been detected in human milk, and a few probable cases of transmission of Zika virus by breastfeeding have been reported, to date there is no consistent evidence that infants acquire Zika virus through breastfeeding. Cases have occurred in areas where Zika virus infection is endemic where mosquito-borne transmission could not be excluded. Current evidence suggests that the benefits of breastfeeding outweigh any the theoretical risks of Zika virus transmission through human milk. The World Health Organization and Centers for Disease Control and Prevention (CDC) recommend infants born to women with suspected, probable, or confirmed Zika virus infection, or to women who live in or have traveled to areas with Zika virus, should be fed according to local infant feeding guidelines. Because of the benefits of breastfeeding, mothers are encouraged to breastfeed even in areas where Zika virus is found.

HUMAN MILK BANKS

Some circumstances, such as preterm delivery, may preclude direct breastfeeding, but infants in these circumstances still may be fed human milk collected from their own mothers or from individual donors. The potential for transmission of infectious agents through donor human milk requires appropriate selection and screening of donors and careful collection, processing, and storage of human milk.[1,2] Currently, US donor milk banks that belong to the Human Milk Banking Association of North America (**www.hmbana.org/**) voluntarily follow pasteurization guidelines drafted in consultation with the US Food and Drug Administration and the CDC. Other pasteurization methods also are acceptable, but use of nonpasteurized donor milk is not recommended. These guidelines include screening of all donors for HBsAg and antibodies to HIV-1, HIV-2, HTLV-1, HTLV-2, hepatitis C virus, and syphilis. Donor milk is dispensed only by prescription after it is heat treated at 62.5°C (144.5°F) for 30 minutes (Holder pasteurization) and no viable bacteria are present after pasteurization.

Although milk banks support hospitalized, high-risk infants, informal human milk sharing is becoming increasingly common. Parents should be informed of the safety risks of milk obtained from unscreened donors and milk that has not been safely

---

[1]American Academy of Pediatrics, Committee on Nutrition, Section on Breastfeeding, Committee on Fetus and Newborn. Donor human milk for the high-risk infant: preparation, safety, and usage options in the United States. *Pediatrics.* 2017;139(1):e20163440

[2]American Academy of Pediatrics, Section on Breastfeeding. Promoting human milk and breastfeeding for the very low birth weight infant. 2021; In press

collected processed, handled, and stored. Parents who decide to use shared milk should be instructed on minimizing risk by screening donors for contraindicated illnesses and medications and ensuring that the milk was safely collected, stored, and delivered. Milk obtained through the internet should be discouraged, as the donors cannot be screened and there are risks of contamination with chemicals and prescription and/or illicit drugs and even adulteration with cow milk.

INADVERTENT HUMAN MILK EXPOSURE

Policies have been developed to deal with occasions when an infant inadvertently is fed expressed human milk not obtained from his or her mother. These policies require documentation, counseling, and observation of the affected infant for signs of infection, and potential testing of the source mother for infections that could be transmitted via human milk. Recommendations for management of a situation involving an accidental exposure may be found on the CDC website (**www.cdc.gov/breastfeeding/recommendations/other_mothers_milk.htm**). Decisions about medical management and diagnostic testing of the infant who received another mother's milk should be based on the details of the individual situation and be determined collaboratively between the infant's physician and parent(s) or guardian(s). A summary of the recommendations includes the following:

1. Inform the donor mother about the inadvertent exposure, and ask:
   - When the milk was expressed and how it was handled?
   - Would she be willing to share information about her current medication use, recent infectious disease history, and presence of cracked or bleeding nipples during milk expression with the other family or the infant's treating physician?
2. Discuss inadvertent administration of the donor milk with the parent(s) of the recipient infant.
   - Inform them that their child was given another mother's expressed human milk.
   - Inform them that the risk of transmission of infectious diseases (eg, HIV, hepatitis B, or hepatitis C) is small.
   - If possible, provide the family with information on when the milk was expressed and how the milk was handled prior to being delivered to the caregiver.
   - Encourage the parent(s) or guardian(s) to notify the infant's treating physician of the situation and share any specific details known.

Antimicrobial Agents and Other Drugs in Human Milk

Antimicrobial agents often are prescribed for lactating women. Although these drugs may be detected in milk, the potential risk to an infant must be weighed against the known benefits of continued breastfeeding. As a general guideline, an antimicrobial agent is safe to administer to a lactating woman if the drug is safe to administer to an infant. Only in rare cases will interruption of breastfeeding be necessary because of maternal antimicrobial use. A breastfed infant who requires antimicrobial therapy should receive the recommended doses, independent of administration of the agent to the mother.

Current information about drugs and lactation can be found on the Toxicology Data Network Web site (**https://toxnet.nlm.nih.gov/newtoxnet/lactmed.htm**). Data for drugs, including antimicrobial agents, administered to lactating women are provided in several categories, including maternal and infant drug concentrations, effects in breastfed infants, possible effects on lactation, alternative drugs to consider, and references. Information on potential risks for drugs and vaccines administered during lactation, including potential effects on the breastfed child, can also be found in US Food and Drug Administration-approved labeling.

Anti-TNF Biologic Response Modifiers in Human Milk

Available evidence supports a lack of any significant transfer of anti-tumor necrosis factor (anti-TNF) drugs to human milk. Anti-TNF drugs include adalimumab, certolizumab pegol, etanercept, golimumab, and infliximab. Women receiving treatment with anti-TNF drugs should be advised to continue breastfeeding. Breastfed infants whose mothers are receiving anti-TNF drugs should receive recommended vaccines, including live virus vaccines, as indicated and according to the recommended schedule unless vaccination is being withheld because of in utero exposure to the biologic response modifier (see Biologic Response-Modifying Drugs Used to Decrease Inflammation, p 82).

CHILDREN IN GROUP CHILD CARE AND SCHOOLS

Infants and young children who are cared for in group child care settings (child care centers and home-based child care) and schools[1] have an increased rate of communicable infectious diseases. Children in group child care settings and schools transmit infections among themselves and spread these infections to their families and child care staff. Risk of communicable diseases decreases gradually as children advance through school, and extends to participants in other group settings such as residential treatment facilities, group homes, and foster care. The illnesses transmitted in these settings primarily reflect what is prevalent in the community. Respiratory infections are more common than gastrointestinal tract infections, and health department interventions are often necessary when outbreaks of infectious diseases occur in these settings.

Children in child care are more likely to receive antimicrobial agents; hence, they may also be colonized or infected with antimicrobial-resistant organisms. Younger age, more time in group child care settings, and exposure to larger group size are all strongly associated with more frequent infections. As children get older and increase their time in group care, they develop lasting immunity to common infections earlier compared with peers with less exposure.

Compared with children in child care, school-aged children experience a lower incidence of infectious diseases because of increased immunity as well as improved infection control measures such as social distancing, hand hygiene, and respiratory etiquette. However, schools remain important sites of transmission of common infectious diseases including rhinovirus infections, influenza, pertussis, and others, including additional vaccine-preventable diseases.

---

[1]American Academy of Pediatrics. *Managing Infectious Diseases in Child Care and Schools: A Quick Reference Guide.* Aronson SS, Shope TR, eds. 5th ed. Itasca, IL: American Academy of Pediatrics; 2019

Modes of Spread of Infectious Diseases

RESPIRATORY TRACT DISEASES

Children, especially young children in child care, spread respiratory pathogens efficiently because of suboptimal social distancing and respiratory etiquette (Table 2.1). Pathogens spread by the respiratory route include bacteria, sometimes associated with invasive infections, and viruses causing acute upper respiratory tract infections. Viral infections of the respiratory tract are common in children in group child care settings. Possible modes of spread of respiratory tract pathogens include aerosols, respiratory droplets, direct contact with secretions, or indirect contact with contaminated fomites. The viral pathogens responsible for respiratory tract disease in child care settings include respiratory syncytial virus (RSV) and human metapneumovirus as well as viruses that also affect children in schools, including parainfluenza virus, influenza virus, adenovirus, and rhinovirus. Respiratory tract viruses are associated with exacerbations of asthma and an increase in the incidence of otitis media and can cause significant complications for children with chronic respiratory tract disease, such as cystic fibrosis, and for children who are immunocompromised.

Seasonal outbreaks of common respiratory infections, such as hand-foot-and-mouth disease (enterovirus) and bronchiolitis, are expected and amplified in group child care settings, and influenza outbreaks occur annually in child care settings and schools. Other respiratory pathogens that can cause sporadic outbreaks include group A streptococcal pharyngitis, *Neisseria meningitidis*, *Mycoplasma pneumoniae* (in schools), and some vaccine-preventable diseases such as pertussis, varicella, measles, mumps, rubella, and, rarely, *Haemophilus influenzae* type b. The incidence of vaccine-preventable diseases has markedly decreased since routine immunizations were implemented, although communities with low vaccination rates continue to be at increased risk for outbreaks. More detailed recommendations for management and exclusion and return to care for these conditions are available in the relevant disease-specific chapters in Section 3 or other resources from the American Academy of Pediatrics (AAP).[1,2]

ENTERIC DISEASES

Diarrheal illness is much more common in child care settings than in schools, because young children and adult caregivers spread enteric diseases primarily by contact with pathogens during diapering and toileting procedures. Enteric diseases can also occur in schools if a person fails to maintain good hygiene after toilet use or if contaminated food is shared among classmates. Organisms spread by the fecal-oral route include common viruses, bacterial pathogens, and parasites. Seasonal enteric pathogens include noroviruses (which are a frequent cause of illness in children), enteric adenoviruses, and astroviruses (see Table 2.1). Rotavirus vaccination has dramatically decreased seasonal outbreaks attributable to this virus, but illness still occurs. Hepatitis

---

[1]American Academy of Pediatrics. *Managing Infectious Diseases in Child Care and Schools: A Quick Reference Guide.* Aronson SS, Shope TR, eds. 5th ed. Itasca, IL: American Academy of Pediatrics; 2019

[2]American Academy of Pediatrics, American Public Health Association, National Resource Center for Health and Safety in Child Care and Early Education. *Caring for Our Children: National Health and Safety Performance Standards: Guidelines for Out-of-Home Child Care.* 4th ed. Itasca, IL: American Academy of Pediatrics; and Washington, DC: American Public Health Association; 2019

Table 2.1. Modes of Transmission of Organisms

Usual Route of Transmission[a]	Bacteria	Viruses	Other[b]
Fecal-oral	*Campylobacter* species, *Salmonella* species; *Shigella* species; Shiga toxin-producing *Escherichia coli*, including *E coli* O157:H7	Astrovirus, enteric adenovirus, enteroviruses, hepatitis A virus, norovirus, rotaviruses, sapovirus	*Cryptosporidium* species, *Enterobius vermicularis*, *Giardia duodenalis*
Respiratory	*Bordetella pertussis*, group A *Streptococcus* species, *Haemophilus influenzae* type b, *Kingella kingae*, *Mycobacterium tuberculosis* (children ≥10 years and adults), *Neisseria meningitidis*, *Streptococcus pneumoniae*	Adenovirus, coronavirus, influenza virus, human metapneumovirus, measles virus, mumps virus, parainfluenza virus, parvovirus B19, respiratory syncytial virus, rhinovirus, rubella virus, SARS-CoV-2, varicella-zoster virus	...
Person-to-person contact	Group A *Streptococcus* species, *Staphylococcus aureus*	Herpes simplex virus, varicella-zoster virus	Agents causing pediculosis, scabies, and ringworm[c]
Contact with blood, urine, and/or saliva	...	Cytomegalovirus, herpes simplex virus, hepatitis C virus	...
Bloodborne	...	Hepatitis B virus, hepatitis C virus, human immunodeficiency virus	...

[a] The potential for transmission of microorganisms in the child care setting by food and animals also exists (see Appendix VI, Clinical Syndromes Associated With Foodborne Diseases, p 1041, and Appendix VII, Diseases Transmitted by Animals [Zoonoses], p 1048).

[b] Parasites, fungi, mites, and lice.

[c] Transmission also may occur from contact with objects in the environment.

A virus can cause outbreaks in child care settings and schools but similarly is much less common since routine implementation of hepatitis A immunization. Bacterial enteropathogens such as *Shigella* species and *Escherichia coli* O157:H7 can cause significant outbreaks in group child care settings and require a very small infective dose of organisms, whereas *Salmonella* species and *Campylobacter* species are less common causes of outbreaks. Parasites like *Giardia duodenalis* and *Cryptosporidium* species can cause outbreaks in child care settings, particularly where shared pools are used in water play activities, because their spores are resistant to chlorination in water sources and to alcohol-based hand sanitizers (see Prevention of Illnesses Associated with Recreational Water Use, p 180). More detailed recommendations for management, exclusion, and return to care for these conditions are available in the relevant disease-specific chapters in Section 3 or other references,[1,2] and local public health authorities should be consulted.

BLOODBORNE INFECTIONS

Bloodborne infections are a potential concern in group child care settings and schools. Hepatitis B virus (HBV) transmission from an infected child biting a susceptible child has occurred in child care, but this is rare, especially given high hepatitis B immunization rates. Human immunodeficiency virus (HIV) transmission in a child care setting has never been documented. School-aged children infected with HIV, HBV, or hepatitis C virus (HCV) do not need to be identified to school personnel. Rather, policies and procedures to manage all potential exposures to blood or blood-containing materials should be established and universally implemented. Care required for school-aged children with physical or intellectual disabilities may expose caregivers to urine, saliva, and in some cases, blood. Therefore, the application of standard precautions and appropriate hand hygiene, as recommended for children in group child care,[1] is the optimal means to prevent spread of infection from these exposures. Parents and students should be educated about the types of exposure that present a risk for school contacts. Although a student's right to privacy should be maintained, decisions about activities at school should be made by parents or guardians together with the child's physician, on a case-by-case basis, keeping the health needs of the infected student and the student's classmates in mind.

Although no prospective studies have been conducted to determine the risk of transmission of HIV, HBV, or HCV during contact sports among high school students, available evidence indicates that the transmission risk is low. Guidelines for management of bleeding injuries have been developed for college and professional athletes in recognition of the possibility of unidentified HIV, HBV, or HCV infection in any athlete. The following are recommendations for prevention of transmission of HIV and other bloodborne pathogens in the athletic setting.

---

[1] American Academy of Pediatrics. *Managing Infectious Diseases in Child Care and Schools: A Quick Reference Guide.* Aronson SS, Shope TR, eds. 5th ed. Itasca, IL: American Academy of Pediatrics; 2019

[2] American Academy of Pediatrics, American Public Health Association, National Resource Center for Health and Safety in Child Care and Early Education. *Caring for Our Children: National Health and Safety Performance Standards: Guidelines for Out-of-Home Child Care.* 4th ed. Itasca, IL: American Academy of Pediatrics; and Washington, DC: American Public Health Association; 2019

- Athletes infected with HIV, HBV, or HCV should be allowed to participate in competitive sports.
- Physicians should respect the rights of infected athletes to confidentiality. The infection status of patients should not be disclosed to other participants or the staff of athletic programs.
- Testing for bloodborne pathogens should not be mandatory for athletes or sports participants.
- Pediatricians are encouraged to counsel athletes who are infected with HIV, HBV, or HCV and to assure them that they have a low risk of infecting other competitors. Infected athletes should consider choosing a sport in which this transmission risk is minimal. This may be protective both for other participants and for the infected athletes themselves, decreasing their possible exposure to bloodborne pathogens other than the one(s) with which they are infected. Wrestling and boxing have the greatest potential for contamination of injured skin by blood. The AAP opposes boxing as a sport for youth for other reasons.[1]
- Athletic programs should inform athletes and their parents that the program is operating under the policies of the aforementioned recommendations and that the athletes have a low risk of becoming infected with a bloodborne pathogen.
- Athletic programs should promote HBV immunization among all athletes, coaches, athletic trainers, equipment handlers, laundry personnel, janitorial staff, and other people who may be exposed to blood as an occupational hazard.
- Each coach and athletic trainer must receive training in first aid and emergency care.
- Coaches and members of the health care team should educate athletes that, in contrast to the assumed low risk of transmission during athletics, there are greater risks of transmission of HIV and other bloodborne pathogens through sexual activity and needle sharing during the use of injection drugs, including anabolic steroids. Athletes should be told not to share personal items, such as razors, toothbrushes, and nail clippers, that might be contaminated with blood.
- Depending on the law in some states, schools may need to comply with Occupational Safety and Health Administration (OSHA) regulations (**www.osha. gov**) for prevention of bloodborne pathogens. The athletic program must determine which OSHA rules are applicable for their enterprise. Compliance with OSHA regulations is a reasonable and recommended precaution even if this is not required specifically by the state.
- The following precautions should be adopted in sports with direct body contact and other sports in which an athlete's blood or other body fluids visibly tinged with blood may contaminate the skin or mucous membranes of other participants or staff members of the athletic program. These precautions will not eliminate the risk that a participant or staff member may become infected with a bloodborne pathogen in the athletic setting but will reduce the risk substantially.
  - Athletes must cover existing cuts, abrasions, wounds, or other areas of broken skin with an occlusive dressing before and during participation. Caregivers should cover their own damaged skin to prevent transmission of infection to or from an injured athlete.

---

[1] American Academy of Pediatrics, Council on Sports Medicine and Fitness; Canadian Paediatric Society, Healthy Active Living and Sports Medicine Committee. Boxing participation by children and adolescents. *Pediatrics*. 2011;128(3):617–623 (Reaffirmed February 2015)

- Disposable, waterproof vinyl or latex gloves should be worn to avoid contact with blood or other body fluids visibly tinged with blood and any objects, such as equipment, bandages, or uniforms, contaminated with these fluids. Hands should be cleaned with soap and water or an alcohol-based antiseptic agent as soon as possible after gloves are removed.
- Athletes with active bleeding should be removed from competition as soon as possible. Wounds should be cleaned with soap and water. Skin antiseptic agents may be used if soap and water are not available. Athletes may return to competition once bleeding has stopped, and cleansed wounds are covered with an occlusive dressing that will remain intact and not become soaked through during further play.
- Athletes should be advised to report injuries and wounds in a timely fashion before or during competition.
- Minor cuts or abrasions that are not bleeding do not require interruption of play but can be cleaned and covered during scheduled breaks. During these breaks, if an athlete's equipment or uniform fabric is wet with blood, the equipment should be cleaned and disinfected (see next bullet), or the uniform should be replaced.
- Equipment and playing areas contaminated with blood must be cleaned using gloves and disposable absorbent material until all visible blood is gone and then disinfected with a product registered with the Environmental Protection Agency and applied in the manner and time recommended.[1] If the disinfecting product is bleach (1:80 dilution of household bleach), the decontaminated equipment or area should be in contact with the bleach solution for at least 30 seconds. The area then may be wiped with a disposable cloth after the minimum contact time or allowed to air dry.
- Emergency care must not be delayed because gloves or other protective equipment are not available. If the responder does not have appropriate protective equipment, a towel may be used to cover the wound until an off-the-field location is reached where gloves can be used during definitive treatment.
- Breathing bags (eg, Ambu manual resuscitators) and oropharyngeal airways should be available for use during resuscitation.
- Equipment handlers, laundry personnel, and janitorial staff must be educated in proper procedures for handling washable or disposable materials contaminated with blood.

OTHER INFECTIONS

Other common infections (Table 2.1) among children in group child care and schools may occur by direct contact with infected lesions, such as *Staphylococcus aureus*, group A *Streptococcus*, and herpes simplex virus. Shared fomites, such as towels, athletic equipment, and razors, have been implicated in the spread of methicillin-resistant *S aureus* (MRSA) within school settings. The AAP has guidance on control and prevention of MRSA and other infections in athletes and other school settings.[2] *Trichophyton tonsurans*,

---

[1]Centers for Disease Control and Prevention. Guidelines for environmental infection control in health-care facilities. Recommendations of CDC and the Healthcare Infection Control Practices Advisory Committee (HICPAC). *MMWR Recomm Rep.* 2003;52(RR-10):1–42

[2]Davies HD, Jackson MA, Rice SG; American Academy of Pediatrics, Committee on Infectious Diseases, Council on Sports Medicine and Fitness. Infectious diseases associated with organized sports and outbreak control. *Pediatrics.* 2017;140(4):e20172477

the predominant cause of tinea capitis (ringworm), remains viable for long periods on combs, hair brushes, furniture, and fabric. Tinea cruris (jock itch) and tinea pedis (athlete's foot) occur in adolescents and young adults. *Sarcoptes scabiei* (scabies) and *Pediculus capitis* (head lice) are transmitted primarily through person-to-person contact. In schools and group child care settings, transmission of scabies is unlikely without prolonged skin-to-skin contact; for lice, transmission occurs by direct head-to-head contact. Transmission of scabies and head lice through shared articles of clothing or hair accessories (combs, hair brushes, hats, and hair ornaments) is possible but uncommon. Cytomegalovirus (CMV) is common in children in child care settings and spreads via contact with infected bodily secretions; it is estimated that up to 70% of children 1 to 3 years of age who attend group child care may shed the virus in saliva or urine. CMV and parvovirus infections can have effects on the fetus of a pregnant child care worker, and those employed or volunteering in child care should discuss this occupational risk with their health care providers. Finally, human-animal contact involving family and classroom pets, animal displays, and petting zoos exposes children to pathogens harbored by these animals. Such animals are commonly colonized with *Salmonella* species, *Campylobacter* species, Shiga toxin-producing *E coli*, lymphocytic choriomeningitis virus, and other viruses that may be transmitted to children via contact (see Appendix VII, Diseases Transmitted by Animals [Zoonoses], p 1048). Detailed recommendations for management and exclusion and return-to-care for these conditions are available in the relevant disease-specific chapters in Section 3 or other references.[1,2]

Management and Prevention of Infectious Diseases

There are 3 primary methods for reducing the transmission of infectious diseases in group child care and school settings: immunization, infection prevention and control, and exclusion and return-to-care policies and practices.

IMMUNIZATION

Immunizations are by far the most effective means of preventing childhood infectious diseases. The United States relies on child care and school entry vaccination requirements to achieve and sustain high levels of vaccination coverage. Most states require vaccination of children entering child care programs, all states require vaccination of children at the time of entry into school, and many states have vaccination requirements for children throughout elementary school and high school and at the time of entry to college. Child care programs should require that all enrollees and staff members receive age-appropriate immunizations as recommended by the AAP and the Advisory Committee on Immunization Practices (ACIP) of the Centers for Disease Control and Prevention (CDC). Parents should be required to report their child's immunization status and programs should keep and review these records. Unless contraindications exist or children have received medical, religious, or philosophic

[1]American Academy of Pediatrics. *Managing Infectious Diseases in Child Care and Schools: A Quick Reference Guide.* Aronson SS, Shope TR, eds. 5th ed. Itasca, IL: American Academy of Pediatrics; 2019

[2]American Academy of Pediatrics, American Public Health Association, National Resource Center for Health and Safety in Child Care and Early Education. *Caring for Our Children: National Health and Safety Performance Standards: Guidelines for Out-of-Home Child Care.* 4th ed. Itasca, IL: American Academy of Pediatrics; and Washington, DC: American Public Health Association; 2019

exemptions (depending on state immunization laws), immunization records should demonstrate complete immunization for age as shown in the recommended childhood and adolescent immunization schedules and be adherent with state vaccine mandates. **(https://redbook.solutions.aap.org/SS/Immunization_Schedules.aspx).** The AAP views these nonmedical exemptions to child care- and school-required immunizations as inappropriate for individual, public health, and ethical reasons and advocates for their elimination.[1] The immunization mandates for children in child care and schools vary by state and can be found online **(www.immunize. org/laws)** and from the National Network for Immunization Information **(www. immunizationinfo.net/).** State requirements often lag behind the AAP and ACIP recommendations.

Children who have not received recommended age-appropriate immunizations before enrollment should be immunized as soon as possible, and the series should be completed according to the recommended childhood and adolescent immunization catch-up schedule as appropriate **(https://redbook.solutions.aap.org/ SS/Immunization_Schedules.aspx).** In the interim, permitting unimmunized or inadequately immunized children to attend child care or school should depend on state and local public health guidance regarding how to handle the risk and whether to inform parents of enrolled infants and children about potential exposure to this risk. Unimmunized or underimmunized children place appropriately immunized children and children with vaccine contraindications at risk of contracting a vaccine-preventable disease. If a vaccine-preventable disease occurs in a child care program or school, all unimmunized and underimmunized children should be excluded for the duration of possible exposure or until they have completed their immunizations. Local public health jurisdictions should be consulted for guidance.

All adults who work in a child care facility or school should receive all vaccines routinely recommended for adults (see adult immunization schedule at **www.cdc. gov/vaccines/schedules/hcp/adult.html**). By being fully immunized, child care providers and teachers protect not only themselves but also vulnerable infants too young to receive or complete immunization series and children who have medical contraindications to immunizations. These children also have the highest morbidity and mortality to infectious diseases such as measles, influenza, and pertussis. More detailed information about adult child care provider and teacher immunization requirements can be found in other references.[2,3]

---

[1] American Academy of Pediatrics, Committee on Practice and Ambulatory Medicine, Committee on Infectious Diseases, Committee on State Government Affairs, Council on School Health, Section on Administration and Practice Management. Medical versus nonmedical immunization exemptions for child care and school attendance. *Pediatrics.* 2016;138(3):e20162145

[2] American Academy of Pediatrics. *Managing Infectious Diseases in Child Care and Schools: A Quick Reference Guide.* Aronson SS, Shope TR, eds. 5th ed. Itasca, IL: American Academy of Pediatrics; 2019

[3] American Academy of Pediatrics, American Public Health Association, National Resource Center for Health and Safety in Child Care and Early Education. *Caring for Our Children: National Health and Safety Performance Standards: Guidelines for Out-of-Home Child Care.* 4th ed. Itasca, IL: American Academy of Pediatrics; and Washington, DC: American Public Health Association; 2019

INFECTION CONTROL AND PREVENTION

Group child care settings and schools both are rich environments for pathogens. However, group child care settings are much more problematic than schools, because young children are in close contact with each other, touching and sharing; they cough and sneeze without proper respiratory etiquette; and they need to be supervised or assisted with toileting and hand hygiene. As a result, viral, bacterial, fungal, and parasitic pathogens can be present in the air, on surfaces, in bodily secretions, and on the skin. Efforts to control the transmission of infectious diseases in child care settings are important but also difficult to implement effectively; as such, infection prevention and control in these settings requires a multifaceted approach. Programs should have written policies and training for staff to be sure they properly implement the best methods. These policies should include procedures for food and medication preparation; diaper changing; cleaning, sanitizing, and disinfecting surfaces; hand hygiene; respiratory etiquette; and other standard precautions.

It is difficult to decrease the spread of respiratory pathogens in group child care settings, with intensive education and infection control measures producing only modest reductions in incidence of respiratory illness, probably because respiratory pathogens are primarily spread by droplets expelled by sneezing and coughing. Young children have difficulty anticipating sneezing and coughing and do not effectively practice respiratory etiquette and hand hygiene. In addition, their social nature causes them to play in close proximity to each other, within the 3-foot radius most contaminated large droplets may travel before contacting another child's mucous membranes. Nevertheless, immunization, hand hygiene, and respiratory etiquette are essential elements of infection control in child care settings, and it is important that staff practice these measures for themselves as well as educate and assist young children to properly do so. Aerosolized droplets that land on surfaces may contain microorganisms capable of causing infections. Therefore, surface cleaning, disinfecting, and sanitizing are important to prevent the spread of respiratory illness. In schools, however, efforts to improve hand hygiene and respiratory etiquette—covering mouth and nose with tissue when coughing or sneezing (if no tissue is available, use the upper arm or elbow area rather than hands)—to reduce transmission of respiratory infections such as influenza are more effective and should be taught and implemented.

Infection control procedures in group child care settings are more effective in reducing diarrheal illness than respiratory illness. Adhering to diaper-changing procedures as recommended by the AAP[1] is a critical step to reduce fecal contamination and should be applied in child care settings as well as in schools that have diapered students with physical and intellectual disabilities. Surface cleaning, sanitizing, and disinfecting are especially important for reducing gastrointestinal tract illnesses. Cleaning removes visible soil to increase the effectiveness of sanitizing or disinfecting agents. Sanitizing reduces the amount of potential pathogens on food preparation surfaces, utensils, tables, countertops, and plastic toys. Disinfection requires stronger concentration or different agents than sanitizing and is used for areas with higher likelihood of pathogens, such as door handles, drinking fountains, and toilet and diaper changing areas.

As with respiratory tract infections, hand hygiene is essential to prevent the fecal-oral spread of gastrointestinal tract pathogens. Hand hygiene should occur for staff and

---

[1] American Academy of Pediatrics. *Managing Infectious Diseases in Child Care and Schools: A Quick Reference Guide.* Aronson SS, Shope TR, eds. 5th ed. Itasca, IL: American Academy of Pediatrics; 2019

children on arrival; when moving from one group to another; before and after contact with food or medication administration; after diaper changing, toileting, and contact with nasal or other body secretions, animals, or garbage; and after playing outside. Hand washing for 20 seconds with soap and water is the preferred method for hand hygiene, should be prioritized in child care and school settings, and is required whenever there is visible particulate matter. However, alcohol-based hand sanitizer may be substituted when soap and water is not available. Alcohol-based hand sanitizers have high alcohol content (60%–95%), which can be ingested or aerosolized; therefore, adult supervision is required. Hand hygiene using soap and water is preferred for *Cryptosporidium* species and norovirus because alcohol-based hand sanitizers are not as effective against these pathogens.

Other important environmental infection control and prevention measures for child care facilities include having adequate air flow in the building; providing enough physical space in the facility and between cots for naps (which may increase social distancing and reduce droplet spread); ensuring physical separation and separate personnel (if possible) involved in food preparation and diaper changing; requiring appropriate handling of animals (and excluding reptiles, turtles, amphibians, birds, primates, live poultry, ferrets, or rodents in the facility), with hand hygiene before and after contact; and adhering to recommended ratios of children to care providers.

Health departments should have plans for responding to reportable and non-reportable outbreaks of communicable diseases in child care programs and schools and should provide training, written information, and technical consultation when requested or alerted. In some instances, administration of appropriate antimicrobial therapy to a patient will limit further spread of infection (eg, *Shigella* species, streptococcal pharyngitis, pertussis). Antimicrobial prophylaxis administered to close contacts of children with infections caused by specific pathogens may be warranted in some circumstances (eg, meningococcal infection [see p 519], invasive *H influenzae* type a or type b [see p 345], and pertussis [see p 578]). Decisions about postexposure prophylaxis after an in-school exposure are best made in conjunction with local public health authorities and the primary pediatrician. Temporary child care program or school closings can be used in limited circumstances: (1) to prevent spread of infection; (2) when an infection is expected to affect a large number of susceptible students and available control measures are considered inadequate; or (3) when an infection is expected to have a high rate of morbidity or mortality. Collaborative efforts of public health officials, teachers, licensing agencies, child care providers, child care health consultants, physicians, nurses, parents, employers, and other members of the community are necessary to address problems of infection prevention and management in child care settings and schools.

Other resources that can assist teachers, caregivers and parents with these issues include the Healthy Child Care website (**www.aap.org/en-us/advocacy-and-policy/aap-health-initiatives/healthy-child-care/Pages/default.aspx**). People involved with early education and child care and schools can use the published national standards[1] related to these topics to provide specific education and implementation measures.

---

[1] American Academy of Pediatrics, American Public Health Association, National Resource Center for Health and Safety in Child Care and Early Education. *Caring for Our Children: National Health and Safety Performance Standards: Guidelines for Out-of-Home Child Care.* 4th ed. Itasca, IL: American Academy of Pediatrics; and Washington, DC: American Public Health Association; 2019

EXCLUSION AND RETURN TO CARE

General recommendations for exclusion of children in group child care and schools are provided in Table 2.2. Exclusions can put a significant economic strain on families, as parents may need to miss work to care for an ill child, and many exclusion decisions made by early child care and education professionals are not evidence-based and are inappropriate. No studies demonstrate that excluding children in group care and schools who are ill with common infectious diseases reduces the likelihood of spread to other children. However, there are some infectious diseases for which exclusion is recommended to try to control environmental contamination and/or spread because the clinical consequences are significant (Table 2.2). Many children are infectious before developing symptoms. Asymptomatic infection, high carriage rates, and prolonged shedding of pathogens in body secretions are common and make it difficult to curb transmission by targeting only symptomatic children. Because mild illness is common among children and most minor illnesses do not constitute a reason for excluding a child from child care or school, decisions about exclusion should be primarily based on the child's behavior. A mildly ill child can remain in child care or school unless the illness prevents the child from participating in normal activities, as determined by the child care staff or teachers, or the illness requires a need for care that is greater than child care staff or teachers can provide.

Each day as the child enters the program or school, and throughout the day as needed, staff members and teachers should evaluate the well-being of the child and observe for signs of illness. Parents should be encouraged to share information with child care staff and teachers about their child's acute and chronic illnesses and medication use utilizing a formal care plan that is signed by the child's health care provider. Examples of illnesses and conditions that do not necessitate exclusion include:

- Common cold.
- Diarrhea, as long as stools are contained in the diaper (for infants), there are no accidents using the toilet (for older children), and stool frequency is no more than 2 stools above normal for that child.
- Rash without fever and without behavioral change.
- Lice, ringworm, and scabies (exclusion and treatment can occur at the end of the day with return the following day). "No-nit" policies have not been effective in controlling head lice transmission and are not recommended.[1]
- Thrush.
- Fifth disease (parvovirus B19 infection) in an immunocompetent child.
- CMV infection.
- Chronic hepatitis B virus (HBV) infection (see p 381 for possible exceptions).
- Conjunctivitis without fever and without behavioral change.
- HIV infection (see p 427 for possible exceptions).
- Colonization with MRSA in children who do not have active lesions or illness that would otherwise require exclusion.

Asymptomatic children who excrete an enteropathogen usually do not need to be excluded (exceptions include children in whom Shiga toxin-producing *E coli*, *Shigella* species, or *Salmonella* serotype Typhi or Paratyphi).

[1] Devore CD, Schutz GE; American Academy of Pediatrics, Council on School Health, Committee on Infectious Diseases. Head lice. *Pediatrics*. 2015;135(5):e1355-e1365

Table 2.2. General Recommendations for Exclusion of Children From Group Child Care and School

Symptom(s)	Management
Illness preventing participation in activities, as determined by child care staff	Exclusion until the child can participate in activities
Illness that requires a level of care that is greater than staff can provide without compromising health and safety of others	Exclusion until the child no longer requires extra care to the extent staff cannot adequately attend to the health and safety of others in their care
Severe illness suggested by fever with behavior changes, lethargy, irritability, persistent crying, difficulty breathing, progressive rash with above symptoms	Medical evaluation and exclusion until severe symptoms have resolved and child can participate in activities and does not require excessive care
Persistent abdominal pain (2 hours or more) or intermittent abdominal pain associated with fever, dehydration, or other systemic signs and symptoms	Medical evaluation and exclusion until severe symptoms have resolved and child can participate and does not require excessive care
Vomiting 2 or more times in preceding 24 hours	Exclusion until symptoms have resolved, unless vomiting is determined to be caused by a noncommunicable condition and child is able to remain hydrated and participate in activities
Diarrhea if stool not contained in diaper or if fecal accidents occur in a child who is normally continent, if stool frequency exceeds 2 stools above normal for that child, or stools contain blood or mucus	Medical evaluation for stools with blood or mucus; exclusion until stools are contained in the diaper or when toilet-trained children no longer have accidents using the toilet, and when stool frequency becomes no more than 2 stools above that child's normal frequency for the time the child is in the program, even if the stools remain loose
Oral lesions	Exclusion if unable to contain drool or if unable to participate because of other symptoms
Skin lesions	Exclusion if lesions are weeping and cannot be covered with a waterproof dressing

Disease- or condition-specific recommendations for exclusion from child care and schools and management of contacts are shown in Table 2.3. Despite the existence of national recommendations for exclusion since 1992,[1,2] states have been slow to

[1] American Academy of Pediatrics. *Managing Infectious Diseases in Child Care and Schools: A Quick Reference Guide.* Aronson SS, Shope TR, eds. 5th ed. Itasca, IL: American Academy of Pediatrics; 2019

[2] American Academy of Pediatrics, American Public Health Association, National Resource Center for Health and Safety in Child Care and Early Education. *Caring for Our Children: National Health and Safety Performance Standards: Guidelines for Out-of-Home Child Care.* 4th ed. Itasca, IL: American Academy of Pediatrics; and Washington, DC: American Public Health Association; 2019

Table 2.3. Disease- or Condition-Specific Recommendations for Exclusion of Children From Group Child Care[a]

Condition	Management of Case	Management of Contacts
Hepatitis A virus (HAV) infection	Serologic testing to confirm HAV infection in suspected cases. Exclusion until 1 week after onset of illness.	In facilities with diapered children, if 1 or more cases confirmed in child or staff attendees or 2 or more cases in households of staff or attendees, hepatitis A vaccine (HepA) or Immune Globulin Intramuscular (IGIM) should be administered within 14 days of exposure to all unimmunized staff and attendees. In centers without diapered children, HepA or IGIM should be administered only to unimmunized classroom contacts of index case. Asymptomatic contacts may return after receipt of IGIM or hepatitis A vaccine (see Hepatitis A, p 373, for further discussion on indications for HepA vaccine or IG).
Impetigo	No exclusion if treatment has been initiated and as long as lesions on exposed skin are covered.	No intervention unless additional lesions develop.
Measles	Exclusion until 4 days after beginning of rash and when the child is able to participate.	In outbreak setting, people without documentation of immunity should be immunized within 72 hours of exposure or excluded. Immediate readmission to group child care may occur following immunization. Unimmunized people and those who do not receive vaccine within 72 hours of exposure should be excluded for at least 21 days after onset of rash in the last case of measles. For use of IG, see Measles (p 503).
Mumps	Exclusion until 5 days after onset of parotid gland swelling.	In outbreak setting, people without documentation of immunity should be immunized or excluded. Immediate readmission to group child care may occur following immunization. Unimmunized people should be excluded until at least 26 days after onset of parotitis in the last person with mumps. A second dose of measles, mumps, and rubella vaccine (MMR) (or measles, mumps, rubella, and varicella vaccine [MMRV], if age appropriate) should be offered to all students (including those in postsecondary school) and to all health care personnel born in or after 1957 who have only received 1 dose of MMR vaccine. A second dose of MMR also may be considered during outbreaks for preschool-aged children who have received 1 MMR dose. People previously vaccinated with 2 doses of a mumps-containing vaccine who are identified by public health as at increased risk for mumps because of an outbreak should receive a third dose of a mumps-containing vaccine to improve protection against mumps disease and related complications (see Mumps, p 538).

Table 2.3. Disease- or Condition-Specific Recommendations for Exclusion of Children From Group Child Care,[a] continued

Condition	Management of Case	Management of Contacts
Pediculosis capitis (head lice) infestation	Treatment at end of program day and readmission on completion of first treatment. Children should not be excluded or sent home early from school because of head lice, because head lice has a low contagion within classrooms.	Household and close contacts should be examined and treated if infested. No exclusion necessary.
Pertussis	Exclusion until completion of 5 days of the recommended course of antimicrobial therapy; if pertussis is suspected; children and providers who refuse treatment should be excluded until 21 days have elapsed from cough onset (see Pertussis, p 578).	Immunization and chemoprophylaxis should be administered as recommended for household and child care contacts. Contacts should be observed for respiratory tract symptoms for 21 days and if they develop symptoms, then they should be treated (see Pertussis, p 578).
Rubella	Exclusion for 7 days after onset of rash for postnatal infection.	In outbreak setting, children without evidence of immunity should be immunized or excluded for 21 days after onset of rash of the last case in the outbreak. Pregnant contacts should be evaluated (see Rubella, p 648).
Infection with *Salmonella* serotypes Typhi or Paratyphi	Exclusion until 3 consecutive stool cultures obtained at least 48 hours after cessation of antimicrobial therapy are negative, stools are contained in the diaper or child is continent, and stool frequency is no more than 2 stools above that child's normal frequency for the time the child is in the program.	When *Salmonella* serotype Typhi infection is identified in a child care staff member, local or state health departments should be consulted regarding regulations for length of exclusion and testing, which may vary by jurisdiction.

Table 2.3. Disease- or Condition-Specific Recommendations for Exclusion of Children From Group Child Care,[a] continued

Condition	Management of Case	Management of Contacts
Infection with nontyphoidal *Salmonella* species, *Salmonella* of unknown serotype	Exclusion until stools are contained in the diaper or child is continent and stool frequency is no more than 2 stools above that child's normal frequency for the time the child is in the program. Stool consistency does not need to return to normal to be able to return to child care. Negative stool culture results generally **not** required for nonserotype Typhi or Paratyphi *Salmonella* species.	Symptomatic contacts should be excluded until stools are contained in the diaper or child is continent and stool frequency is no more than 2 stools above that child's normal frequency for the time the child is in the program. Stool cultures are not required for asymptomatic contacts.
Scabies	Treatment at end of program day and readmission on completion of first treatment. Children should not be excluded or sent home early from school because of scabies, because scabies has a low contagion within classrooms.	Close contacts with prolonged skin-to-skin contact should receive prophylactic therapy. Bedding and clothing in contact with skin of infected people should be laundered (see Scabies, p 663).
Infection with Shiga toxin-producing *Escherichia coli* (STEC), including *E coli* O157:H7	Exclusion until 2 stool cultures (obtained at least 48 hours after any antimicrobial therapy, if administered, has been discontinued) are negative, and stools are contained in the diaper or child is continent, and stool frequency is no more than 2 stools above that child's normal frequency. Report to and consult with local or state public health officials. Some state health departments have less stringent exclusion policies for children who have recovered from less virulent STEC infection.	Meticulous hand hygiene; stool cultures should be performed for any symptomatic contacts. In outbreak situations involving virulent STEC strains, stool cultures of asymptomatic contacts may aid controlling spread. Center(s) with cases should be closed to new admissions during STEC outbreak (see *Escherichia coli* Diarrhea, p 322).

Table 2.3. Disease- or Condition-Specific Recommendations for Exclusion of Children From Group Child Care,[a] continued

Condition	Management of Case	Management of Contacts
Shigellosis	Exclusion until the state or local health department has deemed it safe to return to work per state or local child care exclusion regulations. Following this, children can return to child care facilities if stools are contained in the diaper or when toilet-trained children are continent and when stool frequency becomes no more than 2 stools above that child's normal baseline for the time the child is in the program, even if the stools remain loose.	Meticulous hand hygiene; stool cultures should be performed for any symptomatic contacts (see *Shigella* Infections, p 668).
Staphylococcus aureus skin infections	Exclusion only if skin lesions are draining and cannot be covered with a watertight dressing.	Meticulous hand hygiene; cultures of contacts are not recommended.
Streptococcal pharyngitis	Exclusion until at least 12 hours after treatment has been initiated.	Symptomatic contacts of documented cases of group A streptococcal infection should be tested and treated if test results are positive.

Table 2.3. Disease- or Condition-Specific Recommendations for Exclusion of Children From Group Child Care,[a] continued

Condition	Management of Case	Management of Contacts
Tuberculosis	Most children younger than 10 years are not considered contagious. For those with active disease, exclusion until determined to be noninfectious by physician or health department authority. No exclusion for latent tuberculosis infection.	Local health department personnel should be informed for contact investigation (see Tuberculosis, p 786).
Varicella (see Varicella-Zoster Infections, p 831)	Exclusion until all lesions have crusted or, in immunized people without crusts, until no new lesions appear within a 24-hour period.	For people without evidence of immunity, varicella vaccine should be administered ideally within 3 days but up to 5 days after exposure. Or when indicated, Varicella-Zoster Immune Globulin (see Varicella Zoster Virus, p 831) should be administered up to 10 days after exposure; if Varicella-Zoster Immune Globulin is not available, Immune Globulin Intravenous (IGIV) should be considered as an alternative. If vaccine cannot be administered and Varicella-Zoster Immune Globulin and IGIV are not indicated, preemptive oral acyclovir or valacyclovir can be considered.

[a] Many of these illnesses also require exclusion from school and other activities. Many of these diseases are reportable to local or state public health authorities, and reporting rules for local jurisdictions should be consulted. Public health authorities should be consulted if there are questions about exclusion criteria.

adopt these. Each state has its own regulations pertaining to exclusion and return to care/school, and these may not be evidence based. Child care programs are required to follow these state-specific guidelines to maintain licensing, which can be found at **https://childcareta.acf.hhs.gov/licensing.** Exclusion and return to care guidelines for schools may be addressed by state departments of health or other public health agencies.

During outbreaks of certain diseases, the responsible local and state public health authorities are helpful for determining the benefits and risks of excluding children from their usual care program or school. All states have laws about reporting and isolation of people with specific communicable diseases. Local or state health departments should be contacted for information about these laws, and public health authorities in these areas should be notified about cases of nationally notifiable infectious diseases and unusual outbreaks of other illnesses involving children or adults in the child care environment or schools (see Appendix III, Nationally Notifiable Infectious Diseases in the United States, p 1033). For most outbreaks of vaccine-preventable illnesses, unvaccinated children should be excluded until they are vaccinated and the risk of transmission no longer exists. In circumstances requiring intervention to prevent spread of infection within the school setting, the privacy of children who are infected should be protected.

INFECTION PREVENTION AND CONTROL FOR HOSPITALIZED CHILDREN

Health care-associated infections (HAIs) are a cause of substantial morbidity and some mortality in hospitalized children, particularly children in intensive care units. Hand hygiene before and after each patient contact remains the single most important practice in prevention and control of HAIs. A comprehensive set of guidelines for preventing and controlling HAIs, including isolation precautions, personnel health recommendations, and guidelines for prevention of postoperative and device-related infections, can be found on the Centers for Disease Control and Prevention (CDC) website **(www.cdc.gov/infectioncontrol/guidelines/index.html).** Additional guidelines are available from the principal infection prevention and control societies in the United States, the Society for Healthcare Epidemiology of America, and the Association for Professionals in Infection Control and Epidemiology, as well as other groups, such as the Occupational Safety and Health Administration and the Cystic Fibrosis Foundation.[1] The investigation and control of outbreaks that occur in special pediatric settings (eg, hematopoietic stem cell transplant units, neurosurgical units) always should involve the infection prevention and control team in each facility. Accrediting organizations, such as The Joint Commission, have established infection prevention and control standards. Pediatricians and infection prevention and control professionals should be familiar with this increasingly complex array of guidelines, regulations, and standards. To accomplish

---

[1]Saiman L, Seigel JD, LiPuma JJ, et al. Infection prevention and control guideline for cystic fibrosis: 2013 update. *Infect Control Hosp Epidemiol.* 2014;35(Suppl 1): S1-S67; **www.cff.org/Care/Clinical-Care-Guidelines/Infection-Prevention-and-Control-Clinical-Care-Guidelines/Infection-Prevention-and-Control-Clinical-Care-Guidelines/**

this goal, infection prevention and control programs led by pediatric infectious diseases specialists increasingly are used in hospital settings. These programs require adequate institutional support to be sustainable over time. Ongoing infection prevention and control programs should include education, implementation, reinforcement, documentation, and evaluation of recommendations on a regular basis (annual or sooner based on circumstance). Such activities should include conducting surveillance for high-risk HAIs, participating in improvement projects to reduce the incidence of HAIs, sharing data describing the incidence of specifically targeted HAIs, and complying with key prevention activities, such as hand hygiene.

Infection preventionists should be knowledgeable of the Targeted Assessment for Prevention (TAP) strategy developed by the CDC. This strategy targets health care facilities and specific units within facilities with a disproportionate burden of HAIs so that gaps in infection prevention in the targeted locations can be addressed. The TAP report uses data in the National Healthcare Safety Network system to calculate a metric called the cumulative attributable difference, which is the number of infections that must be prevented within a group, facility, or unit to achieve an HAI reduction goal (**www.cdc.gov/hai/prevent/tap.html**).

Infection Prevention and Control Precautions

Infection prevention and control precautions are designed to protect hospitalized children, health care personnel, and visitors by limiting transmission of potential pathogens within the health care setting. The Healthcare Infection Control Practices Advisory Committee (HICPAC) of the CDC in 2007 updated its evidence-based guidelines for preventing transmission of infectious agents in health care settings (**www.cdc.gov/hicpac/pdf/isolation/Isolation2007.pdf** with updates at **www.cdc.gov/infectioncontrol/guidelines/isolation/updates.html**). Adherence to these policies, supplemented by health care facility policies and procedures for other aspects of infection and environmental control and occupational health, should result in reduced transmission and safer patient care. Adaptations should be made according to the conditions and populations served by each facility, especially in the setting of an emerging infectious disease.

Routine and optimal performance of **Standard Precautions** is appropriate for care of **all** patients, regardless of diagnosis or suspected or confirmed infection status. In addition to Standard Precautions, **Transmission-Based Precautions** are used when caring for patients who are infected or colonized with pathogens transmitted by airborne, droplet, or contact routes. Table 2.4 lists syndromes and conditions that are suggestive of contagious infection and require empiric isolation precautions pending identification of a specific pathogen. When the specific pathogen is known, isolation recommendations and duration of isolation are provided in the pathogen- or disease-specific chapters in Section 3 and can be found in the HICPAC guidelines (**www.cdc.gov/infectioncontrol/guidelines/isolation/appendix/type-duration-precautions.html**).

STANDARD PRECAUTIONS

Standard Precautions are used to prevent transmission of all infectious agents through contact with nonintact skin, mucous membranes, or any body fluid except sweat (regardless of whether these fluids contain visible blood). Barrier techniques (eg, gloves or nonsterile gowns, as described below) are recommended to decrease exposure

Table 2.4. Clinical Syndromes or Conditions Warranting Precautions in Addition to Standard Precautions to Prevent Transmission of Epidemiologically Important Pathogens Pending Confirmation of Diagnosis[a]

Clinical Syndrome or Condition[b]	Potential Pathogens[c]	Empiric Precautions[d]
Diarrhea		
Acute diarrhea with a likely infectious cause	Enteric pathogens[e]	Contact
Diarrhea in patient with a history of recent antimicrobial use	*Clostridioides difficile*	Contact; use soap and water for handwashing
Meningitis	*Neisseria meningitidis, Haemophilus influenzae* type b	Droplet
	Enteroviruses	Contact
Rash or exanthems, generalized, cause unknown		
Petechial or ecchymotic with fever	*Neisseria meningitidis*	Droplet
	Hemorrhagic fever viruses	Contact plus Airborne
	Enteroviruses	Contact
Vesicular	Varicella-zoster virus	Airborne and Contact
Maculopapular with coryza and fever	Measles virus	Airborne
Respiratory tract infections		
Pulmonary cavitary disease	*Mycobacterium tuberculosis*	Airborne
Paroxysmal or severe persistent cough during periods of pertussis activity in the community	*Bordetella pertussis*	Droplet
Viral infections, particularly bronchiolitis and croup, in infants and young children	Respiratory viral pathogens	Contact and Droplet
Risk of multidrug-resistant microorganisms[f]		
Infection or colonization with multidrug-resistant organisms	Resistant bacteria, *Candida auris*	Contact
Skin, wound, or urinary tract infection in a patient with a recent stay in a hospital or chronic care facility	Resistant bacteria	Contact until resistant organism is excluded by cultures

Table 2.4. Clinical Syndromes or Conditions Warranting Precautions in Addition to Standard Precautions to Prevent Transmission of Epidemiologically Important Pathogens Pending Confirmation of Diagnosis,[a] continued

Clinical Syndrome or Condition[b]	Potential Pathogens[c]	Empiric Precautions[d]
Skin or wound infection		
Abscess or draining wound that cannot be covered	*Staphylococcus aureus,* group A *Streptococcus* species	Contact

[a] Infection control professionals are encouraged to modify or adapt this table according to local conditions. To ensure that appropriate empiric precautions are implemented, hospitals must have systems in place to evaluate patients routinely according to these criteria as part of their preadmission and admission care.

[b] Patients with the syndromes or conditions listed may have atypical signs or symptoms (eg, pertussis in neonates may present with apnea; paroxysmal or severe cough may be absent in pertussis in adults). The clinician's index of suspicion should be guided by the prevalence of specific conditions in the community and clinical judgment.

[c] The organisms listed in this column are not intended to represent the complete or even most likely diagnoses but, rather, possible causative agents that require additional precautions beyond **Standard Precautions** until a causative agent can be excluded.

[d] Duration of isolation varies by agent and the antimicrobial treatment administered.

[e] These pathogens include Shiga toxin-producing *Escherichia coli* including *E coli* O157:H7, *Shigella* organisms, *Salmonella* organisms, *Campylobacter* organisms, hepatitis A virus, enteric viruses including rotavirus, *Cryptosporidium* organisms, and *Giardia* organisms. Use masks when cleaning vomitus or stool during norovirus outbreak.

[f] Resistant organisms judged by the infection control program on the basis of current state, regional, or national recommendations to be of special clinical or epidemiologic significance.

of health care personnel to body fluids. Standard Precautions are used with all patients and during all contacts, even when exposure to blood and body fluids is not anticipated. Standard Precautions are designed to decrease transmission of microorganisms from patients who are not recognized as harboring potential pathogens, such as bloodborne pathogens and antibiotic-resistant bacteria. Standard Precautions include the following practices:

- **Respiratory hygiene/cough etiquette (www.cdc.gov/flu/professionals/ infectioncontrol/resphygiene.htm)** includes source containment of infectious respiratory tract secretions in symptomatic patients beginning at the initial point of encounter (eg, triage and reception areas in emergency departments). Symptomatic children should cover mouth/nose when sneezing/coughing; use tissues and dispose in no-touch receptacle; observe hand hygiene after soiling of hands with respiratory tract secretions; and wear a surgical mask if tolerated or maintain spatial separation more than 3 feet, if possible.
- **Hand hygiene (www.cdc.gov/handhygiene/)** is necessary before and after all patient contact and after touching blood, body fluids, secretions, excretions, and contaminated items, whether gloves are worn or not. Hand hygiene should also be performed after contact with the patient environment to ensure that the health care provider is not transmitting potential pathogens from contaminated surfaces that surround the patient. Hand hygiene should be performed either with alcohol-based agents or with soap and water before donning and immediately after removing (doffing) gloves (even if visible soiling did not occur) and when otherwise indicated to avoid transfer of microorganisms to other patients and to items in the

environment. A helpful reference is the World Health Organization's 5 Moments for Hand Hygiene (**www.who.int/gpsc/5may/Hand_Hygiene_Why_How_and_When_Brochure.pdf**). When hands are visibly dirty or contaminated with proteinaceous material, such as blood or other body fluids, hands should be washed with soap and water for at least 20 seconds. The best means of preventing transmission of spores (eg, *Clostridioides difficile*) or norovirus is not clear, but handwashing with soap and water is preferred over alcohol-based agents.

- **Gloves** (clean, nonsterile, single use) should be worn when touching blood, body fluids, secretions, excretions, and items contaminated with these fluids, except for wiping a child's tears or nose or for routine wet diaper changing for the well child. Clean gloves should be used by health care providers before touching mucous membranes and nonintact skin or if contact with body fluids is possible. Gloves should be changed after contact with potentially infectious material (eg, purulent drainage) and between tasks and procedures on the same patient.
- **Masks, eye protection, and face shields** should be worn to protect mucous membranes of the eyes, nose, and mouth during procedures and patient care activities likely to generate splashes or sprays of blood, body fluids, secretions, or excretions. Surgical masks should be worn when placing a catheter or injecting material into the spinal canal or subdural space (eg, during myelograms and spinal or epidural anesthesia).
- **Nonsterile gowns** that are fluid-resistant will protect skin and prevent soiling of clothing during procedures and patient care activities likely to generate splashes or sprays of blood, body fluids, secretions, or excretions. Soiled gowns should be removed promptly and carefully to avoid contamination of clothing.
- **Patient care equipment** that has been used should be handled in a manner that prevents skin or mucous membrane exposures and contamination of clothing or the environment and should be cleaned according to manufacturer's recommendations.
- **All used textiles (linens)** are considered to be contaminated and should be handled, transported, and processed in a manner that prevents aerosolization of microorganisms, skin and mucous membrane exposure, and contamination of clothing.
- **Care of the environment,** which includes shared toys and high-touch surfaces, requires that policies and procedures are established for routine and targeted cleaning of environmental surfaces as indicated by the level of patient contact and degree of soiling. A product registered by the Environmental Protection Agency that has activity against the organisms most likely present in the environment should be used.
- **Safe injection practices** should be followed to prevent risks to patients and health care providers. Syringes should *never* be reused for more than one patient or to access shared medication containers. Likewise, insulin pens and lancing devices must not be used for multiple patients. Do not use medications packaged as single-dose or single-use for more than one patient. Limit the use of multidose vials and dedicate them to a single patient whenever possible. More information is available from the CDC at **www.cdc.gov/injectionsafety.** Bloodborne pathogen exposure of health care personnel should be avoided by taking precautions to prevent injuries caused by needles, scalpels, and other sharp instruments or devices during procedures; when handling sharp instruments after procedures; when cleaning used instruments; and during disposal of used needles. To prevent needlestick injuries, safety devices should be used whenever they are available. Needles should not be

recapped, purposely bent or broken by hand, removed from disposable syringes, or otherwise manipulated by hand. After use, disposable syringes and needles, scalpel blades, and other sharp items should be placed in puncture-resistant containers for disposal; puncture-resistant containers should be located as close as practical to the use area. Large-bore reusable needles should be placed in a puncture-resistant container located close to the site of use for transport to the reprocessing area to ensure maximal patient safety. Sharp devices with safety features are preferred whenever such devices have equivalent function to conventional sharp devices.

- **Mouthpieces, resuscitation bags, and other ventilation devices** should be available in all patient care areas and used instead of mouth-to-mouth resuscitation.
- **Point-of-use equipment cleaning** (eg, stethoscopes, otoscopes) should be performed.

TRANSMISSION-BASED PRECAUTIONS

Transmission-Based Precautions are designed for patients documented or suspected to have colonization or infection with pathogens for which additional precautions beyond **Standard Precautions** are recommended to prevent transmission. The 3 types of transmission routes on which these precautions are based are airborne, droplet, and contact.

- **Airborne transmission** occurs by dissemination of airborne droplet nuclei (small-particle residue [≤5 μm in size] of evaporated droplets containing microorganisms that remain suspended in the air for long periods) or small respirable particles containing the infectious agent or spores. Microorganisms transmitted by the airborne route can be dispersed widely by air currents and can be inhaled by a susceptible host within the same room or a long distance from the source patient, depending on environmental factors. Special air handling and ventilation are required to prevent airborne transmission. Some examples of microorganisms transmitted by airborne droplet nuclei are *Mycobacterium tuberculosis*, measles virus, and varicella-zoster virus. Specific recommendations for **Airborne Precautions** are as follows:
  - Patients with infection or colonization should be provided with a single-patient room (if unavailable, consult an infection preventionist), and the door should be kept closed at all times.
  - Special ventilation should be used, including 6 to 12 air changes per hour, air flow direction from the surrounding area to the room ("negative pressure"), and room air exhausted directly to the outside or recirculated through a high-efficiency particulate air (HEPA) filter.
  - If infectious pulmonary tuberculosis is suspected or proven, respiratory protective devices (ie, National Institute for Occupational Safety and Health-certified personally "fitted" and "sealing" respirator, such as N95 or N100 respirators, or powered air-purifying respirators) should be worn while inside the patient's room. Respirators should be removed after leaving the patient's room.
  - Susceptible health care personnel should not enter rooms of patients with measles or varicella-zoster virus infections. If susceptible people must enter the room of a patient with measles or varicella infection or an immunocompromised patient with local or disseminated zoster infection, a respiratory protective device, such as an N95 (fit-tested) or a powered air-purifying respirator, should be worn. People with proven immunity to varicella need not wear a mask, but in caring for patients with

measles, *all* health care personnel, including those immunized, must wear respiratory protective devices.

  ◆ Airborne, droplet, and contact precautions are recommended for patients with suspected or known SARS-CoV-2 or MERS-CoV infection (including eye protection [face shield or goggles], N95 or higher respirator [or medical mask if not available], gown, and gloves; for aerosol-generating procedures, an N95 or higher respirator should be used). Airborne infection isolation rooms should be prioritized for aerosol-generating procedures. A well-ventilated single-occupancy room with a closed door may be used if aerosol-generating procedures are not performed. Detailed guidance is available on the CDC website (**www.cdc.gov/coronavirus/2019-ncov/hcp/infection-control-recommendations.html**).

• **Droplet transmission** occurs when respiratory droplets containing microorganisms are generated from an infected person, primarily during coughing, sneezing, or talking, and during the performance of certain procedures, such as suctioning and bronchoscopy, and are propelled a short distance (generally less than 3 feet, but in some cases may be more) and deposited into conjunctivae, nasal mucosa, or the mouth of a susceptible person. Because these relatively large droplets do not remain suspended in air, special air handling and ventilation are not required to prevent droplet transmission. Droplet transmission should not be confused with airborne transmission via droplet nuclei, which are much smaller. A few of examples of the many microorganisms transmitted by droplets are *Bordetella pertussis*, group A *Streptococcus* species, rhinovirus, influenza virus, and *Neisseria meningitidis* (see **www.cdc.gov/infectioncontrol/guidelines/isolation/appendix/type-duration-precautions.html#C**). Specific recommendations for **Droplet Precautions** are as follows:

  ◆ The patient should be provided with a single-patient room, if possible. If unavailable, the facility may consider cohorting patients infected with the same organism. Spatial separation of more than 6 feet should be maintained between the bed of the infected patient and the beds of the other patients in multiple-bed rooms. Standard precautions plus a mask should be used.

  ◆ A mask and eye protection or face shield should be worn on entry into the room or into the cubical space, and droplet precautions should be maintained when within 3 to 6 feet of the patient.

  ◆ Masks and other personal protective equipment (PPE) should be removed before leaving the room or caring for another patient in the same room. Hand hygiene should be performed after PPE removal.

  ◆ Children being transported within the health care facility who are old enough to tolerate wearing a mask should wear one; no mask is needed for people transporting the patient.

• **Contact transmission** is the most common route of transmission of HAIs. *Direct contact* transmission involves the physical transfer of microorganisms from a person with infection or colonization to a susceptible host through direct contact with infectious agents, such as occurs when a health care professional examines a patient or performs other patient care activities that require direct personal contact. Direct contact transmission also can occur between 2 patients when one serves as the source of the infectious microorganisms and the other serves as a susceptible host. *Indirect contact* transmission involves contact of a susceptible host with a contaminated intermediate object ("fomite"), usually inanimate, such as contaminated instruments, needles, dressings, toys, or contaminated hands that are not cleansed or gloves that are not changed between patients. A few examples of the many microorganisms transmitted by contact include respiratory syncytial virus, *C difficile,* enterovirus, *Salmonella* species, *Shigella* species, and Shiga toxin-producing *Escherichia coli.* In addition, specific illnesses requiring **Contact Precautions** include the following:

+ Conjunctivitis, viral, and hemorrhagic.
+ Colonization or infection with a specific multidrug-resistant organism (MDRO), as determined by the facility's infection prevention and control program on the basis of current state, regional, or national recommendations to be of special clinical and epidemiologic significance (eg, carbapenemase-producing gram-negative bacilli, *Candida auris,* other MDROs), or another epidemiologically important organism (which may or may not be an MDRO). Information on the containment strategy by the CDC for responding to emerging antibiotic resistant threats is available on the CDC website (**www.cdc.gov/hai/containment/index.html**).

Specific recommendations for **Contact Precautions** are as follows:
+ The patient should be provided with a single-patient room if possible. If unavailable, cohorting patients likely to be infected with the same organism and use of Standard Precautions and Contact Precautions are permissible.
+ Gloves (clean, nonsterile, single use) should be used at all times.
+ Gown and gloves should be used on entry into a patient room and during direct contact with a patient, environmental surfaces, or items in the patient room and should be removed before leaving the patient's room or area.
+ When transport or movement in any health care facility is necessary, infected or colonized areas of the patient's body should be contained and covered.
+ Disposable noncritical patient-care equipment (eg, blood pressure cuffs) should be used, or patient-dedicated use of such equipment should be implemented. If common use of equipment for multiple patients is unavoidable, such equipment should be cleaned and disinfected per manufacturer's recommendations before use on another patient.

Airborne, Droplet, and **Contact Precautions** should be combined for diseases caused by organisms that have multiple routes of transmission. If available testing cannot differentiate between 2 organisms, the recommended precautions for each organism should be combined. When used alone or in combination, these **Transmission-Based Precautions** always are to be used in addition to **Standard Precautions,** which are recommended for all patients. The care of patients with a few highly transmissible and highly lethal infections, such as Ebola virus, requires extensive infection prevention and control measures (**www.cdc.gov/vhf/ebola/clinicians/evd/infection-control.html**).

PEDIATRIC CONSIDERATIONS

Unique differences in pediatric care necessitate modifications of these guidelines, including the following: (1) diaper changing and wiping a child's tears or nose; (2) use of single-patient room isolation; and (3) use of common areas, such as hospital waiting rooms, playrooms, and schoolrooms. More patients and their sibling visitors with transmissible infections may be present in pediatric health care settings, especially during seasonal epidemics.

Because diapering or wiping a child's nose or tears does not soil hands routinely, wearing gloves is not mandatory except when gloves are required as part of **Transmission-Based Precautions.** Meticulous hand hygiene recommendations should always be followed.

Single-patient rooms are recommended for all patients for **Transmission-Based Precautions** (ie, **Airborne, Droplet,** and **Contact**). Single-patient rooms can also be prioritized if the patient is at increased risk of acquiring infection or developing an adverse outcome following infection. Patients placed on **Transmission-Based Precautions** should not leave their rooms to use common areas on the unit, such as child life playrooms, schoolrooms, or waiting areas, or elsewhere in the hospital, such as cafeteria or gift shop, except under special circumstances as defined by the facility's infection preventionist. The guidelines for **Standard Precautions** state that patients who cannot control body excretions should be in single-patient rooms. Because most young children are incontinent, this recommendation does not apply to routine care of uninfected children.

The Society for Healthcare Epidemiology of America has published infection prevention and control guidelines for pediatric residential facilities. Although older adults are the typical residents in long-term care facilities, children may receive long-term care. In these settings, precautions may be modified to "as least restrictive" for activities of daily living of the resident. For specific questions, consultation with a pediatric infection prevention and control specialist is advised. The CDC has developed guidance for containment of novel or targeted MDROs in the long-term care setting (**www.cdc.gov/hai/containment/PPE-Nursing-Homes.html**). Information about infections and the need for precautions should be communicated clearly when patients are transferred between health care facilities.

Strategies to Prevent Health Care-Associated Infections

HAIs in patients in acute care hospitals are associated with substantial morbidity. Important infections include central line-associated bloodstream infections, central nervous system shunt infections, surgical site infections, urinary catheter-associated urinary tract infections, ventilator-associated pneumonias, infections caused by viruses (eg, respiratory syncytial virus, rotavirus), and colitis attributable to *C difficile*. Infection prevention strategies exist for each of these infections. Evidence-based protocols have been shown to reduce HAIs by using "bundled strategies" (when multiple prevention activities are implemented simultaneously) and with multidisciplinary participation from members of the health care team, including administrators, physicians, nurses, therapists, and housekeeping services. Studies in pediatrics have demonstrated bundles to be effective in reducing central line-associated bloodstream infections, surgical site infections, and ventilator-associated pneumonias. Recommendations are available (**www.solutionsforpatientsafety.org/wp-content/uploads/SPS-Prevention-Bundles.pdf** and **www.cdc.gov/infectioncontrol/guidelines/BSI/index.html**).

Occupational Health

Transmission of infectious agents within health care settings is facilitated by close contact between patients and health care personnel and by lack of hygienic practices by infants and young children. **Standard Precautions** and **Transmission-Based Precautions** are designed to prevent transmission of infectious agents in health care settings among patients and health care personnel. To further limit risks of transmission of organisms between children and health care personnel, health care facilities should have established personnel health policies and services. Specifically, personnel should be protected against vaccine-preventable diseases by establishing appropriate screening and immunization policies. Guidelines for immunization of health care personnel are available (**www.cdc.gov/vaccines/adults/rec-vac/hcw.html**).

For infections that are not vaccine preventable, personnel should be counseled about exposures and the possible need for leave from work if they are exposed to, ill with, or a carrier of a specific pathogen, whether the exposure occurs in the home, community, or health care setting.

The frequency and need for screening of health care personnel for tuberculosis should be determined by local epidemiologic data; the CDC has published guidance for the prevention of transmission of tuberculosis in health care settings (**www.cdc.gov/tb/default.htm** and **www.cdc.gov/tb/publications/guidelines/infectioncontrol.htm**). People with commonly occurring infections, such as gastroenteritis, dermatitis, herpes simplex virus lesions on exposed skin, or upper respiratory tract infections, should be evaluated to determine the risk of transmission to patients or to other health care personnel.

Health care personnel education, including understanding of hospital policies, is of paramount importance in infection prevention and control. Pediatric health care personnel should be knowledgeable about the modes of transmission of infectious agents, proper hand hygiene techniques, and serious risks to children from certain mild infections in adults. Frequent educational sessions will reinforce safe techniques and the importance of infection prevention and control policies. Written policies and procedures relating to needlestick or sharp injuries are mandated by the Occupational Safety and Health Administration (**www.osha.gov**).

Pregnant health care personnel who follow recommended precautions should not be at increased risk of infections that have possible adverse effects on the fetus (eg, parvovirus B19, cytomegalovirus, rubella, varicella, and Zika). Pregnant personnel should not care for immunocompromised patients with chronic parvovirus B19 infection or for those with parvovirus B19-associated aplastic crisis, because both groups are likely to be contagious. Pregnant personnel should avoid caring for those receiving aerosolized ribavirin therapy (risk of teratogenicity). The risk of severe influenza infection for pregnant health care personnel can be reduced by influenza immunization and adherence to appropriate infection prevention and control precautions.

Personnel who are immunocompromised and at increased risk of severe infection (eg, *M tuberculosis*, measles virus, herpes simplex virus, and varicella-zoster virus) should seek advice from their primary health care professional.

The consequences to pediatric patients of acquiring infections from adults can be significant. Mild illnesses in adults, such as viral gastroenteritis, upper respiratory tract viral infection, pertussis, or herpes simplex virus infection, can cause life-threatening disease in infants and children. People at greatest risk are preterm infants, children who have heart disease or chronic pulmonary disease, and people who are immunocompromised.

Sibling Visitation

Sibling visits to birthing centers, postpartum rooms, pediatric wards, and intensive care units are encouraged, although some institutions restrict visitation of young children during times of peak respiratory viral activity because of their relatively high frequency of asymptomatic viral shedding and difficulties adhering to basic respiratory etiquette and hand hygiene practices. Neonatal intensive care often results in long hospital stays for the preterm or sick newborn infant, making family visits important.

Sibling visits may benefit hospitalized children. Guidelines for sibling visits should be established to maximize opportunities for visiting and to minimize the risks of transmission of pathogens brought into the hospital setting by young visitors. Guidelines may need to be modified by local nursing, pediatric, obstetric, and infectious diseases staff members to address specific issues in their hospital settings. Basic guidelines for sibling visits to pediatric patients are as follows:

- Before the visit, a trained health care professional should interview the parents at a site outside the unit to assess the health of each sibling visitor. These interviews should be documented, and approval for each sibling visit should be noted. No child with fever or symptoms of an acute infection, including upper respiratory tract infection, gastroenteritis, or cellulitis, should be allowed to visit. Siblings who recently have been exposed to a person with a known communicable disease and are susceptible should not be allowed to visit.
- Siblings who are visiting should have received all recommended immunizations for their age. Before and during influenza season, siblings who visit should have received influenza vaccine.
- Asymptomatic siblings who recently have been exposed to varicella but have been immunized previously can be assumed to be immune.
- The visiting sibling should visit only his or her sibling and not be allowed in playrooms with groups of patients.
- Children should perform recommended hand hygiene before entry into the health care setting and before and after any patient contact, and as otherwise recommended (after toilet, before eating, etc).
- Throughout the visit, sibling activity should be supervised by parents or a responsible adult and limited to the mother's or patient's room or other designated areas where other patients are not present.

Adult Visitation

Guidelines should be established for visits by other relatives and close friends. Guidelines may need to be modified by hospital staff to address specific issues. People with fever or contagious illnesses should not visit. Medical and nursing staff members should be vigilant about potential communicable diseases in parents and other adult visitors (eg, a relative with a cough who may have pertussis or tuberculosis; a parent with a cold visiting a highly immunosuppressed child). Before and during influenza season, all visitors should be encouraged to have received the influenza vaccine. Adherence to these guidelines is especially important for areas of hospitals such as oncology, hematopoietic stem cell transplant, and neonatal intensive care units.

Pet Visitation

- Pet visitation in the health care setting includes visits by a child's personal pet and pet visitation as a part of child life therapeutic programs. Guidelines for pet visitation should be established to minimize risks of transmission of pathogens from pets to humans or injury from animals. The specific health care setting and the level of concern for zoonotic disease will influence establishment of pet visitation policies. The pet visitation policy should be developed in consultation with pediatricians, infection preventionists, nursing staff, the hospital epidemiologist, and veterinarians. Resources for such policies are available.[1]
- Patients having contact with pets must have approval from the patient's physician, nurse, and the facility's infection prevention and control program prior to the visit. For patients who are immunodeficient or for people receiving immunosuppressive therapy, the risks of exposure to the microflora of pets may outweigh the benefits of contact. Contact of children with pets should be approved on a case-by-case basis.
- Personal pets other than dogs should be excluded from the hospital. Pets should be housebroken and at least 1 year of age. Exceptions may be made for end-of-life patients who are in single-patient rooms.
- Visiting pets should have a certificate of immunization from a licensed veterinarian and verification that the pet is healthy. Some institutions require an assessment of temperament (eg, Canine Good Citizen certificate).
- The pet should be bathed and groomed for the visit.
- Pet visitation should be discouraged in an intensive care unit or hematology-oncology unit, but individual circumstances can be considered; involvement with the infection control and prevention team is recommended.
- The visit of a pet should also be approved by an appropriate personnel member (eg, the director of the child life therapy program), who should observe the pet for temperament and general health at the time of visit. The pet should be free of obvious bacterial skin infections, infections caused by superficial dermatophytes, and ectoparasites (fleas and ticks).
- Pet visitation should be confined to designated areas. Contact should be confined to the petting and holding of animals, as appropriate. All contact should be supervised throughout the visit by appropriate personnel and should be followed by hand hygiene performed by the patient and all who had contact with the pet. Supervisors should be familiar with institutional policies for managing animal bites and cleaning pet urine, feces, or vomitus.
- Care should be taken to protect all indwelling devices, including catheter exit sites (eg, central venous catheters, peritoneal dialysis catheters). These sites should have

---

[1]Murthy R, Bearman G, Brown S, et al. SHEA Expert Guidance. Animals in healthcare facilities: recommendations to minimize potential risks. *Infect Control Hosp Epidemiol.* 2015;36(50):495-516. Available at: **www.shea-online.org/index.php/practice-resources/41-current-guidelines/421-expert-guidance-animals-in-healthcare-facilities-recommendations-to-minimize-potential-risks**

semi-occlusive dressings whenever possible that will provide an effective barrier to pet contact, including licking, and be covered with clothing or gown. Concern for contamination of other body sites should be considered on a case-by-case basis.

- The pet policy should not apply to professionally trained service animals. These animals are not pets and separate policies should govern their uses and presence in the hospital, according to the requirements of the Americans with Disabilities Act.

INFECTION PREVENTION AND CONTROL IN AMBULATORY SETTINGS

Infection prevention and control is an integral part of pediatric practice in ambulatory care settings.[1] All health care personnel should be aware of the routes of transmission and techniques to prevent transmission of infectious agents. Written policies and procedures for infection prevention and control should be readily available, implemented, updated regularly, and enforced. Facilities should have ready access to an individual with training in infection prevention and control. **Standard Precautions,** as outlined for the hospitalized child (see Infection Prevention and Control for Hospitalized Children, p 133) and by the Centers for Disease Prevention and Control (CDC),[2] with a modification by the American Academy of Pediatrics exempting the use of gloves for routine diaper changes and wiping a child's nose or eyes,[1] are appropriate for most patient encounters. The CDC has created a guideline and a checklist (**www. cdc.gov/infectioncontrol/pdf/outpatient/guide.pdf** and **www.cdc.gov/ infectioncontrol/pdf/outpatient/guidechecklist.pdf**) that health care professionals can use to ensure that appropriate infection-control practices are being followed and, thus, reduce ambulatory health care-associated infections. Key principles of infection prevention and control in an outpatient setting are as follows:

- Infection prevention and control should begin when the child's appointment is scheduled (eg, triage questions, such as travel, exposures, and symptoms, may guide additional precautions for when the patient arrives) and initiated when the child enters the office or clinic.
- **Standard Precautions** should be used when caring for all patients. **Standard Precautions** are supplemented by **Transmission-Based Precautions** and should include instructions to health care personnel on the proper donning and removal (doffing) of personal protective equipment (gowns, masks, protective eyewear [or face shield], and gloves). Any individual on the care team entering the room should follow the appropriate precautions, regardless of whether the patient is being examined. Contact between contagious children and uninfected children should be minimized. Children who are suspected of having highly contagious infections, such as varicella or measles, should be promptly isolated by removing them

[1]Rathore MH, Jackson MA; American Academy of Pediatrics, Committee on Infectious Diseases. Infection prevention and control in pediatric ambulatory settings. *Pediatrics.* 2017;140(5):e20172857

[2]Centers for Disease Control and Prevention. Guideline for isolation precautions: preventing transmission of infectious agents in health care settings 2007. Recommendations of the Healthcare Infection Control Practices Advisory Committee. Atlanta, GA: Centers for Disease Control and Prevention; 2007. Available at: **www.cdc.gov/hicpac/2007IP/2007isolationPrecautions.html**

from the waiting room and placing them in an examination room with the door closed. Neonates and immunocompromised children should be promptly placed in a room and kept away from people with potentially contagious infections.

- In waiting rooms of ambulatory care facilities, respiratory hygiene/cough etiquette and use of masks should be implemented for patients and accompanying people with suspected respiratory tract infection.[1]
  - Patients with cystic fibrosis who are in the waiting room should be masked (mask may be removed in the examination room). If it is not feasible to use separate waiting areas to prevent contact between patients with cystic fibrosis, a minimum of 6 feet should be used to ensure their separation (this does not apply to members of the same household). It is recommended that patients with cystic fibrosis be taken directly to an examination room after arrival, whenever possible.[2] Health care providers should use contact precautions (gown and gloves) when taking care of a patient with cystic fibrosis.
- All health care personnel should perform hand hygiene before and after each patient contact. In health care settings, alcohol-based hand products are preferred for decontaminating hands routinely. Soap and water are preferred when hands are visibly dirty or contaminated with proteinaceous material, such as blood or other body fluids, and after caring for a patient with known or suspected infectious diarrhea (eg, *Clostridioides difficile* or norovirus). Parents and children should be taught the importance of hand hygiene. Guidelines on hand hygiene can be found on the CDC website (**www.cdc.gov/handhygiene/providers/guideline.html**).
- Health care personnel should receive influenza vaccination annually as well as vaccinations against other vaccine-preventable infections that can be transmitted in an ambulatory setting to patients or to other health care personnel. Recommended vaccines include influenza; tetanus toxoid, reduced diphtheria toxoid, and acellular pertussis (Tdap); measles, mumps, and rubella (MMR); varicella; and hepatitis B. The latest recommendations can be found at **www.cdc.gov/vaccines/adults/rec-vac/hcw.html.** Health care personnel do not need to take additional action regarding measles vaccination if they have written documentation of 2 doses of MMR or laboratory-confirmed measles or laboratory evidence of immunity (positive immunoglobulin G [IgG] titers). Those who were born before 1957 are generally considered immune; however, if no other evidence of immunity exists, administering 2 doses of MMR should be considered and is recommended in an outbreak.
- Depending on the setting where they work, health care personnel should be familiar with aseptic technique, particularly regarding insertion or manipulation of intravascular catheters, performance of other invasive procedures, and preparation and administration of parenteral medications. Aseptic technique includes selection and use of appropriate skin antiseptics. The preferred skin-preparation agent for

---

[1] Centers for Disease Control and Prevention. Respiratory Hygiene/Cough Etiquette in Healthcare Settings. Available at: **www.cdc.gov/flu/professionals/infectioncontrol/resphygiene.htm**

[2] Saiman L, Seigel JD, LiPuma JJ, et al. Infection prevention and control guideline for cystic fibrosis: 2013 update. Infect Control Hosp Epidemiol. 2014;35(Suppl 1): S1-S67. Available at: **www.cff.org/Care/Clinical-Care-Guidelines/Infection-Prevention-and-Control-Clinical-Care-Guidelines/Infection-Prevention-and-Control-Clinical-Care-Guidelines/**

immunization and venipuncture for routine blood collection is 70% isopropyl alcohol. For incision, suture, and collection of blood for culture, skin preparation with either 2% chlorhexidine gluconate (CHG) in 70% isopropyl alcohol–based solutions (for children older than 2 months) or iodine (1% or 2% tincture of iodine, 2% povidone-iodine) should be used.

- Whenever available, medical devices designed to reduce the risk of needle sticks should be used. Sharps disposal containers that are impermeable and puncture resistant should be placed immediately adjacent to the areas where sharps are used (eg, areas where injections or venipunctures are performed). Sharps containers should be replaced when they are two-thirds full and kept out of reach of young children. Policies should be established for removal and the disposal of sharps containers consistent with state and local regulations. Guidance on safe injection practices is available on the CDC website (**www.cdc.gov/injectionsafety/**).

- Appropriate handling of medical waste should be outlined (**www.cdc.gov/infectioncontrol/pdf/outpatient/guide.pdf**).

- A written bloodborne pathogen exposure control plan that includes policies for management of exposures to blood and body fluids, such as through needlesticks and exposures of nonintact skin and mucous membranes, should be developed, readily available to all staff, and updated and reviewed with staff regularly (at least annually) (see Hepatitis B, p 381; Hepatitis C, p 399; and Human Immunodeficiency Virus Infection, p 427, and **www.cdc.gov/niosh/topics/bbp/guidelines.html**).

- Manufacturer's guidelines for processing of medical devices and equipment, including decontamination, disinfection, and sterilization, should be followed meticulously. Once sterilized, devices and equipment should be kept in their sterile packaging until immediately prior to use.

- Cleaning of point-of-use equipment (eg, stethoscopes, otoscopes) should be performed.

- Policies and procedures should be established for cleaning and disinfection of environmental surfaces and general housekeeping. Patients can be encouraged to bring their own toys. If toys are available in waiting areas, they should be disposable or able to be cleaned and disinfected or sanitized between each use.[1]

- Appropriate use of antimicrobial agents is essential to limit the emergence and spread of drug-resistant bacteria (see Antimicrobial Stewardship, p 868).

- Policies and procedures should be developed for communication with local and state health authorities about reportable diseases and suspected outbreaks (**wwwn.cdc.gov/nndss/ and www.cdc.gov/hai/outbreaks/**).

- Educational programs for health care personnel that encompass appropriate aspects of infection control should be implemented, reinforced, documented, and evaluated on a regular basis.

- Outpatient facilities and practices should have access to an individual with training in infection prevention who manages the infection prevention program.

- Physicians should be aware of requirements of government agencies, such as the Occupational Safety and Health Administration (OSHA), as well as state and federal regulations that may apply to the operation of physicians' offices.

[1]Rathore MH, Jackson MA; American Academy of Pediatrics, Committee on Infectious Diseases. Infection prevention and control in pediatric ambulatory settings. *Pediatrics*. 2017;140(5):e20172857

SEXUALLY TRANSMITTED INFECTIONS IN ADOLESCENTS AND CHILDREN

Physicians and other health care professionals perform a critical role in preventing and treating sexually transmitted infections (STIs) in the pediatric and adolescent population. STIs are a major problem for adolescents; an estimated 25% of adolescent females will acquire an STI by 19 years of age. Although an STI in an infant or child early in life can be the result of vertical transmission, nonabusive horizontal transmission, or autoinoculation, STIs (eg, gonorrhea, syphilis, chlamydia, genital herpes, human immunodeficiency virus [HIV] infection, trichomoniasis, or anogenital warts) should raise suspicion of sexual abuse if acquired after the neonatal period. Whenever sexual abuse is suspected, appropriate social service and law enforcement agencies must be involved to evaluate the situation further, to ensure the child or adolescent's protection, and to provide appropriate counseling. When available, consultation with a child abuse pediatrician can help guide further evaluation, aid in decision making on reporting suspected abuse, and assist with rendering an opinion on the etiology of the STI.

STIs During Preventive Health Care of Adolescents

EPIDEMIOLOGY OF STIs IN ADOLESCENTS

Adolescents and young adults have the highest rates of several STIs when compared with any other age group. Adolescents are at greater risk of STIs because of their sexual behavior, access to health care, lack of education, and increased biologic susceptibility. In addition, adolescents may face several potential obstacles in accessing confidential reproductive health care services.[1] Young men, particularly men of color, men who have sex with men (MSM), and transgender women, are at particularly high risk of STIs, including HIV infection. Health care professionals frequently fail to confidentially ask adolescents and young adults about sexual behaviors, assess for STI risks, counsel about risk reduction, and screen for STIs.[2]

EVALUATION OF STIs IN ADOLESCENTS

At each health care visit, the health care provider should allow some private time, apart from the parent(s) or guardian(s), to speak with the adolescent confidentially.[3] Health care professionals should become familiar with local statutes on minors' consent for HIV and STI services to prepare patients and families by educating both parents and preadolescents about the need for confidentiality as adolescence approaches. Pediatricians should screen for STI risk by *routinely* asking all adolescent and young adult patients—apart from their parents—whether they ever have had

---

[1]Centers for Disease Control and Prevention. *Sexually Transmitted Disease Surveillance 2018*. Atlanta, GA: US Department of Health and Human Services; 2019

[2] US Preventive Services Task Force. Behavioral counseling interventions to prevent sexually transmitted infections: US Preventive Services Task Force recommendation statement. *JAMA*. 2020;324(7):674-681. doi:10.1001/jama.2020.13095

[3]The Society for Adolescent Health and Medicine and the American Academy of Pediatrics. Position paper: confidentiality protections for adolescents and young adults in the health care billing and insurance claims process. *J Adolesc Health*. 2016;58(3):374-377

sexual intercourse, currently are sexually active, or are planning to be sexually active in the near future, as well as about gender identity and sexual orientation. Pediatricians must be sure to define the terms "sexual intercourse," "gender identity," "sexual orientation," and "sexually active," because these terms can have different meanings for adolescents. It is important that adolescents and young adults are educated to recognize that noncoital practices (oral/genital contact, anal intercourse, and hand/genital contact), as well as vaginal intercourse, put them at risk of STIs. If a patient indicates a history of sexual activity, the health care professional must further ascertain the particular types of sexual contact, partner gender, and number of partners to determine what type(s) of STI testing to perform. More detailed recommendations for preventive health care for adolescents and young adults are available from the American Academy of Pediatrics (AAP)[1] and Centers for Disease Control and Prevention (CDC).[2]

TREATMENT OF STIs IN ADOLESCENTS

All 50 states allow minors to give their own consent for confidential STI testing and treatment. Pediatricians should consult their own state laws for further guidance. For specific STI treatment recommendations, see the disease-specific chapters in Section 3 and Tables 4.4 (p 898) and 4.5 (p 903). Single-dose therapies are available for many STIs, offering the advantage of high patient adherence; directly observed therapy should be provided where feasible. Patients and their partners treated for *Neisseria gonorrhoeae* infection and *Chlamydia trachomatis* infection should be advised to refrain from sexual intercourse for at least 7 days after completion of appropriate treatment.

Partner treatment is essential, both from a public health perspective and to protect the infected patient from reinfection. Sexual partners during the past 60 days should be informed of exposure to the infection and encouraged to seek comprehensive STI evaluation and treatment. Health departments typically attempt to notify sex partners of patients infected with HIV or syphilis and bring them in for treatment. Depending on health department resources, partner services may be offered for some gonorrhea cases and occasionally for chlamydia. If it appears unlikely that partners of patients treated for gonococcal or chlamydial infections will seek care, pediatricians may consider providing expedited partner therapy (EPT) to patients in states where EPT is permissible.[2] EPT is the clinical practice of treating the sex partners of patients with diagnosed chlamydia or gonorrhea by providing prescriptions or medications to the patient to take to his or her partner without the health care professional first examining the partner. Information should include warning about the low risk of potential adverse events with EPT, with instructions to seek medical attention in the event that an adverse reaction occurs. Published studies suggest that >5% of MSM without a previous HIV diagnosis have a new diagnosis of HIV infection when evaluated as a partner of patients with gonorrhea or chlamydia. Hence, EPT should not be considered a routine partner management strategy in MSM because of the high risk of coexisting undiagnosed STIs or HIV infection. Guidance on the legal status of EPT by jurisdiction is available from the CDC (**www.cdc.gov/std/ept/legal/**).

---

[1]American Academy of Pediatrics, Committee on Adolescence; Society for Adolescent Health and Medicine. Screening for nonviral sexually transmitted infections in adolescents and young adults. *Pediatrics.* 2014;134(1):e302-e311

[2]Centers for Disease Control and Prevention. Sexually transmitted infections treatment guidelines, 2021. *MMWR Recomm Rep.* 2021; in press. Available at: **www.cdc.gov/std/treatment**

PREVENTION OF STIs IN ADOLESCENTS

Pediatricians and other health care professionals can contribute to STI primary prevention by encouraging and supporting a teenager's decision to postpone initiating sexual intercourse. For teenagers who become sexually active or are planning to be sexually active in the near future, pediatricians should discuss methods of protecting against STIs and pregnancies, including the correct and consistent use of male and female condoms with all forms of sexual intercourse (vaginal, oral, and anal). Enhanced risk counseling should be targeted for teenagers who engage in illicit drug use or who are in juvenile detention facilities, for whom consent abilities may be compromised or absent and risk of assault may be increased. Teenagers need to be specifically counseled to consider the association between alcohol or drug use and failure to appropriately use barrier methods correctly when either partner is impaired. Health care professionals should discuss other ways to decrease risk of acquiring STIs, including limiting the number of sex partners and choosing to abstain even if initiation of sexual intercourse already has occurred. Pediatricians should educate parents and adolescents how to recognize symptoms of STIs and to contact their provider for evaluation and treatment when symptoms occur. Adolescents and young adults who have not previously been vaccinated against human papillomavirus (HPV) or hepatitis B virus should complete those immunization series.

Pediatricians should counsel their adolescent and young adult patients at substantial risk for HIV infection about preexposure prophylaxis (PrEP) as an effective strategy to prevent HIV infection. A combination of 2 HIV antiretroviral medications (tenofovir and emtricitabine), sold under the name Truvada, is approved for daily use as PrEP to help prevent an HIV-negative person from acquiring HIV from an HIV-positive sexual or injection-drug-using partner. The indications for PrEP, initial and follow-up prescribing, and laboratory testing recommendations are the same for adolescents and adults. The American Academy of Pediatrics recommends that youth at substantial risk for HIV acquisition be routinely offered HIV pre-exposure prophylaxis.[1] Guidelines for PrEP from the CDC can be found at **www.cdc.gov/hiv/pdf/risk/prep/cdc-hiv-prep-guide-lines-2017.pdf.** When taken consistently, PrEP has been shown to reduce the risk of HIV infection in people who are at high risk by up to 92%.[2] For sexual transmission, those at substantial risk include MSM, transgender women, or heterosexual males or females whose sexual partner(s) are either HIV positive or at high risk of being infected with HIV, such as people who inject drugs, have bisexual male partners, or engage in prostitution.

Sexual Assault and Abuse in Children and Adolescents/ Young Adults

SUSPECTED SEXUAL VICTIMIZATION

When the suspicion of sexual abuse or assault is raised, pediatricians should know how to respond to and evaluate the child, when to refer the child for evaluation by other professionals, when to report the case to the appropriate investigative agency, and how

---

[1]Hsu KK, Rakhmanina NY; American Academy of Pediatrics, Committee on Pediatric AIDS. Clinical report: Adolescents and young adults: the pediatrician's role in HIV testing and pre- and post-exposure HIV prophylaxis. *Pediatrics*. 2021; In press

[2]Centers for Disease Control and Prevention. US Public Health Service: Preexposure prophylaxis for the prevention of HIV infection in the United States—2017 Update: a clinical practice guideline. Atlanta, GA: Centers for Disease Control and Prevention; March 2018. Available at: **www.cdc.gov/hiv/pdf/risk/prep/cdc-hiv-prep-guidelines-2017.pdf**

Table 2.5. Implications of Commonly Encountered Sexually Transmitted (ST) or Sexually Associated (SA) Infections for Diagnosis and Reporting of Sexual Abuse Among Infants and Prepubertal Children

ST/SA Confirmed	Evidence for Sexual Abuse	Suggested Action
Neisseria gonorrhoeae[a]	Diagnostic	Report[b]
Syphilis[a]	Diagnostic	Report[b]
Human immunodeficiency virus[c]	Diagnostic	Report[b]
Chlamydia trachomatis[a]	Diagnostic	Report[b]
Trichomonas vaginalis[a]	Diagnostic	Report[b]
Anogenital herpes	Suspicious	Consider report[b,d]
Condylomata acuminata (anogenital warts)[a]	Suspicious	Consider report[b,d,e]
Anogenital molluscum contagiosum	Inconclusive	Medical follow-up
Bacterial vaginosis	Inconclusive	Medical follow-up

[a] If not likely to be perinatally acquired and rare vertical transmission is excluded.
[b] Reports should be made to the local or state agency mandated to receive reports of suspected child abuse or neglect.
[c] If not likely to be acquired perinatally or through transfusion.
[d] Unless a clear history of autoinoculation exists.
[e] Report if evidence exists to suspect abuse, including history, physical examination, or other identified infections. Lesions appearing for first time in child >5 years old are more likely due to sexual transmission.
Table adapted from Kellogg N; American Academy of Pediatrics, Committee on Child Abuse and Neglect. The evaluation of sexual abuse in children. *Pediatrics.* 2005;116(2):506–512 (Updated 2013 clinical report [reaffirmed August 2018] available at **http://pediatrics.aappublications.org/content/132/2/e558**) and Centers for Disease Control and Prevention. Sexually transmitted infections treatment guidelines, 2021. *MMWR Recomm Rep.* 2021; in press

to counsel parents to decrease long-term deleterious effects of the abuse.[1] Factors to be considered in assessing the likelihood of sexual abuse in a child with an STI include the biological characteristics of the STI in question, the age of the child, and whether the child reports a history of sexual victimization (see Table 2.5). Preferably, children with concerns about possible sexual abuse would be referred for evaluation and management to a specialized clinic or child advocacy center. In areas without specialized abuse-related services, pediatricians can educate themselves about childhood genital and anal examinations and about how to interview children to get enough information to make appropriate decisions about reporting to child protective service or law enforcement agencies, referring to counseling facilities, or referring to pediatric clinics

[1] Jenny C, Crawford-Jakubiak JE; American Academy of Pediatrics, Committee on Child Abuse and Neglect. The evaluation of children in the primary care setting when sexual abuse is suspected. *Pediatrics.* 2013;132(2):e558-e567 (Reaffirmed August 2018)

specializing in abuse evaluations. The AAP offers a variety of educational materials on child abuse to physicians.[1]

WHEN TO SCREEN FOR STIs IN PREPUBERTAL VICTIMS

STIs are not common in **prepubertal** children evaluated for abuse. Therefore, testing all sites for all pathogens is not recommended if the **prepubertal** child is asymptomatic. Examinations and collection of genital specimens in prepubertal children should be performed by an experienced clinician. Factors that would lead clinicians to consider testing for STI include:

1. Child has experienced penetration or has evidence of recent or healed penetrative injury to the genitals, anus, or oropharynx.
2. Child has been abused by a stranger.
3. Child has been abused by a perpetrator known to be infected with an STI or at high risk for STIs (eg, intravenous drug abusers, MSM, people with multiple sexual partners, and people with a history of STIs).
4. Child has a sibling, other relative, or another person in the household with an STI.
5. Child has signs or symptoms of STIs (eg, vaginal discharge or pain, genital itching or odor, urinary symptoms, and genital lesions or ulcers).
6. Child or parent requests STI testing.
7. Child is unable to verbalize details of assault.

STI EVALUATION OF PREPUBERTAL VICTIMS

When STI screening is performed, it should focus on likely anatomic sites of infection as determined by the patient's history and physical examination. A chaperone should be present at the time of evaluation. In the evaluation of prepubertal children for suspected sexual abuse/assault, the CDC offers the following recommendations[2]:

- Physical examination: Visually inspect the genital, perianal, and oropharyngeal areas for genital discharge, odor, bleeding, irritation, warts, and ulcerative lesions. In addition, if STI testing is indicated, then the following laboratory assessments should be performed.
  - Testing for *N gonorrhoeae* and *C trachomatis* should be performed from specimens collected from the pharynx and anus, as well as the vagina in girls, and urine in boys. Cervical specimens are not recommended for prepubertal girls. For boys with a urethral discharge, a meatal specimen discharge is an adequate substitute for an intraurethral swab specimen. Culture or a nucleic acid amplification test (NAAT) can be used to test for *N gonorrhoeae* and *C trachomatis*. Only an FDA-approved NAAT should be used. Consultation with an expert is necessary before using a NAAT in this context, both to minimize the possibility of cross-reaction with nongonococcal *Neisseria* species and other commensals (eg, *N meningitidis*, *Neisseria sicca*, *Neisseria lactamica*, *Neisseria cinerea*, and *Moraxella catarrhalis*) and to ensure appropriate interpretation of results. If culture for isolation of *N gonorrhoeae* or *C*

---

[1] www.aap.org/en-us/advocacy-and-policy/aap-health-initiatives/Child-Abuse-and-Neglect/Pages/Child-Abuse-and-Neglect.aspx

[2] Centers for Disease Control and Prevention. Sexually transmitted infections treatment guidelines, 2021. *MMWR Recomm Rep.* 2021; in press. Available at: www.cdc.gov/std/treatment

trachomatis is performed, only standard culture procedures should be performed. Specimens from the vagina, urethra, pharynx, or rectum should be streaked onto selective media for isolation of *N gonorrhoeae*, and all presumptive isolates of *N gonorrhoeae* should be identified definitively by at least 2 tests that involve different approaches (eg, biochemical, enzyme substrate, or molecular probes). Gram stains are inadequate to evaluate prepubertal children for gonorrhea and should not be used to diagnose or exclude gonorrhea. Every effort should be made to preserve specimens (either NAAT or culture including any isolates) obtained before treatment for further validation if needed. In the case of a positive specimen, the result should be confirmed either by retesting the original specimen or obtaining another. Given the overall low prevalence of *N gonorrhoeae* and *C trachomatis* in children, false-positive results may occur, and all specimens that are initially positive should be confirmed.

- Testing for *Trichomonas vaginalis* should not be limited to girls with vaginal discharge if other indications for vaginal testing exist, because there is some evidence to indicate that asymptomatic sexually abused children might be infected with *T vaginalis* and might benefit from treatment. A NAAT can be used as an alternative or in addition to culture and wet mount, especially in situations in which culture and wet mount of vaginal swab specimens are not obtainable. Consultation with an expert is necessary before using a NAAT in this context to ensure appropriate interpretation of results. Because of the implications of a diagnosis of *T vaginalis* infection in a child, only a validated, FDA-approved NAAT should be used. Point-of-care tests for *T vaginalis* have not been validated for prepubertal children and should not be used. In the case of a positive specimen, the result should be confirmed either by retesting the original specimen or obtaining another. Given the overall low prevalence of *T vaginalis* in children, false-positive results may occur, and all specimens that are initially positive should be confirmed.

- Because herpes simplex virus (HSV) can be indicative of sexual abuse, specimens should be obtained from all vesicular or ulcerative genital or perianal lesions and then sent for NAAT or viral culture.

- Wet mount of a vaginal swab specimen for bacterial vaginosis (BV) should be performed, if discharge is present.

- Serum samples should be collected to be evaluated, preserved for subsequent analysis, and used as a baseline for comparison with follow-up serologic tests. Sera can be tested for antibodies to *Treponema pallidum*, HIV, and hepatitis B virus (HBV). Decisions regarding the infectious agents for which to perform serologic tests should be made on a case-by-case basis.

TESTING SEXUALLY VICTIMIZED POSTPUBERTAL PATIENTS FOR STIs

In the evaluation of the sexual assault victim of **postpubertal** age, if a decision to perform STI testing is made, gonorrhea and chlamydia diagnostic evaluation from any sites of penetration or attempted penetration should be performed, per CDC guidance.[1] The CDC recommends *C trachomatis* and *N gonorrhoeae* NAATs from

---

[1]Centers for Disease Control and Prevention. Sexually transmitted infections treatment guidelines, 2021. *MMWR Recomm Rep.* 2021; in press. Available at: **www.cdc.gov/std/treatment**

specimens at the sites of penetration as the preferred diagnostic evaluation of the **postpubertal** sexual assault victims (Table 2.6). Females should be offered testing for *T vaginalis* using NAATs from a urine or vaginal specimen. Point-of-care testing and/or wet mount with measurement of vaginal pH and KOH application for the whiff test from vaginal secretions should be done for evidence of BV and candidiasis,

Table 2.6. Sexually Transmitted Infection (STI) Testing[a] When Sexual Abuse or Assault Is Suspected

Organism/Syndrome	Specimens
Neisseria gonorrhoeae and *Chlamydia trachomatis*	Prepubertal: Culture or NAAT from pharynx, anus, vagina (in girls), and urine (in boys). For boys with a urethral discharge, a meatus swab specimen is adequate substitute for intraurethral swab specimen. Postpubertal: NAAT from sites of penetration or attempted penetration. May include rectum, throat, vagina or cervix (female), urethra (male).
Syphilis	Darkfield examination (if available) of chancre fluid; blood for serologic tests at time of abuse and 4–6 weeks and 3 months later.
Human immunodeficiency virus	Serologic testing of abuser (if possible); serologic testing of child at time of abuse and 6 weeks and 3 months later.
Hepatitis B virus	Serum hepatitis B surface antigen testing of abuser or hepatitis B surface antibody testing of child, unless the child has received 3 doses of hepatitis B vaccine. See Table 3.22 (p 398) for management.
Herpes simplex virus (HSV)	Culture or NAAT of lesion specimen; all virologic specimens should be typed (HSV-1 vs HSV-2).
Bacterial vaginosis (females only)	Prepubertal: Wet mount of a vaginal swab specimen for BV, if discharge is present. Postpubertal: Point-of-care testing and/or wet mount with measurement of vaginal pH and KOH application for the whiff test from vaginal secretions should be done for evidence of BV, especially if vaginal discharge, malodor, or itching is present.
Human papillomavirus	Clinical examination, with biopsy of lesion specimen, if diagnosis unclear.
Trichomonas vaginalis	Prepubertal: NAAT and/or culture and wet mount. Testing for *T vaginalis* should not be limited to girls with vaginal discharge if other indications for vaginal testing exist. Postpubertal: NAAT from vagina or urine.
Pediculosis pubis	Identification of eggs, nymphs, and lice with naked eye or using hand lens.

NAAT indicates nucleic acid amplification test.

[a]See text for examples of indications for testing for STIs.

Table 2.7. Prophylaxis After Sexual Victimization: Postpubertal Patients

Antimicrobial prophylaxis is recommended to include an empiric regimen to prevent chlamydia, gonorrhea, and trichomoniasis. Vaccination against hepatitis B and HPV is recommended if not fully immunized.

For chlamydia, gonorrhea, and trichomoniasis	Ceftriaxone, 500 mg, intramuscularly, in a single dose **PLUS** Doxycycline, 100 mg, orally, twice daily for 7 days **PLUS (IF FEMALE)** Metronidazole, 500 mg, orally, twice daily for 7 days
For hepatitis B virus infection	See Table 3.22, p 398
For human immunodeficiency virus (HIV) infection	See Figure 2.1, p 157, and text.
For HPV	HPV vaccine series should be initiated at ≥9 y if not already begun or completed if not fully immunized (2 or 3 doses depending on age of initiation of vaccine)

HBIG indicates Hepatitis B Immune Globulin; HBsAg, hepatitis B surface antigen; HPV, human papillomavirus.
Source: Centers for Disease Control and Prevention. Sexually transmitted infections treatment guidelines, 2021. *MMWR Recomm Rep.* 2021; in press. Available at: **www.cdc.gov/std/treatment**

especially if vaginal discharge, malodor, or itching is present. Men who have sex with men should be offered screening for *C trachomatis* and *N gonorrhoeae*, regardless of whether there was sexual contact with these anatomic sites during the assault, if they report receptive oral or anal sex during the preceding year. Anoscopy should be considered in instances of reported anal penetration. Baseline and follow-up serum samples for evaluation for HIV infection, hepatitis B, and syphilis should be obtained (Table. 2.7).

PROPHYLAXIS OF CHILDREN AND ADOLESCENTS AFTER SEXUAL VICTIMIZATION

Antimicrobial therapy should be withheld until the STI diagnostic testing has been performed in cases of suspected sexual abuse/assault.

Presumptive treatment for **prepubertal** children who have been sexually assaulted or abused is not recommended, because their incidence of STIs is low, the risk of spread to the upper genital tract in prepubertal females is low, and follow-up usually can be ensured. Some children or parents/guardians might be concerned about the possibility of an STI. In that circumstance, it might be appropriate to pre-sumptively treat after all relevant diagnostic test specimens have been collected. If the result of an STI test is positive and confirmed with additional testing, treatment then should be given. Factors that may increase the likelihood of infection or that constitute an indication for prophylaxis are as listed under When to Screen for STIs in Prepubertal Victims (p 152).

In contrast, many experts believe that STI prophylaxis, after baseline testing has been performed, is warranted for **postpubertal** female patients who seek care after an episode of sexual victimization. This is recommended in this population because of the greater possibility of a preexisting asymptomatic infection, the potential risk for acquisition of new infections with the assault, the substantial risk of pelvic inflammatory disease after untreated STIs in females of this age group, and established data demonstrating poor compliance with follow-up visits after sexual assault.[1] Regimens for prophylaxis are presented in Table 2.7. The need for emergency contraception should be considered as well.

For more detailed diagnosis and treatment recommendations for specific STIs, see the disease-specific chapters in Section 3 and Tables 4.4 (p 898) and 4.5 (p 903). Completion of the HPV immunization series for children and adolescents 9 years and older should be documented.

HIV infection has been reported in children and adolescents for whom sexual abuse was the only known risk factor. Because of the demonstrated effectiveness of nonoccupational postexposure prophylaxis (PEP) to prevent HIV infection, the question arises whether HIV prophylaxis is warranted for children and adolescents after sexual assault (see Figure 2.1). The risk of HIV transmission from a single sexual assault that involves transfer of secretions and/or blood is low. Prophylaxis may be considered for patients who seek care within 72 hours after an assault if the assault involved mucosal exposure to secretions; repeated abuse; multiple assailants; and oral, vaginal, and/or anal trauma and particularly if the alleged perpetrator(s) is known to have or is at high risk of having HIV infection (see Human Immunodeficiency Virus Infection, p 427).[2]

The following are recommendations for postexposure HIV assessment within 72 hours of sexual assault[3]:

- Assess risk for HIV infection in the assailant, and test that person for HIV whenever possible.
- Use Figure 2.1 to evaluate the survivor for the need for HIV PEP.
- Consult with a specialist in HIV treatment if PEP is being considered.
- If the survivor appears to be at risk for acquiring HIV from the assault, discuss PEP, including benefits and risks.
- If the survivor chooses to start PEP, provide an initial course of 3 to 7 days of medication (ie, a starter pack) with a prescription for the remainder of the course, or provide a prescription for an entire 28-day course. Schedule an early follow-up visit to discuss test results and provide additional counseling.
- If PEP is started, perform serum creatinine, AST and ALT at baseline.
- Perform an HIV antibody test at original assessment; repeat at 6 weeks and 3 months.
- Counsel individuals with ongoing risk of HIV acquisition about HIV pre-exposure prophylaxis, and provide referrals to a PrEP provider.

---

[1]Crawford-Jakubiak JE, Alderman EM, Leventhal JM; American Academy of Pediatrics, Committee on Adolescence. Care of the adolescent after an acute sexual assault. *Pediatrics*. 2017;139(3):e20164243

[2]Centers for Disease Control and Prevention. Updated Guidelines for Antiretroviral Postexposure Prophylaxis after Sexual, Injection Drug Use, or Other Nonoccupational Exposure to HIV—United States, 2016. Atlanta, GA: Centers for Disease Control and Prevention; 2016. Available at: **www.cdc.gov/hiv/ pdf/programresources/cdc-hiv-npep-guidelines.pdf**

[3]Centers for Disease Control and Prevention. Sexually transmitted infections treatment guidelines, 2021. *MMWR Recomm Rep*. 2021; in press. Available at: **www.cdc.gov/std/treatment**

FIGURE 2.1. ALGORITHM FOR EVALUATION AND TREATMENT OF POSSIBLE NONOCCUPATIONAL HIV EXPOSURES[1]

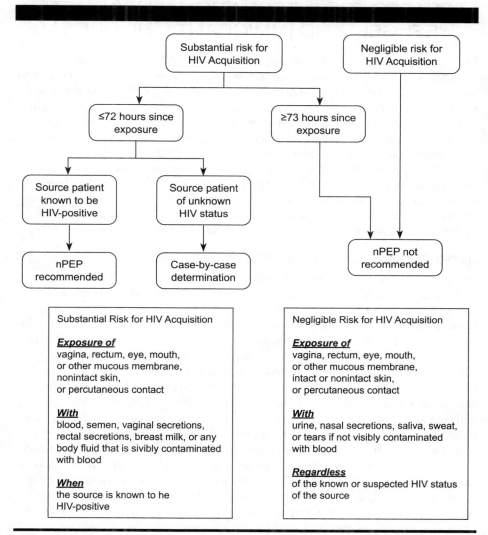

[1]Dominguez, KL, Smith DK, Thomas V, Crepaz N, Lang KS, et al. Updated Guidelines for Antiretroviral Postexposure Prophylaxis After Sexual, Injection Drug Use, or Other Nonoccupational Exposures to HIV—United States, 2016. Atlanta, GA: Centers for Disease Control and Prevention; 2016. Available at: **https://stacks.cdc.gov/view/cdc/38856**

Assistance with PEP-related decisions can be obtained by calling the National Clinician's Post Exposure Prophylaxis Hotline (PEP Line) (telephone: 888-448-4911).

A follow-up visit approximately 4 to 6 weeks after the most recent sexual exposure may include a repeat physical examination and collection of additional specimens. Additional follow-up visits at 3 and 6 months after the most recent sexual exposure may be necessary to obtain convalescent sera to test for hepatitis B (if indicated), hepatitis C (if indicated), syphilis, and HIV infection.

MEDICAL EVALUATION FOR INFECTIOUS DISEASES FOR INTERNATIONALLY ADOPTED, REFUGEE, AND IMMIGRANT CHILDREN[1,2]

Every year, thousands of children arrive in the United States from other countries. They arrive as immigrants, nonimmigrants, refugees or asylum seekers, adoptees, or as undocumented. The medical evaluation of these children is a challenging and important task and is influenced by multiple factors, including the child's country of origin, socioeconomic status, and health history; availability of reliable health care in the country of origin; and the migration route, including type of travel (eg, by foot or by air), countries passed through, and the conditions during the journey.

Children arriving in the United States should be evaluated as soon as possible after arrival to begin medical assessment and preventive health services, including immunizations. Screening for infectious diseases is important to identify infections with a long latency period that may not be prevalent in children born in the United States. Each of the groups mentioned previously has its own characteristics and special needs.

INTERNATIONALLY ADOPTED CHILDREN

There is a great deal of information available to guide management of children adopted internationally. Some health concerns may be addressed before adoption, although some are apparent to the adoptive family only after arrival. Many adoptive families interact with the health care system before the child arrives and make arrangements for the child to have health insurance at the time of arrival in the United States. There often are opportunities to provide advice to the family and to optimize immunizations that the family may need before traveling to pick up the child and for family members and caregivers who will interact with the child after arrival. These immunizations serve to protect the child from diseases that might be transmitted from family and community members (eg, pertussis, influenza) and to protect the family and community from diseases that might be transmitted by the child (eg, hepatitis A). Access to and quality of medical care for international adoptees before arrival in the United States can be variable. Internationally adopted children are required to have a medical examination performed by a physician designated by the US Department of State in their country of origin. This examination usually is limited to completing legal requirements for screening for certain communicable diseases and to examine for serious physical or mental disorders that would prevent issuance of an immigrant visa. Such an evaluation is not a comprehensive assessment of the child's health. During preadoption visits, pediatricians can stress to prospective parents the importance of acquiring immunization and other health records. Parents who have not met with a physician before adoption should notify their physician when their child arrives so that a timely

---

[1]For additional information, see Canadian Paediatric Society (**www.kidsnewtocanada.ca**), the Centers for Disease Control and Prevention (**wwwnc.cdc.gov/travel/yellowbook/2020/family-travel/international-adoption** and **wwwnc.cdc.gov/travel/yellowbook/2020/posttravel-evaluation/newly-arrived-immigrants-and-refugees**), and World Health Organization (**www.who.int**) websites.

[2]Information for parents can be found at **www.cdc.gov/immigrantrefugeehealth/adoption/index.html/**.

medical evaluation can be arranged. Guidance on comprehensive assessment of a newly adopted child is available from the American Academy of Pediatrics (AAP).[1]

REFUGEES AND ASYLEES

Refugees and asylees have legal status in the United States and are required to undergo the same medical examination as immigrants before arrival (with the exception of the vaccination component). The Centers for Disease Control and Prevention (CDC) has issued recommendations for screening of refugees after arrival, and various states have different protocols for the initial evaluation of a refugee (**www.cdc.gov/immigrantrefugeehealth/guidelines/domestic/domestic-guidelines.html**).

IMMIGRANTS

In recent years, the number of immigrant children has increased to represent the largest and most diverse group of new arrivals to the United States. Most pediatricians will encounter immigrant children in their practice. Evaluation is individual to each case, depending on whether the child is documented or has insurance coverage, the circumstances of immigration, country of origin, medical history, and socioeconomic status. Recommendations for refugees and internationally adopted children can guide the pediatrician in evaluating new immigrants. The AAP has developed a toolkit for the evaluation of the health of immigrant children (**www.aap.org/en-us/Documents/cocp_toolkit_full.pdf**).

Most immigrant children have received some immunizations but may have received them on schedules different from those used in the United States or may have missed essential immunizations. Written documentation of immunizations that includes month and year of administration is accepted as valid if the vaccinations conform to the US schedule. See Children Who Received Immunizations Outside the United States or Whose Immunization Status is Unknown or Uncertain (p 96) for recommendations regarding immunizations.

Consideration for Testing for Infectious Agents

Infectious diseases are among the most common medical diagnoses identified in immigrant, refugee, and internationally adopted children after arrival in the United States, including diseases of long latency in asymptomatic children. Because of inconsistent use of the birth dose of hepatitis B vaccine (HepB); inconsistent perinatal screening for hepatitis B virus (HBV), syphilis, and human immunodeficiency virus (HIV); and the high prevalence of certain intestinal parasites and tuberculosis (TB), screening for these diseases should be considered for all immigrant children. Screening for other diseases can be considered on an individual basis, as discussed in the following paragraphs (see Table 2.8) and in the disease-specific chapters in Section 3.

HEPATITIS A

Hepatitis A virus (HAV) is endemic in most countries of origin of internationally adopted, refugee, and immigrant children. Some children may have acquired HAV infection early in life in their country of origin and may be immune, but others may be incubating HAV or remain susceptible at the time of entry into the United States.

---

[1] Jones VF, Schulte EE; American Academy of Pediatrics, Council on Foster Care, Adoption, and Kinship Care. Comprehensive health evaluation of the newly adopted child. *Pediatrics*. 2019;143(5):e20190657

Table 2.8. Suggested Screening Tests for Infectious Diseases in International Adoptees, Refugees, and Immigrants[a]

Hepatitis B virus serologic testing:
Hepatitis B surface antigen (HBsAg); some experts include hepatitis B surface antibody (anti-HBs) and hepatitis B core antibody (anti-HBc)[b]

Hepatitis C virus serologic testing when indicated (see text)

Syphilis serologic testing:
Nontreponemal test (eg, RPR or VDRL)
Treponemal test (eg, MHA-TP, FTA-ABS, EIA, CIA, or TPPA)

Human immunodeficiency virus (HIV) 1 and 2 serologic testing; consider combination rapid antigen/antibody testing

Complete blood cell count with red blood cell indices and differential

Stool examination for ova and parasites (1–3 specimens) with specific request for *Giardia duodenalis* and *Cryptosporidium* species testing by direct fluorescent antibody or EIA testing

Interferon-gamma release assay or tuberculin skin test

In children from countries with endemic infection[c]:
Trypanosoma cruzi serologic testing

In children with eosinophilia (absolute eosinophil count exceeding 450 cells/mm^3) and negative stool ova and parasite examinations[d] can consider:
Toxocara canis serologic testing
Strongyloides species serologic testing
Schistosoma species serologic testing for children from sub-Saharan African, Southeast Asian, and certain Latin American countries

Lymphatic filariasis serologic testing for children older than 2 years from countries with endemic infection

---

CIA indicates chemiluminescence assay; EIA, enzyme immunoassay; FTA-ABS, fluorescent treponemal antibody absorption; MHA-TP, microhemagglutination test for *Treponema pallidum;* RPR indicates rapid plasma reagin; TPPA, *T pallidum* particle agglutination; VDRL, Venereal Disease Research Laboratories.

[a] For evaluation of noninfectious disease conditions, see Linton JM, Green A; American Academy of Pediatrics, Council on Community Pediatrics. Providing care for children in immigrant families. *Pediatrics.* 2019;144(3):e20192077.

[b] Passively acquired maternal anti-HBc may be detected in infant born to HBV-infected mothers up to age 24 months.

[c] Argentina, Belize, Bolivia, Brazil, Chile, Colombia, Costa Rica, Ecuador, El Salvador, French Guiana, Guatemala, Guyana, Honduras, Mexico, Nicaragua, Panama, Paraguay, Peru, Suriname, Uruguay, and Venezuela.

[d] Some experts would perform serologic tests for schistosomiasis in children from areas with high endemicity regardless of eosinophil count because of its poor positive- and negative-predictive values.

Serologic testing for acute infection (hepatitis A immunoglobulin [Ig] M) and immunity (total hepatitis A IgG and IgM antibody) can be considered at the initial visit to determine whether the child is susceptible to HAV, has current HAV infection, or is immune, but testing is not recommended routinely. Children incubating HAV infection could transmit the virus to others on arrival in the United States. In the case of adoption, hepatitis A vaccine (HepA) is recommended for all previously unvaccinated people who anticipate close personal contact (eg, household contact or other regular caregiver) with a child adopted from a country with high or intermediate HAV prevalence during the first 60 days after arrival of the adoptee in the United States. Adoptive parents and accompanying family members traveling to adopt the child should ensure that they themselves are immunized or otherwise immune to HAV infection before traveling to a country of high or intermediate prevalence. After arrival, adopted children without HAV immunity who are 12 months and older should receive HepA according to routine immunization schedules.

HEPATITIS B

More studies evaluating the prevalence of hepatitis B are conducted in internationally adopted and refugee children than in immigrant children. In studies conducted primarily during the 1990s, prevalence of hepatitis B surface antigen (HBsAg) ranged from 1% to 5% in internationally adopted children and from 4% to 7% in refugee children, depending on the country of origin and the year studied. Hepatitis B virus (HBV) infection was associated with country of origin and was most common in children from Asia and Africa, and from some countries of central and eastern Europe (eg, Romania, Bulgaria, Russia, and Ukraine). The number of countries with routine infant hepatitis B immunization programs has increased markedly in the past decade, and many countries have introduced a birth dose of hepatitis B vaccine (HepB; **www.who.int/hepatitis/publications/global-hepatitis-report2017/en/**).

Despite the number of countries that have added the birth dose of HepB, vaccination coverage among infants can be suboptimal. Even when a birth dose of HepB is administered, efficacy of postexposure prophylaxis is lower among infants born to pregnant women with high HBV viral load and hepatitis B e antigen (HBeAg) positivity. All children who were born in or have lived in countries with intermediate (2%–7%) or high (≥8%) (see Fig 3.2, p 383) should be tested to identify cases of chronic infection, regardless of immunization status (see Hepatitis B, p 381). Although HBV serologic tests may be performed in the country of origin, testing is not required for the immigration examination, testing may be incomplete, and children may become infected after testing. Appropriate screening tests are those for hepatitis B surface antigen (HBsAg), antibody (anti-HBs), and core antibody (anti-HBc). Unimmunized children with negative HBsAg and negative HBsAb test results should be immunized according to the recommended childhood and adolescent immunization schedules (also see Children Who Received Immunizations Outside the United States or Whose Immunization Status is Unknown or Uncertain, p 96).

Children with a positive HBsAg test result should be reported to the local or state health department. To distinguish between acute and chronic HBV infection, HBsAg-positive children should be evaluated further. Persistence of HBsAg for at least 6 months indicates chronic HBV infection (**www.cdc.gov/hepatitis/hbv/pdfs/serologicchartv8.pdf;** see Hepatitis B, p 381). Children with chronic HBV infection should be tested for biochemical evidence of liver disease and followed by a specialist who cares for patients with chronic HBV infection (see Hepatitis B, p 381). All unimmunized household contacts of children with chronic HBV infection should be immunized (see Hepatitis B, p 381).

HEPATITIS C

Hepatitis C virus (HCV) screening for refugee and immigrant children is not recommended routinely during the new arrival medical examination unless individuals have risk factors, including an HCV-positive mother, overseas surgery, transfusion, major dental work, intravenous drug use, tattoos, sexual activity/abuse, female genital cutting, and other traditional cutting. Testing for HCV infection also can be considered for internationally adopted children, given that most international adoptees in recent years have been adopted from countries with elevated rates of prevalence (eg, China, Russia, southeast Asia) and because risk factors for infection rarely are known. A serum IgG antibody enzyme immunoassay (EIA) should be used as the initial screening test for children ≥18 months of age.

NAAT for HCV RNA detection can be performed between 2 and 6 months of age. Regardless of NAAT test result, serologic testing also should be performed at 18 months of age for more definitive diagnosis (see Hepatitis C, p 399).

INTESTINAL PATHOGENS

Serial fecal examinations for ova and parasites tested in a laboratory experienced in parasitology will identify a pathogen in 15% to 35% of internationally adopted and refugee children. Presence or absence of symptoms is not predictive of parasitosis. Prevalence of intestinal parasites varies by age of the child and by country of origin. For refugees, guidelines differ depending on whether the child received presumptive therapy before departure (**www.cdc.gov/immigrantrefugeehealth/guidelines/overseas/interventions/interventions.html**). The most common pathogens identified are *Giardia duodenalis, Dientamoeba fragilis, Hymenolepis* species, some *Schistosoma* species, *Strongyloides stercoralis,* and other soil-transmitted helminths including *Ascaris lumbricoides, Trichuris trichiura,* and hookworm *(Necator americanus). Entamoeba histolytica* and *Cryptosporidium* species are recovered less commonly. Regardless of nutritional status or presence of symptoms, 1 to 3 stool specimens collected on separate days (the CDC recommends 2 or more specimens for asymptomatic refugees from Asia, the Middle East, and Africa if they received no or incomplete predeparture treatment) may be examined for ova and parasites, and direct fluorescent antibody testing or EIA may be performed for *Giardia* species and *Cryptosporidium* species. Some clinicians prefer to administer presumptive therapy for helminth infection with albendazole. Studies in children as young as 1 year suggest that albendazole can be administered safely to this population. Therapy for intestinal parasites generally is successful, but complete eradication may not occur. Proof of eradication is not recommended for individuals who are asymptomatic following therapy. If symptoms persist after treatment, however, ova and parasite testing should be repeated to ensure successful elimination of parasites. Children who fail to demonstrate adequate catch-up growth, who have unexplained anemia, or who have gastrointestinal tract symptoms or signs that occur or recur months or even years after arrival in the United States should be reevaluated for intestinal parasites. When newly arrived children have acute onset of bloody diarrhea, stool specimens should be tested for *Salmonella* species, *Shigella* species, *Campylobacter* species, Shiga toxin-producing *Escherichia coli* including *E coli* O157:H7, and *Entamoeba histolytica*. If a bacterial pathogen is detected by a nonculture method, confirmation with culture and antimicrobial susceptibility testing are helpful for informing decisions regarding possible treatment and public health measures.

TISSUE PARASITES/EOSINOPHILIA

Eosinophilia is commonly but not universally present in people with tissue parasites. Refugee children may have received presumptive treatment of intestinal helminths overseas before departure to the United States (**www.cdc.gov/immigrantrefugeehealth/guidelines/overseas/intestinal-parasites-overseas.html**). In children who did not receive albendazole or ivermectin for presumptive therapy of intestinal helminths, who have negative stool ova and parasite test results, and in whom eosinophilia (absolute eosinophil count exceeding 450 cells/mm^3) is found on review of complete blood cell count, serologic testing for *Toxocara canis*, strongyloidiasis, schistosomiasis, and lymphatic filariasis should be considered. Although logistically attractive to perform all tests at first encounter, predictive values of many serologic tests for parasites are suboptimal; common treatable causes of eosinophilia usually should be considered first. Because *T canis* is prevalent worldwide, screening is warranted in children who have no identified cause of eosinophilia. For all immigrant children with eosinophilia and no identified pathogen commonly associated with an increased eosinophil count, serologic testing for *S stercoralis* is reasonable regardless of country of origin, and testing for *Schistosoma* species should be performed for all children who are from sub-Saharan Africa, southeast Asia, or areas of the Caribbean and South America, where schistosomiasis is endemic. Serologic testing for lymphatic filariasis should be considered in children older than 2 years with eosinophilia who are from countries with endemic lymphatic filariasis (**www.cdc.gov/parasites/lymphaticfilariasis/index.html**). A positive serologic result should be confirmed by testing in a reference laboratory (CDC or National Institutes of Health) for release of drugs for treatment of lymphatic filariasis.

SEXUALLY TRANSMITTED INFECTIONS

Congenital syphilis, especially with involvement of the central nervous system, may not have been diagnosed or may have been treated inadequately in children from some resource-limited countries. Immigrant, adoptee, and refugee children 15 years and older are required to have testing for syphilis and gonorrhea as part of the required overseas medical assessment. Younger children are required to be tested for the respective infections if there is a reason to suspect or a history of syphilis or gonorrhea. Children who had positive test results are required to complete treatment before arrival in the United States (**www.cdc.gov/immigrantrefugeehealth/guidelines/domestic/sexually-transmitted-diseases/index.html**). Children who have not undergone predeparture testing and treatment should be tested for syphilis after arrival in the United States by reliable nontreponemal and treponemal serologic tests, regardless of history or a report of treatment (see Syphilis, p 729). Children with positive nontreponemal or treponemal serologic test results should be evaluated by a health care professional with specific expertise to assess the differential diagnosis of pinta, yaws, and syphilis and to determine the stage of infection so that appropriate treatment can be administered (see Syphilis, p 729). Children should also be assessed for other sexually transmitted infections (STIs) as determined by medical history and physical examination findings. Screening of refugees for chlamydia and gonorrhea after arrival is encouraged, as is human immunodeficiency virus (HIV) testing, especially for those with another confirmed STI.

TUBERCULOSIS

Infection with an organism of the *Mycobacterium tuberculosis* complex commonly is encountered in immigrant and refugee children, although incidence rates of TB vary by country and by age within countries. Predeparture screening requirements for immigrants, adoptees, refugees, and other applicants ≥15 years of age include: chest radiograph; 3 sputum smears and cultures for people with an abnormal chest radiograph, signs and symptoms of tuberculosis disease, or known HIV infection; drug susceptibility testing for people with positive cultures; and treatment with a standard CDC-recommended regimen delivered as directly observed therapy to cure before travel to the United States for people with tuberculosis disease. Refugees and immigrant children 2 to 14 years of age from countries with tuberculosis incidence ≥20 cases per 100 000 population (**www.who.int/tb/publications/global_report/en/**) also must have an interferon-gamma release assay (IGRA) performed if IGRA is licensed in the country. Children with a positive IGRA result are required to undergo chest radiography before departure. Children younger than 2 years are not tested unless it is brought to attention of screening physicians outside the United States that they are a known contact of an active case, have known HIV infection, or have signs or symptoms suggestive of tuberculosis disease. Information about the screening and implementation requirements is available at **www.cdc.gov/immigrantrefugeehealth/exams/ ti/panel/tuberculosis-panel-technical-instructions.html.**

Testing for *M tuberculosis* infection after arrival in the United States in the population of high-risk immigrants, adoptees, and refugees is important, because TB can be more severe in young children and can reactivate in later years. Presence or absence of a bacille Calmette-Guérin (BCG) vaccine scar should be noted, but approximately 10% of children who received BCG vaccine as infants will not have a scar. BCG coverage in most countries where the vaccine is used is very high, but BCG vaccination has limitations. Efficacy of BCG vaccine against lethal forms of TB (eg, meningitis) in children is approximately 80%, but efficacy against pulmonary TB disease or TB infection is much lower. Receipt of BCG vaccine is not a contraindication to a tuberculin skin test (TST). TST is the preferred method for detection of *M tuberculosis* infection for children younger than 2 years. Either TST or IGRA can be used for children 2 years and older, but in people previously vaccinated with BCG, IGRA is preferred to avoid a false-positive TST result caused by a previous vaccination with BCG (see Tuberculosis, p 786, for further guidance). Some immigrants may be anergic initially because of malnutrition, stress, or untreated HIV infection and, thus, have falsely negative TST results or indeterminant or falsely negative IGRA test results and, therefore, may require repeat testing. Routine chest radiography is not indicated in asymptomatic children in whom the TST or IGRA result is negative. In children with a positive TST or IGRA, further investigation, including chest radiography and a complete physical examination, is necessary to determine whether tuberculosis disease is present (see Tuberculosis, p 786). When tuberculosis disease is suspected in an immigrant child, efforts to isolate and test the organism for drug susceptibilities are imperative because of the high prevalence of drug resistance in many countries. TB disease, whether suspected or confirmed, is a reportable condition in all US jurisdictions regardless of a patient's immigration status; tuberculosis infection is reportable in some states. Physicians who are experts in the management of TB should be consulted when therapy for TB infection or disease is indicated for children from countries with prevalent isoniazid resistance.

HIV INFECTION

The risk of HIV infection in newly arrived children depends on the country of origin and on individual risk factors. Screening for HIV should be performed for all internationally adopted children, because adoptees may come from populations at high risk of infection. Although some children will have HIV test results documented in their referral information, test results from the child's country of origin may not be reliable. Refugees and immigrants have not been required to have HIV testing routinely as part of the immigration medical assessment since 2010. HIV testing still is recommended for people who are diagnosed with tuberculosis disease as part of this medical assessment, and for any refugee diagnosed with another STI. HIV testing after arrival in the United States is recommended for refugees 13 through 64 years of age and is encouraged for refugees 12 years or younger and older than 64 years of age (**www.cdc.gov/ immigrantrefugeehealth/guidelines/domestic/screening-hiv-infection-domestic.html**). The decision to screen immigrant children for HIV after arrival in the United States should depend on history and risk factors (eg, receipt of blood products, maternal drug use), sexual activity (consensual or nonconsensual), physical examination findings, and prevalence of HIV infection in the child's country of origin. If there is a suspicion of HIV infection, testing should be performed before administration of live-antigen vaccines. Some experts believe HIV testing may be appropriate for most immigrant children.

CHAGAS DISEASE (AMERICAN TRYPANOSOMIASIS)

Chagas disease is found throughout much of Mexico and Central and South America (see American Trypanosomiasis, p 783). Countries with endemic Chagas disease include Argentina, Belize, Bolivia, Brazil, Chile, Colombia, Costa Rica, Ecuador, El Salvador, French Guiana, Guatemala, Guyana, Honduras, Mexico, Nicaragua, Panama, Paraguay, Peru, Suriname, Uruguay, and Venezuela. Transmission within countries with endemic infection is focal, but if a child comes from, or received a blood transfusion in, a country with endemic Chagas disease, testing for *Trypanosoma cruzi* should be considered. Treatment of children with Chagas disease is highly effective. Screening using serologic testing should be performed only in children 12 months or older because of the potential presence of maternal antibody.

OTHER INFECTIOUS DISEASES

Skin infections that may occur in immigrant children include bacterial (eg, impetigo), fungal (eg, candidiasis and tinea corporis and capitis), viral (molluscum contagiosum), and ectoparasitic infestations (eg, scabies and pediculosis). New adoptive parents may need to be instructed on how to examine their child for signs of scabies, pediculosis, and tinea so that treatment can be initiated and transmission to others can be prevented (see Scabies, p 663, and Pediculosis chapters, p 567–574).

Diseases such as typhoid fever, leprosy, or melioidosis are encountered infrequently in immigrant children; routine screening for these diseases is not recommended. Findings of fever, splenomegaly, respiratory tract infection, anemia, or eosinophilia should prompt an appropriate evaluation on the basis of the epidemiology of infectious diseases that occur in the child's country of origin.

Routine screening for malaria is not recommended for immigrants, refugees, or internationally adopted children. Testing for malaria (thick and thin blood films) should be performed immediately for any febrile child who has arrived from an area with endemic malaria (see Malaria, p 493). Malaria also should be considered as a cause of asymptomatic splenomegaly (hyperreactive malaria splenomegaly) in a child from an area with endemic malaria; evaluation should include antibody titers and polymerase chain reaction (PCR) assay for malaria, because asymptomatic children with splenomegaly attributable to a history of repeated malaria infections may have high titers or positive PCR assay results but negative smears. If the malaria IgM or PCR assay result is positive, the child should be treated with antimalarial drugs. Refugee children from Sub-Saharan Africa may have received presumptive treatment for malaria before departure to the United States (**www.cdc.gov/immigrantrefugeehealth/guidelines/overseas/malaria-guidelines-overseas.html;** see Malaria, p 493).

In the United States, multiple outbreaks of measles have been reported in children adopted from China and in their US contacts. Measles transmission continues in many parts of the world. Prospective parents who are traveling internationally to adopt children, as well as their household contacts, should ensure that they have a history of natural disease or have been immunized adequately for measles according to US recommendations. If born after 1957, and in the absence of documented measles infection or contraindication to the vaccine, prospective parents and household contacts of adopted children should receive 2 doses of measles-containing vaccine after the age of 12 months and separated by at least 28 days (see Measles, p 503).

Although one of the major purposes of screening is to identify asymptomatic diseases with long latency, screening should not be performed for all such diseases; an example is neurocysticercosis, which may not be clinically apparent for many years.

For all immigrant children, establishing a medical home with a primary care provider is of prime importance. The child's country of birth and migration history will remain an important health determinant throughout his or her life.

INJURIES FROM NEEDLES DISCARDED IN THE COMMUNITY

Contact with and injuries from hypodermic needles and syringes improperly discarded in public places pose a risk of transmission of bloodborne pathogens, including human immunodeficiency virus (HIV), hepatitis B virus (HBV), and hepatitis C virus (HCV). However, a review of 14 studies of children exposed to needlesticks in the community documented no transmissions with follow-up of 613 children for HIV, 575 for HBV, and 394 for HCV. Infection risks and options for postexposure prophylaxis (PEP) vary depending on the virus and type and extent of exposure. Risk of infection also depends on the nature of the wound, the ability of the pathogens to survive on environmental surfaces, the volume of source material, the concentration of virus in the source material, infection prevalence rates among local persons with a substance use disorder, the probability that the syringe and needle were used by a person with a substance use disorder, and the immunization status of the person with the needle-stick. Although nonoccupational needlestick injuries may pose a lower risk of infection transmission than occupational needlestick injuries, a person injured by a needle in a nonoccupational setting should be evaluated and counseled and, in some cases, should receive PEP. A person who was injured by or exposed to a needlestick should be assessed even if the potential for the discarded syringe to contain a specific bloodborne pathogen is estimated to be low from the background prevalence rates of these infections in the local community.

Wound Care and Tetanus Prophylaxis

Management of people with needlestick injuries includes acute wound care and consideration of the need for antimicrobial prophylaxis. Standard wound cleansing and care is indicated; such wounds rarely require closure. A tetanus toxoid-containing vaccine, with or without Tetanus Immune Globulin, should be considered as appropriate for the patient's age, severity of injury, immunization status, and potential for dirt or soil contamination of the needle (see Tetanus, p 750). Tetanus and diphtheria toxoids vaccine (Td) or tetanus toxoid, reduced diphtheria toxoid, and acellular pertussis vaccine (Tdap) may be used. If the patient's pertussis vaccination status is not current or is unknown, Tdap should be used (see Pertussis, p 578).

Bloodborne Pathogens

Bloodborne pathogens of primary concern in needlestick exposure are HIV, HBV, and HCV. Consideration of the need for PEP for HBV and HIV is the next step in exposure management; currently, there is no recommended PEP for HCV. Unlike an occupational blood or body fluid exposure, in which the status of the exposure source for HBV, HCV, and HIV often is known, these data usually are not available to help in the decision-making process in a nonoccupational exposure.

HEPATITIS B VIRUS

HBV retains infectivity when held at room temperature for at least 7 days after drying. Transmission to health care personnel with needlestick injury occurs at a rate of 23% to 62% from hepatitis B surface antigen (HBsAg)-positive and hepatitis B envelope antigen (HBeAg)-positive sources and at a rate of 1% to 6% for HBsAg-positive and HBeAg-negative sources. Prompt and appropriate PEP intervention reduces this risk.[1] The effectiveness of PEP diminishes the longer it is delayed after exposure. Management following a needlestick is predicated on whether the source of the needle is known to be HBsAg-positive and on the immunization status of the person receiving the needlestick and is detailed in Table 3.22 (p 398).

[1]Schillie S, Murphy TV, Sawyer M, et al. CDC guidance for evaluating health-care personnel for hepatitis B virus protection and for administering postexposure management. *MMWR Recomm Rep*. 2013;62(RR-10):1-19

HUMAN IMMUNODEFICIENCY VIRUS

The risk of HIV transmission from a needle discarded in public is lower than the 0.3% risk of HIV transmission by needlestick from a person with known HIV infection to a health care worker, and no cases of HIV transmission by needlestick outside of health care settings have been reported to date in the United States. HIV is susceptible to drying. When HIV is exposed to air, the 50% tissue culture infective dose decreases by approximately 1 log every 9 hours. In addition, most syringes do not contain transmissible HIV even after being used to draw blood from a person with HIV infection. In injuries from discarded needles in public, viruses that may have been present has been exposed to drying and environmental temperatures. In addition, injury does not generally occur immediately after the needle was used, needles rarely contain fresh blood, and injuries are usually superficial.

Testing for HIV, if indicated, is performed at baseline and 4 to 6 weeks and again 3 months after the injury (see Human Immunodeficiency Virus Infection, p 427). The decision to test for HIV does not compel the initiation of PEP, with treatment decisions based on a case-by-case consideration as detailed below. Because concurrent infection with HCV and HIV may be associated with delayed HIV seroconversion, a person whose HCV antibody test result is negative at baseline but seroconverts to positive after exposure should undergo an additional HIV test at 6 months. Testing also is indicated if an illness consistent with acute HIV-related syndrome develops before the 4- to 6-week testing and should include HIV RNA viral load. An alternative is to save a baseline serum specimen to be tested later for HIV if indicated. Counseling is necessary before and after testing (see Human Immunodeficiency Virus Infection, p 427). A positive initial test result in a pediatric patient requires further investigation of the cause, such as perinatal transmission, sexual abuse or activity, or drug use.

With needlestick injuries, a case-by-case assessment of risk of HIV transmission and of risks and benefits of PEP is indicated. In deciding whether or not to initiate PEP, higher-risk situations in which PEP should be recommended include the source being known to be HIV positive, the injury occurring in an area with a high prevalence of HIV infection and injection drug use (some sources suggest >15% prevalence as a threshold), the needle being a large lumen device with visible blood on it or in the syringe, or the injury involving deeper penetration of the needle or involving a mucosal membrane. In some lower-risk situations, it still may be appropriate to consider PEP on the basis of the specifics of a given case.

An HIV specialist or the CDC PEP Consultation Service for Clinicians (PEPline 888-448-4911) should be consulted before deciding whether to initiate PEP. Other PEP consultation services, such as the New York City PEP Hotline (844-373-7692) and the University of California San Francisco's Clinician Consultation Center (888-448-4911) are also available. For a needlestick with high risk for HIV exposure, PEP should begin within 72 hours. If the needlestick is determined to warrant the 28-day course of PEP, a combination antiretroviral regimen that is appropriate for the patient's age and medical conditions should be selected, and the recommended schedule of laboratory tests should be followed[1] (see Human Immunodeficiency Virus Infection, p 427). Testing the needle for HIV is not practical or reliable and is not recommended.

---

[1]Dominguez KL, Smith DK, Vasavi T, et al. Updated guidelines for antiretroviral postexposure prophylaxis after sexual, injection drug use, or other nonoccupational exposure to HIV—United States, 2016. Atlanta, GA: Centers for Disease Control and Prevention; 2016. Available at: **https://stacks.cdc.gov/view/cdc/38856**

HEPATITIS C VIRUS

HCV retains infectivity in blood in syringes stored for days to weeks, depending on syringe residual volume and ambient temperature. Although HCV transmission by sharing syringes among injection drug users is efficient, the risk of transmission from a discarded syringe is likely to be low. Testing for HCV is not recommended routinely in the absence of a risk factor for infection or a known exposure to HCV. Anti-HCV antibody can be detected in 80% of newly infected patients within 15 weeks after exposure and in 97% by 6 months after exposure. For earlier diagnosis, testing for HCV RNA may be performed at 4 to 6 weeks after exposure. An HCV RNA test should be followed by anti-HCV antibody test at 6 months or later after exposure. Positive antibody results should be confirmed by HCV RNA, but a negative antibody result should be repeated at 6 months after exposure (see Hepatitis C, p 399). There is no recommended PEP for HCV using antiviral drugs. Immune Globulin preparations for HCV are not available, because anti-HCV antibody-positive donors are excluded from the pool from which Immune Globulin products are prepared.

Preventing Needlestick Injuries

Needlestick injuries can be minimized by implementing public health programs on safe needle disposal and comprehensive syringe services programs including sterile needle access or exchange for used syringes and needles from people who use injection drugs. Nearly 30 years of research has shown that comprehensive syringe services programs are safe, effective, and cost-saving; do not increase illegal drug use or crime; and play an important role in reducing the transmission of viral hepatitis, HIV, and other infections. On that basis, the American Academy of Pediatrics supports syringe service programs in conjunction with drug treatment and ongoing evaluation to ensure their effectiveness. Children should be cautioned to avoid playing in areas known to be frequented by people who use injection drugs and to notify a responsible adult parent, teacher, or other caregiver if a discarded syringe or needle is found. Adults should handle used injection paraphernalia with caution; guidance on safe disposal of discarded syringes and needles can be obtained from the local health department.

BITE WOUNDS

An estimated 5 million human or animal bite wounds occur annually in the United States; dog bites account for approximately 90% of those wounds. The rate of infection after a bite varies but can be as high as 50% after a cat bite and 5% to 20% after a dog or human bite. Although postinjury rates of infection can be minimized through early administration of proper wound care, the bites of humans, wild animals, or nontraditional pets are potential sources of serious morbidity. Parents should teach children to avoid contact with wild animals and to secure garbage containers so that raccoons and other animals will not be attracted to the home and places where children play. Nontraditional pets, including ferrets, iguanas and other reptiles, and wild animals also pose infection and injury risks for children, and their ownership should be discouraged in households with young children. Health care professionals should be knowledgeable about and offer counseling to parents whose children will have wild animal contact at petting zoos and exotic animal summer camps. The Centers for Disease Control and Prevention (CDC) has websites that provide information on healthy interactions with pets and other animals.[1] Potential transmission of rabies is increased when a bite is from a wild animal (especially a bat or a carnivore) or from a domestic animal with uncertain immunization status that cannot be captured for adequate quarantine (see Rabies, p 619). Dead animals should be avoided, because saliva from recently deceased mammals can contain active rabies virus, which can be transmitted via physical contact with virus-containing saliva.

Recommendations for bite wound management are provided in Table 2.9. Current guidelines from the Infectious Diseases Society of America (IDSA) state that primary wound closure is not recommended for animal bite wounds, with the exception of those to the face, which should be managed with copious irrigation, cautious débridement, and preemptive antibiotics; other wounds may be approximated.[2] Bite wounds on the face carry a relatively low rate of secondary infection, perhaps because of the generous vascular supply to the area or because these wounds likely receive prompt medical attention; an exception is an injury that causes crushed tissue. Cranial penetrating bite wounds to the scalp and skull sustained from large dogs (eg, Mastiff) can be at increased risk for intracranial infection. Head imaging is recommended to examine possible skull penetration for these bite wounds. The IDSA guidelines note that reports of infection following primary closure on regions other than the face have major limitations including lack of a control group; lack of standardization of the type, severity, and location of the wound; and circumstances surrounding the injury. In addition, thorough wound cleansing before surgical closure has brought the rate of secondary infection of these wounds to well below 10%, no matter the species of animal that inflicted the wound. These factors combine to suggest that, following thoughtful deliberation, primary closure of nonfacial wounds can be considered in some cases. Approximation of margins and closure by delayed primary or secondary intention is prudent for most infected nonfacial wounds. When surgical closures are required, they can be performed at the time of initial management (primary) or delayed until the patient has received a brief course of antibiotic therapy (delayed primary closure). High-pressure irrigation might drive infectious agents into deeper tissue locations and should be avoided. Smaller, cosmetically unimportant wounds can be cleansed and allowed to heal by secondary intention. Hand and foot wounds have a higher risk of infection. This is especially true of deeper wounds that penetrate multiple tissue planes and are more difficult to clean effectively. Injuries that are more complicated should be managed in consultation with an appropriate surgical specialist. To minimize risk of infection, bite wounds should not be sealed with a tissue adhesive, no matter their age or appearance.

Published evidence indicates that most infected mammalian bite wounds are polymicrobial in nature, often involving a mixture of mouth flora from the biting animal and, likely, skin flora from the victim (see Table 2.10). It takes at least 12 hours for signs of infection to manifest clinically. Patients with mild injuries in which the skin is abraded do not need to be treated with antimicrobial agents. For those injuries, cleansing is sufficient.

---

[1] **www.cdc.gov/healthypets/index.html**

[2] Stevens DL, Bisno AL, Chambers HF, et al. Practice guidelines for the diagnosis and management of skin and soft tissue infections: 2014 update by the Infectious Diseases Society of America. *Clin Infect Dis.* 2014;59(2):e10–e52

Table 2.9. Management of Human or Animal Bite Wounds

Category of Management	Management
Cleansing	Remove visible foreign material. Cleanse the wound surface with clean water or saline. Cleansers such as 1% povidone–iodine or 1% benzalkonium chloride can be used for particularly soiled wounds. Irrigate open wounds with a copious volume of sterile water or saline solution by moderate-pressure irrigation.[a] Avoid blind high-pressure irrigation of puncture wounds.
Wound culture	No, for fresh wounds,[b] unless signs of infection exist. Yes, for wounds that appear infected.[c]
Diagnostic imaging	Indicated for penetrating injuries overlying bones or joints, for suspected fracture, or to assess foreign body inoculation.
Débridement	Remove superficial devitalized tissue and foreign material.
Operative débridement and exploration	Yes, if any of the following: • Extensive wounds with devitalized tissue or mechanical dysfunction. • Penetration of joints (eg, clenched fist injury) or cranium. • Plastic or other repairs requiring general anesthesia.
Assess mechanical function	Assess and address mechanical function of injured structures.
Wound closure	Yes, for selected fresh,[b] nonpuncture bite wounds (see text).
Assess tetanus immunization status[d]	Yes, for all wounds.
Assess risk of rabies	Yes, if bite by any rabies-prone, unobservable wild or domestic animal with unknown immunization status.[e]
Assess risk of hepatitis B virus infection	Yes, for human bite wounds.[f]
Assess risk of human immunodeficiency virus (HIV)	Yes, for human bite wounds.[g] An HIV test in the person bitten or in the biter should be considered if bloody saliva from the biter came into contact with abraded or broken skin or if either person involved in the bite incident is HIV infected or at risk for HIV infection. Guidance on initiating nonoccupational HIV postexposure prophylaxis (PEP) as soon as possible but no later than 72 hours after a risky exposure is available from the Centers for Disease Control and Prevention.[h]

Table 2.9. Management of Human or Animal Bite Wounds, continued

Category of Management	Management
Initiate antimicrobial therapy[i]	Yes, for: • Moderate or severe bite wounds, especially if edema or crush injury is present. • Puncture wounds, especially if penetration of bone, tendon sheath, or joint has occurred. • Deep or surgically closed facial bite wounds. • Hand and foot bite wounds. • Genital area bite wounds. • Wounds in immunocompromised and asplenic people. • Wounds with signs of infection. • Cat bite wounds.
Follow-up	Inspect wound for signs of infection within 48 hours.

[a] Use of an 18-gauge needle with a large-volume syringe is effective. Antimicrobial or anti-infective solutions offer no advantage and may increase tissue irritation.
[b] Wounds less than 12 hours old.
[c] Both aerobic and anaerobic bacterial culture should be performed.
[d] See Tetanus, p 750.
[e] See Rabies, p 619.
[f] See Hepatitis B, p 381.
[g] See Human Immunodeficiency Virus Infection, p 427.
[h] Dominguez KL, Smith DK, Vasavi T, et al. Updated Guidelines for Antiretroviral Postexposure Prophylaxis After Sexual, Injection Drug Use, or Other Nonoccupational Exposure to HIV—United States, 2016. Atlanta, GA: Centers for Disease Control and Prevention; 2016. Available at: **https://stacks.cdc.gov/view/cdc/38856**
[i] See Table 2.10 for suggested drug choices.

Specimens for both aerobic and anaerobic culture should be obtained from wounds that appear infected. Limited data exist to guide short-term antimicrobial therapy for patients with wounds that do not appear infected. Preemptive early antimicrobial therapy for 3 to 5 days is recommended for patients who (a) are immunocompromised; (b) are asplenic; (c) have advanced liver disease; (d) have preexisting or resultant edema of the affected area; (e) have moderate to severe injuries, especially to the hand or face; or (f) have injuries that may have penetrated the periosteum or joint capsule.[1] Given the frequency of infection associated with them, antimicrobial therapy is recommended following cat bites. In certain cases, postexposure prophylaxis for rabies may be indicated. Assume that bats, skunks, raccoons, foxes, and woodchucks are rabid unless the geographic area is known to be rabies-free or until the animal tests negative (see Rabies, p 619). Tetanus toxoid should be administered to patients with animal bite wounds who have not had toxoid vaccination within the prior 10 years (see Tetanus, p 750). Routine antiviral prophylaxis following bite wounds is not indicated, although risks for transmission of hepatitis B virus and human immunodeficiency virus (HIV) should be assessed in human bite injuries (see Table 2.9).

Guidelines for initial choice of antimicrobial therapy for human and animal bites are provided in Table 2.10. The treatment of choice following most bite wounds for which therapy is provided is amoxicillin-clavulanic acid (Table 2.10). For a child with

[1] Stevens DL, Bisno AL, Chambers HF, et al. Practice guidelines for the diagnosis and management of skin and soft tissue infections: 2014 update by the Infectious Diseases Society of America. *Clin Infect Dis.* 2014;59(2):e10–e52

Table 2.10. Antimicrobial Agents for Human or Animal Bite Wounds

Source of Bite	Organism(s) Likely to Cause Infection	Antimicrobial Agent			
		Oral Route	Oral Alternatives for Penicillin-Allergic Patients[a]	Intravenous Route[b,c]	Intravenous Alternatives for Penicillin-Allergic Patients[a,b,c]
Dog, cat, or mammal[d]	Pasteurella species, Staphylococcus aureus, streptococci, anaerobes, Capnocytophaga species, Moraxella species, Corynebacterium species, Neisseria species	Amoxicillin-clavulanate	Extended-spectrum cephalosporin or trimethoprim-sulfamethoxazole[e] **PLUS** Clindamycin	Ampicillin-sulbactam[f]	Extended-spectrum cephalosporin or trimethoprim-sulfamethoxazole **PLUS** Clindamycin **OR** Carbapenem
Reptile[g]	Enteric gram-negative bacteria, anaerobes	Amoxicillin-clavulanate	Extended-spectrum cephalosporin or trimethoprim-sulfamethoxazole[e] **PLUS** Clindamycin	Ampicillin-sulbactam[f] **PLUS** Gentamicin	Clindamycin **PLUS** Extended spectrum cephalosporin or gentamicin or aztreonam or quinolone **OR** Carbapenem

Table 2.10. Antimicrobial Agents for Human or Animal Bite Wounds, continued

Source of Bite	Organism(s) Likely to Cause Infection	Antimicrobial Agent			
		Oral Route	Oral Alternatives for Penicillin-Allergic Patients[a]	Intravenous Route[b,c]	Intravenous Alternatives for Penicillin-Allergic Patients[a,b,c]
Human	Streptococci, *S aureus, Eikenella corrodens, Haemophilus* species, anaerobes	Amoxicillin-clavulanate	Extended-spectrum cephalosporin or trimethoprim-sulfamethoxazole[e] PLUS Clindamycin	Ampicillin-sulbactam[f]	Extended spectrum cephalosporin or trimethoprim-sulfamethoxazole PLUS Clindamycin OR Carbapenem

[a]For patients with history of significant allergy or drug reaction to penicillin or one of its congeners, alternative drugs are recommended (see text).

[b]Coverage for methicillin-resistant *Staphylococcus aureus* (MRSA) with vancomycin should be considered for severe bite wounds.

[c]Note that use of ampicillin-sulbactam or carbapenem monotherapy will not include activity against MRSA.

[d]Data are lacking to guide antimicrobial use for bites that are not overtly infected from small mammals, such as guinea pigs and hamsters.

[e]Doxycycline is alternative coverage for *Pasteurella multocida.*

[f]Piperacillin-tazobactam can be used as an alternative.

[g]The role of empirical antimicrobial use for noninfected snake bite wounds is not well-defined. Therapy should be chosen on the basis of results of cultures from infected wounds.

a significant allergy to penicillin, oral or parenteral treatment with trimethoprim-sulfamethoxazole, which is effective against *Staphylococcus aureus* (including methicillin-resistant *S aureus* [MRSA]), *Pasteurella multocida,* and *Eikenella corrodens,* in conjunction with clindamycin, which is active in vitro against anaerobic bacteria, streptococci, and many strains of *S aureus,* may be effective for preventing or treating bite wound infections. Extended-spectrum cephalosporins, such as parenteral ceftriaxone or oral cefpodoxime, do not have good anaerobic activity but can be used in conjunction with clindamycin as alternative therapy for penicillin-allergic patients who can tolerate cephalosporins. Doxycycline is an alternative agent that has activity against *p multocida* and can be used for short durations without regard to patient age (see Antimicrobial Agents and Related Therapy, p 863). Azithromycin and fluoroquinolones display good in vitro activity against organisms that commonly cause bite wound infections, but clinical data are lacking. Carbapenems are an option for children with penicillin allergy. A 5-day course of treatment usually is sufficient for soft tissue infections, but the duration of treatment for bite wound-associated bone infections is based on location, severity, and pathogens isolated.

In the child with a confirmed bite wound-associated infection, initial therapy should be modified when culture results become available. MRSA is a potential but uncommon bite wound pathogen; empiric therapy may require modification in cases of known colonization or when MRSA is isolated from an infected wound (see *Staphylococcus aureus,* p 678). Coverage for MRSA should be considered in severe bite wound infections while cultures are pending.

PREVENTION OF MOSQUITOBORNE AND TICKBORNE INFECTIONS

Mosquitoborne diseases in the continental United States are caused by arboviruses (eg, West Nile, La Crosse, Jamestown Canyon, St. Louis encephalitis, and eastern equine encephalitis [see Arboviruses, p 202]). Local transmission of other mosquitoborne viruses (eg, dengue, chikungunya, and Zika viruses) occurs in US territories (eg, Puerto Rico, US Virgin Islands, American Samoa) and occasionally in the continental United States. International travelers may encounter similar or different arboviruses (eg, yellow fever, Japanese encephalitis) or other mosquitoborne infections (eg, malaria) during travel (also see disease-specific chapters in Section 3).

Tickborne infectious diseases in the United States include diseases caused by spirochetes, rickettsiae, bacteria, protozoa, and viruses. Different species of ticks transmit different infectious agents. *Dermacentor variabilis* (American dog tick), *Dermacentor andersoni* (Rocky Mountain wood tick), and *Rhipicephalus sanguineus* (brown dog tick) are the primary vectors of *Rickettsia rickettsii* (Rocky Mountain spotted fever). *Dermacentor andersoni* also transmits Colorado tick fever virus. *Ixodes scapularis* (deer or blacklegged tick) and *Ixodes pacificus* (western blacklegged tick) transmit *Borrelia burgdorferi* (Lyme disease) and *Anaplasma phagocytophilum* (anaplasmosis). *Ixodes* ticks also transmit *Babesia microti* (babesiosis), *Borrelia miyamotoi, Borrelia mayonii, Ehrlichia muris eauclairensis,* and Powassan virus. *Amblyomma americanum* (lone star tick) transmits *Ehrlichia chaffeensis, Ehrlichia ewingii* (ehrlichiosis), and Heartland virus and is associated with southern tick-associated rash illness (STARI). *Francisella tularensis* (tularemia) can be transmitted by *D andersoni, D variabilis*, or *A americanum*. Soft-bodied ticks (*Ornithodoros* species) transmit *Borrelia hermsii* and other spirochetes causing tickborne relapsing fever.

Prevention of infection depends on avoiding known areas of disease, reducing arthropod habitats, using repellents and clothing to protect against biting arthropods, and limiting the amount of time that ticks are attached to the skin. Vaccines for yellow fever and Japanese encephalitis are licensed and available in the United States for use in travelers. A dengue vaccine is licensed in the United States for use in children 9 to 16 years of age living in areas with endemic infection, but it is not yet available. Chemoprophylactic drugs are available to protect against malaria.

General Protective Measures

Pediatricians can educate about taking the following measures to reduce exposures to vectorborne diseases:

- **Avoid exposure to mosquitoes and ticks**. Physicians need to be aware of the burden of arthropod-related infections in their local areas. Local health departments can provide information about domestic disease risks and patterns. Travelers, to the extent possible, should avoid known areas of disease transmission. The Centers for Disease Control and Prevention (CDC) Travelers' Health website provides updates on regional disease transmission patterns and outbreaks (**wwwnc.cdc.gov/travel/**).

- **Eliminate standing water sources that attract mosquitoes.** Mosquitoes lay eggs on or near standing water, and large numbers of mosquitoes can arise from sources standing water at or near the home. Measures to limit places where mosquitoes can lay eggs around the home include drainage or removal of receptacles for standing water (eg, tires, toys, flower pots, cans, buckets, barrels, other containers that collect rain water); keeping swimming pools, decorative pools, and children's wading pools in working condition so that water does not become stagnant; replacing water in bird baths several times weekly; and clearing clogged rain gutters. Under certain circumstances, large-scale mosquito-control measures may be conducted by community or public health officials. These efforts include drainage of standing water, use of larvicides in waters that are sources of mosquitoes, and use of adulticides to control adult mosquitoes.

- **Reduce exposure to mosquitoes.** Mosquitoes may bite at any time, but different species of mosquitoes have different peak biting times. Peak biting time for vectors of malaria and West Nile virus are from dusk to dawn, and for others (such as those carrying dengue, chikungunya, and Zika viruses) peak times are at dawn and dusk. Limiting outdoor activities at times of peak mosquito biting activity can help reduce exposure to infections. Bed nets, screens, and nets tucked around strollers and other confined spaces where young children play are important barriers against mosquitoes. Mosquito traps, electrocutors (bug zappers), ultrasonic repellers, and other devices marketed to prevent mosquitoes from biting people should not be relied on to reduce mosquito bites.

- **Reduce exposure to ticks.** Ticks generally live in grassy, brushy, or wooded areas. People are more likely to come in contact with ticks while with animals or when camping, gardening or hunting. The residential backyard is a primary environment where people in the Northeast are bitten by ticks that transmit diseases including *B burgdorferi* infection (Lyme disease). Tick-infested areas should be avoided whenever possible. When hiking, using the center of trails would reduce exposure. Risk of exposure to some ticks can be reduced by locating play equipment in sunny, dry areas away from forest edges; creating a barrier of dry wood chips or gravel between recreation areas and forest; regularly mowing of vegetation; and keeping leaves raked and underbrush cleared. The brown dog tick, a concern in the southwestern United States, can survive in more arid environments and can be introduced indoors where it may be found in cracks and crevices in the house; on walls, carpet, and furniture; or in animal housing or bedding. Control of tick populations in the community often is not practical but can be effective in more defined areas, such as around places where children play. Using acaricides (pesticides targeting ticks) on a property or pets can reduce tick populations and possibly the risk of tickborne disease.

- **Wear appropriate protective clothing.** Whenever possible when entering mosquito or tick habitats, clothing should be worn that covers the arms, legs, head, and other exposed skin areas. Tucking in shirts and wearing closed shoes instead of sandals may reduce exposure to ticks.

- **Consider treatment of clothing and gear.** Permethrin (a synthetic pyrethroid) is both a pesticide and a repellent that can be sprayed onto clothes and gear. Permethrin repels both mosquitoes and ticks. For ticks, clothing and gear should be treated with products containing 0.5% permethrin. Permethrin should not be sprayed directly onto skin, and treated clothing should be dried before wearing. The US Environmental Protection Agency (EPA) has registered the commercial sale of permethrin-treated outdoor clothing, hats, bed nets, and camping gear, which is safe for children and for pregnant women. Adverse reactions to permethrin are mild and transient and may include skin rash, burning, stinging, erythema, tingling, or numbness. Permethrin-treated clothing remains effective through multiple launderings but may need retreatment over time. Permethrin or repellents should not be used on clothing or mosquito nets where children may chew or suck on the material.

Repellents for Use on Skin

The EPA regulates repellent products in the United States. The CDC, US Food and Drug Administration (FDA), and American Academy of Pediatrics (AAP) recommend that people use repellent products that have been registered by the EPA, which indicates that the materials have been reviewed for both efficacy and human safety when applied according to the instructions on the label.

Arthropods are attracted to people by body heat, odors on the skin, and carbon dioxide and other volatile chemicals from the breath. The active ingredients in repellents, with the exception of permethrin-based repellents, help ward off mosquitoes or ticks but do not kill them. Repellents should be used during outdoor activities when mosquitoes or ticks are present and should always be used according to the label instructions. Protection times listed below generally are against mosquitoes; duration of protection generally is shorter against ticks. Protection also varies by type and concentration of active ingredient, product formulation, ambient temperatures, and types of activity (eg, protection time is reduced by perspiration, washing of skin, and involvement in water recreation). Product labels should be followed for application and reapplication recommendations. Repellents should not be reapplied more frequently than recommended on the label. Guidelines are available from the EPA (**www.epa.gov/ insect-repellents/find-insect-repellent-right-you**).

EPA-REGISTERED REPELLENTS

Several types of EPA-registered products provide repellent activity sufficient to help people reduce the bites of disease-carrying mosquitoes and ticks (**www.epa.gov/ insect-repellents** and **wwwnc.cdc.gov/travel/yellowbook/2020/noninfectious-health-risks/mosquitoes-ticks-and-other-arthropods**). At this time, products containing the following active ingredients typically provide reasonably long-lasting protection from mosquitoes and ticks when applied directly to the skin.

DEET. Chemical name: N,N-diethyl-meta-toluamide or N,N-diethyl-3-methyl-benzamide. Commercial products registered for direct application to human skin contain from 5% to 99% DEET (**www.epa.gov/insect-repellents/deet**). DEET repels both mosquitoes and ticks. In general, higher concentrations of active ingredient provide longer duration of protection. Protection times for DEET against mosquitoes range from 1 to 2 hours for products containing 5% concentrations (which may not protect against ticks) to 10 hours or more for products containing 40% or more DEET. There does not appear to be a meaningful increase in protection time for products containing >50% DEET. Time-released DEET formulations are available that provide 11 to 12 hours of protection with concentrations of 20% to 30% DEET.

    DEET does not present a health problem if used appropriately. Adverse effects related to DEET are rare; most often are associated with ingestions or chronic or excessive use and do not appear to be related to DEET concentration used. Urticaria and contact dermatitis have been reported in a small number of people. Although rare, adverse systemic effects including encephalopathy have been reported after excessive skin application in children and after unintentional ingestion. DEET is irritating to eyes and mucous membranes. Highly concentrated formulations can damage plastic and certain synthetic fabrics.

PICARIDIN (KBR 3023). Chemical name: 2-(2-hydroxyethyl)-1-piperidinecarboxylic acid 1-methylpropyl ester. Picaridin has concentration-related efficacy and ages for use similar to DEET. Products containing 5% picaridin provide 3 to 4 hours of protection against mosquitoes and ticks, and products with 20% picaridin can provide protection for 8 to 12 hours. Although experience is less extensive than with DEET, no serious toxicity has been reported. Picaridin-containing compounds have been used as repellents for 2 decades in Europe and Australia and for more than 10 years in the United States as a 20% formulation with no serious toxicity reported.

OIL OF LEMON EUCALYPTUS. Chemical name: para-menthane-3,8-diol (PMD). PMD is the synthesized version of oil of lemon eucalyptus (OLE). Only EPA-registered repellent products containing the active ingredient OLE or PMD should be used. "Pure" oil of lemon eucalyptus has not been tested for safety and efficacy and is not registered with the EPA as an insect repellent. Products with 8% to 10% PMD protect for up to 2 hours, and products containing 30% to 40% OLE provide 6 hours of protection. These products should not be used on children younger than 3 years.

IR3535. Chemical name: 3-(N-butyl-N-acetyl)-aminopropionic acid. IR3535 is available in formulations ranging from 7.5% to 20%, with estimated protection times ranging from 2 hours to up to 10 hours depending on concentration.

2-UNDECANONE. Chemical name: methyl nonyl ketone. 2-undecanone is a synthetic version of an organic compound that can also be extracted from oil of rue, a perennial shrub. It can also be found naturally in wild-grown tomatoes, cloves, and other plant sources. 2-undecanone products contain 7.75% active ingredient and provides protection for up to 5 hours for mosquitoes and 2 hours for ticks.

NONREGISTERED PRODUCTS

Topical products based on citronella, catnip oil, and other essential plant oils provide minimal protection and are not recommended. Ingestion of garlic or vitamin B_1 and wearing devices that emit sounds or impregnated wristbands are ineffective.

APPLICATION OF REPELLENTS

The following are recommended precautions for use of repellents:

- Apply repellents only to exposed skin or clothing, as directed on the product label. Do not apply repellents under clothing.
- Never use repellents over cuts, wounds, or irritated skin.
- When using sprays, do not spray directly on face—spray on hands first and then apply to face. Do not apply repellents to eyes or mouth, and apply sparingly around ears.
- Children should not handle repellents. Adults should apply repellents to their own hands first, and then gently spread on the child's exposed skin. Adults should avoid applying directly to children's hands, because children frequently put fingers and hands into their mouths.
- Use just enough repellent to cover exposed skin or clothing.
- Sprays should not be applied in enclosed areas or near food.
- Wash hands after application to avoid accidental exposure to eyes or ingestion.

REPELLENTS AND SUNSCREEN. Sunscreen should be applied first when using both products simultaneously. Repellents that are applied according to label instructions may be used with sunscreen with no reduction in repellent activity; limited data show a one-third decrease in the sun protection factor (SPF) of sunscreens when DEET-containing insect repellents are used after a sunscreen is applied. Reapplication of sunscreen or repellent may be needed depending on the duration of protection needed and type of activity. Products that combine sunscreen and repellent are not recommended.

Tick Inspection and Removal

Parents or caregivers should promptly inspect children's bodies, clothing, and equipment they used during and after possible tick exposure ("tick check"). When conducting tick checks, special attention should be given to the exposed regions of the body where ticks often attach, including the head, neck, and around the ears. Ticks also may attach at areas of tighter clothing (eg, sock line, belt line, axillae, groin). Timely tick checks increase the likelihood of finding and removing ticks before they can transmit an infectious agent. Longer periods of attachment increase the probability of transmission of tickborne pathogens significantly. It is important to remove clothes as soon as possible after potential tick exposure, because they may harbor crawling ticks. Bathing or showering after coming indoors (preferably within 2 hours) can be an opportunity to locate attached or crawling ticks and has been shown to be an important personal protective measure for several tickborne diseases. Unattached ticks can enter the home by hiding in or on clothing. Placing dry clothing in a dryer on high heat for at least 10 min (damp clothes can take up to 1 hour) has been used effectively to kill unattached ticks on clothes.

TICK REMOVAL

Ticks should be removed from skin as soon as possible. Do not wait for the tick to detach itself from the skin by "painting" it with petroleum jelly or using heat. Use fine-tipped forceps or tweezers to grasp the tick as close to the skin as possible and gently pull straight out without twisting motions. Be careful not to break mouthparts as the tick is removed. Tweezers should be cleaned of any potential tick body tissue or fluids that may have been left after pulling on the attached tick. Tweezers then can be used to remove mouthparts or cement (an adhesive secretion that anchors tick mouthparts to the skin) left on the skin. Avoid cutting or digging into skin to remove small remnants; if unable to remove the mouth parts easily, leave them alone and let the skin heal. If fingers are used to remove ticks, they should be protected with a barrier, such as tissue or plastic gloves, and washed after removal of the tick. The bite site should be washed with soap and water to reduce the risk of secondary skin infections.

TESTING TICKS

Testing ticks removed from animals or humans for infectious pathogens is unnecessary, because it is not diagnostically informative.

Other Preventive Measures

PETS

Maintaining tick-free pets also will decrease tick exposure in and around the home. Daily inspection of pets, removal of ticks, and use of appropriate veterinary products to prevent ticks on pets are indicated. Consult a veterinarian for information on effective products. Apply recommended products as instructed.

CHEMOPROPHYLAXIS

Chemoprophylaxis with a single dose of doxycycline to prevent Lyme disease after tick bites may be considered in areas with endemic Lyme disease (see Lyme Disease, p 482). Chemoprophylaxis is not recommended for other tickborne diseases, including rickettsiae.

....

PREVENTION OF ILLNESSES ASSOCIATED WITH RECREATIONAL WATER USE

Pathogen transmission via recreational water (eg, swimming pools, water playgrounds, lakes, oceans) is an increasingly recognized source of illness in the United States. Since the mid-1980s, the annual number of reported outbreaks associated with recreational water—particularly in treated recreational water venues (eg, swimming pools)—has increased significantly.[1] Therefore, preventing recreational water–associated illness (RWI) and promoting healthy swimming is becoming increasingly important for children and adults. RWIs can be caused by pathogens transmitted by ingesting, inhaling aerosols of, or having contact with contaminated water from swimming pools, water

[1]Hlavsa MC, Roberts VA, Kahler AM, et al. Outbreaks of illness associated with recreational water—United States, 2011–2012. *MMWR Morb Mortal Wkly Rep*. 2015;64(24):668-672

playgrounds, hot tubs/spas, lakes, rivers, or oceans. RWIs also can be caused by chemicals or toxins via ingestion, inhalation, or contact. Illnesses associated with recreational water can involve the gastrointestinal tract, respiratory tract, central nervous system, skin, ears, or eyes. Between 2000 and 2014, more than 630 outbreaks of RWIs were reported to the Centers for Disease Control and Prevention (CDC).[1,2] These outbreaks resulted in more than 32 000 cases of illness and 10 deaths. The vast majority of these outbreaks (almost 500) were associated with treated recreational water venues (eg, pools, hot tubs/spas, water playgrounds), of which 43% were caused by *Cryptosporidium* species. Cryptosporidiosis can cause life-threatening infection in immunocompromised children and adolescents (see Cryptosporidiosis, p 288). Other common causes included *Legionella* species (see *Legionella pneumophila* Infections, p 465) and *Pseudomonas* species (folliculitis ["hot tub rash"] or acute otitis externa ["swimmer's ear"]). Among 140 outbreaks associated with untreated recreational water venues (eg, lakes, reservoirs, ponds), common causes included norovirus (see Norovirus and Sapovirus Infections, p 548), pathogenic *Escherichia coli* (see *Escherichia coli* Diarrhea, p 322), *Shigella* species (see *Shigella* infections, p 668), and *Cryptosporidium* species (see Cryptosporidiosis, p 288). Two deaths were attributed to primary amoebic meningoencephalitis (PAM) caused by *Naegleria fowleri*, a free-living amoeba found in natural or ambient bodies of freshwater.

Although rare (0–8 infections per year), *N fowleri* infection is nearly always fatal (>97% fatality rate). Infection primarily affects healthy young males and can occur during swimming in warm, freshwater lakes, ponds, reservoirs, rivers, or streams, although cases have also been associated with inadequately chlorinated swimming pools, an artificial whitewater river, and an inland surf park. After the amebae enter the nasal cavity, they migrate to the brain via the olfactory nerve. Signs and symptoms of *N fowleri* infection are clinically similar to bacterial meningitis.

Cyanobacteria and some other types of algae can produce toxins that cause a range of illnesses, from skin or eye irritation to respiratory, gastrointestinal, or neurologic symptoms depending on type of toxin and the route of exposure. Cyanobacterial toxins from harmful algal blooms were the suspected or confirmed etiology in 15 outbreaks associated with exposure to untreated recreational water reported for 2000–2014.[3,4] Harmful algal blooms result from the rapid growth of algae that can cause harm to animals, people, or the local environment. They appear as foam, scum, or mats on the surface of water, may be different colors, and can occur in warm fresh, marine, or brackish waters with abundant nutrients. Many different organisms with different names produce harmful algal blooms.

Swimming is a communal bathing activity by which the same water is shared by a few individuals to thousands of people each day, depending on venue size (eg, from small, inflatable or hard plastic wading pools [**www.cdc.gov/healthywater/ swimming/swimmers/inflatable-plastic-pools.html**] to pools in water parks).

---

[1]Hlavsa MC, Cikesh BL, Roberts VA, et al. Outbreaks associated with treated recreational water—United States, 2000–2014. *MMWR Morb Mortal Wkly Rep.* 2018;67(19):547-551

[2]Graciaa DS, Cope JR, Roberts VA, et al. Outbreaks associated with untreated recreational water—United States, 2000–2014. *MMWR Morb Mortal Wkly Rep.* 2018;67(25):701-706

[3]Hilborn ED, Roberts VA, Backer L, et al, Algal bloom-associated disease outbreaks among users of freshwater lakes—United States, 2009–2010. *MMWR Morb Mortal Wkly Rep.* 2014;63(1):11-15

[4]Hlavsa MC, Roberts VA, Kahler A, et al. Outbreaks of illness associated with recreational water—United States, 2011–2012. *MMWR Morb Mortal Wkly Rep.* 2015;64(24):668-672

Fecal contamination of recreational water venues is a common occurrence because of the high prevalence of diarrhea and fecal incontinence (particularly in young children [ie, age <5 years]) and the presence of residual fecal material on bodies of swimmers (up to 10 g on young children). Reported recreational water–associated outbreaks can disproportionally affect young children, usually occur during the summer months, and most frequently manifest as gastroenteritis. In addition to fecal contamination by swimmers, untreated recreational waters can be impacted by sewage treatment plant discharges, septic systems, or agricultural waste, which might contain a wide range of potentially infectious pathogens (eg, norovirus, *E coli*, *Shigella* species, *Cryptosporidium* species). Other microorganisms in untreated recreational waters might also cause infection (eg, *Vibrio vulnificus* and *Vibrio parahaemolyticus*) or allergic rashes (eg, cercarial dermatitis attributable to avian schistosomes).

To protect swimmers from infectious pathogens, water in treated recreational water venues is chlorinated. Maintaining pH and disinfectant concentration as recommended by the CDC (**www.cdc.gov/healthywater/swimming/index.html**) is sufficient to inactivate most infectious pathogens within minutes. However, some infectious pathogens are moderately to extremely chlorine tolerant and can survive for extended periods of time, even in properly chlorinated pools. *Giardia duodenalis* has been shown to survive for up to 45 minutes. *Legionella* and *Pseudomonas* species are effectively controlled by chlorination, but because they persist in biofilms, they can proliferate when proper disinfectant concentrations are not maintained. *Cryptosporidium* oocysts can survive for more than 7 days even in properly chlorinated pools, thus contributing to the role of *Cryptosporidium* species as the leading cause of recreational water–associated outbreaks. Additional water treatments (eg, ultraviolet light, ozone) can more efficiently inactivate *Cryptosporidium* oocysts.

Recreational water use is a major route for *Cryptosporidium* transmission because of the organism's extreme chlorine tolerance, low infectious dose, immediate infectiousness upon excretion and high pathogen excretion volume, in addition to poor swimmer hygiene (eg, swimming when ill with diarrhea) and swimmer behavior (eg, ingesting recreational water). One or more swimmers who are ill with diarrhea can contaminate large volumes of water and expose large numbers of swimmers to *Cryptosporidium* species and other pathogens, particularly if pool disinfection is inadequate. Outbreaks associated with treated recreational water venues generally can be prevented and controlled through a combination of proper pH, adequate disinfectant concentration, and improved swimmer hygiene and behavior. Pediatricians and parents of young children can learn more about healthy swimming at **www.cdc.gov/healthyswimming.** Over-the-counter test strips can be purchased to check the free chlorine level and pH of a public swimming pool or hot tub.

CONTROL MEASURES

Swimming is generally a safe and effective means of physical activity. Transmission of infectious pathogens that cause most RWIs can be prevented by reducing contamination of swimming venues and limiting exposure to contaminated water. Pediatricians should counsel families as follows:

- Regularly test home pools to ensure that the water's free chlorine or bromine (another commonly used disinfectant) concentration and the pH are correct and safe:
  - Free chlorine concentration should be at least 1 parts per million (ppm).

- Bromine concentration should be at least 3 ppm.
- pH should be 7.2 to 7.8.
- Do not go into recreational water (eg, swim) when ill with diarrhea.
  - After cessation of symptoms, people who had diarrhea attributable to *Cryptosporidium* species also should avoid recreational water activities for an additional 2 weeks. This is because of prolonged excretion of infectious *Cryptosporidium* oocysts after cessation of symptoms, the potential for intermittent exacerbations of diarrhea, and the increased transmission potential in treated recreational water venues (eg, swimming pools) because of the organism's high chlorine tolerance.
  - After cessation of symptoms, children who had diarrhea attributable to other potential waterborne pathogens (eg, *Shigella* species) and who are incontinent should avoid recreational water activities for 1 additional week (or as advised by local public health authorities).
- Avoid ingestion of recreational water.
- Do not go into recreational water (eg, swim) with open wounds (eg, from surgery or a piercing), because wounds can serve as portals of entry for pathogens.
- Stay out of the water in lakes, rivers, or oceans if:
  - Beaches are closed or an advisory is posted for high bacterial levels or other conditions, such as sewage spills or harmful algal blooms.
  - Recent heavy rainfall has occurred in the previous 48 to 72 hours (rain can wash contaminants from the land, like septic tank overflows or animal feces, into the water).
  - A discharge pipe can be seen from the beach.
  - Fish or other animals in or near the water are dead.
  - Water is discolored, smelly, foamy, or scummy.
- The only certain way to prevent *N fowleri* infection caused by swimming is to refrain from water-related activities in warm freshwater. To reduce exposure risk to *N fowleri:*
  - Use nose clips, hold nose shut, or keep head above water when taking part in water-related activities in bodies of warm freshwater.
  - Avoid putting your head under water in hot springs or other untreated thermal waters.
  - Avoid water-related activities in warm freshwater during periods of high temperature.
- To reduce exposure risk to harmful algal blooms:
  - Avoid water that contains harmful algal blooms (when in doubt, stay out).
  - Keep children and pets from drinking or playing in discolored, smelly, foamy, or scummy water.
  - Get out and rinse off with clean tap water as soon as possible after swimming in water that might contain a harmful algal bloom.
  - Rinse off pets, especially dogs, immediately if they swim in discolored, smelly, foamy, or scummy water. Do not let pets lick the algae off their fur.
- Practice good swimmer hygiene:
  - Shower with soap and water for at least 1 minute before entering recreational water.
  - Instruct children not to urinate or defecate in the water.
  - Take children to the bathroom every hour. Check diapered children every hour and change diapers in a bathroom or diaper changing area—not waterside—to keep infectious agents, urine, and feces out of the water. Swim diapers and swim

pants, although able to hold in some solid feces, do not prevent leakage of pathogens such as *Cryptosporidium* species into the water.
- Wash hands with soap and water after using the bathroom and changing diapers and before consumption of food and drink.

Healthy swimming promotion materials are available at **www.cdc.gov/ healthywater/swimming/materials/index.html.** Healthy swimming brochures and other printed materials are available at **wwwn.cdc.gov/pubs/ cdcInfoOnDemand.aspx?ProgramID=93.**

"SWIMMER'S EAR"/ACUTE OTITIS EXTERNA

Participation in recreational water activities can predispose children to infections of the external auditory canal. Acute otitis externa (AOE) or "swimmer's ear," one of the most common infections encountered by clinicians, is a diffuse inflammation of the external auditory canal and is usually attributable to bacterial infection. Recreational water activities, showering, and bathing can introduce water into the ear canal, wash away protective ear wax, increase the pH, and cause maceration of the thin skin of the ear canal, thus predisposing the ear canal to infection. AOE is most common among children 5 to 14 years of age but can occur in all age groups, including adults. A marked seasonality is observed, with cases peaking during the summer months. Warm, humid environments and frequent submersion of the head while swimming are risk factors for AOE.

Bacterial infections cause 90% of AOE cases. The 2 bacteria that most commonly cause AOE are *Pseudomonas aeruginosa* and *Staphylococcus aureus*. Many cases are polymicrobial. Fungal infections, for example, *Aspergillus* species and *Candida* species, are responsible for a minority (10%) of AOE cases. Cultures of swab specimens taken from the external ear canal in AOE may not be entirely diagnostic because these can reflect normal ear canal flora or pathogenic organisms.

AOE readily responds to treatment with topical antimicrobial agents with or without a topical steroid. Unless the infection has spread to surrounding tissues or the patient has complicating factors (eg, has diabetes or is immunocompromised), topical treatment alone should be sufficient, and systemic antimicrobials usually are not required. Polymyxin B sulfate/neomycin sulfate, gentamicin sulfate, and ciprofloxacin for 7 to 10 days are topical antibiotic agents used commonly. If clinical improvement is not noted by 48 to 72 hours, the patient should be reevaluated for possible foreign body obstruction of the canal, noncompliance with therapy, or alternate diagnoses, such as contact dermatitis or traumatic cellulitis. If delivery of topical antibiotics is being impeded by drainage obstructing the external auditory canal, placement of a cellulose wick or referral to an otolaryngologist for aural toilet should be considered. Topical agents that have the potential for ototoxicity (eg, gentamicin, neomycin, agents with a low pH, hydrocortisone-neomycin-polymyxin) should not be used in children with tympanostomy tubes or a perforated tympanic membrane. Patients with AOE should avoid submerging their head in water for 7 to 10 days, but competitive swimmers might be able to return to the pool if pain has resolved and they use well-fitting ear plugs.

All swimmers should be instructed to keep their ear canals as dry as possible. This can be accomplished by covering the opening of the external auditory canal with a bathing cap or by using ear plugs or molds. Following swimming or showering, the ears should be dried thoroughly using a towel or a hairdryer on the lowest heat and fan setting.

If a person experiences recurring episodes of AOE, consideration can be given to use of antimicrobial otic drops after recreational water exposure as an additional preventive measure. Commercial ear-drying agents are available for use as directed, or a 1:1 mixture of acetic acid (white vinegar) and isopropanol (rubbing alcohol) may be placed in the external ear canal after swimming or showering to restore the proper acidic pH to the ear canal and to dry residual water. Otic drying agents should not be used in the presence of tympanostomy tubes, tympanic membrane perforation, AOE infection, or ear drainage.

Additional information on prevention of otitis externa is available at **www.cdc. gov/healthywater/swimming/swimmers/rwi/ear-infections.html.**

Summaries of Infectious Diseases

Actinomycosis

CLINICAL MANIFESTATIONS: Actinomycosis results from pathogen introduction following a breakdown in mucocutaneous protective barriers. Spread within the host is by direct invasion of adjacent tissues, typically forming sinus tracts that cross tissue planes. The most common species causing human disease is *Actinomyces israelii*.

There are 3 common anatomic sites of infection. **Cervicofacial** is most common, often occurring after tooth extraction, oral surgery, or other oral/facial trauma or even from carious teeth. Localized pain and induration may progress to cervical abscess and "woody hard" nodular lesions ("lumpy jaw"), which can develop draining sinus tracts, usually at the angle of the jaw or in the submandibular region. Infection may contribute to recurrent or persistent tonsillitis. **Thoracic** disease most commonly is secondary to aspiration of oropharyngeal secretions but may be an extension of cervicofacial infection. It occurs rarely after esophageal disruption secondary to surgery or nonpenetrating trauma. Thoracic presentation includes pneumonia, which can be complicated by abscesses, empyema, and rarely, pleurodermal sinuses. Focal or multifocal mediastinal and pulmonary masses may be mistaken for tumors. **Abdominal** actinomycosis usually is attributable to penetrating trauma or intestinal perforation. The appendix and cecum are the most common sites; symptoms are similar to appendicitis. Slowly developing masses may simulate abdominal or retroperitoneal neoplasms. Intra-abdominal abscesses and peritoneal-dermal draining sinuses occur eventually. Chronic localized disease often forms draining sinus tracts with purulent discharge. **Other sites** of infection include the liver, pelvis (which, in some cases, has been linked to use of intrauterine devices), heart, testicles, and brain (which usually is associated with a primary pulmonary focus). Noninvasive primary cutaneous actinomycosis has occurred.

ETIOLOGY: *A israelii* and at least 5 other *Actinomyces* species cause human disease. All are slow-growing, microaerophilic or facultative anaerobic, gram-positive, filamentous branching bacilli. They can be part of normal oral, gastrointestinal tract, or vaginal flora. *Actinomyces* species frequently are copathogens in tissues harboring multiple other anaerobic and/or aerobic species. Isolation of *Aggregatibacter (Actinobacillus) actinomycetemcomitans*, frequently detected with *Actinomyces* species, may predict the presence of actinomycosis.

EPIDEMIOLOGY: *Actinomyces* species occur worldwide, being components of endogenous oral and gastrointestinal tract flora. *Actinomyces* species are opportunistic pathogens in the setting of disrupted mucosal barriers. Infection is uncommon in infants and children, with 80% of cases occurring in adults. The male-to-female ratio in children is 1.5:1. Although microbiologically confirmed infections caused by *Actinomyces* species now are less common, there are reports in patients who have undergone transplantation or are receiving biologics.

The **incubation period** varies from several days to several years.

DIAGNOSTIC TESTS: Microscopic demonstration of beaded, branched, gram-positive bacilli in purulent material or tissue specimens suggests the diagnosis. Only specimens from normally sterile sites should be submitted for culture. Specimens must be obtained, transported, and cultured anaerobically on semiselective (kanamycin/vancomycin) media such as the modified Thayer-Martin agar or buffered charcoal yeast extract (BCYE) agar. Acid-fast testing can distinguish *Actinomyces* species, which are acid-fast negative, from *Nocardia* species, which are variably acid-fast positive staining. Yellow "sulfur granules" visualized microscopically or macroscopically in drainage or loculations of purulent material suggest the diagnosis. A Gram stain of "sulfur granules" discloses a dense aggregate of bacterial filaments mixed with inflammatory debris. *A israelii* forms "spiderlike" microcolonies on culture medium after 48 hours. *Actinomyces* species can be identified in tissue specimens using polymerase chain reaction assay and sequencing of the 16s rRNA.

TREATMENT: Initial therapy should include intravenous penicillin G or ampicillin for 4 to 6 weeks followed by high doses of oral penicillin (up to 2 g/day for adults), usually for a total of 6 to 12 months depending on the extent of disease and success of surgical management (when indicated). Treatment for mild disease can be initiated with oral therapy. Amoxicillin and doxycycline are alternative antimicrobial choices. Amoxicillin/clavulanate, piperacillin/tazobactam, ceftriaxone, clarithromycin, linezolid, and imipenem/meropenem also show high activity in vitro, but the latter antimicrobials have extended spectrums, which may not always be required. All *Actinomyces* species appear to be resistant to ciprofloxacin and metronidazole. Doxycycline is not typically recommended for children younger than 8 years when therapy will continue beyond 21 days (see Tetracyclines, p 866).

Surgical drainage often is a necessary adjunct to medical management and may shorten but does not obviate antimicrobial therapy.

ISOLATION OF THE HOSPITALIZED PATIENT: Standard precautions are recommended. There is no person-to-person spread.

CONTROL MEASURES: Appropriate oral hygiene, regular dental care, and careful cleansing of wounds, including human bite wounds, can prevent infection.

Adenovirus Infections

CLINICAL MANIFESTATIONS: Adenovirus infections of the upper respiratory tract are common and often subclinical; when symptomatic, adenoviruses may cause common cold symptoms, pharyngitis, tonsillitis, otitis media, and pharyngoconjunctival fever. Adenoviruses occasionally cause a pertussis-like syndrome, croup, bronchiolitis, influenza-like illness, exudative tonsillitis, and hemorrhagic cystitis. Ocular adenovirus infections may present as follicular conjunctivitis or as epidemic keratoconjunctivitis. Enteric adenoviruses are an important cause of childhood gastroenteritis. Life-threatening disseminated infection, lower respiratory infection (eg, severe pneumonia, bronchiolitis obliterans), hepatitis, meningitis, and encephalitis occur occasionally, especially among young infants and immunocompromised people.

ETIOLOGY: Adenoviruses are double-stranded, nonenveloped DNA viruses of the *Adenoviridae* family and *Mastadenovirus* genus, with more than 80 recognized types and multiple genetic variants divided into 7 species (A–G) that infect humans. Some adenovirus types are associated primarily with respiratory tract disease (types 1–5, 7, 14, and 21), epidemic keratoconjunctivitis (types 8, 19, and 37), or gastroenteritis (types 40 and 41).

EPIDEMIOLOGY: Infection in children can occur at any age. Adenoviruses causing respiratory tract infections usually are transmitted by respiratory tract secretions through person-to-person contact, airborne droplets, and fomites. Adenoviruses are hardy viruses, can survive on environmental surfaces for long periods, and are not easily inactivated by many disinfectants. Outbreaks of febrile respiratory tract illness attributable to adenoviruses can be a significant problem in military trainees, college students, and residents of long-term care facilities. Community outbreaks of adenovirus-associated pharyngoconjunctival fever have been attributed to water exposure from contaminated swimming pools and fomites, such as shared towels. Health care-associated transmission of adenoviral infections can occur in hospitals, residential institutions, and nursing homes from exposures to infected health care personnel, patients, or contaminated equipment. Adenovirus infections in solid organ transplant recipients can occur from donor tissues. Epidemic keratoconjunctivitis commonly occurs by direct contact and has been associated with equipment used during eye examinations. Enteric strains of adenoviruses are transmitted by the fecal-oral route. Adenoviruses do not demonstrate the marked seasonality of other respiratory tract viruses and instead circulate throughout the year. Enteric disease occurs year-round and primarily affects children younger than 4 years. Adenovirus infections are most communicable during the first few days of an acute illness, but persistent and intermittent shedding for longer periods, even months, can occur especially among people with weakened immune systems. In healthy people, infection with one adenovirus type should confer type-specific immunity or at least lessen symptoms associated with reinfection, which forms the basis of adenovirus vaccines used in new military recruits (see Control Measures).

The **incubation period** for respiratory tract infection varies from 2 to 14 days; for gastroenteritis, the **incubation period** is 3 to 10 days.

DIAGNOSTIC TESTS: Methods for diagnosis of adenovirus infection include molecular detection, isolation in cell culture, and antigen detection. Molecular assays (eg, polymerase chain reaction-PCR) are the preferred diagnostic method for detection of adenoviruses, and these assays are widely available commercially. However, the persistent and intermittent shedding that commonly follows an acute adenoviral infection can complicate the clinical interpretation of a positive molecular test result. Quantitative adenovirus assays can be useful for management of immunocompromised patients, such as hematopoietic stem cell and solid organ transplant recipients. Adenoviruses associated with respiratory tract and ocular disease can be isolated by culture from respiratory specimens (eg, nasopharyngeal swab, oropharyngeal swab, nasal wash, sputum) and eye secretions in standard susceptible cell lines. Enteric adenoviruses types 40 and 41 usually require specialized cell lines for successful isolation. Rapid antigen-detection techniques, including immunofluorescence and enzyme immunoassay, have been used to detect virus in respiratory tract secretions, conjunctival swab specimens, and stool, but these methods lack sensitivity. Adenovirus typing by molecular methods is available from some reference laboratories. Although its clinical utility is limited, typing can help establish an etiologic association with disease and to investigate clusters of adenovirus-associated illness. Serodiagnosis is used primarily for epidemiologic studies and has no clinical utility.

TREATMENT: Treatment of adenovirus infection is primarily supportive. In immunocompromised patients, immunosuppressive therapy should be reduced whenever possible. There are no antivirals approved by the US Food and Drug Administration for the treatment of adenovirus infections. Reports on the successful use of cidofovir and ribavirin in immunocompromised patients with severe adenoviral disease have been published. Although cidofovir is used for treatment of severe, progressive, or disseminated adenovirus diseases in immunocompromised hosts, its utilization is limited by its associated nephrotoxicity and myelotoxicity. Brincidofovir, an oral prodrug of cidofovir, was evaluated in a randomized controlled trial of pediatric and adult hematopoietic stem cell transplant recipients, and although brincidofovir-treated subjects had lower odds of treatment failure and all-cause mortality compared with the placebo group, the observed difference was not statistically significant. Transplant patients with severe hypogammaglobulinemia at the time of active adenovirus infection might benefit from immunoglobulin administration. Adoptive transfer of adenovirus-specific T-lymphocytes is under investigation for the treatment of severe adenovirus diseases in hematopoietic stem cell transplant recipients, but there are limited data in solid organ transplant recipients or other populations.

ISOLATION OF THE HOSPITALIZED PATIENT: In addition to standard precautions for young children with respiratory tract infections, contact and droplet precautions are indicated for the duration of hospitalization. In immunocompromised patients, contact and droplet precautions should be extended because of possible prolonged shedding of the virus. For patients with conjunctivitis and for diapered and incontinent children with adenoviral gastroenteritis, contact precautions are indicated for the duration of illness.

CONTROL MEASURES: Appropriate hand hygiene, respiratory hygiene, and cough etiquette should be followed. Children who are in group child care, particularly children from 6 months through 2 years of age, are at increased risk of adenoviral respiratory tract infections and gastroenteritis. Effective measures for preventing spread of adenovirus infection in group child care settings have not been determined, but frequent hand hygiene is recommended. If 2 or more children in a group child care setting develop conjunctivitis in the same period of time, advice should be sought from the health consultant of the program or the state health department.

Adequate chlorination of swimming pools is recommended to prevent pharyngoconjunctival fever. Epidemic keratoconjunctivitis associated with ophthalmologic practice can be difficult to control and requires use of single-dose medication dispensing and strict attention to hand hygiene and instrument sterilization procedures. Health care professionals with known or suspected adenoviral conjunctivitis should avoid direct patient contact until symptoms have resolved. Adenoviruses are difficult to inactivate with alcohol-based gels, because they lack an envelope and they may remain viable on skin, fomites, and environmental surfaces for extended periods. Thus, assiduous adherence to hand hygiene and use of disposable gloves when caring for infected patients are recommended.

A live, nonattenuated, oral adenovirus vaccine for types 4 and 7 (2 oral tablets, 1 for each of the 2 strains) has been licensed by the US Food and Drug Administration for prevention of febrile acute respiratory tract disease in the US military.

Amebiasis

CLINICAL MANIFESTATIONS: The majority of individuals with *Entamoeba histolytica* have asymptomatic noninvasive intestinal tract infection. When present, symptoms associated with *E histolytica* infection generally include cramps, watery or bloody diarrhea, and weight loss. Occasionally, the parasite may spread to other organs, most commonly the liver (liver abscess), and cause fever and right upper quadrant pain. Disease is more severe in the very young, the elderly, malnourished people, pregnant women, and people who receive corticosteroids. People with symptomatic intestinal amebiasis generally have gradual onset of symptoms over 1 to 3 weeks. The mildest form of intestinal tract disease is nondysenteric colitis. Amebic dysentery is the most common clinical manifestation of amebiasis and generally includes diarrhea with either gross or microscopic blood or mucous in the stool, lower abdominal pain, and tenesmus. Weight loss is common because of the gradual onset, but fever occurs in a minority of patients (8%–38%). Symptoms may be chronic, with periods of diarrhea and intestinal spasms alternating with periods of constipation. The presentation may mimic that of inflammatory bowel disease. Progressive involvement of the colon may produce toxic megacolon, fulminant colitis, ulceration of the colon and perianal area, and rarely, perforation. Colonic progression may occur at multiple sites and has a high fatality rate. Progression may occur in patients inappropriately treated with corticosteroids or antimotility drugs. An amebic granuloma (ameboma) may form as an annular lesion of the colon and may present as a palpable mass on physical examination. Amebomas can occur in any area of the colon but are most common in the cecum and may be mistaken for colonic carcinoma. Amebomas usually resolve with antiamebic therapy and do not require surgery.

Extraintestinal disease occurs in a small proportion of patients. The liver is the most common extraintestinal site, and infection may spread from there to the pleural space, lungs, and pericardium. Liver abscess may be acute, with fever, abdominal pain, tachypnea, liver tenderness, and hepatomegaly, or may be chronic, with weight loss and vague abdominal symptoms. Liver abscess can also be asymptomatic and only discovered on abdominal imaging that is performed for other reasons. Rupture of abscesses into the abdomen or chest may lead to death. Evidence of recent or concurrent intestinal tract infection usually is absent in extraintestinal disease. Infection may spread from the colon to the genitourinary tract and the skin. The organism may spread hematogenously to the brain and other areas of the body.

ETIOLOGY: The genus *Entamoeba* includes 6 species that live in the human intestine. Four of these species are identical morphologically: *E histolytica, Entamoeba dispar, Entamoeba moshkovskii,* and *Entamoeba bangladeshi. Dientamoeba fragilis* also can lead to asymptomatic infection and intraluminal intestinal disease. Not all *Entamoeba* species are virulent. *E dispar* and *Entamoeba coli* generally are recognized as commensals, and although *E moshkovskii* generally was believed to be nonpathogenic, it may be associated with diarrhea in infants. The pathogenic potential of *E bangladeshi* is not clear. *Entamoeba* and *Dientamoeba* organisms are excreted as cysts or trophozoites in stool of infected people.

EPIDEMIOLOGY: *E histolytica* can be found worldwide but is more prevalent in people of lower socioeconomic status who live in resource-limited countries, where prevalence of amebic infection may be as high as 50% in some communities. Groups at increased risk of infection in industrialized countries include immigrants from or long-term visitors to areas with endemic infection, institutionalized people, and men who have sex with men. Intestinal and asymptomatic infection are distributed equally across the sexes, but incidence of invasive disease, especially liver abscess, is significantly higher in adult males.

E histolytica is transmitted via ingestion of infective amebic cysts, through fecally contaminated food or water, or oral-anal sexual practices. Transmission also can occur via direct rectal inoculation through colonic irrigation devices. Ingested cysts, which are unaffected by gastric acid, undergo excystation in the alkaline small intestine and produce trophozoites that can cause invasive disease in the colon. Cysts that develop subsequently are the source of transmission, especially from asymptomatic cyst excreters. Infected patients excrete cysts intermittently, sometimes for years if untreated. Cysts can remain viable in the environment for weeks to months, are relatively resistant to chlorine, and ingestion of a single cyst is sufficient to cause disease.

The **incubation period** is variable, ranging from a few days to months or years, but commonly is 2 to 4 weeks.

DIAGNOSTIC TESTS: Intestinal amebiasis can be diagnosed by molecular tests, direct microscopy, and antigen detection tests. Stool polymerase chain reaction (PCR) tests have the highest sensitivity and specificity, are available in US Food and Drug Administration (FDA)-approved multiplex assays, and can differentiate *E histolytica* from other *Entamoeba* species. Traditionally, diagnosis of intestinal tract infection was made by identifying trophozoites or cysts in stool specimens, either on wet mount or after fixing and staining. This technique is still used in some laboratories but is labor intensive and suffers from sensitivity lower than for PCR and the requirement to review multiple stool samples. Microscopy also does not differentiate between *E histolytica* and less pathogenic species, although trophozoites containing ingested red blood cells are more likely to be *E histolytica*. Antigen test kits are available in some clinical laboratories for testing of *E histolytica* directly from stool specimens. Examination of biopsy specimens, endoscopy scrapings (not swabs), and abscess aspirates using microscopy or antigen detection is not typically fruitful; PCR assay is preferred, when available, but is only FDA approved for stool specimens. Some monoclonal antibody-based antigen detection assays also can differentiate *E histolytica* from other *Entamoeba* species. *D fragilis* is diagnosed by microscopy.

The indirect hemagglutination (IHA) test has been replaced by commercially available enzyme immunoassay (EIA) kits for routine serodiagnosis of amebiasis, especially in countries without endemic disease. The EIA detects antibody specific for *E histolytica* in approximately 95% or more of patients with extraintestinal amebiasis, 70% of patients with active intestinal tract infection, and 10% of asymptomatic people who are passing cysts of *E histolytica*. Patients may continue to have positive serologic test results even after adequate therapy. Diagnosis of an *E histolytica* liver abscess and other extraintestinal infections is aided by serologic testing, because stool tests and abscess aspirates frequently are nondiagnostic.

Ultrasonography, computed tomography, and magnetic resonance imaging can identify liver abscesses presumptively; those caused by *E histolytica* typically are solitary and smooth walled. Imaging also can identify other extraintestinal sites of infection.

TREATMENT: Treatment should be prioritized for all patients with *E histolytica*, including those who are asymptomatic, given the propensity of this organism to spread among family members and other contacts and to cause invasive infection. In settings where tests to distinguish species are not available, treatment should be administered to symptomatic people on the basis of positive results of microscopic examination. A treatment plan should include directed therapy to eliminate invading trophozoites as well as organisms carried in the intestinal lumen, including cysts. Corticosteroids and antimotility drugs should not be used as they can worsen symptoms and aggravate the disease process. The following treatment regimens and follow-up are recommended:

- **Asymptomatic cyst excreters (intraluminal infections):** treat with an intraluminal amebicide alone (paromomycin, diiodohydroxyquinoline/iodoquinol, or diloxanide furoate [the latter is not currently available in the United States]).

(See Table 4.11, Drugs for Parasitic Infections, p 958–959). Metronidazole and tinidazole are not effective against cysts.

- **Patients with invasive colitis manifesting as mild, moderate, or severe intestinal tract symptoms or extraintestinal disease (including liver abscess):** treat with metronidazole or tinidazole, followed by an intraluminal amebicide: diiodohydroxyquinoline/iodoquinol, diloxanide furoate, or, in absence of intestinal obstruction, paromomycin. Nitazoxanide may be effective for mild to moderate intestinal amebiasis, although it is not approved by the FDA for this indication.
- **Additional considerations in patients with hepatic abscess, pleural or pericardial abscess, or other severe complications:** Percutaneous or surgical aspiration of large liver abscesses occasionally may be required when response of the abscess to medical therapy is unsatisfactory or there is risk of rupture. In most cases of liver abscess, however, drainage is not required and does not speed recovery. Although patients typically improve symptomatically within days, it may take months for a liver abscess to resolve on ultrasonography. Rupture into the peritoneal or pleural space usually requires drainage. For patients who have peritonitis attributable to intestinal perforation, broad-spectrum antibacterial therapy should be used in addition to an amebicide. In cases with toxic megacolon, colectomy may be necessary.

Follow-up stool examination is recommended after completion of therapy for intestinal disease, because no pharmacologic regimen is completely effective in eradicating intestinal tract infection. Household members and other suspected contacts should have adequate stool examinations performed and should be treated if results are positive for *E histolytica*.

E dispar and *Entamoeba coli* generally are considered nonpathogenic and do not necessarily require treatment. The pathogenic significance of finding *E moshkovskii* and *E bangladeshi* is unclear; treatment of symptomatic infection is reasonable. *D fragilis* is treated with iodoquinol, paromomycin, or metronidazole.

ISOLATION OF THE HOSPITALIZED PATIENT: Standard precautions are considered adequate for hospitalized patients; nosocomial transmission is rare.

CONTROL MEASURES: Careful hand hygiene after defecation, sanitary disposal of fecal material, and treatment of drinking water will control spread of infection. Sexual transmission may be controlled by use of condoms and avoidance of sexual activity with those who have diarrhea or who recently recovered from diarrhea. Because of the risk of shedding infectious cysts, people diagnosed with amebiasis should refrain from using recreational water venues (eg, swimming pools, water parks) until after their course of luminal chemotherapy is completed and diarrhea has resolved. Some states prohibit return to work or school for food handlers or children until symptoms have resolved.

Amebic Meningoencephalitis and Keratitis
(*Naegleria fowleri*, *Acanthamoeba* species, and *Balamuthia mandrillaris*)

CLINICAL MANIFESTATIONS: *Naegleria fowleri* can cause a rapidly progressive, almost always fatal, primary amebic meningoencephalitis (PAM). Early symptoms include fever, headache, vomiting, and sometimes disturbances of smell and taste. The illness progresses rapidly to signs of meningoencephalitis, including nuchal rigidity, lethargy, confusion, personality changes, and altered level of consciousness. Seizures are common, and death generally occurs within a week of onset of symptoms. No distinct clinical features differentiate this disease from fulminant bacterial meningitis.

Granulomatous amebic encephalitis (GAE) caused by *Acanthamoeba* species and *Balamuthia mandrillaris* has a more insidious onset than PAM and develops as a subacute or chronic disease. In general, patients with GAE die several weeks to months after onset of symptoms. Signs and symptoms may include altered mental status, personality changes, seizures, headaches, ataxia, cranial nerve palsies, hemiparesis, and other focal neurologic deficits. Fever often is low grade and intermittent. The course may resemble that of a bacterial brain abscess or a brain tumor. Chronic granulomatous skin lesions (pustules, nodules, ulcers) may be present without central nervous system (CNS) involvement, particularly in patients with acquired immunodeficiency syndrome, and lesions may be present for months before brain involvement in immunocompetent hosts.

The most common symptoms of amebic keratitis, a vision-threatening infection usually caused by *Acanthamoeba* species, are pain (often out of proportion to clinical signs), photophobia, tearing, and foreign body sensation. Characteristic clinical findings include radial keratoneuritis and stromal ring infiltrate. *Acanthamoeba* keratitis generally follows an indolent course and initially may resemble herpes simplex or bacterial keratitis; delay in diagnosis is associated with worse outcomes.

ETIOLOGY: *N fowleri, Acanthamoeba* species, and *B mandrillaris* are free-living amebae that exist as motile, infectious trophozoites and environmentally hardy cysts.

EPIDEMIOLOGY: *N fowleri* is found in warm fresh water and moist soil. Most infections with *N fowleri* have been associated with swimming in natural bodies of warm fresh water, such as ponds, lakes, and hot springs, but other sources have included tap water from household plumbing systems and geothermal sources as well as poorly chlorinated swimming pools and municipal water. Disease has been reported worldwide but is uncommon. In the United States, infection occurs primarily in the summer and usually affects children and young adults. The recent northward extension of reported cases may be the result of climatic changes. Disease has followed use of tap water for sinus rinses or exposures related to recreational activities (eg, tap water used for a backyard waterslide). Trophozoites of the amebae invade the brain directly from the nose along the olfactory nerves via the cribriform plate. *Acanthamoeba* species are distributed worldwide and are found in soil; dust; cooling towers of electric and nuclear power plants; heating, ventilating, and air conditioning units; fresh and brackish water; whirlpool baths; and physiotherapy pools. The environmental niche of *B mandrillaris* is not delineated clearly, although it has been isolated from soil. CNS infection attributable to *Acanthamoeba* occurs primarily in debilitated and immunocompromised people. Some patients, and all reported children infected with *B mandrillaris*, have had no demonstrable underlying disease or defect. CNS infection by both amebae probably occurs most commonly by inhalation or direct contact with contaminated soil or water. The primary foci of these infections most likely are respiratory tract or skin, followed by hematogenous spread to the brain. Fatal encephalitis caused by *Balamuthia* species transmitted by the donated organ has been reported in recipients of organ transplants. *Acanthamoeba* keratitis occurs primarily in people who wear contact lenses,[1] although it also has been associated with corneal trauma. Poor contact lens hygiene and/or disinfection practices as well as swimming with contact lenses are risk factors.

---

[1]Centers for Disease Control and Prevention. Contact lens–related corneal infections—United States, 2005–2015. *MMWR Morb Mortal Wkly Rep.* 2016;65(32):817–820

The **incubation period** for *N fowleri* infection typically is 3 to 7 days.

The **incubation periods** for *Acanthamoeba* and *Balamuthia* GAE are unknown. It is believed to take several weeks or months to develop the first symptoms of CNS disease following exposure to the amebae. Chronic progression (1–2 years) to CNS symptoms has been reported in children. Patients exposed to *Balamuthia* through solid organ transplantation can develop symptoms of *Balamuthia* GAE more quickly—within a few weeks.

The **incubation period** for *Acanthamoeba* keratitis is unknown but believed to range from several days to several weeks.

DIAGNOSTIC TESTS: In *N fowleri* infection, computed tomography scans of the head without contrast are unremarkable or show only cerebral edema, but with contrast might show meningeal enhancement of the basilar cisterns and sulci. These changes, however, are not specific for amebic infection. Cerebrospinal fluid (CSF) pressure usually is elevated (300 to >600 mm water), and CSF indices may show a polymorphonuclear pleocytosis, an increased protein concentration, and a normal to very low glucose concentration. Motile trophozoites may be visualized by microscopic examination of CSF on a wet mount. If structures resembling trophozoites are seen but no motility is observed, smears of CSF should be stained with Giemsa, Trichrome, or Wright stains to verify the trophozoites. Gram stain is negative in *N fowleri* CNS infection. Trophozoites, but not cysts, can be visualized in sections of brain during autopsy. Microscopic images containing suspicious amebic structures can be evaluated by the morphology experts at the Centers for Disease Control and Prevention (CDC)'s DPDx (Laboratory Identification of Parasites of Public Health Concern; **www.cdc.gov/dpdx/index.html**). Polymerase chain reaction (PCR) and immunofluorescence assays performed on CSF and biopsy material to identify the organism are available through the CDC, as are consultation services for diagnosis and management (telephone: 770-488-7100).

In infection with *Acanthamoeba* species and *B mandrillaris*, trophozoites and cysts can be visualized in sections of brain, lungs, and skin; in cases of *Acanthamoeba* keratitis, they also can be visualized in corneal scrapings and by confocal microscopy in vivo in the cornea on examination by an expert ophthalmologist. In GAE infections, CSF indices typically reveal a lymphocytic pleocytosis and an increased protein concentration, with normal or low glucose but no organisms. Computed tomography and magnetic resonance imaging of the head may show single or multiple space-occupying, ring-enhancing lesions that can mimic brain abscesses, neurocysticercosis, tumors, cerebrovascular accidents, or other diseases. Like *N fowleri*, PCR and immunofluorescence assays can be performed on clinical specimens to identify *Acanthamoeba* species and *Balamuthia* species; these tests are available through the CDC.

TREATMENT: The most current guidance for treatment of PAM can be found on the CDC website (**www.cdc.gov/parasites/naegleria/treatment-hcp.html**) or by contacting the CDC (telephone: 770-488-7100). Early diagnosis and institution of combination high-dose drug therapy is believed to be important for optimizing outcome. If meningoencephalitis possibly caused by *N fowleri* is suspected, treatment should not be withheld pending confirmation. Presence of amebic organisms in CSF is valuable for probable diagnosis, but confirmatory diagnostic tests still should be performed. Although an effective treatment regimen for PAM has not been identified, amphotericin B is the drug of choice in combination with other agents. In vitro testing indicates that *N fowleri* is highly susceptible to amphotericin B. Miltefosine, which is approved for treatment of leishmaniasis, has been used successfully to treat PAM caused by *N fowleri*. The CDC no longer provides miltefosine for treatment of free-living ameba infections; miltefosine is available commercially in the United States (**impavido.com**). There have been 4 US survivors of PAM and on the basis of most recent cases, treatment with the combination of amphotericin B, azithromycin, fluconazole, miltefosine, and rifampin is recommended. These patients also received dexamethasone to control cerebral edema.

Effective treatment for infections caused by *Acanthamoeba* species and *B mandrillaris* has not been established. Several patients with *Acanthamoeba* GAE and *Acanthamoeba* cutaneous infections without CNS involvement have been treated successfully with a multidrug regimen consisting of various combinations of pentamidine, sulfadiazine, flucytosine, either fluconazole or itraconazole (voriconazole is not active against *Balamuthia* species), trimethoprim-sulfamethoxazole, and topical application of chlorhexidine gluconate and ketoconazole for skin lesions. Voriconazole, miltefosine, and azithromycin also might be of some value in treating *Acanthamoeba* infections. For patients with *B mandrillaris* infection, combination therapy, such as with pentamidine, sulfadiazine, fluconazole, either azithromycin or clarithromycin, and flucytosine, in addition to surgical resection of the CNS lesions, has been reported to be successful. Miltefosine has amebicidal activity against *B mandrillaris* in vitro.

Patients with *Acanthamoeba* keratitis should be evaluated by an ophthalmologist. Early diagnosis and therapy are important for a good outcome.

ISOLATION OF THE HOSPITALIZED PATIENT: Standard precautions are recommended.

CONTROL MEASURES: People should assume that there is always a slight risk of developing PAM caused by *N fowleri* when entering warm fresh water. Only avoidance of such water-related activities can prevent *Naegleria* infection, although the risk might be reduced by taking measures to limit water exposure through known routes of entry, such as getting water up the nose (eg, diving, swimming underwater, doing handstands in water). Using tap water for sinus rinses generally is discouraged, but when used should be either previously boiled or properly filtered or labeled as sterile or distilled (additional information available at **www.cdc.gov/naegleria**). Presently, no clearly defined recommendations are available to prevent GAE attributable to *Acanthamoeba* species or *B mandrillaris*. To prevent *Acanthamoeba* keratitis, steps should be taken to avoid corneal trauma, such as the use of protective eyewear during high-risk activities, and contact lens users should maintain good contact lens hygiene and disinfection practices, use only sterile solutions as applicable, change lens cases frequently, and avoid swimming and showering while wearing contact lenses. Advice for people who wear contact lenses can be found on the CDC website (**www.cdc.gov/contactlenses**).[1]

Anthrax[2]

CLINICAL MANIFESTATIONS: Anthrax resulting from natural infection or secondary to a bioterror event can occur in multiple forms, depending on the route of infection: cutaneous, inhalation, ingestion, or injection.

Manifestations of anthrax are mainly from the 2 primary toxins, lethal toxin and edema toxin. **Cutaneous** anthrax accounts for 95% of all human infections and begins

---

[1]Centers for Disease Control and Prevention. Estimated burden of keratitis—United States, 2010. *MMWR Morb Mortal Wkly Rep.* 2014;63(45):1027-1030

[2]**www.cdc.gov/anthrax/index.html**

as a pruritic papule or vesicle that progresses over 2 to 6 days to an ulcerated lesion with subsequent formation of a central black eschar. The lesion is characteristically painless and has surrounding edema and hyperemia. Patients may have associated fever.

Inhalation anthrax is a frequently lethal form of the disease and is a medical emergency. The initial presentation is nonspecific and usually includes fever, malaise, and nonproductive cough. Many patients also complain of chest pain, headache, nausea, vomiting, and abdominal pain; sweating may be profuse. Illness usually progresses to the fulminant phase within 2 to 5 days. Illness has been noted to sometimes be biphasic, with a period of improvement between prodromal symptoms and overwhelming illness. Significant vital sign abnormalities are often present early, and fulminant manifestations include hypotension, dyspnea, hypoxia, cyanosis, and shock. Most patients with inhalation anthrax fulfill sepsis criteria, and up to half develop meningitis. Imaging abnormalities noted at presentation include pleural effusions in most, widened mediastinum in up to half, and infiltrates in many.

Ingestion anthrax can present as one of 2 distinct clinical syndromes—gastrointestinal or oropharyngeal. Patients with the gastrointestinal form often have nausea, anorexia, vomiting, and fever that progress to severe abdominal pain, often accompanied by marked ascites. Vomiting and diarrhea, which are not always present, may be bloody. Although gastrointestinal tract involvement at multiple sites may occur following hematogenous spread, the cecum and terminal ileum often are involved when the disease is primary. Patients with oropharyngeal anthrax may have dysphagia accompanied by posterior oropharyngeal necrotic ulcers. There may be marked, often unilateral neck swelling, regional lymphadenopathy, fever, and sepsis. Evidence of coagulopathy is common.

Injection anthrax occurs primarily among adult injecting drug users, associated with anthrax-contaminated heroin, and has not been reported in children. Smoking and snorting contaminated heroin also have been identified as exposure routes.

Any route of infection can lead to bacteremia and sepsis. Patients with inhalation, ingestion, or injection anthrax should be considered to have systemic illness. Patients with cutaneous anthrax should be considered to have systemic illness if they have tachycardia, tachypnea, hypotension, hyperthermia, hypothermia, or leukocytosis or have lesions that involve the head, neck, or upper torso or that are large, bullous, multiple, or surrounded by edema. Anthrax meningitis or hemorrhagic meningoencephalitis can occur in any patient with systemic illness and in patients without other apparent route of infection. Therefore, lumbar puncture should be performed to rule out central nervous system (CNS) infection whenever clinically indicated. With appropriate treatment and supportive care, case fatality rates range from <2% for cutaneous anthrax to 45% for inhalation anthrax and 92% for anthrax meningitis.

ETIOLOGY: *Bacillus anthracis* is an aerobic, gram-positive, encapsulated, spore-forming, nonhemolytic, nonmotile rod. *B anthracis* has 3 major virulence factors: an antiphagocytic capsule and 2 exotoxins, called lethal toxin and edema toxin. The toxins are responsible for most of the morbidity associated with anthrax and clinical manifestations of hemorrhage, edema, and necrosis.

EPIDEMIOLOGY: Anthrax is a zoonotic disease that most commonly affects domestic and wild herbivores and occurs in many rural regions of the world. *B anthracis* spores can remain viable in the soil for decades, representing a potential source of infection for livestock or wildlife through ingestion of spore-contaminated vegetation or water. In susceptible hosts, spores germinate to become viable bacteria. Natural infection of humans occurs through contact with infected animals or contaminated animal products, including carcasses, hides, hair, wool, meat, and bone meal. Outbreaks of ingestion anthrax have occurred after consumption of meat from infected animals. Historically, more than 95% of anthrax cases in the United States were cutaneous infections among animal handlers or mill workers. The incidence of naturally occurring human anthrax decreased in the United States from an estimated 130 cases annually in the early 1900s to 0 to 2 cases per year from 1979 through 2011. Only one anthrax case (cutaneous) was confirmed in the United States from 2012–2018. Cases of inhalation, cutaneous, and ingestion (gastrointestinal) anthrax have occurred in drum makers working with animal hides contaminated with B anthracis spores and in people participating in events where spore-contaminated drums were played. Severe soft tissue infections among injection heroin users, including cases with disseminated systemic infection, have been reported in Europe.

B anthracis is one of the agents most likely to be used as a biological weapon, because (1) its spores are highly stable; (2) spores can infect via the respiratory route; and (3) the resulting inhalation anthrax has a high mortality rate. In 1979, an accidental release of B anthracis spores from a military microbiology facility in the former Soviet Union resulted in at least 68 deaths. In 2001, 22 cases of anthrax (11 inhalation, 11 cutaneous) were identified in the United States after intentional contamination of the mail; 5 (45%) of the inhalation anthrax cases were fatal. In addition to aerosolization, B anthracis spores introduced into food products or water supplies could theoretically pose a risk to the public's health. Use of B anthracis in a biological attack would require immediate response and mobilization of public health resources (**www.cdc.gov/anthrax/bioterrorism/index.html**).[1]

Although the **incubation periods** for both cutaneous and ingestion anthrax are typically less than 1 week, rare cases for both have been reported more than 2 weeks after exposure. Because of spore dormancy (persistence of viable spores that have not yet germinated) and slow clearance of spores from the lungs, the **incubation period** for inhalation anthrax may be prolonged and has been reported to range from 2 days to 6 weeks in humans and up to 2 months in experimental nonhuman primates. Discharge from cutaneous lesions is potentially infectious, but person-to-person transmission has only rarely been reported, and other forms of anthrax are not associated with person-to-person transmission. Both inhalation and cutaneous anthrax have occurred in laboratory workers.

DIAGNOSTIC TESTS: Depending on the clinical presentation, Gram stain, culture, and polymerase chain reaction (PCR) testing for B anthracis should be performed with the assistance of state or local health departments on specimens of blood, pleural fluid, cerebrospinal fluid (CSF), and tissue biopsy specimens and on swabs of vesicular fluid or eschar material from cutaneous or oropharyngeal lesions, rectal swabs, or stool (**www.cdc.gov/anthrax/lab-testing/index.html**). Acute sera may be tested for lethal factor (one of the two exotoxins of anthrax). Whenever possible, specimens for these tests should be obtained before initiating antimicrobial therapy because previous treatment with antimicrobial agents makes isolation by culture unlikely and decreases the sensitivity of PCR testing on both blood and tissue samples. Traditional microbiologic methods can

---

[1]Centers for Disease Control and Prevention. Clinical framework and medical countermeasure use during an anthrax mass-casualty incident: CDC recommendations. *MMWR Recomm Rep.* 2015;64(RR-4):1-22

presumptively identify *B anthracis* isolated readily on routine agar media (blood and chocolate) used in clinical laboratories. Definitive identification of suspect *B anthracis* isolates can be performed via the Laboratory Response Network (LRN) in each state, accessed through state and local health departments. Additional diagnostic tests for anthrax are available through state health departments and the Centers for Disease Control and Prevention (CDC), including bacterial DNA detection in specimens by PCR assay, tissue immunohistochemistry, an enzyme immunoassay that measures immunoglobulin G antibodies against *B anthracis* protective antigen in paired sera, and a MALDI-TOF (matrix-assisted laser desorption/ionization–time-of-flight) mass spectrometry assay measuring lethal factor activity in sera. A commercially available enzyme-linked immunosorbent assay (QuickELISA Anthrax-PA kit) can be used for screening but not for definitive diagnosis. This assay detects antibodies to protective antigen protein of *B anthracis* in human serum from individuals with clinical history or symptoms consistent with anthrax infection. Clinical evaluation of patients with suspected inhalation anthrax should include a chest radiograph and/or computed tomography scan to evaluate for widened mediastinum, pleural effusion, and/or pulmonary infiltrates. Lumbar punctures should be performed whenever feasible on systemically ill patients with any type of anthrax to rule out meningitis and to guide therapy.

TREATMENT[1,2]: A high index of suspicion and rapid administration of appropriate antimicrobial therapy to people suspected of being infected, along with access to critical care support, are essential for effective treatment of anthrax. No controlled trials in humans have been performed to validate current treatment recommendations for anthrax, and there is limited clinical experience. Case reports suggest that naturally occurring localized or uncomplicated cutaneous disease can be treated effectively with 7 to 10 days of a single oral antimicrobial agent. First-line agents include a fluoroquinolone or doxycycline. Clindamycin is an alternative, as are penicillins, if the isolate is known to be penicillin susceptible, which is likely to occur with environmental isolates. For bioterrorism-associated cutaneous disease in adults or children lacking signs and symptoms of systemic illness (ie, localized cutaneous disease), either oral ciprofloxacin or oral doxycycline is recommended for initial treatment until antimicrobial susceptibility data are available (see Table 4.3, Antibacterial Drugs for Pediatric Patients Beyond the Newborn Period, p 887). Doxycycline can be used regardless of patient age (see Tetracyclines, p 866). Because of the risk of concomitant inhalational exposure and subsequent spore dormancy in the lungs, the antimicrobial regimen for patients with bioterrorism-associated cutaneous anthrax or who were exposed to other sources of aerosolized spores should be continued for a total of 60 days to provide postexposure prophylaxis (PEP), in conjunction with administration of vaccine if available (see Control Measures).

On the basis of in vitro data and animal studies, parenteral ciprofloxacin is recommended as the primary antimicrobial component of an initial multidrug regimen for treatment of all forms of systemic anthrax until results of antimicrobial susceptibility testing are known (see Table 4.3, Antibacterial Drugs for Pediatric Patients Beyond the

[1]Bradley JS, Peacock G, Krug SE, et al; American Academy of Pediatrics, Committee on Infectious Diseases, Disaster Preparedness Advisory Council. Clinical report: Pediatric anthrax clinical management. *Pediatrics.* 2014;133(5):e1411-e1436

[2]Hendricks KA, Wright ME, Shadomy SV, et al. Centers for Disease Control and Prevention expert panel meetings on prevention and treatment of anthrax in adults. *Emerg Infect Dis.* 2014;20(2). Available at: **wwwnc.cdc. gov/eid/article/20/2/13-0687_intro**

Newborn Period, p 882).[1,2] Levofloxacin and moxifloxacin are considered equivalent alternatives to ciprofloxacin. CNS involvement should be suspected in all cases of inhalation anthrax and other systemic anthrax infections; thus, until this has been ruled out, treatment of systemic anthrax should include at least 2 other agents with known CNS penetration in conjunction with ciprofloxacin. There appears to be benefit to the use of a second bactericidal agent and a theoretical benefit to the use of protein synthesis-inhibiting agent as the additional drugs in this combination. Meropenem is recommended as the second bactericidal antimicrobial, and if meropenem is not available, imipenem/cilastatin or meropenem/vaborbactam are considered alternatives; if the strain is known to be susceptible, penicillin G or ampicillin are equivalent alternatives. Linezolid is recommended as the preferred protein synthesis inhibitor if CNS involvement is suspected. Clindamycin and rifampin are alternatives.

If CNS penetration is less important because meningitis has been ruled out, treatment may consist of 2 antimicrobial agents, including a bactericidal and a protein synthesis-inhibiting agent. Ciprofloxacin is the preferred bactericidal agent, with meropenem, levofloxacin, imipenem/cilastatin, and vancomycin being alternatives; if the strain is known to be susceptible, penicillin G or ampicillin are equivalent alternatives. In such an instance, clindamycin is the preferred protein synthesis inhibitor, and linezolid, doxycycline, and rifampin are acceptable alternatives. Because of intrinsic resistance, cephalosporins and trimethoprim-sulfamethoxazole should not be used.

For patients with systemic disease, treatment should continue for at least 14 days or longer, depending on patient condition. Intravenous therapy can be changed to oral therapy when progression of symptoms ceases and clinical symptoms are improving. There is the risk of spore dormancy in the lungs in people with bioterrorism-associated cutaneous or systemic anthrax or people who were exposed to other sources of aerosolized spores. In these cases, one of the PEP antimicrobials mentioned below should be continued for a total of 60 days, in conjunction with administration of vaccine (see Control Measures).

For patients with anthrax and evidence of systemic illness, such as fever, tachypnea, tachycardia, or shock, polyclonal Anthrax Immune Globulin Intravenous or either of the monoclonal *B anthracis* antitoxins, obiltoxaximab or raxibacumab, should be considered in consultation with the CDC. Supportive symptomatic (intensive care) treatment is important. Aggressive pleural fluid or ascites drainage is critical if effusions exist, because drainage appears to be associated with improved survival. Obstructive airway disease resulting from associated edema may complicate cutaneous anthrax of the face or neck and can require aggressive monitoring for airway compromise.

ISOLATION OF THE HOSPITALIZED PATIENT: Standard precautions are recommended. In addition, contact precautions should be implemented when draining cutaneous lesions are present. Cutaneous lesions become sterile within 24 hours of starting appropriate antimicrobial therapy. Patients with cutaneous illness pose minimal risk for transmission if the wound is kept covered during the first day of antimicrobial therapy. Contaminated dressings and bedclothes should be incinerated or steam sterilized (121°C for 30 minutes)

---

[1]Hendricks KA, Wright ME, Shadomy SV, et al. Centers for Disease Control and Prevention expert panel meetings on prevention and treatment of anthrax in adults. *Emerg Infect Dis.* 2014;20(2). Available at: **wwwnc.cdc.gov/eid/article/20/2/13-0687_intro**

[2]Bradley JS, Peacock G, Krug SE, et al; American Academy of Pediatrics, Committee on Infectious Diseases, Disaster Preparedness Advisory Council. Clinical report: pediatric anthrax clinical management. *Pediatrics.* 2014;133(5):e1411-e1436

to destroy spores. Terminal cleaning of the patient's room can be accomplished with an Environmental Protection Agency-registered hospital-grade disinfectant and should follow standard facility practices typically used for all patients. Autopsies performed on patients with systemic anthrax require special precautions.

CONTROL MEASURES: BioThrax (Anthrax Vaccine Adsorbed [AVA]), the only anthrax vaccine currently licensed in the United States for use in humans, is prepared from a cell-free culture filtrate. The vaccine's efficacy for prevention of anthrax is based on animal studies, a single placebo-controlled human trial of the alum-precipitated precursor of the current AVA, observational data from humans, and immunogenicity data from humans and other mammals. In a human trial in adult mill workers, the alum-precipitated precursor to AVA demonstrated 93% efficacy for preventing cutaneous and inhalation anthrax. Multiple reviews and publications evaluating AVA safety have found adverse events usually are local injection site reactions, with rare systemic symptoms, including fever, chills, muscle aches, and hypersensitivity.

Recommendations for the response to possible exposure to anthrax through bioterrorism are available on the CDC's website at **www.cdc.gov/anthrax/bioterrorism/index.html.** In the event of a bioterrorism event, information for health care professionals and the public relevant to that exposure will be posted on the CDC anthrax website (**www.cdc.gov/anthrax/index.html**). Within 48 hours of exposure to *B anthracis* spores, public health authorities plan to provide a 10-day course of antimicrobial prophylaxis to the local population, including children likely to have been exposed to spores. Within 10 days of exposure, public health authorities plan to further define those who have had a clear and significant exposure and will require additional antimicrobial PEP and a 3-dose anthrax vaccine (AVA) series.

Preexposure prophylaxis is only recommended for select groups of workers at continued risk of infection.

PEP for previously unvaccinated people older than 18 years who have been exposed to aerosolized *B anthracis* spores consists of up to 60 days of appropriate antimicrobial prophylaxis combined with 3 subcutaneous doses of AVA (administered at 0, 2, and 4 weeks postexposure). AVA is not licensed for use in pregnant women; however, in a postevent setting that poses a high risk of exposure to aerosolized *B anthracis* spores, pregnancy is neither a precaution nor a contraindication to its use in PEP. Similarly, AVA is not licensed for use in pediatric populations and has not been studied in children. Until there are sufficient data to support US Food and Drug Administration (FDA) approval, AVA is likely to be made available for children at the time of an event as an investigational vaccine under an appropriate regulatory mechanism that will require institutional review board approval, including the use of appropriate informed consent documents. Information on the process required for use of AVA in children will be available on the CDC website at the time of an event (**www.cdc.gov/anthrax/index.html**), as well as through the American Academy of Pediatrics (AAP) and the FDA. All exposed children 6 weeks and older should receive 3 doses of AVA at 0, 2, and 4 weeks in addition to 60 days of antimicrobial chemoprophylaxis. The recommended route of vaccine administration in children is subcutaneous. Children younger than 6 weeks should immediately begin antimicrobial prophylaxis, but initiation of the vaccine series should be delayed until they reach 6 weeks of age.

When no information is available about antimicrobial susceptibility of the implicated strain of *B anthracis*, ciprofloxacin and doxycycline are equivalent first-line antimicrobial agents for initial PEP for adults or children (see Tetracyclines, p 866). Levofloxacin and clindamycin are second-line antimicrobial agents for PEP. Safety data on extended use of levofloxacin in any population for longer than 28 days are limited; however the benefits of using levofloxacin as PEP for anthrax likely outweigh the risk. When the antimicrobial susceptibility profile demonstrates appropriate sensitivity to amoxicillin (minimum inhibitory concentration ≤0.125 µg/mL), public health authorities may recommend changing PEP antimicrobial therapy for children to oral amoxicillin. Because of the lack of data on amoxicillin dosages for treating anthrax (and the associated high mortality rate), the AAP recommends a higher-than-usual dosage of oral amoxicillin, 75 mg/kg per day, divided into 3 daily doses administered every 8 hours (each dose not to exceed 1 g). Because of intrinsic resistance, cephalosporins and trimethoprim-sulfamethoxazole should not be used for prophylaxis.

Case Reporting. Anthrax meets the definition of a nationally and immediately notifiable condition, as specified by the US Council of State and Territorial Epidemiologists; therefore, every suspected case should be reported **immediately** to the state or local health department.

Arboviruses (also see Chikungunya, p 254, Dengue, p 301, West Nile Virus, p 848, and Zika Virus, p 854)

(Including Colorado tick fever, eastern equine encephalitis, Heartland, Jamestown Canyon, Japanese encephalitis, La Crosse, Powassan, St. Louis encephalitis, tickborne encephalitis, and yellow fever viruses)

CLINICAL MANIFESTATIONS: Most infections with arthropodborne viruses (arboviruses) are subclinical. Symptomatic illness usually manifests as 1 of 3 primary clinical syndromes: generalized febrile illness, neuroinvasive disease, or hemorrhagic fever (Table 3.1).

- **Generalized febrile illness.** Most arboviruses are capable of causing a nonspecific febrile illness that often includes headache, arthralgia, myalgia, and rash. Some arboviruses can cause more characteristic clinical manifestations, such as neuroinvasive disease (see West Nile Virus, p 848), severe polyarthralgia (see Chikungunya Virus, p 254), thrombocytopenia and leukopenia (eg, Heartland virus), or jaundice (eg, yellow fever virus). With some arboviruses, fatigue, malaise, and weakness can linger for weeks following the initial infection.
- **Neuroinvasive disease.** Many arboviruses cause neuroinvasive disease, including aseptic meningitis, encephalitis, or myelitis. Less common neurologic manifestations (eg, Guillain-Barré syndrome) also can occur. Illness often presents with a prodrome similar to the systemic febrile illness followed by neurologic symptoms, although in some cases neurologic findings may be the initial indication of infection. Specific symptoms vary by virus but can include vomiting, stiff neck, mental status changes, seizures, or focal neurologic deficits. Some viruses (eg, West Nile and Japanese encephalitis viruses) can cause a syndrome of acute flaccid paralysis, either in conjunction with meningoencephalitis or as an isolated finding. Severity and long-term outcome of the illness vary by etiologic agent and the underlying characteristics of the host, such as age, immune status, and preexisting medical conditions.
- **Hemorrhagic fever.** Hemorrhagic fever can be caused by some arboviruses, such as dengue (see Dengue, p 301) and yellow fever viruses. After several days of nonspecific

Table 3.1. Clinical Manifestations for Selected Domestic and International Arboviral Diseases

Virus	Generalized Febrile Illness	Neuroinvasive Disease[a]	Hemorrhagic Fever
Domestic			
Colorado tick fever	Yes	Rare	No
Eastern equine encephalitis	Yes	Yes	No
Heartland[b]	Yes	No	No
Jamestown Canyon	Yes	Yes	No
La Crosse	Yes	Yes	No
Powassan	Yes	Yes	No
St. Louis encephalitis	Yes	Yes	No
West Nile	Yes	Yes	No
International			
Chikungunya[c]	Yes	Rare	No
Dengue[c]	Yes	Rare	Yes
Japanese encephalitis	Yes	Yes	No
Tickborne encephalitis	Yes	Yes	No
Yellow fever	Yes	No	Yes
Zika[c]	Yes	Yes	No

[a]Meningitis, encephalitis, or myelitis.
[b]As of 2019, no pediatric infections documented; however, testing of children has been limited.
[c]Endemic with periodic outbreaks in US territories (Puerto Rico, US Virgin Islands, American Samoa); local mosquitoborne transmission of chikungunya, dengue, and Zika viruses previously identified in Florida and Texas; local transmission of dengue virus also previously identified in Hawaii.

febrile illness, the patient may develop overt signs of hemorrhage (eg, petechiae, ecchymoses, bleeding from the nose and gums, hematemesis, melena) and shock (eg, decreased peripheral circulation, azotemia, tachycardia, hypotension). Hemorrhagic fever and shock caused by yellow fever virus has a high mortality rate and may be confused with other viral hemorrhagic fevers that can occur in the same geographic areas (eg, Argentine hemorrhagic fever, Bolivian hemorrhagic fever, Ebola, Lassa fever, or Marburg). Although dengue may be associated with severe hemorrhage, the shock is attributable primarily to a capillary leak syndrome, which, if properly treated with fluids, has a good prognosis. For information on other potential infections causing hemorrhagic manifestations, see Dengue (p 301), Hemorrhagic Fevers Caused by Arenaviruses (p 362), Hemorrhagic Fevers and Related Syndromes Caused by Bunyaviruses (p 365), and Hemorrhagic Fevers Caused by Filoviruses: Ebola and Marburg (p 368).

ETIOLOGY: Arboviruses are RNA viruses that are transmitted to humans primarily through bites of infected arthropods (mosquitoes, ticks, sand flies, and biting midges). More than 100 arboviruses are known to cause human disease. The viral families responsible for most arboviral infections in humans are *Flaviviridae* (genus *Flavivirus*), *Togaviridae* (genus *Alphavirus*), *Peribunyaviridae* (genus *Orthobunyavirus*), and *Phenuiviridae* (genus *Phlebovirus*). *Reoviridae* (genus *Coltivirus*) also are responsible for a smaller number of human arboviral infections (eg, Colorado tick fever) (Table 3.2).

EPIDEMIOLOGY: Most arboviruses maintain enzootic cycles of transmission between birds or small mammals and arthropod vectors. Humans and domestic animals usually are infected incidentally as "dead-end" hosts. Important exceptions are chikungunya, dengue, yellow fever, and Zika viruses, which can be spread from person-to-arthropod-to-person (anthroponotic transmission). For other arboviruses, humans usually do not develop a sustained or high enough level of viremia to infect biting arthropod vectors. Direct person-to-person spread of some arboviruses has been documented to occur through blood transfusion, organ transplantation, sexual transmission, intrauterine transmission, perinatal transmission, and human milk (see Breastfeeding and Human Milk, p 107). Transmission through percutaneous, mucosal, or aerosol exposure to some arboviruses has occurred rarely in laboratory and occupational settings.

Arboviral infections occur in the United States primarily from late spring through early fall, when mosquitoes and ticks are most active. The number of domestic or imported arboviral disease cases reported in the United States varies greatly by specific etiology and year. Underdiagnosis of milder disease makes an accurate determination of the number of cases difficult.

In general, the risk of developing severe clinical disease for most arboviral infections in the United States is higher among adults than among children. One notable exception is La Crosse virus infection, for which children are at highest risk of severe neurologic disease and possible long-term sequelae. Eastern equine encephalitis virus causes a low incidence of disease but high case fatality rate (40%) across all age groups.

The **incubation periods** for arboviral diseases typically range between 2 and 15 days. Longer incubation periods can occur in immunocompromised people and with tickborne viruses, such as Colorado tick fever, Powassan, and tickborne encephalitis viruses.

DIAGNOSTIC TESTS: Arboviral infections are confirmed most frequently by detection of virus-specific antibody in serum or cerebrospinal fluid (CSF). Acute-phase serum specimens should be tested for virus-specific immunoglobulin (Ig) M antibody. With clinical and epidemiologic correlation, a positive IgM test result has good diagnostic predictive value, but cross-reaction between related arboviruses from the same viral family can occur (eg, West Nile and St. Louis encephalitis viruses, which both are flaviviruses). For most arboviral infections, IgM is detectable within a week after onset of illness and persists for 30 to 90 days, but longer persistence has been documented, especially with West Nile and Zika viruses. Therefore, a positive serum IgM test result occasionally may reflect a prior infection. Serum collected within 10 days of illness onset may not have detectable IgM, and the test should be repeated on a convalescent-phase serum sample. IgG antibody generally is detectable in serum shortly after IgM and persists for years. A plaque-reduction neutralization test can be performed to measure virus-specific neutralizing antibodies and to discriminate between cross-reacting antibodies in primary arboviral infections. Either seroconversion or a fourfold or greater increase in virus-specific neutralizing antibodies between acute- and convalescent-phase serum specimens collected 2 to 3 weeks apart is diagnostic of recent infection. In patients who have been immunized against or infected

Table 3.2. Genus, Geographic Location, and Vectors for Selected Domestic and International Arboviral Diseases

Virus	Genus	Predominant Geographic locations		Vector
		United States	Non-United States	
Domestic				
Colorado tick fever	*Coltivirus*	Rocky Mountain and western states	Western Canada	Ticks
Eastern equine encephalitis	*Alphavirus*	Eastern and Gulf coast states	Americas	Mosquitoes
Heartland	*Phlebovirus*	Central and Southeast	None	Ticks
Jamestown Canyon	*Orthobunyavirus*	Widespread	Canada	Mosquitoes
La Crosse	*Orthobunyavirus*	Midwest and Appalachia	Canada	Mosquitoes
Powassan	*Flavivirus*	Northeast and Midwest	Canada, Russia	Ticks
St. Louis encephalitis	*Flavivirus*	Widespread	Americas	Mosquitoes
West Nile	*Flavivirus*	Widespread	Americas, Europe, Africa, Asia	Mosquitoes
International				
Chikungunya	*Alphavirus*	Imported and periodic local transmission[a]	Worldwide in tropical and subtropical areas	Mosquitoes
Dengue	*Flavivirus*	Imported and periodic local transmission[a]	Worldwide in tropical and subtropical areas	Mosquitoes
Japanese encephalitis	*Flavivirus*	Imported only	Asia	Mosquitoes
Tickborne encephalitis	*Flavivirus*	Imported only	Europe, northern Asia	Ticks
Yellow fever	*Flavivirus*	Imported only	South America, Africa	Mosquitoes
Zika	*Flavivirus*	Imported and periodic local transmission[a]	Worldwide in tropical and subtropical areas	Mosquitoes

[a]Endemic with periodic outbreaks in US territories (Puerto Rico, US Virgin Islands, American Samoa); local mosquitoborne transmission of chikungunya, dengue, and Zika viruses previously identified in Florida and Texas; local transmission of dengue virus also previously identified in Hawaii.

with another arbovirus from the same virus family in the past (ie, secondary infection), cross-reactive antibodies in both the IgM and neutralizing antibody assays might make it difficult to identify which arbovirus is causing the patient's current illness. For some arboviral infections (eg, Colorado tick fever or Heartland virus disease), the immune response may be delayed, with IgM antibodies not appearing until 2 to 3 weeks after onset of illness and neutralizing antibodies taking up to a month to develop. Patients with significant immunosuppression (eg, patients who have received a solid organ transplant or recent chemotherapy) may have a delayed or blunted serologic response, and nucleic acid amplification tests (NAATs) may be indicated in these cases. Immunization and travel history, date of symptom onset, and information regarding other arboviruses known to circulate in the geographic area that may cross-react in serologic assays should be considered when interpreting results.

Viral culture and NAATs for RNA detection can be performed on acute-phase serum, CSF, or tissue specimens. Arboviruses that are more likely to be detected using culture or NAATs early in the illness include Colorado tick fever, dengue, Heartland, yellow fever, and Zika viruses. For other arboviruses, results of these tests often are negative even early in the clinical course because of the relatively short duration of viremia. Immunohistochemical staining (IHC) can detect specific viral antigen in fixed tissue.

Antibody testing for common domestic arboviral diseases is performed in most state public health laboratories and many commercial laboratories. Confirmatory plaque reduction neutralization tests, viral culture, NAATs, immunohistochemical staining, and testing for less common domestic and international arboviruses are performed at the Centers for Disease Control and Prevention (CDC; telephone: 970-221-6400) and selected other reference laboratories. Confirmatory testing typically is arranged through local and state health departments.

TREATMENT: The primary treatment for all arboviral disease is supportive care. Although various antiviral and immunologic therapies have been evaluated for several arboviral diseases, none has shown clear benefit.

ISOLATION OF THE HOSPITALIZED PATIENT: Standard precautions are recommended.

CONTROL MEASURES: Reduction of vectors in areas with endemic transmission is important to reduce risk of infection. Use of personal protective methods, such as using insect repellent, wearing long pants and long-sleeved shirts while outdoors, conducting a full-body check for ticks after outdoor activities, staying in screened or air-conditioned dwellings, and limiting outdoor activities during peak vector feeding times, can help decrease risk of human infection (see Prevention of Mosquitoborne and Tickborne Infections, p 175). Some arboviral infections also can be prevented through screening of blood donations or through immunization. The blood supply in the United States is screened routinely for West Nile and Zika viruses. Some arboviruses can be transmitted through human milk, although transmission appears rare. Mothers should be encouraged to breastfeed even in areas of active arboviral transmission because benefits of breastfeeding seem to outweigh the low risk of illness in breastfeeding infants (see Breastfeeding and Human Milk, p 107). The CDC has issued guidance for prevention of sexual transmission (see Zika, p 854).

Vaccines are available in the United States to protect against travel-related yellow fever and Japanese encephalitis.

Yellow Fever Vaccine.[1] Live attenuated (17D strain) yellow fever vaccine is available from state-approved clinics or immunization providers. Unless contraindicated, yellow fever immunization is recommended for all people 9 months or older living in or traveling to areas with endemic disease, and is required by international regulations for travel to and from certain countries (**wwwnc.cdc.gov/travel/**). Infants younger than 6 months should not be immunized with yellow fever vaccine, because they have an increased risk of vaccine-associated encephalitis. The decision to immunize infants between 6 and 9 months of age must balance the infant's risk of exposure with risk of vaccine-associated encephalitis.

Booster doses of yellow fever vaccine are no longer recommended for most travelers, because a single dose of yellow fever vaccine provides long-lasting protection. Additional doses are recommended for certain populations (ie, women initially vaccinated when they were pregnant, patients who received a hematopoietic stem cell transplant after their initial vaccination, and people infected with human immunodeficiency virus [HIV]), as they might not have a robust or sustained immune response to yellow fever vaccine compared with other recipients. Additional doses may be administered to certain groups believed to be at increased risk for yellow fever disease because of their itinerary and duration of travel or because of more consistent exposure to virulent virus (ie, laboratory workers).

Yellow fever vaccine is a live-virus vaccine produced in chicken eggs and, thus, is contraindicated in people who have a history of acute hypersensitivity to eggs or egg products and in people who are immunocompromised. Procedures for immunizing people with severe egg allergy are described in the vaccine package insert. Generally, people who are able to eat eggs or egg products may receive the vaccine. Pregnancy and breastfeeding are precautions to yellow fever vaccine administration, because rare cases of transmission of the vaccine virus in utero or through breastfeeding have been documented (see Immunization in Pregnancy, p 69, and Breastfeeding and Human Milk, p 107). Whenever possible, pregnant and breastfeeding women should defer travel to areas where yellow fever is endemic. If travel to an area with endemic disease is unavoidable and risks for yellow fever virus exposure are believed to outweigh the vaccination risks, a pregnant or breastfeeding woman should be vaccinated. If risks of vaccination are believed to outweigh risks for yellow fever virus exposure, a pregnant or breastfeeding woman should be excused from immunization and issued a medical waiver letter to fulfill health regulations. For more detailed information on the yellow fever vaccine, including adverse events, precautions, and contraindications, visit **wwwnc.cdc.gov/travel/** or **www.cdc.gov/yellowfever/healthcareproviders/vaccine-info.html** or see Travel-Related Immunizations (p 101).

As of December 2020, the only yellow fever vaccine licensed in the United States (YF-VAX) is not available because of manufacturing issues. A new manufacturing facility is being built and should alleviate the production problems. In the interim, the manufacturer of YF-VAX (Sanofi Pasteur) has worked with the US Food and Drug Administration to import Stamaril yellow fever vaccine under an investigational new drug (IND) application and distribute it in the United States in an Expanded Access Program. Stamaril is manufactured by Sanofi Pasteur in France and uses the 17D-204 strain of yellow fever virus, which is the same strain as in YF-VAX. More than 430 million doses have been distributed worldwide, and its safety and efficacy profile is comparable to YF-VAX vaccine.

---

[1]Centers for Disease Control and Prevention. Yellow Fever ACIP Vaccine Recommendations. Available at: **www.cdc.gov/vaccines/hcp/acip-recs/vacc-specific/yf.html**

During this period of shortage of YF-VAX, health care providers of yellow fever vaccine can direct their patients to Stamaril vaccine sites (**wwwnc.cdc.gov/travel/page/ search-for-stamaril-clinics**).

Japanese Encephalitis Vaccine.[1] Risk of Japanese encephalitis for most travelers to Asia is very low but varies based on destination, duration of travel, season, activities, and accommodations. All travelers to countries with endemic Japanese encephalitis should be informed of the potential for infection and should use personal protective measures to reduce risk of mosquito bites. For some travelers who might be at increased risk for Japanese encephalitis, Japanese encephalitis vaccine can further reduce the risk for infection. The CDC recommends Japanese encephalitis vaccine for those taking up residence in an endemic country, longer-term travelers (eg, a month or longer), and frequent travelers to endemic areas (**www.cdc.gov/vaccines/hcp/acip-recs/vacc-specific/ je.html**). Japanese encephalitis vaccine also should be considered for shorter-term travelers if they plan to travel outside of an urban area and have an itinerary or activities that will increase their risk of mosquito exposure in an endemic area. Information on the location of Japanese encephalitis virus transmission and detailed information on vaccine recommendations and adverse events can be obtained from the CDC (**wwwnc.cdc. gov/travel/**).

The Japanese encephalitis vaccine licensed in the United States is an inactivated Vero cell culture-derived vaccine (Ixiaro [JE-VC]) available for use in adults and children 2 months and older. The primary vaccination series is 2 doses administered 28 days apart for those younger than 18 years and older than 65 years of age, and 7–28 days apart for those 18 to 65 years of age. The dose is 0.25 mL for children 2 months through 2 years of age and 0.5 mL for adults and children 3 years and older. For adults and children, a booster dose may be administered at 1 year or longer after the primary series if ongoing exposure or reexposure is expected.

No efficacy data exist for JE-VC. The vaccine was licensed on the basis of its ability to induce Japanese encephalitis virus neutralizing antibodies as a surrogate for protection, and because of its safety profile. No safety concerns have been identified in passive post-marketing surveillance of more than 1 million doses distributed in the United States.

Other Arboviral Vaccines. A live attenuated tetravalent dengue vaccine (Dengvaxia) is licensed in multiple countries in Asia, Latin America, and Europe. In 2018, the World Health Organization issued a revised recommendation that the vaccine should be given only to patients with prior exposure to dengue virus based on serologic testing. In 2019, the US Food and Drug Administration approved Dengvaxia for use in people 9 through 16 years of age who have laboratory evidence of previous dengue virus infection and who live in areas with endemic infection (see Dengue, p 301).

Several tickborne encephalitis virus vaccines are available in some countries in Europe and Asia where the disease is endemic, but the vaccines are not available in the United States. Chikungunya and Zika virus vaccines are under development.

REPORTING: Most arboviral diseases are nationally notifiable conditions and should be reported to the appropriate local and state health authorities. Underdiagnosis of these diseases because of challenges with laboratory confirmation and lack of active surveillance

---

[1]Hills SL, Walter EB, Atmar RL, Fischer M. Japanese encephalitis vaccine: Recommendations of the Advisory Committee on Immunization Practices (ACIP). *MMWR Recomm Rep* 2019;68(RR-2):1–33. Available at: **www. cdc.gov/vaccines/hcp/acip-recs/vacc-specific/je.html**

is common, suggesting that the actual numbers of cases is likely significantly higher. For select arboviruses (eg, chikungunya, dengue, Zika, and yellow fever viruses), patients may remain viremic during their acute illness. Such patients pose a risk for further person-to-mosquito-to-person transmission, increasing the importance of timely reporting.

Arcanobacterium haemolyticum Infections

CLINICAL MANIFESTATIONS: Acute pharyngitis attributable to *Arcanobacterium haemolyticum* often is indistinguishable from group A streptococcal pharyngitis. *A haemolyticum* has been associated with fever, pharyngeal erythema and exudates, cervical lymphadenopathy, and rash but not with palatal petechiae and strawberry tongue. A morbilliform or scarlatiniform exanthem is present in half of cases, beginning on extensor surfaces of the distal extremities, spreading to the torso, back, and neck, sparing the face, palms, and soles. Rash typically develops 1 to 4 days after onset of sore throat, although rash preceding pharyngitis can occur; desquamation can occur. Respiratory tract infections that mimic diphtheria, including membranous pharyngitis, peritonsillar and pharyngeal abscesses. Skin and soft tissue infections, including chronic ulcers, cellulitis, paronychia, and wound infection, have been attributed to *A haemolyticum*. Rarely, invasive infections have been reported, including Lemierre syndrome, bacteremia, sepsis, endocarditis, brain abscess, orbital cellulitis, and pyogenic arthritis. Nonsuppurative sequelae have not been reported.

ETIOLOGY: *A haemolyticum* is a catalase-negative, weakly acid-fast, facultatively anaerobic, hemolytic, gram-positive to gram-variable, slender, sometimes club-shaped bacillus.

EPIDEMIOLOGY: Humans are the primary reservoir of *A haemolyticum*, and spread is person to person, presumably via droplet respiratory secretions. Severe disease occurs almost exclusively among immunocompromised people. *Arcanobacterium* pharyngitis occurs primarily in adolescents and young adults and only rarely in young children. *A haemolyticum* accounts for approximately 0.5% of pharyngeal infections overall and up to 2.5% of pharyngeal infections in 15- to 25-year-olds. Isolation of the bacterium from the nasopharynx of asymptomatic people is rare. Person-to-person spread is inferred from family studies.

The **incubation period** is unknown.

DIAGNOSTIC TESTS: *A haemolyticum* grows on blood-enriched agar, but colonies are small, have narrow bands of beta hemolysis, and may not be visible for 48 to 72 hours. The organism is not detected by rapid antigen tests for group A streptococci. Detection is enhanced by culture on rabbit or human blood agar rather than on sheep blood agar, which yields larger colony size and wider zones of hemolysis. Presence of 5% carbon dioxide enhances growth. *A haemolyticum* may be missed in routine throat cultures on sheep blood agar if laboratory personnel are not trained specifically to identify the organism. Pits characteristically form under colonies on blood agar plates. Two biotypes of *A haemolyticum* have been identified: a rough colonial biotype predominates in respiratory tract infections, and a smooth biotype typically in skin and soft tissue infections.

TREATMENT: Optimal management of patients with *A haemolyticum* pharyngitis has not been determined, and symptoms can resolve without antibiotic treatment. Erythromycin and azithromycin are drugs of choice for *A haemolyticum* tonsillopharyngitis, but no controlled trials have been performed. *A haemolyticum* generally is susceptible in vitro to macrolides, clindamycin, cephalosporins, ciprofloxacin, vancomycin, and gentamicin. Treatment failures with penicillin despite predicted susceptibility from in vitro testing occur and may be attributable to tolerance. Resistance to trimethoprim-sulfamethoxazole is common. In rare cases of invasive infection, susceptibility tests should be performed and treatment should be individualized. While awaiting results, initial empiric combination therapy can be initiated using a parenteral beta lactam agent, with or without gentamicin or a macrolide, and with consideration of metronidazole if *Fusobacterium* infection is suspected.

ISOLATION OF THE HOSPITALIZED PATIENT: Standard precautions are recommended.

CONTROL MEASURES: None.

Ascaris lumbricoides Infections

CLINICAL MANIFESTATIONS: Most infections with *Ascaris lumbricoides* are asymptomatic, although moderate to heavy infections may lead to nonspecific gastrointestinal tract symptoms, malnutrition, and growth delay. During the larval migratory phase, an acute transient pneumonitis (Löffler syndrome) associated with cough, substernal discomfort, shortness of breath, fever, and marked eosinophilia may occur. Acute intestinal obstruction has been associated with heavy infections. Children are prone to this complication because of the small diameter of the intestinal lumen and their propensity to acquire large worm burdens. Heavy worm burdens also can affect nutritional status, intellectual development, cognitive performance, and growth. Worm migration can cause peritonitis secondary to intestinal wall perforation as well as appendicitis or common bile duct obstruction resulting in biliary colic, cholangitis, or pancreatitis. Adult worms can be stimulated to migrate by stressful conditions (eg, fever, illness, or anesthesia) and by some anthelmintic drugs.

ETIOLOGY: Following ingestion of embryonated eggs, usually from contaminated soil, larvae hatch in the small intestine, penetrate the mucosa, and are transported passively by portal blood to the liver and lungs. After migrating from alveolar capillaries into the small airways, larvae ascend through the tracheobronchial tree to the pharynx, are swallowed, and mature into adults in the small intestine. Female worms produce approximately 200 000 eggs per day, which are excreted in stool and must incubate in soil to become infectious. Adult worms can live in the lumen of the small intestine for up to 18 months. Female worms are longer than male worms and can measure 40 cm (more than 15 inches) in length and 6 mm in diameter.

EPIDEMIOLOGY: *A lumbricoides* is the most prevalent of all human intestinal nematodes (roundworms), with approximately 800 million people infected worldwide. Infection with *A lumbricoides* is most common in resource-limited countries, including rural and urban communities characterized by poor sanitation. Direct person-to-person transmission does not occur. *Ascaris suum*, a pig roundworm similar to *A lumbricoides*, also causes human disease and is associated with raising pigs and use of their stool for fertilizer.

The **incubation period** (interval between ingestion of eggs and development of egg-laying adults) is approximately 9 to 11 weeks.

DIAGNOSTIC TESTS: Ascariasis is diagnosed by examining a fresh or preserved stool specimen for eggs using light microscopy. Adult worms also may be passed from the rectum, through the nares, or from the mouth, usually in vomitus. Imaging of the gastrointestinal tract or biliary tree using computed tomography or ultrasonography may detect adult *Ascaris* worms, which can cause filling defects following administration of oral contrast.

TREATMENT: Albendazole (taken with food in a single dose), mebendazole (in a single dose or taken twice daily for 3 days), and pyrantel pamoate are first-line agents for treatment of ascariasis. Ivermectin (taken on an empty stomach in a single dose) and nitazoxanide are alternative therapies. Cure rates range from 90% with pyrantel pamoate to 100% with albendazole (see Drugs for Parasitic Infections, p 951). Albendazole, pyrantel pamoate, ivermectin, and nitazoxanide are not approved by the US Food and Drug Administration for treatment of ascariasis, although albendazole has become the drug of choice for most soil-transmitted nematode infections, including ascariasis. Studies in children as young as 1 year of age suggest that albendazole can be administered safely to this population. The safety of ivermectin in children weighing less than 15 kg and in pregnant women has not been established. Reexamination of stool specimens may be performed at approximately 2 weeks after deworming to document cure and again at 2 to 3 months to account for migrating larvae from new infections (which are resistant to anthelmintics) at the time of treatment. Patients who remain infected should be retreated, preferably with albendazole or the multidose regimen of mebendazole, and the reasons for the repeated infections should be explored and addressed.

Conservative management of small bowel obstruction, including nasogastric suction, intravenous fluids, and repletion of electrolytes, may alleviate symptoms before administration of anthelmintic therapy. Use of mineral oil or diatrizoate meglumine and diatrizoate sodium solution, either orally or by nasogastric tube, also may cause relaxation of a bolus of worms. Endoscopic retrograde cholangiopancreatography has been used successfully for extraction of worms from the biliary tree. Surgical intervention (eg, laparotomy) is indicated for intestinal or biliary tract obstruction that does not resolve with conservative therapy or for patients with volvulus or peritonitis secondary to perforation.

ISOLATION OF THE HOSPITALIZED PATIENT: Standard precautions are recommended.

CONTROL MEASURES: Sanitary disposal of human feces prevents transmission. Vegetables cultivated in areas where human feces are used as fertilizer must be washed thoroughly and cooked before eating.

Preventive chemotherapy (deworming) (once or twice annually with albendazole or single-dose mebendazole) targeting high-risk groups, most notably preschool and school-aged children and pregnant women (after the first trimester), is recommended by the World Health Organization for control of *A lumbricoides* and other soil-transmitted nematodes in communities with 20% or more baseline prevalence of infection. Reinfection is common in high-prevalence areas, and additional public health measures, including improved sanitation, safe drinking water, and health education, likely will be required to eliminate these infections.

Aspergillosis

CLINICAL MANIFESTATIONS: Aspergillosis manifests as 5 principal clinical entities: invasive aspergillosis, aspergilloma, allergic bronchopulmonary aspergillosis, allergic sinusitis, and chronic pulmonary aspergillosis. Colonization of the respiratory tract is common. The clinical manifestations and severity depend on host immune status (either immunocompromised or atopic).

- Invasive aspergillosis occurs mostly in immunocompromised patients with prolonged neutropenia, graft-versus-host disease, or impaired phagocyte function (eg, chronic granulomatous disease) or those who have received T-lymphocyte immunosuppressive therapy (eg, corticosteroids, calcineurin inhibitors, tumor necrosis factor [TNF]-alpha inhibitors). Children at highest risk include those with new-onset acute myelogenous leukemia, relapse of hematologic malignancy, aplastic anemia, chronic granulomatous disease, and recipients of allogeneic hematopoietic stem cell and certain types (eg, heart, lung) of solid organ transplants. Invasive infection usually involves pulmonary, sinus, cerebral, or cutaneous sites. Rarely, endocarditis, osteomyelitis, meningitis, peritonitis, infection of the eye or orbit, and esophagitis occur. The hallmark of invasive aspergillosis is angioinvasion with resulting thrombosis, dissemination to other organs, and occasionally erosion of the blood vessel wall with catastrophic hemorrhage. Invasive aspergillosis in patients with chronic granulomatous disease is unique in that it is more indolent and displays a general lack of angioinvasion. Invasive aspergillosis also has been described among intensive care patients with severe influenza, with and without underlying immunocompromise.

- Aspergillomas and otomycosis are 2 syndromes of nonallergic colonization by *Aspergillus* species in immunocompetent children. Aspergillomas ("fungal balls") grow in preexisting pulmonary cavities or bronchogenic cysts without invading pulmonary tissue; almost all patients have underlying lung disease, such as cystic fibrosis or tuberculosis. Patients with otomycosis have chronic otitis media with colonization of the external auditory canal by a fungal mat that produces a dark discharge.

- Allergic bronchopulmonary aspergillosis is a hypersensitivity lung disease that manifests as episodic wheezing, expectoration of brown mucus plugs, low-grade fever, eosinophilia, and transient pulmonary infiltrates. This form of aspergillosis occurs most commonly in immunocompetent children with asthma or cystic fibrosis and can be a trigger for asthmatic flares.

- Allergic sinusitis is a far less common allergic response to colonization by *Aspergillus* species than is allergic bronchopulmonary aspergillosis. Allergic sinusitis occurs in children with nasal polyps or previous episodes of sinusitis or in children who have undergone sinus surgery. Allergic sinusitis is characterized by symptoms of chronic sinusitis with dark plugs of nasal discharge and is different from invasive *Aspergillus* sinusitis.

- Chronic aspergillosis typically affects patients who are not immunocompromised or are less immunocompromised, although exposure to corticosteroids is common, and patients often have underlying pulmonary conditions. Diagnosis of chronic aspergillosis requires at least 3 months of chronic pulmonary symptoms or chronic illness or progressive radiologic abnormalities, along with an elevated *Aspergillus* immunoglobulin (Ig) G concentration or other microbiological evidence. Because of the ubiquitous nature of *Aspergillus* species, a positive sputum culture alone is not diagnostic.

ETIOLOGY: *Aspergillus* species are molds that grow on decaying vegetation and in soil and are very common in the environment. *Aspergillus fumigatus* is the most common (>75%) cause of invasive aspergillosis, with *Aspergillus flavus* being the next most common. Several other major species, including *Aspergillus terreus, Aspergillus nidulans,* and *Aspergillus niger,* also cause invasive human infections. *A nidulans* is the second most encountered mold in patients with chronic granulomatous disease, causing almost exclusively invasive infections in this specific host characterized by its aggressive behavior including lung infection that invades the chest wall with contiguous osteomyelitis and chest wall abscesses. Of increasing concern are emerging *Aspergillus* species that are resistant to antifungals, such as *Aspergillus fumigatus,* which harbors environmentally acquired resistance mutations to azole antifungals; *A terreus*, which is intrinsically resistant to amphotericin B; and *Aspergillus calidoustus*, which is often resistant to most antifungals (see Table 4.7, p 909).

EPIDEMIOLOGY: The principal route of transmission is inhalation of conidia (spores) originating from multiple environmental sources (eg, plants, vegetables, dust from construction or demolition), soil, and water supplies (eg, shower heads). Incidence of disease in hematopoietic stem cell transplant recipients is highest during periods of neutropenia or during treatment for graft-versus-host disease. In solid organ transplant recipients, the risk is highest approximately 6 months after transplantation or during periods of increased immunosuppression. Disease has followed use of contaminated marijuana in the immunocompromised host. Health care-associated outbreaks of invasive pulmonary aspergillosis in susceptible hosts have occurred in which the probable source of the fungus was a nearby construction site or faulty ventilation system, but the source of health care-associated aspergillosis frequently is not known. Cutaneous aspergillosis occurs less frequently and usually involves sites of skin injury, such as intravenous catheter sites (including in neonates), sites of traumatic inoculation, and sites associated with occlusive dressings, burns, or surgery. Transmission by direct inoculation of skin abrasions or wounds is less likely. Person-to-person spread does not occur.

The **incubation period** is unknown and may be variable.

DIAGNOSTIC TESTS: Dichotomously branched and septate hyphae, identified by microscopic examination of 10% potassium hydroxide wet preparations or of Gomori methenamine-silver nitrate stain of tissue or bronchoalveolar lavage specimens, are suggestive of the diagnosis. Isolation of *Aspergillus* species or molecular testing with specific reagents is required for definitive diagnosis. The organism usually is not recoverable from blood (except in catheter-related infections) but is isolated readily from lung, sinus, and skin biopsy specimens when cultured on Sabouraud dextrose agar or brain-heart infusion media (without cycloheximide). *Aspergillus* species can be associated with colonization or may be a laboratory contaminant, but when evaluating results from immunocompromised patients, recovery of this organism frequently indicates infection. Biopsy can be used to establish the diagnosis, but *Aspergillus* hyphae are similar to other hyaline molds (eg, *Fusarium*). Care should be taken to distinguish aspergillosis from mucormycosis, which can appear similar by diagnostic imaging studies but is pauci-septate (few septa) and requires a different treatment regimen.

An enzyme immunosorbent assay for detection of galactomannan, a molecule found in the cell wall of *Aspergillus* species, from serum or bronchoalveolar lavage (BAL) fluid is available commercially and may be useful in children and adults with hematologic malignancies or hematopoietic stem cell transplants. A test result of ≥ 0.5 from the serum or ≥ 1.0 from BAL fluid supports a diagnosis of invasive aspergillosis, and monitoring of serum antigen concentrations twice weekly in periods of highest risk (eg, neutropenia and active graft-versus-host disease) if the patient is not receiving mold-active antifungal prophylaxis may be useful for early detection of invasive aspergillosis in these patients. False-positive test results have been reported and can be related to consumption of food products containing galactomannan (eg, rice and pasta), other invasive fungal infections (eg, *Fusarium, Histoplasma capsulatum*), and colonization of the gut of neonates with *Bifidobacterium* species. Previous cross-reactivity with antimicrobial agents derived from fungi, especially piperacillin-tazobactam, no longer occurs because of manufacturing changes.

A negative galactomannan test result does not exclude diagnosis of invasive aspergillosis, and its greatest utility may be in monitoring response to disease rather than in its use as a diagnostic marker. False-negative galactomannan test results consistently occur in patients with chronic granulomatous disease, so the test should not be used in these patients. Galactomannan is not recommended for routine screening in patients receiving mold-active antifungal therapy or prophylaxis (see Table 4.7, p 909). Galactomannan is not recommended for screening in solid organ transplant recipients because of very poor sensitivity.

Limited data suggest that testing for other nonspecific fungal biomarkers, such as 1,3-β-D glucan, may be useful in the diagnosis of aspergillosis. This test is not specific for aspergillosis, and specificity may be reduced in a variety of clinical settings, including exposure to certain antibiotics, hemodialysis, and coinfection with certain bacteria. *Aspergillus* polymerase chain reaction testing is promising, but its clinical utility remains controversial. Unlike adults, children frequently do not manifest cavitation or the air crescent or halo signs on chest radiography, and lack of these characteristic signs does not exclude the diagnosis of invasive aspergillosis.

In allergic aspergillosis, diagnosis is suggested by a typical clinical syndrome with elevated total concentrations of IgE ($\geq$1000 ng/mL) and *Aspergillus*-specific serum IgE, eosinophilia, and a positive result from a skin test for *Aspergillus* antigens. In people with cystic fibrosis, the diagnosis is more difficult because wheezing, eosinophilia, and a positive skin test result not associated with allergic bronchopulmonary aspergillosis often are present.

TREATMENT[1]**:** Voriconazole is the drug of choice for all clinical forms of invasive aspergillosis (see Antifungal Drugs for Systemic Fungal Infections, p 905), except in neonates, for whom amphotericin B deoxycholate in high doses is recommended because of voriconazole's potential visual adverse effects, and perhaps in patients with chronic granulomatous disease, in whom posaconazole appears to be superior to voriconazole. Voriconazole has been shown to be superior to amphotericin B in a large, randomized trial in adults. Immune reconstitution is paramount; decreasing immunosuppression, if possible (specifically corticosteroid dose), is critical to disease control. The diagnostic workup needs to be aggressive to confirm disease, but it should never delay antifungal therapy in the setting of true concern for invasive aspergillosis. Therapy is continued for a minimum of 6 to 12 weeks, but treatment duration should be individualized on the basis of degree and duration of immunosuppression. Monitoring of serum galactomannan concentrations in those with significant elevation at onset may be useful to assess response to therapy concomitant with clinical and radiologic evaluation.

Close monitoring of voriconazole serum trough concentrations is critical for both efficacy and safety, and most experts agree that for children, voriconazole trough concentrations should be between 2 μg/mL and 6 μg/mL. It is important to individualize dosing in patients following initiation of voriconazole therapy, because there is high interpatient variability in metabolism. Certain *Aspergillus* species (*A calidoustus*) are inherently resistant to azoles, and isolation of azole-resistant *A fumigatus* is increasing and may be related to environmental acquisition through use of agricultural fungicides in previously azole-naïve patients. Resistance can also develop in patients on long-term azole therapy.

Alternative therapies include liposomal amphotericin B, isavuconazole, posaconazole, or other lipid formulations of amphotericin B. Primary therapy with an echinocandin alone (caspofungin, micafungin) is not recommended, but an echinocandin can be used in

---

[1]Patterson TF, Thompson GR III, Denning DW. Practice guidelines for the diagnosis and management of aspergillosis: 2016 update by the Infectious Diseases Society of America. *Clin Infect Dis*. 2016;63(4):e1-e60

settings in which an azole or amphotericin B are contraindicated. The pharmacokinetics and safety of posaconazole have not been evaluated fully in younger children. Posaconazole absorption is improved significantly with use of the extended-release tablet rather than the oral suspension. Isavuconazole is an alternative therapy in adults but has not been studied in children. Combination antifungal therapy with voriconazole and an echinocandin may be considered in select patients with documented invasive aspergillosis. In areas with high azole resistance, empiric therapy until antifungal susceptibilities are obtained should include voriconazole plus an echinocandin, or liposomal amphotericin B monotherapy.

If primary antifungal therapy fails, general strategies for salvage therapy include (a) changing the class of antifungal, (b) tapering or reversal of underlying immunosuppression when feasible, (c) susceptibility testing of any *Aspergillus* isolates recovered, and (d) surgical resection of necrotic lesions in selected cases. In pulmonary disease, surgery is indicated only when a mass is impinging on a great vessel.

Allergic bronchopulmonary aspergillosis is treated with antifungal therapy, usually with itraconazole or another mold-active azole; in addition, corticosteroids are a cornerstone of therapy for exacerbations. Itraconazole has a demonstrable corticosteroid-sparing effect. Allergic sinus aspergillosis also is treated with corticosteroids, and surgery has been reported to be beneficial in many cases. Antifungal therapy has not been found to be useful, but could be considered for refractory infection and/or relapsing disease. There may be an emerging role for immunotherapy. Guidelines specific to treatment of allergic bronchopulmonary aspergillosis in patients with cystic fibrosis are available (**www.cff.org/Care/Clinical-Care-Guidelines/Infection-Prevention-and-Control-Clinical-Care-Guidelines/Allergic-Bronchopulmonary-Aspergillosis-Clinical-Care-Guidelines/**).

ISOLATION OF THE HOSPITALIZED PATIENT: Standard precautions are recommended.

CONTROL MEASURES: Outbreaks of invasive aspergillosis and *Aspergillus* colonization have occurred among hospitalized patients during construction in hospitals and at nearby sites. Environmental measures reported to be effective include erecting suitable barriers between patient care areas and construction sites, routine cleaning of air-handling systems, repair of faulty air flow, and replacement of contaminated air filters. High-efficiency particulate air filters and laminar flow rooms markedly decrease the risk of exposure to conidia in patient care areas. Plants and flowers may be reservoirs for *Aspergillus* and should be avoided in intensive care units and immunocompromised patient care settings. Use of high-efficiency respirators during transport away from protective environment rooms has been associated with reduced incidence of invasive pulmonary aspergillosis incidence during hospital construction.

Posaconazole has been shown to be effective in 2 randomized controlled trials as prophylaxis against invasive aspergillosis for patients 13 years and older who have undergone hematopoietic stem cell transplantation and have graft-versus-host disease as well as in patients with hematologic malignancies with prolonged neutropenia, although breakthrough disease has been reported in those with gastrointestinal tract issues (eg, graft-versus-host disease) affecting drug bioavailability. Low-dose amphotericin B, itraconazole, voriconazole, or posaconazole prophylaxis have been reported for other high-risk patients, but controlled trials have not been completed in pediatric patients.

Patients at risk of invasive infection should avoid high environmental exposure (eg, gardening) following discharge from the hospital. People with allergic aspergillosis should take measures to reduce exposure to *Aspergillus* species in the home.

Astrovirus Infections

CLINICAL MANIFESTATIONS: Astrovirus illness is most commonly manifested as 2 to 5 days of acute watery diarrhea accompanied by low-grade fever, malaise, and nausea, and less commonly, vomiting and mild dehydration. Illness in an immunocompetent host is self-limited, lasting a median of 5 to 6 days. Asymptomatic infections are common. Astrovirus infections also have been associated with encephalitis and meningitis, particularly in immunocompromised individuals.

ETIOLOGY: Members of the family *Astroviridae*, astroviruses are nonenveloped, single-stranded RNA viruses with a subset of particles (10%) having a characteristic star-like appearance when visualized by electron microscopy. Astroviruses are classified into 2 genera: *Mamastrovirus* (MAstV) and *Avastrovirus*, which infect mammals and birds, respectively. Four MAstV species have been identified in humans: MAstV 1, MAstV 6, MAstV 8, and MAstV 9. MAstV 1 includes the 8 antigenic types of classic human astroviruses (HAstV types 1–8), whereas MAstV 6, MAstV 8, and MAstV 9 are novel astroviruses that have been identified in recent years and include Melbourne (MLB) and Virginia/human-mink-ovine-like (VA/HMO) strains.

EPIDEMIOLOGY: Human astroviruses (HAstVs) have a worldwide distribution. Multiple antigenic types co-circulate in the same geographic region. HAstVs have been detected in as many as 5% to 17% of sporadic cases of nonbacterial gastroenteritis among young children in the community but appear to cause a lower proportion of cases of more severe childhood gastroenteritis requiring hospitalization (2.5%–9%). HAstV infections occur predominantly in children younger than 4 years and have a seasonal peak during the late winter and spring in the United States. Transmission is via the fecal-oral route through contaminated food or water, person-to-person contact, or contaminated surfaces. Outbreaks tend to occur in closed populations of the young and the elderly, particularly among hospitalized children (health care-associated infections) and children in child care centers. In general, virus is shed 1 to 2 days before illness and lasts a median of 5 days after onset of symptoms, but asymptomatic excretion after illness can last for several weeks in healthy children. Persistent excretion may occur in immunocompromised hosts. MAstV 6, MAstV 8, and MAstV 9 have been detected sporadically in stool samples, blood, respiratory samples, cerebrospinal fluid, and brain tissue of immunocompromised patients with acute encephalitis.

The **incubation period** is 3 to 4 days.

DIAGNOSTIC TESTS: Commercial tests for diagnosis have not been available in the United States until recently, although enzyme immunoassays are available in many other countries. There are several US Food and Drug Administration (FDA) approved multiplex nucleic acid-based assays for the detection of gastrointestinal tract pathogens, at least 2 of which include astrovirus (MAstV 1). These multiplex tests are more sensitive and are replacing traditional tests to detect fecal viral pathogens. Interpretation of assay results may be complicated by the frequent detection of viruses in fecal samples from asymptomatic children and the detection of multiple viruses in a single sample. A few research and reference laboratories test stool samples by enzyme immunoassay for detection of viral antigen and/or real-time reverse transcriptase-quantitative polymerase chain reaction (RT-qPCR) assay for detection of viral RNA in stool.

TREATMENT: No specific antiviral therapy is available. Oral or parenteral fluids and electrolytes are given to prevent and correct dehydration.

ISOLATION OF THE HOSPITALIZED PATIENT: In addition to standard precautions, contact precautions are recommended for diapered children or incontinent people for the duration of illness or to control institutional outbreaks.

CONTROL MEASURES: No specific control measures are available. The spread of infection in child care settings can be decreased by using general measures for control of diarrhea, such as training care providers in infection-control procedures, maintaining cleanliness of surfaces, keeping food preparation duties and areas separate from child care activities, exercising adequate hand hygiene, cohorting ill children, and excluding ill child care providers, food handlers, and children (see Children in Group Child Care and Schools, p 116).

Babesiosis

CLINICAL MANIFESTATIONS: *Babesia* infection often is asymptomatic or associated with mild, nonspecific symptoms. The infection also can be severe and life threatening, particularly in people who are asplenic, immunocompromised, or elderly. When symptomatic, babesiosis, like malaria, is characterized by the presence of fever and hemolytic anemia. Clinical manifestations of babesiosis include malaise, anorexia, and fatigue, followed by fever, chills, sweats, myalgia, arthralgia, headache, and nausea. Severe babesiosis may require hospitalization for management of marked anemia, adult respiratory distress syndrome, disseminated intravascular coagulation, renal impairment, shock, or splenic rupture. Congenital infection with nonspecific manifestations suggestive of sepsis has been reported.

Babesiosis should be considered in a patient who resides in or traveled to an endemic area and develops compatible symptoms and characteristic laboratory abnormalities, including anemia, thrombocytopenia, and evidence of intravascular hemolysis (abnormal aspartate aminotransferase [AST], alanine aminotransferase [ALT], alkaline phosphatase, lactate dehydrogenase [LDH], total and direct bilirubin concentrations, and reduced haptoglobin).

ETIOLOGY: *Babesia* species are intraerythrocytic protozoa that are transmitted mostly by the bite of a hard-bodied tick. The etiologic agents of human babesiosis in the United States include *Babesia microti*, which is the cause of most reported cases, and less commonly *Babesia duncani* and *Babesia divergens*.

EPIDEMIOLOGY: Babesiosis predominantly is a tickborne zoonosis. *Babesia* parasites also can be transmitted via blood transfusion, via organ transplantation, and perinatally. The primary reservoir host for *B microti* in the United States is the white-footed mouse *(Peromyscus leucopus)*, and the tick vector is *Ixodes scapularis*, which can transmit other pathogens, such as *Borrelia burgdorferi*, the causative agent of Lyme disease, and *Anaplasma phagocytophilum*, the causative agent of human granulocytic anaplasmosis. The tick bite often is not noticed, in part because the nymphal stage of the tick is approximately the size of a poppy seed. White-tailed deer *(Odocoileus virginianus)* serve as hosts for blood meals by the tick but are not reservoir hosts of *B microti*. An increase in the deer population in some geographic regions, including in some suburban areas, during the past few decades is thought to be a major factor in the spread of *I scapularis*. The reported vectorborne cases of *B microti* infection have been acquired in the Northeast (in parts of Connecticut, Massachusetts, New Jersey, New York, and Rhode Island, as well as other states, including Maine and New Hampshire) and in the upper Midwest (Wisconsin and Minnesota). The majority of cases are in the New England and Mid-Atlantic regions (**www.cdc.gov/parasites/babesiosis/data-statistics/maps/maps.html**). Occasional human cases of babesiosis caused by other species have been described in various regions of the United States; tick vectors and reservoir hosts for these agents typically have not yet been identified. Most US vectorborne cases of babesiosis occur during late spring, summer, or fall; transfusion-associated cases can occur year round. More than 2000 cases of babesiosis are reported annually to the Centers for Disease Control and Prevention, but the number of cases is likely to be higher.

The **incubation period** typically ranges from approximately 1 week to 5 weeks following a tick bite. A study of transfusion-associated cases found a median incubation period following a contaminated blood transfusion of 37 days (range, 11 to 176 days), but it may be longer (eg, latent infection might become symptomatic after splenectomy).

DIAGNOSTIC TESTS[1]: Acute, symptomatic cases of babesiosis typically are diagnosed by microscopic identification of *Babesia* parasites on Giemsa- or Wright-stained blood smears. If the diagnosis of babesiosis is being considered, manual (nonautomated) review of blood smears for parasites should be requested explicitly. If seen, the tetrad (Maltese-cross) form is pathognomonic. *B microti* and other *Babesia* species can be difficult to distinguish from the *Plasmodium falciparum* trophozoite; examination of blood smears by a reference laboratory should be considered for confirmation of the diagnosis. Blood smear examination is rapid and inexpensive.

In cases in which blood smear examination is negative but index of suspicion for babesiosis remains high, molecular testing by polymerase chain reaction (PCR) offers increased sensitivity in settings of low-level *B microti* parasitemia; PCR results may remain positive for several months after successful treatment. PCR testing is now available at some clinical and public health laboratories as well as at the Centers for Disease Control and Prevention.

Serologic tests for *Babesia* antibody detection on a single serum specimen should not be used to diagnose acute disease because of difficulty distinguishing acute disease from previous infection. Real-time PCR assays are typically species specific, but most laboratories only offer *B microti* PCR (**www.cdc.gov/dpdx/babesiosis/index.html**). In geographic areas where both *B microti* and *B burgdorferi* are endemic, approximately one tenth of early Lyme disease patients experience concurrent babesiosis coinfection and approximately half of patients with babesiosis are coinfected with *B burgdorferi*. Other tickborne coinfections, such as anaplasmosis, should be considered in patients with babesiosis with clinical signs of Lyme disease; people with laboratory abnormalities, such as neutropenia, that suggest anaplasmosis; or people who do not respond as expected to treatment. When coinfection is documented, patients should receive therapies appropriate for each infection.

TREATMENT[1]: Atovaquone (administered orally) plus azithromycin (administered orally in ambulatory patients with mild to moderate disease and intravenously in hospitalized patients with severe disease) for 7 to 10 days is the regimen of choice (see Drugs for Parasitic Infections, p 952). Oral or intravenous clindamycin plus oral quinine may be

---

[1]Krause PJ, Auwaerter PG, Bannuru RR, et al. Clinical practice guidelines by the Infectious Diseases Society of America (IDSA): 2020 Guideline on diagnosis and management of babesiosis. *Clin Infect Dis.* 2020; Epub ahead of print November 30, 2020. DOI: 10.1093/cid/ciaa1216

used for patients who do not respond to atovaquone and azithromycin, although quinine commonly causes severe adverse effects. Severe babesiosis can be life-threatening despite antimicrobial therapy. Limited data suggest exchange transfusion has potential benefits that may outweigh potential adverse effects, particularly in patients with high levels of parasitemia. In severely immunocompromised patients, treatment for at least 6 weeks or longer, with negative blood smears for 2 weeks or longer before discontinuing therapy, is recommended. Higher doses of azithromycin (500 to 1000 mg per day, orally, in adolescents/adults) should be considered when treating a highly immunocompromised patient. Limited data are available for treatment of infection caused by *B duncani* or *B divergens*, but most reported patients have been treated with intravenous clindamycin plus oral quinine. Efficacy of atovaquone plus azithromycin in treating *B duncani* infection has not been evaluated.

ISOLATION OF THE HOSPITALIZED PATIENT: Standard precautions are recommended.

CONTROL MEASURES: Babesiosis is a nationally notifiable disease and a reportable disease in many states. Recommendations for prevention of tick bites are similar to those for prevention of Lyme disease and other tickborne infections (see Prevention of Mosquitoborne and Tickborne Infections, p 175). People with a known history of *Babesia* infection are deferred indefinitely from donating blood. In 2019, the US Food and Drug Administration (FDA) issued guidance to industry for regional, year-round testing using a licensed nucleic acid amplification test for *Babesia* infection or use of an FDA approved pathogen reduction device in the 14 highest-risk states (**www. fda.gov/regulatory-information/search-fda-guidance-documents/ recommendations-reducing-risk-transfusion-transmitted-babesiosis**).

Bacillus cereus Infections and Intoxications

CLINICAL MANIFESTATIONS: *Bacillus cereus* is associated primarily with 2 toxin-mediated foodborne illnesses, emetic and diarrheal, but it also can cause invasive extraintestinal infection. The **emetic syndrome** develops after a short incubation period, similar to staphylococcal foodborne illness. It is characterized by nausea, vomiting, and abdominal cramps, and diarrhea may follow in up to one third of patients. The **diarrheal syndrome** has a longer incubation period, is more severe, and resembles *Clostridium perfringens* foodborne illness. It is characterized by moderate to severe abdominal cramps and watery diarrhea, vomiting in approximately 25% of patients, and occasionally low-grade fever. Both illnesses usually are short-lived, about 24 hours, but the emetic toxin is occasionally associated with fulminant liver failure.

Invasive extraintestinal infection can be severe and includes wound and soft tissue infections; sepsis and bacteremia, including central line-associated bloodstream infection; endocarditis; osteomyelitis; purulent meningitis and ventricular shunt infection; pneumonia; and ocular infections (ie, endophthalmitis and keratitis). Infection can be acquired through use of contaminated blood products, especially platelets. *B cereus* is a leading cause of bacterial endophthalmitis following penetrating ocular trauma. Endogenous endophthalmitis can result from bacteremic seeding. Other ocular manifestations include an indolent keratitis related to corneal abrasions and may be seen in contact lens users or those who have undergone cataract surgery.

Rare infections attributable to *B cereus* strains that express anthrax toxin genes, which clinically resemble anthrax, have been reported.

ETIOLOGY: *B cereus* is an aerobic and facultative anaerobic, spore-forming, gram-positive or gram-variable bacillus.

EPIDEMIOLOGY: *B cereus* is ubiquitous in the environment because of the high resistance of its endospores to extreme conditions, including heat, cold, desiccation, salinity, and radiation, and commonly is present in small numbers in raw, dried, and processed foods and in the feces of healthy people. The organism is a common cause of foodborne illness in the United States but may be underrecognized, because few people seek care for mild illness and physicians and clinical laboratories do not routinely test for *B cereus*. Several confirmed outbreaks were reported to the Centers for Disease Control and Prevention (CDC) in recent years. A wide variety of food vehicles has been implicated.

Spores of *B cereus* are heat resistant and can survive pasteurization, brief cooking, boiling, and high saline concentrations. Spores germinate to vegetative forms that produce enterotoxins over a wide range of temperatures, both in foods and in the gastrointestinal tract. The diarrheal syndrome is caused by several distinct toxins that are ingested preformed or are produced after spores germinate in the gastrointestinal tract. The diarrheal toxins are heat labile and can be destroyed by heating. The emetic syndrome occurs after eating contaminated food containing a preformed toxin called cereulide. The best known association of the emetic syndrome is with ingestion of fried rice made from boiled rice stored at room temperature overnight, because *B cereus* can be present in uncooked rice. However, a wide variety of foods, especially starchy foods (including cereals), cheese products, meats, and vegetables, has been implicated. The toxin is elaborated by vegetative forms that germinate from spores when the food is reheated; it is heat stable and gastric acid resistant. Foodborne illness caused by *B cereus* is not transmissible from person to person.

Risk factors for invasive disease attributable to *B cereus* include history of injection drug use, presence of indwelling intravascular catheters or implanted devices, neutropenia or immunosuppression, and preterm birth. *B cereus* endophthalmitis has occurred after penetrating ocular trauma and injection drug use. Hospital outbreaks have been associated with contaminated medical equipment, but pseudoepidemics are more common and refer to sharp increases in contamination rates of clinical specimens associated with common source contamination — for example, ethanol pads or solutions, linen, and blood culture media.

The **incubation period** for foodborne illness is 0.5 to 6 hours for the emetic syndrome and 6 to 15 hours for the diarrheal syndrome.

DIAGNOSTIC TESTS: Diagnostic testing is not recommended for sporadic cases. For foodborne outbreaks, isolation of *B cereus* from the stool or vomitus of 2 or more ill people and not from control patients, or isolation of 10^5 colony-forming units/g or greater from epidemiologically implicated food, suggests that *B cereus* is the cause of the outbreak. Because the organism can be recovered from stool specimens from some well people, the presence of *B cereus* in feces or vomitus of ill people is not definitive evidence of infection. Food samples must be tested for both types of diarrheal enterotoxins, because either alone can cause illness. Although there is currently no commercial kit that detects the cereulide emetic toxin, *B cereus* colonies isolated from food or specimens of ill individuals may be tested by polymerase chain reaction assay for the emetic toxin gene in diagnostic laboratories.

In patients with risk factors for invasive disease (eg, preterm infants, people with immunosuppressing conditions), isolation of *B cereus* from wounds or from blood or other sterile body fluids is significant. The common perception of *Bacillus* species as "contaminants" may delay recognition and treatment of serious *B cereus* infections.

TREATMENT: *B cereus* foodborne illness usually requires only supportive treatment, including rehydration. Antimicrobial therapy is indicated for patients with invasive disease. Prompt removal of any potentially infected foreign bodies, such as central lines or implants, is essential. For intraocular infections, an ophthalmologist should be consulted regarding surgical management and use of intravitreal antimicrobial therapy in addition to systemic therapy. *B cereus* is usually resistant to beta-lactam antibiotics and often to clindamycin but is susceptible to vancomycin, which is the drug of choice. Alternative drugs, including linezolid, clindamycin, aminoglycosides, erythromycin, tetracyclines, and fluoroquinolones, may be considered depending on susceptibility results.

ISOLATION OF THE HOSPITALIZED PATIENT: Standard precautions are recommended.

CONTROL MEASURES: Proper cooking and appropriate storage of foods will help prevent foodborne illness attributable to *B cereus*. For example, rice cooked for later use should not be held at room temperature. Information on recommended safe food handling practices, including time and temperature requirements during cooking, storage, and reheating, can be found at **www.foodsafety.gov.** Hand hygiene and strict aseptic technique in caring for immunocompromised patients or patients with indwelling intravascular catheters are important to minimize the risk of invasive disease. The organism can survive in high concentrations of ethanol, but hand washing and use of 2% chlorhexidine are effective preventive measures.

Bacterial Vaginosis

CLINICAL MANIFESTATIONS: Bacterial vaginosis (BV) is a polymicrobial clinical syndrome characterized by changes in vaginal flora, with a reduction in normally abundant *Lactobacillus* species and acquisition of a diverse community of anaerobic and facultative bacteria. Vaginal lactobacilli act as an important host-defense mechanism by secreting substances that inhibit the growth of microbial pathogens and indigenous anaerobes. BV is diagnosed primarily in sexually active postpubertal females. Symptoms may include vaginal irritation, vaginal discharge, and/or vaginal odor. However, studies have shown that up to 50% of females who meet microbiologic criteria for a diagnosis of BV are asymptomatic. Classic signs, when present, include a thin white or grey, homogenous, adherent vaginal discharge with a fishy odor. Symptoms of pruritus, dysuria, or abdominal pain are not typically associated with BV but can be suggestive of mixed vaginitis. In pregnant females, BV has been associated with adverse outcomes, including chorioamnionitis, premature rupture of membranes, preterm delivery, and postpartum endometritis.

Vaginitis and vulvitis in prepubertal girls rarely, if ever, are manifestations of BV. Vaginitis in prepubertal girls frequently is nonspecific. Possible causes of vaginitis in this population include foreign bodies and infections attributable to group A streptococci, *Escherichia coli*, herpes simplex virus, *Neisseria gonorrhoeae*, *Chlamydia trachomatis*, *Trichomonas vaginalis*, or enteric bacteria, including *Shigella* species. In any prepubertal girl who has symptoms of BV, a full history and workup should be considered to rule out sexual abuse and/or a sexually transmitted infection (STI [see Sexual Assault and Abuse in Children and Adolescents/Young Adults, p 150]). If sexual abuse is suspected, those who are mandated to report need to follow their state's regulations for immediate reporting.

ETIOLOGY: The microbiologic cause of BV has not been delineated fully. Hydrogen peroxide and lactic acid-producing *Lactobacillus* species, particularly *Lactobacillus crispatus*, predominate among vaginal flora and play a protective role by maintaining a low vaginal pH. In females with BV, these species largely are replaced by commensal facultative and strict anaerobes. Increased concentrations of *Gardnerella vaginalis*, *Prevotella bivia*, *Atopobium vaginae*, *Mycoplasma hominis*, *Megasphaera* types, and *Mobiluncus* species, along with numerous other fastidious organisms, have been identified in women with BV.

G vaginalis, present in 95% to 100% of BV cases, was originally believed to be the primary BV pathogen. However, *G vaginalis* is also found in sexually active women with normal vaginal flora, and colonization with *G vaginalis* does not always lead to BV. Thus, microbiologic identification of *G vaginalis* is not, by itself, sufficient for the diagnosis of BV, even in a symptomatic individual.

EPIDEMIOLOGY: BV is the most common cause of vaginal discharge in sexually active adolescent and adult females. BV occurs more frequently in females with a new sexual partner or a higher number of sexual partners and is also associated with douching and not using condoms. BV may be the sole cause of the symptoms or it may accompany other conditions associated with vaginal discharge, such as trichomoniasis or cervicitis secondary to other STIs. BV can increase the risk of acquisition of other STIs, including human immunodeficiency virus (HIV), herpes simplex virus, *Mycoplasma genitalium*, *N gonorrhoeae*, *C trachomatis*, and *Trichomonas vaginalis*, and increase the risk of infectious complications following gynecologic surgeries. It can also increase the risk of HIV transmission to male partners.

Although the exact etiology of BV remains unknown, an **incubation period** of around 4 days (similar to other bacterial STIs such as *N gonorrhoeae*) has been suggested in recent studies. Recurrence is common, with more than 50% of women experiencing BV within 12 months after treatment.

DIAGNOSTIC TESTS: BV most commonly is diagnosed clinically using the Amsel criteria, requiring that 3 or more of the following symptoms or signs are present:
- Homogenous, thin grey or white vaginal discharge that smoothly coats the vaginal walls;
- Vaginal fluid pH greater than 4.5;
- A fishy (amine) odor of vaginal discharge before or after addition of 10% potassium hydroxide (ie, the "whiff test"); or
- Presence of clue cells (squamous vaginal epithelial cells covered with bacteria, which cause a stippled or granular appearance and ragged "moth-eaten" borders) representing at least 20% of the total vaginal epithelial cells seen on microscopic evaluation of vaginal fluid.

An alternative method for diagnosing BV is the Nugent score, which is used widely as the gold standard for making the diagnosis in the research setting and is commonly a standard against which newer diagnostic tests for BV are measured. A Gram stain of the vaginal fluid is evaluated, and a numerical score is generated on the basis of the apparent quantity of lactobacilli relative to BV-associated bacteria (*G vaginalis* and *Mobiluncus* species). The score is interpreted as normal (0–3), intermediate (4–6), or BV (7–10). Douching, recent intercourse, menstruation, and coexisting infection can alter findings on Gram stain.

Over-the-counter vaginal pH test kits have been marketed as home screening or testing options for BV. Despite diagnostic claims for such basic pH test kits, formal clinical evaluation and targeted laboratory-based diagnostic testing are warranted for patients reporting a positive home test result before any therapeutic interventions are instituted. Similarly, persistent symptoms despite a negative result on a home test kit warrants more sensitive laboratory evaluation.

There are a wide variety of diagnostic laboratory assays available to diagnose BV, ranging from point-of-care tests that typically identify a single agent, commonly *G vaginalis*, to multiplex molecular assays in which diagnosis is based on algorithms of relative quantifications of both favorable and detrimental vaginal organisms. Clinicians need to consider costs, result turnaround time, and accuracy in their decision to select a particular assay to test for BV among symptomatic females. No recommendations exist to screen asymptomatic females for BV. Culture for *G vaginalis* is not recommended as a diagnostic tool, because it is not specific, and Papanicolaou (Pap) testing is not recommended because of its extremely low sensitivity. Although the microscopy-based wet mount is advantageous for its low cost and immediate results, the multiplex polymerase chain reaction (PCR) assays might be more useful, particularly in the diagnostic workup of symptomatic females with recurrent or refractory vaginitis.

Sexually active females with BV should be evaluated for coinfection with other STIs, including syphilis, gonorrhea, chlamydia, trichomoniasis, and HIV infection. If the hepatitis B and human papillomavirus vaccine series have not been completed, these immunizations should be offered.

TREATMENT[1]: Symptomatic patients with BV should be treated. The goals of treatment are to relieve the symptoms and signs of infection and potentially to decrease the risk of acquiring other STIs. Treatment considerations should include patient preference for oral versus intravaginal treatment, possible adverse effects, and the presence of coinfections.

Nonpregnant females may be treated orally with metronidazole or topically with metronidazole gel 0.75% or clindamycin cream 2% (see Table 4.4, p 899, and Table 4.5, p 903). Alternative regimens include oral tinidazole, oral clindamycin, oral secnidazole, or clindamycin intravaginal ovules.[1] Patients should refrain from sexual intercourse or use condoms appropriately during treatment, keeping in mind that clindamycin cream is oil-based and can weaken latex condoms and diaphragms for up to 5 days after completion of therapy. There is no evidence that treatment of sexual partners effects treatment response or risk of recurrence. Follow-up is not necessary if symptoms resolve.

Pregnant females with symptoms of BV should be treated since they are at high risk of having preterm or low birth weight infants, premature rupture of membranes, intra-amniotic infections, and postpartum endometriosis. Metronidazole crosses the placenta. However, there are no studies showing any teratogenic evidence. Because oral therapy has not been shown to be superior to topical therapy for treating symptomatic BV in effecting cure or preventing adverse outcomes of pregnancy, symptomatic pregnant females can be treated with either the oral or vaginal metronidazole or clindamycin regimens recommended for nonpregnant females. Tinidazole should be avoided during pregnancy, as animal studies have shown teratogenic effects.

Breastfeeding mothers with symptoms of BV should be treated. Metronidazole is secreted in human milk, so topical metronidazole is preferred for treating breastfeeding

---

[1]Centers for Disease Control and Prevention. Sexually transmitted infections treatment guidelines, 2021. *MMWR Recomm Rep*. 2021; in press

mothers. Some clinicians advise deferring breastfeeding for 12 to 24 hours following oral maternal treatment with systemic metronidazole. Because information on safety of tinidazole in breastfeeding mothers is limited, it should only be used in difficult to treat cases. Interruption of breastfeeding is recommended during treatment and for 3 days after the last dose of tinidazole.

Approximately 30% of appropriately treated females have a recurrence within 3 months. Retreatment with the same regimen or an alternative regimen are both reasonable options for treating persistent or recurrent BV after the first occurrence. For females with multiple recurrences (more than 3 in the previous 12 months), either 0.75% metronidazole gel or 750 mg metronidazole vaginal suppository twice weekly for at least 3 months has been shown to reduce recurrences, although this benefit does not persist when suppressive therapy is discontinued. Limited data suggest an oral nitroimidazole (metronidazole or tinidazole 500 mg twice daily for 7 days) followed by intravaginal boric acid 600 mg daily for 21 days and suppressive 0.75% metronidazole gel twice weekly for 4 to 6 months might be an option for women with multiple recurrences of BV. Boric acid can cause death if ingested orally; it should be stored in a secure place inaccessible to children. Monthly oral metronidazole, 2 g, administered with fluconazole, 150 mg, has also been evaluated as suppressive therapy; this regimen reduced the incidence of BV and promoted colonization with normal vaginal microbiota. A randomized controlled trial of Astodrimer 1% vaginal gel (a dendrimer-based microbicide) also found favorable results in prolonging the time to BV recurrence compared with placebo. Studies thus far do not support currently available *Lactobacillus* formulations or probiotics as an adjunctive or replacement therapy for BV management.

ISOLATION OF THE HOSPITALIZED PATIENT: Standard precautions are recommended.

CONTROL MEASURES: None.

Bacteroides, Prevotella, and Other Anaerobic Gram-Negative Bacilli Infections

CLINICAL MANIFESTATIONS: *Bacteroides, Prevotella,* and other anaerobic gram-negative bacilli (AGNB) organisms from the oral cavity can cause chronic sinusitis, chronic otitis media, parotitis, dental infection, peritonsillar abscess, cervical adenitis, retropharyngeal space infection, aspiration pneumonia, lung abscess, pleural empyema, or necrotizing pneumonia. Species from the gastrointestinal tract are recovered in patients with peritonitis, intra-abdominal abscess, pelvic inflammatory disease, Bartholin cyst abscess, tubo-ovarian abscess, endometritis, acute and chronic prostatitis, prostatic and scrotal abscesses, scrotal gangrene, postoperative wound infection, and vulvovaginal and perianal infections. Invasion of the bloodstream from the oral cavity or intestinal tract can lead to brain abscess, meningitis, endocarditis, arthritis, or osteomyelitis. Skin and soft tissue infections include bacterial gangrene and necrotizing fasciitis; omphalitis in newborn infants; cellulitis at the site of fetal monitors, human bite wounds, or burns; infections adjacent to the mouth or rectum; and infected decubitus ulcers. Neonatal infections, including conjunctivitis, pneumonia, bacteremia, or meningitis, rarely occur. In most cases in which *Bacteroides, Prevotella,* and other AGNB are implicated, the infections are polymicrobial, with between 5 and 10 different organisms being present.

ETIOLOGY: Most *Bacteroides, Prevotella, Porphyromonas,* and *Fusobacterium* organisms associated with human disease are pleomorphic, non–spore-forming, facultatively anaerobic, gram-negative bacilli.

EPIDEMIOLOGY: *Bacteroides, Prevotella,* and other AGNB are part of the normal flora of the mouth, gastrointestinal tract, and female and male genital tracts. Members of the *Bacteroides fragilis* group predominate in the gastrointestinal tract flora; enterotoxigenic *B fragilis* may be a cause of diarrhea. Members of the *Prevotella melaninogenica* (formerly *Bacteroides melaninogenicus*) and *Prevotella oralis* (formerly *Bacteroides oralis*) groups are more common in the oral cavity. These species cause infection as opportunists, usually after an alteration in skin or mucosal membranes in conjunction with other endogenous species, and often are associated with chronic injury. Rates of upper respiratory tract, head, and neck infections associated with AGNB are higher in children. Endogenous infection results from aspiration, bowel perforation, or damage to mucosal surfaces from trauma, surgery, or chemotherapy. Mucosal injury or granulocytopenia predispose to infection. Except in infections resulting from human bites, no evidence of person-to-person transmission exists.

The **incubation period** is variable and depends on the inoculum and the site of involvement but usually is 1 to 5 days.

DIAGNOSTIC TESTS: Anaerobic culture media are necessary for recovery of *Bacteroides, Prevotella,* and other AGNB species. Because infections usually are polymicrobial, aerobic and anaerobic cultures should be obtained. A putrid odor, with or without gas in the infected site, suggests anaerobic infection. Use of an anaerobic transport tube or a sealed syringe is recommended for collection of clinical specimens.

TREATMENT: Abscesses should be drained when feasible; abscesses involving the brain, liver, and lungs may resolve with effective antimicrobial therapy alone. Necrotizing soft tissue lesions should be débrided surgically.

The choice of antimicrobial agent(s) is based on anticipated or known in vitro susceptibility testing and local antimicrobial resistance patterns. *Bacteroides* infections of the mouth and respiratory tract generally are susceptible to penicillin G, ampicillin, and clindamycin. However, some species of *Bacteroides* and almost 50% of *Prevotella* species produce beta-lactamase, and penicillin treatment failure has emerged as a consequence, so penicillin is not recommended for empirical coverage or for treatment of severe oropharyngeal or pleuropulmonary infections or for any abdominopelvic infections. A beta-lactam penicillin active against *Bacteroides* species combined with a beta-lactamase inhibitor (ampicillin-sulbactam, amoxicillin-clavulanate, or piperacillin-tazobactam) can be used to treat these infections. *Bacteroides* species of the gastrointestinal tract are often resistant to penicillin G but typically susceptible to metronidazole, beta-lactam plus beta-lactamase inhibitors, carbapenems, and chloramphenicol, but resistance is emerging to clindamycin. More than 80% of isolates are susceptible to cefoxitin and linezolid. Tigecycline has demonstrated in vitro activity against *Prevotella* and *Bacteroides* species but has limited pediatric dosing and safety data available, particularly for children younger than 8 years. Moxifloxacin may be an alternative for anaerobic infections in children with severe beta-lactam allergies, although emerging resistance to *Bacteroides* species is a concern. Cefuroxime, cefotaxime, and ceftriaxone are not reliably effective.

ISOLATION OF THE HOSPITALIZED PATIENT: Standard precautions are recommended.

CONTROL MEASURES: None.

Balantidium coli Infections
(Balantidiasis)

CLINICAL MANIFESTATIONS: Most human infections are asymptomatic. Symptomatic infection is characterized either by acute onset of bloody or watery mucoid diarrhea with abdominal pain or with chronic or intermittent episodes of diarrhea, anorexia, and weight loss. Inflammation of the gastrointestinal tract and local lymphatic vessels can result in bowel dilation, ulceration, perforation, and extraintestinal spread or secondary bacterial invasion. Colitis produced by *Balantidium coli* can mimic that of *Entamoeba histolytica* or noninfectious causes. Fulminant disease can occur in malnourished or otherwise debilitated or immunocompromised patients.

ETIOLOGY: *B coli*, a ciliated protozoan, is the largest pathogenic protozoan known to infect humans.

EPIDEMIOLOGY: Pigs are the primary host reservoir of *B coli*, but the parasite has also been found in other primates and domestic animals. Infections have been reported in most areas of the world but are more common in tropical and subtropical areas or areas with poor sanitation systems. Cysts excreted in feces can be transmitted directly from hand to mouth or indirectly through fecally contaminated water or food. Excysted trophozoites infect the colon. A person is infectious as long as cysts are excreted in stool. Cysts may remain viable in the environment for months.

The **incubation period** is not established but may be several days.

DIAGNOSTIC TESTS: Diagnosis usually is made by demonstrating trophozoites (or less frequently, cysts) in stool or tissue by scraping lesions via sigmoidoscopy or colonoscopy, histologic examination of intestinal biopsy specimens, or ova and parasite examination of stool. Stool examination is less sensitive; repeated examination may be necessary, because shedding of organisms can be intermittent. Because trophozoites degenerate rapidly, fresh diarrheal stools require either prompt microscopic examination or placement in stool fixation medium.

TREATMENT: The drug of choice is tetracycline (see Drugs for Parasitic Infections, p 953). Alternative drugs are metronidazole (or tinidazole), iodoquinol, and nitazoxanide.

ISOLATION OF THE HOSPITALIZED PATIENT: Standard and contact precautions are recommended, because human-to-human transmission can occur rarely.

CONTROL MEASURES: Control measures include sanitary disposal of human and porcine feces and good handwashing. Cysts are resistant to the levels of chlorination used for drinking water; waterborne outbreaks of disease have occurred despite chlorination.

Bartonella henselae (Cat-Scratch Disease)

CLINICAL MANIFESTATIONS: Cat scratch disease, the predominant clinical manifestation of *Bartonella henselae* infection, presents in 85 to 90% of children as a localized cutaneous and regional lymphadenopathy disorder. A skin papule or pustule develops within 12 days at the presumed site of inoculation in approximately two thirds of cases and usually precedes development of lymphadenopathy by 1 to 2 weeks (range, 7–60 days). Lymphadenopathy occurs in nodes that drain the site of inoculation, typically axillary, but cervical, submandibular, submental, epitrochlear, or inguinal nodes can be involved. Low-grade fever lasting several days develops in 30% of patients. The skin overlying affected lymph nodes can be normal or tender, warm, erythematous, and indurated, and approximately 10% to 20% of affected nodes suppurate. Typically, lymphadenopathy resolves spontaneously in 2 to 4 months.

Less common manifestations of *B henselae* infection likely reflect bloodborne disseminated disease and include culture-negative endocarditis, encephalopathy, osteolytic lesions, glomerulonephritis, pneumonia, thrombocytopenic purpura, erythema nodosum, and prolonged fever with granulomata in the liver and spleen. Chronic *Bartonella* infection in nonimmunocompromised children has not been substantiated scientifically.

Ocular manifestations occur in 5% to 10% of patients. The most classic and frequent presentation of ocular *B henselae* infection is Parinaud oculoglandular syndrome, which consists of follicular conjunctivitis and ipsilateral preauricular lymphadenopathy. Another occasional ocular manifestation is neuroretinitis, which is characterized by abrupt unilateral (and rarely bilateral) painless vision impairment, granulomatous optic disc swelling, and macular edema, with lipid exudates (macular star). Rare presentations include retinochoroiditis, anterior uveitis, vitritis, pars planitis, retinal vasculitis, retinitis, branch retinal arteriolar or venular occlusions, macular hole, or retinal detachments (extraordinarily rare).

ETIOLOGY: *B henselae* is a fastidious, slow-growing, gram-negative bacillus that also is the causative agent of bacillary angiomatosis (vascular proliferative lesions of skin and subcutaneous tissue) and bacillary peliosis (reticuloendothelial lesions in visceral organs, primarily the liver). The latter 2 manifestations of infection are reported among immunocompromised patients, primarily those with human immunodeficiency virus infection. Additional species, such as *Bartonella clarridgeiae*, also have been found to cause cat scratch disease (CSD). *B henselae* is related closely to *Bartonella quintana*, the agent of human body louseborne trench fever that caused significant disease among troops during World War I and now affects homeless people lacking adequate sanitation and hygiene. *B quintana* also can cause bacillary angiomatosis and endocarditis.

EPIDEMIOLOGY: *B henselae* is a common cause of regional lymphadenopathy in children. The highest incidence (9 per 100 000 population) is found in children 5 to 9 years of age; infections occur more often during the fall and winter. Cats are the natural reservoir for *B henselae*, with a seroprevalence of 30% to 40% in domestic and adopted shelter cats in the United States. Other animals, including dogs, can be infected and are rarely associated with human illness. Cat-to-cat transmission occurs via the cat flea *(Ctenocephalides felis)*, with feline infection resulting in bacteremia that usually is asymptomatic and lasts weeks to months. Fleas acquire the organism when feeding on a bacteremic cat and then shed infectious organisms in their feces. The bacteria are transmitted to humans by inoculation through a scratch, lick, or bite from a bacteremic cat. Most patients with CSD have a history of recent contact with apparently healthy cats, especially kittens. Kittens are nearly 5 times as likely to be bacteremic with *B henselae* than are older cats. Cats obtained from shelters or adopted as strays also have high rates of bacteremia. There is no convincing evidence that ticks are a competent vector for transmission of *Bartonella* organisms to humans. No evidence of person-to-person transmission exists.

The **incubation period** from the time of the scratch to appearance of the primary cutaneous lesion is 3 to 12 days; the median period from the appearance of the primary lesion to the appearance of lymphadenopathy is 12 days (range, 7 to 60 days).

DIAGNOSTIC TESTS: Both enzyme immunoassay (EIA) and indirect immunofluorescent antibody (IFA) platforms for detection of IgM and IgG serum antibodies to antigens of *Bartonella* species are available for diagnosis of CSD. Both formats have limitations in sensitivity and specificity. With both types of tests, cross-reactivity with other infectious agents (such as *Chlamydia pneumoniae, Coxiella burnetii,* and especially other *Bartonella* species) is common. Elevated immunoglobulin (Ig) M titers may suggest recent infection, but both false-positive and false-negative IgM test results occur. In adults, there is a high rate of anti-*B henselae* IgG seroprevalence in the general population attributable to prior exposure. Generally speaking, if an IFA or EIA IgG titer is <1:64, the patient does not have acute infection. Titers between 1:64 and 1:256 may represent past or acute infection, and follow-up titers in 2 to 4 weeks should be considered. An IgG titer of ≥1:256 or a fourfold increase in IgG titer is consistent with acute infection.

Polymerase chain reaction (PCR) assays are available in some commercial and research laboratories for testing of tissue or body fluids. *Bartonella* PCR assay is highly specific and fairly sensitive for use on tissue, although some assays do not distinguish between the various *Bartonella* species. *Bartonella* PCR assay is very insensitive when testing blood, however, and it is not generally recommended for this specimen.

B henselae is a fastidious organism; recovery by routine culture requires prolonged incubation (>10 days) and rarely is successful.

If tissue (eg, lymph node) specimens are available, bacilli occasionally may be visualized using a silver stain (eg, Warthin-Starry or Steiner stain); however, these stains are not specific for *B henselae.* Early histologic changes in lymph node specimens consist of lymphocytic infiltration with epithelioid granuloma formation. Later changes consist of polymorphonuclear leukocyte infiltration with granulomas that become necrotic and resemble granulomas from patients with tularemia, brucellosis, or mycobacterial infections.

TREATMENT: Management of localized uncomplicated CSD primarily is aimed at relief of symptoms, because the disease is self-limited, resolving spontaneously in 2 to 4 months. No antibiotic regimen has been shown to be beneficial in improving the clinical cure rate, and in most cases, antibiotic therapy is not indicated. Painful suppurative nodes can be treated with needle aspiration for relief of symptoms. Incision and drainage should be avoided, because this may facilitate fistula formation; surgical excision generally is unnecessary.

Some experts recommend antimicrobial therapy in acutely or severely ill immunocompetent patients with systemic symptoms, particularly people with retinitis, hepatic or splenic involvement, osteomyelitis, or painful adenitis. Several antimicrobial agents (azithromycin, clarithromycin, ciprofloxacin, doxycycline, trimethoprim-sulfamethoxazole, ceftriaxone, gentamicin, and rifampin) have in vitro activity against *B henselae.* However, outcomes for most forms of CSD are generally excellent with or without therapy.

Doxycycline plus rifampin are often used for patients with neuroretinitis. Doxycycline may be used regardless of patient age (see Tetracyclines, p 866). Reports in the literature note that a large majority of such patients experience significant visual recovery to 20/40 or better. Corticosteroids should be considered in conjunction with ophthalmology consultation.

Antimicrobial therapy is recommended for all immunocompromised people, because treatment of bacillary angiomatosis and bacillary peliosis has been shown to be beneficial. Azithromycin or doxycycline is effective for treatment of these conditions; therapy should be administered for 3 months for bacillary angiomatosis and for 4 months for bacillary peliosis to prevent relapse. In these patients, doxycycline can be used for short durations (ie, 21 days or less) without regard to patient age; for the longer treatment durations required for treatment of *Bartonella* infection in immunocompromised people, for whom the alternative treatment of azithromycin exists, doxycycline is not recommended in children younger than 8 years (see Tetracyclines, p 866).

For patients with unusual manifestations of *Bartonella* infection (eg, culture-negative endocarditis, neuroretinitis, disease in immunocompromised patients), consultation with a pediatric infectious diseases expert is recommended.

ISOLATION OF THE HOSPITALIZED PATIENT: Standard precautions are recommended.

CONTROL MEASURES: CSD is a preventable infection. All cats >8 weeks of age should be treated topically for fleas and ticks regularly. Effort should be undertaken to avoid scratches and bites from cats or kittens. Sites of cat scratches or bites should be washed immediately, and cats should not be allowed to lick open cuts or wounds. Immunocompromised people should avoid contact with cats younger than 1 year, stray cats, and cats that scratch or bite. Testing or treatment of cats for *Bartonella* infection is not recommended, nor is declawing or removal of the cat from the household.

Baylisascaris Infections

CLINICAL MANIFESTATIONS: Infection with *Baylisascaris procyonis*, a raccoon roundworm, can present with nonspecific signs such as nausea, fever, and fatigue. Other clinical presentations include neural larval migrans, ocular larva migrans, and visceral larval migrans. Acute central nervous system (CNS) disease (eg, altered mental status and seizures) accompanied by peripheral and/or cerebrospinal fluid (CSF) eosinophilia are manifestations of neural larval migrans (eosinophilic meningoencephalitis) and can occur 2 to 4 weeks after infection. Severe neurologic sequelae or death are usual outcomes. Ocular larva migrans can result in diffuse unilateral subacute neuroretinitis; direct visualization of larvae in the retina sometimes is possible. Visceral larval migrans can present with nonspecific signs, such as macular rash, pneumonitis, and hepatomegaly. Similar to visceral larva migrans caused by *Toxocara* species, subclinical or asymptomatic infection is thought to be the most common outcome of infection.

ETIOLOGY: *B procyonis* is a 10- to 25-cm long roundworm (nematode) with a direct life cycle usually limited to its definitive host, the raccoon. Domestic dogs and some less commonly owned pets, such as kinkajous and ringtails, can serve as definitive hosts and are potential sources of human disease.

EPIDEMIOLOGY: *B procyonis* is distributed focally throughout the United States; in areas where disease is endemic, 22% to 80% of raccoons can harbor the parasite in their intestines. Reports of infections in dogs raise concern that infected dogs may be able to spread the disease. Embryonated eggs containing infective larvae are ingested from the soil by raccoons, rodents, and birds. When infective eggs or an infected host is eaten by a raccoon, the larvae grow to maturity in the small intestine, where adult female worms shed millions of eggs per day. Eggs become infective after 2 to 4 weeks in the environment and may persist long-term in the soil. Cases of raccoon infection have been reported in many parts of the United States. Risk of human infection is greatest in areas where significant raccoon populations live in peridomestic settings. Fewer than 30 cases of *Baylisascaris* CNS disease have been documented in the United States, although cases may be undiagnosed or underreported.

Risk factors for *Baylisascaris* infection include contact with raccoon latrines (communal defecation sites often found at or on the base of trees; raised flat surfaces such as tree stumps, logs, rocks, decks, and rooftops; or unsealed attics or garages), geophagia/pica, age younger than 4 years, and, in older children, developmental delay. Most reported cases of CNS disease have been in males.

The **incubation period** is usually 1 to 4 weeks.

DIAGNOSTIC TESTS: *Baylisascaris* infection is confirmed by identification of larvae in biopsy specimens. A presumptive diagnosis of CNS disease can be made on the basis of clinical (meningoencephalitis, diffuse unilateral subacute neuroretinitis, pseudotumor), epidemiologic (raccoon exposure), and laboratory (blood and CSF eosinophilia) findings. Serologic testing (serum, CSF) for patients with clinical symptoms is available at the Centers for Disease Control and Prevention. Neuroimaging results can be normal initially, but as larvae grow and migrate through CNS tissue, focal abnormalities are found in periventricular white matter and elsewhere. In ocular disease, ophthalmologic examination can reveal chorioretinal lesions or rarely larvae. Stool examination is not helpful because eggs are not shed in human feces. The disease is not transmitted from person to person.

TREATMENT: Albendazole, in conjunction with high-dose corticosteroids, has been advocated most widely on the basis of CNS and CSF penetration and in vitro activity (see Drugs for Parasitic Infections, p 953). Treatment with anthelmintic agents and corticosteroids may not affect clinical outcome once severe CNS disease manifestations are evident. Treatment should be initiated while the diagnostic evaluation is being completed if infection is suspected. Preventive therapy with albendazole should be considered for children with a history of ingestion of soil potentially contaminated with raccoon feces but no definitive preventive dosing regimen has been established. Studies in children as young as 1 year of age suggest that albendazole can be administered safely to this population. Limited data are available regarding safety and efficacy of alternate anthelmintic therapies in children though mebendazole and ivermectin have been proposed as alternatives if albendazole is unavailable. The safety of ivermectin in children weighing less than 15 kg and in pregnant women has not been established. Larvae localized to the retina may be killed by direct photocoagulation.

ISOLATION OF THE HOSPITALIZED PATIENT: Standard precautions are recommended.

CONTROL MEASURES: *Baylisascaris* infections are prevented by avoiding ingestion of soil contaminated with stool of infected animal reservoirs, primarily raccoons; avoiding raccoon defecation sites (latrines); washing hands after contact with soil or with pets or other animals; discouraging raccoon presence by limiting access to human or pet food sources; and decontaminating raccoon latrines (especially if located near homes) by treating the area with boiling water or a propane torch, in keeping with local fire safety regulations, or through proper removal if located within the home (eg, attic).

Infections With *Blastocystis* Species

CLINICAL MANIFESTATIONS: The importance of *Blastocystis* species as a cause of gastrointestinal tract disease is controversial. The asymptomatic carrier state is well documented. Clinical symptoms reported include bloating, flatulence, acute or chronic watery diarrhea without fecal leukocytes or blood, constipation, abdominal pain, nausea, anorexia, weight loss, and poor growth; fever is generally absent. Some case series and reports have noted an association between infection with *Blastocystis* and chronic urticaria and irritable bowel syndrome. When *Blastocystis* organisms are identified in stool from symptomatic patients, other causes of this symptom complex, particularly *Giardia duodenalis* and *Cryptosporidium parvum*, should be investigated before assuming that blastocystosis is the cause of the signs and symptoms. Polymerase chain reaction fingerprinting suggests that some *Blastocystis* subtypes are disease associated and others are not. On the other hand, an emerging literature proposes that rather than a cause of disease, *Blastocystis* may be a marker of gastrointestinal health.

ETIOLOGY: *Blastocystis* species (previously referred to as *Blastocystis hominis)* consists of several species that reside in the gastrointestinal tracts of humans as well as other mammals, reptiles, amphibians, and fish. Some *Blastocystis* species believed to be specific to other animals are now recognized as being able to be transmitted to humans. Previously classified as a protozoan, more recent molecular studies have led the organism to be characterized as a stramenopile (a eukaryote). Multiple forms have been described: vacuolar, which is observed most commonly in clinical specimens; granular, which is seen rarely in fresh stools; amoeboid; and cystic.

EPIDEMIOLOGY: *Blastocystis* infection is observed commonly throughout the world, although prevalence among countries and communities varies. In the United States, Europe, and Japan, *Blastocystis* species are recovered from 1% to 20% of stool specimens examined for ova and parasites, whereas prevalence of 100% has been observed among school-aged children in countries without modern sanitation. Because transmission is believed to occur via the fecal-oral route, presence of the organism may be a marker for presence of other pathogens spread by fecal contamination. *Blastocystis* infection is more common among people with pets or living near farm animals; however, exposure is not sufficient for infection as pathogenicity appears related to subtype, host immunocompetence and other factors. Organisms may remain in the gastrointestinal tract for years.

The **incubation period** has not been established.

DIAGNOSTIC TESTS: Stool specimens should be preserved in polyvinyl alcohol and stained with trichrome or iron-hematoxylin before microscopic examination. The trophozoite stage of the parasite is very difficult to identify and rarely is seen. Small round cysts, the most common form, vary markedly in size from 6 to 40 μm and are characterized by a large central body (similar to large vacuole) surrounded by multiple nuclei. The parasite may be present in varying numbers, and infections may be reported as light to heavy. The presence of 5 or more organisms per high-power (x400 magnification) field can indicate heavy infection, which to some experts suggests causation when other enteropathogens are absent. Other experts consider the presence of 10 or more organisms per 10 oil immersion fields (x1000 magnification) to represent heavy infection. A serum antibody test is available, but its diagnostic utility is still unclear.

TREATMENT: Indications for treatment are not established. Some experts recommend that treatment should be reserved for patients who have persistent symptoms and in whom no other pathogen or process is found to explain the gastrointestinal tract symptoms. Randomized controlled treatment trials with both metronidazole and nitazoxanide have demonstrated benefit in symptomatic patients, although microbiologic resolution does not always occur. Tinidazole is an alternative that may be tolerated better than metronidazole. Case series suggest high resolution of symptoms in symptomatic patients treated with trimethoprim-sulfamethoxazole but less success in clearing the organism.

Case reports or small series indicate paromomycin, iodoquinol, and ketoconazole alone or in combination have varying success (see Drugs for Parasitic Infections, p 954). Other experts believe that *Blastocystis* infection does not cause symptomatic disease and recommend only a careful search for other causes of symptoms.

ISOLATION OF THE HOSPITALIZED PATIENT: Standard precautions should be followed; contact precautions also recommended for diapered or incontinent children.

CONTROL MEASURES: Personal hygiene measures, including hand washing with soap and warm water after using the toilet, after changing diapers, and before preparing food, should be practiced.

Blastomycosis

CLINICAL MANIFESTATIONS: Infections can be acute, chronic, or fulminant but are asymptomatic in up to 50% of infected people. The most common clinical manifestation of blastomycosis in children is cough (often productive) accompanying pulmonary disease, with fever, chest pain, and nonspecific symptoms such as fatigue and myalgia. Rarely, patients may develop acute respiratory distress syndrome (ARDS). Typical radiographic patterns include consolidation, patchy pneumonitis, a mass-like infiltrate, or nodules. Blastomycosis can be misdiagnosed as bacterial pneumonia, tuberculosis, sarcoidosis, or malignant neoplasm. Disseminated blastomycosis, which can occur in up to 25% of symptomatic cases, most commonly involves the skin and osteoarticular structures. Cutaneous manifestations can be verrucous, nodular, ulcerative, or pustular. Abscesses usually are subcutaneous but can involve any organ. Erythema nodosum, which is common in patients with histoplasmosis and coccidioidomycosis, is rare in blastomycosis. Central nervous system infection is less common, and intrauterine or congenital infection is rare.

ETIOLOGY: Blastomycosis is caused by *Blastomyces* species *(Blastomyces dermatitidis, Blastomyces gilchristii,* and *Blastomyces helicus),* which are thermally dimorphic fungi existing in the yeast form at 37°C (98°F) in infected tissues and in a mycelial form at room temperature and in soil. Conidia, produced from hyphae of the mycelial form, are infectious.

EPIDEMIOLOGY: Infection is acquired through inhalation of conidia from the environment. Increased mortality rates for patients with pulmonary blastomycosis have been associated with advanced age, chronic obstructive pulmonary disease, cancer, and Black race. Person-to-person transmission does not occur. In the United States, blastomycosis is endemic in the central states, with most cases occurring in the Ohio and Mississippi river valleys, the southeastern states, and states that border the Great Lakes; however, sporadic cases have occurred outside these areas. Similar to *Histoplasma capsulatum, Blastomyces* species can grow in bird and animal excreta. Occupational and recreational activities associated with infection often involve environmental disruption such as construction of homes or roads, boating and canoeing, tubing on a river, fishing, exploration of beaver dams and underground forts, and a community compost pile.

The **incubation period** ranges from approximately 2 weeks to 3 months.

DIAGNOSTIC TESTS: Definitive diagnosis of blastomycosis is based on microscopic identification of characteristic thick-walled, broad-based, single budding yeast cells either by culture at 37°C or in histopathologic specimens. The organism may be seen in sputum, tracheal aspirates, cerebrospinal fluid, urine, or histopathologic specimens from lesions processed with 10% potassium hydroxide or a silver stain. Children with pneumonia who are unable to produce sputum may require bronchoalveolar lavage or open biopsy to establish the diagnosis. Bronchoalveolar lavage is high yield, even in patients with bone or skin manifestations. Organisms can be cultured on brain-heart infusion media and Sabouraud dextrose agar at 25°C to 30°C as a mold; identification can be confirmed by conversion to yeast phase at 37°C. Chemiluminescent DNA probes are available for identification of *B dermatitidis;* rare false-positive identification attributable to cross-reactivity with other endemic fungi has been reported. Polymerase chain reaction assay can be used directly on certain clinical specimens but is not widely performed.

Because serologic tests (immunodiffusion and complement fixation) lack adequate sensitivity, they are generally not useful for diagnosis. An enzyme immunoassay that detects *Blastomyces* antigen in urine has replaced classic serologic studies and performs well for the diagnosis of disseminated and pulmonary disease as well as for monitoring response to antifungal therapy. Antigen testing in urine performs better than antigen testing of serum, and antigen testing in bronchoalveolar lavage fluid or cerebrospinal fluid is also available. Significant cross-reactivity occurs in patients with other endemic mycoses (specifically, *H capsulatum, Paracoccidioides brasiliensis*, and *Talaromyces marneffei*); clinical and epidemiologic considerations often aid with interpretation.

TREATMENT[1]**:** Because of the high risk of dissemination, some experts recommend that all cases of blastomycosis in children should be treated. Amphotericin B deoxycholate or an amphotericin B lipid formulation is recommended for initial therapy of severe pulmonary disease for 1 to 2 weeks or until improvement, followed by 6 to 12 months of itraconazole therapy. Oral itraconazole is recommended for 6 to 12 months for mild to moderate infection (see Table 4.7, p 910). Some experts suggest 12 months of therapy for patients with osteoarticular disease. For central nervous system infection, a lipid formulation of amphotericin B is recommended for 4 to 6 weeks, followed by an azole for at least 12 months and until resolution of all cerebrospinal fluid abnormalities. The preferred azole for prolonged central nervous system infection treatment is voriconazole, given the limited central nervous system penetration of itraconazole. Itraconazole is indicated for treatment of non–life-threatening infection outside the central nervous system in adults and is recommended in children. Serum trough concentrations of itraconazole should be 1 to 2 µg/mL. Concentrations should be checked after several days of therapy to ensure adequate drug exposure. When measured by high-pressure liquid chromatography, both itraconazole and its bioactive hydroxyitraconazole metabolite are reported, the sum of which should be considered in assessing drug concentrations. The itraconazole oral solution formulation is preferred because of improved absorption and should be taken on an empty stomach.

ISOLATION OF THE HOSPITALIZED PATIENT: Standard precautions are recommended.

CONTROL MEASURES: None.

Bocavirus

CLINICAL MANIFESTATIONS: Human bocavirus (HBoV) first was identified in 2005 from a cohort of children with acute respiratory tract symptoms. Pneumonia, bronchiolitis, exacerbations of asthma, the common cold, and acute otitis media have been attributed

---

[1]Chapman SW, Dismukes WE, Proia LA, et al. Clinical guidelines for the management of blastomycosis: 2008 update by the Infectious Diseases Society of America. *Clin Infect Dis.* 2008;46(12):1801–1812

to HBoV. Symptoms may include cough, rhinorrhea, wheezing, and fever. HBoV has been identified in 5% to 33% of all children with acute respiratory tract infections in various settings (eg, inpatient facilities, outpatient facilities, child care centers). High rates of HBoV subclinical infections have been documented, complicating etiologic association with disease. The role of HBoV as a pathogen in human infection is further confounded by simultaneous detection of other viral pathogens in patients in whom HBoV is identified, with coinfection rates ranging from 20% to as high as 80%. However, a number of lines of evidence support the role of HBoV as a pathogen, at least during primary infection. These include longitudinal cohort studies showing an association of primary infection with symptomatic illness and case-control studies showing associations of illness with monoinfection, high viral load, and detection of HBoV mRNA.

HBoV has been detected in stool samples from children with acute gastroenteritis; however, further studies are needed to better understand the role of HBoV in gastroenteritis. Infection with HBoV appears to be ubiquitous, because nearly all children develop serologic evidence of previous HBoV infection by 5 years of age.

ETIOLOGY: HBoV is a nonenveloped, single-stranded DNA virus classified in the family *Parvoviridae*, subfamily *Parvovirinae*, genus *Bocaparvovirus*, on the basis of its genetic similarity to the closely related **bo**vine parvovirus 1 and **ca**nine minute virus, from which the name "**boca**virus" was derived. Four distinct genotypes have been described (HBoV types 1–4), although there are no data regarding antigenic variation or distinct serotypes. HBoV1 replicates primarily in the respiratory tract and has been associated with upper and lower respiratory tract illness. HBoV2, HBoV3, and HBoV4 have been found predominantly in stool, without clear association with any clinical illness except a few reports that have associated HBoV2 with gastroenteritis.

EPIDEMIOLOGY: Detection of HBoV has been described only in humans. Transmission is presumed to be from respiratory tract secretions, although fecal-oral transmission may be possible because of finding of HBoV in stool specimens from children, including symptomatic children with diarrhea.

The frequent codetection of other viral pathogens of the respiratory tract in association with HBoV has led to speculation about the pathologic role played by HBoV; it may be a true pathogen or copathogen, and emerging evidence seems to support both roles. Codetection of HBoV with other respiratory viruses is more common when HBoV is present at lower viral loads ($\leq 10^4$ copies/mL). Extended and intermittent shedding of HBoV has been reported for up to a year after initial detection, with median shedding duration of approximately 2 months. Because HBoV may be shed for long periods after primary infection and because of the possibility of reactivation during subsequent viral infections and the high rate of detection in healthy people, clinical interpretation of HBoV detection is difficult.

HBoV circulates worldwide and throughout the year. In temperate climates, seasonal clustering in the spring associated with increased transmission of other respiratory tract viruses has been reported.

DIAGNOSTIC TESTS: Commercial molecular diagnostic assays for HBoV are available. HBoV quantitative polymerase chain reaction (respiratory and serum specimens), detection of HBoV mRNA in the respiratory tract, and detection of HBoV-specific immunoglobulin (Ig) M and IgG antibody also are used by research laboratories to detect the presence of virus and infection. A positive laboratory test does not necessarily imply etiology, in part because of prolonged shedding and codetection of other respiratory pathogens.

TREATMENT: No specific therapy is available.

ISOLATION OF THE HOSPITALIZED PATIENT: The presence of virus in respiratory tract secretions and stool suggests that, in addition to standard precautions, contact precautions should be initiated to limit the spread of infection for the duration of the symptomatic illness in infants and young children. Prolonged shedding of virus in respiratory tract secretions and in stool may occur after resolution of symptoms, particularly in immuno-compromised hosts; therefore, the duration of contact precautions should be extended in these situations.

CONTROL MEASURES: Appropriate respiratory hygiene and cough etiquette should be followed. Although possible health care-associated transmission of HBoV has been described, investigations of transmissibility of HBoV in community or health care settings have not been published. Appropriate hand hygiene, particularly when handling respiratory tract secretions or diapers of ill children, is recommended. The presence of HBoV DNA in serum also raises the possibility of transmission by transfusion, although this mode of transmission has not been documented.

Borrelia Infections Other Than Lyme Disease
(Relapsing Fever)

CLINICAL MANIFESTATIONS: Two types of relapsing fever occur in humans: tickborne and louseborne. Both are characterized by sudden onset of high fever, shaking chills, sweats, headache, muscle and joint pain, altered sensorium, and nausea. A fleeting macular rash of the trunk and petechiae of the skin and mucous membranes sometimes occur but are not common. Findings and complications can differ between types of relapsing fever and include hepatosplenomegaly, jaundice, thrombocytopenia, iridocyclitis, cough with pleuritic pain, pneumonitis, Bell's palsy, meningitis, and myocarditis. Mortality rates are 10 to 70% in untreated louseborne relapsing fever (possibly related to comorbidities in refugee-type settings, where this disease typically is found) and 4% to 10% in untreated tickborne relapsing fever. Death occurs predominantly in infants, older adults, and people with underlying illnesses. Early treatment reduces mortality to less than 5%. Untreated, an initial febrile period of 2 to 6 days terminates spontaneously and is followed by an afebrile period of several days to weeks, then by 1 relapse or more (0–13 for tickborne, 1–5 for louseborne). Relapses typically become shorter and progressively milder as afebrile periods lengthen. Relapse is associated with expression of new borrelial antigens, and resolution of symptoms is associated with production of antibody specific to those new antigenic determinants. Infection during pregnancy often is severe and can result in spontaneous abortion, preterm birth, stillbirth, or neonatal infection.

ETIOLOGY: Relapsing fever is caused by certain spirochetes of the genus *Borrelia*. Worldwide, at least 14 *Borrelia* species cause tickborne (endemic) relapsing fever, including *Borrelia hermsii*, *Borrelia turicatae*, and *Borrelia parkeri* in North America. *Borrelia miyamotoi* is associated with a similar but distinct tick-borne acute febrile illness in the United States. Louseborne (epidemic) relapsing fever is cause by *Borrelia recurrentis*. Lyme disease, caused by more distantly related *Borrelia* species (predominantly *Borrelia burgdorferi* in the United States), is discussed in the Lyme Disease chapter (p 482).

EPIDEMIOLOGY: Endemic tickborne relapsing fever is distributed widely throughout the world. Most species, including *B hermsii*, *B turicatae*, and *B parkeri*, are transmitted through the bite of soft-bodied ticks (*Ornithodoros* species). *B miyamotoi*, which only recently has been recognized as a cause of human illness, is transmitted through the bite of hard-bodied ticks (*Ixodes* species). Vector ticks become infected by feeding on rodents or other small mammals and transmit infection via their saliva during subsequent blood meals. Ticks may serve as reservoirs of infection through transovarial and trans-stadial transmission. Because of differences in the distribution, life cycle, and feeding habits of soft- and hard-bodied ticks, the epidemiology differs somewhat for infections transmitted by these 2 classes of ticks.

Soft-bodied ticks typically live within rodent nests. They inflict painless bites and feed briefly (seconds to 30 minutes), usually at night, so that people often are unaware of having been bitten. In the United States, vector soft-bodied ticks are found most often in mountainous areas of the West. Human infection typically follows sleeping in rustic, rodent-infested cabins, although cases have been associated with primary residences and luxurious rental properties. Cases occur sporadically or in small clusters among families or cohabiting groups. *B hermsii* is the most common cause of these infections. *B turicatae* infections occur less frequently; most cases have been reported from Texas and are associated with tick exposures in rodent-infested caves. Clinically apparent human infections with *B parkeri* in the United States are rare; the tick infected with this *Borrelia* species is associated with arid areas or grasslands in the western United States.

The hard-bodied ticks *Ixodes scapularis* and *Ixodes pacificus* transmit *B miyamotoi* in North America. These ticks are better known as vectors of Lyme disease, anaplasmosis, and babesiosis; coinfections have been reported. It is likely that risk factors described for Lyme disease are similar for *B miyamotoi*. Unlike Lyme disease, *B miyamotoi* can be transmitted within the first 24 hours of tick attachment, and probability of transmission increases with prolonged attachment. Most known cases of *B miyamotoi* infection have occurred in July or August, later than most Lyme disease cases. This suggests that *B miyamotoi* transmission more often occurs through the bite of larval, rather than nymphal, *Ixodes* ticks.

Louseborne epidemic relapsing fever had previously been widespread but is now mainly restricted to Ethiopia, Eritrea, Somalia, and Sudan, especially in refugee and displaced populations. Epidemic transmission occurs when body lice *(Pediculus humanus)* become infected by feeding on humans with spirochetemia; infection is transmitted when infected lice are crushed and their body fluids contaminate a bite wound or skin abraded by scratching.

Infected body lice and ticks may remain alive and infectious for several years to decades without feeding. Relapsing fever is not transmitted between individual humans, but perinatal transmission from an infected mother to her infant occurs and can result in preterm birth, stillbirth, and neonatal death.

The **incubation period** is 2 to 18 days, with a mean of 7 days.

DIAGNOSTIC TESTS: Spirochetes can be observed by dark-field microscopy and in Wright-, Giemsa-, or acridine orange-stained preparations of thin or dehemoglobinized thick smears of peripheral blood or in stained buffy-coat preparations. Organisms often can be visualized in blood obtained while the person is febrile, particularly during initial febrile episodes; organisms are less likely to be recovered from subsequent relapses. Direct detection by polymerase chain reaction (PCR) is available at some commercial and reference laboratories. Spirochetes can be cultured in specialized media from blood obtained before treatment. Serum antibodies to *Borrelia* species can be detected by enzyme immunoassay and Western immunoblot analysis at some reference and commercial specialty laboratories. Serum tested early in infection may be negative, so it is important to also obtain a serum sample for serologic testing during the convalescent period (at least 21 days after symptom onset); development of an immunoglobulin (Ig) G response in the convalescent sample is supportive of a tickborne relapsing fever diagnosis. Early antibiotic treatment may limit the antibody response. Antibody tests are not standardized and are affected by antigenic variations among and within *Borrelia* species and strains. Serologic cross-reactions can occur with other spirochetes, including *B burgdorferi, Treponema pallidum,* and *Leptospira* species. For inquiries about laboratory testing at the Centers for Disease Control and Prevention, visit **www.cdc.gov/laboratory/specimen-submission/ list.html.**

Serologic tests for *B miyamotoi* are under development and not widely available commercially but may be ordered from a limited number of laboratories approved under the Clinical Laboratory Improvement Amendments (CLIA).

TREATMENT: Treatment of tickborne relapsing fever with a 5- to 10-day course of doxycycline produces prompt clearance of spirochetes and remission of symptoms; doxycycline can be used regardless of patient age (see Tetracyclines, p 866). For pregnant women, penicillin and erythromycin are the preferred drugs. Penicillin G procaine or intravenous penicillin G is recommended as initial therapy for people who cannot tolerate oral therapy, although low-dose penicillin G has been associated with a higher frequency of relapse. A Jarisch-Herxheimer reaction (an acute febrile reaction accompanied by headache, myalgia, respiratory distress in some cases, and an aggravated clinical picture lasting less than 24 hours) commonly is observed during the first few hours after initiating antimicrobial therapy. Because this reaction sometimes is associated with transient hypotension attributable to decreased effective circulating blood volume (especially in louseborne relapsing fever), patients should be hospitalized and monitored closely, particularly during the first 4 hours of treatment. The Jarisch-Herxheimer reaction in children may be milder and typically can be managed with antipyretic agents alone.

Physicians have treated patients infected with *B miyamotoi* successfully with a 2- to 4-week course of doxycycline. Amoxicillin and ceftriaxone also have been used.

For louseborne relapsing fever, single-dose treatment using doxycycline, penicillin, or erythromycin is effective.

ISOLATION OF THE HOSPITALIZED PATIENT: Standard precautions are recommended. If louse infestation is present, contact precautions are indicated until delousing (see Pediculosis, p 567–574).

CONTROL MEASURES: Soft ticks often can be found in rodent nests; exposure is reduced most effectively by preventing rodent infestations of homes or cabins by blocking rodent access to foundations and attics and using other forms of rodent control. Dwellings infested with soft ticks should be rodent proofed and treated professionally with chemical agents. When in a louse-infested environment, body lice can be controlled by bathing, washing clothing at frequent intervals, and use of pediculicides (see Pediculosis, p 567–574). Reporting of suspected cases of relapsing fever to health authorities is required in most western states and is important for initiation of prompt investigation and institution of control measures.

Brucellosis

CLINICAL MANIFESTATIONS: Onset of brucellosis in children can be acute or insidious. Manifestations are nonspecific and include fever, night sweats, weakness, malaise, anorexia, weight loss, arthralgia, myalgia, back pain, abdominal pain, and headache. Physical findings may include lymphadenopathy, hepatosplenomegaly, and arthritis. Abdominal pain and peripheral arthritis are reported more frequently in children than in adults. Neurologic deficits, ocular involvement, epididymo-orchitis, and liver or spleen abscesses are reported. Anemia, leukopenia, thrombocytopenia, or less frequently, pancytopenia and hemophagocytosis are hematologic findings that might suggest the diagnosis. Serious complications include meningitis, endocarditis, spondylitis, osteomyelitis, and less frequently, pneumonitis and aortic involvement. A detailed history including travel, exposure to animals, and food habits, including ingestion of unpasteurized milk or cheese, and occupational history should be obtained if brucellosis is considered. Chronic disease is less common among children than among adults, although the rate of relapse has been found to be similar. Brucellosis in pregnancy is associated with risk of spontaneous abortion, preterm delivery, miscarriage, and intrauterine infection with fetal death.

ETIOLOGY: *Brucella* bacteria are small, nonmotile, gram-negative coccobacilli. The species that are commonly known to infect humans are *Brucella abortus*, *Brucella melitensis*, *Brucella suis*, and rarely, *Brucella canis*. However, human infections with *Brucella ceti*, *Brucella pinnipedialis*, *Brucella inopinata*, and *Brucella neotomae* also have been identified. *B abortus* strain RB51 is a live attenuated cattle vaccine strain that can be shed in milk and can cause infections in humans.

EPIDEMIOLOGY: Brucellosis is a zoonotic disease of wild and domestic animals. It is transmissible to humans by direct or indirect exposure to aborted fetuses or to tissues or fluids of infected animals. Transmission occurs by inoculation through mucous membranes or cuts and abrasions in the skin, inhalation of contaminated aerosols, or ingestion of unpasteurized dairy products.[1] People in occupations such as farming, ranching, and veterinary medicine, as well as abattoir workers, meat inspectors, and laboratory personnel, are at increased risk. Clinicians should alert the laboratory if they anticipate *Brucella* organisms might grow from microbiologic specimens so that appropriate laboratory precautions can be taken. In the United States, approximately 100 to 120 cases of brucellosis are reported annually, and 3% to 10% of cases occur in people younger than 19 years. The majority of pediatric cases reported in the United States result from ingestion of unpasteurized dairy products, commonly acquired from outside the United States. Human-to-human transmission is rare. Mother-to-child transmission is possible by transplacental transmission or via human milk. Other less common modes of transmission include blood transfusion, hematopoietic stem cell transplant, and sexual transmission.

The **incubation period** varies from 5 days to 6 months, but most people become ill within 2 to 4 weeks of exposure.

DIAGNOSTIC TESTS: A definitive diagnosis is established by recovery of *Brucella* species from blood, bone marrow, or other tissue specimens. A variety of media will support growth of *Brucella* species, but the physician should contact laboratory personnel and

---

[1] American Academy of Pediatrics, Committee on Infectious Diseases, Committee on Nutrition. Consumption of raw or unpasteurized milk and milk products by pregnant women and children. *Pediatrics*. 2014;133(1):175-179 (Reaffirmed November 2019)

ask that cultures be incubated for a minimum of 14 days. Newer BACTEC systems have greater reliability and can detect *Brucella* species within 7 days with no need to prolong incubation. Caution should be taken with isolation of this organism because of the high risk of laboratory-acquired infection.

In patients with a clinically compatible illness, serologic testing using the serum agglutination test can confirm the diagnosis with a fourfold or greater increase in antibody titers between acute and convalescent phase serum specimens collected at least 2 weeks apart. The serum agglutination test, the gold standard test for serologic diagnosis, will detect antibodies against *B abortus, B suis,* and *B melitensis* but not *B canis* or *B abortus* strain RB51. Although a single titer is not diagnostic, most patients with active infection in an area where brucellosis is not endemic will have a titer of 1:160 or greater within 2 to 4 weeks of clinical disease onset. Lower titers may be found early in the course of infection. Enzyme immunoassay is a sensitive method for determining total or specific immunoglobulin (Ig) G, IgA, and IgM anti-*Brucella* antibody titers. Until better standardization is established, enzyme immunoassay should be used only for suspected cases with negative serum agglutination test results or for evaluation of patients with suspected chronic brucellosis, reinfection, or complicated cases.

When interpreting serologic results, it is important to take into consideration exposure history, because a serologic response for *B canis* and *B abortus* strain RB51 will not be detected by commercially available tests. *Brucella* antibodies also cross-react with antibodies against other gram-negative bacteria, such as *Yersinia enterocolitica* serotype 09, *Francisella tularensis, Escherichia coli* O116 and O157, *Salmonella urbana, Vibrio cholerae, Xanthomonas maltophilia,* and *Afipia clevelandensis.* The timing of exposure and symptom development will assist in determining the classes of antibodies expected. IgM antibodies are produced within the first week, followed by a gradual increase in IgG synthesis. Low IgM titers may persist for months or years after initial infection. Increased concentrations of IgG agglutinins are found in acute infection, chronic infection, and relapse.

Polymerase chain reaction tests that can be performed in blood and body tissue samples have been developed but are not yet available in most clinical laboratories, as improved standardization and better understanding of their clinical applicability are needed. If a laboratory is not available to perform diagnostic testing for *Brucella* species, the physician should contact the local or state health department for assistance.

TREATMENT: Prolonged antimicrobial therapy is imperative for achieving a cure. Relapses generally are not associated with development of *Brucella* resistance but rather with premature discontinuation of therapy, localized infection, or monotherapy. Because monotherapy is associated with a high rate of relapse, combination therapy is recommended as standard treatment. Most combination regimens include oral doxycycline or trimethoprim-sulfamethoxazole plus rifampin.

Oral doxycycline is the drug of choice and should be administered for a minimum of 6 weeks. Because of this prolonged duration of therapy, doxycycline is not recommended for children younger than 8 years (see Tetracyclines, p 866); these younger children (under 8 years) should receive oral trimethoprim-sulfamethoxazole for at least 6 weeks. Rifampin should be added to doxycycline or trimethoprim-sulfamethoxazole. See Table 4.3 (p 882) for antibiotic dosages. Failure to complete the full 6-week course of therapy may result in relapse.

For treatment of serious infections or complications, including endocarditis, meningitis, spondylitis, and osteomyelitis, a 3-drug regimen should be used, with gentamicin included for the first 7 to 14 days of therapy, in addition to doxycycline (or trimethoprim-sulfamethoxazole, if doxycycline is not used) and rifampin for a minimum of 6 weeks. For life-threatening complications of brucellosis, such as meningitis or endocarditis, the duration of therapy often is extended for 4 to 6 months. Surgical intervention should be considered in patients with complications, such as deep tissue abscesses, endocarditis, mycotic aneurysm, and foreign body infections.

Because of antibiotic resistance with *B abortus* strain RB51, rifampin and penicillin should not be used for treatment of infection caused by this cattle vaccine strain (see Control Measures).

The benefit of corticosteroids for people with neurobrucellosis is unproven. Occasionally, a Jarisch-Herxheimer-like reaction (an acute febrile reaction accompanied by headache, myalgia, and an aggravated clinical picture lasting less than 24 hours) occurs shortly after initiation of antimicrobial therapy, but this reaction rarely is severe enough to require corticosteroids.

ISOLATION OF THE HOSPITALIZED PATIENT: In addition to standard precautions, contact precautions are indicated for patients with draining wounds. If aerosol-generating procedures are performed, respiratory protection (eg, use of N95 respirators) also is indicated.

CONTROL MEASURES: The control of human brucellosis depends on control of transmission of *Brucella* species from cattle, goats, swine, and other animals. Vaccination of cattle, sheep, and goats can be effective but needs to be sustained over several years. Contact with infected animals should be avoided, especially female animals that have aborted or are giving birth.

Mothers with active brucellosis should not breastfeed their infants until their infection is cleared. Breastfeeding infants of mothers diagnosed with brucellosis should be closely monitored for evidence of infection. Pasteurization of dairy products for human consumption is important in preventing disease. The certification of unpasteurized milk does not eliminate the risk of transmission of *Brucella* organisms.

People who have consumed raw milk or raw milk products that are potentially contaminated with the live attenuated cattle vaccine strain *B abortus* strain RB51 are at high risk for brucellosis. For these people, postexposure prophylaxis (PEP) with doxycycline plus trimethoprim-sulfamethoxazole is recommended for 21 days, in addition to symptom monitoring for 6 months following the last exposure. Because of antibiotic resistance with *B abortus* strain RB51, rifampin and penicillin should not be used (see **https://emergency.cdc.gov/han/han00417.asp**).

Burkholderia Infections

CLINICAL MANIFESTATIONS: Species within the *Burkholderia cepacia* complex have been primarily associated with infections in individuals with cystic fibrosis (CF) or chronic granulomatous disease (CGD). Infections have also been reported in people with hemoglobinopathies and malignant neoplasms and in preterm infants. Airway infections of *B cepacia* in people with cystic fibrosis usually occur later in the course of disease, after respiratory epithelial damage and bronchiectasis have occurred. Patients with cystic fibrosis can become chronically infected with little change in the rate of pulmonary decompensation, or can experience an accelerated decline in pulmonary function or an unexpectedly rapid deterioration in clinical status that results in death. In patients with chronic granulomatous disease, pneumonia is the most common manifestation of *B cepacia* complex infection; lymphadenitis also occurs. Disease onset is insidious, with low-grade fever early in the course and systemic effects occurring 3 to 4 weeks later. Pleural effusions are common, and lung abscesses can occur. Health care-associated infections including wound and urinary tract infections and pneumonia have been reported, and clusters of disease have been associated with contaminated pharmaceutical products, including nasal sprays, mouthwash, sublingual probes, prefilled saline flush syringes, and oral docusate sodium.

Burkholderia pseudomallei is the cause of melioidosis. Its geographic range is expanding, and disease now is known to be endemic in Southeast Asia, northern Australia, areas of the Indian Subcontinent, southern China, Hong Kong, Taiwan, several Pacific and Indian Ocean Islands, and some areas of South and Central America. Melioidosis can occur in patients in the United States, usually among travelers returning from areas with endemic disease. Melioidosis can be asymptomatic or can manifest as a localized infection or as fulminant septicemia with or without pneumonia. Approximately 50% of adults with melioidosis are bacteremic on admission to hospital; bacteremia is less common in children. Pneumonia is the most commonly reported clinical manifestation of melioidosis in adults. Localized cutaneous disease is the most common presentation in immunocompetent children. Genitourinary infections including prostatic abscesses, septic arthritis and osteomyelitis, and central nervous system involvement, including brain abscesses, also occur. Acute suppurative parotitis is a manifestation that occurs frequently in children in Thailand and Cambodia but is less commonly seen in other areas with endemic infection. In severe cutaneous infection, necrotizing fasciitis has been reported. In disseminated infection, hepatic and splenic abscesses can occur, as can disseminated cutaneous abscesses, and relapses are common without prolonged therapy.

ETIOLOGY: The Burkholderia genus comprises more than 115 diverse species that are oxidase- and catalase-producing, non–lactose-fermenting, gram-negative bacilli. B cepacia complex comprises at least 22 species. Additional members of the complex continue to be identified but are rare human pathogens. Other clinically important species of Burkholderia include B pseudomallei, Burkholderia mallei (the agent responsible for glanders), Burkholderia gladioli, Burkholderia thailandensis, and Burkholderia oklahomensis.

EPIDEMIOLOGY: Burkholderia species are environmentally derived waterborne and soilborne organisms that can survive for prolonged periods in a moist environment. Depending on the species, transmission may occur from other people (person to person), from contact with contaminated fomites, and from exposure to environmental sources. Epidemiologic studies of recreational camps and social events attended by people with cystic fibrosis from different geographic areas have documented person-to-person spread of B cepacia complex. The source of acquisition of B cepacia complex by patients with chronic granulomatous disease has not been clearly identified, although environmental sources seem likely. B cepacia complex can persist in the environment and spread through lapses in infection control, including indirect contact via environmental surfaces. Health care-associated spread of B cepacia complex has been associated with contamination of disinfectant solutions used to clean reusable patient equipment, such as bronchoscopes and pressure transducers, or to disinfect skin. Its intrinsic resistance to preservatives enables it to contaminate many types of aqueous medical and personal care products leading to large outbreaks. Contaminated mouthwash, liquid docusate sodium, and inhaled medications have been identified as causes of multistate outbreaks of colonization and infection. B gladioli also is isolated from sputum of people with cystic fibrosis and may be mistaken for B cepacia. B gladioli may be associated with transient or more prolonged, chronic infection in patients with cystic fibrosis; poor outcomes have been noted in lung transplant recipients who have *B gladioli* infection.

In areas of high endemicity, children may be exposed to *B pseudomallei* early in life, with the highest seroconversion rates occurring between 6 months and 4 years of age. Melioidosis is seasonal in countries with endemic infection, with more than 75% of cases occurring during the rainy season. Disease can be acquired by direct inhalation of aerosolized organisms or dust particles containing organisms, by percutaneous or wound inoculation with contaminated soil or water, or by ingestion of contaminated soil, water, or food. People also can become infected as a result of laboratory exposures when proper techniques and/or proper personal protective equipment guidelines are not followed. Symptomatic infection can occur in children 1 year or younger, with pneumonia and parotitis reported in infants as young as 8 months; in addition, 2 cases of human milk transmission from mothers with mastitis have been reported. Risk factors for melioidosis include frequent contact with soil and water as well as underlying chronic disease, such as diabetes mellitus, renal insufficiency, chronic pulmonary disease, thalassemia, and immunosuppression not related to human immunodeficiency virus (HIV) infection. *B pseudomallei* also has been reported to cause pulmonary infection in people with cystic fibrosis and septicemia in children with chronic granulomatous disease.

The **incubation period** for melioidosis is 1 to 21 days, with a median of 9 days, but can be prolonged (years).

DIAGNOSTIC TESTS: Culture is the appropriate method to diagnose *B cepacia* complex infection. In cystic fibrosis airway infection, culture of sputum on selective agar is recommended to decrease the potential for overgrowth by mucoid *Pseudomonas aeruginosa*. Confirmation of identification of *B cepacia* complex species by mass spectrometry or by polymerase chain reaction assay is recommended.

Definitive diagnosis of melioidosis is made by isolation of *B pseudomallei* from blood or other specimens. The likelihood of successfully isolating the organism is increased by culture of sputum, throat, rectum, and ulcer or skin lesion specimens, in addition to blood. Serologic testing is not adequate for diagnosis in areas with endemic infection because of high background seropositivity. However, a positive result by the indirect hemagglutination assay for a traveler who has returned from an area with endemic infection may support the diagnosis of melioidosis; definitive diagnosis still requires isolation of *B pseudomallei* from blood or other specimens. Other rapid assays are being developed for diagnosis of melioidosis but are not yet commercially available.

Suspected isolates of *B mallei* and *B pseudomallei* should be referred to local or state Public Health Laboratory Response Network Laboratories. If laboratory personnel are suspected to have been exposed to these pathogens while conducting initial diagnostic testing, occupational exposure in the original clinical laboratory should be reviewed and evaluated.

TREATMENT: Drugs that may have activity against *B cepacia* complex include trimethoprim-sulfamethoxazole, ceftazidime, minocycline, fluoroquinolones, carbapenems, and newer beta-lactam/beta-lactamase inhibitor combinations. Some experts recommend combinations of antimicrobial agents that provide synergistic activity against *B cepacia* complex in vitro. The majority of *B cepacia* complex isolates are intrinsically resistant to aminoglycosides and polymyxins and are resistant to many beta lactam agents such as penicillin, ampicillin, carboxypenicillins, and first- and second-generation cephalosporins.

The drugs of choice for initial treatment of melioidosis depend on the type of clinical infection, susceptibility testing, and presence of comorbidities in the patient (eg, diabetes mellitus, liver or renal disease, cancer, hemoglobinopathies, cystic fibrosis). Treatment of severe invasive infection should include meropenem or ceftazidime (rare resistance) for a minimum of 10 to 14 days, with prolonged therapy (>4 weeks) for deep-seated and complicated infections. After acute therapy is completed, oral eradication therapy with trimethoprim-sulfamethoxazole for 3 to 6 months is recommended to reduce recurrence. Amoxicillin clavulanate is considered a second-line oral agent and may be associated with a higher rate of relapse.

ISOLATION OF THE HOSPITALIZED PATIENT: The Cystic Fibrosis Foundation recommends implementation of contact precautions in addition to standard precautions for care of all patients with cystic fibrosis in inpatient or ambulatory care settings, regardless of respiratory tract cultures. Human-to-human transmission is extremely rare for *B pseudomallei*, and standard precautions are recommended.

CONTROL MEASURES: Because some strains of *B cepacia* complex cause a highly virulent course in some patients with new acquisition, the Cystic Fibrosis Foundation recommends that all cystic fibrosis care centers limit contact between patients. This includes inpatient, outpatient, and social settings. When in a health care setting, patients with cystic fibrosis should wear a mask while outside of a clinic examination room or a hospital room. Education of patients and families about hand hygiene and appropriate personal hygiene is recommended.

Prevention of infection with *B pseudomallei* in areas with endemic disease can be difficult because contact with contaminated water and soil is common. People with diabetes mellitus, renal insufficiency, or general immunocompromising conditions should avoid contact with soil and standing water in areas suspected to be contaminated. Wearing boots and gloves during agricultural work in areas with endemic disease and thorough cleaning and protecting of skin wounds is recommended. Patients with cystic fibrosis and diabetes should be educated regarding their risk of infection when traveling to regions where *B pseudomallei* is endemic. A human vaccine is not available, but research is ongoing. Cases of melioidosis are notifiable in many states, and reporting cases to local or state health departments is prudent.

Campylobacter Infections

CLINICAL MANIFESTATIONS: Predominant symptoms of *Campylobacter* infection include diarrhea, abdominal pain, malaise, and fever. Stools can contain visible or occult blood. In neonates and young infants, bloody diarrhea without fever can be the only manifestation of infection. Pronounced fevers in children can result in febrile seizures that can occur before gastrointestinal tract symptoms. Abdominal pain can mimic appendicitis or intussusception. Mild infection lasts 1 or 2 days and resembles viral gastroenteritis. Most patients recover in less than 1 week, but 10% to 20% have a relapse or a prolonged or severe illness. Severe or persistent infection can mimic acute inflammatory bowel disease. Bacteremia is uncommon but can occur in elderly patients and in patients with underlying conditions. Immunocompromised hosts can have prolonged, relapsing, or extraintestinal infections, especially with *Campylobacter fetus* and other *Campylobacter* species. Immunoreactive complications, such as Guillain-Barré syndrome (occurring in 1:1000), Miller Fisher variant of Guillain-Barré syndrome (ophthalmoplegia, areflexia, ataxia), reactive arthritis (with the classic triad, formerly known as Reiter syndrome, consisting of arthritis, urethritis, and bilateral conjunctivitis), myocarditis, pericarditis, and erythema nodosum, can occur during convalescence.

ETIOLOGY: *Campylobacter* species are motile, comma-shaped, gram-negative bacilli that cause gastroenteritis. There are 25 species within the genus *Campylobacter*, but *Campylobacter jejuni* and *Campylobacter coli* are the species isolated most commonly from patients with diarrhea. *C fetus* predominantly causes systemic illness in neonates and debilitated hosts. Other *Campylobacter* species, including *Campylobacter upsaliensis*, *Campylobacter lari*, and *Campylobacter hyointestinalis*, can cause similar diarrheal or systemic illnesses in children.

EPIDEMIOLOGY: *Campylobacter* is associated with an estimated 1.3 million illnesses each year in the United States. Although incidence decreased in the early 2000s, data from the Foodborne Diseases Active Surveillance Network indicate that in recent years the incidence has increased and the 2018 incidence of infections with *Campylobacter* was 19.6 infections per 100 000 population.[1] This increased incidence likely resulted from the increased use and sensitivity of culture-independent diagnostic tests (CIDTs). The highest rates of infection occur in children younger than 5 years. The majority of *Campylobacter* infections are acquired domestically, but it is also a very common cause of laboratory-confirmed diarrhea in returning international travelers. In susceptible people, as few as 500 *Campylobacter* organisms can cause infection.

The gastrointestinal tracts of domestic and wild birds and animals are reservoirs of the bacteria. *C jejuni* and *C coli* have been isolated from feces of 30% to 100% of healthy chickens, turkeys, and waterfowl. Poultry carcasses commonly are contaminated. Many farm animals, pets, and meat sources can harbor the organism and are potential sources of infection. Transmission of *C jejuni* and *C coli* occurs by ingestion of contaminated food or water or by direct contact with fecal material from infected animals or people. Improperly cooked poultry, untreated or contaminated water, and unpasteurized milk have been the main vehicles of transmission. *Campylobacter* infections usually are sporadic; outbreaks are rare but have occurred among school children participants in field trips to dairy farms where they consumed unpasteurized milk, and among people who had contact with pet store puppies (**www.cdc.gov/campylobacter/outbreaks/outbreaks. html**). Person-to-person spread occurs occasionally, particularly among very young children, and risk is greatest during the acute phase of illness. Person-to-person transmission has occurred in neonates of infected mothers and has resulted in health care-associated outbreaks in nurseries. In perinatal infection, *C jejuni* and *C coli* usually cause neonatal gastroenteritis, whereas *C fetus* often causes neonatal septicemia or meningitis. Enteritis occurs in people of all ages. Excretion of *Campylobacter* organisms typically lasts 2 to 3 weeks without antimicrobial treatment but can be as long as 7 weeks.

The **incubation period** usually is 2 to 5 days but can be longer.

DIAGNOSTIC TESTS: *C jejuni* and *C coli* can be recovered from feces, and *Campylobacter* species, including *C fetus*, can be recovered from blood. Isolation of *C jejuni* and *C coli* from stool specimens requires selective media, microaerobic conditions, and an incubation temperature of 42°C. Additional methods may be necessary to isolate other species of *Campylobacter*, such as hydrogen-rich microaerobic conditions and filter plating on

---

[1]Centers for Disease Control and Prevention. Preliminary incidence and trends of infections with pathogens transmitted commonly through food—Foodborne Diseases Active Surveillance Network, 10 U.S. sites, 2015–2018. *MMWR Morb Mortal Wkly Rep.* 2019;68(16):369-373

media not containing antibiotic supplements. Notably, not all clinical laboratories identify *Campylobacter* to the species level; clinicians can consult state public health laboratories for further identification. Molecular and antigen CIDTs can provide rapid diagnostic testing; however, these tests will not provide antibiotic susceptibilities. It should be noted that false-positive results from antigen-based tests have been reported, and molecular tests detect bacterial DNA, which may not reflect viable organism; therefore, clinical correlation is advised. Additionally, some of these tests may not distinguish between *C jejuni* and *C coli* and may not detect other *Campylobacter* species. Referral of isolates and CIDT positive specimens to state public health laboratories is based on state regulations. Molecular analysis of isolates is important for national *Campylobacter* surveillance and outbreak monitoring.

TREATMENT: Rehydration is the mainstay of treatment for all children with diarrhea. Most patients do not require antimicrobial therapy. Azithromycin and erythromycin shorten the duration of illness and excretion of susceptible organisms (2% of *C jejuni* isolates are resistant to erythromycin and azithromycin, and 17% and 18% of *C coli* are resistant to erythromycin and azithromycin, respectively) and may prevent relapse when administered early in gastrointestinal tract infection. Treatment with azithromycin (10 mg/kg/day, for 3 days) or erythromycin (40 mg/kg/day, in 4 divided doses, for 5 days) usually eradicates the organism from stool within 2 or 3 days. A fluoroquinolone, such as ciprofloxacin, may be effective, but resistance to ciprofloxacin is common (found in 28% of isolates in 2017 [**www.cdc.gov/DrugResistance/Biggest-Threats.html**]; see also **www.cdc.gov/NARMS** and Fluoroquinolones, p 864). Resistance to fluoroquinolones is more common in low- to middle-income countries. Antimicrobial susceptibility testing of the isolate or epidemiologic data from the location of acquisition can help guide appropriate therapy. If antimicrobial therapy is administered for treatment of gastroenteritis, the recommended duration is 3 to 5 days. *C fetus* generally is susceptible to aminoglycosides, extended-spectrum cephalosporins, meropenem, imipenem, ampicillin, and erythromycin. Antimotility agents are generally not recommended in children because of their limited benefit and reports of adverse outcomes in those who received these agents as monotherapy.

ISOLATION OF THE HOSPITALIZED PATIENT: In addition to standard precautions, contact precautions are recommended for diapered and incontinent children for the duration of illness.

CONTROL MEASURES:

- Hand hygiene should be performed after handling raw poultry and cutting boards, and utensils should be washed with soap and hot water after contact with raw poultry. Food preparation areas and cutting boards used for raw poultry should be separate from all other foods, especially fruits and vegetables.
- Poultry should be cooked thoroughly.
- Hand hygiene should be performed after contact with feces of dogs, cats, and farm animals.
- People should not drink raw milk.[1] The certification of raw milk does not eliminate the risk of transmission of *Campylobacter* organisms.

---

[1] American Academy of Pediatrics, Committee on Infectious Diseases, Committee on Nutrition. Consumption of raw or unpasteurized milk and milk products by pregnant women and children. *Pediatrics*. 2014;133(1):175-179 (Reaffirmed November 2019)

- Chlorination of water supplies is important.
- People with diarrhea should be excluded from food handling, care of patients in hospitals, and care of people in custodial care and child care centers.
- Infected food handlers and hospital employees who are asymptomatic need not be excluded from work if proper personal hygiene measures, including hand hygiene, are maintained.
- People with diarrhea should not go into recreational water (see Prevention of Illnesses Associated With Recreational Water, p 180). Incontinent children should abstain from recreational water for 1 week after resolution of symptoms (or as advised by local public health authorities).
- Outbreaks of campylobacteriosis are uncommon in child care centers. General measures for interrupting enteric transmission in child care centers are recommended (see Children in Group Child Care and Schools, p 116). Infants and children should be excluded from child care centers until stools are contained in the diaper or when continent children no longer have fecal accidents and when stool frequency becomes no more than 2 stools above that child's normal frequency for the time the child is in the program, even if the stools remain loose. Although antibiotics are not generally recommended in most cases, azithromycin or erythromycin treatment may reduce the potential for person-person transmission.
- Diagnostic testing of asymptomatic exposed children is not recommended.
- Campylobacteriosis is a nationally notifiable condition and should be reported to the local or state health department.

Candidiasis

CLINICAL MANIFESTATIONS: Mucocutaneous infection results in oral-pharyngeal (thrush) or vaginal or cervical candidiasis; intertriginous lesions of the gluteal folds, buttocks, neck, groin, and axilla; paronychia; and onychia. Dysfunction of T lymphocytes, other immunologic disorders, and endocrinologic diseases are associated with chronic mucocutaneous candidiasis. Chronic or recurrent oral candidiasis can be the presenting sign of human immunodeficiency virus (HIV) infection or primary immunodeficiency. Esophageal and laryngeal candidiasis can occur in immunocompromised patients. Disseminated candidiasis has a predilection for extremely preterm neonates and immunocompromised or debilitated hosts, can involve virtually any organ or anatomic site, and can be rapidly fatal. Candidemia can occur with or without associated end-organ disease in patients with indwelling central vascular catheters, especially in patients receiving prolonged intravenous infusions with parenteral alimentation or lipids. Peritonitis can occur in patients undergoing peritoneal dialysis, especially in patients receiving prolonged broad-spectrum antimicrobial therapy. Candiduria can occur in patients with indwelling urinary catheters, focal renal infection, or disseminated disease.

ETIOLOGY: *Candida* species are yeasts that reproduce by budding. *Candida albicans* and several other species form long chains of elongated yeast forms called pseudohyphae. *C albicans* causes most infections, but in some regions and patient populations, non-*albicans Candida* species now account for more than half of invasive infections. Other species, including *Candida tropicalis, Candida parapsilosis, Candida glabrata, Candida krusei, Candida guilliermondii, Candida lusitaniae,* and *Candida dubliniensis,* can cause serious infections, especially in immunocompromised and debilitated hosts. *C parapsilosis* is second only to *C albicans* as a cause of systemic candidiasis in pediatric and neonatal populations. *Candida auris*, a *Candida* species that is often multidrug resistant, is found virtually always in immunocompromised hosts or those requiring high acuity care. It generally is acquired in health care settings, especially high acuity postacute care settings such as long-term acute care hospitals and skilled nursing facilities that provide care for patients on ventilators.

EPIDEMIOLOGY: Like other *Candida* species, *C albicans* is present on skin and in the mouth, intestinal tract, and vagina of immunocompetent people. Vulvovaginal candidiasis is associated with pregnancy, and newborn infants can acquire the organism in utero, during passage through the vagina, or postnatally. Mild mucocutaneous infection is common in healthy infants. Person-to-person transmission occurs rarely for most *Candida* species but is common for *C auris*. Invasive disease typically occurs in those with impaired immunity, with infection usually arising endogenously from colonized sites. Factors such as extreme prematurity, neutropenia, or treatment with corticosteroids or cytotoxic chemotherapy increase the risk of invasive infection. People with diabetes mellitus generally have localized mucocutaneous lesions. People with neutrophil defects, such as chronic granulomatous disease or myeloperoxidase deficiency, are at increased risk. People undergoing intravenous alimentation or receiving broad-spectrum antimicrobial agents, especially extended-spectrum cephalosporins, carbapenems, and vancomycin, or requiring long-term indwelling central venous or peritoneal dialysis catheters, have increased susceptibility to infection. Postsurgical patients can be at risk, particularly after cardiothoracic or abdominal procedures.

The **incubation period** is unknown.

DIAGNOSTIC TESTS: Presumptive diagnosis of mucocutaneous candidiasis or thrush usually can be made clinically, but other organisms or trauma can cause clinically similar lesions. Yeast cells and pseudohyphae can be found in *C albicans*-infected tissue and are identifiable by microscopic examination of scrapings prepared with Gram, calcofluor white, or fluorescent antibody stains or in a 10% to 20% potassium hydroxide suspension. Endoscopy is useful for diagnosis of esophagitis. Although ophthalmologic examination can reveal typical retinal lesions attributable to hematogenous dissemination, the yield of routine ophthalmologic evaluation in affected patients is low. Lesions in the brain, kidney, liver, heart, or spleen can be detected by ultrasonography, computed tomography (CT), or magnetic resonance imaging, but these lesions typically are not detected by imaging until late in the course of disease or after neutropenia has resolved.

A definitive diagnosis of invasive candidiasis requires isolation of the organism from a normally sterile body site (eg, blood, cerebrospinal fluid, bone marrow) or demonstration of organisms in a tissue biopsy specimen. Negative results of culture for *Candida* species do not exclude invasive infection in immunocompromised hosts; in some settings, blood culture is <50% sensitive. Special fungal culture media are not needed to grow *Candida* species. A presumptive species identification of *C albicans* can be made by demonstrating germ tube formation, and molecular fluorescence in situ hybridization testing rapidly can distinguish *C albicans* from non-*albicans Candida* species. *C auris* may be misidentified as another *Candida* species. Recovery of the organism is expedited using automated blood culture systems or a lysis-centrifugation method. Peptide nucleic acid fluorescent in situ hybridization (PNA FISH) probes cleared by the US Food and Drug Administration (FDA) and multiplex polymerase chain reaction (PCR) assays have been developed for rapid detection of *Candida* species directly from positive blood culture bottles.

Patient serum can be tested using the assay for (1,3)-beta-D-glucan from fungal cell walls, which does not distinguish *Candida* species from other fungi. Data on use of this assay for children are more limited than for adult patients, and there are a significant number of false-positive results. The diagnostic cut-point for this assay is not well established in children. A molecular assay (T2Candida) cleared by the FDA uses magnetic resonance technology to identify 5 different *Candida* species, but data on this assay are very limited in children.

Testing for azole susceptibility is recommended for all bloodstream and other clinically relevant *Candida* isolates. Testing for echinocandin susceptibility should be considered in patients who have had prior treatment with an echinocandin and among those who have infection with *C glabrata, C parapsilosis,* or confirmed or suspected *C auris.*

TREATMENT[1]:

Mucous Membrane and Skin Infections. Oral candidiasis in immunocompetent hosts is treated with oral nystatin suspension, clotrimazole troches applied to lesions, or miconazole mucoadhesive buccal tablets. Troches should not be used in infants. Fluconazole may be more effective than oral nystatin or clotrimazole troches and may be considered if other treatments fail. Fluconazole can be beneficial for immunocompromised patients with oropharyngeal candidiasis. For fluconazole-refractory disease, itraconazole, voriconazole, posaconazole, amphotericin B deoxycholate oral suspension, or intravenous echinocandins (caspofungin, micafungin) are alternatives.

Esophagitis caused by *Candida* species generally is treated with oral fluconazole. Intravenous fluconazole, an echinocandin, or amphotericin B should be used for patients who cannot tolerate oral therapy. For disease refractory to fluconazole, itraconazole solution, voriconazole, posaconazole, or an echinocandin is recommended. The recommended duration of therapy is 14 to 21 days but depends on severity of illness and patient factors, such as age and degree of immunocompromise. Changing from intravenous to oral therapy with fluconazole is recommended when the patient is able to tolerate oral intake. Suppressive therapy with fluconazole (3 times weekly) is recommended for recurrent infections.

Skin infections are treated with topical nystatin, miconazole, clotrimazole, naftifine, ketoconazole, econazole, or ciclopirox (see Topical Drugs for Superficial Fungal Infections, p 922). Nystatin usually is effective and is the least expensive of these drugs.

Vulvovaginal candidiasis is treated effectively with many topical formulations, including clotrimazole or miconazole (available over the counter). Such topically applied azole drugs are more effective than nystatin. Oral azole agents also are effective and should be considered for recurrent or refractory cases (see Recommended Doses of Parenteral and Oral Antifungal Drugs, p 913). Azole treatment of *C glabrata* vulvovaginal candidiasis is not effective; nystatin intravaginal suppositories have been effective.

Nipple and ductal breast infections with candidiasis have been described in breast-feeding mothers. Topical treatment as above may be adequate for nipple infection, but systemic treatment with fluconazole is often used in breast infections, with continuation of breastfeeding.

For chronic mucocutaneous candidiasis, fluconazole, itraconazole, and voriconazole are effective drugs. Low-dose amphotericin B administered intravenously is effective in

[1]Pappas PG, Kauffman CA, Andes DR, et al. Clinical practice guideline for the management of candidiasis: 2016 update by the Infectious Diseases Society of America. *Clin Infect Dis.* 2016;62(4):e1-e50

severe cases. Relapses are common with any of these agents once therapy is terminated, and treatment should be viewed as a lifelong process that generally requires intermittent pulses of antifungal agents. Invasive infections in patients with this condition are rare.

For management of asymptomatic candiduria, elimination of predisposing factors, such as indwelling bladder catheters, is strongly recommended. Antifungal treatment is not recommended unless patients are at high risk of candidemia, such as neutropenic patients and preterm infants. If candiduria occurs in a preterm infant, evaluation should be performed (blood cultures, cerebrospinal fluid evaluation, ophthalmologic examination, brain imaging, and abdominal ultrasonography) and treatment should be initiated. For patients with symptomatic *Candida* cystitis, elimination of predisposing factors, such as indwelling bladder catheters, is strongly recommended, in addition to use of fluconazole for 2 weeks. Repeated bladder irrigations with amphotericin B (50 µg/mL of sterile water) have been used to treat patients with candidal cystitis, but this procedure does not treat disease beyond the bladder and is not recommended routinely. Urinary catheters, if not able to be removed, should be replaced promptly in patients with candidiasis. Echinocandins have poor urinary concentration.

Keratomycosis is treated with corneal baths of voriconazole (1%) and always in conjunction with systemic therapy. Vision-threatening infections (near the macula or into the vitreous) require intravitreal injection of antifungal agents, usually amphotericin B or voriconazole, with or without vitrectomy, in addition to systemic antifungal agents.

Invasive Disease

General Recommendations. Most *Candida* species are susceptible to amphotericin B, although *C lusitaniae, C auris,* and some strains of *C glabrata* and *C krusei* exhibit decreased susceptibility or resistance (see Table 4.7, p 909). *C auris* is often drug resistant, and echinocandins should be used as initial therapy because most *C auris* strains have been susceptible to echinocandins; susceptibility testing should be performed and patients should be monitored carefully for treatment effectiveness. Investigation for a deep focus of infection should be conducted for all patients with candidemia, regardless of species, when candidemia persists despite appropriate therapy.

C krusei is resistant to fluconazole, and more than 50% of *C glabrata* and approximately 90% of *C auris* isolates can be resistant. Although voriconazole is effective against *C krusei*, it often is ineffective against *C glabrata* and *C auris*. The echinocandins (caspofungin, micafungin, and anidulafungin) all are active in vitro against most *Candida* species and are recommended first-line drugs for *Candida* infections in severely ill or neutropenic patients (see Antifungal Drugs for Systemic Fungal Infections, p 905). Earlier studies suggested the echinocandins should be used with caution against *C parapsilosis* infection because some decreased in vitro susceptibility was initially reported, but data now suggest echinocandin resistance is extremely rare. If an echinocandin is initiated empirically and *C parapsilosis* is isolated in a patient who is recovering, then the echinocandin can be continued. Removal of infected devices (eg, ventriculostomy drains, shunts, nerve stimulators, prosthetic reconstructive devices) is absolutely necessary in addition to antifungal treatment. Breastfeeding may continue during maternal treatment for candidiasis.

Neonatal Candidiasis. Infants are more likely than older children and adults to have meningitis as a manifestation of candidiasis. Although meningitis can occur in association with candidemia, approximately half of infants with *Candida* meningitis do not have a positive blood culture. Central nervous system disease in the infant typically manifests as meningoencephalitis and should be assumed to be present in the infant with candidemia and signs and symptoms of meningoencephalitis because of the high incidence of this complication. Lumbar puncture, brain imaging, and dilated retinal examination are recommended for all infants with cultures positive for *Candida* in the blood and/or urine. CT or ultrasonography of the genitourinary tract, liver, and spleen also should be performed.

Amphotericin B deoxycholate (first choice for infants), fluconazole (for infants who have not been on fluconazole prophylaxis), or an echinocandin (generally reserved for salvage therapy) can be used in infants with systemic candidiasis. Amphotericin B deoxycholate, 1 mg/kg, intravenously, daily, is recommended for initial treatment. Fluconazole, 25 mg/kg loading dose followed by 12 mg/kg daily, may be used for isolates susceptible to fluconazole. Therapy for candidemia without metastatic disease should continue for 2 weeks after documented clearance of *Candida* species from the bloodstream and resolution of signs attributable to candidemia. Therapy for central nervous system infection is at least 3 weeks and should be continued until all signs, symptoms, and cerebrospinal fluid and radiologic abnormalities, if present, have resolved. CT or ultrasonography of the genitourinary tract, liver, heart, and spleen should be performed or repeated if blood cultures are persistently positive for *Candida* species.

Lipid formulations of amphotericin B should be used with caution in infants, particularly in infants with urinary tract involvement. Retrospective evidence suggests that treatment of infants with lipid formulations of amphotericin may be associated with worse outcomes when compared with amphotericin B deoxycholate or fluconazole. Published reports in adults and anecdotal reports in preterm infants indicate that lipid-associated amphotericin B preparations have failed to eradicate renal candidiasis, because these large-molecule drugs may not penetrate well into the renal parenchyma. It is unclear whether this is the reason for the inferior outcomes reported with the lipid formulations. Flucytosine is not recommended routinely for infants because of concerns regarding toxicity.

Older Children and Adolescents. In neutropenic or nonneutropenic children and adults, an echinocandin (caspofungin, micafungin, anidulafungin) is preferred according to guidelines, but fluconazole may be considered in those who are considered clinically stable and also are unlikely to have a fluconazole-resistant isolate. Transition from an echinocandin to fluconazole (usually in 5 to 7 days) is indicated in patients who are clinically stable, have isolates that are susceptible to fluconazole, and have negative blood cultures since initiation of antifungal therapy. Amphotericin B deoxycholate or lipid formulations are alternative therapies (see Antifungal Drugs for Systemic Fungal Infections, p 905). In nonneutropenic patients with candidemia and no metastatic complications, treatment should continue for 2 weeks after documented clearance of *Candida* organisms from the bloodstream and resolution of clinical manifestations associated with candidemia.

In neutropenic patients who are not critically ill, fluconazole is the alternative treatment for patients who have not had recent azole exposure, but voriconazole can be considered in situations in which additional mold coverage is desired. Duration of treatment for candidemia without metastatic complications is 2 weeks after documented clearance of *Candida* organisms from the bloodstream and resolution of symptoms attributable to candidemia. Avoidance or reduction of systemic immunosuppression is advised when feasible.

For chronic disseminated candidiasis (hepatosplenic infection), initial therapy with lipid formulation amphotericin B or an echinocandin for several weeks is recommended, followed by oral fluconazole (only for patients who are unlikely to have a fluconazole-resistant isolate). Discontinuation of therapy is recommended once lesions have resolved on repeated imaging.

Management of Indwelling Catheters. Prompt removal of any infected vascular or peritoneal catheters is strongly recommended, although this recommendation is weaker for neutropenic children, because the source of candidemia in these patients is more likely to be gastrointestinal and it is difficult to determine the relative contribution of the catheter. Immediate replacement of a catheter over a wire in the same catheter site is not recommended. Replacement can be attempted once the infection is controlled.

Additional Assessments. Nonneutropenic patients with candidemia should have a dilated ophthalmologic examination within the first week after diagnosis. In neutropenic patients, dilated fundoscopic examinations should be performed within the first week after counts have recovered because ophthalmologic findings of choroidal and vitreal infection are minimal until recovery from neutropenia is achieved.

ISOLATION OF THE HOSPITALIZED PATIENT: Standard precautions are recommended for all *Candida* species except *C auris*, for which both Standard and Contact Precautions are recommended because of the high transmissibility of this species.

CONTROL MEASURES: Prolonged broad-spectrum antimicrobial therapy and use of systemic corticosteroids in susceptible patients promote overgrowth of *Candida* and predispose to invasive infection. Meticulous care of central intravascular catheters is recommended for any patient requiring long-term intravenous access.

Additional control measures are recommended for *C auris*, because this organism is spread easily in health care facilities. Patients with *C auris* should be placed in a single room whenever possible and Standard and Contact Precautions implemented. Hand hygiene should be performed diligently, and the patient care environment and reusable equipment should be cleaned and disinfected thoroughly using products effective against *C auris*. Communication of the patient's *C auris* status should be clear to associated health care personnel and, if the patient is transferred, to the receiving health care facility. Surveillance and screening of other patients also should be considered to identify transmission so that infection control measures can be implemented for any other patients who may have *C auris*.

Chemoprophylaxis. Invasive candidiasis in infants is associated with prolonged hospitalization and neurodevelopmental impairment or death in almost 75% of affected infants with extremely low birth weight (less than 1000 g). The poor outcomes, despite prompt diagnosis and therapy, make prevention of invasive candidiasis in this population desirable. A number of randomized controlled trials of fungal prophylaxis in extremely preterm infants have demonstrated significant reduction of invasive candidiasis in nurseries with a moderate or high incidence of invasive candidiasis. Risk factors for invasive candidiasis in infants also include inadequate infection prevention practices and prolonged exposure to broad-spectrum antibiotic agents. Adherence to optimal infection control practices, including "bundles" for intravascular catheter insertion and maintenance and antimicrobial stewardship, can diminish infection rates and should be optimized before implementation of chemoprophylaxis as standard practice in a neonatal intensive care unit. Fluconazole is the preferred agent for prophylaxis and is recommended for extremely low birth weight infants (<1000 g) cared for in neonatal intensive care units with high (≥10%) rates of invasive candidiasis. The recommended regimen for extremely low birth weight infants is to initiate fluconazole treatment intravenously during the first 48 to 72 hours after birth at a dose of 6 mg/kg and then to administer it twice a week for 6 weeks. Once infants tolerate enteral feeds, fluconazole oral absorption is good, even in preterm infants. This chemoprophylaxis dosage, dosing interval, and duration has not been associated with emergence of fluconazole-resistant *Candida* species in randomized trials.

Fluconazole prophylaxis can decrease the risk of mucosal (eg, oropharyngeal and esophageal) candidiasis in patients with advanced HIV disease. Adults undergoing allogeneic hematopoietic stem cell transplantation have significantly fewer *Candida* infections when receiving fluconazole, but limited data are available for children. Micafungin has been used for prophylaxis. Among patients without HIV infection receiving prophylaxis with fluconazole, an increased incidence of infections attributable to *C krusei* (which intrinsically is resistant to fluconazole) has been reported. Prophylaxis should be considered for children undergoing allogenic hematopoietic stem cell transplantation and other highly myelosuppressive chemotherapy during the period of neutropenia. Prophylaxis is not recommended routinely for other immunocompromised children, including children with HIV infection.

Chancroid and Cutaneous Ulcers

CLINICAL MANIFESTATIONS: Chancroid is an acute ulcerative disease of the genitalia that occurs primarily in sexually active adolescents and adults. A clinical presentation with a painful genital ulcer and tender suppurative inguinal lymphadenopathy should raise suspicion for chancroid. An ulcer begins as an erythematous papule that becomes pustular and erodes over several days, forming a sharply demarcated, somewhat superficial lesion with a serpiginous border. The base of the ulcer is friable and can be covered with a gray or yellow, purulent exudate. Single or multiple ulcers can be present. Unlike a syphilitic chancre, which is painless and indurated, the chancroidal ulcer often is painful and non-indurated and can be associated with painful, inguinal suppurative adenitis (bubo) ipsilateral to the lesion. Without treatment, ulcer(s) can spontaneously resolve, cause extensive erosion of the genitalia, or lead to scarring and, in men, phimosis, a painful inability to retract the foreskin.

In most males, chancroid manifests as a genital ulcer with or without inguinal tenderness; edema of the prepuce is common. In females, most lesions are at the vaginal introitus, and symptoms include dysuria, dyspareunia, and vaginal discharge. Both men and women with anal infection may have pain on defecation or anal bleeding. Constitutional symptoms are unusual.

ETIOLOGY: Chancroid and cutaneous ulcers are caused by *Haemophilus ducreyi*, a gram-negative coccobacillus.

EPIDEMIOLOGY: Chancroid is a sexually transmitted infection. Chancroid is prevalent in some parts of Africa and the tropics but is uncommon in the United States, and when it does occur, it is usually imported from areas with endemic infection. Thus, recent travel to or from an area with endemic infection should raise suspicion for this diagnosis. Coinfection with syphilis or herpes simplex virus (HSV) occurs in as many as 17% of patients. Chancroid is a well-established cofactor for acquisition and transmission of human immunodeficiency virus (HIV).

Because sexual contact is the major primary route of transmission in the United States, the diagnosis of chancroid ulcers in infants and young adults, especially in the genital or perineal region, is highly suspicious of sexual abuse. However, *H ducreyi* is recognized as a major cause of non–sexually transmitted cutaneous ulcers in children in tropical regions and, specifically, countries with endemic yaws. The acquisition of a lower extremity ulcer attributable to *H ducreyi* in a child or young adult without genital ulcers and reported travel to a region with endemic yaws should not be considered evidence of sexual abuse.

For both chancroid and cutaneous ulcers, the **incubation period** is 1 to 10 days.

DIAGNOSTIC TESTS: Chancroid usually is diagnosed on the basis of clinical findings (1 or more painful genital ulcers with tender suppurative inguinal adenopathy) and by excluding other genital ulcerative diseases, such as syphilis, herpes simplex virus infection, or lymphogranuloma venereum. Cutaneous ulcers can be diagnosed on the basis of clinical findings described, but clinical findings overlap, and mixed infections with *H ducreyi* and *T pallidum* subspecies *pertenue* are common. Confirmation is made by isolation of *H ducreyi* from an ulcer or lymph node aspirate, although culture sensitivity is less than 80%. Because special culture media and conditions are required for isolation, laboratory personnel should be informed of the suspicion of *H ducreyi*. Approximately 30% to 40% of lymph node aspirates are culture positive. Polymerase chain reaction (PCR) assays can provide a specific diagnosis but are not widely available. No PCR test cleared by the US Food and Drug Administration for *H ducreyi* is available in the United States. Such testing can be performed by clinical laboratories that have developed their own PCR test and have conducted Clinical Laboratory Improvement Amendments verification studies.

TREATMENT: Genital strains of *H ducreyi* have been uniformly susceptible only to third-generation cephalosporins, macrolides, and quinolones. The prevalence of antibiotic resistance is unknown because of syndromic management of genital ulcers and the lack of diagnostic testing. Recommended regimens include azithromycin orally in a single dose, ceftriaxone intramuscularly in a single dose, erythromycin orally for 7 days, or ciprofloxacin orally for 3 days (see Table 4.4, p 901, and Table 4.5, p 904). Patients with HIV infection and uncircumcised men do not respond as well to treatment and may need repeated or longer courses of therapy. In syndromic management approaches to genital ulcer disease, treatment will typically include syphilis as a target as well as chancroid.

Clinical improvement occurs 3 to 7 days after initiation of therapy, and healing is complete in approximately 2 weeks. Adenitis often is slow to resolve and can require needle aspiration or surgical incision. Patients should be reexamined 3 to 7 days after initiating therapy to verify healing. If healing has not begun, the diagnosis may be incorrect or the patient may have an additional sexually transmitted infection, both of which necessitate further testing. Slow clinical improvement and relapses can occur after therapy, especially in HIV-infected people. Close clinical follow-up is recommended; retreatment with the original regimen usually is effective in patients who experience a relapse.

Patients with chancroid should be evaluated for other sexually transmitted infections, including syphilis, herpes simplex virus, chlamydia, gonorrhea, and HIV infection, at the time of diagnosis. Because chancroid is a risk factor for HIV infection and facilitates HIV transmission, if the initial HIV test result is negative, it should be repeated 3 months after the diagnosis of chancroid. If the hepatitis B and human papillomavirus vaccine series have not been completed, these immunizations should be offered if appropriate for age. Because syphilis and *H ducreyi* are frequently cotransmitted, serologic testing for syphilis also should be repeated 3 months after the diagnosis of chancroid. All people who had sexual contact with patients with chancroid within 10 days before onset of the patient's symptoms need to be examined and treated, even if they are asymptomatic.

Penicillin has long been used as empiric therapy for cutaneous ulcers in the tropics, but several beta-lactamase–producing cutaneous *H ducreyi* strains have been recovered. Cutaneous ulcers, therefore, should be treated with single-dose azithromycin (30 mg/kg, maximum 2 g) to cover both *T pallidum* subspecies *pertenue* and *H ducreyi*. Cutaneous ulcers attributable to *H ducreyi* respond to single-dose azithromycin within 14 days. Given the environmental sources, it is unclear whether contacts of people with leg ulcers should be treated.

ISOLATION OF THE HOSPITALIZED PATIENT: Standard precautions are recommended.

CONTROL MEASURES: Identification, examination, and treatment of sexual partners of patients with chancroid are important control measures. Regular condom use may decrease transmission, and male circumcision is believed to be partially protective.

Chikungunya

CLINICAL MANIFESTATIONS: Most people infected with chikungunya virus become symptomatic. The disease most often is characterized by acute onset of high fever (typically >39°C [102°F]) and polyarthralgia. Other symptoms may include headache, myalgia, arthritis, conjunctivitis, nausea, vomiting, or maculopapular rash. Fever typically lasts for several days to a week and can be biphasic. Rash usually occurs after onset of fever, can be pruritic, and typically involves the trunk and extremities, but the palms, soles, and face may be affected. Joint symptoms are often severe and debilitating, usually are bilateral and symmetric, and occur most commonly in the hands and feet but can affect more proximal joints. The name "chikungunya" derives from a word in the Kimakonde language meaning "to become contorted," in reference to the stooped appearance of sufferers attributable to the joint pain. Clinical laboratory findings can include lymphopenia, thrombocytopenia, elevated creatinine, and elevated hepatic aminotransferases. Acute symptoms typically resolve within 7 to 10 days. Meningoencephalitis, myelitis, Guillain-Barré syndrome, and cranial nerve palsies occur rarely but appear to be the most common severe complications of chikungunya virus infection. Other rare complications include uveitis, retinitis, myocarditis, hepatitis, nephritis, bullous skin lesions, and hemorrhage. In infants, acrocyanosis without hemodynamic instability, symmetrical vesicobullous lesions, and edema of the lower extremities may occur. People at risk for severe disease include neonates exposed perinatally, older adults (eg, >65 years), and people with underlying medical conditions (eg, hypertension, diabetes, cardiovascular, and kidney disease). Some patients might have relapse of rheumatologic symptoms (polyarthralgia, polyarthritis, and tenosynovitis) in the months following acute illness. Arthralgia is the most frequent chronic symptom. Studies report variable proportions of patients with persistent joint pains for months to years. Risk factors for chronic arthralgia are age >50 years, arthritis during the acute phase, and severe or prolonged initial infection. Mortality is rare.

The similar epidemiology and possible cocirculation of Zika, chikungunya, and dengue viruses demonstrate the increasing need to consider the differential diagnosis in travelers returning from tropical and subtropical regions of the Americas presenting with acute febrile syndrome.

ETIOLOGY: Chikungunya virus is a single-stranded RNA virus in the *Alphavirus* genus of the *Togaviridae* family.

EPIDEMIOLOGY: Chikungunya virus primarily is transmitted to humans through the bites of infected mosquitoes, predominantly *Aedes aegypti* and *Aedes albopictus*. Humans are the primary host of chikungunya virus during epidemic periods. Once a person has been infected, he or she is likely to be protected from future infections. Bloodborne transmission is possible; cases have been documented among laboratory personnel handling infected blood and a health care worker drawing blood from an infected patient. To date, there are no known reports of virus transmission through a blood transfusion. Rare in utero transmission has been documented, mostly during the second trimester. Intrapartum transmission also has been documented when the mother was viremic around the time of delivery. There are no reports of infants infected with chikungunya virus through breastfeeding.

Before 2013, outbreaks of chikungunya infection were reported from countries in Africa, Asia, Europe, and the Indian and Pacific Oceans. In 2013, chikungunya virus was found for the first time in the Americas on islands in the Caribbean. The virus then spread rapidly throughout the Americas, with local transmission reported from 44 countries and territories, and more than 1 million suspected cases reported by the end of 2014. Chikungunya virus disease cases were reported among US travelers returning from affected areas in the Americas beginning in 2014, and local transmission was identified in Florida, Puerto Rico, Texas, and the US Virgin Islands. Chikungunya virus disease became a nationally notifiable condition in the United States in 2015. Since then, sporadic outbreaks have continued to occur in many areas of the world. In 2018, 90 chikungunya virus disease cases were reported from 23 US states, all in travelers returning from affected areas; 2 locally transmitted cases were reported from Puerto Rico. Updated reports of cases in the United States can be found at **www.cdc.gov/chikungunya/geo/index.html.**

The **incubation period** typically is between 3 and 7 days (range, 1–12 days).

DIAGNOSTIC TESTS: Preliminary diagnosis is based on the patient's clinical features, places and dates of travel, and activities. Laboratory diagnosis generally is accomplished by testing serum to detect virus, viral nucleic acid, or virus-specific immunoglobulin (Ig) M and neutralizing antibodies. During the first week after onset of symptoms, chikungunya virus infection often can be diagnosed by performing reverse transcriptase-polymerase chain reaction (RT-PCR) on serum. Chikungunya virus-specific IgM and neutralizing antibodies normally develop toward the end of the first week of illness. A plaque-reduction neutralization test can be performed to quantitate virus-specific neutralizing antibodies and to discriminate between cross-reacting antibodies (eg, Mayaro and o'nyong nyong viruses). IgM antibodies usually persist for 30 to 90 days, but longer persistence has been documented. Therefore, a positive IgM test result on serum occasionally may reflect a past infection. Immunohistochemical staining can detect specific viral antigen in fixed tissue.

Routine molecular and serologic testing for chikungunya virus is performed at commercial laboratories, several state health department laboratories, and Centers for Disease Control and Prevention (CDC) laboratories. Plaque-reduction neutralization tests and immunohistochemical staining are performed at CDC and selected other reference laboratories.

TREATMENT: There is no antiviral treatment available for chikungunya. The primary treatment is supportive care and includes rest, fluids, analgesics, and antipyretics. In areas where dengue is endemic, acetaminophen is the preferred treatment for fever and joint pain. Nonsteroidal anti-inflammatory drugs should be avoided initially until a dengue diagnosis is ruled out to reduce the risk of hemorrhagic complications if the patient were to have dengue. Patients with persistent joint pain may benefit from the use of nonsteroidal anti-inflammatory drugs, corticosteroids, and physiotherapy. Methotrexate and hydroxychloroquine have been used in some patients with severe persistent arthritis.

ISOLATION OF THE HOSPITALIZED PATIENT: Standard precautions are recommended.

CONTROL MEASURES: No vaccines or preventive drugs are available. Reduction of vectors in areas with endemic transmission is important to reduce risk of infection. Symptomatic febrile patients should be protected from mosquito bites to reduce further spread. Use of certain personal protective measures can help decrease the risk of human infection, including using insect repellent, wearing long pants and long-sleeved shirts, staying in screened or air-conditioned dwellings, and limiting outdoor activities during peak vector feeding times (see Prevention of Mosquitoborne and Tickborne Infections, p 175). Chikungunya also can be prevented through screening of blood and organ donations.

Breastfeeding. Although chikungunya viral RNA has been documented in human milk of one woman acutely infected with chikungunya virus, no infants have been found to be infected through breastfeeding.

REPORTING: Health care professionals should report suspected chikungunya cases to their state or local health departments to facilitate diagnosis and mitigate the risk of local transmission. As a nationally notifiable disease, state health departments should report laboratory-confirmed cases to the CDC through ArboNET, the national surveillance system for arboviral diseases.

CHLAMYDIAL INFECTIONS

Chlamydia pneumoniae

CLINICAL MANIFESTATIONS: Patients may be asymptomatic or mildly to moderately ill with a variety of respiratory tract diseases caused by *Chlamydia pneumoniae,* including pneumonia, acute bronchitis, prolonged cough, and less commonly, pharyngitis, laryngitis, otitis media, and sinusitis. In some patients, a sore throat precedes the onset of cough by a week or more. The clinical course can be biphasic, culminating in atypical pneumonia. *C pneumoniae* can present as severe community-acquired pneumonia in immunocompromised hosts and has been associated with onset or acute exacerbation of respiratory symptoms in patients with asthma, cystic fibrosis, and acute chest syndrome in children with sickle cell disease. Rare cases of meningoencephalitis and myocarditis have been attributed to *C pneumoniae.*

Physical examination may reveal nonexudative pharyngitis, pulmonary rales, and bronchospasm. Chest radiography may reveal a variety of findings ranging from pleural effusion and bilateral infiltrates to a single patchy subsegmental infiltrate. Illness can be prolonged and cough can persist for 2 to 6 weeks or longer.

ETIOLOGY: *C pneumoniae* is an obligate intracellular bacterium for which entry into mucosal epithelial cells is necessary for intracellular survival and growth. It exists in both an infectious nonreplicating extracellular form called an elementary body and a replicating intracellular form called a reticulate body. Reticulate bodies replicate within a protective intracellular membrane-bound vesicle called an inclusion.

EPIDEMIOLOGY: *C pneumoniae* infection is presumed to be transmitted from person-to-person via infected respiratory tract secretions. It is unknown whether there is an animal reservoir. The disease occurs worldwide but is earlier in life in tropical and less developed areas than in industrialized countries in temperate climates. The timing of initial infection peaks between 5 and 15 years of age; however, studies have shown that the prevalence rate of infection in children beyond early infancy is similar to that in adults. In the United States, approximately 50% of adults have *C pneumoniae*-specific serum antibody by 20 years of age, indicating previous infection by the organism. Recurrent infection is common, especially in adults. Clusters of infection have been reported in groups of children and adults. There is no evidence of seasonality.

The mean **incubation period** is 21 days.

DIAGNOSTIC TESTS: Nucleic acid amplification tests (NAATs), such as real-time polymerase chain reaction (PCR) assays, are the preferred method for the diagnosis of an acute *C pneumoniae* infection because of their utility for rapid and accurate detection. Specimen types that can be assayed may vary according to the laboratory; thus, acceptable and preferred specimen types should be confirmed with the laboratory prior to testing. Multiplex PCR assays have been cleared by the US Food and Drug Administration for the diagnosis of *C pneumoniae* using nasopharyngeal swab samples. The tests appear to have high sensitivity and specificity. However, nasopharyngeal shedding can occur for months after acute disease, even with treatment.

Serologic testing for *C pneumoniae* is problematic. The microimmunofluorescent antibody test is the most sensitive and specific serologic test for acute infection, but it is technically complex and interpretation is subjective. A fourfold increase in immunoglobulin (Ig) G titer between acute and convalescent sera provides evidence of acute infection. Use of a single IgG titer in diagnosis of acute infection is not recommended, because IgG antibody may not appear until 6 to 8 weeks after onset of illness during primary infection and increases within 1 to 2 weeks with reinfection. In primary infection, IgM antibody appears approximately 2 to 3 weeks after onset of illness, and an IgM titer of 1:16 or greater is supportive of an acute infection. However, caution is advised when interpreting a single IgM antibody titer for diagnosis because a single result can be either falsely positive because of cross-reactivity with other *Chlamydia* species or falsely negative in cases of reinfection, when IgM may not appear. Early antimicrobial therapy may suppress antibody response. Past exposure is indicated by a stable IgG titer of 1:16 or greater.

C pneumoniae is difficult to culture but can be isolated from swab specimens obtained from the nasopharynx or oropharynx or from sputum, bronchoalveolar lavage, or tissue biopsy specimens. Specimens should be placed into appropriate transport media and stored at 4°C until inoculation into cell culture; specimens that cannot be processed within 24 hours should be frozen and stored at −70°C. Immunohistochemistry, used to detect *C pneumoniae* in tissue specimens, requires control antibodies and tissues in addition to skill in recognizing staining artifacts to avoid false-positive results.

TREATMENT: Most respiratory tract infections believed to be caused by *C pneumoniae* are treated empirically. For suspected *C pneumoniae* infections, treatment with macrolides (eg, azithromycin, erythromycin, or clarithromycin) is recommended. Doxycycline can be used for short durations (ie, 21 days or less) without regard to patient age. Tetracycline may be used but should not be administered routinely to children younger than 8 years (see Tetracyclines, p 866). Fluoroquinolones (levofloxacin and moxifloxacin) are alternative drugs for patients who are unable to tolerate macrolide antibiotic agents but should not be used as first-line treatment. In vitro data suggest that *C pneumoniae* is not susceptible to sulfonamides.

Duration of therapy typically is 10 to 14 days for erythromycin, clarithromycin, tetracycline, or doxycycline. With azithromycin, the treatment duration typically is 5 days. Duration of therapy for levofloxacin is 7 to 14 days and for moxifloxacin is 10 days. However, with all these antimicrobial agents, the optimal duration of therapy has not been established.

ISOLATION OF THE HOSPITALIZED PATIENT: Standard precautions.

CONTROL MEASURES: Recommended prevention measures include minimizing crowding, employing respiratory hygiene (or cough etiquette), and frequent hand hygiene.

Chlamydia psittaci
(Psittacosis, Ornithosis, Parrot Fever)

CLINICAL MANIFESTATIONS: Psittacosis (ornithosis) is an acute respiratory tract infection with systemic symptoms and signs that often include fever, nonproductive cough, dyspnea, headache, myalgia, chills, and malaise. Less common symptoms include pharyngitis, diarrhea, constipation, nausea and vomiting, abdominal pain, arthralgia, rash, and altered mental status. Extensive interstitial pneumonia can occur, with radiographic changes characteristically more severe than would be expected from physical examination findings. Rarely, infection with *Chlamydia psittaci* has been reported to affect organ systems other than the respiratory tract, resulting in arthritis, endocarditis, myocarditis, pericarditis, dilated cardiomyopathy, thrombophlebitis, nephritis, hepatitis, cranial nerve palsy (including sensorineural hearing loss), transverse myelitis, meningitis, and encephalitis. Infection in pregnancy may be life-threatening to the mother and cause fetal loss. There are conflicting reports regarding an association of psittacosis with ocular adnexal marginal zone lymphomas involving orbital soft tissue, lacrimal glands, and conjunctiva.

ETIOLOGY: *C psittaci* is a gram-negative, obligate intracellular bacterial pathogen that exists in 2 forms. The extracellular form is called an elementary body and is infectious. The elementary body enters the epithelial host cell through receptor-mediated endocytosis, then differentiates into a replicating reticulate body within a membrane-bound vesicle called an inclusion. Reticulate bodies require host cell nutrients to multiply and later differentiate to produce new elementary bodies that are released from the host cell to infect neighboring cells.

EPIDEMIOLOGY: Birds are the major reservoir of *C psittaci*. The term psittacosis commonly is used, although the term ornithosis more accurately describes the potential for nearly all domestic and wild birds to spread this infection, not just psittacine birds (eg, parakeets, parrots, macaws, cockatoos). In the United States, a variety of birds including psittacine birds, poultry birds (eg, chickens, ducks, turkeys, pheasants), and pigeons have been reported as sources of human disease. Infected birds, whether they appear healthy or ill, may transmit the organism. Infection usually is acquired by direct contact or inhaling aerosolized excrement or respiratory secretions from the eyes or beaks of infected birds. Once dry, the organism remains viable for months, particularly at room temperature. Importation and illegal trafficking of exotic birds may be associated with disease in humans, because shipping, crowding, and other stress factors may increase shedding of the organism among birds with latent infection. Handling of plumage and mouth-to-beak contact are the modes of exposure described most frequently, although transmission has been reported through exposure to aviaries, poultry slaughter plants, bird exhibits, and lawn mowing. Excretion of *C psittaci* from birds may be intermittent or continuous for weeks or months. Pet bird owners and breeders, veterinarians, and workers at poultry slaughter plants, poultry farms, and pet shops may be at increased risk of infection. Laboratory personnel working with *C psittaci* also are at risk. Psittacosis is worldwide in distribution and tends to occur sporadically in any season.

The **incubation period** usually is 5 to 14 days but may be longer.

DIAGNOSTIC TESTS: The diagnosis of *C psittaci* disease historically has been based on clinical presentation and a positive serologic test result using microimmunofluorescence (MIF) with paired sera. Although the MIF test generally is more sensitive and specific than complement fixation (CF) tests, MIF still displays cross-reactivity with other *Chlamydia* species in some instances. Because of this, a titer less than 1:128 should be interpreted with caution. Paired acute- and convalescent-phase serum specimens obtained at least 2 to 4 weeks apart should be obtained and performed simultaneously within a single laboratory to ensure consistency of results.[1] Treatment with antimicrobial agents may suppress the antibody response, and in such cases, a third serum sample obtained 4 to 6 weeks after the acute-phase sample may be useful in confirming the diagnosis. Although serologic testing is more commonly used and available than molecular testing, serologic test results can often be ambiguous, subjective in their interpretation, and misleading because of the inherent limitations of this approach. If possible, serologic testing should be considered a supportive test that augments the findings of other more reliable assays, such as nucleic acid-based tests.

Nucleic acid amplification tests (NAATs) have been developed that can distinguish *C psittaci* from other chlamydial species. Real-time polymerase chain reaction (PCR) assays are now available within specialized laboratories (**www.cdc.gov/laboratory/specimen-submission/detail.html?CDCTestCode=CDC-10153**). Currently, there are no NAATs cleared by the US Food and Drug Administration for detection of *C psittaci* in clinical specimens. Because the organism is difficult to recover in culture and laboratory-acquired cases have been reported, culture generally is not recommended and should be attempted only by experienced personnel in laboratories in which strict containment measures to prevent spread of the organism are used. *C psittaci* currently is classified as an organism requiring biological safety level-3 biocontainment practices.

TREATMENT: Doxycycline is the drug of choice and can be used for short durations (ie, 21 days or less) without regard to patient age. Erythromycin and azithromycin are alternative agents and are recommended for pregnant women. Therapy should continue for 10 to 14 days after fever abates. Most *C psittaci* infections are responsive to antimicrobial agents within 1 to 2 days. In patients with severe infection, intravenous doxycycline may be considered.

---

[1]National Association of State Public Health Veterinarians. Compendium of measures to control *Chlamydia psittaci* infection among humans (psittacosis) and pet birds (avian chlamydiosis). *J Avian Med Surg*. 2017;31(3). Available at: **www.nasphv.org/Documents/PsittacosisCompendium.pdf**

ISOLATION OF THE HOSPITALIZED PATIENT: Standard precautions are recommended. Person-to-person transmission is believed to be rare but has been reported.

CONTROL MEASURES: Human psittacosis is a nationally notifiable disease and should be reported to public health authorities. All birds suspected to be the source of human infection should be seen by a veterinarian for evaluation and management. Birds with *C psittaci* infection should be isolated and treated with appropriate antimicrobial agents.[1] Birds suspected of dying from *C psittaci* infection should be transported to an animal diagnostic laboratory for testing as directed by the laboratory. Birds exposed to psittacosis should be also isolated and monitored by a veterinarian for signs of illness even if they do not appear ill. All potentially contaminated caging and housing areas should be disinfected thoroughly before reuse to eliminate any infectious organisms. People cleaning cages, handling birds confirmed with *C psittaci*, or handling birds exposed to those confirmed with *C psittaci* should wear personal protective equipment including a smock or coveralls, gloves, eyewear, designated footwear or shoe covers, a disposable hat, and disposable particulate respirator (N95 mask). *C psittaci* is susceptible to many but not all household disinfectants and detergents. Effective disinfectants include 1:1000 dilutions of quaternary ammonium compounds, 1% Lysol, freshly prepared 1:32 dilutions of household bleach (1/2 cup per gallon), or other oxidizing agents such as accelerated hydrogen peroxide-based disinfectants.

Chlamydia trachomatis

CLINICAL MANIFESTATIONS: *Chlamydia trachomatis* is associated with a range of clinical manifestations, including neonatal conjunctivitis, nasopharyngitis, and pneumonia in young infants as well as genital tract infection, lymphogranuloma venereum (LGV), and trachoma in children, adolescents, and adults.

- **Neonatal chlamydial conjunctivitis** is characterized by ocular congestion, edema, and discharge developing a few days to several weeks after birth and lasting for 1 to 2 weeks and sometimes longer. In contrast to trachoma, scars and pannus formation (vascularization of the normally avascular cornea) are rare.
- **Pneumonia** in young infants usually is an afebrile illness of insidious onset occurring between 2 and 19 weeks after birth. A repetitive staccato cough, tachypnea, and rales in an afebrile 1-month-old infant are characteristic but not always present. Wheezing is uncommon. Hyperinflation usually accompanies infiltrates seen on chest radiographs. Nasal stuffiness and otitis media may occur. Untreated disease can linger or recur. Severe chlamydial pneumonia has occurred in infants and some immunocompromised adults.
- **Genitourinary tract** manifestations, such as vaginitis in prepubertal females; urethritis, cervicitis, endometritis, salpingitis, and pelvic inflammatory disease, with or without perihepatitis (Fitz-Hugh-Curtis syndrome) in postpubertal females; urethritis and epididymitis in males; and reactive arthritis (with the classic triad, formerly known as Reiter syndrome, consisting of arthritis, urethritis, and bilateral conjunctivitis) can occur. Infection can persist for months to years. Reinfection is common.

---

[1]National Association of State Public Health Veterinarians. Compendium of measures to control *Chlamydia psittaci* infection among humans (psittacosis) and pet birds (avian chlamydiosis). *J Avian Med Surg.* 2017;31(3). Available at: **www.nasphv.org/Documents/PsittacosisCompendium.pdf**

- **Proctocolitis** may occur in women or men who engage in receptive anal intercourse. Symptoms can resemble those of inflammatory bowel disease, including mucoid or hemorrhagic rectal discharge, constipation, tenesmus, and/or anorectal pain. Stricture or fistula formation can follow severe or inadequately treated infection. Infection often is asymptomatic in females.
- **LGV** classically is an invasive lymphatic infection with an initial ulcerative lesion on the genitalia accompanied by tender, suppurative inguinal and/or femoral lymphadenopathy that typically is unilateral. The ulcerative lesion often resolves by the time the patient seeks care for the adenopathy.
- **Trachoma** is a chronic follicular keratoconjunctivitis with pannus formation that results from repeated and chronic infection. Blindness secondary to extensive local scarring and inflammation occurs in 1% to 15% of people with trachoma.

ETIOLOGY: *C trachomatis* is an obligate intracellular bacterial agent with at least 15 serologic variants (serovars) divided between the following biologic variants (biovars): oculogenital (serovars A–K) and LGV (serovars L1, L2, and L3). Trachoma usually is caused by serovars A through C, and genital and perinatal infections are caused by serovars B and D through K.

EPIDEMIOLOGY: *C trachomatis* is the most commonly reported notifiable condition in the United States, with highest rates among sexually active adolescents and young adult females (ages 15–24 years). A significant proportion of female patients are asymptomatic, providing an ongoing reservoir for infection. Among sexually active 14- to 24-year-old females participating in the 2013–2016 cycles of the National Health and Nutrition Examination Survey, the estimated prevalence was 4.3% (5.5% among 14- to 19-year-olds and 3.6% among 20- to 24-year-olds). Among men, infection rates are highest in those 20 to 24 years of age. Among men who have sex with men (MSM) tested for chlamydial infection through the STD Surveillance Network of the Centers for Disease Control and Prevention (CDC), 27.8% of those 19 years and younger and 26.1% of 20- to 24-year-olds tested positive for *C trachomatis*. Racial disparities are significant, with higher rates in Black, American Indian/Alaska Native, Native Hawaiian/Other Pacific Islander, and Hispanic populations compared with white people.[1]

Oculogenital serovars of *C trachomatis* can be transmitted from the genital tract of infected mothers to their infants during birth. Acquisition occurs in approximately 50% of infants born vaginally to infected mothers and in some infants born by cesarean delivery with membranes intact. In infants who contract *C trachomatis*, the risk of conjunctivitis is 25% to 50% and the risk of pneumonia is 5% to 30%. The nasopharynx is the anatomic site most commonly infected. Asymptomatic infection of the nasopharynx, conjunctivae, vagina, and rectum can be acquired at birth, and cultures from these sites of perinatal infection may remain positive for 2 to 3 years. Infection is not known to be communicable among infants and children. The degree of contagiousness of pulmonary disease is unknown but seems to be low.

Genital tract infection in adolescents and adults is sexually transmitted. The possibility of sexual abuse always should be considered in prepubertal children beyond infancy who have vaginal, urethral, or rectal chlamydial infection (see Table 2.5, p 151). Health

---

[1]Centers for Disease Control and Prevention. Sexually Transmitted Disease Surveillance 2018. Atlanta, GA: US Department of Health and Human Services; 2019. Available at: **www.cdc.gov/std/stats18/default.htm**

care professionals are mandated to report suspected sexual abuse to their state child protective services agency.

LGV biovars are worldwide in distribution but are particularly prevalent in tropical and subtropical areas. Although disease occurs rarely in the United States, reports of outbreaks of LGV proctocolitis have been increasing among MSM. Perinatal transmission is rare. LGV is infectious during active disease. Little is known about the prevalence or duration of asymptomatic carriage.

Although rarely observed in the United States since the 1950s, trachoma is the leading infectious cause of blindness worldwide, causing up to 3% of the world's blindness. Trachoma is transmitted by transfer of ocular discharge and is generally confined to poor populations in resource-limited nations in Africa, the Middle East, Asia, and Latin America; the Pacific Islands; and remote aboriginal communities in Australia.

The **incubation period** of chlamydial illness is variable, depending on the type of infection, but usually is at least 1 week.

DIAGNOSTIC TESTS[1]: Among **postpubertal individuals,** *C trachomatis* nucleic acid amplification tests (NAATs) are the most sensitive tests and are recommended for laboratory diagnosis. Commercial NAATs have been cleared by the US Food and Drug Administration (FDA) for testing vaginal (provider or patient collected), endocervical, male intraurethral, throat, and rectal swab specimens; male and female first-catch urine specimens placed in appropriate transport devices; and liquid cytology specimens. The CDC recommends that *C trachomatis* urogenital infection be diagnosed in women by vaginal or cervical swab specimens or first-catch urine. Patient-collected vaginal swab specimens are equivalent in sensitivity and specificity to those collected by a clinician using NAATs. Diagnosis of *C trachomatis* urethral infection in men can be made by testing first-catch urine or a urethral swab specimen. Patient collection of a meatal swab for *C trachomatis* testing may be a reasonable approach for men who are either unable to provide urine or prefer to collect their own meatal swab over providing urine. NAATs have been demonstrated to have improved sensitivity and specificity compared with culture for the detection of *C trachomatis* at rectal and oropharyngeal sites. Data indicate that performance of NAATs on self-collected rectal swab specimens is comparable to those with clinician-collected rectal swab specimens. Most people with *C trachomatis* detected at oropharyngeal sites do not have oropharyngeal symptoms, and the clinical significance of oropharyngeal *C trachomatis* infection is unclear.

Specimen collection for diagnosis of **neonatal chlamydial ophthalmia** must contain conjunctival cells, not eye discharge alone. Sensitive and specific methods used for diagnosis include both cell culture and nonculture tests (eg, DFA and NAAT). DFA is the only culture-independent method that is FDA approved for the detection of chlamydia from conjunctival swab specimens; NAATs are not FDA cleared for the detection of chlamydia from conjunctival swab specimens, but clinical laboratories may offer such testing once they have verified the use of such specimens according to regulations of the Clinical Laboratory Improvement Amendments (CLIA). Specimens for culture isolation and nonculture tests should be obtained from the everted eyelid using a dacron-tipped swab or the swab specified by the manufacturer's test kit; for culture and DFA, specimens must contain conjunctival cells, not exudate alone.

---

[1]Centers for Disease Control and Prevention. Sexually transmitted infections treatment guidelines, 2021. *MMWR Recomm Rep.* 2021; in press

For diagnosing **infant pneumonia** caused by *C trachomatis*, specimens for chlamydial testing should be collected from the posterior nasopharynx. Isolation of the organism in cell culture is the definitive standard diagnostic test for chlamydial pneumonia. Culture-independent tests (eg, DFA and NAAT) can be used. DFA is the only culture-independent FDA-approved test for the detection of *C trachomatis* from nasopharyngeal specimens. DFA testing of nasopharyngeal specimens has a lower sensitivity and specificity than culture. If NAATs are to be used for the detection of *C trachomatis* from nasopharyngeal specimens, the clinical laboratories must verify the procedure according to CLIA regulations. Tracheal aspirates and lung biopsy specimens, if collected, should be tested for *C trachomatis* by cell culture.

For the **evaluation of prepubertal children for suspected sexual abuse,** see STI Evaluation of Prepubertal Victims, p 152. Diagnosis of genitourinary tract chlamydial disease in a child should prompt examination for **other STIs,** including syphilis, gonorrhea, trichomoniasis, human immunodeficiency virus (HIV), hepatitis B virus, hepatitis C virus, and investigation of sexual abuse.

Serologic testing has little, if any, value in diagnosing uncomplicated genital *C trachomatis* infection. In **children with pneumonia,** an acute microimmunofluorescent (MIF) serum titer of *C trachomatis*-specific immunoglobulin (Ig) M of 1:32 or greater is diagnostic.

A definitive **diagnosis of LGV** can be made only with LGV-specific molecular testing. (eg, PCR-based genotyping). These tests can differentiate LGV from non-LGV *C trachomatis* in rectal swab specimens. Genital or oral lesions, rectal swab, and lymph node specimens (ie, lesion swab or bubo aspirate) can be tested for *C trachomatis* by NAAT or culture. NAAT is the preferred approach to testing as these tests can detect both LGV strains and non-LGV *C trachomatis* strains. *Chlamydia* serology (complement fixation or microimmunofluorescence) should not be routinely used to make a diagnosis of LGV because the diagnostic utility of these serologic methods has not been established, interpretation has not been standardized, and validation for clinical proctitis presentation has not been done.

Diagnosis of **ocular trachoma** usually is made clinically in countries with endemic infection.

TREATMENT[1]:

* **Infants with chlamydial conjunctivitis or pneumonia** are treated with oral erythromycin base or ethylsuccinate (50 mg/kg/day in 4 divided doses daily) for 14 days or with azithromycin (20 mg/kg as a single daily dose) for 3 days. Because the efficacy of erythromycin treatment for either disease is approximately 80%, a second course of therapy might be required. Data on the efficacy of azithromycin for ophthalmia neonatorum or pneumonia are limited. Clinical follow-up of infants treated with either drug is recommended to determine whether initial treatment was effective. A diagnosis of *C trachomatis* infection in an infant should prompt treatment of the mother and her sexual partner(s). Neonates with documented chlamydial infection should be evaluated for possible gonococcal infection. An association between orally administered erythromycin and azithromycin and infantile hypertrophic pyloric stenosis (IHPS) has

---

[1]Centers for Disease Control and Prevention. Sexually transmitted infections treatment guidelines, 2021. *MMWR Recomm Rep.* 2021; in press

been reported in infants younger than 6 weeks. Infants treated with either of these anti-microbial agents should be followed for signs and symptoms of IHPS.

- Infants born to mothers known to have untreated chlamydial infection are at high risk of infection; however, prophylactic antimicrobial treatment is not indicated, because the efficacy of such treatment is unknown. Infants should be monitored clinically to ensure appropriate treatment if infection develops. If adequate follow-up cannot be ensured, preemptive therapy should be considered.
- For treatment of **chlamydial infections in infants and children: For children who weigh <45 kg,** the recommended regimen is oral erythromycin base or ethylsuc-cinate, 50 mg/kg/day, divided into 4 doses daily for 14 days. Data are limited on the effectiveness and optimal dose of azithromycin for treatment of chlamydial infections in infants and children who weigh <45 kg. **For children who weigh ≥45 kg but who are younger than 8 years,** the recommended regimen is azithromycin, 1 g, orally, in a single dose. **For children 8 years and older,** the recommended regimen is azithro-mycin, 1 g, orally, in a single dose, or doxycycline, 100 mg, orally, twice a day for 7 days.
- For uncomplicated *C trachomatis* **anogenital tract infection in adolescents or adults,** oral doxycycline (100 mg, twice daily) for 7 days is recommended (see Table 4.4, p 898). Alternatives include oral azithromycin in a single 1-g dose, or levo-floxacin (500 mg orally, once daily) for 7 days. **For pregnant females,** the recom-mended treatment is azithromycin (1 g, orally, as a single dose), with amoxicillin (500 mg, orally, 3 times/day for 7 days) as an alternative regimen.

Follow-up Testing. Test of cure immediately following treatment is not recommended for **nonpregnant adult or adolescent** patients treated for uncomplicated chlamydial infection unless compliance is in question, symptoms persist, or reinfection is suspected. Reinfection is common after initial infection and treatment, and all infected adolescents and adults should be retested for *C trachomatis* approximately 3 months following initial treatment, regardless of whether patients believe their sexual partners were treated. If retesting at 3 months is not possible, patients should be retested when they next present for health care in the 12 months after initial treatment. Test of cure (preferably by NAAT) is recommended approximately 4 weeks after treatment of **pregnant females.** In addi-tion, all pregnant females who have diagnosed chlamydia should be retested 3 months after treatment.

- For **LGV,** doxycycline (100 mg, orally, twice daily for 21 days) is the preferred treat-ment. Azithromycin (1 g, once weekly for 3 weeks) and erythromycin (500 mg, orally, 4 times daily for 21 days) are alternative regimens. Because azithromycin has not been rigorously validated, a test-of-cure with *C trachomatis* NAAT 4 weeks after completion of treatment can be considered.
- Treatment for **trachoma** is azithromycin, orally, as a single dose of 20 mg/kg (maxi-mum dose of 1 g), as recommended by the World Health Organization for all people diagnosed with trachoma as well as for all of their household contacts.

ISOLATION OF THE HOSPITALIZED PATIENT: Standard precautions are recommended.

CONTROL MEASURES:

Pregnancy. Identification and treatment of females with *C trachomatis* genital tract infection during pregnancy, before delivery, can prevent peripartum acquisition of disease in the infant. The CDC and US Preventive Services Task Force (USPSTF) recommend routine screening of pregnant women ≤24 years of age and screening of women ≥25 years of age at increased risk of chlamydia (eg, women who have a new sex partner, more than one sex partner, a sex partner with concurrent sex partners, or a sex partner who has a sexually transmitted infection (STI) at the first prenatal visit and advise retesting of all pregnant females ≤24 years and those ≥25 years of age who remain at increased risk during the third trimester to prevent perinatal complications. Discussion of partner treatment is important in this setting.

Neonatal Chlamydial Conjunctivitis. Recommended topical prophylaxis with erythromycin or tetracycline for all newborn infants for prevention of gonococcal ophthalmia will not prevent neonatal chlamydial conjunctivitis or extraocular infection (see Prevention of Neonatal Ophthalmia, p 1023).

Contacts of Infants With C trachomatis *Conjunctivitis or Pneumonia*. Mothers of infected infants and mothers' sexual partners should be treated for *C trachomatis*.

Routine Screening.[1] All sexually active females (≤24 years) should be tested at least annually for chlamydial infection, even if no symptoms are present or barrier contraception is reported. Although evidence is insufficient to recommend routine screening for *C trachoma* in sexually active males, annual screening should be considered in clinical settings serving populations of young males with high prevalence of chlamydia (eg, correctional facilities, national job training programs, military recruits, STI clinics, high school clinics, adolescent clinics) or in populations with high burden of infection. Sexually active MSM should be screened at least annually for rectal and urethral chlamydia if they engaged in receptive or insertive anal intercourse, respectively (regardless of condom use during exposure). MSM should be screened every 3 to 6 months if at high risk for STI because of multiple or anonymous sex partners, sex in conjunction with illicit drug use, or sex with partners who participate in these activities.

Management of Sex Partners. All people with sexual contact in the 60 days preceding diagnosis or onset of symptoms of patients with *C trachomatis* infection (whether symptomatic or asymptomatic), nongonococcal urethritis, mucopurulent cervicitis, epididymitis, or pelvic inflammatory disease should be evaluated and treated for *C trachomatis* infection. The patient's last sex partner should be treated even if last sexual contact was more than 60 days before diagnosis in the index case. Among females or heterosexual male patients, if concerns exist that sex partners who are referred for evaluation and treatment will not seek care, expedited partner therapy (EPT), which is the practice of treating the sex partners of patients with chlamydia or gonorrhea by providing prescriptions or medications to the index patient to take to his or her partner without the health care provider first examining the partner, can be considered. To clarify the legal status of EPT in each state, refer to the CDC website (**www.cdc.gov/std/ept/legal/**). Efforts should be made to educate partners about symptoms of chlamydia and gonorrhea and to encourage partners to seek clinical evaluation. Published studies suggest that >5% of MSM without a previous HIV diagnosis have a new diagnosis of HIV infection when evaluated as a partner of patients with gonorrhea or chlamydia. Hence, EPT should not be considered a routine partner management strategy in MSM because of the high risk of coexisting undiagnosed STIs or HIV infection.

---

[1]American Academy of Pediatrics, Committee on Adolescence; Society for Adolescent Health and Medicine. Screening for nonviral sexually transmitted infections in adolescents and young adults. *Pediatrics*. 2014;134(1):e302-e311

Patients and contacts should abstain from unprotected intercourse until treatment of both partners is complete (ie, after completion of a multiple-dose treatment or for 7 days after single-dose therapy).

LGV. Nonspecific preventive measures for LGV are the same as measures for STIs in general and include education, case reporting, condom use, and avoidance of sexual contact with infected people. Partners exposed to an LGV-infected person within the 60 days before the patient's symptom onset should be tested and presumptively treated with a chlamydia regimen.

Trachoma. Prevention methods recommended by the World Health Organization for global elimination of blindness attributable to trachoma by 2020 include surgery, antimicrobial agents, face washing, and environmental improvement (SAFE). Azithromycin (20 mg/kg, maximum 1 g), once a year as a single oral dose, is used in mass drug administration campaigns for trachoma control.

CLOSTRIDIAL INFECTIONS

Botulism and Infant Botulism
(Clostridium botulinum)

CLINICAL MANIFESTATIONS: Botulism is a neuroparalytic disorder characterized by an acute, afebrile, symmetric, descending, flaccid paralysis that can progress to respiratory distress or failure. Paralysis is caused by blockade of neurotransmitter release at the voluntary motor and autonomic neuromuscular junctions. Four naturally occurring forms of human botulism exist: infant, foodborne, wound, and adult intestinal colonization. Cases of iatrogenic botulism, which result from injection of excess therapeutic or cosmetic botulinum toxin, have been reported, and botulinum neurotoxins are considered a potential agent of bioterrorism. Symptoms of botulism can occur abruptly, within hours of exposure, or evolve gradually over several days and may include diplopia, dysphagia, dysphonia, and dysarthria. Cranial nerve palsies are followed by symmetric, descending, flaccid paralysis of somatic musculature in patients who remain fully alert. Infant botulism, which occurs predominantly in infants younger than 6 months (range, 1 day–12 months), is preceded by or begins with constipation and manifests as decreased movement, loss of facial expression, poor feeding, weak cry, diminished gag reflex, ocular palsies, loss of head control, and progressive descending generalized weakness and hypotonia. Some reports suggest that sudden infant death could result from rapidly progressing infant botulism.

ETIOLOGY: Botulism occurs after absorption of botulinum toxin into the circulation from a mucosal or wound surface. At least 7 antigenic toxin types (A–G) of *Clostridium botulinum* are known. An eighth toxin type (H) has been reported, but its identity as a distinct serotype remains controversial. Non-*botulinum* species of *Clostridium* may rarely produce these neurotoxins and cause disease. The most common botulinum toxin serotypes associated with naturally occurring illness are types A, B, E, and rarely, F. Most cases of infant botulism result from toxin types A and B, but a few cases of types E and F have been caused by *Clostridium butyricum* (type E), *C botulinum* (type E), and *Clostridium baratii* (type F). *C botulinum* spores are ubiquitous in soils and dust worldwide and have been isolated from the home environment and vacuum cleaner dust of infant botulism cases.

EPIDEMIOLOGY: Infant botulism results after ingested spores of *C botulinum* or related neurotoxigenic clostridial species germinate, multiply, and produce botulinum toxin in the large intestine through transient colonization of the intestinal microflora. Cases may occur in breastfed infants before or after the first introduction of nonhuman milk substances; the source of spores usually is not identified. Honey has been identified as an avoidable source of spores. No case of infant botulism has been proven to be from consumption of corn syrup. Rarely, intestinal botulism can occur in older children and adults, usually after intestinal surgery and exposure to antimicrobial agents.

Foodborne botulism results when food that carries spores of *C botulinum* is preserved or stored improperly under anaerobic conditions that permit germination, multiplication, and toxin production. Illness follows ingestion of the food containing preformed botulinum toxin. Home processing of foods is the most common cause of foodborne botulism in the United States, followed by rare outbreaks associated with commercially processed foods, restaurant-associated foods, and wine produced in prisons ("pruno" and "hooch").

Wound botulism results when *C botulinum* contaminates traumatized tissue, germinates, multiplies, and produces toxin. Gross trauma or crush injury can be a predisposing event. In recent years, "skin popping" and self-injection of contaminated black tar heroin have been associated with most cases.

Immunity to botulinum toxin does not develop in botulism. Botulism is not transmitted from person to person. The usual **incubation period** for foodborne botulism is 12 to 48 hours (range, 6 hours–10 days). In infant botulism, the **incubation period** is estimated at 3 to 30 days from the time of ingestion of spores. For wound botulism, the **incubation period** is 4 to 14 days from time of injury until onset of symptoms.

DIAGNOSTIC TESTS: A toxin neutralization bioassay in mice[1] and an in vitro mass spectrometry assay can used to detect botulinum toxin in serum, stool, enema fluid, gastric aspirate, or suspect foods. Enriched selective media are required to isolate *C botulinum* from stool and foods. The diagnosis of infant botulism is made by demonstrating botulinum toxin in serum or feces or botulinum toxin-producing organisms in feces or enema fluid. Wound botulism is confirmed by demonstrating botulinum toxin-producing organisms in the wound or tissue or toxin in the serum. Foodborne botulism is confirmed by demonstrating botulinum toxin in food, serum, or stool or botulinum toxin-producing organism in stool. Confirmation can also occur when a symptomatic patient consumed the same food as a laboratory-confirmed patient. To increase the likelihood of diagnosis in foodborne botulism, all suspect foods should be collected, and serum and stool or enema specimens should be obtained from all people with suspected illness. In foodborne cases, the length of time serum specimens may be positive for toxin varies, and in some cases can be longer than 10 days after illness onset. Although toxin can be demonstrated in serum in some infants with botulism (13% in one large study), stool is the best specimen for diagnosis; enema effluent also can be useful. If constipation makes obtaining a stool specimen difficult, an enema of sterile, nonbacteriostatic water should be administered promptly. Because results of laboratory testing may require several days, treatment with antitoxin should be initiated urgently for all forms of botulism on the basis of clinical suspicion. The most prominent electromyographic finding is an incremental increase of evoked muscle potentials at high-frequency nerve stimulation (20–50 Hz). In addition, a

---

[1]For information on testing for botulinum toxin, consult your state health department.

characteristic pattern of brief, small-amplitude, overly abundant motor action potentials may be seen after stimulation of muscle, but its absence does not exclude the diagnosis; this test sometimes is needed to assist with diagnosis.

TREATMENT:

Meticulous Supportive Care. Meticulous supportive care, in particular respiratory and nutritional support, constitutes a fundamental aspect of therapy in all forms of botulism. Recovery from botulism may take weeks to months.

Antitoxin for Infant Botulism. Human-derived antitoxin should be administered immediately. Human Botulism Immune Globulin for intravenous use (BIG-IV, which goes by the brand name BabyBIG) is licensed by the US Food and Drug Administration (FDA) for treatment of infant botulism caused by *C botulinum* type A or type B. BabyBIG is produced and distributed by the California Department of Public Health (24-hour telephone number: 510-231-7600; **www.infantbotulism.org**). BabyBIG significantly decreases days of mechanical ventilation, days of intensive care unit stay, and total length of hospital stay by almost 1 month and is cost saving. BabyBIG is first-line therapy for naturally occurring infant botulism. Equine-derived heptavalent botulinum antitoxin (BAT; see below) was licensed by the FDA in 2013 for treatment of adult and pediatric botulism and is available through the Centers for Disease Control and Prevention (CDC). BAT has been used, on a case by case basis, to treat type F infant botulism patients, where the antitoxin is not contained in BabyBIG.

As with other Immune Globulin Intravenous preparations, routine live-virus vaccines should be delayed for 6 months after receipt of BabyBIG because of potential interference with immune responses (see Table 1.11, p 40).

Antitoxin for Noninfant Forms of Botulism. Immediate administration of antitoxin is the key to successful therapy, because antitoxin treatment ends the toxemia and stops further uptake of toxin. However, because botulinum neurotoxin becomes internalized in the nerve ending, administration of antitoxin does not reverse paralysis. If foodborne or other botulism is suspected, the state health department should be contacted immediately to discuss and report the case; all states maintain a 24-hour telephone service. If contact cannot be made with the state health department, the CDC Emergency Operations Center should be contacted at 770-488-7100 for botulism case consultation and antitoxin. Since 2010, BAT is the only botulinum antitoxin released in the United States for treatment of noninfant botulism. BAT contains antitoxins against botulinum toxin types A–G and has been "despeciated" by enzymatic removal of the Fc immunoglobulin fragment, resulting in a product that is >90% Fab and F(ab')₂ immunoglobulin fragments. BAT is provided by the CDC with the product information that includes specific, detailed instructions for intravenous administration of antitoxin. Additional information may be found on the CDC website (**www.cdc.gov/botulism/**).

Antimicrobial Agents. Antimicrobial therapy is not prescribed in infant botulism unless clearly indicated for a concurrent infection. Aminoglycoside agents can potentiate the paralytic effects of the toxin and should be avoided. Given theoretical concerns of toxin release from antibiotic-induced bacterial cell death, providers should consider delaying the use of antibiotics in wound botulism until after antitoxin is administered, depending on the clinical situation. The role for antimicrobial therapy in the adult intestinal colonization form of botulism, if any, has not been established.

ISOLATION OF THE HOSPITALIZED PATIENT: Standard precautions are recommended.

CONTROL MEASURES:

- Any case of suspected botulism is a nationally notifiable disease and is required by law to be reported immediately to local and state health departments. Immediate reporting of suspected cases is particularly important, because a single case could be the harbinger of many more cases, as with foodborne botulism, and because of possible use of botulinum toxin as a bioterrorism weapon.

- Honey should not be given to children younger than 12 months because of the possibility of contaminating *C botulinum* spores. Many foods and commercial products contain honey, and the honey is included in a variety of ways. Because the details of each manufacturing process vary, the California Department of Public Health is unable to comment on the likelihood that the honey-containing food product may contain viable *C botulinum* spores (**www.infantbotulism.org/general/faq.php**). Prudence would dictate that these types of foods also should be avoided during the first 12 months of life. Botulism is not transmitted by human milk, and nursing mothers may consume honey.

- Prophylactic antitoxin is not recommended for asymptomatic people who have ingested a food known to contain botulinum toxin. Physicians treating a patient who has been exposed to toxin or is suspected of having any type of botulism should contact their state health department immediately. People exposed to toxin who are asymptomatic should have close medical observation in nonsolitary settings.

- Education regarding safe practices in food preparation and home-canning methods should be promoted. Use of a pressure cooker (at 116°C [240.8°F]) is necessary to kill spores of *C botulinum*. Bringing the internal temperature of foods to 85°C (185°F) for 10 minutes will destroy the toxin. Time, temperature, and pressure requirements vary with altitude and the product being heated. Food containers that appear to bulge may contain gas produced by *C botulinum* and should be discarded. Other foods that appear to have spoiled should not be eaten or tasted (**https://nchfp.uga.edu/publications/publications_usda.html**).

Clostridial Myonecrosis
(Gas Gangrene)

CLINICAL MANIFESTATIONS: Disease onset is heralded by acute and progressive pain at the site of the wound, followed by edema, increasing exquisite tenderness, and exudate. Systemic findings initially include tachycardia disproportionate to the degree of fever, pallor, and diaphoresis. Crepitus is suggestive but not pathognomonic of *Clostridium* infection and is not always present. Tense bullae containing thin, serosanguineous or dark fluid develop in the overlying skin and areas of green-black cutaneous necrosis appear. Fluid in the bullae has a foul odor. Disease can progress rapidly with development of hypotension, renal failure, and alterations in mental status. Diagnosis is based on clinical manifestations, including the characteristic appearance of necrotic muscle at surgery. Untreated clostridial myonecrosis, also known as gas gangrene, can lead to disseminated myonecrosis, suppurative visceral infection, septicemia, and death within hours.

Nontraumatic gas gangrene usually is caused by *Clostridium septicum* and is a complication of bacteremia, which is the result of an occult gastrointestinal mucosal lesion (most commonly colon cancer) or a complication of neutropenic colitis, leukemia, or diabetes mellitus.

ETIOLOGY: Clostridial myonecrosis is caused by *Clostridium* species, most often *Clostridium perfringens*. Other *Clostridium* species (eg, *Clostridium sordellii, C septicum, Clostridium novyi*) have also been associated with myonecrosis. These organisms are large, gram-positive, spore-forming, anaerobic bacilli with blunt ends. Disease manifestations are caused by potent clostridial exotoxins. Mixed infection with other gram-positive and gram-negative bacteria is common.

EPIDEMIOLOGY: Clostridial myonecrosis usually results from contamination of deep open wounds. The sources of *Clostridium* species are soil, contaminated foreign bodies, and human and animal feces. Dirty surgical or traumatic wounds, particularly those with retained foreign bodies or significant amounts of devitalized tissue, predispose to disease. Cases have occurred in people who inject drugs, in association with contaminated black tar heroin. Rarely, nontraumatic gas gangrene occurs in immunocompromised people, most frequently in those with underlying malignancy, neutrophil dysfunction, or diseases associated with bowel ischemia.

The **incubation period** from the time of injury is 6 hours to 4 days.

DIAGNOSTIC TESTS: Anaerobic cultures of wound exudate, involved soft tissue and muscle, and blood should be performed. Matrix-assisted laser desorption/ionization–time-of-flight (MALDI-TOF) devices have an approved indication from the US Food and Drug Administration to identify *C perfringens*. Because *Clostridium* species are ubiquitous, their recovery from a wound is not diagnostic unless typical clinical manifestations are present. A Gram-stained smear of wound discharge demonstrating characteristic gram-positive bacilli and few, if any, polymorphonuclear leukocytes suggests clostridial infection. Tissue specimens (not swab specimens) for anaerobic culture must be obtained to confirm the diagnosis. Because some pathogenic *Clostridium* species are exquisitely sensitive to oxygen, care should be taken during the collection and processing of a sample to optimize anaerobic growth conditions. A radiograph of the affected site might demonstrate gas in the tissue, but this is a nonspecific finding that is not always present. Occasionally, blood cultures are positive and are considered diagnostic.

TREATMENT:

- Prompt and complete surgical excision of necrotic tissue and removal of foreign material is essential. Repeated surgical débridement may be required to ensure complete removal of all infected tissue. Vacuum-assisted wound closure can be used following multiple débridements.
- Management of shock, fluid and electrolyte imbalance, hemolytic anemia, and other complications is crucial.
- High-dose penicillin G should be administered intravenously (see Table 4.3, p 892). Clindamycin, metronidazole, meropenem, ertapenem, and chloramphenicol can be considered as alternative drugs for patients with a serious penicillin allergy or for treatment of polymicrobial infections. The combination of penicillin G and clindamycin may be superior to penicillin alone because of the theoretical benefit of clindamycin inhibiting toxin synthesis.
- Hyperbaric oxygen may be beneficial, but efficacy data from adequately controlled clinical studies are not available.

ISOLATION OF THE HOSPITALIZED PATIENT: Standard precautions are recommended.

CONTROL MEASURES: Prompt and careful débridement, flushing of contaminated wounds, and removal of foreign material should be performed.

Penicillin G (50 000 U/kg per day) or clindamycin (20–30 mg/kg per day) has been used for prophylaxis in patients with grossly contaminated wounds, but there are no data on recommended duration or the effectiveness of treatment.

Clostridioides difficile (formerly Clostridium difficile)

CLINICAL MANIFESTATIONS: *Clostridioides difficile* (formerly *Clostridium difficile*) is associated with a spectrum of gastrointestinal illness as well as with asymptomatic colonization that is common, especially in young infants. Mild to moderate illness is characterized by watery diarrhea, low-grade fever, and abdominal pain. In the past, hospital onset of symptoms was believed to be the most common presentation. However, recent studies have found that *C difficile* often is diagnosed in nonhospitalized children. Pseudomembranous colitis is characterized by diarrhea with mucus in feces, abdominal cramps and pain, fever, and systemic toxicity. Toxic megacolon (acute dilatation of the colon) should be considered in children who develop marked abdominal tenderness and distension with minimal diarrhea and may be associated with hemodynamic instability. Other complications of *C difficile* disease include intestinal perforation, hypotension, shock, and death. Complicated infections are less common in children than adults. Severe or fatal disease is more likely to occur in neutropenic children with leukemia, infants with Hirschsprung disease, and patients with inflammatory bowel disease. Extraintestinal manifestations of *C difficile* infection are uncommon but can include bacteremia, wound infections, and reactive arthritis. Clinical illness attributable to *C difficile* is considered very rare in children younger than 12 months. In infants, *C difficile* should not be considered until other infectious and noninfectious causes of diarrhea have been excluded.

C difficile colonization occurs when there are no attributable clinical symptoms, but tests are positive for *C difficile* organism or its toxins. *C difficile* disease occurs when attributable clinical symptoms are present in the setting of tests which are positive for *C difficile* organisms or its toxins.

ETIOLOGY: *C difficile* is a spore-forming, obligate anaerobic, gram-positive bacillus. Some strains produce exotoxins (toxins A and B), which are responsible for the clinical manifestations of disease when there is overgrowth of *C difficile* in the intestine.

EPIDEMIOLOGY: *C difficile* is shed in feces. People can acquire infection from the stool of other colonized or infected people through the fecal-oral route. Any surface (including hands), device, or material that has become contaminated with feces may also transmit *C difficile* spores. Hospitals, nursing homes, and child care facilities are major reservoirs for *C difficile*. Risk factors for acquisition of the bacterium include prolonged hospitalization and exposure to an infected person either in the hospital or the community. Risk factors for *C difficile* disease include antimicrobial therapy, repeated enemas, proton pump inhibitor therapy, prolonged nasogastric tube placement, gastrostomy and jejunostomy tube placement, underlying bowel disease, gastrointestinal tract surgery, renal insufficiency, and immunocompromised state. *C difficile* colitis has been associated with exposure to almost every antimicrobial agent; cephalosporins and fluoroquinolones are considered to be the highest-risk antibiotic agents, particularly for recurrent *C difficile* disease and infections with epidemic strains. The ribotype 027 (formerly known as NAP-1) strain is a virulent strain of *C difficile* because of increased toxin production and is associated with an increased risk of severe disease. Ribotype 027 strains of *C difficile* have emerged as a cause of outbreaks among adults and are reported sporadically in children.

Recent data reveal that overall *C difficile disease* and associated hospitalizations among children ≥1 year of age and adults in the United States decreased 24% from 2011 to 2017, after adjusting the data for the use of a more sensitive type of test called a nucleic acid amplification test (NAAT). The overall decrease was driven by a 36% decrease in health care-associated cases, while community-associated cases did not change. The incidence of pediatric community-associated *C difficile* disease may be twice as frequent as health care-associated disease.

Asymptomatic intestinal colonization with *C difficile* (including toxin-producing strains) is common in children younger than 2 years and is most common in infants younger than 1 year. Epidemiologic studies show that up to 50% of healthy infants have colonization. Colonization rates drop to less than 5% in healthy children older than 5 years and adults. The rate of asymptomatic colonization with *C difficile* in hospitalized adults is reported to be 3% to 26%

The **incubation period** is unknown; colitis usually develops 5 to 10 days after initiation of antimicrobial therapy but can occur on the first day of treatment and up to 10 weeks after therapy cessation.

DIAGNOSTIC TESTS: Endoscopic findings of pseudomembranes (2- to 5-mm, raised yellowish plaques) and hyperemic, friable rectal mucosa suggesting pseudomembranous colitis are highly correlated with *C difficile* disease. More commonly, the diagnosis of *C difficile* disease is based on laboratory methods including the detection of *C difficile* toxin(s) or toxin gene(s) in a diarrheal stool specimen. In general, laboratory tests for *C difficile* should not be ordered on a patient who is having formed stools unless ileus or toxic megacolon is suspected. Similarly, *C difficile* tests should not be ordered on a patient who is receiving laxatives or stool softeners or has evidence suggestive of a viral or noninfectious cause of diarrhea. Notwithstanding the availability of several test methods, there presently is no generally agreed on gold standard laboratory test method for the diagnosis of *C difficile* disease.

Molecular assays using nucleic acid amplification tests (NAATs) are commonly used for toxigenic strains of *C difficile* toxins in both adult and pediatric hospitals. NAATs detect genes responsible for the production of toxins A and B, rather than free toxins A and B in the stool, which are detected by enzyme immunoassay (EIA). EIAs are rapid, performed easily, and highly specific for diagnosis of *C difficile* disease, but their sensitivity is relatively low. The cell culture cytotoxicity assay, which also tests for toxin in stool, is more sensitive than the EIA but is labor intensive and has a long turnaround time, limiting its usefulness in the clinical setting.

NAATs combine excellent sensitivity and analytic specificity and provide results to clinicians in times comparable to EIAs. However, detecting toxin gene(s) in patients who are only colonized with *C difficile* is common and likely contributes to misdiagnosis of *C difficile* disease in children with other causes of diarrhea, leading to unnecessary antibiotic treatment for *C difficile*. Several steps can be taken to reduce the likelihood of misdiagnosis of *C difficile* disease related to use of highly sensitive NAATs. Age should be considered, because colonization with *C difficile* in infants is common and symptomatic infection in this age group is not believed to occur; therefore, *C difficile* diagnostic testing on samples from children younger than 12 months is discouraged. Likewise, testing should not be performed routinely in toddlers with diarrhea who are 1 to 2 years of age unless other infectious or noninfectious causes have been excluded. For children older than 2 years, testing is recommended if there is new onset of prolonged and worsening diarrhea and risk factors (eg, inflammatory bowel disease, immunocompromising condition) or recent course of antibiotics or health care exposures. Because shedding of *C difficile* in the stool can persist for several months after treatment and symptom resolution and because sensitivity of NAAT testing is nearly 100%, tests of cure are discouraged. Patients should be screened carefully for clinical symptoms likely associated with *C difficile* disease (eg, unexplained and new onset of at least 3 loose or unformed stools in ≤24 hours, no history of patient taking laxatives) prior to testing for infection when a highly sensitive test such as a NAAT is used.

A 2- or 3-stage approach increases the positive predictive value versus 1-stage testing. Multistep algorithms have been suggested by the Infectious Diseases Society of America guidelines[1] that incorporate testing for stool toxin (EIA), testing for glutamate dehydrogenase (GDH), an enzyme expressed by both toxigenic and nontoxigenic strains of *C difficile* and NAAT depending on whether the laboratory has a policy with screening symptoms incorporated. In the case of such a policy, the testing could include NAAT alone or EIA as part of a multistep algorithm (GDH plus EIA, GDH plus EIA arbitrated by NAAT, or NAAT plus toxin). If a screening policy is not incorporated, the testing would include EIA as part of a multistep algorithm as outlined above (and not NAAT alone).

TREATMENT: A central tenet to control *C difficile* disease is the discontinuation of precipitating antimicrobial therapy. Stopping these agents will allow competing gut flora to reemerge and, thus, crowd out *C difficile* within the intestine. A variety of therapies are available; use of a particular treatment modality is dependent on severity of illness, the number of recurrences of infection, tolerability of adverse effects, and cost. Recommended therapies for first occurrence, first recurrence, and second recurrence are provided in Table 3.3. Drugs that decrease intestinal motility should not be administered. Asymptomatic patients should not be treated.

To reduce costs, some experts recommend oral administration of the intravenous formulation of vancomycin. The intravenous formulation is less expensive than the product available for oral use. Intravenously administered vancomycin is not effective for *C difficile* disease.

Fidaxomicin is approved for treatment of *C difficile*-associated diarrhea in adults and children 6 months and older. Studies have demonstrated equivalent efficacy to oral vancomycin, although subjects with life-threatening and fulminant infection, hypotension, septic shock, peritoneal signs, significant dehydration, or toxic megacolon were excluded. No comparative data of fidaxomicin to metronidazole are available.

There are limited data on the use of nitazoxanide in the treatment of recurrent *C difficile* disease in adults, but it has not been approved for this indication and no pediatric data are available.

Up to 20% of patients experience a recurrence after discontinuing therapy, but infection usually responds to a second course of the same treatment. Metronidazole should not be used for treatment of a second recurrence or for prolonged therapy, because neurotoxicity is possible. A variety of tapered or pulsed regimens of vancomycin have been used to treat recurrent disease, including the following regimens:

---

[1]McDonald LC, Gerding DN, Johnson S, et al. Clinical practice guidelines for *Clostridium difficile* infection in adults and children: 2017 update by the Infectious Diseases Society of America (IDSA) and Society for Healthcare Epidemiology of America (SHEA). *Clin Infect Dis.* 2018;66(7):e1-e48

Table 3.3. Treatments for *Clostridioides difficile* Disease

Severity	Recommendation
First Occurrence	
Mild-moderate	Metronidazole, 30 mg/kg/day, PO, every 6 h (preferred), or IV, every 6 h for 10 days (maximum 500 mg/dose)
	If failure to respond in 5–7 days: Consider switch to vancomycin, 40 mg/kg/day, PO, every 6 h for 10 days (maximum 125 mg/dose)
	For pregnant/breastfeeding or metronidazole-intolerant patients: Vancomycin, 40 mg/kg/day, PO, every 6 h for 10 days (maximum 125 mg/dose)
	In patients for whom oral therapy cannot reach colon: To above regimen, **ADD** vancomycin, 500 mg/100 mL normal saline, enema, as needed every 8 h until improvement
Severe[a]	Vancomycin, 40 mg/kg/day, PO, every 6 h for 10 days (maximum 125 mg/dose)
Severe and complicated[b]	If no abdominal distension (use both for 10 days): Vancomycin, 40 mg/kg/day, PO, every 6 h (maximum 125 mg/dose) **PLUS** metronidazole, 30 mg/kg/day, IV, every 6 h (maximum 500 mg/dose)
	If complicated with ileus or toxic colitis and/or significant abdominal distension (use all for 10 days): Vancomycin, 40 mg/kg/day, PO, every 6 h (maximum 500 mg/dose) **PLUS** metronidazole, 30 mg/kg/day, IV, every 6h (maximum 500 mg/dose) **PLUS** vancomycin, 500 mg/100 mL normal saline enema, as needed every 8 h until improvement

Severity	Recommendation
First Recurrence	
Mild-moderate	Same regimen as for first occurrence (see above)
Severe	Vancomycin, 40 mg/kg/day, PO, every 6 h (maximum 125 mg/dose)
Second Recurrence	
All	DO NOT USE METRONIDAZOLE Vancomycin, PO, as pulsed or prolonged tapered dose (see text for options)

PO indicates orally; IV, intravenously.

[a] Severe: not well defined in children, but should be considered in the presence of leukocytosis, leukopenia, or worsening renal function.

[b] Severe and complicated: intensive care unit admission, hypotension or shock, pseudomembranous colitis by endoscopy, ileus, toxic megacolon.

- Vancomycin, orally, 10 mg/kg/dose (maximum 125 mg/dose), 4 times a day for 7 days, then 3 times a day for 7 days, then twice a day for 7 days, then once daily for 7 days, then once every other day for 7 days, then every 72 hours for 7 days.
- Vancomycin, orally, 10 mg/kg/dose (maximum 125 mg/dose) 4 times a day for 14 days, then twice a day for 7 to 14 days, then once daily for 7 to 14 days, then every 2 to 3 days for 2 to 8 weeks.
- Vancomycin, orally, 10 mg/kg/dose (maximum 125 mg/dose) 4 times a day for 14 days, then either:
  - Rifaximin, orally, 400 mg, 3 times a day for 14 days (note that rifaximin dosing in pediatric patients is not well described; it is poorly water-soluble and minimally absorbed and should be avoided if the patient recently has received rifaximin for *C difficile* disease or another indication).

    OR
  - Nitazoxanide, orally, 100 mg, twice a day (1–3 years of age), 200 mg, twice a day (4–11 years of age), or 500 mg, twice a day (≥12 years of age) for 10 days.

Fecal transplant (intestinal microbiota transplantation) appears to be effective in adults, but there are limited data in pediatrics. No pediatric data are available evaluating use of human monoclonal antibodies (against toxin A and B); a lower rate of recurrent disease in adult patients receiving antibiotic therapy for primary or recurrent *C difficile* disease is reported in those receiving human monoclonal antibodies. These or other therapies may be appropriate for third recurrences of disease, especially in consultation with an infectious disease or gastroenterology expert. Cholestyramine is not recommended. Other potential adjunctive therapies of unclear efficacy include immune globulin therapy and probiotics (particularly *Saccharomyces boulardii* and kefir).

ISOLATION OF THE HOSPITALIZED PATIENT: In addition to standard precautions, contact precautions and a private room (if feasible) are recommended at the time that disease is suspected through resolution of diarrhea.

CONTROL MEASURES: Exercising meticulous hand hygiene, properly handling contaminated waste (including diapers), disinfecting fomites, and limiting use of antimicrobial agents are the best available methods for control of *C difficile* infection. Gloves should be worn for all in-room care to prevent hand contamination and hand hygiene should be performed immediately after glove removal. Alcohol-based hand hygiene products do not inactivate *C difficile* spores. Washing hands with soap and water is considered to be more effective in removing *C difficile* spores from contaminated hands. There is disagreement among experts about when and whether soap-and-water hand hygiene should be used preferentially over alcohol hand gel in non-outbreak settings. However, in outbreak settings or an increased *C difficile* infection rate,[1] washing hands with soap and water is the preferred method of hand hygiene after each contact with a *C difficile*-infected patient.

Thorough cleaning of hospital rooms and bathrooms of patients with *C difficile* disease, as well as reusable equipment with which infected patients had contact, is essential. Because *C difficile* spores are difficult to kill with standard hospital disinfectants approved by the US Environmental Protection Agency, many health care facilities have instituted the use of disinfectants with sporicidal activity (eg, hypochlorite).

[1]McDonald LC, Gerding DN, Johnson S, et al. Clinical practice guidelines for *Clostridium difficile* infection in adults and children: 2017 update by the Infectious Diseases Society of America (IDSA) and Society for Healthcare Epidemiology of America (SHEA). *Clin Infect Dis.* 2018;66(7):e1-e48

Children with *C difficile* diarrhea should be excluded from child care settings until stools are contained in the diaper or the child is continent and stool frequency is no more than 2 stools above that child's normal frequency for the time the child is in the program, and infection-control measures should be enforced.

Clostridium perfringens Foodborne Illness

CLINICAL MANIFESTATIONS: *Clostridium perfringens* foodborne illness is characterized by a sudden onset of watery diarrhea and moderate-to-severe crampy, mid-epigastric pain. Symptoms usually resolve within 24 hours. The shorter incubation period, shorter duration of illness, and absence of fever in most patients differentiates *C perfringens* foodborne disease from shigellosis and salmonellosis. As compared with foodborne illnesses associated with heavy metals, *Staphylococcus aureus* enterotoxins, *Bacillus cereus* emetic toxin, and fish and shellfish toxins, *C perfringens* foodborne illness is infrequently associated with vomiting. Diarrheal illness caused by *B cereus* diarrheal enterotoxins can be indistinguishable from that caused by *C perfringens* (see Appendix VI, Clinical Syndromes Associated With Foodborne Diseases, p 1041). Necrotizing colitis and death have been described in patients with disease attributable to type A *C perfringens* who received antidiarrheal medications resulting in constipation. Enteritis necroticans (also known as pigbel) results from hemorrhagic necrosis of the midgut and is a cause of severe illness and death attributable to *C perfringens* infection caused by contamination with *Clostridium* strains carrying a β toxin. Rare cases have been reported in the highlands of Papua New Guinea and in Thailand; protein malnutrition is an important risk factor. Additionally, enteritis necroticans has been reported in a child with poorly controlled diabetes in the United States who consumed chitterlings (pig intestine).

ETIOLOGY: Typical infection is caused by a heat-labile *C perfringens* enterotoxin, produced during sporulation in the small intestine. *C perfringens* type F (formerly *cpe*-positive type A), which produces α toxin and enterotoxin, commonly causes foodborne illness. Enteritis necroticans is caused by *C perfringens* type C, which produces a β toxin that causes necrotizing small bowel inflammation.

EPIDEMIOLOGY: *C perfringens* is a gram-positive, spore-forming bacillus that is ubiquitous in the environment and the intestinal tracts of humans and animals and is commonly present in raw meat and poultry. Spores of *C perfringens* that survive cooking can germinate and multiply rapidly during slow cooling, when stored at temperatures from 20°C to 60°C (68°F–140°F), and during inadequate reheating. At an optimum temperature, *C perfringens* has one of the fastest rates of growth of any bacterium. Illness results from consumption of food containing high numbers of vegetative organisms ($>10^5$ colony forming units/g) that produce enterotoxin in the intestine of the consumer.

Ingestion of the organism is most commonly associated with foods prepared by restaurants or caterers or in institutional settings (eg, schools and camps) where food is prepared in large quantities, cooled slowly, and stored inappropriately for prolonged periods. Beef, poultry, gravies, and dried or precooked foods are the most commonly implicated sources. Illness is not transmissible from person to person.

The **incubation period** is 6 to 24 hours, usually 8 to 12 hours.

DIAGNOSTIC TESTS: Because the fecal flora of healthy people commonly includes *C perfringens*, counts of *C perfringens* of 10^6 colony-forming units (CFU)/g of feces or greater obtained within 48 hours of onset of illness support the diagnosis in ill people. The diagnosis also can be supported by detection of enterotoxin in stool. *C perfringens* can be confirmed as the cause of an outbreak if 10^6 CFU/g are isolated from stool, enterotoxin is demonstrated in the stool of 2 or more ill people, or the concentration of organisms is at least 10^5 CFU/g in the implicated food. Although *C perfringens* is an anaerobe, special transport conditions are unnecessary. Whole stool, rather than rectal swab specimens, should be obtained, transported in ice packs, and tested within 24 hours. For enumeration and enterotoxin testing, obtaining stool specimens in bulk without added transport media is required.

TREATMENT: *C perfringens* foodborne illness is typically self-limited. Oral rehydration or, occasionally, intravenous fluid and electrolyte replacement may be indicated to prevent or treat dehydration. Antimicrobial agents are not indicated.

ISOLATION OF THE HOSPITALIZED PATIENT: Standard precautions are recommended.

CONTROL MEASURES: Preventive measures depend on limiting proliferation of *C perfringens* in foods by cooking foods thoroughly and maintaining food at warmer than 60°C (140°F) or cooler than 7°C (45°F). Meat dishes should be served hot. Foods should never be held at room temperature to cool; they should be refrigerated in shallow containers after removal from warming devices or serving tables as soon as possible and within 2 hours of preparation. Information on recommended safe food handling practices, including time and temperature requirements during cooking, storage, and reheating, can be found at **www.foodsafety.gov.**

Coccidioidomycosis

CLINICAL MANIFESTATIONS: Coccidioidomycosis, also called valley fever, is an infection caused by the fungus *Coccidioides*. Primary pulmonary infection is acquired by inhaling fungal conidia and is asymptomatic or self-limited in 60% to 65% of infected children and adults. Constitutional symptoms, including extreme fatigue and weight loss, are common and can persist for weeks or months. Symptomatic disease can resemble influenza or community-acquired pneumonia, with malaise, fever, cough, myalgia, arthralgia, headache, and chest pain. Pleural effusion, empyema, and mediastinal involvement are more common in children.

Acute infection may be associated only with cutaneous abnormalities, such as erythema multiforme, an erythematous maculopapular rash, or erythema nodosum manifesting as bilateral symmetrical violaceous nodules usually overlying the shins. Chronic pulmonary lesions are rare, but approximately 5% of infected people develop asymptomatic pulmonary radiographic residua (eg, cysts, nodules, cavitary lesions, coin lesions).

Nonpulmonary primary infection is rare and usually follows trauma associated with contamination of wounds by arthroconidia. Cutaneous lesions and soft tissue infections often are accompanied by regional lymphadenitis.

Disseminated (extrapulmonary) infection occurs in less than 0.5% of infected people; common sites of dissemination include skin, bones, joints, and the central nervous system (CNS). Meningitis is invariably fatal if untreated. Congenital infection is rare.

ETIOLOGY: *Coccidioides* species are dimorphic fungi. In soil, *Coccidioides* organisms exist in the mycelial phase as mold that grows as branching, septate hyphae. Infectious arthroconidia (ie, spores) produced from hyphae become airborne, infecting the host after inhalation or, rarely, inoculation. In tissues, arthroconidia enlarge to form spherules; mature spherules release hundreds to thousands of endospores that develop into new spherules and continue the tissue cycle. Molecular studies have divided the genus *Coccidioides* into 2 species: *Coccidioides immitis,* confined mainly to California, and *Coccidioides posadasii,* encompassing the remaining areas of distribution of the fungus within certain deserts of the southwestern United States, northern Mexico, and areas of Central and South America.

EPIDEMIOLOGY: *Coccidioides* species are found mostly in soil in areas of the southwestern United States with endemic infection, including California, Arizona, New Mexico, west and south Texas, southern Nevada, and Utah; northern Mexico; and throughout certain parts of Central and South America. Areas of endemicity may extend beyond traditionally defined ranges.

In areas with endemic coccidioidomycosis, clusters of cases can follow dust-generating events, such as storms, seismic events, archaeological digging, and recreational and construction activities, including building of solar farms. The majority of cases occur without a known preceding event.

Infection is believed to provide lifelong immunity. Person-to-person transmission of coccidioidomycosis does not occur except in rare instances of cutaneous infection with actively draining lesions, donor-derived transmission via an infected organ, or congenital infection following in utero exposure. People with impairment of T-lymphocyte–mediated immunity caused by a congenital immune defect or HIV infection or those receiving immune-modulating medications (eg, tumor necrosis factor [TNF] alpha antagonists) are at major risk for severe primary coccidioidomycosis, disseminated disease, or relapse of past infection. Other people at elevated risk for severe or disseminated disease include people of African or Filipino ancestry, women in the third trimester of pregnancy and those postpartum, and children younger than 1 year. Cases may occur in people who do not reside in regions with endemic infection but who previously have visited these areas, including months or even years previously. In regions without endemic infection, careful travel histories should be obtained from people with symptoms or findings compatible with coccidioidomycosis.

The **incubation period** typically is 1 to 3 weeks in primary infection. Disseminated infection may develop years after primary infection.

DIAGNOSTIC TESTS: Diagnosis of coccidioidomycosis is best established using serologic, histopathologic, and culture methods. Nucleic acid amplification tests have been developed but are not widely available.

Serologic tests are useful in the diagnosis and management of infection. One approach is to test first with EIA, then perform immunodiffusion testing if the EIA result is positive. The former is more sensitive, the latter more specific. The immunoglobulin (Ig) M response can be detected by enzyme immunoassay (EIA) or immunodiffusion methods. IgM is detected in the first and third weeks, respectively, in approximately 50% and 90% of primary infections, but an EIA positive result by IgM alone should be interpreted with caution because of the low specificity of this test. IgG response can be detected by immunodiffusion, EIA, or complement fixation (CF) tests. Immunodiffusion is considered more specific, whereas CF is more sensitive. A combination of both CF and immunodiffusion tests is often helpful in diagnosis, although both immunodiffusion and especially CF are known to cross-react with *Histoplasma* organisms. Serum antibodies detected by CF usually are of low titer and are transient if the disease is asymptomatic or mild; persistent high titers (≥1:16) occur with severe disease and are almost always seen in disseminated infection. Cerebrospinal fluid (CSF) antibodies also are detectable by immunodiffusion or CF testing. Increasing serum and CSF titers indicate progressive disease, and decreasing titers usually suggest improvement. Antibody titers detected by CF may not be reliable in immunocompromised patients; low or nondetectable titers in immunocompromised patients should be interpreted with caution.

Spherules are as large as 80 μm in diameter and can be visualized with 100x to 400x magnification in infected body fluid specimens (eg, pleural fluid, bronchoalveolar lavage) and biopsy specimens of skin lesions or organs. Use of silver or period-acid Schiff staining is helpful for biopsy specimens. The presence of a mature spherule with endospores is pathognomonic of infection. Isolation of *Coccidioides* species in culture establishes the diagnosis, even in patients with mild symptoms. When a specimen from a patient suspected of having coccidioidomycosis is sent for culture, the diagnostic laboratory should be alerted. Culture of organisms is possible on a variety of artificial media but is hazardous to laboratory personnel, because spherules can convert to arthroconidia-bearing mycelia on culture plates. Suspect cultures should be sealed and handled using appropriate safety equipment and procedures. A DNA probe can identify *Coccidioides* species in cultures.

At least one commercial laboratory offers an EIA test for urine, serum, plasma, CSF, or bronchoalveolar lavage fluid for detection of *Coccidioides* antigen. Antigen may be positive in patients with more severe forms of disease (sensitivity 71%) in a study of immunosuppressed patients. Cross-reactions occur in patients with histoplasmosis, blastomycosis, or paracoccidioidomycosis.

TREATMENT[1]: Antifungal therapy is not recommended routinely for uncomplicated asymptomatic primary infection in people without risk factors for severe disease. Although most mild cases will resolve without therapy, some experts believe that treatment may reduce illness duration or risk of severe complications. Most experts recommend treatment of coccidioidomycosis with fluconazole for 3 to 6 months for people at risk of severe disease or people with severe primary infection. During pregnancy, amphotericin B (including lipid formulations) is the treatment of choice over fluconazole and other azole antifungals, as fluconazole has been demonstrated to be a teratogen in early pregnancy. Follow-up every 1 to 3 months for up to 2 years, either to document radiographic resolution or to identify residual abnormalities or pulmonary or extrapulmonary complications, is recommended. For diffuse pneumonia, defined as bilateral reticulonodular or miliary infiltrates, amphotericin B or high-dose fluconazole is recommended. Amphotericin B is used more frequently in the presence of severe hypoxemia or rapid clinical deterioration. The total length of therapy for diffuse pneumonia is 1 year.

Oral fluconazole or itraconazole is the recommended initial therapy for disseminated infection not involving the CNS. Amphotericin B is recommended as alternative therapy if lesions are progressing or are in critical locations, such as the vertebral column, or in fulminant infections because it is believed to result in more rapid improvement.

Consultation with a specialist for treatment of patients with CNS disease caused by *Coccidioides* species is recommended. High-dose oral fluconazole (adult dose: 400–1200 mg/day) is recommended for treatment of patients with CNS infection. Patients who respond to azole therapy should continue this treatment indefinitely (for the remainder of life). For CNS infections that are unresponsive to oral azoles or are associated with severe

[1]Galgiani JN, Ampel NM, Blair JE, et al. 2016 Infectious Diseases Society of America (IDSA) clinical practice guideline for the treatment of coccidioidomycosis. *Clin Infect Dis.* 2016;63(6):e112-e146. Available at: **https:// doi.org/10.1093/cid/ciw360**

basilar inflammation, intrathecal amphotericin B deoxycholate therapy can be used to augment the azole therapy. A subcutaneous reservoir can facilitate administration into the cisternal space or lateral ventricle. Hydrocephalus is a common complication of coccidioidal meningitis and nearly always requires a shunt for decompression.

There are reports of success with voriconazole, posaconazole, and isavuconazole in treatment of coccidioidomycosis, but this has not been established in children. These newer agents may be administered in certain clinical settings, such as therapeutic failure in severe coccidioidal disease (eg, meningitis). When used, these newer azoles should be administered in consultation with experts experienced with their use in treatment of coccidioidomycosis.

The duration of antifungal therapy is variable and depends on the site(s) of involvement, clinical response, and mycologic and immunologic test results. In general, therapy is continued until clinical and laboratory evidence indicates that active infection has resolved. Treatment for disseminated coccidioidomycosis is at least 6 months but for some patients may be extended to 1 year or longer. The role of subsequent suppressive azole therapy is uncertain, except for patients with CNS infection, osteomyelitis, or underlying human immunodeficiency virus (HIV) infection or for solid organ transplant recipients. Coccidioidal meningitis requires lifelong therapy. The duration of suppressive therapy also may be lifelong for other high-risk groups.[1] Women should be advised to avoid pregnancy while receiving fluconazole, which is known to be teratogenic.

Surgical débridement or excision of lesions in bone, pericardium, and lung has been advocated for localized, symptomatic, persistent, resistant, or progressive lesions. In some localized infections with sinuses, fistulae, or abscesses, amphotericin B has been instilled locally or used for irrigation of wounds. Antifungal prophylaxis for solid organ transplant recipients may be considered if they reside in areas with endemicity and have prior serologic evidence or a history of coccidioidomycosis.

ISOLATION OF THE HOSPITALIZED PATIENT: Standard precautions are recommended. Care should be taken in handling, changing, and discarding dressings, casts, and similar materials through which arthroconidial contamination could occur.

CONTROL MEASURES: Coccidioidomycosis is a reportable disease in many states and some countries. Measures to control dust are recommended in areas with endemic infection, including construction sites, archaeological project sites, or other locations where activities cause excessive soil disturbance. Immunocompromised people residing in or traveling to areas with endemic infection should be counseled to avoid exposure to activities that may aerosolize spores in contaminated soil.

Coronaviruses, Including SARS-CoV-2 and MERS-CoV

CLINICAL MANIFESTATIONS: Novel coronavirus disease 2019 (COVID-19), caused by severe acute respiratory syndrome coronavirus 2 (SARS-CoV-2), emerged in China in late 2019. The most common presenting symptoms of COVID-19 in children are fever and cough; other symptoms can include shortness of breath, sore throat, headache, myalgia, fatigue, and, less frequently, rhinorrhea. Gastrointestinal symptoms such as nausea,

---

[1]Panel on Opportunistic Infections in HIV-Exposed and HIV-Infected Children. Guidelines for the Prevention and Treatment of Opportunistic Infections in HIV-Exposed and HIV-Infected Children. Department of Health and Human Services. Available at: **https://clinicalinfo.hiv.gov/sites/default/files/inline-files/oi_guidelines_pediatrics.pdf**

vomiting, diarrhea, and poor appetite may occur, with or without respiratory symptoms. Less frequently, infected people can experience anosmia (loss of smell) or ageusia (loss of taste); these occur more commonly in adolescents than in younger children. Conjunctivitis and rashes also have been reported. Children generally have mild disease or may be asymptomatic, although severe and even fatal cases have occurred. Children with obesity or medical comorbidities are at risk for more severe disease. Children from racial or ethnic minority groups may be at higher risk for severe illness. Complications include respiratory failure, acute cardiac injury, acute kidney injury, shock, coagulopathy, and multiorgan failure. Diabetic ketoacidosis and intussusception also have been reported. Laboratory findings may be normal or may include lymphopenia, leukopenia, elevated C-reactive protein or procalcitonin, and elevated alanine aminotransferase and aspartate aminotransferase. Chest imaging may be normal or there may be unilateral or bilateral lung involvement with multiple areas of consolidation and ground glass opacities.

Multisystem inflammatory syndrome in children (MIS-C) may present during or weeks following SARS-CoV-2 infection. Children present with fever, severe disease of ≥2 organ systems (cardiac, gastrointestinal tract, skin, kidney, neurologic, hematologic, or respiratory tract), and laboratory evidence of inflammation. The case definition from the Centers for Disease Control and Prevention (CDC; **www.cdc.gov/mis-c/ hcp/**) includes no alternative diagnosis in addition to evidence of recent or concurrent SARS-CoV-2 infection or exposure to someone with known or suspected COVID-19 within the past 4 weeks. Children with MIS-C often present with severe abdominal pain, and many have features that can be similar to Kawasaki disease. Children with MIS-C may have echocardiographic abnormalities, including myocarditis and coronary artery abnormalities.

Human coronaviruses (HCoVs) 229E, OC43, NL63, and HKU1 are associated most frequently with an upper respiratory tract infection characterized by rhinorrhea, nasal congestion, sore throat, sneezing, and cough that may be associated with mild fever. Symptoms are self-limited and typically peak on day 3 or 4 of illness. These HCoV infections also may be associated with acute otitis media or asthma exacerbations. Less frequently, they are associated with lower respiratory tract infections, including bronchiolitis, croup, and pneumonia, primarily in infants and children and adults who are immunocompromised.

MERS-CoV, the virus associated with the Middle East respiratory syndrome (MERS), can cause severe disease, but asymptomatic infections and mild disease may occur. Most cases have been identified in adult males with comorbidities. Infections in children are uncommon and typically are milder. Patients initially present with fever, myalgia, and chills followed by a nonproductive cough and dyspnea a few days later. Approximately 25% of patients may experience vomiting, diarrhea, or abdominal pain. Rapid deterioration of oxygenation with progressive unilateral or bilateral airspace infiltrates on chest imaging may follow, requiring mechanical ventilation and often associated with acute renal failure. The case fatality rate is high, estimated at 36%, but may partially reflect surveillance bias for more severe disease. Surprisingly, this case-fatality rate for hospitalized patients has remained higher than 30% for all new cases since 2012 despite improved diagnostics and supportive care. Laboratory abnormalities may include thrombocytopenia, lymphopenia, and increased lactate dehydrogenase (LDH) concentration, particularly among severely infected individuals.

SARS-CoV-1 was responsible for the 2002–2003 global outbreak of SARS, which was associated with severe symptoms, although a spectrum of disease including asymptomatic infections and mild disease occurred. Infections in children were less severe than in adults and typically presented with fever, cough, and rhinorrhea. Adolescents with SARS had clinical courses more closely resembling those of adult disease, presenting with fever, myalgia, headache, and chills. No deaths in children or adolescents from SARS-CoV-1 infection were documented.

ETIOLOGY: Coronaviruses are enveloped, nonsegmented, single-stranded, positive-sense RNA viruses named after their crown- or Latin "corona"-like surface projections observed on electron microscopy that correspond to large surface spike proteins. Coronaviruses are classified in the *Nidovirales* order. Coronaviruses are host specific and can infect humans as well as a variety of different animals, causing diverse clinical syndromes. Four distinct genera have been described: *Alphacoronavirus*, *Betacoronavirus*, *Gammacoronavirus*, and *Deltacoronavirus*. HCoVs 229E and NL63 belong to the genus *Alphacoronavirus*. HCoVs OC43 and HKU1 belong to lineage A, SARS-CoV-1 and SARS-CoV-2 belong to lineage B, and MERS-CoV belongs to lineage C of the genus *Betacoronavirus*.

EPIDEMIOLOGY: SARS-CoV-2 emerged in Wuhan, China, near the end of 2019. Infection rapidly spread throughout Hubei province and across China. In January 2020, cases were detected outside of China (the first US case was reported on January 21, 2020). The World Health Organization (WHO) declared SARS-CoV-2 a "public health emergency of international concern" on January 30, 2020, and the United States declared a "public health emergency" the following day. A global pandemic was declared by the WHO on March 11, 2020. By March 2021, more than 112 million cases and 2.5 million deaths were reported globally, with approximately 28 million cases and 500 000 deaths in the United States. Children constitute approximately 10% of US cases. MIS-C is a rare diagnosis, with just over 2000 cases and approximately 30 deaths in the US by early February 2021; most cases occurred in children age 1-14 years, with an average age of 8 years. Additional information on COVID-19 and the fast-moving pandemic can be found at **www.cdc.gov/coronavirus/2019-ncov/index.html.**

SARS-CoV-2 is transmitted efficiently between people, including from presymptomatic, symptomatic, and asymptomatic people. Infection is believed to be primarily through transmission of large and small respiratory droplets and particles among people in close proximity (generally within 6 feet), although transmission can occur at larger distances. Aerosol transmission, which essentially is spread from very small droplets that can remain suspended in the air for longer periods of time, also can occur. Crowded, enclosed, and poorly ventilated spaces are particularly concerning environments for the transmission of SARS-CoV-2. Infected people are believed to be infectious 2 days prior to symptom onset through 10 days after symptom onset, with viral loads being higher earlier in the course of infection and with decreasing infectivity as time progresses. Patients with severe disease or who are severely immunocompromised may shed viable virus for longer than 10 days. Health care-associated transmission occurs with SARS-CoV-2, and strict adherence to infection prevention guidance is necessary. Outbreaks of SARS-CoV-2 infection occur readily in congregate settings (eg, long-term care facilities, group homes, prisons, shelters, congregate workplaces, dormitories) and households.

HCoVs 229E, OC43, NL63, and HKU1 can be found worldwide. They cause most disease in the winter and spring months in temperate climates. Seroprevalence data for these HCoVs suggest that exposure is common in early childhood, with approximately 90% of adults being seropositive for HCoVs 229E, OC43, and NL63 and 60% being seropositive for HCoV HKU1. The modes of transmission for HCoVs 229E, OC43, NL63, and HKU1 have not been well studied. However, on the basis of studies of other respiratory tract viruses, it is likely that transmission occurs primarily via a combination of droplet and direct and indirect contact spread. HCoVs 229E and OC43 are most likely to be transmitted during the first few days of illness, when symptoms and respiratory viral loads are at their highest.

MERS-CoV likely evolved from bat coronaviruses and infected dromedary camels, which now demonstrate seroprevalence and infection with MERS-CoV in parts of the Middle East and Africa. MERS-CoV cases continue mostly in the Middle East, primarily linked to close contact with camels or an infected person. Human-to-human transmission occurs generally in health care settings and less frequently in household settings and is believed to occur most commonly through droplet and contact spread, although airborne spread may occur. Updated figures on global cases can be found on the WHO website (**www.who.int/emergencies/mers-cov/en/**).

SARS-CoV-1 likely evolved from a natural reservoir of SARS-CoV-like viruses in horseshoe bats through civet cats or intermediate animal hosts in wet markets of China. Public health interventions ultimately aborted the epidemic. SARS-CoV-1 was last reported with human disease in 2004 from laboratory acquired infections.

The **incubation period** for SARS-CoV-2 is 2 to 14 days (median, 5 days). The **incubation period** for HCoV-229E is 2 to 5 days (median, 3 days). Further study is needed to confirm the incubation periods for HCoVs OC43, NL63, and HKU1. The **incubation period** for MERS-CoV is estimated to be 2 to 14 days (median 5 days).

DIAGNOSTIC TESTS: Acute SARS-CoV-2 infection can be diagnosed by detection of viral RNA from a respiratory source from the upper or lower airway (eg, nasopharynx, oropharynx, nose, saliva, trachea) through reverse transcriptase-polymerase chain reaction (RT-PCR) assay (some may be multiplex assays) or through direct antigen testing for SARS-CoV-2 from a nasopharyngeal or nasal specimen. Serologic testing is not helpful for the diagnosis of acute SARS-CoV-2 infection but can be used in the diagnosis of MIS-C. Additional information on SARS-CoV-2 assays can be found on the CDC and Food and Drug Administration (FDA) websites (**www.cdc.gov/coronavirus/2019-ncov/ hcp/testing-overview.html** and **www.fda.gov/medical-devices/coronavirus-disease-2019-covid-19-emergency-use-authorizations-medical-devices/ vitro-diagnostics-euas**).

Multiplex assays for respiratory pathogens are commercially available that include HCoVs 229E, OC43, NL63, and HKU1 as targets. State public health departments should be contacted for evaluation of suspected cases of MERS-CoV using RT-PCR assay. Guidance regarding testing for MERS-CoV (including specimen collection, typically upper respiratory, lower respiratory and serum) is available on the CDC MERS website (**www.cdc.gov/coronavirus/mers/guidelines-clinical-specimens.html**).

TREATMENT: Treatment of COVID-19 is evolving rapidly. The National Institutes of Health (**www.covid19treatmentguidelines.nih.gov/**) and the Infectious Diseases Society of America (**www.idsociety.org/practice-guideline/covid-19-guideline-treatment-and-management/**) have updated information on treatment for

COVID-19 on their websites. As of the end of February 2021, remdesivir has received FDA approval for use in children ≥12 years (≥40 kg) and adults who are hospitalized with COVID-19, in whom the medication shortens hospitalization, and has received emergency use authorization (EUA) for use in younger children. In adults, use of dexamethasone in COVID-19 hospitalized patients requiring oxygen or invasive mechanical ventilation has improved survival. Use of convalescent plasma in children with COVID-19 is under investigation. A number of monoclonal antibody therapies are under investigation, with at least 3 (bamlanivimab, as monotherapy or in combination with etesevimab, and the combination of casirivimab and imdevimab) receiving EUA for use in infected nonhospitalized children ≥12 years (≥40 kg) and adults who are at high risk of severe COVID-19.

For the treatment of MIS-C, the American Academy of Pediatrics (**https://services.aap.org/en/pages/2019-novel-coronavirus-covid-19-infections/clinical-guidance/multisystem-inflammatory-syndrome-in-children-mis-c-interim-guidance/**), CDC (**www.cdc.gov/mis-c/hcp/**), and American College of Rheumatology[1] have developed interim guidance. As of March 2021, there are no trials evaluating efficacy of treatment options. A multidisciplinary approach, with the involvement of pediatric specialists in cardiology, rheumatology, infectious disease, hematology, immunology, and critical care, is recommended to guide individual management. In addition to supportive care, therapies have included Immune Globulin Intravenous (1–2 g/kg), steroids, biologics (anakinra), and prophylaxis or treatment of thromboses.

Infections attributable to HCoVs HKU1, OC43, 229E, and NL63 are treated with supportive care. No controlled trials have been conducted for treatment of MERS-CoV.

ISOLATION OF THE HOSPITALIZED PATIENT: Airborne, droplet, and contact precautions are recommended for patients with suspected or known SARS-CoV-2 or MERS-CoV infection (including eye protection [face shield or goggles], N95 or higher respirator [or medical mask if not available], gown, and gloves; for aerosol-generating procedures, an N95 or higher respirator should be used). Airborne infection isolation rooms should be prioritized for aerosol-generating procedures. A well-ventilated single-occupancy room with a closed door may be used if aerosol-generating procedures are not performed. Detailed guidance is available on the CDC website (**www.cdc.gov/coronavirus/2019-ncov/hcp/infection-control-recommendations.html**).

For other HCoV infections, in addition to standard precautions, health care professionals should use droplet and contact precautions when examining and caring for infants and young children.

CONTROL MEASURES: When SARS-CoV-2 is circulating in a community, control measures include use of face masks for children 2 years and older and for adults (**www.cdc.gov/coronavirus/2019-ncov/more/masking-science-sars-cov2.html**), keeping a 6-foot or greater distance from other people whenever possible, and hand hygiene. During the COVID-19 pandemic, jurisdictions have specific guidance and policies regarding community mitigation, and referral to state, local, and CDC websites is recommended. The AAP (**https://services.aap.org/en/**

---

[1] Henderson LA, Canna SW, Friedman KG, et al. American College of Rheumatology Clinical Guidance for Multisystem Inflammatory Syndrome in Children Associated With SARS–CoV-2 and Hyperinflammation in Pediatric COVID-19: Version 1. *Arthritis Rheumatol*. 2020;72(11):1791-1805. Available at: **https://doi.org/10.1002/art.41454**

pages/2019-novel-coronavirus-covid-19-infections/clinical-guidance/) and other professional organizations have also developed guidance. Practicing appropriate hand and respiratory hygiene can help curb spread of all respiratory tract viruses, including coronaviruses. Cleaning and disinfection of high-touch environmental surfaces using standard disinfectants should decrease the potential for indirect transmission of coronaviruses via fomites.

As of February 2021, 2 mRNA vaccines and 1 nonreplicating viral vector vaccine for SARS-CoV-2 have received EUA status from the FDA. Numerous additional vaccines using different platforms are in varying stages of development. Pediatric vaccine studies are underway. Recommendations for use of these vaccines in children will be issued by the CDC Advisory Committee on Immunization Practices (**www.cdc.gov/vaccines/hcp/acip-recs**) and the AAP.

MERS-CoV transmission within hospitals and households can be averted with case identification and the use of infection control and public health measures, including contact tracing. However, preventing the transmission of MERS-CoV from camels to humans is more challenging, given the prevalent use of camels in some Middle East countries. Most experts believe that sporadic transmission will continue until an effective MERS-CoV vaccine is found. Several candidate vaccines are currently in human trials.

Cryptococcus neoformans and *Cryptococcus gattii* Infections (Cryptococcosis)

CLINICAL MANIFESTATIONS: Primary pulmonary infection is acquired by inhalation of aerosolized *Cryptococcus* fungal propagules found in contaminated soil or organic material (eg, trees, rotting wood, and bird guano), and infection often is asymptomatic or mild. Pulmonary disease, when symptomatic, is characterized by cough, chest pain, and constitutional symptoms. Chest radiographs may reveal solitary or multiple masses; patchy, segmental, or lobar consolidation, which often is multifocal; or a nodular or reticulonodular pattern with interstitial changes. Pulmonary cryptococcosis may present as acute respiratory distress syndrome (ARDS) and can mimic *Pneumocystis* pneumonia. Hematogenous dissemination occurs particularly to the central nervous system (CNS) but also to bones, skin, and other body sites. Disseminated cryptococcosis is generally rare in children and almost always occurs in children with defects in T-lymphocyte–mediated immunity, including children with leukemia or lymphoma, those taking corticosteroids, children with congenital immunodeficiency such as hyperimmunoglobulin M syndrome or severe combined immunodeficiency syndrome, those with acquired immunodeficiency syndrome (AIDS), or those who have undergone solid organ transplantation. Several sites usually are infected, but manifestations of involvement at one site predominate. Cryptococcal meningitis, the most common and serious form of cryptococcal disease, often follows an indolent course but symptoms can be more acute in severely immunosuppressed patients. Symptoms are often typical of those of meningitis, meningoencephalitis, or space-occupying lesions, but sometimes manifest only as subtle, nonspecific findings such as fever, headache, or behavioral changes. Cryptococcal fungemia without apparent organ involvement occurs in patients with human immunodeficiency virus (HIV) infection but is rare in children.

ETIOLOGY: There are more than 30 species of *Cryptococcus*, but only 2, *Cryptococcus neoformans* (var *neoformans* and var *grubii*) and *Cryptococcus gattii*, are regarded as human pathogens. These 2 species have been divided into approximately 10 genotypes or sibling species. Further taxonomic studies and disease correlations are anticipated to aid in understanding the clinical relevance of these groups.

EPIDEMIOLOGY: *C neoformans* var *neoformans* and *C neoformans* var *grubii* are isolated primarily from soil contaminated with pigeon or other bird droppings and cause most human infections, especially infections in immunocompromised hosts. *C neoformans* infects 5% to 10% of adults with AIDS, but cryptococcal disease is rare in HIV-infected and non–HIV-infected children. *C gattii* is associated with certain trees and the surrounding soil and has emerged as a pathogen producing a respiratory syndrome with or without neurologic findings in individuals from British Columbia, Canada, the Pacific Northwest region of the United States, and occasionally other regions of the United States. A high frequency of disease also has been reported in Aboriginal people in Australia and in the central province of Papua New Guinea. *C gattii* causes disease in both immunocompetent and immunocompromised individuals, and cases have been reported in children. Person-to-person transmission generally does not occur with cryptococcal species.

The **incubation period** for *C neoformans* is unknown but likely variable; dissemination often represents reactivation of latent disease acquired previously. The **incubation period** for *C gattii* is estimated at 8 weeks to 13 months based on outbreak investigations, but these figures also are imprecise.

DIAGNOSTIC TESTS: The cerebrospinal fluid (CSF) profile of cryptococcal meningoencephalitis is characterized by low cell counts, low glucose, and elevated protein. Opening pressure may be markedly elevated, especially in HIV-infected individuals. Laboratory diagnosis of cryptococcal infection is best performed using cryptococcal antigen (CRAG) detection methods or by culture. The latex agglutination test, lateral flow immunoassay, and enzyme immunoassay for detection of cryptococcal capsular polysaccharide antigen (galactoxylomannan) in serum or CSF specimens are excellent rapid diagnostic tests for those with suspected meningitis. CRAG is detected in CSF or serum specimens from more than 95% of patients with cryptococcal meningitis. Antigen test results can be falsely negative when antigen concentrations are very high (prozone effect), which can be addressed by dilution of samples. CRAG assays are less useful in following response to therapy than they are in diagnosis. Accuracy, ease of use, and cost have made the lateral flow immunoassay, which shows good agreement with standard CRAG testing, a common test in both resource-available and resource-limited settings and has allowed pre-emptive management strategies for adults in high incidence areas of HIV infection.

Definitive diagnosis requires isolation of the yeast from body fluid or tissue specimens. Encapsulated yeast cells can be visualized using India ink or other stains of CSF and bronchoalveolar lavage specimens, but this method has limited sensitivity and is not recommended as a stand-alone rapid test. CSF specimens may contain only a few organisms, and a large quantity of CSF may be needed to recover the organism. Automated blood culture systems are acceptable for growing *Cryptococcus*. Sabouraud dextrose agar is useful for isolation of *Cryptococcus* organisms from sputum, bronchopulmonary lavage, tissue, or CSF specimens. Differentiation between *C neoformans* and *C gattii* can be made by the use of the selective medium L-canavanine, glycine, bromothymol blue (CGB) agar. A MALDI-TOF (matrix-assisted laser desorption/ionization time-of-flight) mass spectrometer can identify yeasts to species level accurately and rapidly. Polymerase chain multiplex reaction assays are available (BioFire) but may miss low burden infections with yeasts. Focal pulmonary or skin lesions can be biopsied for fungal staining and culture. Although there are Clinical & Laboratory Standards Institute standards for in vitro cryptococcal susceptibility testing, there are no break point interpretations; therefore, generally, a three-fold change in minimum inhibitory concentration is evidence for direct resistance.

TREATMENT: Practice management guidelines for cryptococcal disease are available.[1,2,3] No trials dedicated to children have been performed, so optimal dosing and duration of therapy for children with cryptococcal infection have not been determined precisely. Amphotericin B deoxycholate (1 mg/kg/day), liposomal amphotericin B (5–7.5 mg/kg/day), or amphotericin B lipid complex (5 mg/kg/day) is indicated in combination with oral flucytosine (25 mg/kg/dose, 4 times/day when renal function is normal) as first-line induction therapy for pediatric patients with meningeal and/or other serious cryptococcal infections (see Antifungal Drugs for Systemic Fungal Infections, p 905). Frequent monitoring of blood counts and/or serum peak flucytosine concentrations (with a target of 40 to 60 µg/mL 2 hours after the dose) are recommended to prevent neutropenia. Patients with meningitis should receive induction combination therapy for at least 2 weeks and until a repeat CSF culture is negative, followed by consolidation therapy with fluconazole (10–12 mg/kg/day in 2 divided daily doses; maximum 800 mg day) for a minimum of 8 weeks. If flucytosine cannot be administered, amphotericin B alone has been successfully used in pediatric cryptococcosis, or amphotericin B can be combined with fluconazole for the induction phase of therapy. A lumbar puncture should be performed after 2 weeks of therapy to document microbiologic clearance. The 20% to 40% of patients in whom culture is positive after 2 weeks of therapy will require a more prolonged induction treatment course. For any relapse, induction antifungal therapy should be restarted for 4 to 10 weeks, CSF cultures should be repeated every 2 weeks until sterile, and antifungal susceptibility of the relapse isolate should be determined and compared to the original isolate. Monitoring of serum CRAG is not useful to determine response to therapy in patients with cryptococcal meningitis.

Increased intracranial pressure occurs frequently despite microbiologic response and often is associated with clinical deterioration. Significant elevation of intracranial pressure is a major source of morbidity and should be managed with frequent repeated lumbar punctures or placement of a lumbar drain in those with high intracranial pressures and symptoms. Immune reconstitution inflammatory syndrome (IRIS) is described in children, and although there are no guidelines for specific management of IRIS in children, a patient should be monitored closely for signs and symptoms associated with symptomatic central nervous system IRIS and a steroid taper should be considered for management. In antiretroviral-naive patients with newly diagnosed cryptococcal meningitis or disseminated disease, delay in potent antiretroviral therapy may be prudent until the end of the first 2 weeks of induction therapy; further delays in initiating combined antiretroviral therapy, especially in resource-limited settings, should be individualized.[3]

[1] Perfect J, Dismukes WE, Dromer F, et al. Clinical practice guidelines for the management of cryptococcal disease: 2010 update by the Infectious Diseases Society of America. *Clin Infect Dis*. 2010;50(3):291-322

[2] Panel on Opportunistic Infections in HIV-Exposed and HIV-Infected Children. Guidelines for the Prevention and Treatment of Opportunistic Infections in HIV-Exposed and HIV-Infected Children. Department of Health and Human Services. Available at: **https://clinicalinfo.hiv.gov/sites/default/files/inline-files/oi_guidelines_pediatrics.pdf**

[3] World Health Organization. Guidelines for the diagnosis, prevention and management of cryptococcal disease in HIV-infected adults, adolescents and children, March, 2018. Available at: **www.who.int/hiv/pub/guidelines/cryptococcal-disease/en/**

Children with HIV infection who have completed initial therapy for cryptococcosis should receive long-term suppressive/maintenance therapy with fluconazole (6 mg/kg daily; maximum dose 400 mg). The safety of discontinuing secondary prophylaxis for cryptococcosis after immune reconstitution with combined antiretroviral therapy (ART) has not been studied in children. On the basis of adult data and experience, discontinuing suppressive/maintenance therapy for cryptococcosis (after receiving secondary prophylaxis for at least 1 year) can be considered for asymptomatic children ≥6 years of age, with increase in their CD4+ T-lymphocyte counts to ≥100 cells/mm^3 and an undetectable viral load after receiving ART for ≥3 months.[1] Suppressive/maintenance therapy should be reinitiated if the CD4+ T-lymphocyte count decreases to <100 cells/mm^3. Most experts would not discontinue secondary prophylaxis for patients younger than age 6 years.

Patients with less severe nonmeningeal disease (pulmonary disease) can be treated with fluconazole alone, but data on use of fluconazole for children with *C neoformans* infection are limited; itraconazole is a potential alternative. Another potential treatment option for patients in whom amphotericin B treatment is not possible is the combination therapy with fluconazole and flucytosine; this combination has superior efficacy compared with fluconazole alone for severe disease. Echinocandins are not active against cryptococcal infections and should not be used.

ISOLATION OF THE HOSPITALIZED PATIENT: Standard precautions are recommended.

CONTROL MEASURES: None.

Cryptosporidiosis

CLINICAL MANIFESTATIONS: Cryptosporidiosis commonly presents with frequent, nonbloody, watery diarrhea, although infection can be asymptomatic. Other symptoms include abdominal cramps, fatigue, fever, vomiting, anorexia, and weight loss. In an immunocompetent person, symptomatic cryptosporidiosis is self-limited, usually resolving within 2 to 3 weeks. Asymptomatic intestinal infection with *Cryptosporidium* is associated with poor childhood growth.

In an immunocompromised person, such as a child who has received a solid organ transplant or has advanced human immunodeficiency virus (HIV) disease, cryptosporidiosis can result in profuse diarrhea lasting weeks to months, leading to severe dehydration, malnutrition, wasting, and death. The diagnosis of cryptosporidiosis should be considered in any immunocompromised person with diarrhea. Extraintestinal (eg, pulmonary or biliary tract) cryptosporidiosis has been reported in immunocompromised people and is associated with CD4+ T-lymphocyte counts less than 50/mm^3.

ETIOLOGY: Cryptosporidia are oocyst-forming coccidian protozoa. Oocysts are excreted in feces of an infected host. Approximately 20 *Cryptosporidium* species or genotypes have been reported to infect humans, but *Cryptosporidium hominis* and *Cryptosporidium parvum* cause more than 90% of cases of human cryptosporidiosis. The organism is highly infectious with 10 or fewer oocysts causing infection. *Cryptosporidium* oocysts can tolerate extreme environmental conditions and can survive in water and soil for several months.

---

[1] Panel on Opportunistic Infections in HIV-Exposed and HIV-Infected Children. Guidelines for the Prevention and Treatment of Opportunistic Infections in HIV-Exposed and HIV-Infected Children. Department of Health and Human Services. Available at: **https://clinicalinfo.hiv.gov/sites/default/files/inline-files/oi_guidelines_pediatrics.pdf**

Even in properly chlorinated pools, *Cryptosporidium* oocysts can survive for more than 7 days.

EPIDEMIOLOGY: *Cryptosporidium* organisms can be transmitted between humans and to humans via contaminated water and food and from animals. Extensive waterborne disease outbreaks have been associated with contamination of drinking water and recreational water (eg, pools, lakes, and water playgrounds). *Cryptosporidium* infection has become the leading cause of outbreaks associated with treated recreational water venues (eg, swimming pools), responsible for 212 (58%) of 363 such outbreaks during 2000–2014 for which an infectious cause was identified.[1]

In children, the incidence of cryptosporidiosis is greatest during summer and early fall, corresponding to the outdoor swimming season. Cases are reported most frequently in children 1 through 4 years of age, followed by those 5 through 9 years.

Foodborne transmission can occur; *Cryptosporidium* organisms have been detected in raw produce and in raw or unpasteurized apple cider and milk. People can acquire infections from pets, livestock, and from animals found in petting zoos, particularly preweaned bovine calves, lambs, and goat kids. *Cryptosporidium* organisms can spread by person-to-person transmission and result in outbreaks in child care settings and are a cause of travelers' diarrhea. (**www.cdc.gov/parasites/crypto/audience-travelers.html**).

The **incubation period** of *Cryptosporidium* species usually is 2 to 10 days. Recurrence of symptoms has been reported frequently. In immunocompetent people, oocyst shedding usually ceases within 2 weeks after symptoms abate. In immunocompromised people, the period of oocyst shedding can continue for months.

DIAGNOSTIC TESTS: Routine laboratory examination of stool for ova and parasites might not include testing for *Cryptosporidium* species, so testing for the organism should be requested specifically. The direct fluorescent antibody (DFA) method for microscopic detection of oocysts in stool and multi-well plate enzyme immunoassays (EIAs) targeting cryptosporidial antigens are widely available and are recommended for laboratory diagnosis of cryptosporidiosis. Some EIAs target *Cryptosporidium* species and *Giardia duodenalis* in a single test format. Rapid point-of-care lateral flow immunochromatographic tests for detecting antigen in stool are available. Specimens positive by these tests should be confirmed by another diagnostic assay because of reported problems with false-positive results and poor positive predictive values. The detection of oocysts on microscopic examination of stool specimens can be accomplished by direct wet mount if concentration of the oocysts is high. Alternatively, the formalin ethyl acetate stool concentration method can be used followed by staining of the stool specimen with a modified Kinyoun acid-fast stain. Oocysts generally are small (4–6 µm in diameter) and can be missed in a rapid scan of a slide.

At least 3 stool specimens collected on separate days should be examined before considering test results to be negative, because shedding can be intermittent. Organisms also can be identified in intestinal biopsy tissue or sampling of intestinal fluid. Molecular methods are being used increasingly for diagnosis of cryptosporidiosis, particularly nucleic acid amplification tests (NAATs) that target multiple gastrointestinal tract pathogens in

[1]Gharpure R, Perez A, Miller AD, Wikswo ME, Silver R, Hlavsa MC. Cryptosporidium outbreaks – United States 2009-2017. *MMWR Morb Mortal Wkly Rep*. 2019;68(25):568–572. Available at: **www.cdc.gov/mmwr/volumes/68/wr/mm6825a3.htm?s_cid=mm6825a3_w**

a single assay and have received clearance from the US Food and Drug Administration (FDA).

TREATMENT: Immunocompetent people might not need specific therapy. If treatment of diarrhea associated with cryptosporidiosis is indicated, a 3-day course of nitazoxanide oral suspension has been approved by the FDA for non–HIV-infected, immunocompetent people 1 year or older. (see Table 4.11, Drugs for Parasitic Infections, p 955). Longer courses of nitazoxanide (up to 14 days or longer) are recommended for immunocompromised children for treatment of diarrhea caused by *Cryptosporidium*, although efficacy is questionable. Disease in immunocompromised children, especially solid organ transplant recipients or those with HIV infection, can be refractory to treatment with nitazoxanide.

In HIV-infected people, improvement in CD4+ T-lymphocyte count associated with antiretroviral therapy can lead to resolution of symptoms and cessation of oocyst shedding. For this reason, administration of combination antiretroviral therapy (ART) is the primary treatment for cryptosporidiosis in patients with HIV infection. In vitro and observational studies suggest ART containing a protease inhibitor could be preferable because of a potential direct effect of the protease inhibitor on the parasite. Given the seriousness of cryptosporidiosis in immunocompromised people, use of nitazoxanide can be considered in immunocompromised HIV-infected children in conjunction with immune restoration with ART. Paromomycin or azithromycin are alternatives for children who do not respond to nitazoxanide.[1]

ISOLATION OF THE HOSPITALIZED PATIENT: In addition to standard precautions, contact precautions are recommended for diapered or incontinent people for the duration of illness. Hydrogen peroxide is preferred over bleach for environmental cleaning because of the organism's high chlorine tolerance.

CONTROL MEASURES: Cryptosporidiosis is a reportable disease to state or local health departments. Suspected or confirmed cases or outbreaks of cryptosporidiosis should be reported promptly and appropriate control and prevention measures implemented to prevent disease spread. In general these measures include the following, and other measures may be indicated depending on suspected source and mode of transmission:

- Wash hands frequently with soap and water. Alcohol-based hand sanitizers are not effective against *Cryptosporidium* species.
- Do not swim or participate in recreational water activities if sick with diarrhea. If cryptosporidiosis is diagnosed, wait 2 weeks after diarrhea has stopped before participating in recreational water activities. Avoid swallowing recreational water. Additional information on healthy swimming can be found at **www.cdc.gov/healthywater/swimming/swimmers/swim-healthy.html.**
- Do not consume food or drink that might be contaminated, such as water from lakes or rivers; inadequately treated water (eg, while traveling in areas with unsafe water); fruits or vegetables washed in water that might be contaminated; and unpasteurized milk or apple cider.
- If immunocompromised, avoid contact with farm animals (see **www.cdc.gov/parasites/crypto/gen_info/prevent_ic.html**).

---

[1]Panel on Opportunistic Infections in HIV-Exposed and HIV-Infected Children. Guidelines for the Prevention and Treatment of Opportunistic Infections in HIV-Exposed and HIV-Infected Children. Department of Health and Human Services. Available at: **https://clinicalinfo.hiv.gov/sites/default/files/inline-files/oi_guidelines_pediatrics.pdf**

Cutaneous Larva Migrans

CLINICAL MANIFESTATIONS: Cutaneous larva migrans is a clinical diagnosis based on advancing serpiginous tracks in the skin with associated intense pruritus. Certain nematode larvae may penetrate intact skin and produce pruritic, reddish papules at the site of skin entry. Signs and symptoms typically develop several days after larval penetration of the skin, but in rare cases onset of disease may be delayed for weeks to months. As the larvae migrate through skin, advancing up to 20 millimeters per day, intensely pruritic serpiginous tracks are formed, a condition also referred to as creeping eruption. Bullae may develop later as a complication of the larval migration. Larval activity can continue for several weeks, but the infection is self-limiting. Rarely, in infections with certain species of parasites, larvae may penetrate deeper tissues and cause pneumonitis (Löffler syndrome), which can be severe. Occasionally, the larvae of *Ancylostoma caninum* can reach the intestine and may cause eosinophilic enteritis.

ETIOLOGY: Infective larvae of cat and dog hookworms (most often *Ancylostoma braziliense*, also *A caninum, Ancylostoma ceylanicum,* and *Uncinaria stenocephala*) cause cutaneous larva migrans. Other skin-penetrating nematodes are occasional causes of similar clinical presentations (eg, larva currens caused by *Strongyloides*).

EPIDEMIOLOGY: Cutaneous larva migrans is a disease of children, utility workers, gardeners, sunbathers, and others who come in contact with soil contaminated with cat and dog feces. Locally acquired cases in the United States are mostly in the Southeast. Most identified cases are not acquired locally but occur among travelers to tropical and subtropical regions, particularly those who have walked barefoot or have unprotected skin contact on beaches.

The **incubation period** typically is short, with signs and symptoms developing several days after larval penetration of the skin.

DIAGNOSTIC TESTS: The diagnosis is made clinically, and biopsies are not indicated. Biopsy specimens typically demonstrate an eosinophilic inflammatory infiltrate, but the migrating parasite is not visualized. Eosinophilia and increased immunoglobulin (Ig) E serum concentrations occur in some cases. Larvae have been detected in sputum and gastric washings in patients with the rare complication of pneumonitis. Enzyme immunoassay or Western blot analysis using antigens of *A caninum* have been developed in research laboratories, but these assays are not available for routine diagnostic use.

TREATMENT: The disease usually is self-limited, with spontaneous cure after several weeks; treatment may hasten resolution of symptoms. Orally administered ivermectin or albendazole is the recommended therapy (see Drugs for Parasitic Infections, p 955). The safety of ivermectin in children weighing less than 15 kg and in pregnant women has not been established. Ingestion of ivermectin with a meal increases its bioavailability. Studies in children as young as 1 year suggest that albendazole can be administered safely to this population. Repeated application of topical 10% albendazole may be useful in young children who cannot take oral medication, but it is not commercially available and must be formulated at a pharmacy. Outside the United States, topical thiabendazole has also been used successfully for treatment of localized larvae.

ISOLATION OF THE HOSPITALIZED PATIENT: Standard precautions are recommended.

CONTROL MEASURES: Skin contact with moist soil contaminated with animal feces should be avoided. Beaches should be kept free of dog and cat feces.

Cyclosporiasis

CLINICAL MANIFESTATIONS: Watery diarrhea is the most common symptom of cyclosporiasis and can be profuse and protracted. Anorexia, nausea, vomiting, substantial weight loss, flatulence, abdominal cramping, myalgia, and prolonged fatigue can occur. Low-grade fever occurs in approximately 50% of patients. Biliary tract disease has been reported. Infection usually is self-limited, but untreated people may have remitting, relapsing symptoms for weeks to months. Asymptomatic infection has been documented most commonly in settings where cyclosporiasis is endemic.

ETIOLOGY: *Cyclospora cayetanensis* is a coccidian protozoan; oocysts (rather than cysts) are passed in stools. These oocysts must then sporulate at temperatures between 22°C and 32°C for days to weeks before they are infectious.

EPIDEMIOLOGY: *C cayetanensis* is endemic in many resource-limited countries and has been reported as a cause of travelers' diarrhea. Foodborne and waterborne outbreaks have been reported. Most outbreaks in the United States and Canada for which a food vehicle and its source have been identified have been associated with consumption of imported fresh produce (eg, basil, cilantro, raspberries, sugar snap peas, lettuce). There has been a trend in the United States of seasonal increases in reported cases from May through August; many cases occurred among people without a history of international travel. The Centers for Disease Control and Prevention (CDC) reported 2299 US cases of cyclosporiasis from May through August 2018 in people without recent international travel, one third of which were associated with 1 of 2 large outbreaks implicating packaged vegetables. This higher incidence (164 cases in 2016, 623 cases in 2017) might be attributable, in part, to increased use of now commercially available molecular testing.

Humans are the only known hosts for *C cayetanensis*. Direct person-to-person transmission is unlikely, because excreted oocysts take days to weeks under favorable environmental conditions to sporulate and become infective. Oocysts are resistant to most disinfectants used in food and water processing and can remain viable for prolonged periods in cool, moist environments.

The **incubation period** typically is 1 week but can range from 2 days to 2 weeks or more.

DIAGNOSTIC TESTS: Diagnosis is made by identification of oocysts (8–10 µm in diameter) in stool, intestinal fluid/aspirates, or intestinal biopsy specimens. Oocysts may be shed at low levels, even by people with profuse diarrhea. This constraint underscores the utility of repeated stool examinations, sensitive recovery methods (eg, concentration procedures including formalin-ethyl acetate sedimentation or sucrose centrifugal flotation), and detection methods that highlight the organism. Oocysts are autofluorescent and are variably acid fast after modified acid-fast staining of stool specimens. Molecular diagnostic assays (eg, polymerase chain reaction) are available commercially as part of a multiplex gastrointestinal panel and at the CDC.

TREATMENT: Trimethoprim-sulfamethoxazole, typically for 7 to 10 days, is the drug of choice (see Drugs for Parasitic Infections, p 949); immunocompromised patients may need longer courses of therapy. No highly effective alternatives have been identified for people who cannot tolerate trimethoprim-sulfamethoxazole (**www.cdc.gov/parasites/ cyclosporiasis/health_professionals/tx.html**), but case reports suggest that nitazoxanide might be an effective alternative for patients who cannot tolerate sulfa drugs.

ISOLATION OF THE HOSPITALIZED PATIENT: In addition to standard precautions, contact precautions are recommended for diapered or incontinent children.

CONTROL MEASURES: Avoiding food or water that may be contaminated with feces is the best known way to prevent cyclosporiasis. Fresh produce should be avoided in high-risk settings or should be washed thoroughly before it is eaten, although this may not completely eliminate risk for transmission. Cyclosporiasis is a nationally notifiable disease and is a reportable disease in many states.

Cystoisosporiasis (formerly Isosporiasis)

CLINICAL MANIFESTATIONS: Watery diarrhea is the most common symptom of cystoisosporiasis and can be profuse and protracted, even in immunocompetent people. Manifestations are similar to those caused by other enteric protozoa (eg, *Cryptosporidium* and *Cyclospora* species) and can include abdominal pain, cramping, anorexia, nausea, vomiting, weight loss, and low-grade fever. The proportion of infected people who are asymptomatic is unknown. Severity of infection ranges from self-limiting in immunocompetent hosts to chronic, debilitating, sometimes life-threatening diarrheal infection with wasting in immunocompromised patients, particularly people infected with human immunodeficiency virus (HIV). Infections of the biliary tract and reactive arthritis also have been reported. Peripheral eosinophilia may occur.

ETIOLOGY: *Cystoisospora belli* (formerly *Isospora belli*) is a coccidian protozoan; oocysts (rather than cysts) are passed in stools.

EPIDEMIOLOGY: Infection occurs predominantly in tropical and subtropical regions of the world and results from ingestion of sporulated oocysts (eg, in food or water contaminated with human feces). Humans are the only known host for *C belli* and shed noninfective oocysts in feces. These oocysts must mature (sporulate) outside the host in the environment to become infective. Under favorable conditions, sporulation can be completed in 1 to 2 days and perhaps more quickly in some settings. Oocysts probably are resistant to most disinfectants and can remain viable for prolonged periods in a cool, moist environment.

The **incubation period** averages 1 week but may range from several days to 2 or more weeks.

DIAGNOSTIC TESTS: Identification of oocysts in feces or in duodenal aspirates or finding developmental stages of the parasite in biopsy specimens (eg, of the small intestine) is diagnostic. Oocysts in stool are elongate and ellipsoidal (length, 25 to 35 µm). Oocysts can be shed in low numbers, even by people with profuse diarrhea. This underscores the utility of repeated stool examinations, sensitive recovery methods (eg, concentration methods), and the need for detection methods that highlight the organism (eg, oocysts stain bright red with modified acid-fast staining techniques and autofluoresce when viewed by ultraviolet fluorescence microscopy). Polymerase chain reaction (PCR) assays have been developed for detecting *Cystoisospora* DNA in feces but are not widely available. Like *Cryptosporidium* and *Cyclospora* species, *Cystoisospora* organisms usually are not detected by routine stool ova and parasite examination. Therefore, the laboratory should be notified specifically when any coccidian parasite is suspected on clinical grounds so that the latter special microscopic methods are used in addition to traditional ova and parasite examination.

TREATMENT: Treatment has been studied predominantly in patients with HIV infection. In the immunocompetent host, treatment may not be necessary, as symptoms are usually self-limited. If symptoms do not start to resolve by 5 to 7 days, and in immunocompromised patients, trimethoprim-sulfamethoxazole typically for 7 to 10 days, is the drug of choice (see Drugs for Parasitic Infections, p 949). Immunocompromised patients may need higher doses and a longer duration of therapy. Pyrimethamine (plus leucovorin, to prevent myelosuppression) is an alternative for people who cannot tolerate (or whose infection does not respond to) trimethoprim-sulfamethoxazole. Ciprofloxacin is less effective than trimethoprim-sulfamethoxazole. Nitazoxanide has been reported to be effective, but data are limited. In adolescents and adults coinfected with HIV with CD4+ T-lymphocyte counts of <200 cells/mm³, maintenance therapy is recommended to prevent recurrent disease. In adults, secondary prophylaxis may be discontinued once the CD4+ T-lymphocyte count is >200 cells/mm³ for >6 months as a result of antiretroviral therapy. In children, a reasonable time to discontinue secondary prophylaxis would be after sustained improvement (for >6 months) in CD4+ T-lymphocyte count or CD4+ T-lymphocyte percentage from CDC immunologic category 3 to 1 or 2, in response to antiretroviral therapy (**https://clinicalinfo.hiv.gov/en/guidelines/pediatric-opportunistic-infection/isosporiasis-cystoisosporiasis** and **www.cdc.gov/mmwr/preview/mmwrhtml/rr6303a1.htm?s_cid=rr6303a1_e**). These individuals should be monitored closely for recurrent symptoms. Supportive treatment for dehydration and/or malnutrition associated with severe diarrheal illness may be required.

ISOLATION OF THE HOSPITALIZED PATIENT: In addition to standard precautions, contact precautions are recommended for diapered and incontinent people.

CONTROL MEASURES: Preventive measures include avoiding fecal exposure (eg, food, water, skin, and fomites contaminated with stool), practicing hand and personal hygiene, and thorough washing of fruits and vegetables before eating.

Cytomegalovirus Infection

CLINICAL MANIFESTATIONS: Manifestations of acquired human cytomegalovirus (CMV) infection vary with the age and immunocompetence of the host. Asymptomatic infections are the most common, particularly in children. An infectious mononucleosis-like syndrome with prolonged fever and mild hepatitis, occurring in the absence of heterophile antibody production ("monospot negative"), may occur in adolescents and adults. End-organ disease, including pneumonia, colitis, retinitis, meningoencephalitis, or transverse myelitis, or a CMV syndrome characterized by fever, thrombocytopenia, leukopenia, and mild hepatitis may occur in immunocompromised hosts, including people receiving treatment for malignant neoplasms, people infected with human immunodeficiency virus (HIV), and people receiving immunosuppressive therapy for solid organ or hematopoietic stem cell transplantation. Less commonly, patients treated with biologic response modifiers (see Biologic Response-Modifying Drugs Used to Decrease Inflammation, p 82) can exhibit CMV end-organ disease, such as retinitis and hepatitis.

Congenital CMV infection has a spectrum of clinical manifestations but usually is not evident at birth (asymptomatic congenital CMV infection). Approximately 10% of infants with congenital CMV infection exhibit clinical findings that are evident at birth (symptomatic congenital CMV disease), with manifestations including jaundice attributable to direct hyperbilirubinemia, petechiae attributable to thrombocytopenia, purpura, hepa-tosplenomegaly, microcephaly, intracerebral (typically periventricular) calcifications, and retinitis; developmental delays can occur among affected infants in later infancy and early childhood. Death attributable to congenital CMV is estimated to occur in 3% to 10% of infants with symptomatic disease or 0.3% to 1.0% of all infants with congenital CMV infection.

Congenital CMV infection is the leading nongenetic cause of sensorineural hear-ing loss (SNHL) in children in the United States. Approximately 20% of all hearing loss at birth and 25% of all hearing loss at 4 years of age is attributable to congenital CMV infection. SNHL is the most common sequela following congenital CMV infection, with SNHL occurring in up to 50% of children with congenital infections that are symptom-atic at birth and up to 15% of those with asymptomatic infections. Approximately 40% of infected children who ultimately develop SNHL will not have hearing loss detectable within the first month of life, illustrating the risk of late-onset SNHL in these populations. Approximately 50% of children with CMV-associated SNHL continue to have further deterioration (progression) of their hearing loss over time.

Infection acquired during the intrapartum period from maternal cervical secretions or in the postpartum period from human milk usually is not associated with clinical illness in term infants. In preterm infants, however, postpartum infection resulting from human milk or from transfusion from CMV-seropositive donors has been associated with hepa-titis, interstitial pneumonia, hematologic abnormalities including thrombocytopenia and leukopenia, and a viral sepsis syndrome.

ETIOLOGY: Human CMV, also known as human herpesvirus 5, is a member of the her-pesvirus family *(Herpesviridae)*, the beta-herpesvirus subfamily *(Betaherpesvirinae)*, and the *Cytomegalovirus* genus. The viral genome contains double-stranded DNA that range in size from 196 000 to 240 000 bp encoding at least 166 proteins and is the largest of the human herpesvirus genomes.

EPIDEMIOLOGY: CMV is highly species-specific, and only human CMV has been shown to infect and cause disease in humans. The virus is ubiquitous, and CMV strains exhibit extensive genetic diversity. Transmission occurs horizontally (by direct person-to-person contact with virus-containing secretions), vertically (from mother to infant before, during, or after birth), and via transfusions of blood, platelets, and white blood cells from infected donors. CMV also can be transmitted with solid organ or hematopoietic stem cell trans-plantation. Infections have no seasonal predilection. CMV persists in leukocytes and tis-sue cells after a primary infection, with intermittent virus shedding; symptomatic infection can occur throughout the lifetime of the infected person, particularly under conditions of immunosuppression. Reinfection with other strains of CMV can occur in seropositive hosts, including pregnant women. In the United States, there appears to be 3 periods in life when there is an increased incidence of CMV acquisition: early childhood, adoles-cence, and the child-bearing years.

Horizontal transmission probably is the result of exposure to saliva, urine, or genital secretions from infected individuals. Spread of CMV in households and child care centers is well documented. Excretion rates from urine or saliva in children 1 to 3 years of age who attend child care centers usually range from 30% to 40% but can be as high as 70%. In addition, children who attend child care frequently excrete large quantities of virus for prolonged periods. Young children can transmit CMV to their parents, including moth-ers who may be pregnant, and other caregivers, including child care staff (see Children in Group Child Care and Schools, p 116). In adolescents and adults, sexual transmission occurs, as evidenced by detection of virus in seminal and cervical fluids. As such, CMV is considered to be a sexually transmitted infection (STI).

CMV-seropositive healthy people have latent CMV in their leukocytes and tissues; hence, blood transfusions and organ transplantation can result in transmission. Severe CMV disease following transfusion or solid organ transplantation is more likely to occur if the recipient is CMV seronegative before transplantation. In contrast, among nonautologous hematopoietic stem cell transplant recipients, CMV-seropositive individuals who receive transplants from seronegative donors are at greatest risk of disease when exposed to CMV after transplantation, likely because of the failure of the transplanted graft to provide immunity to the recipient. Latent CMV may reactivate in immunosuppressed individuals and result in disease if immunosuppression is severe (eg, in patients with acquired immunodeficiency syndrome [AIDS] or solid organ or hematopoietic stem cell transplant recipients).

Vertical transmission of CMV to an infant occurs in one of the following time periods: (1) in utero, by transplacental passage of maternal bloodborne virus; or (2) at birth, by passage through an infected maternal genital tract. Postnatal acquisition occurs via ingestion of CMV-positive human milk. Approximately 5 per 1000 live-born infants are infected in utero and excrete CMV at birth, making this the most common congenital viral infection in the United States. Significant racial and ethnic differences exist in the prevalence of congenital CMV, with the highest prevalence of CMV in Black newborn infants (9.5/1000 live births) and lower prevalence in non-Hispanic white infants (2.7/1000 live births) and Hispanic white infants (3.0/1000 live births). In utero fetal infection can occur in women with no preexisting CMV immunity (maternal primary infection) or in women with preexisting antibody to CMV (maternal nonprimary infection) either by acquisition of a different viral strain during pregnancy or by reactivation of an existing maternal infection. Congenital infection and associated sequelae can occur irrespective of the trimester of pregnancy when the mother is infected, but severe sequelae are associated more commonly with maternal infection acquired during the first trimester. Damaging fetal infections and sequelae can occur following both primary and nonprimary maternal infections. It is estimated that more than three quarters of infants with congenital CMV infection in the United States are born to women with nonprimary infection, and in populations with higher maternal CMV seroprevalence than the United States, most damaging congenital CMV infections occur in infants born to women with nonprimary infection.

Among infants who acquire infection from maternal cervical secretions or human milk, preterm infants born before 32 weeks' gestation and with a birth weight less than 1500 g are at greater risk of developing CMV disease than are full-term infants. Most infants who acquire CMV from ingestion of human milk from CMV-seropositive mothers do not develop clinical illness or sequelae, likely because of the presence of passively transferred maternal antibody.

The **incubation period** for horizontally transmitted CMV infections is highly variable. Infection usually manifests 3 to 12 weeks after blood transfusions and between 1 and 4 months after organ transplantation. For vertical transmission through human milk in preterm infants, the median time to onset of CMV viruria is 7 weeks (range, 3–24 weeks).

DIAGNOSTIC TESTS: The diagnosis of CMV disease is confounded by the ubiquity of the virus, the high rate of asymptomatic excretion, the frequency of reactivated infections, reinfection with different strains of CMV, the development of serum immunoglobulin

(Ig) M CMV-specific antibody in some episodes of reactivation and reinfection, and concurrent infection with other pathogens.

Viral DNA can be detected by polymerase chain reaction (PCR) and other nucleic acid amplification assay methods in tissues and some fluids, including cerebrospinal fluid (CSF), amniotic fluid, human milk, aqueous and vitreous humor fluids, urine, saliva and other respiratory secretions, and peripheral blood. Detection of CMV DNA by PCR assay in blood does not necessarily indicate acute infection or disease, especially in immunocompetent people. Several quantitative PCR assays for detection of CMV have been cleared by the US Food and Drug Administration (FDA). These assays are sensitive, use standardized international units for reporting, provide rapid results compared with culture, and generally are the preferred method for detecting viremia. The same specimen type should always be used when testing any given patient over time. Antigenemia assays also have been cleared by the FDA, but they are labor intensive and require timely processing of specimens to obtain accurate results. Because of these drawbacks, molecular assays are preferred.

CMV can be isolated in conventional cell culture from urine, saliva, peripheral blood leukocytes, human milk, semen, cervical secretions, and other tissues and body fluids. Recovery of virus from a target organ provides strong evidence that the disease is caused by CMV infection. Standard viral cultures must be maintained for more than 28 days before considering such cultures negative. Shell vial culture coupled with staining of cells using immunofluorescence antibody techniques for immediate early antigen provides results within 24 to 36 hours but is not available in many laboratories.

Various serologic assays, including immunofluorescence assays, latex agglutination assays, and enzyme immunoassays, are available for detecting both IgG and IgM CMV-specific antibodies. Single serum specimens for IgG antibody testing are useful in screening for past infection in individuals at risk for CMV reactivation or for screening potential organ transplant donors and recipients. For diagnosis of suspected recent infection, testing for CMV IgG in paired sera obtained at least 2 weeks apart and testing for IgM in a single serum specimen may be useful. Determination of low-avidity CMV IgG in the presence of CMV IgM in pregnant women can suggest more recent infection.

Fetal CMV infection can be diagnosed by detection of CMV DNA in amniotic fluid. Congenital infection with CMV requires detection of CMV or CMV DNA in urine, saliva, blood, or CSF obtained within 3 weeks of birth; detection beyond this initial period of life could reflect postnatal acquisition of virus. PCR testing of saliva swab specimens from neonates has been shown to be >95% sensitive for the identification of congenital CMV infection. Positive saliva swab specimen test results may require confirmation with testing of urine because of potential contamination of saliva with CMV in human milk. The analytical sensitivity of CMV PCR of dried blood spots is low, limiting use of this type of specimen for widespread screening for congenital CMV infection. A positive PCR assay result from a neonatal dried blood spot confirms congenital infection, but a negative result does not rule out congenital infection. Differentiation between congenital and perinatal infection is difficult at later than 2 to 4 weeks of age unless clinical manifestations of the former, such as chorioretinitis or intracranial calcifications, are present. At least 1 commercial assay has been cleared by the FDA for detection of CMV DNA from saliva of neonates within the first 3 weeks of life. IgM serologic methods commonly have reduced specificity and may yield false-positive results, making serologic diagnosis of congenital CMV infection problematic.

TREATMENT: Intravenous ganciclovir (see Non-HIV Antiviral Drugs, p 930) is approved for induction and maintenance treatment of retinitis caused by acquired or recurrent CMV infection in immunocompromised adult patients, including HIV-infected patients, and for prophylaxis and treatment of CMV disease in adult transplant recipients. Valganciclovir, the oral prodrug of ganciclovir, is approved for treatment (induction and maintenance) of CMV retinitis in immunocompromised adult patients, including HIV-infected patients, and for prevention of CMV disease in kidney, kidney-pancreas, or heart transplant recipients at high risk of CMV disease. Valganciclovir also is approved for prevention of CMV disease in pediatric kidney transplant patients 4 months and older and for pediatric heart transplant patients 1 month and older. Ganciclovir and valganciclovir are used to treat CMV infections of other sites (esophagus, colon, lungs) and for preemptive treatment of immunosuppressed adults with CMV antigenemia or viremia. Valganciclovir is available in both tablet and powder for oral solution formulations. Oral ganciclovir and ganciclovir ocular implants are no longer available in the United States.

Neonates with symptomatic congenital CMV disease with or without central nervous system (CNS) involvement have improved audiologic and neurodevelopmental outcomes at 2 years of age when treated with oral valganciclovir for 6 months (see Non-HIV Antiviral Drugs, p 930). The dose should be adjusted each month to account for weight gain. Therapy can be accomplished using oral valganciclovir for the entire treatment course, because drug exposure following appropriate dosing of valganciclovir is the same as that achieved with intravenous ganciclovir. If an infant is unable to absorb medications reliably from the gastrointestinal tract (eg, because of necrotizing enterocolitis or other bowel disorders), intravenous ganciclovir can be used initially. Significant neutropenia occurs in one fifth of infants treated with oral valganciclovir and in two thirds of infants treated with parenteral ganciclovir. Absolute neutrophil counts should be performed weekly for 6 weeks, then at 8 weeks, then monthly for the duration of antiviral treatment; serum alanine aminotransferase concentration should be measured monthly during treatment. When it occurs, neutropenia is more common during the first 4 to 6 weeks of therapy; if the absolute neutrophil count reproducibly drops below 500 cells/mm^3, either treatment can be held until counts recover above 750 cells/mm^3, or granulocyte colony-stimulating factor can be administered once daily for 1 to 3 consecutive days. Antiviral therapy should be limited to patients with moderate to severe symptomatic congenital CMV disease who are able to start treatment within the first month of life. Infants with asymptomatic congenital CMV infection should not receive antiviral treatment outside the confines of a research study. Neonates with mild symptomatic disease or with isolated SNHL and no other disease manifestations should not routinely receive antiviral treatment because of a lack of data suggesting benefit in this less severely affected population. International consensus recommendations for congenital CMV diagnosis and management have been published.[1]

Patients with symptomatic or asymptomatic congenital CMV infection should have serial audiologic assessments throughout childhood. The American Academy of Pediatrics *Bright Futures: Guidelines for Health Supervision of Infants, Children, and Adolescents*, 4th Edition, recommends hearing testing at 4, 6, 9, 12, 15, 18, 24, and 30 months of age of

---

[1] Rawlinson W, Boppana S, Fowler KB, et al. Congenital cytomegalovirus infection in pregnancy and the neonate: consensus recommendations for prevention, diagnosis, and therapy. *Lancet Infect Dis.* 2017;17(6):e177-e188

children with congenital CMV, in addition to the standard hearing assessments recommended for all children at 4, 5, 6, 8, and 10 years of age.

Preterm infants with perinatally acquired CMV infection can have symptomatic, end-organ disease (eg, pneumonitis, hepatitis, thrombocytopenia). Antiviral treatment has not been studied in this population. If such patients are treated with parenteral ganciclovir, a reasonable approach is to treat for 2 weeks and then reassess responsiveness to therapy. If clinical data suggest benefit of treatment, an additional 1 to 2 weeks of parenteral ganciclovir can be considered if symptoms and signs have not resolved. Valganciclovir generally is not a reasonable alternative in this setting, given the degree of illness these infants are experiencing and the corresponding effect that this potentially could have on gastrointestinal tract absorption of valganciclovir and first-pass hepatic metabolism to ganciclovir.

In hematopoietic stem cell transplant recipients, the combination of Immune Globulin Intravenous (IGIV) or CMV Immune Globulin Intravenous (CMV-IGIV) and intravenous ganciclovir has been reported to be synergistic in treatment of CMV pneumonia. Unlike CMV-IGIV, IGIV products have varying anti-CMV antibody concentrations from lot to lot, are not tested routinely for their quantities of anti-CMV antibodies, and do not have a specified titer of antibodies to CMV that have correlated with efficacy. Valganciclovir and foscarnet have been approved for treatment and maintenance therapy of CMV retinitis in adults with acquired immunodeficiency syndrome, and letermovir has been approved for prophylaxis of CMV infection and disease in adult CMV-seropositive recipients of an allogeneic hematopoietic stem cell transplant (see Non-HIV Antiviral Drugs, p 930). Foscarnet is more toxic (with high rates of limiting nephrotoxicity) but may be advantageous for some patients with HIV infection, including people with disease caused by ganciclovir-resistant virus or people who are unable to tolerate ganciclovir. Cidofovir is efficacious for CMV retinitis in adults with AIDS but is associated with significant nephrotoxicity.

CMV establishes lifelong persistent infection, and as such, it is not eliminated from the body with antiviral treatment of CMV disease. Until immune reconstitution is achieved with antiretroviral therapy, chronic suppressive therapy should be administered to HIV-infected patients with a history of CMV end-organ disease (eg, retinitis, colitis, pneumonitis) to prevent recurrence. Discontinuing prophylaxis may be considered for pediatric patients 6 years and older with CD4+ T-lymphocyte counts of >100 cells/mm^3 for >6 consecutive months and for children younger than 6 years with CD4+ T-lymphocyte percentages of >15% for >6 consecutive months. For immunocompromised children with CMV retinitis, such decisions should be made in close consultation with an ophthalmologist and should take into account such factors as magnitude and duration of CD4+ T-lymphocyte increase, anatomic location of the retinal lesion, vision in the contralateral eye, and the feasibility of regular ophthalmologic monitoring. All patients who have had anti-CMV maintenance therapy discontinued should continue to undergo regular ophthalmologic monitoring at 3- to 6-month intervals for early detection of CMV relapse as well as immune reconstitution uveitis.[1]

ISOLATION OF THE HOSPITALIZED PATIENT: Standard precautions are recommended.

---

[1]Panel on Opportunistic Infections in HIV-Exposed and HIV-Infected Children. Guidelines for the Prevention and Treatment of Opportunistic Infections in HIV-Exposed and HIV-Infected Children. Department of Health and Human Services. Available at: **https://clinicalinfo.hiv.gov/sites/default/files/inline-files/oi_guidelines_pediatrics.pdf**

CONTROL MEASURES:

Care of Exposed People. When caring for children, hand hygiene, particularly after changing diapers, is advised to decrease transmission of CMV. Because asymptomatic excretion of CMV is common in people of all ages, a child with congenital CMV infection should not be treated differently from other children.

Although unrecognized exposure to people who are shedding CMV likely is common, concern may arise when immunocompromised patients or nonimmune pregnant women, including health care professionals, are exposed to patients with clinically recognizable CMV infection. Standard precautions should be sufficient to interrupt transmission of CMV (see Infection Prevention and Control for Hospitalized Children, p 133).

Child Care. Female child care workers in child care centers should be aware of CMV and its potential risks and should have access to appropriate hand hygiene measures to minimize occupationally acquired infection (**www.cdc.gov/cmv/index.html**).

Immunoprophylaxis. CMV-IGIV has been developed for prophylaxis of CMV disease in seronegative kidney, lung, liver, pancreas, and heart transplant recipients. CMV-IGIV seems to be moderately effective in kidney and liver transplant recipients and has been used in combination with antiviral agents. The use of CMV-IGIV in pregnant women to prevent CMV transmission to the fetus is not recommended because of lack of effectiveness in randomized controlled clinical trials. Evaluation of investigational vaccines in healthy volunteers and renal transplant recipients is in progress, but to date only inconsistent evidence of efficacy has been reported.

Prevention of Transmission by Blood Transfusion. Transmission of CMV by blood transfusion to newborn infants or other immune-compromised hosts virtually has been eliminated by use of CMV antibody-negative donors, by freezing red blood cells in glycerol before administration, by removal of the buffy coat, or by filtration to remove white blood cells.

Prevention of Transmission by Human Milk. Pasteurization of donated human milk can decrease the likelihood of CMV transmission. Holder pasteurization (62.5°C [144.5°F] for 30 minutes) and short-term pasteurization (72°C [161.6°F] for 5 seconds) of human milk appear to inactivate CMV; short-term pasteurization may be less harmful to the beneficial constituents of human milk. Freezing human milk at −20°C (−4°F) for the sole purpose of reducing CMV infectivity is not advised because, although it may reduce the viral load of CMV, it does not change the risk of CMV sepsis-like syndrome and freezing reduces the bioactivity of mother's milk. If fresh donated human milk is needed for infants born to CMV antibody-negative mothers, providing these infants with milk from only CMV antibody-negative women should be considered. For infants already infected with CMV, either congenitally or postnatally, the benefits of human milk from their mothers likely outweigh any risk of additional CMV exposure. For further information on human milk banks, see Breastfeeding and Human Milk (p 107).

Prevention of Transmission in Transplant Recipients. CMV-seronegative recipients of tissue from CMV-seropositive donors are at high risk of CMV disease. If such circumstances cannot be avoided, prophylactic administration of antiviral therapy or monitoring for viremia and administering preemptive antiviral therapy are options to decrease the incidence of CMV disease. Monitoring and preemptive therapy result in lower risk for drug associated toxicity. Among CMV-negative recipients of a liver transplant from a CMV-positive donor, preemptive therapy recently has been shown to significantly reduce CMV disease compared with prophylaxis.

Dengue

CLINICAL MANIFESTATIONS: Dengue infection may be asymptomatic or, if symptomatic, may have a wide range of clinical presentations. The 2009 World Health Organization classification for dengue severity is divided into: (1) **Dengue without warning signs:** fever plus 2 of the following: nausea/vomiting, rash, aches and pains, leukopenia, or positive tourniquet test; (2) **Dengue with warning signs:** dengue as defined above plus any of the following: abdominal pain or tenderness, persistent vomiting, clinical fluid accumulation (ascites, pleural effusion), mucosal bleeding, lethargy, restlessness, or liver enlargement >2 cm; and (3) **Severe dengue:** dengue with at least one of the following criteria: severe plasma leakage leading to shock or fluid accumulation with respiratory distress, severe bleeding as evaluated by a clinician, or severe organ involvement (eg, aspartate aminotransferase [AST] or alanine aminotransferase [ALT] ≥1000 IU/L, impaired consciousness, failure of heart and other organs). Less common clinical syndromes include myocarditis, pancreatitis, hepatitis, hemophagocytic lymphohistiocytosis, and neurologic disease, including acute meningoencephalitis and post-dengue acute disseminated encephalomyelitis (ADEM).

Dengue begins abruptly with a nonspecific, acute febrile illness lasting 2 to 7 days **(febrile phase),** often accompanied by muscle, joint, and/or bone pain, headache, retro-orbital pain, facial erythema, injected oropharynx, macular or maculopapular rash, leukopenia, and petechiae or other minor bleeding manifestations. During defervescence, usually on days 3 through 7 of illness, an increase in vascular permeability in parallel with increasing hematocrit (hemoconcentration) may occur. The period of clinically significant plasma leakage usually lasts 24 to 48 hours **(critical phase),** followed by a **convalescent phase** with gradual improvement and stabilization of the hemodynamic status. Warning signs of progression to severe dengue occur in the late febrile phase and include persistent vomiting, severe abdominal pain, mucosal bleeding, difficulty breathing, early signs of shock, and a rapid decline in platelet count with an increase in hematocrit. Patients with nonsevere disease begin to improve during the critical phase, but people with clinically significant plasma leakage attributable to increased vascular permeability develop severe disease that may include pleural effusions, ascites, hypovolemic shock, and hemorrhage.

ETIOLOGY: Four related RNA viruses of the genus *Flavivirus* (see Arboviruses, p 202), dengue viruses 1, 2, 3, and 4, cause symptomatic (approximately 25%) and asymptomatic (approximately 75%) infections. Infection with one dengue virus serotype most often produces lifelong immunity against that serotype, and a period of cross-protection (often lasting 1 to 3 years) against infection with the other 3 serotypes can be observed. After this period of cross-protection, infection with a different serotype may predispose to more severe disease. A person has a lifetime risk of up to 4 dengue virus infections.

EPIDEMIOLOGY: Dengue virus primarily is transmitted to humans through the bite of infected *Aedes aegypti* (and less commonly, *Aedes albopictus* or *Aedes polynesiensis*) mosquitoes. Humans are the main amplifying host of dengue virus and the main source of virus for *Aedes* mosquitoes. A sylvatic nonhuman primate dengue virus transmission cycle exists in parts of Africa and Southeast Asia but rarely crosses to humans. Other forms of transmission are relatively rare and include vertical transmission; transmission via breastfeeding, blood, or organ donation; and health care-associated transmission via needlestick or mucocutaneous exposure. The rate of vertical transmission is around 20% and is even higher when maternal dengue occurs late in pregnancy near delivery. Sexual transmission is also possible but is considered a rare route of infection, and the risk (both among men who have sex with men and heterosexual people) is considered extremely low.

Dengue is a major public health problem in the tropics and subtropics; around 3.9 billion people in 128 countries are at risk of infection with dengue viruses. Approximately 390 million dengue infections occur annually worldwide, of which 96 million have clinical manifestations, including 500 000 hospitalizations and 20 000 deaths every year. Dengue is endemic in the United States territories of Puerto Rico, the US Virgin Islands, and American Samoa. Puerto Rico has the highest incidence of dengue among all US territories (3000 to 27 000 cases per year). Incidence rates are highest from July to September, and vary significantly by geographic locale, affected by factors such as population density, elevation, and mosquito breeding and water supply patterns. Outbreaks with local dengue virus transmission have occurred in Texas, Hawaii, and Florida and in Mexican cities bordering Yuma, Arizona (San Luis Rio Colorado, Sonora), and Calexico, California (Mexicali, Baja California) (see Table 3.2, p 205). Although up to 28 states now have *A aegypti* and 40 states have *A albopictus* mosquitoes, local dengue virus transmission is uncommon because of infrequent contact between people and infected mosquitoes. Millions of US travelers, including children, are at risk; dengue is the leading cause of febrile illness among travelers returning from the Caribbean, Latin America, and South Asia. Dengue occurs in people of all ages but occurs at higher rates in healthy adolescents and young adults and is most likely to cause severe disease in infants, pregnant women, and patients with chronic diseases (eg, asthma, sickle cell anemia, and diabetes mellitus). Severe dengue disease is most likely to occur with second, heterologous dengue serotype infections and although less likely, it can occur with a third or fourth heterologous dengue serotype infections.

The **incubation period** for dengue virus replication in mosquitoes is 8 to 12 days (extrinsic incubation); mosquitoes remain infectious for the remainder of their life cycle. In humans, the **incubation period** is 3 to 14 days before symptom onset (intrinsic incubation). Infected people, both symptomatic and asymptomatic, can transmit dengue virus to mosquitoes 1 to 2 days before symptoms develop and throughout the approximately 7-day viremic period.

DIAGNOSTIC TESTS: Laboratory confirmation of the clinical diagnosis of dengue can be made on a single serum specimen obtained during the febrile phase of the illness by testing both virologically (either by detection of dengue virus RNA by reverse transcriptase-polymerase chain reaction [RT-PCR] assay or detection of dengue virus nonstructural protein 1 [NS-1] antigen by immunoassay) and serologically (anti-dengue virus immunoglobulin [Ig] M antibodies by enzyme immunoassay [EIA]). Dengue virus is detectable by RT-PCR or NS1 antigen EIAs from the beginning of the febrile phase until day 7 to 10 after illness onset. Anti-dengue virus IgM antibodies are detectable beginning 3 to 5 days after illness onset; 99% of patients have IgM antibodies by day 10. IgM levels peak after 2 weeks and then often decline to undetectable levels over 2 to 3 months but can cross-react with IgM antibodies against Zika virus and other closely related flaviviruses. Testing for NS-1 antigen and anti-dengue IgM in a single serum specimen collected during the first 10 days of illness accurately identifies ≥90% of dengue primary and secondary cases. Anti-dengue virus IgG antibody remains elevated for life after dengue virus infection. Anti-dengue virus IgG antibody may be falsely positive in people with previous infection with or immunization against other flaviviruses (eg, West Nile, Japanese encephalitis, yellow fever, or Zika viruses). A fourfold or greater increase in anti-dengue virus IgG antibody titers between the acute (≤5 days after onset of symptoms) and convalescent (>15 days after onset of symptoms) samples confirms recent infection. Conventional serologic tests may be less reliable for diagnosis of acute dengue virus infection in individuals who have been vaccinated with a dengue vaccine within the previous several months. Dengue diagnostic testing is available through commercial reference laboratories and some state public health laboratories; reference testing is available from the Dengue Branch of the Centers for Disease Control and Prevention (**www.cdc.gov/dengue/**).

TREATMENT: No specific antiviral therapy exists for dengue. During the febrile phase, patients should stay well hydrated and avoid use of aspirin (acetylsalicylic acid), salicylate-containing drugs, and other nonsteroidal anti-inflammatory drugs (eg, ibuprofen) to minimize potential for bleeding. Additional supportive care is required if the patient becomes dehydrated or develops warning signs of severe disease at or around the time of defervescence.

Early recognition of shock and intensive supportive therapy can reduce risk of death from severe dengue from approximately 5% to 10% to less than 1%. During the critical phase, maintenance of fluid volume and hemodynamic status is crucial to management of severe cases. Patients should be monitored for early signs of shock, occult bleeding, and plasma leak to avoid prolonged shock, end-organ damage, and fluid overload. Patients with refractory shock may require intravenous colloids and/or blood or blood products after an initial trial of intravenous crystalloids. Reabsorption of extravascular fluid occurs during the convalescent phase with stabilization of hemodynamic status and diuresis. It is important to watch for signs of fluid overload, which may manifest as a decrease in the patient's hematocrit as a result of the dilutional effect of reabsorbed fluid.

ISOLATION OF THE HOSPITALIZED PATIENT: Standard precautions are recommended, with attention to the potential for bloodborne transmission. When indicated, attention should be given to control of *Aedes* mosquitoes to prevent secondary transmission of dengue virus from infected patients to others.

CONTROL MEASURES: Vector control can reduce dengue transiently, when applied rigorously. A recombinant live attenuated tetravalent dengue vaccine, CYD-TDV (chimeric yellow fever dengue-tetravalent dengue vaccine) (Dengvaxia) with a 3-dose schedule administered at 0, 6, and 12 months has been approved for use in individuals aged 9 to 45 years of age in approximately 17 countries with endemic dengue as of 2019. CYD-TDV was approved by the US Food and Drug Administration (FDA) in 2019 for use in individuals 9 through 16 years of age who reside in areas with endemic dengue and who have laboratory confirmation of a previous dengue infection (**www.fda.gov/ vaccines-blood-biologics/dengvaxia**).

Analyses of data from clinical trials revealed an increased hazard ratio for severe dengue in seronegative vaccine recipients compared with seropositive vaccine recipients, while confirming efficacy in preventing dengue cases attributable to any serotype in seropositive individuals. For this reason, CYD-TDV is not approved for use in individuals not infected previously by any dengue virus serotype or for whom this information is unknown, because those not infected previously are at increased risk for severe dengue disease when vaccinated and subsequently infected with a different dengue virus serotype. Previous dengue infection can be assessed through a medical record of a previous laboratory-confirmed dengue infection or through serological testing before vaccination.

However, there is no FDA-cleared test available to determine a previous dengue infection, and available non–FDA-cleared tests may yield false-positive results. Safety and effectiveness of CYD-TDV have not been established in individuals living in areas where dengue is not endemic but who travel to areas with endemic infection.

People traveling to areas with endemic dengue (see DengueMap: **www.healthmap. org/dengue/**) are at risk of dengue and should take precautions to protect themselves from mosquito bites. Travelers should select accommodations that are air conditioned and/or have screened windows and doors. *Aedes* mosquitoes bite most often during the daytime, so bed nets are indicated for children sleeping during the day. Travelers should wear clothing that fully covers arms and legs whenever possible, especially during early morning and late afternoon, and use mosquito repellents registered by the US Environmental Protection Agency (see Prevention of Mosquitoborne and Tickborne Infections, p 175).

Dengue, acquired locally in the United States and during travel, became a nationally notifiable disease in 2010. Suspected cases should be reported to local or state health departments.

Diphtheria

CLINICAL MANIFESTATIONS: Respiratory tract diphtheria usually presents as membranous nasopharyngitis, obstructive laryngotracheitis, or bloody nasal discharge. Local infections are associated with low-grade fever and gradual onset of manifestations over 1 to 2 days. Less commonly, diphtheria presents as cutaneous, vaginal, conjunctival, or otic infection. Cutaneous diphtheria is more common in tropical areas and among urban homeless. Extensive neck swelling with cervical lymphadenitis (bull neck) is a sign of severe disease. Life-threatening complications of respiratory diphtheria include upper airway obstruction caused by membrane formation; myocarditis, with heart block; and cranial and peripheral neuropathies. Palatal palsy, noted by nasal speech, frequently occurs in pharyngeal diphtheria. Case fatality rates are 5% to 10%, and up to 50% in untreated people.

ETIOLOGY: Diphtheria is caused by toxigenic strains of *Corynebacterium diphtheriae*. Toxigenic strains of *Corynebacterium ulcerans* also have emerged as an important cause of diphtheria-like illness. *C diphtheriae* is an irregularly staining, gram-positive, non–spore-forming, nonmotile, pleomorphic bacillus with 4 biotypes (*mitis*, *intermedius*, *gravis*, and *belfanti*). All biotypes of *C diphtheriae* may be toxigenic or nontoxigenic. Bacteria remain confined to superficial layers of skin or mucosal surfaces, inducing a local inflammatory reaction. Within several days of respiratory tract infection, a dense pseudomembrane forms, becoming adherent to tissue. Toxigenic strains produce an exotoxin that consists of an enzymatically active A domain and a binding B domain, which promotes the entry of A into the cell. The toxin, an ADP-ribosylase toxin, inhibits protein synthesis in all cells, including myocardial, renal, and peripheral nerve cells, resulting in myocarditis, acute tubular necrosis, and delayed peripheral nerve conduction. Nontoxigenic strains of *C diphtheriae* can cause sore throat and, rarely, other invasive infections, including endocarditis and infections related to foreign bodies.

EPIDEMIOLOGY: Humans are the sole reservoir of *C diphtheriae*. Infection is spread by respiratory tract droplets and by contact with discharges from skin lesions. In untreated people, organisms can be present in discharges from the nose and throat and from eye and skin lesions for 2 to 6 weeks after infection. Patients treated with an appropriate antimicrobial agent usually are not infectious 48 hours after treatment is initiated. Transmission results from close contact with patients or carriers. People traveling to areas with endemic diphtheria or people who come into contact with infected travelers from such areas are at increased risk of being infected; rarely, fomites or milk products can serve as vehicles of transmission. Severe disease occurs more often in people who are unimmunized or inadequately immunized. Fully immunized people may be asymptomatic carriers or have mild sore throat.

Prior to 2019, respiratory disease caused by *C diphtheriae*, regardless of toxigenicity status, was nationally notifiable. Beginning in 2019, national notifications were restricted to disease caused by toxigenic *C diphtheriae* but could originate from respiratory or nonrespiratory sites. From 2000 through 2018, 6 cases of respiratory diphtheria were reported in the United States; however, the last bacteriologically confirmed case caused by toxigenic *C diphtheriae* occurred in 1997. There has been increasing recognition of cutaneous diphtheria; 4 toxigenic cases were identified from 2015 to 2018 among travelers to areas with endemic diphtheria. The incidence of respiratory diphtheria is greatest during fall and winter, but summer epidemics may occur in warm climates where skin infections are prevalent. Globally, endemic diphtheria occurs in Africa, Latin American, Asia, the Middle East, and parts of Europe where immunization coverage with diphtheria toxoid-containing vaccines is suboptimal. Since 2011, large outbreaks have been reported in Indonesia, Laos, Haiti, Venezuela, Yemen, and Bangladesh. In 2017, the World Health Organization reported 8819 global cases of diphtheria.

The **incubation period** usually is 2 to 5 days (range, 1–10 days).

DIAGNOSTIC TESTS: Laboratory personnel should be notified that *C diphtheriae* is suspected. Specimens for culture should be obtained from the nares and throat or any mucosal or cutaneous lesion. Obtaining multiple samples from respiratory sites increases yield of culture. Material should be obtained for culture from beneath the membrane (if present) or a portion of the membrane. Specimens collected for culture can be placed in any transport medium or in a sterile container and transported at 4°C. All isolates of *C diphtheriae* should be sent through the state health department to the Centers for Disease Control and Prevention (CDC) to verify toxigenicity status.

TREATMENT:

Antitoxin. Because patients can deteriorate rapidly, a single dose of diphtheria (equine) antitoxin (DAT) should be administered on the basis of clinical presentation, history of travel, and vaccination status before culture results are available. DAT, its indications for use, suggested dosage, and instructions for administration are available through the CDC (CDC Emergency Operations Center [telephone: 770-488-7100] or at **www.cdc.gov/ diphtheria/dat.html**). DAT is not available from any commercial source. To neutralize toxin as rapidly as possible, intravenous administration of antitoxin is preferred. Before intravenous administration of antitoxin, tests for sensitivity to horse serum should be performed according to instructions provided with the material. Allergic reactions to horse serum varying from anaphylaxis to rash can be expected in 5% to 20% of patients. The dose of antitoxin depends on the site and size of the membrane, duration of illness, and degree of toxic effects and specific recommendations are available from CDC.

Antimicrobial Therapy. Erythromycin administered orally or parenterally for 14 days, aqueous penicillin G administered intravenously for 14 days, or penicillin G procaine administered intramuscularly for 14 days constitute acceptable therapy (see Table 4.3, p 882). Antimicrobial therapy is required to stop toxin production, eradicate *C diphtheriae* organism, and prevent transmission but is not a substitute for antitoxin. Elimination of the organisms should be documented 24 hours after completion of treatment by 2 consecutive negative cultures from specimens taken 24 hours apart.

Immunization. Active immunization against diphtheria should be undertaken during convalescence from diphtheria, because disease does not necessarily confer immunity.

Cutaneous Diphtheria. Thorough cleansing of the lesion with soap and water and administration of an appropriate antimicrobial agent for 10 days are recommended.

Carriers (Regardless of Toxigenic Strain or Not). If not immunized, carriers should receive active immunization promptly and measures should be taken to ensure completion of the immunization schedule. If a carrier has been immunized previously but has not received a booster of diphtheria toxoid within 5 years, a booster dose of age-appropriate vaccine containing diphtheria toxoid (DTaP, Tdap, DT, or Td) should be administered. Carriers should receive oral erythromycin for 10 to 14 days or a single intramuscular dose of penicillin G benzathine (600 000 U for children weighing <30 kg, and 1.2 million U for children weighing ≥30 kg or adults). Two follow-up cultures should be performed after completing antimicrobial treatment to detect persistence of carriage, which occurs following erythromycin treatment in some cases. The first culture should be performed 24 hours after completing treatment. If results of cultures are positive, an additional 10-day course of oral erythromycin should be administered, and follow-up cultures should be performed again. Erythromycin-resistant strains have been identified, but their epidemiologic significance is undetermined. Fluoroquinolones (see Fluoroquinolones, p 864), rifampin, clarithromycin, and azithromycin have good in vitro activity and may be better tolerated than erythromycin, but these drugs have not been evaluated in clinical infection or in carriers.

ISOLATION OF THE HOSPITALIZED PATIENT: In addition to standard precautions, droplet precautions are recommended for patients and carriers with respiratory diphtheria until 2 cultures from both the nose and throat collected 24 hours after completing antimicrobial treatment are negative for *C diphtheriae*. Contact precautions are recommended for patients with cutaneous diphtheria until 2 cultures of skin lesions taken at least 24 hours apart and 24 hours after cessation of antimicrobial therapy are negative.

CONTROL MEASURES:

Care of Exposed People. Whenever respiratory diphtheria is suspected or proven, local public health officials should be notified promptly. Toxigenic *C diphtheriae* isolated from a cutaneous lesion requires investigation and prophylaxis of close contacts, as with respiratory diphtheria. Cases of cutaneous or respiratory diphtheria caused by infections with nontoxigenic strains of *C diphtheriae* are not nationally notifiable and do not require routine investigation or prophylaxis of contacts. Management of exposed people is based on individual circumstances, including immunization status and likelihood of adherence to follow-up and prophylaxis. Close contacts of a person suspected to have diphtheria should be identified, and the following are recommended:

- Contact tracing usually can be limited to household members and people with direct, habitual close contact or health care personnel exposed to nasopharyngeal secretions, people sharing kitchen facilities, or people caring for infected children.

- For close contacts, *regardless of their immunization status,* the following measures should be taken: (1) surveillance for evidence of disease for 7 days from last exposure to an untreated patient; (2) culture for *C diphtheriae;* and (3) antimicrobial prophylaxis with oral erythromycin (40–50 mg/kg per day for 7 to 10 days, maximum 1 g/day) or a single intramuscular injection of penicillin G benzathine (600 000 U for children weighing <30 kg, and 1.2 million U for children weighing ≥30 kg and for adults). Follow-up cultures of pharyngeal specimens should be performed after completion of therapy for contacts proven to be carriers. If cultures are positive, an additional 10-day course of erythromycin should be administered, and follow-up cultures of pharyngeal specimens again should be performed.
- Asymptomatic, previously immunized close contacts should receive a booster dose of an age-appropriate diphtheria toxoid-containing vaccine (DTaP [or DT], Tdap, or Td) if they have not received a booster dose of a diphtheria toxoid-containing vaccine within 5 years.
- Asymptomatic close contacts who have had fewer than 3 doses of a diphtheria toxoid-containing vaccine, children younger than 7 years in need of their fourth dose of DTaP (or DT), or people whose immunization status is not known should be immunized with an age-appropriate diphtheria toxoid-containing vaccine (DTaP, DT, Tdap, or Td, as indicated).
- Contacts who cannot be kept under surveillance should receive penicillin G benzathine rather than erythromycin, and if not fully immunized or if immunization status is not known, they should be immunized with DTaP, Tdap, DT, or Td vaccine, as appropriate for age.
- Use of equine diphtheria antitoxin in unimmunized close contacts is not recommended, because there is no evidence that antitoxin provides additional benefit.

Immunization. Universal immunization with a diphtheria toxoid-containing vaccine is the only effective control measure. The schedules for immunization against diphtheria are presented in the childhood and adolescent (**http://aapredbook.aappublications. org/site/resources/izschedules.xhtml**) and adult (**www.cdc.gov/vaccines**) immunization schedules.

Immunization of children from 2 months of age through 6 years of age (to the seventh birthday) routinely consists of 5 doses of diphtheria and tetanus toxoid-containing and acellular pertussis vaccine (DTaP). Regular booster injections of diphtheria toxoid as Td or Tdap are required every 10 years after completion of the initial immunization series. Immunization against diphtheria and tetanus for children younger than 7 years in whom pertussis immunization is contraindicated (see Pertussis, p 578) should be accomplished with DT. Other recommendations for diphtheria immunization, including recommendations for older children (7 through 18 years of age) and adults, can be found in Tetanus (p 750) as well as the childhood and adolescent and adult immunization schedules. When children and adults require booster tetanus toxoid for wound management (see Tetanus, p 750), Tdap or Td is used. Tetanus toxoid no longer is available as a single-antigen preparation in the United States.

Travelers to countries with endemic or epidemic diphtheria should have their diphtheria immunization status reviewed and updated when necessary.

Pneumococcal and meningococcal conjugate vaccines containing inactivated diphtheria toxoid or CRM_{197} protein, a nontoxic variant of diphtheria toxin, are not substitutes for diphtheria toxoid immunization.

Ehrlichia, Anaplasma, and Related Infections
(Human Ehrlichiosis, Anaplasmosis, and Related Infections Attributable to Bacteria in the Family Anaplasmataceae)

CLINICAL MANIFESTATIONS: Early signs and symptoms of infections by members of the bacterial family *Anaplasmataceae* can be nonspecific. All are acute febrile illnesses with common systemic manifestations including fever, headache, chills, rigors, malaise, myalgia, and nausea. More variable symptoms include arthralgia, vomiting, diarrhea, anorexia, cough, and confusion. Severe manifestations of these diseases can include acute respiratory distress syndrome, encephalopathy, meningitis, disseminated intravascular coagulation, toxic shock-like or septic shock-like syndromes, spontaneous hemorrhage, hepatic failure, and renal failure. Symptoms typically last 1 to 2 weeks, but prompt treatment with doxycycline shortens duration of illness and reduces the risk of serious manifestations and sequelae. Fatigue can last several weeks, and neurologic sequelae have been reported in some children after severe disease, more commonly with *Ehrlichia* infections.

A maculopapular rash is seen in up to 60% of ***Ehrlichia chaffeensis* infections** in children but in less than 30% of adults. The rash typically begins 5 days after symptom onset (notably fever). In adults, skin rash is reported more often for *Ehrlichia* infections than for *Anaplasma* infections. Severe disease and fatal outcome is more common in *E chaffeensis* infections (approximately 1%–3% case fatality) than with *Anaplasma phagocytophilum* infection.

Coinfections of ***Anaplasma*** with other tickborne diseases, including babesiosis and Lyme disease, can cause illness that is more severe or of longer duration than a single infection. Case fatality is uncommon (<1%).

Significant laboratory findings in **both *Anaplasma* and *Ehrlichia* infections** may include leukopenia with neutropenia (anaplasmosis) or lymphopenia (ehrlichiosis), thrombocytopenia, hyponatremia, and elevated serum hepatic aminotransferase concentrations. Cerebrospinal fluid abnormalities (eg, pleocytosis with a predominance of lymphocytes and increased total protein concentration) are common. People with underlying immunosuppression are at greater risk of severe disease. Severe disease has been reported in people who initially received trimethoprim-sulfamethoxazole before a correct diagnosis was made.

Because of the nonspecific presenting symptoms, Rocky Mountain spotted fever should be considered in the differential diagnosis in the United States. Heartland virus infection also manifests with similar clinical features and should be considered in patients without a more likely explanation who have tested negative for *Ehrlichia* and *Anaplasma* infection or have not responded to doxycycline therapy.

ETIOLOGY: *Ehrlichia* and *Anaplasma* species are obligate intracellular bacteria, which appear as gram-negative cocci that measure 0.5 to 1.5 μm in diameter. Although genetically different, *Anaplasma* and *Ehrlichia* infections often are grouped with rickettsia because of overlapping clinical presentation and their vectorborne spread (Table 3.4). Ehrlichiosis is the manifestation of (predominately) *E chaffeensis*, although *Ehrlichia ewingii* and *Ehrlichia muris eauclairensis* also are found in the United States (Table 3.5). Anaplasmosis is predominately caused by *A phagocytophilum* in the United States.

EPIDEMIOLOGY: Reported and suspected cases of ehrlichiosis and anaplasmosis are confined to geographic regions where their vectors are prevalent. Increased incidence is observed with heightened tick activity (mostly warm summer months) as well as with human activities with high levels of exposure to ticks. Similar to other tickborne diseases, patients often have no memory of being bitten by a tick.

Table 3.4. Taxonomy of *Rickettsiales*

Order	*Rickettsiales*			
Family	*Rickettsiaceae*		*Anaplasmataceae*	
Genera	*Rickettsiae*		*Anaplasma*	*Ehrlichia*
Species	Spotted fever group (SFG): Rocky Mountain spotted fever, Mediterranean spotted fever, Japanese spotted fever, etc	Typhus group: endemic, epidemic	*Anaplasma phagocytophilum*	*Ehrlichia chaffeensis, Ehrlichia ewingii, Ehrlichia muris eauclairensis*

Table 3.5. Human Ehrlichiosis, Anaplasmosis, and Related Infections in the United States

Disease	Causal Agent	Major Target Cell	Tick Vector	Geographic Distribution
Ehrlichiosis caused by *Ehrlichia chaffeensis*	*E chaffeensis*	Usually monocytes	Lone star tick (US) *(Amblyomma americanum)*	Predominantly southeast, south-central, from the East Coast extending westward to Texas; has been reported outside USA
Anaplasmosis	*Anaplasma phagocytophilum*	Usually granulocytes	Blacklegged tick *(Ixodes scapularis)* or Western blacklegged tick *(Ixodes pacificus)* (US)	Northeastern and upper Midwestern states and northern California; Europe and Asia
Ehrlichiosis caused by *Ehrlichia ewingii*	*E ewingii*	Usually granulocytes	Lone star tick (US) *(A americanum)*	Southeastern, south-central, and Midwestern states; Africa, Asia
Ehrlichiosis caused by *Ehrlichia muris eauclairensis*	*E muris eauclairensis*	Unknown, suspected in monocytes	Blacklegged tick *(Ixodes scapularis)*	Minnesota, Wisconsin

The reported incidence of **E chaffeensis infection** in the United States in 2017 was 5.2 cases per million population. Reported incidence of *E ewingii* infection in 2017 was 0.1 cases per million population, but the incidence is believed to be underreported because of nonspecific illness similar to *E chaffeensis* infections. Ehrlichiosis caused by *E chaffeensis* and *E ewingii* is reported most commonly from the south-central and southeastern United States, from the East Coast extending westward to Texas. *E chaffeensis* and *E ewingii* is transmitted by the bite of the lone star tick *(Amblyomma americanum)* and is reported from states within its geographic range. Cases attributable to *E muris eauclairensis* have been reported only from Minnesota and Wisconsin and are transmitted by the black-legged tick *(Ixodes scapularis)*. Cases of ehrlichiosis have occurred after blood transfusion or solid organ donation from asymptomatic donors.

The reported incidence of **Anaplasma infections** in the United States in 2017 was 18.3 cases per million population. Cases of human anaplasmosis are reported most frequently from the northeastern and upper midwestern United States. Cases of anaplasmosis also have been reported in northern California. In most of the United States, *A phagocytophilum* is transmitted by *Ixodes scapularis*, which also is the vector for ehrlichiosis caused by *E muris eauclairensis,* Lyme disease *(Borrelia burgdorferi),* Powassan virus infection, and babesiosis *(Babesia microti)*. In the western United States, the western blacklegged tick *(Ixodes pacificus)* is the main vector for *A phagocytophilum*. Cases of *Anaplasmataceae* infections have occurred after blood transfusion or solid organ donation from asymptomatic donors. Possible perinatal transmission of *A phagocytophilum* has been reported.

The **incubation period** usually is 5 to 14 days for both *E chaffeensis* and *A phagocytophilum.*

DIAGNOSTIC TESTS: Treatment of ehrlichiosis or anaplasmosis with doxycycline should not be delayed while awaiting confirmation of the diagnosis. Polymerase chain reaction (PCR) testing of whole blood for the organism is most sensitive for anaplasmosis and ehrlichiosis. Sensitivity of PCR testing decreases rapidly following administration of doxycycline, and a negative result does not rule out the diagnosis.

Tissue biopsies may be analyzed by PCR or immunohistochemistry. Because of the hazardous nature of these organisms, tissues should be fixed in paraffin or formalin before testing. Tissue analysis is available at specialized laboratories.

Serologic testing may be used to demonstrate a fourfold change in immunoglobulin (Ig) G-specific antibody titer by indirect immunofluorescence antibody (IFA) assay between paired acute and convalescent specimens taken 2 to 4 weeks apart. A single mildly elevated IgG titer may not be diagnostic, particularly in regions with high prevalence. IgM serologic assays are prone to false-positive reactions, and IgM can remain elevated for lengthy periods of time, reducing its diagnostic utility. Specific antigens are available for serologic testing of *E chaffeensis* and *A phagocytophilum* infections, although cross-reactivity between species can make interpretation difficult in areas where geographic distributions overlap.

Occasionally, *Anaplasmataceae* and *Ehrlichia* bacteria can be identified in Giemsa or Wright-stained peripheral blood smears or buffy coat leukocyte preparations in the first week of illness. Bacteria enter the host cell via phagocytosis, and these compartments provide a protective environment for bacterial replication. These morulae can be seen within granulocytes (targeted by *Anaplasma*) or monocytes (targeted by *Ehrlichia*). Culture for isolation of these pathogens is not performed routinely given requirement for biosafety-level 3 facilities to prevent accidental inoculation and aerosolization from culture.

TREATMENT: Doxycycline is the treatment of choice for all tickborne rickettsial diseases, including ehrlichiosis and anaplasmosis, and all other tickborne rickettsial diseases (see Table 4.3, p 895). Early initiation of therapy can minimize complications and should not be delayed awaiting laboratory confirmation. Treatment with doxycycline is recommended in patients of all ages, including children younger than 8 years, when rickettsial diseases are being considered (see Tetracyclines, p 866). After doxycycline is initiated, fever generally subsides within 24 to 48 hours.

Patients with suspected **ehrlichiosis** should be treated with doxycycline until at least 3 days after defervescence and until evidence of clinical improvement, typically 5 to 7 days. Patients with suspected **anaplasmosis** should be treated with doxycycline for 10 to 14 days to provide appropriate length of therapy for possible concurrent *Borrelia burgdorferi* (Lyme disease) infection.

Rifampin may provide an alternative to doxycycline in patients with anaplasmosis who demonstrate hypersensitivity to doxycycline. Rifampin has been used successfully in several pregnant women with anaplasmosis, and studies suggest that this drug appears effective against *A phagocytophilum*. Small numbers of children younger than 8 years of age have also been treated successfully for anaplasmosis with rifampin for a 7- to 10-day course. Rifampin has been shown to be effective against *E chaffeensis* in a laboratory setting but has not been evaluated as an alternative therapy in a clinical setting.

Treatment with trimethoprim-sulfamethoxazole has been linked to more severe outcomes and is contraindicated.

ISOLATION OF THE HOSPITALIZED PATIENT: Standard precautions are recommended. Human-to-human transmission via direct contact has not been documented.

CONTROL MEASURES: Limiting exposures to ticks and tick bites is the primary means of prevention (see Prevention of Mosquitoborne and Tickborne Infections, p 175). Risk of transmission through blood transfusion or organ transplantation should be considered in areas with endemic infection. Prophylactic administration of doxycycline after a tick bite is not indicated because of the low risk of infection and lack of proven effectiveness. Cases of ehrlichiosis and anaplasmosis are notifiable diseases in the United States and should be reported to the local or state health department. Additional information is available on the CDC website (**www.cdc.gov/ehrlichiosis, www.cdc.gov/anaplasmosis,** and **www.cdc.gov/ticks**), including a collaborative report providing recommendations for the diagnosis and management of tickborne rickettsial diseases.[1]

Serious Neonatal Bacterial Infections Caused by *Enterobacteriaceae*
(Including Septicemia and Meningitis)

CLINICAL MANIFESTATIONS: Neonatal septicemia or meningitis caused by *Escherichia coli* and other gram-negative bacilli cannot be differentiated clinically from septicemia or meningitis caused by other organisms. The early signs of sepsis can be subtle and similar to signs observed in noninfectious processes. Signs of septicemia include fever,

---

[1] Biggs HM, Behravesh CB, Bradley KK, et al. Diagnosis and management of tickborne rickettsial diseases: Rocky Mountain spotted fever and other spotted fever group rickettsioses, ehrlichioses, and anaplasmosis—United States. *MMWR Recomm Rep*. 2016;65(RR-2):1–44. Available at: **www.cdc.gov/mmwr/volumes/65/rr/rr6502a1.htm**

temperature instability, heart rate abnormalities, grunting respirations, apnea, cyanosis, lethargy, irritability, anorexia, vomiting, jaundice, abdominal distention, cellulitis, and diarrhea. Meningitis, especially early in the course, can occur without overt signs suggesting central nervous system involvement. Some gram-negative bacilli, such as *Citrobacter koseri*, *Cronobacter* (formerly *Enterobacter*) *sakazakii*, *Serratia marcescens*, and *Salmonella* species, are associated with increased risk for brain abscesses in infants with meningitis caused by these organisms.

ETIOLOGY: *Enterobacteriaceae* are a large family of gram-negative, facultatively anaerobic, rod-shaped bacteria that include *Escherichia* species, *Klebsiella* species, *Enterobacter* species, *Proteus* species, *Providencia* species, and *Serratia* species, among many others. *E coli* strains, often those with the K1 capsular polysaccharide antigen, are the most common cause of septicemia and meningitis in neonates. Other important gram-negative bacilli causing neonatal septicemia include *Klebsiella* species, *Enterobacter* species, *Proteus* species, *Citrobacter* species, *Salmonella* species, and *Serratia* species. Nonencapsulated strains of *Haemophilus influenzae* and anaerobic gram-negative bacilli are rare causes. *Elizabethkingia meningoseptica* has been associated with outbreaks of neonatal meningitis, with infections in immunocompromised people or with other health care-associated outbreaks related to environmental contamination. *Elizabethkingia anophelis* has been reported as a recent cause of health care-associated infection in adults older than 65 years, with rare cases reported in neonates.

EPIDEMIOLOGY: The source of *E coli* and other *Enterobacteriaceae* in neonatal infections during the first days of life typically is the maternal genital tract. Reservoirs for gram-negative bacilli can be present within the health care environment. Acquisition of gram-negative organisms can occur through person-to-person transmission from hospital nursery personnel as well as from nursery environmental sites such as sinks, countertops, powdered infant formula, and respiratory therapy equipment, especially among very preterm infants who require prolonged neonatal intensive care management. Predisposing factors in neonatal gram-negative bacterial infections include maternal intrapartum infection, gestation less than 37 weeks, low birth weight, and prolonged rupture of membranes. Metabolic abnormalities (eg, galactosemia), fetal hypoxia, and acidosis have been implicated as predisposing factors. Neonates with defects in the integrity of skin or mucosa (eg, myelomeningocele) or abnormalities of gastrointestinal or genitourinary tracts are at increased risk of gram-negative bacterial infections. In neonatal intensive care units, systems for respiratory and metabolic support, invasive or surgical procedures, and indwelling vascular catheters are risk factors for infection. Frequent use of broad-spectrum antimicrobial agents enables selection and proliferation of strains of gram-negative bacilli that may be resistant to multiple antimicrobial agents.

Multiple mechanisms of resistance in gram-negative bacilli can be present simultaneously. Resistance resulting from production of chromosomally encoded or plasmid-derived AmpC beta-lactamases or from plasmid-mediated extended-spectrum beta-lactamases (ESBLs) occurs primarily in *E coli*, *Klebsiella* species, and *Enterobacter* species but has been reported in many other gram-negative species. Resistant gram-negative infections have been associated with nursery outbreaks, especially in very low birth weight infants. Additional risk factors for neonatal infection with ESBL-producing organisms include prolonged mechanical ventilation, extended hospital stay, use of invasive devices, and use of antimicrobial agents. Infants born to mothers colonized with ESBL-producing *E coli* are themselves at an increased risk of becoming colonized with ESBL-producing *E coli* compared with infants born to noncolonized mothers. Organisms that produce ESBLs typically are resistant to penicillins, cephalosporins, and monobactams and can be resistant to aminoglycosides. Carbapenemase-producing *Enterobacteriaceae* also have emerged, especially *Klebsiella pneumoniae, E coli,* and *Enterobacter cloacae.* ESBL- and carbapenemase-producing bacteria often carry additional plasmid-borne genes that encode for high-level resistance to aminoglycosides, fluoroquinolones, and trimethoprim-sulfamethoxazole.

The **incubation period** is variable; time of onset of infection ranges from birth to several weeks after birth or longer in very low birth weight, preterm infants with prolonged hospitalizations.

DIAGNOSTIC TESTS: Diagnosis is established by growth of *E coli* or other gram-negative bacilli from blood, cerebrospinal fluid (CSF), or other usually sterile sites. Isolates may be identified by traditional biochemical tests, commercially available biochemical test systems, mass spectrometry of bacterial cell components, or molecular methods. Multiplexed molecular tests capable of rapidly identifying a variety of gram-negative rods including *E coli* directly in positive blood culture bottles have been cleared by the US Food and Drug Administration. Special screening and confirmatory laboratory procedures are required to detect some multidrug-resistant gram-negative organisms. Molecular diagnostics are being used increasingly for identification of pathogens; specimens should be saved for resistance testing.

TREATMENT[1,2]:

- Initial empiric treatment for suspected early-onset gram-negative sepsis in neonates should be based on local and regional antimicrobial susceptibility data. The proportion of *E coli* bloodstream infections with onset within 72 hours of life that are resistant to ampicillin is high (approximately two-thirds) among very low birth weight infants. These *E coli* infections almost invariably are susceptible to gentamicin, although monotherapy with an aminoglycoside is not recommended.
- Ampicillin and an aminoglycoside may be first-line therapy for neonatal sepsis in areas with low ampicillin resistance. An alternative regimen of ampicillin and an extended-spectrum cephalosporin (such as cefotaxime or, if that is unavailable, ceftazidime or cefepime) can be used, but rapid emergence of cephalosporin-resistant organisms, especially *Enterobacter* species, *Klebsiella* species, and *Serratia* species and increased risk of colonization or infection with ESBL-producing *Enterobacteriaceae* can occur when cephalosporin use is routine in a neonatal unit. The empiric addition of broader-spectrum antibiotic therapy may be considered until culture results are available if patient is a severely ill preterm infant at the highest risk for early-onset gram-negative sepsis (such as infants with very low birth weight born after prolonged premature rupture of membranes and infants exposed to prolonged courses of antepartum antibiotic therapy) or a term neonate who is critically ill. When there is a concern for gram-negative meningitis, an extended-spectrum cephalosporin (eg, cefotaxime or, if that is unavailable, ceftazidime or cefepime) should be used unless local resistance profiles increase the likelihood

[1]Puopolo KM, Benitz WE, Zaoutis TE; American Academy of Pediatrics, Committee on Fetus and Newborn; Committee on Infectious Diseases. Management of neonates born at ≤34 6/7 weeks' gestation with suspected or proven early-onset bacterial sepsis. *Pediatrics.* 2018;142(6):e20182896

[2]Puopolo KM, Benitz WE, Zaoutis TE; American Academy of Pediatrics, Committee on Fetus and Newborn; Committee on Infectious Diseases. Management of neonates born at ≥35 0/7 weeks' gestation with suspected or proven early-onset bacterial sepsis. *Pediatrics.* 2018;142(6):e20182894

of a multidrug-resistant gram-negative organism, in which case a carbapenem is the preferred choice for empiric therapy.
- Once the causative agent and its in vitro antimicrobial susceptibility pattern are known, nonmeningeal infections should be treated with ampicillin, an appropriate aminoglycoside, or an extended-spectrum cephalosporin (such as cefotaxime) on the basis of the susceptibility results. Some experts treat nonmeningeal infections caused by *Enterobacter* species, *Serratia* species, and some other less commonly occurring gram-negative bacilli with a beta-lactam antimicrobial agent and an aminoglycoside.
- For ampicillin-susceptible CSF isolates of *E coli*, meningitis can be treated with ampicillin or cefotaxime; meningitis caused by an ampicillin-resistant, cefotaxime-susceptible isolate can be treated with cefotaxime. Combination therapy of ampicillin or cefotaxime with an aminoglycoside is used until CSF is sterile. Expert advice from an infectious disease specialist is helpful for management of meningitis.
- A carbapenem is the drug of choice for treatment of *Enterobacteriaceae* infections caused by ESBL-producing organisms, especially certain *K pneumoniae* isolates. Of the aminoglycosides, amikacin retains the most activity against ESBL-producing strains. An aminoglycoside or cefepime can be used if the organism is susceptible, because cefepime does not induce chromosomal AmpC enzymes.
- *E meningoseptica* intrinsically is resistant to most beta-lactams, including carbapenems, and has variable susceptibility to trimethoprim-sulfamethoxazole and fluoroquinolones; most are susceptible to piperacillin-tazobactam and rifampin. Expert advice from an infectious disease specialist is helpful in management of multidrug-resistant infection (eg, *E meningoseptica*) and ESBL-producing gram-negative infections in neonates.
- The treatment of infections caused by carbapenemase-producing gram-negative organisms is guided by the susceptibility profile, which depends in part on the carbapenemase type. Treatment can include an aminoglycoside, especially amikacin; trimethoprim-sulfamethoxazole; or colistin. Isolates often are susceptible to tigecycline, fluoroquinolones, and polymyxin B, for which experience in neonates is limited. Ceftazidime-avibactam may be effective in some cases and is approved for children 3 months to 18 years of age for the treatment of complicated urinary tract infection or complicated intrabdominal infection (in the latter case, additional therapy such as metronidazole is needed for anaerobic coverage). Some carbapenemase-producing isolates may retain susceptibility to aztreonam. Combination therapy often is used. Treatment regimens using carbapenems may be an option if the carbapenem minimal inhibitory concentration is in the intermediate range or lower, and with a second antibiotic agent being added or when a prolonged infusion regimen is used. Expert advice from an infectious disease specialist is helpful in management of carbapenemase-producing gram-negative infections.
- All neonates with gram-negative meningitis should undergo repeat lumbar puncture to ensure sterility of the CSF after 24 to 48 hours of therapy. If CSF remains culture positive, choice and doses of antimicrobial agents should be reevaluated, and another lumbar puncture should be performed after another 48 to 72 hours.
- Duration of therapy is based on clinical and bacteriologic response of the patient and the site(s) of infection; the usual duration of therapy for uncomplicated bacteremia is 10 to 14 days, and for meningitis, minimum duration is 21 days.
- All infants with gram-negative meningitis should undergo careful follow-up examinations, including testing for hearing loss, neurologic abnormalities, and developmental delay.

- Immune Globulin Intravenous (IGIV) therapy for newborn infants receiving antimicrobial agents for suspected or proven serious infection has been shown to have no effect on outcomes measured and is not recommended.

ISOLATION OF THE HOSPITALIZED PATIENT: Standard precautions are recommended. Exceptions include hospital nursery epidemics, infants with *Salmonella* infection, and infants with infection caused by gram-negative bacilli that are resistant to multiple antimicrobial agents, including ESBL-producing strains and carbapenemase-producing *Enterobacteriaceae;* in these situations, contact precautions also are indicated.[1]

CONTROL MEASURES: Infection-control personnel should be aware of pathogens causing infections in infants so that clusters of infections are recognized and investigated appropriately. Several cases of infection caused by the same genus and species of bacteria occurring in infants in physical proximity or caused by an unusual pathogen indicate the need for an epidemiologic investigation (see Infection Prevention and Control for Hospitalized Children, p 133). Periodic review of in vitro antimicrobial susceptibility patterns of clinically important bacterial isolates from newborn infants, especially infants in the neonatal intensive care unit, can provide useful epidemiologic and therapeutic information.

Enterovirus (Nonpoliovirus)
(Group A and B Coxsackieviruses, Echoviruses, Numbered Enteroviruses)

CLINICAL MANIFESTATIONS: Nonpolio enteroviruses are responsible for significant and frequent illnesses in infants and children and result in protean clinical manifestations. The most common manifestation is nonspecific febrile illness, which in young infants may lead to evaluation for bacterial sepsis. Other manifestations can include: (1) respiratory: coryza, pharyngitis, herpangina, stomatitis, parotitis, croup, bronchiolitis, pneumonia, pleurodynia, and bronchospasm; (2) skin: hand-foot-and-mouth disease, onychomadesis (shedding of nails), and nonspecific exanthems (particularly associated with echoviruses); (3) neurologic: aseptic meningitis, encephalitis, and motor paralysis (acute flaccid myelitis); (4) gastrointestinal/genitourinary: vomiting, diarrhea, abdominal pain, hepatitis, pancreatitis, and orchitis; (5) eye: acute hemorrhagic conjunctivitis and uveitis; (6) heart: myopericarditis; and (7) muscle: pleurodynia and other skeletal myositis. Neonates, especially those who acquire infection in the absence of type-specific maternal antibody, are at risk of severe and life-threatening disease, including viral sepsis, meningoencephalitis, myocarditis, hepatitis, coagulopathy, and pneumonitis. Acute flaccid myelitis (AFM) is a rare but serious neurologic illness that presents with acute onset of limb weakness, most often accompanied by cerebrospinal fluid pleocytosis and nonenhancing lesions localized to the gray matter of the spinal cord on magnetic resonance imaging. Multiple viruses are known to cause this condition, including enteroviruses.

Infection with enterovirus A71 is associated with hand-foot-and-mouth disease, herpangina, and in a small proportion of cases, severe neurologic disease, including brainstem encephalomyelitis and acute flaccid myelitis; secondary pulmonary edema/hemorrhage and cardiopulmonary collapse can occur, resulting in fatalities and sequelae among survivors.

---

[1]Centers for Disease Control and Prevention. Facility Guidance for Control of Carbapenem Resistant Enterobacteriaceae (CRE) November 2015 Update. Available at: **www.cdc.gov/hai/pdfs/cre/CRE-guidance-508.pdf**

Other noteworthy but not exclusive clinical associations include coxsackieviruses A6, A10, and A16 with hand-foot-and-mouth disease (including severe hand-foot-and-mouth disease, "eczema coxsackium," and atypical cutaneous involvement with coxsackievirus A6); coxsackievirus A24 variant and enterovirus D70 with acute hemorrhagic conjunctivitis; and coxsackieviruses B1 through B5 with pleurodynia and myopericarditis. Enterovirus D68 (EV-D68) is associated with mild to severe respiratory illness in infants, children, and teenagers and has been responsible for localized and large multinational outbreaks of respiratory disease. Disease is usually characterized by exacerbation of preexisting asthma or new-onset wheezing in children without history of asthma, often requiring hospitalization and, in some patients, intensive supportive care. Enterovirus D-68 has also been epidemiologically linked to biennial outbreaks of AFM beginning in 2014, although this pattern was disrupted during the pandemic year 2020.

Patients with humoral and combined immune deficiencies can develop persistent central nervous system infections, a dermatomyositis-like syndrome, arthritis, hepatitis, and/or disseminated infection. Severe and/or chronic neurologic or multisystem disease is reported in hematopoietic stem cell and solid organ transplant recipients, children with malignancies, and patients treated with anti-CD20 monoclonal antibody (eg, rituximab).

ETIOLOGY: The enteroviruses, along with the rhinoviruses, comprise a genus of small, nonenveloped, single-stranded, positive-sense RNA viruses in the *Picornaviridae* family. The nonpolio enteroviruses include more than 110 distinct types formerly subclassified as group A coxsackieviruses, group B coxsackieviruses, echoviruses, and newer numbered enteroviruses. A more recent classification system groups the enteroviruses into 4 species (enterovirus [EV] A, B, C, and D) on the basis of genetic similarity, although traditional serotype names are retained for some individual types. Echoviruses 22 and 23 have been reclassified as parechoviruses 1 and 2, respectively (see Parechovirus Infections, p 561).

EPIDEMIOLOGY: Humans are the principal reservoir for enteroviruses, although some primates can become infected. Enterovirus infections are common and are distributed worldwide; the majority of infections are asymptomatic. Enteroviruses are spread by fecal-oral and respiratory routes and from mother to infant prenatally, in the peripartum period, and rarely via breastfeeding. EV-D68 is believed to be spread primarily by respiratory transmission. Enteroviruses may survive on environmental surfaces for periods long enough to allow transmission from fomites, and transmission via contaminated water and food can occur. Hospital nursery and other institutional outbreaks may occur. Infection incidence, clinical attack rates, and disease severity typically are greatest in infants and young children, and infections occur more frequently in tropical areas and where poor sanitation, poor hygiene, and high population density are present. Most enterovirus infections in temperate climates occur in the summer and fall (June through October in the northern hemisphere), but seasonal patterns are less evident in the tropics. Fecal shedding of most enteroviruses can persist for several weeks or months after onset of infection, but respiratory tract shedding usually is limited to 1 to 3 weeks or less. Fecal shedding is uncommon with EV-D68 infection. Enterovirus infection and viral transmission can occur without signs of clinical illness.

The usual **incubation period** for enterovirus infections is 3 to 6 days, except for acute hemorrhagic conjunctivitis, in which the **incubation period** is 24 to 72 hours.

DIAGNOSTIC TESTS: Enteroviruses generally can be detected by qualitative reverse transcriptase-polymerase chain reaction (RT-PCR) assay and culture from a variety of specimens, including stool, rectal swab specimens, throat swab specimens, nasopharyn-geal aspirates, conjunctival swab specimens, tracheal aspirates, vesicle fluid, blood, urine, tissue biopsy specimens, and cerebrospinal fluid (CSF). RT-PCR assay is rapid and more sensitive than isolation of enteroviruses in cell culture and can detect all enteroviruses, including types that are difficult or impossible to cultivate in cell cultures. RT-PCR assays for detection of enterovirus RNA are available at many reference and commercial labo-ratories for CSF, blood, and other specimens. Enterovirus PCR assays will not detect parechoviruses (and vice versa).

Patients with enterovirus A71 neurologic disease often have negative results of RT-PCR assay and culture of CSF (even in the presence of CSF pleocytosis) and blood; RT-PCR assay and culture of throat or rectal swab and/or vesicle fluid specimens (in cases of hand-foot-and-mouth disease) are more frequently positive.

EV-D68 is demonstrated primarily in respiratory tract specimens and can be detected with multiplex respiratory RT-PCR assays, but these assays do not distinguish entero-viruses from rhinoviruses. Definitive identification of EV-D68 requires partial genomic sequencing or amplification with an EV-D68-specific RT-PCR assay.

Sensitivity of culture ranges from 0% to 80% depending on type and cell lines used. Many group A coxsackieviruses grow poorly or not at all in vitro. Culture usually requires 3 to 8 days to detect growth. The type of enterovirus may be identified by genomic sequencing. Typing may be indicated in cases of special clinical interest or for epidemio-logic purposes (eg, for investigation of disease clusters or outbreaks). Acute infection with a known enterovirus type can be determined at reference laboratories by demonstration of a change in neutralizing antibody titer between acute and convalescent serum speci-mens or by detection of type-specific immunoglobulin (Ig) M, but serologic assays are rel-atively insensitive, may lack specificity, and are rarely used for diagnosis of acute infection. Antigen detection assays for enterovirus A71 have been developed but are not routinely available.

TREATMENT: No specific therapy is available for enteroviruses infections. Immune Globulin Intravenous (IGIV), administered intravenously or via intraventricular admin-istration, may be beneficial for chronic enterovirus meningoencephalitis in immunodefi-cient patients. However, IGIV is not approved for intraventricular administration. IGIV also has been used for life-threatening neonatal enterovirus infections (maternal convales-cent plasma also has been used), severe enterovirus infections in transplant recipients and people with malignancies, suspected viral myocarditis, enterovirus A71 neurologic disease, and for patients with AFM, but proof of efficacy for these uses is lacking. The CDC has provided interim guidance on the clinical management of children with AFM (**www. cdc.gov/acute-flaccid-myelitis/hcp/clinical-management.html**) with no specific therapy recommended. Interferons occasionally have been used for treatment of enterovirus-associated myocarditis and chronic enterovirus meningoencephalitis, without definitive proof of efficacy.

The antiviral drug pleconaril has activity against many enteroviruses but is not avail-able commercially. Pocapavir is another antiviral drug that is being developed primarily for the treatment of chronic poliovirus infection in patients with a primary immunodefi-ciency and has some activity in vitro against some nonpolio enteroviruses. Like pleconaril, pocapavir is not commercially available but may be accessible under a compassionate use mechanism. Fluoxetine has in vitro activity against group B and D enteroviruses (includ-ing EV-D68), but studies have not proven clinical benefit.

ISOLATION OF THE HOSPITALIZED PATIENT: In addition to standard precautions, contact precautions are indicated for infants and young children for the duration of enterovirus illness. Droplet precautions also are indicated for EV-D68 respiratory infections. Cohorting of infected neonates has been effective in controlling hospital nursery enterovirus outbreaks.

CONTROL MEASURES: Hand hygiene, especially after diaper changing, and respiratory hygiene (particularly for EV-D68) are important in decreasing spread of enteroviruses within families, child care facilities, and other institutions. Other measures include avoidance of contaminated utensils and fomites, and disinfection of surfaces. Isolation of symptomatic children or temporary closure may be required to control hand-foot-and-mouth disease outbreaks in child care facilities (see Children in Group Child Care and Schools, p 116). Recommended chlorination treatment of drinking water and swimming pools may help prevent transmission.

Maintenance administration of IGIV in patients with severe deficits of B-lymphocyte function (eg, severe combined immunodeficiency syndrome, X-linked agammaglobulinemia) may prevent chronic enterovirus infection of the central nervous system. Enterovirus A71 vaccines have been licensed in China and are being evaluated in other Asian countries; vaccines for other enterovirus serotypes associated with more severe disease also are under investigation.

Epstein-Barr Virus Infections
(Infectious Mononucleosis)

CLINICAL MANIFESTATIONS: Infectious mononucleosis is the most common presentation of primary symptomatic Epstein-Barr virus (EBV) infection. It manifests typically as fever, pharyngitis with or without petechiae, exudative pharyngitis, lymphadenopathy, hepatosplenomegaly, and atypical lymphocytosis. The spectrum of disease is wide, ranging from asymptomatic to fatal infection. Infections are unrecognized or nonspecific in infants and young children. Rash can occur in up to 20% of patients and is more common in patients treated with antibiotics, most commonly ampicillin or amoxicillin as well as with other penicillins. Central nervous system (CNS) manifestations include aseptic meningitis, encephalitis, myelitis, optic neuritis, cranial nerve palsies, transverse myelitis, Alice in Wonderland syndrome, and Guillain-Barré syndrome. Hematologic complications include splenic rupture, thrombocytopenia, agranulocytosis, hemolytic anemia, and hemophagocytic lymphohistiocytosis (HLH, or hemophagocytic syndrome). Pneumonia, orchitis, and myocarditis are observed infrequently. Early in the course of primary infection, 1% to 10% of circulating B lymphocytes are infected with EBV, and EBV-specific cytotoxic/suppressor T lymphocytes account for up to 50% of the CD8+ T lymphocytes in the blood. Replication of EBV in B lymphocytes results in T-lymphocyte proliferation and inhibition of B-lymphocyte proliferation by T-lymphocyte cytotoxic responses, natural killer (NK) cell activation, and the production of neutralizing antibodies. Fatal disseminated infection or B-lymphocyte, T-lymphocyte, or NK-cell lymphomas rarely occur in children with no detectable immunologic abnormality as well as in children with congenital or acquired cellular immune deficiencies.

EBV is associated with several other distinct disorders, including X-linked lymphoproliferative syndrome, post-transplantation lymphoproliferative disorders, Burkitt lymphoma, nasopharyngeal carcinoma, undifferentiated B- or T-lymphocyte lymphomas, and leiomyosarcoma. X-linked lymphoproliferative syndrome occurs most often in people with an inherited, maternally derived, recessive genetic defect in the SH2DIA or XIAP/BIRC4 genes, which are important in several lymphocyte signaling pathways. The syndrome is characterized by several phenotypic expressions, including occurrence of fatal infectious mononucleosis early in life among boys; HLH; nodular B-lymphocyte lymphomas, often with CNS involvement; and profound pancytopenia. Similarly, X-linked immunodeficiency with magnesium defect, EBV infection, and neoplasia (XMEN) disease is characterized by loss-of-function mutations in the gene encoding magnesium transporter 1 (MAGT1), chronic high-level EBV DNAemia with increased EBV-infected B cells, and heightened susceptibility to EBV-associated lymphomas. Several other genetic mutations associated with the failure to control EBV infection because of changes in T lymphocyte and NK cell function have also been described.

EBV-associated lymphoproliferative disorders can also occur in patients who are immunocompromised, such as transplant recipients or people infected with human immunodeficiency virus (HIV). The highest incidence of these disorders occurs in small intestine transplant recipients, with moderate risk in liver, pancreas, lung, and heart transplant recipients. Proliferative states range from benign lymph node hypertrophy to monoclonal lymphomas. Other EBV-associated lymphoproliferative syndromes are of greater importance outside the United States, such as Burkitt lymphoma, which can be endemic or sporadic. EBV is present in virtually 100% of endemic Burkitt lymphoma (a B-lymphocyte tumor predominantly found in head and neck lymph nodes primarily in Central Africa) versus 20% in sporadic Burkitt lymphoma (a B-lymphocyte tumor of abdominal lymphoid tissue predominantly in North America and Europe). EBV is found in nearly 100% of nasopharyngeal carcinoma in Southeast Asia and the Inuit populations. EBV also has been associated with Hodgkin disease (a B-lymphocyte tumor), non-Hodgkin lymphomas (both B and T lymphocyte types), gastric carcinoma "lymphoepitheliomas," and a variety of other epithelial malignancies.

Chronic fatigue syndrome is not directly caused by EBV infection; however, fatigue lasting 6 months or more may follow approximately 10% of cases of classic infectious mononucleosis.

ETIOLOGY: EBV (also known as human herpesvirus 4) is a gamma herpesvirus of the *Lymphocryptovirus* genus and is the most common cause of infectious mononucleosis (>90% of cases).

EPIDEMIOLOGY: Humans are the only known reservoir of EBV, and approximately 90% of US adults have been infected. Close personal contact usually is required for transmission. The virus is viable in saliva for several hours outside the body; the role of fomites in transmission is unknown. EBV may be transmitted by blood transfusion or transplantation. Infection commonly is contracted early in life, particularly among members of lower socioeconomic groups, where crowding and intrafamilial spread is common. Endemic infectious mononucleosis is common in group settings of adolescents, such as in educational or military institutions. No seasonal pattern has been clearly documented. Intermittent excretion in saliva is lifelong after infection and likely explains viral spread and persistence in the population.

The **incubation period** of infectious mononucleosis is estimated to be 30 to 50 days.

Table 3.6. Serum Epstein-Barr Virus (EBV) Antibodies in EBV Infection

Infection	VCA IgG	VCA IgM	EA (D)	EBNA
No previous infection	–	–	–	–
Acute infection	+	+	+/–	–
Recent infection	+	+/–	+/–	+/–
Past infection	+	–	+/–	+

VCA IgG indicates immunoglobulin (Ig) G class antibody to viral capsid antigen; VCA IgM, IgM class antibody to VCA; EA (D), early antigen diffuse staining; and EBNA, EBV nuclear antigen.

DIAGNOSTIC TESTS: Routine diagnosis depends on serologic testing. Nonspecific tests for heterophile antibody, including the Paul-Bunnell test and slide agglutination reaction test, are available most commonly and are approximately 90% sensitive and specific. The heterophile antibody response primarily is immunoglobulin (Ig) M, which appears during the first 2 weeks of illness and usually disappears over 6 months. The results of heterophile antibody tests often are negative in children younger than 4 years of age with EBV infection, but heterophile antibody tests identify at least 85% of cases of classic infectious mononucleosis in older children and adults during the second week of illness. An absolute increase in atypical lymphocytes during the second week of illness with infectious mononucleosis is another characteristic but nonspecific finding.

Multiple specific serologic antibody tests for EBV infection are available (see Table 3.6 and Fig 3.1). The most commonly performed test is for antibody against the viral capsid antigen (VCA) of EBV. Because IgG antibodies against VCA occur in high titer early in infection and persist for life at modest levels, testing of acute and convalescent serum specimens for IgG anti-VCA alone is not useful for establishing the presence of active infection. In contrast, testing for the presence of IgM anti-VCA antibody and the absence or very low titers of antibodies to Epstein-Barr nuclear antigen (EBNA) is useful for identifying active and recent infections. Because serum antibody against EBNA is not present until several weeks to months after onset of infection and rises with convalescence, a very elevated anti-EBNA antibody concentration typically excludes active primary infection. Testing for antibodies against early antigen (EA) is not usually required to assess EBV-associated mononucleosis. Typical patterns of antibody responses to EBV infection are illustrated in Table 3.6 and Fig 3.1.

Serologic testing for EBV is useful, particularly for evaluating patients who have heterophile-negative infectious mononucleosis, are younger than 4 years, or in whom the infectious mononucleosis syndrome is not classic. Testing for other agents, especially cytomegalovirus, *Toxoplasma*, human herpesvirus 6, adenovirus, and HIV (in those with HIV risk factors), may be indicated for some patients. Diagnosis of the entire range of EBV-associated illness requires use of additional molecular and antibody techniques, particularly for patients with immune deficiencies.

Polymerase chain reaction (PCR) assay for detection of EBV DNA in serum, plasma, and tissue and reverse transcriptase-PCR assay for detection of EBV RNA in lymphoid cells, tissue, and/or body fluids are available and can be useful in evaluation of immunocompromised patients and in complex clinical situations.

FIG 3.1. SCHEMATIC REPRESENTATION OF THE EVOLUTION OF ANTIBODIES TO VARIOUS EPSTEIN-BARR VIRUS ANTIGENS IN PATIENTS WITH INFECTIOUS MONONUCLEOSIS.

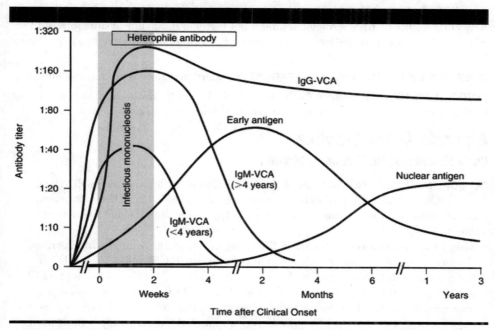

Source: *Manual of Clinical Laboratory Immunology.* Washington, DC: American Society for Microbiology; 1997:636. © 1997 American Society for Microbiology. Used with permission. No further reproduction or distribution is permitted without the prior written permission of American Society for Microbiology.

TREATMENT: Currently, there is no antiviral treatment approved for EBV infection. Patients suspected to have infectious mononucleosis should not receive ampicillin or amoxicillin, which may cause nonallergic morbilliform rashes in a proportion of patients with active EBV infection. Although therapy with short-course corticosteroids may have a beneficial effect on some acute symptoms, because of potential adverse effects, their use is usually considered only for patients with marked tonsillar inflammation with impending airway obstruction, massive splenomegaly, myocarditis, hemolytic anemia, or HLH. The dosage of prednisone usually is 1 mg/kg per day, orally (maximum 60 mg/day), for 5 to 7 days, in some cases with tapering. Life-threatening HLH has been treated with cytotoxic agents and immunomodulators, including etoposide, cyclosporine, and/or corticosteroids. Although acyclovir and valacyclovir have in vitro antiviral activity against EBV and reduce viral replication, they produce no clinical benefit in infectious mononucleosis but are occasionally used in immunocompromised patients. Decreasing immunosuppressive therapy often is beneficial for patients with EBV-induced post-transplant lymphoproliferative disorders (PTLD). Rituximab, a monoclonal antibody directed against CD20+ B lymphocytes, also is used both preemptively and for treatment of PTLD in hematopoietic stem cell and solid organ transplant patients, respectively.

Strenuous activity and contact sports should be avoided for at least 21 days after onset of symptoms of infectious mononucleosis. After 21 days, limited noncontact aerobic activity can be allowed if there are no symptoms and there is no overt splenomegaly. Clearance to participate in contact sports is appropriate after 4 to 7 weeks following the onset of symptoms if the athlete is asymptomatic and has no overt splenomegaly. Imaging modalities rarely are helpful in decisions about clearance to return to contact sports. Repeat monospot or EBV serologic testing is not useful in most clinical situations. It may take 3 to 6 months or longer following mononucleosis for an athlete to return to preillness fitness.

ISOLATION OF THE HOSPITALIZED PATIENT: Standard precautions are recommended.

CONTROL MEASURES: None in the hospital or clinic. Avoid salivary exchange or sharing food or drink with someone who recently had infectious mononucleosis.

Escherichia coli Diarrhea
(Including Hemolytic-Uremic Syndrome)

CLINICAL MANIFESTATIONS: *Escherichia coli* is a common bacterial cause of diarrheal illness. At least 5 pathotypes of diarrhea-producing *E coli* strains have been identified. Clinical features of disease caused by each pathotype are summarized as follows (see Table 3.7):

- **Shiga toxin-producing *E coli* (STEC)** organisms are associated with diarrhea, hemorrhagic colitis, and hemolytic-uremic syndrome (HUS). STEC O157:H7 is the serotype most often implicated in outbreaks and consistently is a virulent STEC serotype, but other serotypes also can cause illness. STEC illness typically begins with nonbloody diarrhea. Stools usually become bloody after 2 or 3 days, representing the onset of hemorrhagic colitis. Severe abdominal pain typically is short lived, and low-grade fever is present in approximately one third of cases. Diseases caused by *E coli* O157:H7 and other STEC organisms should be considered in people with presumptive diagnoses of intussusception, appendicitis, inflammatory bowel disease, or ischemic colitis. There are 2 types of Shiga toxin (Stx), Stx1 and Stx2; several variants of each type exist. In general, STEC strains that produce Stx2, especially variants Stx2a, Stx2c, and Stx2d, are more virulent than strains that only produce Stx1. However, in the clinical setting, there is limited ability to differentiate between Stx variants.
- Diarrhea caused by **enteropathogenic *E coli* (EPEC)** is watery. Illness occurs almost exclusively in children younger than 2 years and predominantly in resource-limited countries, either sporadically or in epidemics, or in travelers to those settings. Although usually mild, diarrhea can result in dehydration and even death, particularly in resource-limited countries. EPEC diarrhea can be persistent and can result in wasting or growth restriction. EPEC infection is uncommon in breastfed infants. Strains known as atypical EPEC have been isolated; their role in causing disease is unclear, but there is evidence supporting an association between some strains of atypical EPEC and prolonged watery diarrhea. EPEC can also cause travelers' diarrhea.
- Diarrhea caused by **enterotoxigenic *E coli* (ETEC)** is a 1- to 5-day, self-limited illness of moderate severity, typically with watery stools and abdominal cramps. ETEC is common in infants in resource-limited countries and in travelers to those countries. ETEC in the United States is most commonly associated with travel; its role in sporadic disease in the United States is unknown. With increasing use of culture-independent tests, ETEC infections may be detected more frequently especially in late summer into fall.

Table 3.7. Classification of *Escherichia coli* Associated With Diarrhea

Pathotype	Epidemiology	Type of Diarrhea	Mechanism of Pathogenesis
Shiga toxin-producing *E coli* (STEC)	Hemorrhagic colitis and hemolytic-uremic syndrome in all ages	Bloody or nonbloody	Shiga toxin production, large bowel adherence, coagulopathy
Enteropathogenic *E coli* (EPEC)	Acute and chronic endemic and epidemic diarrhea in infants in resource-limited countries; certain atypical strains in industrialized countries may cause disease	Watery	Small bowel adherence and effacement
Enterotoxigenic *E coli* (ETEC)	Infant diarrhea in resource-limited countries, travelers' diarrhea in all ages, and some cases in nontravelers	Watery	Small bowel adherence, heat stable and/or heat-labile enterotoxin production
Enteroinvasive *E coli* (EIEC)	Diarrhea with fever in all ages	Bloody or nonbloody; dysentery	Mucosal invasion and inflammation of large bowel
Enteroaggregative *E coli* (EAEC)	Acute and chronic diarrhea in all ages	Watery, occasionally bloody	Small and large bowel adherence, enterotoxin and cytotoxin production

- Diarrhea caused by **enteroinvasive *E coli* (EIEC)** is similar clinically to diarrhea caused by *Shigella* species. Although dysentery can occur, diarrhea usually is watery without blood or mucus. Patients often are febrile, and stools can contain leukocytes. Hospitalization, including to an intensive care unit, can occur.
- **Enteroaggregative *E coli* (EAEC)** organisms cause watery diarrhea and are common in people of all ages in industrialized as well as resource-limited countries. EAEC is a common cause of childhood diarrhea in developing countries, acute diarrhea in travelers, and persistent diarrhea in children or HIV-infected patients. EAEC has been associated with prolonged diarrhea (14 days or longer). Asymptomatic infection can be accompanied by subclinical inflammatory enteritis, which can cause linear growth faltering.

Sequelae of STEC Infection. HUS is a serious sequela of STEC enteric infection. STEC O157:H7, particularly strains producing Stx2, are most commonly associated with HUS, which is defined by the triad of microangiopathic hemolytic anemia, thrombocytopenia, and acute renal dysfunction. HUS occurs in approximately 15% of children younger than 5 years (children 1 through 4 years of age are at higher risk than are infants) with laboratory-confirmed *E coli* O157 infection, as compared with approximately 6% among people of all ages. HUS occurs in approximately 1% of patients of all ages with laboratory confirmed non-O157 STEC infection. HUS typically develops 7 days (up to 2 weeks, and rarely 2–3 weeks) after onset of diarrhea. The risk of developing HUS is lower in children who have a longer interval between diarrhea onset and presentation to the emergency department. More than 50% of children with HUS require dialysis, and 3% to 5% die. Patients with HUS can develop neurologic complications (eg, seizures, coma, or cerebral vessel thrombosis). Children presenting with an increased white blood cell count (>20 x 10^9/mL) or oliguria or anuria are at higher risk of poor outcome, as are, seemingly paradoxically, children with hematocrit close to normal rather than low. Most patients who survive have a very good prognosis, which can be predicted by normal creatinine clearance and no proteinuria or hypertension 1 year or more after HUS.

ETIOLOGY: The 5 pathotypes of diarrhea-producing *E coli* have been distinguished by genetic, pathogenic, and clinical characteristics. Each pathotype is defined by the presence of virulence-related genes, and each comprises characteristic serotypes, indicated by somatic (O) and flagellar (H) antigens. Diarrhea is caused by the direct effects of the pathogens in the intestine. HUS is an infectious sequelae believed to follow Stx-induced vasculitis and systemic complement cascade activation.

EPIDEMIOLOGY: Transmission of most diarrhea-associated *E coli* strains is from food or water contaminated with human or animal feces or from infected symptomatic people. STEC is shed in feces of cattle and, to a lesser extent, sheep, deer, and other ruminants. Human infection is acquired via contaminated food or water or via contact with an infected person, a fomite, or a carrier animal or its environment. Many foods have caused *E coli* O157 outbreaks, including raw leafy vegetables, undercooked ground beef, and unpasteurized milk and juice (see *Red Book* Online outbreaks page for information on current outbreaks, **https://redbook.solutions.aap.org/selfserve/sspage.asp x?selfservecontentid=outbreaks**). Outbreak investigations have implicated petting zoos, drinking water, and ingestion of recreational water. The infectious dose is low; thus, person-to-person transmission is common in households and child care centers. Less is known about the epidemiology of STEC strains other than O157, although the number of infections reported annually to the US laboratory-based enteric disease system of the Centers for Disease Control and Prevention (CDC) has increased in recent years. The non-O157 STEC serogroups most commonly linked to illness in the United States are O26, O111, O103, O121, O45, and O145. Outbreaks from these serogroups are uncommon and are generally attributable to contaminated food or person-to-person transmission (often in a child care setting). A severe outbreak of bloody diarrhea and HUS occurred in Europe in 2011; the outbreak was attributed to an EAEC strain of serotype O104:H4 that had acquired the Stx2a-encoding phage. This experience highlights the importance of considering serogroups other than O157 in outbreaks and cases of HUS.

With the exception of EAEC, non-STEC pathotypes most commonly are associated with disease in resource-limited countries, where food and water supplies commonly are contaminated and facilities and supplies for hand hygiene are suboptimal. For young children in resource-limited countries, transmission of ETEC, EPEC, and other diarrheal pathogens via contaminated weaning foods (sometimes by use of untreated drinking water in the foods) is common. ETEC diarrhea occurs in people of all ages but is especially frequent and severe in infants in resource-limited countries. Breastfeeding is protective in such settings. ETEC is a major cause of travelers' diarrhea. An increasing number of various *E coli* pathotypes are being reported as nucleic acid amplification tests (NAATs) that detect genes encoding putative virulence factors associated with non-STEC *E coli* pathotypes (ETEC, EPEC, EAEC, EIEC) have become available. However, the combination of virulence factors necessary for a strain to be a pathogen has not been determined for all pathotypes.

The **incubation period** for most diarrhea-associated *E coli* strains is 10 hours to 6 days; for *E coli* O157:H7, the **incubation period** usually is 3 to 4 days (range, 1–10 days).

DIAGNOSTIC TESTS: Several US Food and Drug Administration (FDA)-cleared multiplex polymerase chain reaction (PCR) assays (usually offered as diagnostic panels) can detect a variety of enteric pathogens, including EAEC, EPEC, ETEC, and STEC, the last by detection of the genes encoding Stx1 and Stx2. Using culture-independent methods, EAEC, EPEC, and ETEC may be detected more frequently than in the past. In the majority of children, EAEC, EPEC, and ETEC are codetected with at least 1 other pathogen, raising questions about the clinical significance of these codetections on multiplex panels.

Several commercially available, sensitive, specific, and rapid immunologic assays for Shiga toxins in stool or broth culture of stool, including enzyme immunoassays (EIA) and immunochromatographic assays, have been approved by the FDA. The Shiga toxin assays performed on broth enriched stool specimens (usually incubated 18–24 hours) generally are more sensitive than those that test stool directly.

Ideally, all stool specimens submitted for routine diagnosis of acute community-acquired diarrhea (regardless of patient age, season, or presence or absence of blood in the stool) should be simultaneously cultured for *E coli* O157 and tested for non-O157 Shiga toxins or the genes encoding these toxins, although the yield will be low in some geographic regions, including the southern United States.

Rapid diagnosis facilitates patient management and prompt institution of fluid rehydration. Hydration is the cornerstone of management for all diarrhea cases and may be particularly protective against the development of nephropathy associated with HUS. Most *E coli* O157 isolates can be identified presumptively when grown on sorbitol-containing selective media because they cannot ferment sorbitol within 24 hours. All presumptive *E coli* O157 isolates and all Shiga toxin-positive stool specimens that did not yield a presumptive *E coli* O157 isolate should be sent to a public health laboratory for further characterization, including selective methods to identify non-O157 STEC, serotyping, and whole genome sequencing.

STEC should be sought in stool specimens from all patients diagnosed with postdiarrheal HUS. However, the absence of STEC does not preclude the diagnosis of probable STEC-associated HUS, because HUS typically is diagnosed a week or more after onset of diarrhea, when the organism may not be detectable by conventional bacteriologic methods. In this setting, the selective enrichment of stool samples followed by immunomagnetic separation can markedly enhance the isolation of *E coli* O157 and other STEC for which immunomagnetic reagents are available. The test is available at some state public health laboratories and, through requests to state health departments, at the CDC. Serologic diagnosis using enzyme immunoassay to detect serum antibodies to *E coli* O157 and O111 lipopolysaccharides is available at the CDC for outbreak investigations and for patients with HUS; the testing can be arranged through state health departments.

TREATMENT: Treatment is primarily supportive for all diarrhea-producing *E coli*. Orally administered electrolyte-containing solutions usually are adequate to prevent or treat dehydration and electrolyte abnormalities.[1] Antimotility agents should not be administered to children with inflammatory or bloody diarrhea. Patients with proven or suspected STEC infection should be rehydrated fully but prudently as soon as clinically feasible. Many experts advocate intravenous volume expansion during the first 4 days of proven STEC infection to maintain renal perfusion and reduce the risk of renal injury. Careful monitoring of patients with hemorrhagic colitis (including complete blood cell count with smear, blood urea nitrogen, and creatinine concentrations) is recommended to detect changes suggestive of HUS. If patients have no laboratory evidence of hemolysis, thrombocytopenia, or nephropathy 3 days after resolution of diarrhea, their risk of developing HUS is low.

In resource-limited countries, nutritional rehabilitation, including supplemental zinc and vitamin A, should be provided as part of case management algorithms for diarrhea where feasible. Feeding, including breastfeeding, should be continued for young children with *E coli* enteric infection.

Bismuth subsalicylate has been approved by the FDA for use in children 12 years and older and may be used in mild cases of travelers' diarrhea. It can cause blackening of the tongue and stool, and patients should be advised to rinse their mouths after each dose. It contains salicylate and should not be used if a viral infection, such as varicella or influenza, also is suspected.

Antimicrobial Therapy. Antimicrobial therapy in patients with STEC infection remains controversial because of its association with an increased risk of developing HUS in some studies. A meta-analysis did not find that children with hemorrhagic colitis caused by STEC have a greater risk of developing HUS if treated with an antimicrobial agent. However, an association was found in analyses restricted to studies with low risk of bias and using the accepted HUS definition. Moreover, a controlled trial has not been performed, and a beneficial effect of antimicrobial treatment has not been proven. The most recently published observational studies found that treatment of diarrhea with at least some classes of antimicrobial agents was associated with HUS development. Most experts advise not prescribing antimicrobial therapy for children with *E coli* O157 enteritis or a clinical or epidemiologic picture strongly suggestive of STEC infection.

Empiric self-treatment of diarrhea for travelers to a resource-limited country can slightly reduce duration of diarrhea; however, the prevalence of antimicrobial-resistant enteric pathogens in resource-limited settings is increasing. Azithromycin or a fluoroquinolone have been the most reliable agents for therapy (see Fluoroquinolones, p 864); the choice of therapy depends on the pathogen and local antibiotic resistance patterns. Rifaximin may be used for people 12 years and older.

Patients with domestically acquired atypical EPEC (ie, that detected only by homology with the *eae* gene on molecular panel), EAEC, or ETEC will generally have self-limited diarrhea that does not require antimicrobial therapy. For patients with moderate or severe illness with persistent (>14 days) diarrhea attributable to diarrheagenic *E coli* and no other pathogen detected, a treatment regimen similar to that used for travelers' diarrhea (azithromycin, a fluoroquinolone, or rifaximin) may be used.

---

[1]Centers for Disease Control and Prevention. Managing acute gastroenteritis among children: oral rehydration, maintenance, and nutritional therapy. *MMWR Recomm Rep.* 2003;52(RR-16):1−16

ISOLATION OF THE HOSPITALIZED PATIENT: In addition to standard precautions, contact precautions are indicated for diapered and incontinent patients with all types of *E coli* diarrhea for the duration of illness. Prolonged shedding has been noted in children younger than 5 years. Patients with postdiarrheal HUS should be presumed to have STEC infection.

CONTROL MEASURES:

Escherichia coli O157:H7 and Other STEC Infection. All meat should be cooked thoroughly. Ground beef should be cooked thoroughly until no pink meat remains and the juices are clear and to an internal temperature of 160°F (71°C). Raw milk should not be ingested, and the certification of raw milk does not eliminate the risk of transmission of *E coli* organisms.[1] Only pasteurized apple juice and cider products should be consumed. Care should be taken to prevent cross-contamination in areas of food preparation. Hands should be washed with soap and water immediately after contact with raw/undercooked meats, animals, the environment around animals, and animal food or treats; adults should supervise hand washing for young children.

Outbreaks in Child Care Centers. If an outbreak of HUS or diarrhea attributable to STEC occurs in a child care center, immediate involvement of public health authorities is critical. Infection caused by STEC is notifiable, and rapid reporting of cases allows intervention to prevent further disease. Ill children with STEC O157 infection or virulent non-O157 STEC infection (such as in the context of another contact case that includes HUS cases or an outbreak of bloody diarrhea) should not be permitted to reenter the child care center until 2 stool cultures (obtained at least 48 hours after any antimicrobial therapy, if administered, has been discontinued) are negative, stools are contained in the diaper or the child is continent, stool frequency is no more than 2 stools above that child's normal frequency for the time the child is in the program, and the health department agrees with the return to child care (see Table 2.3, p 128). Some state health departments have less stringent exclusion policies for children who have recovered from less virulent STEC infection. Stool cultures should be performed for any symptomatic contacts, and these children should be excluded from child care while symptomatic and the evaluation is pending. In outbreak situations involving virulent STEC strains, stool cultures of asymptomatic contacts may aid controlling spread; consultation with public health authorities is advised. Strict attention to hand hygiene is important but can be insufficient to prevent transmission. The child care center should be closed to new admissions during an outbreak, and care should be exercised to prevent transfer of exposed children to other centers.

Nursery and Other Institutional Outbreaks. Strict attention to hand hygiene is essential for limiting spread. Exposed patients should be observed closely, their stools should be cultured for the causative organism, and they should be separated from unexposed infants.

Travelers' Diarrhea. Travelers' diarrhea usually is acquired by ingestion of contaminated food or water or contact with fomites and is a significant problem for people traveling in resource-limited countries. Diarrhea commonly is caused by ETEC and EAEC. Diarrhea attributable to *E coli* O157 is rare in US travelers; a much higher proportion

---

[1]American Academy of Pediatrics, Committee on Infectious Diseases, Committee on Nutrition. Consumption of raw or unpasteurized milk and milk products by pregnant women and children. *Pediatrics.* 2014;133(1): 175–179 (Reaffirmed November 2019)

of patients with non-O157 STEC infection have traveled internationally in the previous week. Travelers should be advised to drink only bottled or canned beverages and boiled or bottled water; travelers should avoid ice, raw produce including salads, and fruit that they have not peeled themselves (only fruits with a thick peel, such as bananas and oranges, should be consumed). Cooked foods should be eaten steaming hot. Hands should be washed carefully before preparing or eating food or feeding another person. Antimicrobial agents are not recommended for prevention of travelers' diarrhea in children. Rehydration is the mainstay of treatment. Packets of oral rehydration salts can be added to boiled or bottled water and ingested to help maintain fluid balance, and breastfeeding should be encouraged and continued for young children. Antimicrobial therapy generally is recommended for travelers in resource-limited areas when diarrhea is moderate to severe or is associated with fever or bloody stools; however, the prevalence of antimicrobial resistance among enteric pathogens is increasing. Several antimicrobial agents, such as azithromycin, fluoroquinolones, and rifaximin can be effective in treatment of travelers' diarrhea. The drug of first choice for travelers' diarrhea in children is azithromycin and in adults is azithromycin, a fluoroquinolone, or rifaximin. Treatment for no more than 3 days is advised.

Recreational Water. People should avoid ingesting recreational water. Because STEC has a low infectious dose and can be waterborne, people with proven or suspected STEC infection should not use recreational water venues (eg, swimming pools, water slides) when ill with diarrhea. As with other causes of diarrhea, children who have diarrhea attributable to STEC and who are incontinent should continue not to use recreational water venues until 1 week after symptoms resolve (or as advised by local or state public health authorities) (see Prevention of Illnesses Associated With Recreational Water Use, p 180). Showering before swimming, taking children to the restroom frequently, changing diapers at designated diapering stations, and then washing hands can limit transmission of diarrheal pathogens through recreational water.

Other Fungal Diseases

Uncommonly encountered fungi can cause infection in infants and children with immunosuppression or other underlying conditions. Fungi can cause invasive mold infections, such as mucormycosis, fusariosis, scedosporiosis, and the phaeohyphomycoses (black molds), as well as invasive yeast infections with organisms such as *Malazzesia*, *Trichosporon*, *Rhodotorula*, and many more (more common mycoses, including aspergillosis, blastomycosis, candidiasis, coccidioidomycosis, cryptococcosis, histoplasmosis, paracoccidioidomycosis, and sporotrichosis, are discussed in individual chapters of Section 3 of the *Red Book*). Children can acquire infection from these fungi through inhalation via the respiratory tract or direct inoculation after traumatic disruption of cutaneous barriers. A list of some of these fungi and the pertinent underlying host conditions, reservoirs or routes of entry, clinical manifestations, diagnostic laboratory tests, and treatments can be found in Table 3.8. Taken as a group, few in vitro antifungal susceptibility data are available on which to base treatment recommendations for these uncommon invasive fungal infections, especially in children (see Antifungal Drugs for Systemic Fungal Infections, p 905, and Table 4.7, p 909). Physicians should consider consultation with a pediatric infectious disease specialist experienced in the diagnosis and treatment of invasive fungal infections when treating a child infected with one of these mycoses.

Table 3.8. Additional Fungal Diseases

Disease and Agent	Underlying Host Condition(s)	Reservoir(s) or Route(s) of Entry	Common Clinical Manifestations	Diagnostic Laboratory Test(s)	Treatment
Hyalohyphomycosis					
Fusarium species	Granulocytopenia; hematopoietic stem cell transplantation; severe immunocompromise; severe neutropenia and/or T-lymphocyte immunodeficiency	Respiratory tract; sinuses; skin; ingestion	Pulmonary infiltrates; cutaneous lesions (eg, ecthyma); sinusitis; disseminated infection	Culture of blood or tissue specimen, histopathologic examination of tissue	Voriconazole, posaconazole,[a,b] isavuconazole,[a,b] or D-AMB[c]
Pseudallescheria boydii/Scedosporium apiospermum complex	None or trauma or immunosuppression; cystic fibrosis; chronic granulomatous disease; chronic glucocorticoid use; hematologic malignancy	Environment; respiratory tract; direct inoculation (eg, skin puncture)	Pneumonia; localized pulmonary process or disseminated infection; osteomyelitis or septic arthritis; mycetoma (immunocompetent patients); endocarditis; keratitis and endophthalmitis; brain abscesses; lesions of the skin, soft tissue, or bone	Culture and histopathologic examination of tissue	Voriconazole or isavuconazole[b]
Lomentospora (formerly *Scedosporium*) *prolificans*					Voriconazole; Consider addition of an echinocandin or terbinafine

Table 3.8. Additional Fungal Diseases, continued

Disease and Agent	Underlying Host Condition(s)	Reservoir(s) or Route(s) of Entry	Common Clinical Manifestations	Diagnostic Laboratory Test(s)	Treatment
Talaromycosis					
Talaromyces (Penicillium) marneffei	Human immunodeficiency virus infection and exposure to southeast Asia	Respiratory tract	Pneumonitis; invasive dermatitis; disseminated infection	Culture of blood, bone marrow, or tissue; histopathologic examination of tissue	Amphotericin B; alternative, itraconazole[b]
Phaeohyphomycosis					
Alternaria species	None, trauma, or immunosuppression	Respiratory tract; skin	Sinusitis; cutaneous lesions	Culture and histopathologic examination of tissue	Voriconazole[b] or D-AMB[c]
Bipolaris species	None, trauma, immunosuppression, or chronic sinusitis	Environment	Sinusitis; cerebral and disseminated infection	Culture and histopathologic examination of tissue	Voriconazole,[b] posaconazole,[b] itraconazole,[d] or D-AMB[c]; surgical excision
Cladophialophora species	None, trauma, or immunosuppression	Environment	Cerebral infection	Culture and histopathologic examination of tissue	Voriconazole,[b] posaconazole,[b] itraconazole,[d] or D-AMB[c]; surgical excision

Table 3.8. Additional Fungal Diseases, continued

Disease and Agent	Underlying Host Condition(s)	Reservoir(s) or Route(s) of Entry	Common Clinical Manifestations	Diagnostic Laboratory Test(s)	Treatment
Curvularia species	Immunosuppression; altered skin integrity; asthma or nasal polyps; chronic sinusitis	Environment	Allergic fungal sinusitis; invasive dermatitis; disseminated infection	Culture and histopathologic examination of tissue	Allergic fungal sinusitis: surgery and corticosteroids Invasive disease: voriconazole,[b] itraconazole,[b,d] or D-AMB[c]
Exophiala species, *Exserohilum* species	None, trauma, or immunosuppression	Environment	Sinusitis; cutaneous lesions; disseminated infection; meningitis associated with contaminated steroid for epidural use	Culture and histopathologic examination of tissue	Voriconazole,[b,e] itraconazole,[b,d] D-AMB, or surgical excision
Invasive Yeasts					
Trichosporon species	Immunosuppression; central venous catheter; hematologic malignancy, often with neutropenia; acquired immunodeficiency syndrome; extensive burns; glucocorticoid treatment; heart valve surgery; exposure to tropical environments	Environment; normal flora of gastrointestinal tract	Bloodstream infection; superficial skin lesions endocarditis; peritonitis; pneumonitis; disseminated infection	Blood culture; histopathologic examination of tissue or nodules; urine, sputum, and cerebrospinal cultures; bronchoscopy with alveolar lavage cultures	For invasive infections, voriconazole or d-AMB[b] For superficial infections, shaving of the hair and application of a topical azole antifungal to the affected areas

Table 3.8. Additional Fungal Diseases, continued

Disease and Agent	Underlying Host Condition(s)	Reservoir(s) or Route(s) of Entry	Common Clinical Manifestations	Diagnostic Laboratory Test(s)	Treatment
Malassezia species	Immunosuppression; preterm birth; exposure to parenteral nutrition that includes fat emulsions	Skin	Pityriasis versicolor, seborrheic dermatitis, central line-associated bloodstream infection; interstitial pneumonitis; urinary tract infection; meningitis	Culture of blood, catheter tip, or tissue specimen (requires special laboratory handling)	Removal of catheters and temporary cessation of lipid infusion; D-AMB, azole therapy
Mucormycosis (formerly Zygomycosis)					
Rhizopus; Mucor; Lichtheimia (formerly *Absidia*) species; *Rhizomucor* species; *Cunninghamella* species	Immunosuppression; hematologic malignant neoplasm; renal failure; diabetes mellitus; iron overload syndromes	Respiratory tract; skin	Rhinocerebral infection; pulmonary infection; disseminated infection; skin (traumatic wounds) and gastrointestinal tract (less commonly)	Histopathologic examination of tissue and culture	D-AMB for initial therapy and consider posaconazole[a] for maintenance therapy; with surgical excision and débridement, as feasible; isavuconazole (voriconazole has no activity); echinocandins (eg, caspofungin) may have clinical utility when combined with AMB

ABLC indicates amphotericin B lipid complex; D-AMB, deoxycholate amphotericin B (if the patient is intolerant of or refractory to D-AMB, L-AMB can be substituted); L-AMB, liposomal amphotericin B.

[a] Demonstrates activity in vitro, but few clinical data are available for children.

[b] No US Food and Drug Administration approval for this indication.

[c] Consider use of a lipid-based formulation of amphotericin B.

[d] Itraconazole has been shown to be effective for cutaneous disease in adults, but safety and efficacy have not been established in children younger than 18 years.

[e] Voriconazole demonstrates activity in vitro, but no clinical data are available.

Fusobacterium Infections
(Including Lemierre Syndrome)

CLINICAL MANIFESTATIONS: *Fusobacterium* species, including *Fusobacterium necrophorum* and *Fusobacterium nucleatum,* can be isolated from oropharyngeal specimens in healthy people and are frequent components of human dental plaque with the potential to lead to periodontal disease. Invasive disease attributable to *Fusobacterium* species has been associated with otitis media, tonsillitis, gingivitis, and oropharyngeal trauma including dental and oropharyngeal surgery such as tonsillectomy. Ten percent of cases of invasive *Fusobacterium* infections are associated with concomitant Epstein-Barr virus infection.

Preceding oropharyngeal infection is the most frequent primary source for invasive infection. Invasive infections can be characterized by peritonsillar abscess, deep neck space infection, mastoiditis, and sinusitis that can be complicated by meningitis, cerebral abscess, and dural sinus venous thrombosis. Otogenic sources of infection have also been reported.

Invasive infection following tonsillitis was described early in the 20th century and was referred to as postanginal sepsis or Lemierre syndrome. The classic syndrome starts with sore throat symptoms, which may improve or may continue to worsen. Fever and sore throat are followed by severe neck pain (anginal pain) that can be accompanied by unilateral neck swelling, trismus, dysphagia, and rigors associated with development of suppurative jugular venous thrombosis (JVT). Patients with classic Lemierre syndrome have a sepsis syndrome with multiple organ dysfunction. Metastatic complications from septic embolic phenomena associated with JVT are common and may manifest as multiple pleural septic emboli, pleural empyema, pyogenic arthritis, osteomyelitis, or disseminated intravascular coagulation. Laboratory abnormalities associated with Lemierre syndrome can include significantly elevated inflammatory markers, thrombocytopenia, elevated aminotransferases, hyperbilirubinemia, and elevated creatinine. Persistent headache or other neurologic signs may indicate the presence of cerebral venous sinus thrombosis (eg, cavernous sinus thrombosis), meningitis, or brain abscess. *Fusobacterium* species (most commonly *F necrophorum)* are often isolated from blood or other normally sterile sites and account for at least 80% of Lemierre syndrome cases. Lemierre-like syndromes also have been reported following infection with *Arcanobacterium haemolyticum, Bacteroides* species, anaerobic *Streptococcus* species, other anaerobic bacteria, and methicillin-susceptible and -resistant strains of *Staphylococcus aureus.*

With respect to thrombosis, the JVT can be completely vaso-occlusive. Some children with JVT associated with Lemierre syndrome have evidence of thrombophilia at diagnosis. These findings often resolve over several months and can indicate response to the inflammatory, prothrombotic process associated with infection rather than an underlying hypercoagulable state.

Fusobacterium species have also been associated with intraabdominal and pelvic infections including acute appendicitis, suppurative portomesenteric vein thrombosis, and suppurative thrombosis of the pelvic vasculature.

ETIOLOGY: *Fusobacterium* species are filamentous, anaerobic, non–spore-forming, gram-negative bacilli. Human infection usually results from *F necrophorum* subspecies *funduliforme,* but infections with other species including *F nucleatum, Fusobacterium gonidiaformans, Fusobacterium naviforme, Fusobacterium mortiferum,* and *Fusobacterium varium* have been reported. Infection with *Fusobacterium* species, alone or in combination with other oral anaerobic bacteria, may result in Lemierre syndrome, but unlike other anaerobic infections, *Fusobacterium* species are frequently the only organisms identified in these infections.

EPIDEMIOLOGY: *Fusobacterium* species commonly are found in soil and in the respiratory tracts of animals, including cattle, dogs, fowl, goats, sheep, and horses, and can be isolated from the oropharynx of healthy people. *Fusobacterium* infections are most common in adolescents and young adults, but infections, including fatal cases of Lemierre syndrome, have been reported in infants and young children.

DIAGNOSTIC TESTS: *Fusobacterium* species can be isolated using conventional liquid anaerobic blood culture media. However, the organism grows best on semisolid media for fastidious anaerobic organisms or blood agar supplemented with vitamin K, hemin, menadione, and a reducing agent. Colonies generally are cream to yellow colored, smooth, and round and may show a narrow zone of alpha or beta-hemolysis on blood agar, depending on the species of blood used in the medium; however, *F nucleatum* may appear as bread crumb-like colonies. Many strains fluoresce chartreuse green under ultraviolet light. Most *Fusobacterium* organisms are indole positive. On gram stain, *F nucleatum* usually exhibits spindle-shaped cells with tapered ends, while *F necrophorum* and other species may be highly pleomorphic with swollen areas. The accurate identification of anaerobes to the species level has become important with the increasing incidence of microorganisms that are resistant to multiple drugs. Conventional and commercial culture-based biochemical test systems are reasonably accurate, at least to the genus level. Sequencing of the 16S rRNA gene and phylogenetic analysis or the use of mass spectrometry of bacterial cell components can accurately identify *Fusobacterium* species to the species level.

Currently, there are no commercially available tests for diagnosing *Fusobacterium necrophorum* pharyngitis. Routine throat cultures for beta-hemolytic streptococci do not generally include screening for the presence of *Fusobacterium* species. Researchers have used special media to grow *F necrophorum* from throat swab specimens or have used polymerase chain reaction techniques to document and describe *F necrophorum* tonsillitis/pharyngitis.

One should consider Lemierre syndrome in ill-appearing febrile children and especially adolescents having a sore throat with exquisite neck pain and swelling over the angle of the jaw, accompanied by rigors. Aerobic and anaerobic blood cultures should be performed to detect invasive *Fusobacterium* species and other possible pathogens. Imaging studies of the internal jugular veins should be obtained, but it is important to note that a significant proportion of patients with a diagnosis of Lemierre syndrome will not have a thrombus detected by imaging. Computed tomography and magnetic resonance imaging are more sensitive than ultrasonography to document thrombosis and thrombophlebitis of the internal jugular vein early in the course of illness and to better identify thrombus extension beyond the areas visible by ultrasound including under the mandible and clavicle.

TREATMENT: Aggressive and prompt antimicrobial therapy is the mainstay of treatment. *Fusobacterium* species generally are susceptible to metronidazole, clindamycin, chloramphenicol, penicillin with beta-lactamase inhibitor combinations (ampicillin-sulbactam or piperacillin-tazobactam), carbapenem, cefoxitin, and ceftriaxone. Antimicrobial resistance has increased in anaerobic bacteria, and susceptibility is no longer predictable. Therefore, susceptibility testing is indicated for all clinically significant anaerobic isolates, including *Fusobacterium* species. Combination therapy with metronidazole or clindamycin, in addition to a beta-lactam agent active against aerobic oral and respiratory tract pathogens (cefotaxime, ceftriaxone, or cefuroxime), is recommended for patients with invasive infection caused by *Fusobacterium* species. Alternatively, some experts recommend monotherapy with a penicillin-beta-lactamase inhibitor combination (ampicillin-sulbactam or piperacillin-tazobactam) or a carbapenem (meropenem, imipenem, or ertapenem). Up to 50% of *F nucleatum* and 20% of *F necrophorum* isolates produce beta-lactamases, rendering them resistant to penicillin, ampicillin, and some cephalosporins. *Fusobacterium* species intrinsically are resistant to gentamicin, fluoroquinolone agents, and typically, macrolides. Tetracyclines have limited activity.

The duration of antimicrobial therapy depends on the anatomic location and severity of infection but usually is several weeks. Surgical intervention involving débridement or incision and drainage of abscesses may be necessary. Anticoagulation therapy has been used in both adults and children with JVT and cavernous sinus thrombosis. However, evidence for the role of anti-coagulation in thrombosis outcome is lacking

ISOLATION OF THE HOSPITALIZED PATIENT: Standard precautions are recommended. Person-to-person transmission of *Fusobacterium* species has not been documented.

CONTROL MEASURES: Oral hygiene and dental cleanings may reduce density of oral colonization with *Fusobacterium* species, prevent gingivitis and dental caries, and reduce the risk of invasive disease.

Giardia duodenalis (formerly *Giardia lamblia* and *Giardia intestinalis*) Infections
(Giardiasis)

CLINICAL MANIFESTATIONS: Symptoms of *Giardia* infection are attributable to dysfunction of the small bowel caused by residing trophozoites and range from asymptomatic carriage to fulminant diarrhea and dehydration. Most infections are asymptomatic, but children are more often symptomatic than adults. Symptomatic patients are mildly to moderately ill and complain frequently of intermittent abdominal cramping and bloating, and almost intolerable foul-smelling flatus and stools. Chronic infection, often with weight loss, is common. A more fulminant presentation with acute and chronic diarrhea, malabsorption, failure to thrive, and weight loss may occur, but systemic symptoms, other than malaise, are uncommon.

Symptoms are also caused by lactose intolerance and malabsorption, which result in voluminous diarrhea often described as "greasy or fatty" and foul smelling. Sometimes atypical upper gastrointestinal symptoms of belching, nausea, and vomiting predominate, causing a delay in diagnosis. Fever, mucus, and blood in stool are distinctly atypical and suggest infection with another agent(s). Chronic symptoms similar to those of irritable bowel may be confused with giardiasis and are also sequelae of giardiasis. The natural history of acquired untreated infections is not well documented, but duration of infection typically is prolonged, can be abnormally longstanding in young people, and can last years in immunosuppressed individuals. In children, development of immunity is poor and repeated infections are common. Patients with cystic fibrosis have an increased prevalence of *G duodenalis* infection. Extraintestinal involvement (eg, arthritis, urticaria, retinal changes, and bile or pancreatic duct involvement) is unusual and its association with *Giardia* infection is suggested but unproven. Giardiasis is not associated with eosinophilia.

ETIOLOGY: *G duodenalis* (syn *Giardia lamblia* and *Giardia intestinalis)* is a flagellate protozoan that exists in trophozoite and cyst forms; the infective form is the cyst. *Giardia* undergoes a simple life cycle alternating between the orally ingested infectious resistant cyst and the motile trophozoite that resides and multiplies in the small intestine. Encystation occurs in the lower small bowel and cysts are infectious when excreted. Infection is limited to the small intestine and biliary tract. *Giardia* cysts are infectious immediately after being excreted in feces and remain viable for 3 months in water at 4°C. A single freeze/thaw cycle kills most *Giardia* cysts; complete killing occurs after multiple freeze/thaw cycles. Heating, drying, and seawater are microcidal to cysts, but this may vary depending on the specific conditions.

EPIDEMIOLOGY: Giardiasis has a worldwide distribution and is the most common intestinal parasitic infection of humans identified in the United States and globally. Highest incidence in the United States is reported among children 1 through 9 years of age, adults 25 to 29 years of age, and adults 55 through 59 years of age and residents of northern states. Peak illness onset occurs from early summer through early fall. High infectivity is a result of the combination of enormous numbers of infectious cysts that may be excreted and the fact that as few as 10 to 100 cysts are able to initiate infection. Transmission of *G duodenalis* is most likely to occur in situations in which exposure to infected feces is likely, including (1) child care centers; (2) areas of the world with endemic disease; (3) close contact, including sexual contact, with infected people; (4) swallowing of contaminated drinking or recreational water; and (5) consumption of unfiltered or untreated water such as during outdoor activities (eg, camping or backpacking). Although less common, outbreaks associated with food or food handlers have been reported. Among the 242 outbreaks of giardiasis in the US between 1971 and 2011, most resulted from waterborne (74.8%), foodborne (15.7%), person-to-person (2.5%), and animal contact (1.2%) transmission. Most (74.6%) of the waterborne outbreaks were associated with drinking water, followed by recreational water (18.2%). Surveys conducted in the United States have identified overall prevalence rates of *Giardia* organisms in stool specimens that range from 5% to 7%, with variations depending on age, geographic location, and seasonality. Duration of cyst excretion is variable but can range from weeks to months. Giardiasis is communicable for as long as the infected person excretes cysts.

The **incubation period** usually is 1 to 3 weeks.

DIAGNOSTIC TESTS: *Giardia* cysts or trophozoites are not seen consistently in the stools of infected patients. Diagnostic sensitivity can be increased by examining up to 3 stool specimens over several days. New molecular enteric panel assays generally include *Giardia* as a target pathogen. Diagnostic techniques include direct fluorescence antibody (DFA; considered the gold standard), rapid immunochromatographic cartridge assays, enzyme immunoassay (EIA) kits, microscopy with trichrome staining, and molecular assays. If there is a suspicion of false-negative results, repeated testing should be performed and use of a different methodology considered. Invasive testing of the duodenal contents or an intestinal biopsy is required only rarely. Molecular testing (such as PCR) can be used to identify the genotypes and subtypes of *Giardia*, but this is not helpful clinically. Retesting is only recommended if symptoms persist after treatment. In the United States, giardiasis is a nationally notifiable disease.

TREATMENT: Some infections are self-limited, and treatment may not be required. Tinidazole, metronidazole, and nitazoxanide are the drugs of choice (see Table 4.11, p 961). Although not FDA approved for this indication, metronidazole is the least expensive of these therapies, but generally has poor palatability when compounded into a suspension. A 5- to 7-day course of metronidazole has an efficacy of 80% to 100% in pediatric patients. A single dose of tinidazole, a nitroimidazole for children 3 years and older, has a median efficacy of 91% in pediatric patients (range, 80%–100%) and has fewer adverse effects than metronidazole. A 3-day course of nitazoxanide oral suspension has similar efficacy to metronidazole and has the advantage(s) of treating other intestinal parasites and of being approved for use in children 1 year and older. If treatment is needed during pregnancy, paromomycin, a poorly absorbed aminoglycoside, is 50% to 70% effective and is the recommended treatment. Metronidazole has been used, but data regarding safety in the first trimester are conflicting.

Symptom recurrence after completing antimicrobial treatment can be attributable to reinfection or recurrence, post-*Giardia* irritable bowel, residual lactose intolerance (occurs in 20%–40% of patients), or symptoms attributable to another process or infection. Recurrences are associated with immunosuppression or poor immunity, insufficient treatment, drug resistance, or reexposure. Because new or residual symptoms are nonspecific, repeated testing should be performed. There is no clear best course for retreatment, but options include treatment with an alternative drug of a different class, a longer course of the first failed drug, or a combined drug regimen consisting of 2 different drug types. One such combination is tinidazole plus quinacrine for at least 2 weeks, which is almost always curative.

Patients who are immunocompromised because of hypogammaglobulinemia or lymphoproliferative disease are at higher risk of giardiasis, and a cure is more difficult for these people. Among human immunodeficiency virus (HIV)-infected children and adults without acquired immunodeficiency syndrome (AIDS), effective combination antiretroviral therapy (ART) and antiparasitic therapy are the major initial treatments for these infections. Patients with AIDS often respond to standard therapy but in some cases, additional treatment is required. If giardiasis is refractory to standard treatment among HIV-infected patients with AIDS, longer treatment duration or combination antiparasitic therapy (eg, tinidazole, nitazoxanide, or metronidazole plus one of the following: paromomycin, albendazole, or quinacrine) may be appropriate. Studies in children as young as 1 year of age suggest that albendazole can be administered safely to this population.

Treatment of asymptomatic carriers is controversial but recommended in the United States and other areas of low prevalence to prevent infection within families or of other children, which is a common scenario. Treatment of children likely to be reinfected, such as those residing in areas of high prevalence, is not recommended unless medically indicated.

ISOLATION OF THE HOSPITALIZED PATIENT: Standard precautions plus contact precautions for the duration of illness are recommended for diapered and incontinent children.

CONTROL MEASURES: Safe water, appropriate sanitation, and handwashing are the most important measures to avoid giardiasis. Avoid drinking and recreational water that may be contaminated. If the safety of drinking water is in doubt (eg, during travel to a location with poor sanitation or lack of water treatment systems), do one of the following:
- Drink commercially bottled water from an unopened factory-sealed container.
- Disinfect tap water by heating it to a rolling boil for 1 minute.
- Use a filter that has been certified for cyst and oocyst reduction.

Boiling is the most reliable method to make water safe for drinking with required boiling time dependent on altitude (1 minute at sea level). Chemical disinfection with iodine is an alternative method of water treatment using either tincture of iodine or tetraglycine hydroperiodide tablets. Chlorine in various forms also has been used for chemical disinfection, but germicidal activity is dependent on several factors, including pH, temperature, and organic content of the water. Chlorination has low to moderate effectiveness in killing *Giardia*. Additional information about water purification, including a traveler's guide for buying water filters, can be found at **www.cdc.gov/parasites/crypto/ gen_info/filters.html.**

Avoid swallowing water while from swimming in pools, hot tubs, interactive fountains, lakes, rivers, springs, ponds, streams, or the ocean or drinking untreated water from lakes, rivers, springs, ponds, streams, or shallow wells.

Infected people and individuals at risk especially should adhere to strict hand-hygiene techniques after contact with feces. Use of gloves before handling infected feces or contaminated diapers is a more stringent approach. For additional prevention guidance, visit the CDC *Giardia* website (**www.cdc.gov/parasites/giardia**).

When an outbreak is suspected in a child care center (also see Children in Group Child Care and Schools, p 116), the local health department should be contacted, and an epidemiologic investigation should be undertaken to identify and treat all symptomatic children, child care providers, and family members infected with *G duodenalis*. Infected children should be excluded until stools are contained in the diaper or the child is continent, stool frequency is no more than 2 stools above that child's normal frequency, and the health department agrees with the return to child care. Testing of asymptomatic individuals and treatment of asymptomatic carriers in a child care center outbreak are controversial.

People with diarrhea caused by *Giardia* species should not use recreational water venues (eg, swimming pools, water slides) while symptomatic. Children who had diarrhea attributable to *Giardia* should avoid recreational water activities and shared bathing for 1 week after cessation of symptoms. People should avoid ingestion of recreational water. For additional information, see Prevention of Illnesses Associated With Recreational Water Use (p 180).

Gonococcal Infections

CLINICAL MANIFESTATIONS: Gonococcal infections are manifested by a spectrum of clinical presentations ranging from asymptomatic carriage, to characteristic localized infections (usually mucosal), to disseminated disease, and should be considered in 3 distinct age groups: newborn infants, prepubertal children, and postpubertal sexually active adolescents and young adults. Multiple sites of infection can occur simultaneously in one individual.

- **Asymptomatic carriage** has been detected in the oropharynx of child sexual abuse survivors, and in the urogenital tract of sexually active females (up to 80% are asymptomatic) and males (around 10% can be asymptomatic). In all age groups, most pharyngeal infections are asymptomatic. Likewise, most rectal infections are asymptomatic; rectal carriage can accompany 20% to 70% of female urogenital infections.
- **Localized disease** presents at the site of inoculation and includes (1) scalp abscess, which can be associated with fetal scalp monitoring; (2) ophthalmia neonatorum in

newborn infants following exposure to an infected birth canal or conjunctivitis in any age group following eye inoculation with infected secretions (eg, through hand transfer from urogenital tract); (3) acute tonsillopharyngitis, accompanied by cervical adenopathy; (4) urethritis(with mucopurulent discharge, dysuria, and/or suprapubic pain) in any age group or gender; (5) genital disease such as vulvitis and/or vaginitis in prepubertal females (with vaginal discharge and/or dysuria), bartholinitis and/or cervicitis in postpubertal females (with mucopurulent discharge, intermenstrual bleeding, and/or dyspareunia), and penile abscess; and (6) proctitis (symptoms range from painless mucopurulent discharge and scant rectal bleeding to overt proctitis with associated rectal pain and tenesmus). Extension to the upper genital tract and beyond (less common in prepubertal children) can result in pelvic inflammatory disease (endometritis and/or salpingitis) and perihepatitis (Fitz-Hugh-Curtis syndrome) in females and epididymitis, prostatitis, and/or seminal vesiculitis in males, with resultant scarring, ectopic pregnancy, impairment of fertility, and chronic pelvic pain, particularly in females (see Sexually Transmitted Infections in Adolescents and Children, p 148). Localized neonatal gonococcal infection of the scalp can also result from internal fetal heart rate monitoring during labor via scalp electrodes, if the mother has an undiagnosed gonococcal infection.

- Disseminated gonococcal infection (DGI) occurs in up to 3% of untreated people with mucosal gonorrhea. DGI can manifest as petechial or pustular skin lesions and as asymmetric polyarthralgia, tenosynovitis, or oligoarticular septic arthritis (arthritis-dermatitis syndrome). In neonates, DGI can present as sepsis, arthritis, or meningitis. Bacteremia can result in a maculopapular rash with necrosis, tenosynovitis, and migratory arthritis. Arthritis may be reactive (sterile) or septic in nature. Meningitis and endocarditis occur rarely.

ETIOLOGY: *Neisseria gonorrhoeae* is a gram-negative, oxidase-positive diplococcus.

EPIDEMIOLOGY: Gonococcal infections occur only in humans. The source of the organism is exudate and secretions from infected mucosal surfaces; *N gonorrhoeae* is communicable as long as a person harbors the organism. Transmission results from intimate contact, such as sexual acts and parturition. Sexual abuse is the most frequent cause of gonococcal infection in prepubertal children beyond the newborn period (see Sexual Assault and Abuse in Children and Adolescents/Young Adults, p 150).

N gonorrhoeae infection is the second most commonly reported sexually transmitted infection (STI) in the United States, following *Chlamydia trachomatis* infection. From Centers for Disease Control and Prevention (CDC) surveillance reports as of October 2019, a total of 583 405 cases of gonorrhea (179 cases per 100 000 population) were reported in the United States for 2018: this represents an increase of 82.6% over the historic low reported in 2009. Reported gonorrhea cases continued to be highest among adolescents and young adults. In 2018, the highest rates among females were observed among those aged 20 through 24 years (702.6 cases per 100 000 females) and 15 through 19 years (548.1 cases per 100 000 females). Among males, the rate was highest among those aged 20 through 24 years (720.9 cases per 100 000 males) and 25 through 29 years (674.0 cases per 100 000 males). Rates of reported gonorrhea are highest in the southern United States and have significant racial/ethnic disparities. In 2018, the rate of reported gonorrhea cases remained highest among Black people (548.9 cases per 100 000 population), a rate 7.7 times the rate among white people (71.1 cases per 100 000 population).

Comparable differences in gonorrhea rates were also seen in other racial/ethnic groups versus white people: 4.6 times higher among American Indian/Alaska Native (AI/AN) people, 2.6 times higher among Native Hawaiian/Other Pacific Islander populations, 1.6 times higher among Hispanic people, and 1.3 times higher among multiracial people. The rate among Asian people, however (35.1 cases per 100 000 population), was half the rate among white people. Disparities in gonorrhea rates also are observed by sexual behavior. Surveillance networks that monitor trends in STI prevalence among men who have sex with men (MSM) have found very high proportions of positive gonorrhea pharyngeal, urethral, and rectal test results as well as coinfection with other STIs. Populations at greater risk for DGI include asymptomatic carriers; neonates; menstruating, pregnant, and postpartum females; MSM; and individuals with complement deficiency.

Diagnosis of genitourinary tract gonorrhea infection should also prompt investigation for other STIs, including chlamydia, trichomoniasis, syphilis, and HIV infection. Concurrent infection with *C trachomatis* is common. This finding has led to the longstanding recommendation that persons treated for gonococcal infection also be treated with a regimen that is effective against uncomplicated genital *C trachomatis* infection.

The **incubation period** usually is 2 to 7 days.

DIAGNOSTIC TESTS[1,2]**:** Microscopic examination of Gram-stained smears of exudate from the conjunctivae, male urethra, skin lesions, synovial fluid, and when clinically warranted, cerebrospinal fluid (CSF) may be useful in the initial evaluation. Identification of gram-negative intracellular diplococci in these smears can be helpful, particularly if the organism is not recovered in culture. However, because of low sensitivity, a negative smear result should not be considered sufficient for ruling out infection. Intracellular gram-negative diplococci identified on Gram stain of conjunctival exudate justify presumptive treatment for gonorrhea after appropriate cultures for *N gonorrhoeae* are performed.

N gonorrhoeae can be isolated from normally sterile sites, such as blood, CSF, or synovial fluid, using nonselective chocolate agar with incubation in 5% to 10% carbon dioxide. Selective media that inhibit normal flora and nonpathogenic *Neisseria* organisms are used for cultures from nonsterile sites, such as the cervix, vagina, rectum, urethra, and pharynx. Specimens for *N gonorrhoeae* culture from mucosal sites should be inoculated immediately onto appropriate agar, because the organism is extremely sensitive to drying and temperature changes. Culture allows for antimicrobial susceptibility testing to aid in management if infection persists following initial therapy.

A nucleic acid amplification test (NAAT) is far superior in overall performance compared with other *N gonorrhoeae* culture and nonculture diagnostic methods to test genital and extragenital specimens.[48] Most commercially available products now are cleared by the US Food and Drug Administration (FDA) for testing male urethral swab specimens, female endocervical or vaginal swab specimens (provider or patient collected), male or female urine specimens, oropharynx or rectal swab specimens, or liquid cytology specimens. Although NAATs are not FDA cleared for *N gonorrhoeae* testing on conjunctival swab specimens, they have been shown to be more sensitive compared with *N gonorrhoeae* culture. Product inserts for each NAAT manufacturer should be reviewed, because approved

---

[1]American Academy of Pediatrics, Committee on Adolescence; Society for Adolescent Health and Medicine. Screening for nonviral sexually transmitted infections in adolescents and young adults. *Pediatrics.* 2014;134(1):e302-e311

[2]Centers for Disease Control and Prevention. Recommendations for the laboratory-based detection of *Chlamydia trachomatis* and *Neisseria gonorrhoeae*—2014. *MMWR Recomm Rep.* 2014;63(RR-2):1-19

collection methods and specimen types vary. Many clinical laboratories have met Clinical Laboratory Improvement Amendment (CLIA) and other regulatory requirements and have validated gonorrhea NAAT performance on extragenital specimens. For urogenital infections, the CDC recommends that optimal specimen types for gonorrhea screening using NAATS include first void urine for men and vaginal swab specimens in women. Patient-collected samples can be used in place of provider-collected samples in clinical settings when testing by NAAT for urine (men and women) and vaginal, rectal, and oropharyngeal swab specimens and appropriate instructions to patients have been provided. Certain NAAT platforms also permit combined testing of specimens for *N gonorrhoeae*, *C trachomatis*, and *Trichomonas vaginalis*.

Infants and Children. Culture can be used to test urogenital and extragenital sites in girls and boys. NAAT can be used to test for *N gonorrhoeae* from vaginal and urine specimens from girls and urine for boys. Although data on NAAT from extragenital sites in children are more limited and performance is test dependent, no evidence suggests that performance of NAAT for detection of *N gonorrhoeae* in children would differ from that in adults. Because of the implications of a diagnosis of *N gonorrhoeae* in a child, only validated FDA-cleared NAAT assays should be used from extragenital specimens. Consultation with an expert is necessary before using NAAT in this context, both to minimize the possibility of cross-reaction with nongonococcal *Neisseria* species and other commensals. Gram stains are inadequate for evaluating prepubertal children for gonorrhea and should not be used to diagnose or exclude gonorrhea. If evidence of disseminated gonococcal infection exists, gonorrhea culture and antimicrobial susceptibility testing should be performed on specimens from relevant clinical sites.

TREATMENT[1]: A single dose of intramuscular ceftriaxone is the recommended treatment for uncomplicated gonorrhea infections of the cervix, urethra, and rectum. If chlamydial infection has not been excluded, treatment for *Chlamydia trachomatis* with oral doxycycline for 7 days should also be provided. Treatment regimens for most syndromes caused by gonococcal infections, including urethritis, cervicitis, pelvic inflammatory disease, epididymitis, and proctitis, are provided in the chapter on Sexually Transmitted Infections (Table 4.4, p 898, and Table 4.5, p 903). A single 500-mg dose of intramuscular ceftriaxone also is recommended for the treatment of uncomplicated gonococcal infections of the pharynx. Gonococcal infections of the pharynx are more difficult to eradicate than are infections at urogenital and anorectal sites.

Resistance to penicillin and tetracycline is widespread, and as of 2007, the CDC no longer recommends the use of fluoroquinolones for gonorrhea because of the increased prevalence of quinolone-resistant *N gonorrhoeae* in the United States. Over the past decade, the minimum inhibitory concentrations (MIC) for cefixime against *N gonorrhoeae* strains circulating in the United States and other countries has increased and treatment failure following the use of cefixime has been described in North America, Europe, and Asia. Therefore, as of 2012, the CDC no longer recommends the use of cefixime as a first-line treatment for gonococcal infection. Dual therapy for gonococcal infection with ceftriaxone and azithromycin was previously recommended in the 2015 CDC STI guidelines as a theoretical strategy to improve treatment efficacy and potentially slow the emergence and spread of ceftriaxone resistance by using 2 antimicrobials with different mechanisms.

---

[1]Centers for Disease Control and Prevention. Sexually transmitted infections treatment guidelines, 2021. *MMWR Recomm Rep.* 2021; in press

Although no increases in ceftriaxone or cefixime MICs were identified since the dual therapy recommendation, significant concerns about azithromycin antimicrobial steward-ship impacting the treatment of chlamydia, *Mycoplasma genitalium*, and other organisms outweighs the rationale for dual therapy. Consequently, only ceftriaxone is recommended currently for treatment of gonorrhea in the United States.

To maximize adherence with recommended therapies and reduce complications and transmission, medication for gonococcal infection should be provided on site and directly observed. If medications are not available when treatment is indicated, linkage to an STI treatment facility should be provided for same-day treatment. To minimize disease trans-mission, people treated for gonorrhea should be instructed to abstain from sexual activity for 7 days after treatment and until all sex partners are adequately treated (7 days after receiving treatment and resolution of symptoms, if present).

Neonatal Infection. Infants with clinical evidence of ophthalmia neonatorum or scalp abscess attributable to *N gonorrhoeae* should be hospitalized, managed in consultation with an infectious disease specialist, and evaluated for disseminated infection (sepsis, arthritis, meningitis).

One dose of ceftriaxone (25–50 mg/kg, IV or IM, not to exceed 250 mg) is adequate therapy for gonococcal ophthalmia. Cefotaxime, 100 mg/kg, IV or IM as a single dose, can be administered for neonates who are unable to receive ceftriaxone because of simul-taneous administration of intravenous calcium. Topical antibiotic therapy alone is inad-equate and unnecessary if systemic treatment is administered.

For gonococcal scalp abscesses and disseminated gonococcal infections in neonates, treatment is with ceftriaxone (25–50 mg/kg/day, IV, in a single daily dose) or cefotaxime (50 mg/kg/day in 2 divided daily doses, IV or IM) for 7 days, with a duration of 10 to 14 days if meningitis is documented.

Ceftriaxone should not be used in neonates (28 days of age and younger) receiving (or expected to receive) calcium-containing intravenous products.

ISOLATION OF THE HOSPITALIZED PATIENT: Standard precautions are recommended, including for newborn infants with ophthalmia.

CONTROL MEASURES: Current control measures consist of counseling on the use of barrier protection during sexual intercourse, close follow-up of cases and their contacts, chemoprophylaxis recommended for specific clinical scenarios, routine screening in accor-dance with guidelines, and case reporting to public health authorities. There is no vaccine to prevent gonococcal infections.

Follow-up. A test-of-cure is not needed for people in whom uncomplicated urogenital or rectal gonorrhea is diagnosed who are treated with a single dose of ceftriaxone. Any per-son with pharyngeal gonorrhea should return between 7 to 14 days after initial treatment for a test-of cure using either culture or NAAT. If the NAAT result is positive, effort should be made to perform a confirmatory culture before retreatment, especially if a culture was not already collected. All positive cultures for test-of-cure should undergo antimicrobial susceptibility testing. Men or women who have been treated for gonorrhea should be retested 3 months after treatment for the possibility of reinfection, regardless of whether they believe their sex partners were treated. If retesting at 3 months is not possible, clini-cians should retest whenever people next present for medical care within 12 months fol-lowing initial treatment. All people in whom gonorrhea is diagnosed should be tested for other STIs, including chlamydia, syphilis, and human immunodeficiency virus.

Management of Sex Partners. Recent sex partners (ie, people having had sexual contact with the infected patient within the 60 days preceding onset of symptoms or gonorrhea diagnosis) should be referred for evaluation, testing, and presumptive treatment. If the patient's last potential sexual exposure was >60 days before onset of symptoms or diagnosis, the most recent sex partner should be treated. To avoid reinfection, sex partners should be instructed to abstain from condomless sexual intercourse for 7 days after they and their sexual partner(s) have completed treatment and after resolution of symptoms, if present.

For people with gonorrhea for whom health department partner-management strategies are impractical or unavailable and whose providers are concerned about partners' access to prompt clinical evaluation and treatment, expedited partner therapy (EPT) can be delivered to the partner by the patient, a disease investigation specialist, or a collaborating pharmacy, as permitted by law. Details are provided in the CDC STI Guidelines.[1]

Prophylaxis.

Neonatal Ophthalmia. If gonorrhea is prevalent in the region and prenatal treatment cannot be ensured, or where required by law, a prophylactic agent of 0.5% erythromycin ointment should be instilled into the eyes of all newborn infants (including those born by cesarean delivery) to prevent sight-threatening gonococcal ophthalmia. Efficacy is unlikely to be influenced by delaying prophylaxis for as long as 1 hour to facilitate parent-infant bonding. Longer delays have not been studied for efficacy (see Prevention of Neonatal Ophthalmia, p 1023). Topical prophylaxis for preventing chlamydial ophthalmia is not effective, likely because colonization of the nasopharynx is not prevented. Erythromycin is the only antibiotic ointment recommended in neonates. Silver nitrate and tetracycline ophthalmic ointment are no longer manufactured in the United States, bacitracin is not effective, and povidone iodine has not been studied adequately. Gentamicin ophthalmic ointment has been associated with severe ocular reactions in neonates and should not be used for ocular prophylaxis. Periodic shortages of erythromycin ointment have occurred in recent years. If erythromycin ointment is not available, azithromycin ophthalmic solution 1% is recommended as an acceptable substitute. If azithromycin ophthalmic solution 1% is not available, ciprofloxacin ophthalmic ointment 0.3% can be considered as a less suitable alternative. In most cases, potential resistance of *N gonorrhoeae* to ciprofloxacin will be overcome by the high concentrations of ciprofloxacin achieved.

Infants Born to Mothers With Gonococcal Infections. Neonates born to mothers who have untreated gonorrhea are at high risk for infection. Neonates should be tested for gonorrhea at exposed sites (eg, conjunctive, vaginal, rectal and oropharynx) and treated presumptively for gonorrhea with 1 dose of ceftriaxone (25–50 mg/kg, IV or IM, not to exceed 250 mg) (see Prevention of Neonatal Ophthalmia, p 1023). Ceftriaxone should be administered cautiously to infants with hyperbilirubinemia, especially those born preterm. For infants in whom ceftriaxone is contraindicated (eg, receiving continuous intravenous calcium, as in parenteral nutrition), then 1 dose of cefotaxime (100 mg/kg, IV or IM) or 1 dose of parenteral gentamicin (2.5 mg/kg, IV or IM) can be substituted for postexposure prophylaxis. Other extended spectrum cephalosporins should be effective, although studies have not been performed. Note that gentamicin should not be used as treatment of neonates with gonococcal ocular disease because of inadequate penetration into the globe

[1]Centers for Disease Control and Prevention. Sexually transmitted infections treatment guidelines, 2021. *MMWR Recomm Rep.* 2021; in press

of the eye. When systemic ceftriaxone therapy is administered prophylactically, topical antimicrobial therapy is not necessary.

Children and Adolescents With Sexual Exposure to a Patient Known to Have Gonorrhea. People sexually exposed within the 60 days preceding onset of symptoms or gonorrhea in the index case (or most recent sexual contact, if last potential sexual exposure was >60 days before onset of symptoms or gonorrhea) should undergo examination and culture and should receive the same treatment as do people known to have gonorrhea.

Routine Screening. Annual screening for *N gonorrhoeae* infection is recommended for all sexually active women younger than 25 years and for older women at increased risk for infection (eg, those who have a new sex partner, more than 1 sex partner, a sex partner with concurrent partners, or a sex partner who has an STI). Additional risk factors for gonorrhea include inconsistent condom use among people who are not in mutually monogamous relationships, previous or coexisting STIs, and exchanging sex for money or drugs. Clinicians should consider the communities they serve and might opt to consult local public health authorities for guidance on identifying groups at increased risk. Gonococcal infection, in particular, is concentrated in specific geographic locations and communities. MSM at high risk for gonorrhea infection (multiple anonymous partners, substance use) or those at risk for HIV acquisition should be screened at all sites of exposure every 3 to 6 months. At least annual screening is recommended for all MSM. Screening for gonorrhea in heterosexual men and older women who are at low risk for infection is not recommended. A recent travel history with sexual contacts outside of the United States should be part of any gonorrhea evaluation.

All pregnant females younger than 25 years should be screened for gonorrhea at the first prenatal visit. Pregnant females 25 years and older should be screened if they are considered at risk (ie, a new sex partner, more than 1 sex partner, a sex partner with concurrent partners, or a sex partner who has an STI or lives in an area with a high rate of gonorrhea). A repeat screen in the third trimester is recommended for females at continued risk of gonococcal infection, including all females younger than 25 years. Pregnant females with a diagnosis of gonorrhea should be treated immediately and rescreened within 3 months.

Case Reporting. All cases of gonorrhea must be reported to local public health officials (see Appendix III, Nationally Notifiable Infectious Diseases in the United States, p 1033). Cases in prepubertal children must be investigated to determine the source of infection (see Sexual Assault and Abuse in Children and Adolescents/Young Adults, p 150).

Granuloma Inguinale
(Donovanosis)

CLINICAL MANIFESTATIONS: Initial lesions of this sexually transmitted genital ulcerative disease are single or multiple painless subcutaneous nodules that gradually ulcerate. These nontender, granulomatous ulcers have raised, rolled margins, are beefy red and highly vascular, and bleed readily on contact. "Kissing" lesions may occur from autoinoculation on adjacent skin. Lesions usually involve the genitalia or perineum without regional adenopathy; however, lesions at both the genitalia and inguinal region occur in 5% to 10% of patients. Subcutaneous granulomas extending into the inguinal area can mimic inguinal adenopathy (ie, "pseudobubo"). Extragenital lesions (eg, face, mouth) account for 6% of cases. Dissemination to intra-abdominal organs and bone is rare.

ETIOLOGY: The disease, donovanosis, is caused by *Klebsiella granulomatis* (formerly known as *Calymmatobacterium granulomatis*), an intracellular gram-negative bacillus.

EPIDEMIOLOGY: Indigenous granuloma inguinale occurs very rarely in the United States and most industrialized nations. The disease is endemic in some tropical and developing areas, including India, Papua New Guinea, the Caribbean, and southern Africa. The incidence of infection seems to correlate with sustained high temperatures and high relative humidity. Infection usually is acquired by sexual contact, most commonly with a person with active infection. Young children and others, however, can, less commonly, acquire infection by contact with infected secretions. The period of communicability extends throughout the duration of active lesions.

The **incubation period** is uncertain; a range of 1 to 360 days has been reported. Experimental production of typical donovanosis lesions was induced in humans 50 days after inoculation.

DIAGNOSTIC TESTS: The causative organism is difficult to culture, and diagnosis requires microscopic demonstration of dark-staining intracytoplasmic Donovan bodies on Wright, Leishman, or Giemsa staining of a crush preparation from subsurface scrapings of a lesion or tissue. The microorganism also can be detected by histologic examination of biopsy specimens. Culture of *K granulomatis* is difficult to perform and is not available routinely. No molecular tests exist that have been cleared by the US Food and Drug Administration for the detection of *K granulomatis*. Diagnosis by polymerase chain reaction assay and serologic testing is only available in research laboratories.

TREATMENT[1]: The recommended treatment regimen is azithromycin (Table 4.4, p 901) for at least 3 weeks and until all lesions have completely healed. Treatment has been shown to halt progression of lesions. Partial healing usually is noted within 7 days of initiation of therapy and typically proceeds inward from the ulcer margins. Prolonged therapy usually is required to permit granulation and re-epithelialization of the ulcers. Relapse can occur, especially if the antimicrobial agent is stopped before the primary lesion has healed completely. In addition, relapse can occur 6 to 18 months after apparently effective therapy. Complicated or long-standing infection can require surgical intervention.

Patients should be evaluated for other sexually transmitted infections, including chlamydia, trichomoniasis, syphilis, and HIV infection.

ISOLATION OF THE HOSPITALIZED PATIENT: Standard precautions are recommended.

CONTROL MEASURES: People who have had sexual contact with a patient who has granuloma inguinale within the 60 days before onset of the patient's symptoms should be examined and offered therapy. However, the value of empiric therapy in the absence of clinical signs and symptoms has not been established.

Haemophilus influenzae Infections

CLINICAL MANIFESTATIONS: *Haemophilus influenzae* type b (Hib) causes pneumonia, bacteremia, meningitis, epiglottitis, septic arthritis, cellulitis, otitis media, purulent pericarditis, and less commonly, endocarditis, endophthalmitis, osteomyelitis, peritonitis, and gangrene. Infections caused by encapsulated but non-type b *H influenzae* present in a similar manner to type b infections. Nonencapsulated strains more commonly cause infections

---

[1]Centers for Disease Control and Prevention. Sexually transmitted infections treatment guidelines, 2021. *MMWR Recomm Rep.* 2021; in press

of the respiratory tract (eg, otitis media, sinusitis, pneumonia, conjunctivitis), but cases of bacteremia, meningitis, chorioamnionitis, and neonatal septicemia are well described.

ETIOLOGY: *H influenzae* is a pleomorphic gram-negative coccobacillus. Encapsulated strains express 1 of 6 antigenically distinct capsular polysaccharides (a through f); nonencapsulated strains lack complete capsule genes and are designated nontypeable.

EPIDEMIOLOGY[1]: The mode of transmission is person to person by inhalation of respiratory tract droplets or by direct contact with respiratory tract secretions. In neonates, infection is acquired intrapartum by aspiration of amniotic fluid or by contact with genital tract secretions containing the organism. Pharyngeal colonization by *H influenzae* is relatively common, especially with nontypeable strains. In the pre-Hib vaccine era, the major reservoir of Hib was young infants and toddlers, who may asymptomatically carry the organism in their upper respiratory tracts.

Before introduction of effective Hib conjugate vaccines, Hib was the most common cause of bacterial meningitis in young children in the United States. The peak incidence of invasive Hib infections occurred between 6 and 18 months of age. In contrast, the peak age for Hib epiglottitis was 2 to 4 years of age.

Unimmunized children younger than 5 years are at increased risk of invasive Hib disease. Other factors that predispose to invasive disease include sickle cell disease, asplenia, human immunodeficiency virus (HIV) infection, certain immunodeficiency syndromes, and chemotherapy for malignant neoplasms. Historically, invasive Hib infection was more common in Black and American Indian/Alaska Native children, boys, child care attendees, children living in crowded conditions, and children who were not breastfed.

Since introduction of Hib conjugate vaccines in the United States, the incidence of invasive Hib disease has decreased by more than 99% in children younger than 5 years. In 2017, 33 cases of invasive type b disease were reported in children younger than 5 years (0.17 cases per 100 000). In the United States, invasive Hib disease occurs primarily in underimmunized children and among infants too young to have completed the primary immunization series. Hib remains an important pathogen in many resource-limited countries where Hib vaccine coverage is suboptimal.

The epidemiology of invasive *H influenzae* disease in the United States has shifted in the post-Hib vaccination era. Nontypeable *H influenzae* is now the most common cause of invasive *H influenzae* disease in all age groups. In 2017, the annual incidence of invasive nontypeable *H influenzae* disease was 1.7/100 000 in children younger than 5 years, and the rate was highest in children younger than 1 year (5.4/100 000). Among the cases in children younger than 1 year, more than half were diagnosed within the first 2 weeks of life; many were in preterm neonates who had a positive culture on the day of birth. In addition to invasive disease, nontypeable *H influenzae* causes approximately 50% of episodes of acute otitis media and sinusitis in children and is a common cause of recurrent otitis media.

H influenzae type a (Hia) has emerged as the most common encapsulated serotype causing invasive disease, with a clinical presentation similar to Hib. In some North American Indigenous populations (eg, Alaska Native children, northern Canadian Indigenous children), the rate of invasive Hia infection has been increasing and there is evidence

---

[1]Centers for Disease Control and Prevention. Prevention and control of *Haemophilus influenzae* type b disease: recommendations of the Advisory Committee on Immunization Practices (ACIP). *MMWR Recomm Rep.* 2014;63(RR-1):1–14

of secondary cases having occurred. Although the incidence of invasive Hia is lower among the general population of US children, it has also been increasing in recent years, with a nearly 300% increase over the last 10 years among children younger than 1 year. Invasive disease may also be caused by other encapsulated non-type b strains c, d, e, and f.

The **incubation period** is unknown.

DIAGNOSTIC TESTS: The diagnosis of invasive disease is established by growth on appropriate media of *H influenzae* from cerebrospinal fluid (CSF), blood, synovial fluid, pleural fluid, or pericardial fluid. Because occult meningitis is known to occur in young children with invasive Hib disease, a lumbar puncture should be strongly considered in the presence of invasive disease, even in the absence of central nervous system signs and symptoms. Gram stain of an infected body fluid specimen can facilitate presumptive diagnosis. Antigen detection methods, which have historically been used on CSF, blood, and urine specimens, are not recommended because they lack sensitivity and specificity. Nucleic acid amplification tests (NAATs) available in multiplexed assays to detect *H influenzae* DNA directly in blood or CSF may be particularly useful in patients whose specimens are obtained after the initiation of antibiotics. Most of these assays do not determine the capsular polysaccharide type, and they all are incapable of determining the antibiotic susceptibilities of the pathogen.

The capsular polysaccharide of *H influenzae* isolates associated with invasive infection should be determined. Serotyping by slide agglutination using polyclonal antisera can have suboptimal sensitivity and specificity depending on reagents used and the experience of the technologist. Capsule typing by molecular methods, such as PCR assay of genes in the *cap* locus are preferred methods for capsule typing. If serotyping or capsule typing by molecular methods are not available locally, isolates should be submitted to the state health department or to a reference laboratory for testing.

TREATMENT:

- Initial therapy for children with *H influenzae* meningitis is cefotaxime or ceftriaxone. Intravenous ampicillin may be substituted if the isolate is found to be susceptible. Beta-lactamase–negative, ampicillin-resistant strains of *H influenzae* have been described, and some experts recommend caution in using ampicillin when minimum inhibitory concentrations (MICs) of 1 to 2 μg/mL are found, especially in the setting of invasive infection or disease in immunocompromised hosts. Treatment of other invasive *H influenzae* infections is similar. Therapy is continued for 7 days by the intravenous route and longer in complicated infections.

- Dexamethasone is beneficial for treatment of infants and children with Hib meningitis to diminish the risk of hearing loss, if administered before or concurrently with the first dose of antimicrobial agent(s).

- Epiglottitis is a medical emergency. An airway must be established promptly via controlled intubation.

- Infected pleural or pericardial fluid should be drained.

- According to clinical practice guidelines of the American Academy of Pediatrics (AAP) and the American Academy of Family Physicians (AAFP) on acute suppurative otitis media (AOM),[1] amoxicillin (80–90 mg/kg/day) is recommended for infants younger than 6 months, for those 6 through 23 months of age with bilateral disease, and for

---

[1]Lieberthal AS, Carroll AE, Chonmaitree T, et al. Clinical practice guideline: diagnosis and management of acute otitis media. *Pediatrics*. 2013;131(3):e964-e999

those older than 6 months with severe signs and symptoms (see *Streptococcus pneumoniae* [Pneumococcal] Infections, p 717, and Appropriate and Judicious Use of Antimicrobial Agents, p 868). A watch-and-wait option can be considered for older children and those with nonsevere disease. Optimal duration of therapy is uncertain. For younger children and children with severe disease at any age, a 10-day course is recommended; for children 6 years and older with mild or moderate disease, a duration of 5 to 7 days is appropriate. Otalgia should be treated symptomatically. Patients who fail to respond to initial management should be reassessed at 48 to 72 hours to confirm the diagnosis of AOM and exclude other causes of illness. If AOM is confirmed in the patient managed initially with observation, amoxicillin should be administered. If the patient has failed initial antibacterial therapy, a change in antibacterial agent is indicated. Suitable alternative agents should be active against penicillin-nonsusceptible pneumococci as well as beta-lactamase–producing *H influenzae* (in the United States, approximately 30%–40% of *H influenzae* isolates produce beta-lactamase) and *Moraxella catarrhalis*. Such agents include high-dose oral amoxicillin-clavulanate; oral cefdinir, cefpodoxime, or cefuroxime; or 3 daily doses of intramuscular ceftriaxone. Patients who continue to fail to respond to therapy with one of the aforementioned oral agents should be treated with a 3-day course of parenteral ceftriaxone. Macrolide resistance among *Streptococcus pneumoniae* is high, so clarithromycin and azithromycin are not considered appropriate alternatives for initial therapy even in patients with a type I (immediate, anaphylactic) reaction to a beta-lactam agent. In such cases, treatment with clindamycin (if susceptibility is known) or levofloxacin is preferred. For patients with a history of non-type I allergic reaction to penicillin, agents such as cefdinir, cefuroxime, or cefpodoxime can be used orally.

ISOLATION OF THE HOSPITALIZED PATIENT: In addition to standard precautions, in patients with invasive Hib disease, droplet precautions are recommended for 24 hours after initiation of effective antimicrobial therapy.

CONTROL MEASURES (FOR INVASIVE HIB DISEASE):

Care of Exposed People. Secondary cases of Hib disease have occurred in unimmunized or incompletely immunized children exposed in a child care or household setting to invasive Hib disease. Such children should be observed carefully for fever or other signs/symptoms of disease. Exposed young children in whom febrile illness develops should receive prompt medical evaluation.

Chemoprophylaxis.[1] The risk of invasive Hib disease is increased among unimmunized household contacts younger than 4 years. Rifampin eradicates Hib from the pharynx in approximately 95% of carriers and decreases the risk of secondary invasive illness in exposed household contacts. Child care center contacts also may be at increased risk of secondary disease, but secondary disease in child care contacts is rare when all contacts are older than 2 years. Indications and guidelines for chemoprophylaxis in different circumstances are summarized in Table 3.9.

- **Household.** See Table 3.9 for details regarding prophylaxis for household members of a person with invasive Hib disease, when at least 1 household member fits the listed criteria. Given that most secondary cases in households occur during the first week

---

[1] Centers for Disease Control and Prevention. Prevention and control of *Haemophilus influenzae* type b disease: recommendations of the Advisory Committee on Immunization Practices (ACIP). *MMWR Recomm Rep.* 2014;63(RR-1):1–14

Table 3.9. Indications and Guidelines for Rifampin Chemoprophylaxis for Contacts of Index Cases of Invasive *Haemophilus influenzae* Type b (Hib) Disease[a]

Chemoprophylaxis Recommended

- For all household contacts[b] in the following circumstances:
  - o Household with at least 1 child younger than 4 years who is unimmunized or incompletely immunized[c]
  - o Household with a child younger than 12 months who has not completed the primary Hib series
  - o Household with an immunocompromised child, regardless of that child's Hib immunization status or age

- For preschool and child care center contacts when 2 or more cases of Hib invasive disease have occurred within 60 days (see text)

- For index patient, if younger than 2 years or member of a household with a susceptible contact and treated with a regimen other than cefotaxime or ceftriaxone, chemoprophylaxis at the end of therapy for invasive infection

Chemoprophylaxis Not Recommended

- For occupants of households with no children younger than 4 years other than the index patient

- For occupants of households when all household contacts are immunocompetent, all household contacts 12 through 48 months of age have completed their Hib immunization series, and when household contacts younger than 12 months have completed their primary series of Hib immunizations

- For preschool and child care contacts of 1 index case

- For pregnant women

[a]Similar criteria may be used for Hia; however, the criteria for Hib immunization are not applicable.
[b]Defined as people residing with the index patient or nonresidents who spent 4 or more hours with the index patient for at least 5 of the 7 days preceding the day of hospital admission of the index case.
[c]Complete immunization is defined as having had at least 1 dose of conjugate vaccine at 15 months of age or older; 2 doses between 12 and 14 months of age; or the 2- or 3-dose primary series when younger than 12 months with a booster dose at 12 months of age or older.

after hospitalization of the index case, when indicated, prophylaxis should be initiated as soon as possible. Because some secondary cases occur later, initiation of prophylaxis 7 days or more after hospitalization of the index patient still may be of some benefit.

- **Child care and preschool.** When 2 or more cases of invasive Hib disease have occurred within 60 days and unimmunized or incompletely immunized children attend the child care facility or preschool, rifampin prophylaxis for all attendees (irrespective of their age and vaccine status) and child care providers should be considered. In addition to these recommendations for chemoprophylaxis, unimmunized or incompletely immunized children should receive a dose of vaccine and should be scheduled for completion of the recommended age-specific immunization schedule (**https://redbook. solutions.aap.org/SS/Immunization_Schedules.aspx**). Data are insufficient on the risk of secondary transmission to recommend chemoprophylaxis for attendees

Table 3.10. *Haemophilus influenzae* Type b (Hib) Conjugate Vaccines Licensed and Available for Use in Infants and Children in the United States[a]

Vaccine	Trade Name	Components	Manufacturer
PRP-T	ActHIB	PRP conjugated to tetanus toxoid	Sanofi Pasteur
PRP-T[a]	Hiberix	PRP conjugated to tetanus toxoid	GlaxoSmithKline Biologicals
PRP-OMP	PedvaxHIB	PRP conjugated to OMP	Merck & Co, Inc
DTaP-IPV-Hib[b]	Pentacel	DTaP-IPV + PRP-T	Sanofi Pasteur
DTaP-IPV-Hib-HepB	Vaxelis	DTaP-IPV + PRP-OMP + HepB	Sanofi Pasteur and Merck & Co, Inc

PRP-T indicates polyribosylribotol phosphate-tetanus toxoid; OMP, outer membrane protein complex from *Neisseria meningitidis;* DTaP, diphtheria and tetanus toxoids and acellular pertussis; IPV, inactivated poliovirus vaccine; HepB, hepatitis B vaccine.

[a]Hib conjugate vaccines may be administered in combination products or as reconstituted products, provided the combination or reconstituted vaccine is licensed by the US Food and Drug Administration (FDA) for the child's age and administration of the other vaccine component(s) also is justified.

[b]The DTaP-IPV liquid component is used to reconstitute a lyophilized ActHIB vaccine component to form Pentacel.

and child care providers when a single case of invasive Hib disease occurs; the decision to provide chemoprophylaxis in this situation is at the discretion of the local or state health department.

- **Index case.** See Table 3.9.
- **Dosage.** For prophylaxis, rifampin should be administered orally, once a day for 4 days (20 mg/kg; maximum dose, 600 mg). The dose for infants younger than 1 month is not established; some experts recommend lowering the dose to 10 mg/kg. For adults, each dose is 600 mg. If rifampin is contraindicated, administering a single dose of ceftriaxone can be considered, although the durability of eradication using this approach has not been well established.
- **Invasive Hia.** Clinicians can consider chemoprophylaxis of household contacts of index cases of invasive Hia disease in those households with a child younger than 4 years or with an immunocompromised child. For these individuals and contacts, chemoprophylaxis recommendations for Hib may be followed; however, because there is not a licensed vaccine for Hia the criteria regarding vaccination do not apply. A similar approach as Hib also may be considered for preschool and child care contacts in consultation with the local or state public health department.

Immunization.[1] Three single-antigen (monovalent) Hib conjugate vaccine products and 2 combination vaccine products that contain Hib conjugate are available in the United States (see Table 3.10). The Hib conjugate vaccine consists of the Hib capsular

---

[1]Centers for Disease Control and Prevention. Prevention and control of *Haemophilus influenzae* type b disease: recommendations of the Advisory Committee on Immunization Practices (ACIP). *MMWR Recomm Rep.* 2014;63(RR-1):1–14.

polysaccharide (polyribosylribotol phosphate [PRP]) covalently linked to a carrier protein. Protective antibodies are directed against PRP.

Depending on the vaccine, the recommended primary series consists of 3 doses administered at 2, 4, and 6 months of age or of 2 doses administered at 2 and 4 months of age (see Recommendations for Immunization, p 352, and Table 3.11). The regimens in Table 3.11 likely are to be equivalent in protection after completion of the recommended primary series. For American Indian/Alaska Native children, optimal immune protection is achieved by administration of PRP-OMP (outer membrane protein complex) Hib vaccine (see American Indian/Alaska Native Children and Adolescents, *Haemophilus influenzae* type b, p 345). Information on immunogenicity after dose 1 of new PRP-OMP containing vaccines is important for assessing their suitability for use in American Indian/Alaska Native children.

Table 3.11. Recommended Regimens for Routine *Haemophilus influenzae* Type b (Hib) Conjugate Immunization for Children Immunized at 2 Months Through 4 Years of Age[a]

Vaccine Product	Primary Series	Booster Dose	Catch-up Doses[b]
PRP-T (ActHIB, Sanofi Pasteur)	2, 4, 6 mo	12 through 15 mo	16 mo through 4 y
PRP-T (Hiberix, GlaxoSmithKline)	2, 4, 6 mo	12 through 15 mo	16 mo through 4 y
PRP-OMP (PedvaxHIB, Merck)[c,d]	2, 4 mo	12 through 15 mo	16 mo through 4 y
Combination vaccine			
DTaP-IPV-Hib (Pentacel, Sanofi Pasteur)	2, 4, 6 mo	12 through 15 mo	16 mo through 4 y
DTaP-IPV-Hib-HepB (Vaxelis, Sanofi Pasteur, Merck & Co, Inc)	2, 4, 6 mo	Use other Hib containing vaccine for booster, at least 6 months after last priming dose	

PRP-T indicates polyribosylribotol phosphate-tetanus toxoid; OMP, outer membrane protein complex from *Neisseria meningitidis;* DTaP, diphtheria and tetanus toxoids and acellular pertussis; IPV, inactivated poliovirus vaccine; Hep B, hepatitis B vaccine.

[a]See text and Table 3.10 for further information about specific vaccines and Table 1.10 (p 37) for information about combination vaccines.

[b]See Catch-up Immunization Schedule (**https://redbook.solutions.aap.org/SS/Immunization_Schedules.aspx**) for additional information.

[c]If a PRP-OMP(PedvaxHIB) vaccine is not administered as both doses in the primary series, a third dose of Hib conjugate vaccine is needed to complete the primary series.

[d]Preferred for American Indian/Alaska Native children.

- **Combination Vaccines.** There are 2 combination vaccines that contain Hib licensed in the United States. DTaP-IPV-Hib (Pentacel) is administered as a 4-dose series at 2, 4, 6, and 15 through 18 months of age, and DTaP-IPV-Hib-HepB (Vaxelis) is given for the 3-dose primary series at 2, 4, and 6 months of age; a different Hib-containing vaccine (other than Vaxelis) should be administered for the booster dose at 15 to 18 months of age. Vaxelis is not recommended as the preferred PRP-OMP Hib vaccine for American Indian/Alaska Native children because of the lack of immunogenicity data after dose 1.

- **Vaccine Interchangeability.** Hib conjugate vaccines licensed within the age range for the primary vaccine series are considered interchangeable as long as recommendations for a total of 3 doses in the first year of life are followed (ie, if 2 doses of Hib-OMP are not administered, 3 doses of a Hib-containing vaccine are required). Data are not available on safety and effectiveness of interchangeability of some vaccines (see package inserts).

- **Dosage and Route of Administration.** The dose of each Hib conjugate vaccine is 0.5 mL, administered intramuscularly.

- **Children With Immunologic Impairment.** Children at increased risk of Hib disease may have impaired anti-PRP antibody responses to conjugate vaccines. Examples include children with functional or anatomic asplenia, HIV infection, or immunoglobulin deficiency (including an isolated immunoglobulin [Ig] G2 subclass deficiency) or early component complement deficiency); recipients of hematopoietic stem cell transplants; and children undergoing chemotherapy for a malignant neoplasm. Some children with immunologic impairment may benefit from more doses of conjugate vaccine than usually indicated (see Recommendations for Immunization: Indications and Schedule).

- **Adverse Reactions.** Adverse reactions to Hib conjugate vaccines are uncommon. Pain, redness, and swelling at the injection site occur in approximately 25% of recipients, but these symptoms typically are mild and last fewer than 24 hours.

Recommendations for Immunization

Indications and Schedule

- All children should be immunized with a Hib conjugate vaccine beginning at approximately 2 months of age (see Table 3.11). Other general recommendations are as follows:
  - Immunization can be initiated as early as 6 weeks of age.
  - Vaccine can be administered during visits for other childhood immunizations (see Simultaneous Administration of Multiple Vaccines, p 36).
- For routine immunization of children younger than 7 months, the following guidelines are recommended:
  - **Primary series.** Table 3.11 lists the options for the primary vaccination series. Doses are administered at approximately 2-month intervals. When sequential doses of different vaccine products are administered or uncertainty exists about which products previously were used, 3 doses of a conjugate vaccine are considered sufficient to complete the primary series, regardless of the regimen used (see package inserts; data are not available for some vaccines on interchangeability).
  - **Booster immunization at 12 through 15 months of age.** For children who have completed a primary series, an additional dose of conjugate vaccine is

recommended at 12 through 15 months of age and at least 2 months after the last dose. Any monovalent or the pentavalent combination (Pentacel) Hib conjugate vaccine is acceptable for this dose.

- Children younger than 5 years who did not receive Hib conjugate vaccine during the first 6 months of life should be immunized according to the recommended catch-up immunization schedule (see **https://redbook.solutions.aap.org/SS/Immunization_Schedules.aspx** and Table 3.11). For accelerated immunization in infants younger than 12 months, a minimum of a 4-week interval between doses can be used.

- Children with invasive Hib infection younger than 24 months can remain at risk of developing a second episode of disease. These children should be immunized according to the age-appropriate schedule for unimmunized children as if they had received no previous Hib vaccine doses (see Table 3.11, and Table 1.10, p 37). Immunization should be initiated 1 month after onset of disease or as soon as possible thereafter.

   Immunologic evaluation should be performed in children who experience invasive Hib disease despite 2 to 3 doses of vaccine and in children with recurrent invasive disease attributable to type b strains.

- See Table 3.12 for special circumstances such as patients undergoing chemotherapy, radiation therapy, hematopoietic stem cell transplant, or splenectomy. Additional details are as follows:
  - **Lapsed immunizations.** Recommendations for children who have had a lapse in the schedule of immunizations are summarized in the annual immunization schedule **(https://redbook.solutions.aap.org/SS/Immunization_Schedules.aspx).**
  - **Preterm infants.** For preterm infants, immunization should be based on chronologic age and should be initiated at 2 months of age according to recommendations in Table 3.11.
  - **Functional/anatomic asplenia.** Children with decreased or absent splenic function who have received a primary series of Hib immunizations and a booster dose at 12 months or older need not be immunized further against Hib.
  - **Other high-risk groups.** Children with HIV infection, IgG2 subclass deficiency, or early component complement deficiency are at increased risk of invasive Hib disease. Whether these children will benefit from additional doses after completion of the primary series of immunizations and the booster dose at 12 months or older is unknown.

- Catch-up immunization for high-risk groups **(https://redbook.solutions.aap.org/SS/Immunization_Schedules.aspx)** (Table 3.12):
  - For children 12 through 59 months of age with an underlying condition predisposing to Hib disease (functional or anatomic asplenia, HIV infection, immunoglobulin deficiency, early component complement deficiency, or receipt of hematopoietic stem cell transplant or chemotherapy for a malignant neoplasm) who are not immunized or have received only 1 dose of conjugate vaccine before 12 months of age, 2 doses of any conjugate vaccine, separated by 2 months, are recommended. For children in this age group who received 2 or more doses before 12 months of age, 1 additional dose of conjugate vaccine is recommended.

Reporting. All cases of *H influenzae* invasive disease, including type b, non-type b, and nontypeable, should be reported to the local or state public health department.

Table 3.12. Use of *Haemophilus influenzae* Type b (Hib) Conjugate Immunization in Special Populations

High-Risk Group	Vaccine Recommendations
Patient <12 mo	Follow routine Hib vaccination recommendations
Patients 12 through 59 mo	If unimmunized or received 0 or 1 dose before age 12 months: 2 doses 2 months apart
	If received 2 or more doses before age 12 months: 1 dose
	If completed a primary series and received a booster dose at age 12 months or older: no additional doses
Patients undergoing chemotherapy or radiation therapy, age <60 mo	If routine Hib doses administered 14 or more days before starting therapy: revaccination not required
	If dose administered within 14 days of starting therapy or during therapy: repeat doses starting at least 3 months following therapy completion of therapy
Patients undergoing elective splenectomy, age ≥15 mo	If unimmunized[a]: 1 dose, preferably at least 14 days prior to procedure
Asplenic patients ≥60 mo and adults	If unimmunized[a]: 1 dose
HIV-infected children ≥60 mo	If unimmunized[a]: 1 dose
HIV-infected adults	Hib vaccination is not recommended
Recipients of hematopoietic stem cell transplant, all ages	Regardless of Hib vaccination history: 3 doses (at least 1 month apart) beginning 6–12 mo after transplant[b]

[a]Patients who have not received a primary series and booster dose or at least 1 dose of Hib vaccine after 14 months of age are considered unimmunized.
[b]The CDC Advisory Committee on Immunizations Practices recommends this, although Hib vaccines are not licensed for individuals older than 5 years.

Hantavirus Pulmonary Syndrome

CLINICAL MANIFESTATIONS: Hantaviruses cause 2 distinct clinical syndromes: (1) hantavirus pulmonary syndrome (HPS), also known as hantavirus cardiopulmonary syndrome (HCPS), characterized by noncardiogenic pulmonary edema, which is observed in the Americas; and (2) hemorrhagic fever with renal syndrome (HFRS), which occurs worldwide (see Hemorrhagic Fevers and Related Syndromes Caused by Bunyaviruses, p 365). After an incubation period of 1 to 6 weeks, the prodromal illness of HPS lasts 3 to 7 days and is characterized by fever, chills, headache, myalgia, nausea, vomiting, diarrhea, dizziness, and sometimes cough. Respiratory tract symptoms or signs usually do not occur during the first 3 to 7 days, but then pulmonary edema and severe hypoxemia appear abruptly and present as cough and dyspnea. The disease then progresses over hours. In severe cases, myocardial dysfunction causes hypotension, which is why the syndrome sometimes is called hantavirus cardiopulmonary syndrome.

Extensive bilateral interstitial and alveolar pulmonary edema with pleural effusions are attributable to diffuse pulmonary capillary leak. Intubation and assisted ventilation usually are required for only 2 to 4 days, with resolution heralded by onset of diuresis and rapid clinical improvement.

The severe myocardial depression is different from that of septic shock, with low cardiac indices and stroke volume index, normal pulmonary wedge pressure, and increased systemic vascular resistance. Poor prognostic indicators include persistent hypotension, marked hemoconcentration, a cardiac index of less than 2, and abrupt onset of lactic acidosis with a serum lactate concentration of >4 mmol/L (36 mg/dL).

The mortality rate for patients with HPS is between 30% and 40%; death usually occurs in the first 1 or 2 days of hospitalization. A disproportionate number of cases occurs in American Indian/Alaska Native populations, and case-fatality rates for these populations (46%) are higher than for non-Native populations. Milder forms of disease have been reported. Limited information suggests that clinical manifestations and prognosis are similar in adults and children. Serious sequelae are uncommon.

ETIOLOGY: Hantaviruses are RNA viruses of the *Hantaviridae* family. Sin Nombre virus (SNV) is the major cause of HPS in the western and central regions of the United States. Bayou virus, Black Creek Canal virus, Monongahela virus, and New York virus are responsible for sporadic cases in Louisiana, Texas, Florida, New York, and other areas of the eastern United States. Andes virus, Oran virus, Laguna Negra virus, and Choclo virus are responsible for cases in South and Central America. There are typically 20 to 40 cases of HPS reported annually in the United States, with the majority (>95%) of cases occurring west of the Mississippi River. Cases in children younger than 10 years are exceedingly rare. Children may be less likely to become infected than adults, because children are less likely to perform tasks that would place them at increased risk. Nonspecific immune mechanisms may reduce the risk of symptoms in children.

EPIDEMIOLOGY: Rodents are natural hosts for hantaviruses and acquire lifelong, asymptomatic, chronic infection with prolonged viruria and virus in saliva and feces. Humans acquire infection through direct contact with infected rodents, rodent droppings, or rodent nests or through the inhalation of aerosolized virus particles from rodent urine, droppings, or saliva. Rarely, infection may be acquired from rodent bites or contamination of broken skin with excreta. At-risk activities include handling or trapping rodents, cleaning or entering closed or rarely used rodent-infested structures, cleaning feed storage or animal shelter areas, hand plowing, and living in a home with an increased density of mice. For backpackers or campers, sleeping in a structure inhabited by rodents has been associated with HPS, with a notable outbreak occurring in 2012 in Yosemite National Park secondary to rodent-infested cabins. Exceptionally heavy rainfall improves rodent food supplies, resulting in an increase in the rodent population with more frequent contact between humans and infected rodents, resulting in more human disease. Most cases occur during the spring and summer, with the geographic location determined by the habitat of the rodent carrier.

SNV is transmitted by the deer mouse, *Peromyscus maniculatus;* Black Creek Canal virus is transmitted by the cotton rat, *Sigmodon hispidus;* Bayou virus is transmitted by the rice rat, *Oryzomys palustris;* and the New York and Monongahela viruses are transmitted by the white-footed mouse, *Peromyscus leucopus* and *Peromyscus maniculatus.*

Andes virus is transmitted by the long-tailed rice rat (*Oligoryzomys longicaudatus*), endemic to most of Argentina and Chile. Unlike all other hantaviruses, Andes virus can also be transmitted person to person.

DIAGNOSTIC TESTS: HPS should be considered when thrombocytopenia occurs with severe pneumonia clinically resembling acute respiratory distress syndrome in the proper epidemiologic setting. Other characteristic laboratory findings include neutrophilic leukocytosis with immature granulocytes, including more than 10% immunoblasts (basophilic cytoplasm, prominent nucleoli, and an increased nuclear-cytoplasmic ratio) and increased hematocrit. In areas where HPS is known to occur, use of a 5-point peripheral blood screen has aided in the early detection of patients with HPS. Elements of the screen are: (1) hemoglobin elevated for gender/age; (2) left shift of granulocytic series; (3) absence of toxic changes; (4) thrombocytopenia; and (5) immunoblasts and plasma cells >10% of lymphocytes. For cases fulfilling 4 of 5 criteria, the positive predictive value of the 5-point screen is >90%.

Molecular detection of virus has been described in peripheral blood mononuclear cells and other clinical specimens from the early phase of the disease but not usually in bronchoalveolar lavage fluids. Viral culture is not useful. Hantavirus-specific immunoglobulin (Ig) M and IgG antibodies often are present at the onset of clinical disease, and serologic testing remains the method of choice for diagnosis. IgG may be negative in rapidly fatal cases. Although some commercial labs offer Hantavirus serologies, any IgM positives are referred to the Centers for Disease Control and Prevention for confirmation. Clinicians can contact the Viral Special Pathogens Branch Clinical Inquiries Line (470-312-0094) for assistance with diagnosis and management.

Immunohistochemical staining of tissues (capillary endothelial cells of the lungs and almost every organ in the body) can establish the diagnosis at autopsy.

TREATMENT: Patients with suspected HPS should be transferred immediately to a tertiary care facility where supportive management of pulmonary edema, severe hypoxemia, and hypotension can occur during the first critical 24 to 48 hours.

In severe forms, early mechanical ventilation and inotropic and pressor support are necessary. Extracorporeal membrane oxygenation (ECMO) should be considered when pulmonary wedge pressure and cardiac indices have deteriorated, and may provide short-term support for the severe capillary leak syndrome in the lungs.

Ribavirin is active in vitro against hantaviruses, including SNV. However, 2 clinical studies of intravenous ribavirin (1 open-label study and 1 randomized, placebo-controlled, double-blind study) failed to show benefit in treatment of HPS in the cardiopulmonary stage. At the present time, ribavirin should not be considered the standard of care.

Cytokine-blocking agents for HPS theoretically may have a role, but these agents have not been evaluated in a systematic fashion. Antibacterial agents are unlikely to offer benefit. However, broad-spectrum antibiotic therapy often is administered until the diagnosis is established, because bacterial shock is far more common than shock attributable to hantavirus.

ISOLATION OF THE HOSPITALIZED PATIENT: Standard precautions are recommended. Health care-associated or person-to-person transmission has not been associated with HPS in the United States but has been reported in Chile and Argentina with the Andes virus.

CONTROL MEASURES:

Care of Exposed People. Serial clinical examinations should be used to monitor individuals at high risk of infection after exposure (see Epidemiology).

Environmental Control. Hantavirus infections of humans occur primarily in adults and are associated with domestic, occupational, or leisure activities facilitating contact with infected rodents, usually in a building in a rural setting. Eradicating the host reservoir is not feasible. Risk reduction includes practices that discourage rodents from colonizing the home and work environment and that minimize aerosolization and contact with rodent saliva and excreta. Tactics include eliminating food sources for rodents, reducing nesting sites by sealing holes, and using "snap traps" and rodenticides. Before entering areas with potential rodent infestations, doors and windows should be opened to ventilate the enclosure. Regionally and culturally appropriate educational materials should be used to direct prevention messages.

Hantaviruses, because of their lipid envelope, are susceptible to diluted bleach solutions, detergents, and most general household disinfectants. Dusty areas or articles should be moistened with 10% bleach or other disinfectant solution before being cleaned. Brooms and vacuum cleaners should not be used to clean rodent-infested areas. Use of a 10% bleach solution to disinfect dead rodents and wearing rubber gloves before handling trapped or dead rodents is recommended. Gloves and traps should be disinfected after use. The cleanup of areas potentially infested with hantavirus-infected rodents should be conducted by knowledgeable professionals using appropriate personal protective equipment. Potentially infected material should be handled according to local regulations for infectious waste.

Public Health Reporting. Possible hantavirus cases should be reported to local and state public health authorities. For state health department contact information, see **www.cdc. gov/hantavirus/surveillance/index.html.** HPS and nonpulmonary hantavirus infections are nationally notifiable diseases, reportable through the Nationally Notifiable Disease Surveillance System.

Helicobacter pylori Infections

CLINICAL MANIFESTATIONS: Most *Helicobacter pylori* infections in children are believed to be asymptomatic. *H pylori* may cause chronic active gastritis and may result in duodenal and, to a lesser extent, gastric ulcers. Persistent infection with *H pylori* also increases the risk for the development of gastric cancers including mucosal-associated lymphoid tissue (MALT) lymphoma and adenocarcinoma in adults. However, complications of infection are infrequent in children. In children, acute *H pylori* infection can result in gastroduodenal inflammation that can manifest as epigastric pain, nausea, vomiting, hematemesis, and guaiac-positive stools. If present, these symptoms usually are self-limited. There is no clear association between infection and recurrent abdominal pain in the absence of peptic ulcer disease. The presence of night-time wakening can distinguish those children with peptic ulcer disease from those with chronic gastritis attributable to *H pylori* infection (for whom nighttime wakening rarely occurs). Endoscopic findings of *H pylori* infection include nodular gastritis, chronic gastritis, and rarely, the presence of gastric or duodenal erosions or ulcers. Extraintestinal conditions in children that have been associated with *H pylori* infection include treatment-refractory iron-deficiency anemia and chronic immune thrombocytopenia purpura (cITP).

ETIOLOGY: *H pylori* is a gram-negative, spiral, curved, or U-shaped microaerobic bacillus that has single or multiple flagella at one end. The organism is positive for catalase, oxidase, and urease activity. The 2 main virulence factors associated with more severe disease including the cytotoxin associated gene (CagA) and the vacuolating cytotoxin (VacA).

EPIDEMIOLOGY: *H pylori* organisms have been isolated from humans and other primates. An animal reservoir for human transmission has not been demonstrated. Organisms are thought to be transmitted from infected humans by the fecal-oral, gastro-oral, and oral-oral routes.

H pylori is estimated to have infected 70% of people living in resource-limited countries and 30% to 40% of people living in industrialized countries. Infection rates in children are low in resource-rich, industrialized countries, except in children from lower socioeconomic groups, immigrants from resource-limited countries, and those living in poor hygienic conditions. Most infections are acquired in the first 8 years of life. The organism can persist in the stomach for years or for life.

Although all infected people have gastritis, over a lifetime, approximately 10% to 15% will develop peptic ulcer disease and less than 1% will develop gastric cancer.

The **incubation period** is unknown.

DIAGNOSTIC TESTS: *H pylori* infection can be diagnosed by culture of gastric biopsy tissue on nonselective media (eg, chocolate agar, brucella agar, brain-heart infusion agar) or selective media (eg, Skirrow agar) at 37°C under microaerophilic conditions (decreased oxygen, increased carbon dioxide, and increased hydrogen concentrations) for 3 to 10 days. Colonies are small, smooth, and translucent and are positive for catalase, oxidase, and urease activity. Antimicrobial susceptibility testing of cultured isolates should be performed to guide therapy. Organisms can be visualized on histologic sections with Warthin-Starry silver, Steiner, Giemsa, or Genta staining. Presence of *H pylori* can be confirmed but not excluded on the basis of hematoxylin-eosin stains. Immunohistologic staining with specific *H pylori* antibodies may improve specificity. Because of production of high levels of urease by these organisms, urease testing of a gastric biopsy specimen can be used to detect the presence of *H pylori*. Urease hydrolyzes urea into ammonia and carbonate; the resulting increase in pH from the production of ammonia is detected in the assay.

Noninvasive, commercially available tests include urea breath tests and stool antigen tests; these tests are designed for detection of active infection and have high sensitivity and specificity. Stool antigen tests by enzyme immunoassay monoclonal antibodies are available commercially and can be used for children of any age. The urea breath test detects labeled carbon dioxide in expired air after oral administration of isotope-labeled urea (^{13}C or ^{14}C). Although urea breath tests are expensive and are not useful in very young children, there is a test approved by the US Food and Drug Administration (FDA) for children 3 to 17 years of age. Patients with identified peptic ulcer disease may benefit from testing and treating for *H pylori* infection. Patients with functional abdominal pain (absence of alarm symptoms by Rome criteria[1]) should not be tested, because there is a lack of evidence that treating *H pylori* infection provides relief. Testing should be used for the initial diagnosis of infection in the case of chronic immune thrombocytopenia

---

[1] Hyams JS, Di Lorenzo C, Saps M, Shulman RJ, Staiano A, van Tilburg M. Functional disorders: children and adolescents. *Gastroenterology*. 2016;150(6):1456-1468

purpura in which endoscopy and biopsy may pose increased risk of bleeding. Testing also is appropriate to confirm eradication of infection following completion of treatment.

H pylori can be detected by polymerase chain reaction (PCR) or fluorescence in situ hybridization (FISH) of gastric biopsy tissue, and PCR also has been applied to detecting the organism in stool specimens. However, none of these assays are currently cleared by the FDA for *H pylori* testing.

Serologic testing for *H pylori* infection by detection of immunoglobulin (Ig) G antibodies specific for *H pylori* should not be used in children for diagnosis or for confirming eradication.

The European Society for Paediatric Gastroenterology, Hepatology and Nutrition and the North American Society for Pediatric Gastroenterology, Hepatology & Nutrition (ESPGHAN/NASPGHAN) joint guideline recommends against a "test and treat" strategy for *H pylori* infection in children. Instead, they recommend the following[1]:

- The diagnosis of *H pylori* infection should be based on either (a) histopathology (*H pylori*–positive gastritis) plus at least 1 other positive biopsy-based test, or (b) positive culture.
- When testing for *H pylori*, wait at least 2 weeks after stopping a proton pump inhibitor (PPI) and 4 weeks after stopping antimicrobial agents.
- Testing for *H pylori* should be performed in children with gastric or duodenal ulcers. If *H pylori* infection is identified, then treatment should be advised and eradication should be confirmed.
- Diagnostic testing for *H pylori* infection should not be performed as part of the initial investigation in children with iron-deficiency anemia. In children with refractory iron deficiency anemia in which other causes have been ruled out, testing for *H pylori* during upper endoscopy may be considered.
- Diagnostic testing for *H pylori* infection should not be performed in children with functional abdominal pain.
- Diagnostic testing for *H pylori* infection should not be performed when investigating causes of short stature.

The 2011 guidelines from the American Society of Hematology (ASH) recommends against routine testing for *H pylori* in children with chronic immune thrombocytopenia purpura (cITP).[2]

TREATMENT[1]**:** Treatment options are detailed in Tables 3.13 and 3.14. Treatment is recommended for infected patients who have peptic ulcer disease, gastric mucosa-associated lymphoid tissue-type lymphoma, or early gastric cancer. Treatment of *H pylori* infection, if found, may be considered for children who have unexplained and refractory iron-deficiency anemia. Additionally, both the ESPGHAN/NASPGHAN and ASH guidelines recommend eradication if infection is associated with chronic immune thrombocytopenia purpura.[1,2] For patients with *H pylori* infection in the absence of clinical or endoscopic evidence of peptic ulcer disease, treatment is not recommended unless the patient is within a risk group or region with high incidence of gastric cancer. Adherence is critical to the success of eradication therapy.

[1]Jones NL, Koletzko S, Goodman K, et al; ESPGHAN, NASPGHAN. Joint ESPGHAN/NASPGHAN guidelines for the management of *Helicobacter pylori* in children and adolescents (update 2016). *J Pediatr Gastroenterol Nutr.* 2017;64(6):991-1003

[2]Neunert C, Lim W, Crowther M, Cohen A, Solberg L Jr, Crowther MA. The American Society of Hematology 2011 evidence-based guideline for immune thrombocytopenia. *Blood.* 2011;117(16):4190–4207

Table 3.13. Recommended Options for First-Line Therapy for *H pylori* Infections[a,b]

H pylori Antimicrobial Susceptibilities	Suggested First-Line Treatment
Susceptible to clarithromycin, susceptible to metronidazole	PPI + amoxicillin + clarithromycin for 14 days[c]
Resistant to clarithromycin, susceptible to metronidazole	PPI + amoxicillin + metronidazole for 14 days OR Bismuth-based therapy as detailed in "Unknown" row below.
Susceptible to clarithromycin, resistant to metronidazole	PPI + amoxicillin + clarithromycin for 14 days
Resistant to clarithromycin, resistant to metronidazole ("double resistant")	<8 y of age: PPI + amoxicillin + metronidazole + bismuth for 14 days ≥8 y of age: PPI + tetracycline + metronidazole + bismuth for 14 days
Susceptibilities not known	<8 y of age: PPI + amoxicillin + metronidazole + bismuth for 14 days ≥8 y of age: PPI + tetracycline + metronidazole + bismuth for 14 days

[a] Adapted from Jones NL, Koletzko S, Goodman K, et al; ESPGHAN, NASPGHAN. Joint ESPGHAN/NASPGHAN guidelines for the management of *Helicobacter pylori* in children and adolescents (update 2016). *J Pediatr Gastroenterol Nutr.* 2017;64(6):991-1003.

[b] Refer to Joint ESPGHAN/NASPGHAN guidelines for antibiotic dosing.

[c] Sequential therapy for 10 days (PPI + amoxicillin for 5 days, followed by PPI + clarithromycin + metronidazole for 5 days) is equally effective, but has the disadvantage of exposing the child to 3 different antibiotics.

The backbone of all recommended therapies includes a PPI and amoxicillin. Additions of metronidazole, clarithromycin, and/or bismuth are based on the patient's previous treatment experience or known susceptibilities to clarithromycin and metronidazole. Reports of increasing prevalence of antibiotic-resistant strains (particularly clarithromycin resistance) as well as increasing failures of triple therapies suggest the need for bismuth-based quadruple therapy regimens (meaning 3 antibiotics and bismuth) and longer durations (14 days) for eradication of *H pylori*. A number of treatment regimens have been evaluated and are approved for use in adults; the safety and efficacy of these regimens in pediatric patients have not been firmly established. There is no current evidence to support the use of probiotics to reduce medication adverse effects or improve eradication of *H pylori*. Limited options exist for penicillin-allergic patients.

Table 3.14. Rescue Therapies in Pediatric Patients Who Fail Therapy[a,b]

Initial Antibiotic Susceptibilities	Past Treatment Regimen	Suggested Rescue Treatment
Susceptible to clarithromycin, susceptible to metronidazole	PPI + amoxicillin + clarithromycin	PPI + amoxicillin + metronidazole
	PPI + amoxicillin + metronidazole	PPI + amoxicillin + clarithromycin
Susceptible to clarithromycin, susceptible to metronidazole	Sequential therapy (see footnote **c** in Table 3.13)	Consider performing a second endoscopy and use a tailored treatment for 14 days OR Treat like double-resistant in Table 3.13
Resistant to clarithromycin	PPI + amoxicillin + metronidazole	Treat like double-resistant in Table 3.13
Resistant to metronidazole	PPI + amoxicillin + clarithromycin	Consider performing a second endoscopy and use a tailored treatment for 14 days OR Treat like double-resistant in Table 3.13
Susceptibilities not known	PPI + amoxicillin + clarithromycin OR PPI + amoxicillin + metronidazole OR Sequential therapy (see footnote c in Table 3.13)	Consider performing a second endoscopy to assess secondary antimicrobial susceptibility OR Treat like double-resistant in Table 3.13

[a]Adapted from Jones NL, Koletzko S, Goodman K, et al; ESPGHAN, NASPGHAN. Joint ESPGHAN/NASPGHAN guidelines for the management of *Helicobacter pylori* in children and adolescents (update 2016). *J Pediatr Gastroenterol Nutr.* 2017;64(6):991-1003.
[b]Refer to Joint ESPGHAN/NASPGHAN guidelines for antibiotic dosing.

Initial Therapy

- In a treatment-naïve patient with *H pylori*, selection of therapeutic regimen is best guided by knowledge of the susceptibilities of that patient's organism.
- Treatment options are detailed in Table 3.13.

- A breath or stool test should be performed to document organism clearance 4 to 6 weeks after completion of initial therapy; relief of clinical symptoms is not an indicator of successful eradication.

Rescue Therapy

- Infection within the first 12 months following treatment is likely a relapse of the previous infection. The reinfection rate within 5 years may be as high as 50%. In contrast to adults, reduced options exist for rescue therapy for children.
- Management and treatment options are detailed in Table 3.14.
- A breath or stool test should be performed to document organism eradication 4 to 6 weeks after completion of rescue therapy.

ISOLATION OF THE HOSPITALIZED PATIENT: Standard precautions are recommended.

CONTROL MEASURES: Disinfection of gastroscopes prevents transmission of the organism between patients.

Hemorrhagic Fevers Caused by Arenaviruses[1]

CLINICAL MANIFESTATIONS: Arenaviruses are responsible for several hemorrhagic fever (HF) syndromes. Arenaviruses are divided into 2 groups: the New World or Tacaribe complex and the Old World or lymphocytic choriomeningitis (LCMV)/Lassa complex (see Etiology). LCMV is discussed in a separate chapter (p 492). Disease associated with arenaviruses ranges from asymptomatic or mild, acute, febrile infections to severe illnesses in which vascular leak, shock, and multiorgan dysfunction are prominent features. Fever, weakness, malaise, headache, arthralgia, myalgia, conjunctival suffusion, retro-orbital pain, facial flushing, anorexia, vomiting, diarrhea, and abdominal pain are common early symptoms in all infections. Thrombocytopenia, leukopenia, petechiae, generalized lymphadenopathy, and encephalopathy usually are present in Argentine HF, Bolivian HF, and Venezuelan HF, and exudative pharyngitis often occurs in Lassa fever. Mucosal bleeding generally occurs in severe cases as a consequence of vascular damage, coagulopathy, thrombocytopenia, and platelet dysfunction. However, hemorrhagic manifestations occur in only one third of patients with Lassa fever. Proteinuria is common, but renal failure is unusual. Increased serum concentrations of aspartate aminotransferase (AST) can portend a severe or possibly fatal outcome of Lassa fever. Shock develops 7 to 9 days after onset of illness in more severely ill patients with these infections. Upper and lower respiratory tract symptoms can develop in people with Lassa fever. Encephalopathic signs, such as tremor, alterations in consciousness, and seizures, can occur in South American HFs and in severe cases of Lassa fever. Transient or permanent deafness is reported in 30% of convalescents of Lassa fever. The overall mortality rate in Lassa fever is 1% to 20% of all infections, but it is highest among hospitalized patients (15%–50%); for South American HFs, the mortality rate is 10% to 35%, and for Lujo virus HF, the mortality rate is 80% (estimated from a small number of patients). Pregnant women are at substantially higher risk of mortality (~80%) and spontaneous abortion with 95% mortality in fetuses of infected mothers. Symptoms resolve 10 to 15 days after disease onset in surviving patients.

---

[1]Does not include lymphocytic choriomeningitis virus, which is reviewed on p 492.

ETIOLOGY: Mammalian arenaviruses (mammarenaviruses) are enveloped, biseg-mented, single-stranded RNA viruses. Old World arenaviruses include LCMV, which causes lymphocytic choriomeningitis, Lassa virus (Lassa HF), and Lujo virus (Lujo HF) in western and southern Africa. New World arenaviruses include Junín virus (Argentine HF) Machupo virus (Bolivian HF), Sabiá virus (Brazilian HF), Guanarito virus (Venezuelan HF), and Chapare virus (Chapare HF). Whitewater Arroyo virus is a rare cause of human disease in North America. Antibodies to Tamiami viruses have been detected in people in North America, but clinical disease has not been con-firmed. Several other arenaviruses are known only from their rodent reservoirs in the Old and New World.

EPIDEMIOLOGY: Arenaviruses are maintained in nature by association with specific rodent hosts, in which they produce chronic viremia and viruria. The principal routes of infec-tion are inhalation and direct contact of mucous membranes and skin (eg, through cuts, scratches, or abrasions) with urine and salivary secretions from these persistently infected rodents. Ingestion of food contaminated by rodent excrement also may cause disease trans-mission. All arenaviruses are infectious as aerosols, and human-to-human transmission may occur in community or hospital settings following unprotected contact or through droplets. Excretion of arenaviruses in urine and semen for several weeks after infection has been documented. Arenaviruses causing HF should be considered highly hazardous to people working with any of these viruses in the laboratory. Laboratory-acquired infections have been documented with Lassa, Machupo, Junín, and Sabiá viruses. The geographic distri-bution and habitats of the specific rodents that serve as reservoir hosts largely determine areas with endemic infection and populations at risk. Before a vaccine became available in Argentina, several hundred cases of Argentine HF occurred annually in agricultural work-ers and inhabitants of the Argentine pampas; the Argentine HF vaccine is not licensed in the United States. Epidemics of Bolivian HF occurred in small towns between 1962 and 1964; sporadic disease activity in the countryside has continued since then. Venezuelan HF first was identified in 1989 and occurs in rural north-central Venezuela. Lassa fever is endemic in most of western Africa, where rodent hosts live in proximity to humans, caus-ing thousands of infections annually. Lassa fever has been reported in the United States and Western Europe in people who have traveled to western Africa.

The **incubation periods** for these HF range from 6 to 21 days.

DIAGNOSTIC TESTS: Viral nucleic acid can be detected in acute disease by reverse transcriptase-polymerase chain reaction assay. These viruses may be isolated from blood of acutely ill patients as well as from various tissues obtained postmortem, but isolation should be attempted only under biosafety level-4 (BSL-4) conditions. Virus antigen is detectable by enzyme immunoassay (EIA) in acute specimens and postmortem tissues. Virus-specific immunoglobulin (Ig) M antibodies are present in the serum during acute stages of illness by immunofluorescent antibody or enzyme-linked immunosorbent assays but may be undetectable in rapidly fatal cases. The IgG antibody response is delayed. Diagnosis can be made retrospectively by immunohistochemical staining of formalin-fixed tissues obtained from autopsy.

If a viral HF is suspected, the state/local health department or Centers for Disease Control and Prevention (CDC) (Viral Special Pathogens Branch: 404-639-1115) should be contacted to assist with case investigation, diagnosis, treatment, and control measures.

TREATMENT: Intravenous ribavirin substantially decreases the mortality rate in patients with severe Lassa fever, particularly if they are treated early, during the first week of illness. For Argentine HF, transfusion of immune plasma in defined doses of neutralizing antibodies is the standard specific treatment when administered during the first 8 days from onset of symptoms and reduces mortality to 1% to 2%. Intravenous ribavirin has been used with success to abort a Sabiá laboratory infection, and to treat Bolivian HF patients and the only known Lujo virus infection survivor. Ribavirin did not reduce mortality when initiated 8 days or more after onset of Argentine HF symptoms. Whether ribavirin treatment initiated early in the course of the disease has a role in the treatment of Argentine HF remains to be seen. Intravenous ribavirin is available only from the manufacturer through an investigational new drug (IND) protocol. Health care providers who need to obtain intravenous ribavirin should contact the US Food and Drug Administration (**www.fda.gov/drugs/investigational-new-drug-ind-application/physicians-how-request-single-patient-expanded-access-compassionate-use**; US Food and Drug Administration 24-hour emergency lines: 866-300-4374 or 301-796-8240). Meticulous fluid and electrolyte balance is an important aspect of supportive care in each of the HFs.

ISOLATION OF THE HOSPITALIZED PATIENT: In addition to standard precautions, contact and droplet precautions, including careful prevention of needlestick injuries and careful handling of clinical specimens for the duration of illness, are recommended for all HFs caused by arenaviruses. A negative-pressure ventilation room is recommended for patients with prominent cough or severe disease, and people entering the room should wear personal protective equipment including respirators and goggles. A negative-pressure room should be used when aerosol-generating procedures are conducted, such as intubation or airway suctioning. The CDC infection prevention recommendations for patients under investigation for Ebola virus disease in US hospitals are applicable in the event that an HF virus is used as a weapon of bioterrorism.[1]

CONTROL MEASURES:

Care of Exposed People. No specific measures are warranted for exposed people unless direct contamination with blood, excretions, or secretions from an infected patient has occurred. If such contamination has occurred, recording body temperature twice daily for 21 days is recommended. Reporting of fever or of symptoms of infection is an indication for intravenous ribavirin treatment for Lassa fever, Bolivian HF, or Sabiá or Lujo virus infections. There is no evidence to support ribavirin for postexposure prophylaxis for Lassa fever.

Immunoprophylaxis. A live attenuated Junín vaccine protects against Argentine HF and probably against Bolivian HF. The vaccine is associated with minimal adverse effects in adults; similar findings have been obtained from limited safety studies in children 4 years and older. The vaccine is not available in the United States. Various vaccines for Lassa fever are currently in development and early phase clinical trials in west Africa.

Environmental. In town-based outbreaks of Bolivian HF, rodent control has proven successful. Area rodent control is not practical for control of Argentine HF or Venezuelan HF.

---

[1]Centers for Disease Control and Prevention. Infection Prevention and Control Recommendations for Hospitalized Patients Under Investigation (PUIs) for Ebola Virus Disease (EVD) in U.S. Hospitals. Atlanta, GA: Centers for Disease Control and Prevention; 2018. Available at: **www.cdc.gov/vhf/ebola/clinicians/evd/infection-control.html**

Intensive rodent control efforts have decreased the rate of peridomestic Lassa virus infection, but rodents eventually reinvade human dwellings, and infection still occurs in rural settings.

Public Health Reporting. Because of the risk of health care-associated transmission, state health departments and the CDC should be contacted for specific advice about management and diagnosis of suspected cases. Lassa fever and New World arenavirus HFs are reportable in the United States according to guidelines of the US Council of State and Territorial Epidemiologists.

Hemorrhagic Fevers Caused by Bunyaviruses[1]

CLINICAL MANIFESTATIONS: Bunyaviruses are arthropod- or rodentborne infections that often result in severe febrile disease with multisystem involvement and may be associated with high rates of morbidity and mortality.

Hemorrhagic fever with renal syndrome (HFRS) is a complex, multiphasic disease characterized by vascular instability and varying degrees of renal insufficiency. Fever, flushing, conjunctival injection, headache, blurred vision, abdominal pain, and lumbar pain are followed by hypotension, oliguria, and subsequently, polyuria. Petechiae are frequent, but more serious bleeding manifestations are rare. Shock and acute renal insufficiency may occur.

Crimean-Congo hemorrhagic fever (CCHF) is a multisystem disease characterized by hepatitis and hemorrhagic manifestations. Fever, headache, and myalgia are followed by signs of a diffuse capillary leak syndrome with facial suffusion, conjunctivitis, icteric hepatitis, proteinuria, and disseminated intravascular coagulation associated with petechiae and purpura on the skin and mucous membranes. A hypotensive crisis often occurs after the appearance of frank hemorrhage from the gastrointestinal tract, nose, mouth, or uterus.

Rift Valley fever (RVF), in most cases, is a self-limited undifferentiated febrile illness. In 8% to 10% of cases, however, hemorrhagic fever with shock and icteric hepatitis, encephalitis, or retinitis develops.

ETIOLOGY: The order *Bunyavirales* includes segmented, single-stranded RNA viruses with different geographic distributions depending on their vector or reservoir. Hemorrhagic fever syndromes are associated with viruses from 3 families: *Hantaviridae* (Old World Hantaviruses), *Nairoviridae* (CCHF virus), and *Phenuiviridae* (RVF virus). Old World hantaviruses (Hantaan, Seoul, Dobrava, and Puumala viruses) cause HFRS, and New World hantaviruses (Sin Nombre and related viruses) cause hantavirus pulmonary syndrome (see Hantavirus Pulmonary Syndrome, p 354).

EPIDEMIOLOGY: The epidemiology of these diseases is a function of the distribution and behavior of their reservoirs and vectors. All families except *Hantaviridae* are associated with arthropod vectors. Hantavirus infections are transmitted via contact with virus shed in rat urine, saliva, or droppings, inhalation of virus in dust from contaminated nesting materials, or being bitten by an infected rat.

Classic HFRS occurs throughout much of Asia and Europe, with up to 100 000 cases per year. The most severe form of the disease is caused by the prototype Hantaan and Dobrava viruses in rural Asia and Europe, respectively; Puumala virus is associated

---

[1]Does not include hantavirus pulmonary syndrome, which is reviewed on p 354.

with milder disease (nephropathia epidemica) in Western Europe. Seoul virus is distributed worldwide in association with brown Norway rat (*Rattus* species) and can cause a disease of variable severity. Cases have been reported in the United States among rat fanciers. Person-to-person transmission has never been reported with HFRS. Fatal outcome is seen in 1% to 15% of cases, depending on the species of virus and the level of care.

CCHF occurs in much of sub-Saharan Africa, the Middle East, northwestern China, part of the Indian subcontinent, Ukraine, Russia, Georgia, Armenia, Central Asia, and Southeast Europe. CCHF virus is transmitted by hard ticks and occasionally by contact with viremic livestock and wild animals at slaughter. Health care-associated transmission of CCHF is a frequent and serious hazard. Fatal outcome is seen in 9% to 50% of hospitalized patients.

RVF occurs and there have been large outbreaks throughout sub-Saharan Africa, Egypt, Saudi Arabia, and Yemen. The virus is mosquitoborne and can also be directly transmitted from domestic livestock to humans via contact with infected aborted tissues or freshly slaughtered infected animal carcasses. Person-to-person transmission has not been reported, but laboratory-acquired cases are well documented. Overall fatal outcome occurs in 1% to 2% of cases but has been reported to be up to 30% in hospitalized patients.

The **incubation periods** for CCHF and RVF range from 2 to 10 days; for HFRS, the **incubation period** usually is longer, ranging from 7 to 42 days.

DIAGNOSTIC TESTS: Viral culture of blood and/or tissue, acute-phase quantitative reverse transcriptase-polymerase chain reaction (qRT-PCR), and serologic testing may facilitate diagnosis (Table 3.15). Immunoglobulin (Ig) M antibodies or increasing IgG titers in paired serum specimens, as demonstrated by enzyme immunoassay (EIA), are diagnostic; neutralizing antibody tests provide greater virus-strain specificity but rarely are used. Serum IgM and IgG virus-specific antibodies typically develop early in convalescence in CCHF and RVF but can be absent in rapidly fatal cases of CCHF. In HFRS, IgM and IgG antibodies usually are detectable at the time of onset of illness or within 48 hours, when it is too late for virus isolation and qRT-PCR assay. Diagnosis can be made retrospectively by immunohistochemical staining of formalin-fixed tissues. Although some commercial labs offer Hantavirus serologies, any positive IgM results

Table 3.15. Diagnostic Tests To Be Performed for Hemorrhagic Fevers Caused by Bunyaviruses

Diagnostic Testing	HFRS	CCHF	RVF
Virus culture of blood or tissue	No (usually not detected at time of illness)	Yes (in biosafety Level 4 [BSL-4] conditions	Yes (in biosafety Level 4 [BSL-4] conditions
Acute phase virus qRT-PCR	Yes, but not routinely done	Yes	Yes
IgM and IgG serology	Yes (at time of illness onset or within 48 h)	Yes (detectable in early convalescence, but could be absent in fatal cases)	Yes (detectable in early convalescence)

are referred to the Centers for Disease Control and Prevention (CDC) for confirmation. CCHF and RVF testing are only available at the CDC. Referrals are made through the state health department.

TREATMENT: Ribavirin, administered intravenously to patients with HFRS within the first 4 days of illness, may be effective in decreasing renal dysfunction, vascular instability, and mortality. However, intravenous ribavirin is not available commercially in the United States and is available only from the manufacturer through an investigational new drug (IND) protocol. Health care providers who need to obtain intravenous ribavirin should contact the US Food and Drug Administration (**www.fda.gov/drugs/investigational-new-drug-ind-application/physicians-how-request-single-patient-expanded-access-compassionate-use**; FDA 24-hour emergency lines: 866-300-4374 or 301-796-8240). Supportive therapy for HFRS should include: (1) treatment of shock; (2) monitoring of fluid balance; (3) dialysis for complications of renal failure; (4) control of hypertension during the oliguric phase; and (5) early recognition of possible myocardial failure with appropriate therapy.

Oral and intravenous ribavirin, when administered early in the course of CCHF, has been associated with milder disease, although no controlled studies have been performed. Ribavirin also may be efficacious as postexposure prophylaxis of CCHF.

During the RVF outbreak in Saudi Arabia in 2000, a clinical trial of ribavirin in patients with confirmed disease was halted because of an increased observation of encephalitis in patients receiving ribavirin (more than expected in RVF patients). Experimental data in hamster, mice, and rats reported the same type of observation when treatment was delayed. Therefore, ribavirin should be avoided in RVF.

ISOLATION OF THE HOSPITALIZED PATIENT: In addition to standard precautions, contact and droplet precautions, including careful prevention of needlestick injuries and management of clinical specimens, are indicated for patients with CCHF for the duration for their illness. Airborne isolation may be required in certain circumstances when patients undergo procedures that stimulate coughing and promote generation of aerosols. Standard precautions should be followed with RVF and HFRS.

CONTROL MEASURES:

Care of Exposed People. People having direct contact with blood or other secretions from patients with CCHF should be observed closely for 21 days with daily monitoring for fever. Immediate therapy with intravenous ribavirin should be considered at the first sign of disease. Ribavirin also may be efficacious as postexposure prophylaxis of CCHF.

Environmental.

Hemorrhagic Fever With Renal Syndrome. Monitoring of laboratory rat colonies, community pet rat colonies, and urban rodent control may be effective for ratborne HFRS.

Crimean-Congo Hemorrhagic Fever. In countries with endemic CCHF, arachnicides for tick control generally have limited benefit but should be used in stockyard settings. Personal protective measures (eg, physical tick removal and protective clothing with permethrin sprays) may be effective for people at-risk (farmers, veterinarians, abattoir workers).

Rift Valley Fever. Regular immunization of domestic animals should have an effect on limiting or preventing RVF outbreaks and protecting humans. Some livestock vaccines are currently in use in areas with endemicity. Personal protective clothing (with permethrin sprays) and insect repellants may be effective for people at risk (farmers, veterinarians, abattoir workers). Mosquito control measures are difficult to implement.

Immunoprophylaxis. No vaccines currently are approved in Europe or the United States for use in humans against HFs caused by Bunyaviruses. In some Asian countries, inactivated vaccines against HFRS are currently in use.

Public Health Reporting. Because of the risk of health care-associated transmission and diagnostic confusion with other hemorrhagic illnesses state health departments and the CDC (Viral Special Pathogens Branch Clinical Inquiries Line: 470-312-0094) should be contacted about any suspected diagnosis of viral hemorrhagic.

Hemorrhagic Fevers Caused by Filoviruses: Ebola and Marburg

CLINICAL MANIFESTATIONS: Data on Ebola and Marburg virus infections primarily are derived from adult populations. More is known about Ebola virus disease (EVD) than Marburg virus disease, although the same principles apply generally to the 2 filoviruses known to cause human disease. Historically, the overall incidence of EVD infections is lower in children compared with adults. However, pediatric mortality is high, with the youngest children having the highest case fatality rates. Symptomatic disease ranges from mild to severe; case fatality rates for severely affected people range from 25% to 90%. After a typical incubation period of 8 to 10 days (range, 2–21 days), disease in children and adults begins with nonspecific signs and symptoms including fever, severe headache, myalgia, fatigue, abdominal pain, and weakness followed several days later by vomiting, diarrhea, and sometimes unexplained bleeding or bruising. Data from the 2014–2016 Ebola outbreak in West Africa, the largest since the virus was identified in 1976, indicate that children may have shorter incubation periods than adults. Respiratory symptoms are more common and central nervous system manifestations are less common in children than in adults. A fleeting maculopapular rash on the torso or face after approximately 4 to 5 days of illness may occur. Hiccups have been reported. Conjunctival injection or subconjunctival hemorrhage may be present. Leukopenia, frequently with lymphopenia, is followed later by elevated neutrophils, a left shift, and thrombocytopenia. Hepatic dysfunction, with elevations in aspartate aminotransferase (AST) at markedly higher concentrations than alanine aminotransferase (ALT), and metabolic derangements, including hypokalemia, hyponatremia, hypocalcemia, and hypomagnesemia, are common. In the most severe cases, microvascular instability ensues around the end of the first week of disease. Although hemostasis is impaired, hemorrhagic manifestations develop in a minority of patients. The most common hemorrhagic manifestations consist of bleeding from the gastrointestinal tract, sometimes with oozing from the mucous membranes or venipuncture sites in late stages. Twenty percent of infected children have no fever at presentation.

Central nervous system manifestations and renal failure are frequent in end-stage disease. In fatal cases, death typically occurs around 10 to 12 days after symptom onset, usually resulting from viral- or bacterial-induced septic shock and multiorgan system failure. Factors associated with pediatric Ebola deaths in the 2014–2016 outbreak were age <5 years, bleeding at any time during hospitalization, and high viral load.

Approximately 30% of pregnant women with EVD present with spontaneous abortion and vaginal bleeding. Maternal mortality approaches 90% when infection occurs during the third trimester. Ebola virus can cross the placenta and pregnant women infected with the virus will likely transmit the virus to the fetus. In infants born to infected mothers, Ebola virus RNA has been detected in amniotic fluid, fetal meconium, umbilical cord, and buccal swab specimens. There has only been 1 report of survival of a neonate born to a mother with active EVD. The neonate was treated with monoclonal antibodies, a buffy coat transfusion from an Ebola survivor, and the antiviral drug remdesivir shortly after birth. The exact mechanism of neonatal deaths is unknown, but high viral loads of Ebola virus have been documented in amniotic fluid, placental tissue, and fetal tissues of stillborn neonates. EVD survivors are at risk for reactivation of disease in immune-privileged sites, such as the eye or the central nervous system, because of persistence of Ebola virus. However, disease reactivation currently is thought to be a rare event. Long-term shedding of virus in semen has been implicated in the origin of several clusters of EVD in West Africa.

ETIOLOGY: Filoviruses (from the Latin filo meaning thread, referring to their filamentous shape) are single-stranded, negative-sense RNA viruses. There are 6 genera in the family *Filoviridae*, but only 2, *Marburgvirus* and *Ebolavirus*, cause disease in humans. This includes 4 of the 6 viruses within the genus *Ebolavirus* and both known viruses within the genus *Marburgvirus*. These filoviruses are endemic only in Africa.

EPIDEMIOLOGY: Fruit bats are believed to be the animal reservoir for most filoviruses. Human infection is believed to occur from inadvertent exposure to infected bat excreta or saliva following entry into roosting areas in caves, mines, and forests. Nonhuman primates, especially gorillas and chimpanzees, and other wild animals (eg, rodents, small antelopes) may become infected from bat contact and serve as intermediate hosts that transmit filoviruses to humans through contact with their blood and bodily fluids, usually associated with hunting and butchering (see Control Measures, Environmental). For unclear reasons, filovirus outbreaks tend to occur after prolonged dry seasons.

Molecular epidemiologic evidence shows that most outbreaks result from a single point introduction (or very few) into humans from wild animals, followed by human-to-human transmission, almost invariably fueled by health care-associated transmission in areas with inadequate infection-control equipment and resources. Filoviruses are the most transmissible of all hemorrhagic fever viruses. The secondary attack rate in households is generally between 10% to 20% in African communities. Risk to household contacts is associated with direct physical contact, with little to no transmission observed otherwise. Human-to-human transmission usually occurs through oral, mucous membrane, or nonintact skin exposure to blood or bodily fluids of a symptomatic person with filovirus disease or by exposure to objects contaminated with infected blood or bodily fluids, most often in the context of providing care to a sick family or community member (community transmission) or patient (health care-associated transmission). Funeral rituals that entail the touching of the corpse also have been implicated. Sexual transmission has been documented and implicated in several clusters of disease. Ebola virus has been detected in human milk; genomic analysis in a case of fatal Ebola in a 9-month-old strongly suggested Ebola virus transmission through human milk (see Control Measures, Breastfeeding). Respiratory spread of virus does not occur. Infection through fomites cannot be excluded. Health care-associated transmission is highly unlikely if rigorous infection-control practices are in place in health care facilities (see Isolation of the Hospitalized Patient). Filoviruses are not spread through the air, by water, or in general by food (with the exception of bushmeat; see Control Measures, Environmental).

Children may be less likely to become infected from interfamilial spread than adults when a primary case occurs in a household, possibly because they are not typically primary caregivers of sick individuals and are less likely to take part in funeral rituals that involve touching and washing of the deceased person's body. Underreporting of Ebola cases in children to health officials also is possible.

The degree of viremia correlates with the clinical state. People are most infectious late in the course of severe disease, especially when copious vomiting, diarrhea, and/or bleeding are present. Disease transmission does not occur during the incubation period, when the person is asymptomatic. Virus may persist in a few sites for several weeks to months after clinical recovery, including in testicles/semen, vaginal fluid, placenta, amniotic fluid, human milk, saliva, the central nervous system (particularly cerebrospinal fluid), joints, conjunctivae, and the chambers of the eye (resulting in transient uveitis and other ocular problems). Because of the proven risk of sexual transmission, abstinence or use of condoms is recommended for at least 12 months after recovery and possibly longer. Guidance for the management of survivors of EVD can be found at **www.cdc.gov/vhf/ebola/ clinicians/evaluating-patients/guidance-for-management-of-survivors- ebola.html.**

Updated information on identification, current management of people traveling from areas of transmission or with contact with a person with Ebola virus infection, and communicating with children about Ebola can be found on the Centers for Disease Control and Prevention (CDC) website (**www.cdc.gov/vhf/ebola/**) and the American Academy of Pediatrics (AAP) website (**www.healthychildren.org/English/health- issues/conditions/infections/Pages/Ebola.aspx** and **www.cdc.gov/vhf/ ebola/pdf/how-talk-children-about-ebola.pdf**).

The **incubation period** for Ebola virus disease is 8 to 10 days (range, 2–21 days).

DIAGNOSTIC TESTS: The diagnosis of filovirus infection should be considered in a person who develops a fever within 21 days of travel to an area with endemic infection. Because initial clinical manifestations are difficult to distinguish from those of more common febrile diseases, prompt laboratory testing is imperative in a suspected case. Malaria, measles, typhoid fever, Lassa fever, dengue, and influenza should be included in the differential diagnosis of a symptomatic person returning from Africa within 21 days and are much more likely than a filovirus to be the cause of fever. Filovirus disease can be diagnosed by testing of blood by reverse transcriptase-polymerase chain reaction (RT-PCR) assay, enzyme-linked immunosorbent assay (ELISA) for viral antigens or immunoglobulin (Ig) M, and virus isolation early in the disease course, with the latter being attempted only under biosafety level-4 conditions. Viral RNA generally is detectable by RT-PCR assay within 3 days after the onset of symptoms. However, if blood is obtained within 3 days of symptom onset, 2 negative RT-PCR test results at least 48 hours apart are required to rule out disease. IgM and IgG antibodies may be used later in disease course or after recovery. Postmortem diagnosis can be made via immunohistochemical staining of skin or liver or spleen tissue. Testing generally is not performed routinely in clinical laboratories. Local and state public health department officials must be contacted and can facilitate testing at a regional certified laboratory or at the CDC. Current information on the most appropriate diagnostic testing for EVD is available on the CDC website (**www.cdc.gov/vhf/ ebola/diagnosis/index.html**).

In October 2019, the US Food and Drug Administration (FDA) allowed marketing of the OraQuick Ebola Rapid Antigen Test, a rapid diagnostic test (RDT) for detecting Ebola virus in both symptomatic patients and recently deceased people. This is the first Ebola RDT that the FDA has allowed for marketing in the United States. The RDT should be used only in cases in which more sensitive molecular testing is not available. All

OraQuick Ebola Rapid Antigen Test results are presumptive; all test results (positive and negative) must be verified through real-time reverse transcriptase polymerase chain reaction (rRT-PCR) testing at a Laboratory Response Network (LRN) laboratory located in 49 states and at the CDC.

TREATMENT: People suspected of having filovirus infection should be placed in isolation immediately, and public health officials should be notified. Management of patients with filovirus disease primarily is supportive, including oral or intravenous fluids with electrolyte repletion, vasopressors, blood products, oxygen, total parenteral nutrition, analgesics, antipyretics, and antimalarial and antimicrobial medications when coinfections are suspected or confirmed (**www.cdc.gov/vhf/ebola/treatment/index.html**). Volume losses can be enormous (10 L/day in adults), and some centers in the United States report better results with repletion using lactated Ringer solution rather than normal saline solution in management of adult patients. When antimicrobial agents are used to treat sepsis, the medications should have coverage for intestinal microbiota based on limited evidence of translocation of gut bacteria into the blood of patients with filovirus disease. Use of needles and aerosol generating procedures should be limited as much as possible.

On October 14, 2020, the FDA approved the first treatment for *Zaire ebolavirus* infection in adult and pediatric patients. Under the brand name Inmazeb, it consists of a mixture of 3 monoclonal antibodies: atoltivimab, maftivimab, and odesivimab-ebgn (**www.accessdata.fda.gov/drugsatfda_docs/label/2020/761169s000lbl. pdf**). On December 21, 2020, a second monoclonal antibody therapy, ansuvimab-zykl, which goes by the brand name Ebanga, received FDA approval, also for use in adult and pediatric patients (**www.accessdata.fda.gov/drugsatfda_docs/ label/2020/761172s000lbl.pdf**). There currently are no specific therapies approved by the FDA for other filovirus infections. Because therapeutic options are likely to change following results from numerous ongoing clinical trials, it would be appropriate to consult with the CDC to determine the most current treatment guidelines (**www.cdc.gov/vhf/ ebola/treatment/index.html**).

ISOLATION OF THE HOSPITALIZED PATIENT: Standard, contact, and droplet precautions are recommended for management of hospitalized patients with known or suspected EVD. Although it is prudent to place the patient in a negative-pressure room as an extra precaution, availability of such a resource should not prevent care because there is no evidence for natural aerosol transmission between humans. A negative pressure room should be used when aerosol-generating procedures are conducted, such as intubation or airway suctioning. Access to the patient should be limited to a small number of designated staff and family members with specific instructions and training on filovirus infection control and on the use of personal protective equipment (PPE). Although experience suggests that standard universal and contact precautions usually are protective, viral hemorrhagic fever precautions consisting of at least 2 pairs of gloves, fit-tested N95 or particulate respirator, impermeable or fluid-resistant gown, face shield (if using N95 respirator), protective apron, and shoe covers or rubber boots are recommended when filovirus infection is confirmed or suspected. Health care workers should have no skin exposed, and a buddy system should be used for supervision of donning and doffing PPE. All health care workers should be knowledgeable with and proficient in donning and doffing PPE prior to participating in management of a patient as detailed on the CDC website (**www.cdc. gov/vhf/ebola/healthcare-us/ppe/guidance.html**). Particulate respirators are recommended when aerosol-generating procedures, such as endotracheal intubation, are performed. The duration of precautions should be determined in consultation with state and federal public health authorities.

The AAP has published a clinical report[1] that provides guidance to health care providers and hospitals on options to consider regarding parental presence at the bedside while caring for a child with suspected or proven EVD or other highly consequential infections.

CONTROL MEASURES:

Contact Tracing. Monitoring and movement of people with potential Ebola virus exposure currently is based on the degree of possible risk. At a minimum, asymptomatic people with any level of risk should self-monitor for fever and other symptoms of Ebola. The individual should immediately notify the public health authority if fever or other symptoms develop. A full description of recommended management for people with consistent signs or symptoms and risk factors for EVD including neonates who are at risk can be found on the following CDC websites: **www.cdc.gov/vhf/ebola/clinicians/ evaluating-patients/index.html** and **www.cdc.gov/vhf/ebola/clinicians/ evd/neonatal-care.html.** Hospitalization of asymptomatic contacts is not warranted, but contacts who develop fever or other manifestations of filovirus disease should be isolated immediately until the diagnosis can be ruled out.

Ebola Vaccine. On December 19, 2019, the FDA approved the world's first Ebola vaccine, ERVEBO, for the prevention of EVD after prior conditional marketing approval from the European Medicines Agency (EMA) and prequalification by the World Health Organization. This vesicular stomatitis platform-based live virus (sVSV-ZEBOV) vaccine has been used under expanded access protocol in the ongoing 2018–2019 outbreak in the Democratic Republic of Congo in a ring vaccination trial of first responders, health care workers, burial providers, and close contacts of cases. In February 2020, the CDC Advisory Committee on Immunization Practices recommended its use for preexposure vaccination of adults 18 years or older in the US population who are at potential risk of exposure to Ebola virus (species *Zaire ebolavirus*) and are responding to an outbreak of Ebola virus disease, work as health care personnel at federally designated Ebola treatment centers in the United States, or work as laboratorians or other staff at biosafety-level 4 facilities.[2] In addition, a number of experimental vaccines and passively transferred immunoglobulins have been shown to be efficacious in nonhuman primate models, including when administered after exposure.

Breastfeeding. Live virus has been cultured from human milk and at least 1 fatal case associated with breastfeeding has been reported. Given what is known about transmission of Ebola virus, regardless of breastfeeding status, infants whose mothers are acutely infected with Ebola virus already are at high risk of acquiring Ebola virus infection through close contact with the mother and are at high risk of death overall. Therefore, mothers with probable or confirmed Ebola virus infection should not have close contact with their infants (including breastfeeding unless there is no alternative method to feed the infant) (see Breastfeeding and Human Milk, p 107). There is not enough evidence

---

[1] American Academy of Pediatrics, Committee on Infectious Diseases. Parental presence during treatment of Ebola or other highly consequential infection. *Pediatrics*. 2016;138(3):e20161891. Available at: **https:// pediatrics.aappublications.org/content/138/3/e20161891**

[2] Choi MJ, Cossaboom CM, Whitesell AN, et al. Use of Ebola vaccine: recommendations of the Advisory Committee on Immunization Practices, United States, 2020. *MMWR Recomm Rep.* 2021;70(RR-1):1–12. DOI: **http://dx.doi.org/10.15585/mmwr.rr7001a1**

to provide guidance on when it is safe to resume breastfeeding after a mother's recovery, unless her milk can be demonstrated to be Ebola virus-free by laboratory testing.

Travelers. Nonessential travel to areas where Ebola outbreaks are occurring is not recommended. Travelers to an area affected by an Ebola outbreak should practice careful hygiene (eg, wash hands with soap and water or a 9:1 water to bleach solution, use an alcohol-based hand sanitizer, and avoid contact with blood and body fluids). Travelers should not handle items that may have come in contact with an infected person's blood or body fluids, such as clothes, bedding, needles, and medical equipment. Funeral or burial rituals that require handling the body of someone who has died from Ebola should be avoided. Travelers should avoid hospitals where Ebola patients are being treated in areas of Africa with endemic disease; the US embassy or consulate often is able to provide advice on facilities that should be avoided. Following return to the United States, travelers should monitor their health closely for 21 days and seek medical care immediately if they develop symptoms of Ebola (see Control Measures, Environmental). State laws mandating confinement or quarantine may apply. Current travel information for countries affected by Ebola can be found on the CDC website (**www.cdc.gov/vhf/ebola/travelers/index.html**).

Environmental. Avoiding contact with bats, primarily by avoiding entry into caves and mines in areas with endemic disease, is a key preventive measure for filoviruses. People also should avoid exposure to blood, bodily fluids, or meat of wild animals (bushmeat), especially nonhuman primates but also bats, porcupines, duikers (a type of antelope), and other mammals, in areas with endemic filovirus disease. In health care settings, detailed guidance for infection control is available at **www.cdc.gov/vhf/ebola/clinicians/cleaning/ hospitals.html.** Disinfectants with a label claim for a nonenveloped virus should be used.

Public Health Reporting. Because of the risk of health care-associated transmission, state/local health departments and the CDC should be contacted immediately for specific advice about confirmation and management of suspected cases. In the United States, Ebola and Marburg hemorrhagic fevers are reportable by guidelines of the Council of State and Territorial Epidemiologists. If a filoviral hemorrhagic fever is suspected, the state/local health department or CDC Emergency Operations Center (telephone: 770-488-7100) should be contacted to assist with case investigation, diagnosis, management, and control measures.

Hepatitis A

CLINICAL MANIFESTATIONS: Hepatitis A is an acute, self-limited illness associated with fever, malaise, jaundice, anorexia, and nausea that typically lasts less than 2 months, although 10% to 15% of symptomatic people have prolonged or relapsing disease that lasts as long as 6 months. Symptomatic hepatitis A virus (HAV) infection occurs in approximately 30% of infected children younger than 6 years of age, but few of these children will have jaundice. Among older children and adults, infection usually is symptomatic, with jaundice occurring in 70% or more of cases. Fulminant hepatitis is rare but is more common in people with underlying liver disease. Chronic infection does not occur.

ETIOLOGY: HAV is a small, nonenveloped, positive-sense RNA virus with an icosahedral capsid and classified as a member of the family *Picornaviridae*, genus *Hepatovirus*.

EPIDEMIOLOGY: The most common mode of transmission is person to person, resulting from fecal contamination and oral ingestion (ie, the fecal-oral route). In resource-limited countries where infection is endemic, most people are infected during the first decade of life. In the United States, rates of HAV infection decreased by 95% from 1996 to 2011 following implementation of universal infant vaccination in 2006. Recently, HAV incidence has increased from a historic low of 1239 cases reported in 2014 to more than 11 000 cases reported in 2018, primarily related to outbreaks associated with contaminated food, men who have sex with men, and people who use drugs or experience homelessness. Hepatitis A vaccination coverage (≥1 dose) for children 19 to 35 months of age was 86% in 2017. Significant decreases in anti-HAV seroprevalence in adults 40 years of age and older have occurred because of reduced exposure to HAV earlier in life since the introduction of universal infant vaccination, resulting in an increased proportion of adults in the United States being susceptible to HAV infection. The majority of HAV infection cases now are in adults 20 years and older.

Recognized risk groups for HAV infection include people who have close personal contact with a person infected with HAV, people with chronic liver disease, people with clotting factor disorders, people with human immunodeficiency virus (HIV) infection, men who have sex with men, people who use injection and noninjection drugs, people who experience homelessness, people traveling to or working in countries that have highly or intermediately endemic HAV, people who anticipate close contact with an adoptee from a country of high or intermediate endemic HAV during the first 60 days following arrival, and people who work with HAV-infected primates or with HAV in a research laboratory setting. Although HAV infections and outbreaks have been associated with food-service establishments and food handlers, health care institutions, institutions for people with developmental disabilities, schools, and child care facilities, they typically reflect transmission in the community.

Outbreaks have been associated with consumption of raw produce (eg, green onions) and fruits (eg, strawberries) and oysters and mussels. Waterborne outbreaks are rare and typically are associated with sewage-contaminated or inadequately treated water.

People with HAV infection are most infectious during the 1 to 2 weeks before onset of jaundice or elevation of liver enzymes, when concentration of virus in the stool is highest. Risk of transmission subsequently diminishes and is minimal by 1 week after onset of jaundice. HAV can be detected in stool for longer periods, especially in neonates and young children.

The **incubation period** is 15 to 50 days, with an average of 28 days.

DIAGNOSTIC TESTS: Serologic tests for HAV-specific total antibody (ie, immunoglobulin [Ig] G plus IgM), IgG-only anti-HAV, and IgM-only anti-HAV are available commercially, primarily in enzyme immunoassay format. A single total or IgG anti-HAV test does not have diagnostic value for acute infection. The presence of serum IgM anti-HAV indicates current or recent infection, although false-positive results may occur, particularly if the person is asymptomatic. IgM anti-HAV generally is included in most acute hepatitis serologic test panels offered by hospital or reference laboratories. IgM anti-HAV is detectable in up to 20% of hepatitis A (HepA) vaccine recipients when measured 2 weeks after vaccination. In most people with HAV infection, serum IgM anti-HAV becomes detectable 5 to 10 days before onset of symptoms and declines to undetectable concentrations within 6 months after infection. People who have positive test results for IgM anti-HAV more than 1 year after infection have been reported. IgG anti-HAV is detectable shortly after appearance of IgM. A positive IgG anti-HAV or total anti-HAV (IgM and IgG) test result with a negative IgM anti-HAV test result indicate immunity from past infection or

Table 3.16. Recommendations for Postexposure Prophylaxis of Hepatitis A Virus (HAV)

Time Since Exposure	Age	Recommended
≤2 wk	<12 mo	IGIM (0.1mL/kg)[a]
	12 mo–40 y	HepA vaccine[b,c,d]
	>40 y	HepA[c,d]; consider IGIM
>2 wk	<12 mo	No prophylaxis
	≥12 mo	No prophylaxis, but HepA may be indicated for ongoing exposure

IGIM: Immune Globulin Intramuscular; HepA: hepatitis A vaccine.

[a] Measles, mumps, and rubella vaccine (MMR) should not be administered for at least 6 months after receipt of IGIM.

[b] People with immunocompromising conditions or chronic liver disease should also receive IGIM.

[c] Although 1 dose of HepA is needed for postexposure prophylaxis, the 2 dose series should be completed according to the recommended schedule.

[d] People with severe allergy to HepA or its components should receive IGIM (0.1 mL/kg) but not HepA.

vaccination. Polymerase chain reaction (PCR) assays for hepatitis A are available but not currently licensed by the US Food and Drug Administration (FDA). PCR assay may be considered for detection of very early infections and to assist with interpretation of questionable IgM anti-HAV results.

TREATMENT: Supportive and management of complications.

ISOLATION OF THE HOSPITALIZED PATIENT: Contact precautions should be practiced in addition to standard precautions for diapered and incontinent patients for at least 1 week after onset of symptoms.

CONTROL MEASURES[1]:

General Measures. The major methods of prevention of HAV infections are improved sanitation (eg, in food preparation and of water sources) and personal hygiene (eg, hand hygiene after toilet use and diaper changes in child care settings). Hepatitis A vaccine (HepA) or Immune Globulin (IG) is effective in preventing infection when administered within 14 days of last exposure (see Table 3.16).

Schools, Child Care, and Work. Children and adults with acute HAV infection who work as food handlers or attend or work in child care settings should be excluded for 1 week after onset of the illness (see Table 2.3, p 128).

Hepatitis A Vaccine. Two inactivated single-antigen HepA vaccines, Havrix and Vaqta, are available in the United States. The vaccines are prepared from cell culture-adapted HAV, which is propagated in human fibroblasts, purified from cell lysates, formalin inactivated, and adsorbed to an aluminum hydroxide adjuvant. Vaqta contains no preservative. Havrix contains 0.5% 2-phenoxyethanol as a preservative. The hepatitis A and hepatitis B combination vaccine (HepA-HepB), Twinrix, can also be used for people 18 years and older.

---

[1] Nelson NP, Weng MK, Hofmeister MG, et al. Prevention of hepatitis A virus infection in the United States: recommendations of the Advisory Committee on Immunization Practices, 2020. *MMWR Recomm Rep.* 2020;69(RR-5):1-38

Table 3.17. Recommended Doses and Schedules for Inactivated Hepatitis A Virus Vaccines

Age	Vaccine	Hepatitis A Antigen Dose	Volume per Dose, mL	No. of Doses	Schedule
6–11 mo, traveling to area with endemic hepatitis A	Havrix or Vaqta	720 ELU/ 25 U	0.5	1	One dose for infants traveling to areas with endemic hepatitis A; this dose does not count toward completing the immunization requirement; 2 doses needed at the routine schedule after 12 mo of age
12 mo–18 y	Havrix	720 ELU	0.5	2	Initial and 6–12 mo later
12 mo–18 y	Vaqta	25 U	0.5	2	Initial and 6–18 mo later
≥19 y	Havrix	1440 ELU	1.0	2	Initial and 6–12 mo later
≥19 y	Vaqta	50 U	1.0	2	Initial and 6–18 mo later
≥18 y	Twinrix[a]	720 ELU	1.0	3 or 4	3-dose series: Initial, 1 mo, and 6 mo 4-dose series: Initial, 7 days, 21–30 days, and 12 mo

ELU indicates enzyme-linked immunosorbent assay units.

[a] A combination of hepatitis B (Engerix-B, 20 µg) and hepatitis A (Havrix, 720 ELU) vaccine (Twinrix) is licensed for use in people age ≥18 years in 3-dose and 4-dose schedules. For pre- and postexposure hepatitis A prophylaxis, the use of single-antigen hepatitis A vaccine, ie, Havrix or Vaqta, is recommended.

Administration, Dosages, and Schedules (see Table 3.17). Both single-antigen HepA vaccines are licensed for people 12 months and older and have pediatric and adult formulations that are administered in a 2-dose schedule. Pediatric formulations are available for ages 12 months through 18 years, and adult formulations for people age 19 years and older. HepA-HepB vaccine can be used for people 18 years and older and can be administered in a 3-dose schedule, or an accelerated 3-dose schedule plus a booster dose 12 months later. HepA and HepA-HepB vaccines are administered intramuscularly. Recommended doses and schedules for these vaccines are listed in Table 3.17.

Immunogenicity. HepA vaccines are highly immunogenic. At least 95% of healthy children, adolescents, and adults have protective antibody concentrations when measured 1 month after receipt of the first dose. One month after a second dose, more than 99% of healthy children, adolescents, and adults have protective antibody concentrations.

Antibody concentrations are lower in infants with passively acquired maternal anti-HAV in comparison with vaccine recipients lacking anti-HAV. Passively acquired maternal anti-HAV antibody is not detectable in most infants by 12 months of age. HepA vaccine is highly immunogenic for children who begin immunization at 12 months or older, regardless of maternal anti-HAV status.

Efficacy. In double-blind, controlled, randomized trials, the protective efficacy in preventing clinical HAV infection was 94% to 100%.

Duration of Protection. For children and adults, detectable antibody persists for at least 20 years after completion of a 2-dose series of HepA vaccine. Kinetic models of antibody decline indicate that protective levels of anti-HAV could be present for 40 years or longer in adults and 14 to 20 years in children. Additional booster doses beyond the 2-dose primary immunization series are not recommended.

Vaccine in Immunocompromised People. Because HepA vaccine is inactivated, no special precautions need to be taken when vaccinating immunocompromised people. The immune response in immunocompromised people, including people with HIV infection, may be suboptimal based on the level of immunosuppression at the time of vaccine administration.

Vaccine Interchangeability. The 2 single-antigen HepA vaccines have similar effectiveness when administered as recommended. Studies among adults have found no difference in the immunogenicity of a vaccine series that mixed the 2 currently available vaccines, compared with using the same vaccine throughout the licensed schedule. Completion of the immunization regimen with the same product is preferable, although interchangeability of products is acceptable if the same product is not available.

Administration With Other Vaccines. Data indicate that HepA vaccine may be administered concurrently with other vaccines. Vaccines should be administered in a separate syringe and at a separate injection site (see Simultaneous Administration of Multiple Vaccines, p 36).

Adverse Events. No serious adverse events attributed definitively to HepA vaccine have been reported. Adverse reactions are mild and include local pain and, less commonly, induration at the injection site. The vaccine can be administered either in the thigh or the arm; the site of injection does not affect the incidence of local reactions.

Precautions and Contraindications to Immunization. The vaccine should not be administered to people with hypersensitivity to any of the vaccine components. A review published in 2014 of Vaccine Adverse Event Reporting System (VAERS) data from January 1, 1996, to April 5, 2013, did not identify any concerning pattern of adverse events in pregnant women or their infants following maternal hepatitis A immunizations during pregnancy. Risk to the fetus is considered to be low or nonexistent because the vaccine contains inactivated, purified virus particles. Hepatitis A vaccination is recommended during pregnancy for women with an additional risk factor for HAV infection.

Preimmunization Serologic Testing. Preimmunization testing for anti-HAV generally is not recommended for children. Testing may be cost-effective for people who have a high likelihood of hepatitis A immunity from previous infection, including people whose childhood was in a country with high endemicity, and people with a history of jaundice potentially caused by HAV.

Postimmunization Serologic Testing. Postimmunization testing for anti-HAV generally is not indicated because of the high seroconversion rates in adults and children. In addition, some commercially available anti-HAV tests may not detect low but protective concentrations of antibody among immunized people.

Immune Globulin. Postexposure prophylaxis (PEP) with Immune Globulin Intramuscular (IGIM), when administered within 2 weeks after exposure to HAV, is more than 85% effective in preventing symptomatic infection. When administered as preexposure prophylaxis (PrEP), a dose of 0.1 mL/kg confers protection against hepatitis A for up to 1 month, and a dose of 0.2 mL/kg protects for up to 2 months. Recommended PrEP and PEP IGIM doses and duration of protection are provided in Tables 3.18 and 3.16, respectively.

PREVENTION MEASURES:

PrEP Against HAV Infection (see Tables 3.18, p 379, and 3.17, p 376). HepA vaccine is recommended routinely for children age 12 through 23 months of age and children and adolescents age 2 to 18 years of age who have not received HepA vaccine previously. HepA vaccine is recommended for people who are at increased risk of infection or severe disease and during outbreaks. Anyone 12 months and older who wants protection against HAV may receive HepA vaccine; no specific risk factor needs to be identified to be eligible for hepatitis A vaccination. The routine childhood immunization schedule (**https://redbook.solutions.aap.org/SS/Immunization_Schedules.aspx**). Table 3.17 (p 375) includes HepA-containing vaccines licensed by the FDA, their doses, and schedules.

People at Increased Risk of HAV Infection or its Consequences Who Should Be Immunized.

- **People with chronic liver disease.** Susceptible people with chronic liver disease (including, but not limited to, those with hepatitis C virus [HCV] and/or hepatitis B virus [HBV] infection, cirrhosis, fatty liver disease, alcoholic liver disease, autoimmune hepatitis, or an alanine aminotransferase [ALT] or aspartate aminotransferase [AST] level greater than twice the upper limit of normal). and people who are unvaccinated and awaiting or have received liver transplants should be immunized.
- **People experiencing homelessness.** Outbreaks of hepatitis A associated with homelessness have occurred in several cities. People 1 year or older experiencing homelessness should be immunized against HAV.
- **People who travel to or work in countries that have high or intermediate endemic hepatitis A** (parts of Africa and Asia, Central and South America, and Eastern Europe) should be protected against HAV infection before departure (see Table 3.18) as follows:
  - Infants aged 6 through 11 months should receive a dose of HepA vaccine. This travel-related dose does not count toward the routine 2-dose series, and the routine 2-dose hepatitis A vaccination series should begin at age 12 months. HepA vaccine does not interfere with the measles-mumps-rubella vaccine (MMR), which is recommended for international travelers 6 months or older.
  - Healthy people 12 months through 40 years of age should receive a dose of HepA as soon as travel is considered and complete the 2-dose series according to the routine schedule.
  - Infants younger than 6 months and travelers for whom vaccine is contraindicated or who choose not to receive vaccine should receive IGIM before travel when protection against HAV is recommended. For travel duration up to 1 month, 1 dose of IGIM at 0.1 mL/kg is recommended; for travel up to 2 months, 1 dose of IGIM at 0.2 mL/kg is recommended, and for travel of ≥2 months, a 0.2-mL/kg dose of IG should be repeated every 2 months for the duration of travel or until the infant is administered HepA vaccine (ie, at age ≥6 months) (see Table 3.18).
  - People older than 40 years, people with immunocompromising conditions, and people with chronic liver disease should receive a single dose of HepA vaccine as soon as travel is considered. People traveling in <2 weeks should receive the initial dose of HepA vaccine and simultaneously may be administered IGIM in a different anatomic injection site. The HepA vaccine series should be completed according to the routine schedule.

Table 3.18. Recommendations for Preexposure Prophylaxis of Hepatitis A Virus (HAV) for Travelers to Countries With High or Intermediate Endemic Rates of Hepatitis A[a]

Age	Recommended	Notes
<6 mo	IGIM[b]	For travel lasting up to 1 mo, 0.1 mL/kg; up to 2 mo, 0.2 mL/kg (repeat 0.2 mL/kg every 2 mo thereafter if risk remains).
6–11 mo	HepA vaccine	This dose does not count toward the routine 2-dose series. Start the hepatitis A vaccination series at age 12 mo.
12 mo–40 y	HepA vaccine	Those with immunocompromising conditions, chronic liver disease, or other chronic medical conditions may also receive IGIM.[b,c]
>40 y	HepA vaccine, consider IGIM	If departure is within 2 wk, may also receive IGIM[c]; those with immunocompromising conditions, or chronic liver disease may also receive IGIM.

HepA indicates hepatitis A vaccine; IGIM, Immune Globulin Intramuscular.

[a]People age 12 months or older should receive HepA vaccine routinely; those who have a severe allergy to HepA or its components should receive IGIM.

[b]Measles, mumps, and rubella vaccine (MMR) should not be administered for at least 6 months after receipt of IGIM. If both MMR and IGIM are indicated and travel will commence in less than 6 months, administer MMR.

[c]HepA vaccine and IGIM should be administered at the same time at different limbs.

- **Close contacts of newly arriving international adoptees.**[1,2] Data from a study conducted at 3 adoption clinics in the United States indicate that 1% to 6% of newly arrived international adoptees have acute HAV infection. Risk of HAV infection among close personal contacts of international adoptees is estimated at 106 (range, 90–819) per 100 000 household contacts of international adoptees within the first 60 days of their arrival in the United States. HepA vaccine should be administered to all unvaccinated people who anticipate close personal contact (eg, household contact or regular babysitting) with an international adoptee from a country with high or intermediate endemic hepatitis A during the first 60 days following arrival of the adoptee in the United States. The first dose of the 2-dose HepA vaccine series should be administered as soon as adoption is planned, ideally 2 or more weeks before the arrival of the adoptee.
- **Men who have sex with men.** Cyclic outbreaks of hepatitis A among men who have sex with men have been reported often, including in urban areas in the United States, Canada, and Australia. Therefore, men (adolescents and adults) who have sex with men should be immunized. Preimmunization serologic testing may be cost-effective for older people in this group.
- **People who use injection or noninjection drugs.** Periodic outbreaks among people who use injection or noninjection drugs have been reported in many parts of

[1]Centers for Disease Control and Prevention. Updated recommendations from the Advisory Committee on Immunization Practices (ACIP) for use of hepatitis A vaccine in close contacts of newly arriving international adoptees. *MMWR Morb Mortal Wkly Rep.* 2009;58(36):1006–1007

[2]American Academy of Pediatrics, Committee on Infectious Diseases. Recommendations for administering hepatitis A vaccine to contacts of international adoptees. *Pediatrics.* 2011;128(4):803–804

the United States and Europe. Adolescents and adults who use injection or noninjection drugs should receive HepA vaccine.

- **People at risk of occupational exposure (eg, handle nonhuman primates infected with HAV or work with HAV in a research laboratory).** Outbreaks of HAV infection have been reported among people who work with nonhuman primates infected with HAV. People working with HAV-infected nonhuman primates or HAV in a research laboratory should receive HepA vaccine.
- **People with clotting-factor disorders** are not considered to be at risk for hepatitis A infection.

Postexposure Prophylaxis (PEP) (see Table 3.16, p 375). Use of HepA vaccine for PEP provides several advantages compared with IGIM, including the induction of active immunity, longer duration of protection, ease of administration, and greater acceptability and availability. In general, people who previously have not received HepA vaccine and have been exposed to HAV should receive a dose of single-antigen HepA vaccine as soon as possible within 14 days of exposure (see Table 3.16, p 375, for prophylaxis guidance and dosages). For people who should not receive HepA vaccine because they are too young or have a severe allergy to the vaccine or its components, IGIM should be used. Efficacy of HepA vaccine or IGIM for PEP when administered more than 2 weeks after exposure has not been established. No data are available for PEP with people who have underlying medical conditions.

- **Healthy people age 12 months and older** who have been exposed to HAV within the past 2 weeks and have not previously completed the HepA vaccine series should receive 1 dose of single-antigen HepA vaccine and complete the 2-dose series according to the recommended schedule. In addition to HepA vaccine, IGIM (0.1 mL/kg) may be administered to people 40 years or older, depending on the provider's risk assessment.
- **Infants younger than age 12 months** and **people who have serious allergy to HepA or its components** should receive IGIM (0.1 mL/kg).
- **People who are immunocompromised or have chronic liver disease** should receive a dose of HepA and IGIM (0.1 mL/kg) at different limbs at the same time. Complete the 2-dose HepA series according to the recommended schedule.

There are other situations for which HepA vaccine and IGIM can be considered. These groups of people or settings include:

- **Newborn infants of HAV-infected mothers.** Perinatal transmission of HAV and severe disease in healthy infants are rare. IGIM (0.1 mL/kg) may be given to an infant if the mother's HAV infection symptoms began between 2 weeks before and 1 week after delivery. Efficacy in this circumstance has not been established.
- **Child care centers.** PEP should be administered to all previously unvaccinated staff members and attendees of child care centers or institutions if (1) one or more cases of HAV infection are recognized in children; or (2) cases are recognized in 2 or more households of center attendees. In centers that do not provide care to children who wear diapers, PEP can be considered only for care center contacts of the index patient (see Table 2.3, p 128).
- **Schools and non–health care work settings.** School- or work-based HAV exposure generally does not pose a risk of infection, and PEP is not indicated when the source of infection is outside the school or work.

- **Hospitals and other health care settings.** Health care-associated transmission of HAV is uncommon when recommended infection control practices are followed. PEP within the health care setting may be considered on a case-by-case basis depending on risk of transmission. Health care workers do not have increased prevalence of HAV infection.
- **Common-source food exposure and food handlers.** Food handlers are not at increased risk for hepatitis A infection based on their occupation. Most food handlers with HAV infection do not transmit HAV to others, but PEP can be considered based on risk of transmission.

Hepatitis B

CLINICAL MANIFESTATIONS: People acutely infected with hepatitis B virus (HBV) may be asymptomatic or symptomatic. The likelihood of developing symptoms of acute hepatitis is age- dependent: less than 1% of infants younger than 1 year, 5% to 15% of children 1 through 5 years of age, and 30% to 50% of people 6 through 30 years are symptomatic. Few data are available for adults older than 30 years. The spectrum of signs and symptoms is varied and includes subacute illness with nonspecific symptoms (eg, anorexia, nausea, or malaise), clinical hepatitis with jaundice, or fulminant hepatitis. Gianotti-Crosti syndrome (papular acrodermatitis), urticaria, macular rash, or purpuric lesions may be seen in acute HBV infection. Extrahepatic manifestations associated with circulating immune complexes that have been reported in HBV-infected children include arthralgias, arthritis, polyarteritis nodosa, thrombocytopenia, and glomerulonephritis. Acute HBV infection cannot be distinguished from other forms of acute viral hepatitis on the basis of clinical signs and symptoms or nonspecific laboratory findings.

Chronic HBV infection is defined as persistence in serum for at least 6 months of any one of the following: hepatitis B surface antigen (HBsAg), HBV DNA, or hepatitis B e antigen (HBeAg). Chronic HBV infection is likely in the presence of HBsAg, HBV DNA, or HBeAg in serum from a person who tests negative for antibody of the immunoglobulin (Ig) M subclass to hepatitis B core antigen (IgM anti-HBc).

Age at the time of infection is the primary determinant of risk of progressing to chronic infection. Up to 90% of infants infected perinatally or in the first year of life will develop chronic HBV infection. Between 25% and 50% of children infected between 1 and 5 years of age become chronically infected, whereas 5% to 10% of infected older children and adults develop chronic HBV infection. Patients who become infected with HBV while immunosuppressed or with an underlying chronic illness (eg, end-stage renal disease) have an increased risk of developing chronic infection. In the absence of treatment, up to 25% of infants and children who acquire chronic HBV infection will die prematurely from HBV-related hepatocellular carcinoma (HCC) or cirrhosis.

The clinical course of untreated chronic HBV infection varies according to the population studied, reflecting differences in age at acquisition, rate of loss of HBeAg, and possibly HBV genotype. Most children have asymptomatic infection. For years to decades after initial infection, perinatally infected children are in an "immune tolerant" phase with normal or minimally elevated alanine aminotransferase (ALT) concentrations and minimal or mild liver histologic abnormalities, detectable HBeAg and high HBV DNA concentrations (≥20 000 IU/mL). Some children with chronic HBV may exhibit growth impairment. Chronic HBV infection acquired during later childhood or adolescence usually is accompanied by more active liver disease and increased serum aminotransferase concentrations. Patients with detectable HBeAg *(HBeAg-positive chronic hepatitis B)* usually have high concentrations of HBV DNA and HBsAg in serum and are more likely to transmit infection. Over time (years to decades), HBeAg becomes undetectable in many chronically infected people. This transition often is accompanied by development of antibody to HBeAg (anti-HBe) and decreases in serum HBV DNA and serum aminotransferase concentrations and may be preceded by a temporary exacerbation of liver disease. These patients have *inactive chronic infection* but still may have exacerbations of hepatitis. Serologic reversion (reappearance of HBeAg) is more common if loss of HBeAg is not accompanied by development of anti-HBe; reversion with loss of anti-HBe also can occur. Because HBV-associated liver injury is thought to be immune-mediated, in people coinfected with human immunodeficiency virus (HIV) and HBV, the return of immune competence with antiretroviral treatment of HIV infection may lead to a reactivation of HBV-related liver inflammation and damage.

Some patients who lose HBeAg may continue to have ongoing histologic evidence of liver damage and moderate to high concentrations of HBV DNA *(HBeAg-negative chronic hepatitis B)*. Patients with histologic evidence of chronic HBV infection, regardless of HBeAg status, remain at higher risk of death attributable to liver failure compared with HBV-infected people with no histologic evidence of liver inflammation and fibrosis.

Resolved hepatitis B is defined as clearance of HBsAg, normalization of serum aminotransferase concentrations, and development of antibody to HBsAg (anti-HBs). Chronically infected adults clear HBsAg and develop anti-HBs at the rate of 1% annually; during childhood, the annual clearance rate is less than 1%. Reactivation of resolved chronic infection in HBsAg-positive patients is possible if these patients become immunosuppressed, receive anti-tumor necrosis factor agents or disease-modifying anti-rheumatic drugs (12% of such patients), and has been reported in patients with chronic HCV infection being treated with direct acting antiviral agents (21%).

ETIOLOGY: HBV is a partially double-stranded DNA-containing 42-nm-diameter enveloped virus in the family *Hepadnaviridae*. Important components of the viral particle include an outer lipoprotein envelope containing HBsAg and an inner nucleocapsid consisting of hepatitis B core antigen (HBcAg).

EPIDEMIOLOGY: HBV is transmitted through infected blood or body fluids. Although HBsAg has been detected in multiple body fluids including human milk, saliva, and tears, the most potentially infectious fluids include blood, serum, semen, vaginal secretions, and cerebrospinal, synovial, pleural, pericardial, peritoneal, and amniotic fluids. People with chronic HBV infection are the primary reservoirs for infection. Common modes of transmission include percutaneous and permucosal exposure to infectious body fluids; sharing or using nonsterilized needles, syringes, or glucose monitoring equipment or devices; sexual contact with an infected person; perinatal exposure to an infected mother; and household exposure to a person with chronic HBV infection. The risks of HBV acquisition when a susceptible child bites a child who has chronic HBV infection or when a susceptible child is bitten by a child with chronic HBV infection are unknown (see Bite Wounds, p 169). A theoretical risk exists if HBsAg-positive blood enters the oral cavity of the biter, but transmission by this route has not been reported. Transmission by transfusion of contaminated blood or blood products is rare in the United States because of routine screening of blood donors and viral inactivation of certain blood products before administration.

FIG 3.2. MAP OF HEPATITIS B PREVALENCE GLOBALLY.

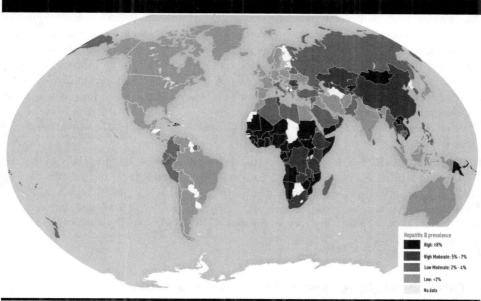

Reproduced from **www.cdc.gov/travel-static/yellowbook/2020/map_4-04.pdf.**

Perinatal transmission of HBV is highly efficient and usually occurs from blood exposures during labor and delivery. In utero transmission accounts for less than 2% of all vertically transmitted HBV infections in most studies. Without postexposure prophylaxis, the risk of an infant acquiring HBV from an infected mother as a result of perinatal exposure is 70% to 90% for infants born to mothers who are HBsAg and HBeAg positive; the risk is 5% to 20% for infants born to HBsAg-positive but HBeAg-negative mothers. Infants born to mothers with very high HBV DNA levels (>200 000 IU/mL) are at high risk of breakthrough infection despite receipt of recommended prophylaxis.

Prevalence of HBV infection and patterns of transmission vary markedly throughout the world (see Fig 3.2). Approximately 80% of people worldwide live in regions of inter-mediate to high HBV endemicity, defined as prevalence of chronic HBV infection of 2% or greater. Historically, most new HBV infections occurred as a result of perinatal or early childhood infections in regions of high HBV endemicity, defined as prevalence of HBV infection of 8% or greater. Infant immunization programs in some of these countries have, in recent years, greatly reduced seroprevalence of HBsAg, but many countries with endemic HBV have yet to implement widespread routine birth-dose and/or childhood hepatitis B immunization programs. In regions of intermediate HBV endemicity (preva-lence of HBV infection 2% to 7%), multiple modes of transmission (ie, perinatal, house-hold, sexual, injection drug use, and health care associated) contribute to the burden of infection. In countries with low endemicity (chronic HBV infection prevalence <2%) and where routine immunization has been adopted, new infections occur most often in age groups where routine immunization is not conducted.

In regions of the world with high prevalence of chronic HBV infection, transmission between children in household settings may account for a substantial amount of transmission. Precise mechanisms of transmission from child to child are unknown, but frequent interpersonal contact of nonintact skin or mucous membranes with blood-containing secretions, open skin lesions, or blood-containing saliva are potential means of transmission. Transmission from sharing inanimate objects, such as razors or toothbrushes, also may occur. HBV can survive in the environment for 7 or more days but is inactivated by commonly used disinfectants, including household bleach diluted 1:10 with water. HBV is not transmitted by the fecal-oral route.

The **incubation period** for acute HBV infection is 45 to 160 days, with an average of 90 days.

DIAGNOSTIC TESTS: Serologic protein antigen tests are available commercially to detect HBsAg and HBeAg. Serologic antibody assays also are available for detection of anti-HBs, total anti-HBc, IgM anti-HBc, and anti-HBe (see Table 3.19, Fig 3.3, and Fig 3.4). Most laboratories now use real-time polymerase chain reaction (PCR) assays for analysis of HBV DNA, with very high sensitivity at low levels and broad dynamic range for quantitation.

Table 3.19. Diagnostic Tests for Hepatitis B Virus (HBV) Antigens and Antibodies

Factors To Be Tested	HBV Antigen or Antibody	Use
HBsAg	Hepatitis B surface antigen	Detection of acutely or chronically infected people; antigen used in hepatitis B vaccine; rarely can be detected for up to 3 weeks after a dose of hepatitis B vaccine
Anti-HBs	Antibody to HBsAg	Identification of people who have resolved infections with HBV; determination of immunity after immunization
HBeAg	Hepatitis B e antigen	Identification of infected people at increased risk of transmitting HBV
Anti-HBe	Antibody to HBeAg	Identification of infected people with lower risk of transmitting HBV
Anti-HBc (total)	Antibody to HBcAg[a]	Identification of people with acute, resolved, or chronic HBV infection (not present after immunization); passively transferred maternal anti-HBc is detectable for as long as 24 months among infants born to HBsAg-positive women
IgM anti-HBc	IgM antibody to HBcAg	Identification of people with acute or recent HBV infections (including HBsAg-negative people during the "window" phase of infection; unreliable for detecting perinatal HBV infection)

HBcAg indicates hepatitis B core antigen; IgM, immunoglobulin M.
[a]No test is available commercially to measure HBcAg.

FIG 3.3. TYPICAL SEROLOGIC COURSE OF ACUTE HEPATITIS B VIRUS INFECTION WITH RECOVERY.

*Hepatitis B e antigen.
§Antibody to hepatitis B core antigen.
¶Hepatitis B surface antigen.
**Immunoglobulin M.
 From Centers for Disease Control and Prevention. Recommendations for identification and public health management of persons with chronic hepatitis B virus infection. *MMWR Recomm Rep.* 2008;57(RR-8):1-20

FIG 3.4. TYPICAL SEROLOGIC COURSE OF ACUTE HEPATITIS B VIRUS (HBV) INFECTION WITH PROGRESSION TO CHRONIC HBV INFECTION

*Hepatitis B e antigen.
§Antibody to hepatitis B core antigen.
¶Hepatitis B surface antigen.
**Immunoglobulin M.
 From Centers for Disease Control and Prevention. Recommendations for identification and public health management of persons with chronic hepatitis B virus infection. *MMWR Recomm Rep.* 2008;57(RR-8):1-20

HBsAg is detectable during acute and chronic infection. If HBV infection is self-limited, HBsAg disappears in most patients within a few weeks to several months after infection, followed by appearance of anti-HBs. The time between disappearance of HBsAg and appearance of anti-HBs is termed the *window period* of infection. During the window period, the only marker of acute infection is IgM anti-HBc. IgM anti-HBc usually is not present in infants infected perinatally. People with chronic HBV infection have circulating HBsAg and circulating total anti-HBc (Fig 3.4); in a minority of chronically infected individuals, anti-HBs also is present. Both anti-HBs and total anti-HBc are present in people with resolved infection, whereas anti-HBs alone is present in people immunized with hepatitis B vaccine. The presence of HBeAg in serum correlates with higher concentrations of HBV DNA and greater infectivity. Tests for HBeAg and HBV DNA are useful in selection of candidates to receive antiviral therapy and to monitor response to therapy.

Transient presence of HBsAg can occur following receipt of HepB vaccine, with HBsAg being detected as early as 24 hours after and up to 3 weeks following administration of the vaccine.

TREATMENT: No therapy for uncomplicated *acute* HBV infection is recommended. Treatment with a nucleoside or nucleotide analogue is indicated if there is concern for severe infection with acute liver failure. Acute HBV infection may be difficult to distinguish from reactivation of HBV. If reactivation is a possibility, referral to a hepatitis specialist would be warranted. Hepatitis B Immune Globulin (HBIG) and corticosteroids are not effective treatment for acute or chronic disease.

The goal of treatment in chronic HBV infection is to prevent progression to cirrhosis, hepatic failure, and hepatocellular carcinoma (HCC), with antibody to HBeAg (anti-HBe) seroconversion as the surrogate endpoint. Current indications for treatment of chronic HBV infection include evidence of ongoing HBV viral replication, as indicated by the presence for longer than 6 months of either serum HBV DNA greater than 20 000 IU/mL with HBeAg positivity or greater than 2000 IU/mL without HBeAg positivity, AND elevated serum ALT concentrations for longer than 6 months or evidence of chronic hepatitis on liver biopsy. Children without necroinflammatory liver disease and children in the immunotolerant phase (ie, normal ALT concentrations despite the presence of HBV DNA) do not warrant antiviral therapy. Treatment response is measured by biochemical, virologic, and histologic response. The American Association for the Study of Liver Diseases and the Centers for Disease Control and Prevention (CDC) recommend that women with viral loads >200 000 IU/mL be offered antiviral therapy to prevent transmission to their child (**www.aasld.org/sites/default/files/2019-06/ HBVGuidance_Terrault_et_al-2018-Hepatology.pdf; www.cdc.gov/mmwr/ volumes/67/rr/rr6701a1.htm**).

The US Food and Drug Administration (FDA) has approved 3 nucleoside analogues (entecavir, lamivudine, and telbivudine), 3 nucleotide analogues (tenofovir disoproxil fumarate, tenofovir alafenamide fumarate, and adefovir), and 2 interferon-alfa drugs (interferon alfa-2b and pegylated interferon alfa-2a) for treatment of chronic HBV infection in adults. An important consideration in choice of treatment is to avoid selection of antiviral-resistant mutations. Tenofovir disoproxil fumarate, tenofovir alafenamide fumarate, entecavir, and pegylated interferon alfa-2a are preferred in adults as first-line therapy because of the lower likelihood of developing antiviral resistance mutations over long-term therapy. FDA licensure in the pediatric population is as follows: interferon alfa-2b, ≥1 year of age; entecavir, ≥2 years of age; tenofovir disoproxil fumarate, ≥2 years of age; and telbivudine, ≥16 years of age (see Non-HIV Antiviral Drugs, p 930). Pegylated interferon alfa-2a is not approved for treatment of children with chronic hepatitis B but is approved for children ≥5 years of age to treat chronic hepatitis C infection. Developments in antiviral therapies of HBV and updated practice guidelines may be found on the American Association for the Study of Liver Diseases website (**www.aasld. org/publications/practice-guidelines-0**). Specific therapy guidelines for children coinfected with HIV and HBV can be accessed online (**https://clinicalinfo.hiv.gov/ en/guidelines**).

Consultation with health care professionals with expertise in treating chronic hepatitis B in children is recommended.

ISOLATION OF THE HOSPITALIZED PATIENT: Standard precautions are indicated for patients with acute or chronic HBV infection. For infants born to HBsAg-positive mothers, no special care in addition to standard precautions, as described under Control Measures, is needed, other than removal of maternal blood by a gloved attendant.

CONTROL MEASURES:

Hepatitis B Immunoprophylaxis. Two types of products are available for immunoprophylaxis.

Hepatitis B Immune Globulin.[1] HBIG provides short-term protection (3–6 months) and is indicated in specific postexposure circumstances (see Care of Exposed People, p 397). HBIG is prepared from the plasma of donors with high concentrations of anti-HBs, with an anti-HBs titer of at least 1:100 000 by radioimmunoassay. Standard Immune Globulin is not effective for postexposure prophylaxis against HBV infection because concentrations of anti-HBs are too low.

Hepatitis B Vaccine. HepB vaccine is used for preexposure and postexposure prophylaxis and provides long-term protection. Preexposure immunization with HepB vaccine is the most effective means to prevent HBV transmission. Highly effective and safe HepB vaccines produced by recombinant DNA technology are licensed in the United States in single-antigen formulations and as components of combination vaccines. Recombinant vaccines contain 10 to 40 μg of HBsAg protein/mL, and a completed vaccine series results in production of anti-HBs of at least 10 mIU/mL in most people, which provides long-term protection for immunocompetent recipients. Single-dose formulations, including all pediatric formulations, contain no thimerosal as a preservative. Although the concentration of recombinant HBsAg protein differs among vaccine products, rates of seroprotection are equivalent when administered to immunocompetent infants, children, adolescents, or young adults in the doses recommended (see Table 3.20). A 2-dose single-antigen hepatitis B vaccine with a novel adjuvant is available for people 18 years and older (HepB-CpG [Heplisav-B]).

High seroconversion rates and protective concentrations of anti-HBs (10 mIU/mL or greater) are achieved when HepB vaccine is administered in any of the recommended schedules, including schedules begun soon after birth in term infants (see Table 3.20). Only single-antigen HepB vaccine can be used for doses administered between birth

---

[1]Dosages recommended for postexposure prophylaxis are for products licensed in the United States. Because concentration of anti-HBs in other products may vary, different dosages may be recommended in other countries.

Table 3.20. Recommended Dosages of Hepatitis B Vaccines

Patients	Single-Dose Vaccines[a]			Combination Vaccines		
	Recombivax HB[b] Dose, μg (mL)	Engerix-B[c] Dose, μg (mL)	Heplisav-B[d] Dose, μg (mL)	Pediarix[e] Dose, μg/mL	Twinrix Dose, μg (mL)[f]	Vaxelis[g] Dose, μg (mL)
Infants, children, and adolescents younger than 20 y (except as noted)	5 (0.5)	10 (0.5)	Not applicable	10 μg HBsAg (0.5) (ages 6 weeks through 6 years only)	Not applicable	10 μg HBsAg (0.5) (ages 6 weeks through 4 years only)
Adolescents 11–15 y of age[b]	10 (1)	Not approved for 2-dose schedule	Not applicable	Not applicable	Not applicable	Not applicable
Adults 18 y or older			20 (0.5)	Not applicable	20 (1)	Not applicable
Adults 20 y or older	10 (1)	20 (1)	Not applicable	Not applicable	20 (1)	Not applicable
Adults undergoing dialysis	40 (1)[h,i]	40 (2)[i,j]	Not applicable	Not applicable	Not applicable	Not applicable

HBIG indicates Hepatitis B Immune Globulin; HBsAg, hepatitis B surface antigen.

[a] Recombivax and Engerix-B vaccines are administered in a 3-dose schedule at 0, 1, and 6 months; 4 doses may be administered if a combination vaccine is used (at 2, 4, and 6 months) to complete the series. Only single-antigen hepatitis B vaccine can be used for the birth dose. Single-antigen or combination vaccine containing hepatitis B vaccine may be used to complete the series. See text for management of infants born to HBsAg positive or HBsAg unknown mothers.

[b] Available from Merck & Co Inc. A 2-dose schedule, administered at 0 months and then 4 to 6 months later, is licensed for adolescents 11 through 15 years of age using the adult formulation of Recombivax HB (10 μg [Merck & Co Inc]).

[c] Available from GlaxoSmithKline Biologicals. The US Food and Drug Administration also has licensed this vaccine for use in an optional 4-dose (0.5-mL/dose for ages birth through 10 years and 1.0 mL/dose for ages 11-19) schedule at 0, 1, 2, and 12 months for all age groups. A 0-, 12-, and 24-month schedule is licensed for children 5 through 10 years of age at a 0.5-mL dose and for children 11 through 16 years of age at a 1.0-mL dose for whom an extended administration schedule is appropriate on the basis of risk of exposure.

[d] Available from Dynavax Technologies Corporation. A 2-dose schedule administered at 0 and 1 month for use in people ≥18 years of age; safety and effectiveness of Heplisav-B have not been established in adults on hemodialysis.

[e] Combination of diphtheria and tetanus toxoids and acellular pertussis (DTaP), inactivated poliovirus (IPV), and hepatitis B (Engerix-B 10 μg) is approved for use at 2, 4, and 6 months of age (Pediarix [GlaxoSmithKline]). This vaccine should not be administered at birth, before 6 weeks of age, or at 7 years of age or older. For additional information, see Pertussis (p 578).

[f] A combination of hepatitis B (Engerix-B, 20 μg) and hepatitis A (Havrix, 720 enzyme-linked immunosorbent assay units [ELU]) vaccine; Twinrix is licensed for use in people 18 years of age and older in a 3-dose schedule at 0, 1, and 6 months. Alternatively, a 4-dose schedule at days 0, 7, and 21 to 30, followed by a booster dose at 12 months, may be used.

[g] Combination of diphtheria and tetanus toxoids and acellular pertussis (DTaP), inactivated poliovirus (IPV), Haemophilus influenzae type b conjugate, and hepatitis B recombinant vaccines approved for use at 2, 4, and 6 months of age to be used from 6 weeks of age through age 4. Not to be used for the birth dose or for children 5 years and older.

[h] Special formulation for adult dialysis patients administered at 0, 1, and 6 months.

[i] When administered to these populations, follow up serologic testing is recommended 1–2 months after completion of 2-dose series.

[j] Two 1-mL doses administered in 1 or 2 injections in a 4-dose schedule at 0, 1, 2, and 6 months of age.

and 6 weeks of age. Single-antigen or combination vaccine may be used to complete the series; 4 doses of vaccine may be administered if a birth dose is administered and a combination vaccine containing a hepatitis B component is used to complete the series.[1] Guidelines for minimum scheduling time between vaccine doses for infants are available in Table 1.9 (p 33).

Recommended schedules for routine and catch-up hepatitis B immunization are available annually from the CDC and American Academy of Pediatrics (**www.cdc. gov/vaccines/schedules/index.html** and **http://redbook.solutions.aap. org/selfserve/ssPage.aspx?SelfServeContentId=Immunization_Schedules**). Alternate administration schedules are available and licensed by the FDA (see Table 3.20). These alternate dosage and administration schedules result in equivalent immunogenicity and can be used when acceptable on the basis of low risk of exposure and to facilitate adherence.

Children and adolescents who have never received HepB vaccine should be immunized routinely at any age with the age-appropriate doses and schedule. The vaccine schedule should be chosen with consideration of the need to achieve completion of the vaccine series. Immunization should be initiated in all settings, even though completion of the vaccine series might not be ensured.

HepB vaccine can be administered concurrently with other vaccines (see Simultaneous Administration of Multiple Vaccines, p 36).

VACCINE INTERCHANGEABILITY. In general, the various brands of age-appropriate HepB vaccines are interchangeable within an immunization series. Until additional data supporting interchangeability of acellular pertussis-containing HepB combination vaccines are available, vaccines from the same manufacturer should be used, whenever feasible, for at least the first 3 doses in the pertussis series (see Pertussis, p 578). Vaccination should not be deferred when the manufacturer of the previously administered vaccine is unknown or when the vaccine from the same manufacturer is unavailable. Data are limited on the safety and immunogenicity effects when 2-dose Heplisav-B (which is licensed only for people 18 years and older) is interchanged with other 3-dose HepB vaccines from other manufacturers.

ROUTES OF ADMINISTRATION. Vaccine is administered intramuscularly in the anterolateral thigh for infants or deltoid area for children and adults (see Vaccine Administration, p 26). Administration in the buttocks or by the intradermal route is not recommended at any age.

EFFICACY AND DURATION OF PROTECTION. HepB vaccines licensed in the United States have a 90% to 95% efficacy for preventing HBV infection and clinical HBV disease among susceptible children and adults. Immunocompetent people who achieve anti-HBs concentration ≥ 10 mIU/mL after preexposure vaccination have virtually complete protection against infection with HBV. Long-term studies of immunocompetent adults and children indicate that immune memory remains intact for 2 decades and protects against symptomatic acute and chronic HBV infection, even though anti-HBs concentrations may become low or undetectable over time. Breakthrough infections (detected by presence of anti-HBc or HBV DNA) have occurred in a limited number of immunized people, but these infections typically are transient and asymptomatic. Chronic HBV infection in immunized people has been documented in dialysis

---

[1] Centers for Disease Control and Prevention. General recommendations on immunization. Recommendations of the Advisory Committee on Immunization Practices (ACIP). *MMWR Recomm Rep.* 2011;60(RR-2):1–64

patients whose anti-HBs concentrations fell below 10 mIU/mL and rarely among people who did not respond to vaccination (eg, adults and infants born to HBsAg-positive mothers).

BOOSTER DOSES. Routine booster doses of HepB vaccine are not recommended for children and adults with normal immune status. For patients undergoing hemodialysis who are at continued risk of infection, immunity should be assessed by annual anti-HBs testing, and a booster dose should be administered when the anti-HBs concentration is <10 mIU/mL. Annual anti-HBs testing and booster doses when anti-HBs concentrations decrease to <10 mIU/mL should be considered for immunocompromised people (eg, HIV-infected people, hematopoietic stem cell transplant recipients, and people receiving chemotherapy) if they have an ongoing risk for HBV exposure. Similar consideration may be given to children with cystic fibrosis, liver disease, or celiac disease if there is an ongoing risk for HBV exposure. Children with HIV and celiac disease may not respond as well to HepB vaccine.

ADVERSE EVENTS. Adverse effects most commonly reported in adults and children are pain at the injection site, reported by 3% to 29% of recipients, and a temperature greater than 37.7°C (99.8°F), reported by 1% to 6% of recipients. Anaphylaxis is uncommon, occurring in less than 1 in 1.3 million recipients. Large, controlled epidemiologic studies and review by the Institute of Medicine,[1] now called the National Academy of Medicine (NAM [see National Academy of Medicine Reviews of Adverse Events After Immunization, p 43]), found no evidence of an association between HepB vaccine and sudden infant death syndrome, type 1 diabetes mellitus, seizures, encephalitis, or autoimmune (eg, vasculitis) or demyelinating disease, including multiple sclerosis.

IMMUNIZATION DURING PREGNANCY OR LACTATION. No adverse effect on the developing fetus has been observed after immunization during pregnancy. Pregnancy and lactation are not contraindications to immunization. Data about safety during pregnancy are not yet available for Heplisav B; until such data are available, other HepB vaccines are recommended for immunization during pregnancy.

SEROLOGIC TESTING. Susceptibility testing before immunization is not indicated routinely for children or adolescents. Serologic testing, the primary purpose of which is to identify HepB infection (positive HBsAg), is indicated in specific circumstances, including for pregnant women (p 391), for infants born to HBsAg positive mothers (p 391), for people in risk groups for hepatitis B infection (p 396), and for foreign-born individuals (p 396). Testing of health care personnel (p 397) and others at increased or ongoing risk of hepatitis B exposure (see Booster Doses, above) may be performed to document presence of protective antibody. Recommendations from the US Preventive Services Task Force released in December 2020 can be found at **https://uspreventiveservicestaskforce.org/uspstf/recommendation/hepatitis-b-virus-infection-screening**.

Pre-Exposure Universal Immunization of Infants, Children, and Adolescents. Immunization with HepB vaccine is recommended for all infants, children, and adolescents (**www.cdc.gov/vaccines/schedules/hcp/imz/catchup.html** and **http://redbook.**

[1]Institute of Medicine. *Adverse Effects of Vaccines: Evidence and Causality.* Washington, DC: National Academies Press; 2011

solutions.aap.org/selfserve/ssPage.aspx?SelfServeContentId=Immunizat ion_Schedules). Age-specific vaccine dosages are provided in Table 3.20 (p 388).

Newborn Immunization, Including Management Based On Maternal HBsAg Status

Serologic Screening of Pregnant Women. Prenatal HBsAg testing of all pregnant women, regardless of HepB vaccination history, is recommended to identify newborn infants who require immediate postexposure prophylaxis. All pregnant women should be tested during an early prenatal visit with every pregnancy. Testing should be repeated at the time of admission to the hospital for delivery for HBsAg-negative women who are at high risk of HBV infection or who have had clinical hepatitis. Women who are HBsAg positive also should receive testing for hepatitis B virus deoxyribonucleic acid (HBV DNA) and be referred to appropriate specialists to assess need for treatment and to ensure follow-up of their infants and immunization of sexual and household contacts.

Birth Dose of Hepatitis B Vaccine and Use of HBIG. The strategy for preventing hepatitis B in newborn infants relies on providing a birth dose of hepatitis B vaccine to all infants and, for some infants, HBIG, and is based on birth weight and maternal HBsAg status. HepB vaccine should be administered to all infants born to HBsAg-negative mothers within 24 hours of birth for infants with birth weight >2000 g and at hospital discharge or 1 month of age (whichever is first) for infants with birth weight <2000 g. HepB vaccine plus HBIG should be administered within 12 hours of birth to all newborn infants born to HBsAg-positive mothers. Appropriate management at birth of these infants and those born to mothers with unknown HBsAg status is described in Fig 3.5 (p 392).

Subsequent Immunization of Newborns of HBsAg Negative Mothers and Those with HBsAg Unknown at Birth Confirmed as Negative (Tables 3.20, p 388, and 3.21, p 393). Infants born to HBsAg negative women and to those with initial unknown HBsAg status confirmed as negative should complete hepatitis B immunization according to routine immunization schedules with either single-antigen (at ages 1–2 months and 6–18 months) or combination hepatitis B-containing (ages 2, 4, and 6 months) vaccine. Minimum intervals of 1 month should occur between doses 1 and 2, and 8 weeks between doses 2 and 3, with a minimum of 16 weeks between doses 1 and 3; when 4 doses are administered, substitute "dose 4" for "dose 3" in these calculations (**www.cdc.gov/vaccines/schedules/hcp/imz/ child-adolescent.html** and **http://redbook.solutions.aap.org/selfserve/ ssPage.aspx?SelfServeContentId=Immunization_Schedules**). Infants born to mothers with unknown status that remains unknown are managed as infants who are born to mothers who are HBsAg positive (see below).

Management of Infants Born to HBsAg-Positive Women. All infants born to HBsAg-positive mothers, including infants weighing less than 2000 g, should receive the initial dose of HepB vaccine within 12 hours of birth (see Table 3.21, p 393, for appropriate dosages), and HBIG (0.5 mL) should be administered concurrently but at a different anatomic site (Fig 3.5, p 392). Infants born to mothers for whom other evidence suggestive of maternal HBV infection exists (eg, presence of HBV DNA, HBeAg positive, or mother known to be chronically infected with HBV) should be managed as if born to an HBsAg-positive mother. Effectiveness of HBIG diminishes the longer after exposure that it is initiated. The interval of effectiveness is unlikely to exceed 7 days. Subsequent doses of vaccine should be administered as recommended in Table 3.21 (p 393). For infants who weigh <2000 g at birth, the initial vaccine dose should not be counted in

FIG 3.5. ADMINISTRATION OF BIRTH DOSE OF HEPATITIS B VACCINE BY BIRTH WEIGHT AND MATERNAL HBsAg STATUS.

Modified from American Academy of Pediatrics, Committee on Infectious Diseases, Committee on Fetus and Newborn. Elimination of perinatal hepatitis b: providing the first vaccine dose within 24 hours of birth. *Pediatrics.* 2017;140(3):e20171870

[a] For newborns with birth weight <2000 grams, this dose will not count toward total doses in series.

the required 3-dose schedule (a total of 4 doses of HepB vaccine should be administered), and the subsequent 3 doses should be administered at months 1, 2 to 3, and 6 months for single-antigen products and months 2, 4, and 6 for hepatitis B-containing combination vaccines (Table 3.21, p 393). By the chronologic age of 1 month, all medically stable preterm infants, regardless of initial birth weight or gestational age, are as likely to respond to HepB immunization as are term and larger infants.

Breastfeeding of an infant by an HBsAg-positive mother poses no additional risk of acquisition of HBV infection by the infant with appropriate administration of HepB vaccine and HBIG (see Breastfeeding and Human Milk, p 107).

Follow-up Management of Infants Born to HBsAg-Positive Mothers. Infants born to HBsAg-positive women should be tested for anti-HBs and HBsAg at 9 to 12 months of age (generally at the next well-child visit after completion of the immunization series).[1,2] Testing should not be performed before 9 months of age to maximize likelihood of detecting late

---

[1] Schillie S, Murphy TV, Fenlon N, et al. Update: shortened interval for postvaccination serologic testing of infants born to hepatitis B-infected mothers. *MMWR Morb Mortal Wkly Rep.* 2015;64(30):1118-1120

[2] American Academy of Pediatrics, Committee on Infectious Diseases. Elimination of perinatal hepatitis B: providing the first vaccine dose within 24 hours of birth. *Pediatrics.* 2017;140(3):e20171870

Table 3.21. Hepatitis B Vaccine Schedules for Infants by Maternal Hepatitis B Surface Antigen (HBsAg) Status and Birth Weight *(continued on next page)*

Maternal HBsAg Status	Single-Antigen Vaccine		Single-Antigen + Combination	
	Dose	Age	Dose	Age
Positive	1[a]	Birth (12 h or less)	1[a] Birth (12 h or less) (Combination vaccine should not be used for birth dose)	
	HBIG[b]	Birth (12 h or less)	HBIG[b]	Birth (12 h or less)
	2	1 through 2 mo for BW ≥2000 g; 1 mo for BW <2000 g	2	2 mo
	3[c]	6 mo for BW ≥2000 g; 2–3 mo for BW <2000 g	3	4 mo
	4 Only if BW <2000 g	6 mo	4[d]	6 mo (Pediarix)
Unknown[e]	1[a]	Birth (12 h or less) BW <2000 g HBIG at birth (12 h or less)	1[a] Birth (12 h or less) (Combination vaccine should not be used for birth dose)	
	2	1 through 2 mo for BW ≥2000 g; 1 mo for BW <2000 g if maternal status remains unknown	2	2 mo
	3[d]	6 mo for BW ≥2000 g; 2–3 mo for BW <2000 g if maternal status remains unknown	3	4 mo
	4 Only if BW <2000 g AND maternal status remains unknown	6 mo	4[d]	6 mo (Pediarix)

Table 3.21. Hepatitis B Vaccine Schedules for Infants by Maternal Hepatitis B Surface Antigen (HBsAg) Status and Birth Weight, continued

Maternal HBsAg Status	Single-Antigen Vaccine		Single-Antigen + Combination	
	Dose	Age	Dose	Age
Negative	1[a]	Birth (12 h or less) for BW ≥2000 g; hospital discharge or age 1 mo for BW <2000 g	1[a]	Birth (24 h or less) (Combination vaccine should not be used for birth dose)
	2	1 through 2 mo	2	2 mo
	3[d]	6 through 18 mo	3	4 mo
	4	Not applicable	4[d]	6 mo (Pediarix)

BW indicates birth weight; HBIG, Hepatitis B Immune Globulin.

[a] Recombivax HB or Engerix-B should be used for the birth dose. Pediarix and Vaxelis should not be administered at birth or before 6 weeks of age.

[b] HBIG (0.5 mL) administered intramuscularly in a separate site from vaccine.

[c] Mothers should have blood drawn and tested for HBsAg as soon as possible after admission for delivery. Infants with birth weight <2000 g should receive HBIG by 12 hours; for infants with birth weight ≥2000 g if the mother is found to be HBsAg positive, the infant should receive HBIG as soon as possible but no later than 7 days of age.

[d] The final dose in the vaccine series should not be administered before 24 weeks (164 days) of age.

Source: Schillie S, Vellozzi C, Reingold A, et al. Prevention of hepatitis B virus infection in the United States: recommendations of the Advisory Committee on Immunization Practices. *MMWR Recomm Rep.* 2018;67(RR-1):1-31.

onset of HBV infections. Immunized infants with anti-HBs concentrations ≥10 mIU/mL and who are HBsAg negative are considered not to be infected and to have adequate vaccine-associated immune protection. Infants with anti-HBs concentrations <10 mIU/mL and who are HBsAg negative following a 3-dose hepatitis B vaccine series should receive 1 additional dose of hepatitis B vaccine followed by testing for anti-HBs and HBsAg 1 to 2 months after the fourth dose. Infants with anti-HBs concentrations ≥10 mIU/mL and who are HBsAg negative after the fourth dose are considered not to be infected and to have adequate vaccine-associated immune protection. Infants with anti-HBs concentrations <10 mIU/mL and who are HBsAg negative after the fourth dose should receive 2 additional doses of vaccine, separated by at least 8 weeks, followed by testing for anti-HBs and HBsAg 1 to 2 months after the sixth dose. An alternate approach for children who have completed a 3-dose series of HepB vaccine but did not achieve anti-HBs titers ≥10 mIU/mL is to give 3 additional doses of HepB vaccine at the same dosing intervals as the first series and then retest for anti-HBs titers 1 to 2 months after the third dose of this second series. Subsequent doses of hepatitis B vaccine when anti-HBs concentrations are <10 mIU/mL after the sixth dose are not indicated.

Management of Infants Born to Mothers with Unknown HBsAg Status or Not Tested During Pregnancy for HBsAg.

TERM INFANTS (WEIGHING ≥2000 g AT BIRTH). Pregnant women whose HBsAg status is unknown at delivery should undergo blood testing as soon as possible to determine their HBsAg status. While awaiting results, the infant should receive the first HepB vaccine dose within 12 hours of birth, as recommended for infants born to HBsAg-positive mothers (see Table 3.21, p 393, and Fig 3.5, p 392). If the woman is found to be HBsAg positive, term infants should receive HBIG (0.5 mL) as soon as possible, but within 7 days of birth, and should complete the HepB immunization series as recommended (see Tables 3.20, p 388, and 3.21, p 393). If the mother is found to be HBsAg negative, HepB immunization in the dose and schedule recommended for term infants born to HBsAg-negative mothers should be completed (see Table 3.20, p 388). If the mother's HBsAg status remains unknown, it is appropriate to administer HBIG within 7 days of birth and complete the HepB immunization series as recommended for infants born to mothers who are HBsAg positive (Table 3.21, p 393, and Fig 3.5, p 392).

INFANTS WEIGHING LESS THAN 2000 g. Maternal HBsAg status should be determined as soon as possible. Infants weighing <2000 g born to mothers whose HBsAg status is unknown should receive HepB vaccine within the first 12 hours of life (Table 3.21, p 393, and Fig 3.5, p 392). Because of the potentially decreased immunogenicity of the HepB vaccine in infants weighing <2000 g at birth, these infants should receive HBIG (0.5 mL) within 12 hours of birth if the mother's HBsAg status cannot be determined by that time (Table 3.21, p 393, and Fig 3.5, p 392). The initial vaccine dose should not be counted toward the 3 doses of hepatitis B vaccine required to complete the immunization series, and the subsequent 3 doses (for a total of 4 doses) are administered according to the HBsAg status of the mother. If the mother is HBsAg positive or the mother's status remains unknown, the infant would receive the subsequent 3 doses administered at months 1, 2 to 3, and 6 months for single antigen products, and months 2, 4, and 6 for hepatitis B-containing combination vaccines (Tables 3.20, p 388, and 3.21, p 393). Serologic testing for both of these groups of infants should be performed as described above for infants born to HBsAg-positive mothers and revaccination performed if necessary.

Routine Immunization of Infants, Children, and Adolescents Who Did Not Begin Immunization at Birth. Serologic testing to identify HBV infection (positive HBsAg) should be performed for people in risk groups with high rates, including people born in countries with intermediate and high HBV endemicity (even if immunized, because the series may have been started after the infection was acquired), users of injection drugs, men who have sex with men, and household and sexual contacts of HBsAg-positive people. The first dose of vaccine may be given at the time of testing so that immunization efforts are not delayed or impeded. Children identified as HBsAg positive should be referred for management and monitoring of hepatitis B infection. Those who are HBsAg and antibody negative should be immunized according to doses and schedules noted in Table 3.20 (p 388). Testing for antibody (anti-HBs) often is performed along with testing for HBsAg. Children who have not completed a 3-dose series of HepB vaccine should complete the series regardless of the anti-HBs test result. Routine postimmunization testing is not recommended.

Lapsed Immunizations. For infants, children, adolescents, and adults with lapsed immunizations (ie, the interval between doses is longer than that in one of the recommended schedules), the vaccine series should be completed without repeating doses, as long as minimum dosing intervals between the remaining doses necessary to complete the series are heeded (see Lapsed Immunizations, p 38).

Negative Anti-HBs in Previously Immunized Children. Providers may be asked to manage children tested for anti-HBs following receipt of hepatitis B immunization given at age-appropriate doses and intervals and found to have anti-HBs <10 mIU/mL. Serologic testing following routine immunization of children is not recommended routinely. If confirming response to vaccine is desired, such as after a needlestick injury, a single dose of vaccine may be administered, followed by testing for anti-HBs 1 to 2 months later. Children with anti-HBs ≥10 mIU/mL can be considered to have adequate vaccine-associated immune protection. Those with anti-HBs <10 mIU/mL may be given 2 more doses of hepatitis B with testing for anti-HBs 1 to 2 months after the last dose. A vaccine nonresponder is defined as a person with anti-HBs <10 mIU/mL after ≥6 doses of HepB vaccine.

SPECIAL CONSIDERATIONS:

Considerations for High-Risk Groups:

Patients Undergoing Hemodialysis. Immunization is recommended for susceptible patients undergoing hemodialysis. Immunization early in the course of renal disease is encouraged, because response is better than in advanced disease. Specific dosage recommendations have not been made for children undergoing hemodialysis. Some experts recommend increased doses of HepB vaccine for children receiving hemodialysis to increase immunogenicity.

People Born in Countries Where the Prevalence of Chronic HBV Infection Is 2% or Greater. Foreign-born people (including immigrants, refugees, asylum seekers, and internationally adopted children) from countries where prevalence of chronic HBV infection is 2% or greater (see Fig 3.2, p 383) should be screened for HBsAg regardless of immunization status (see Medical Evaluation for Infectious Diseases for Internationally Adopted, Refugee, and Immigrant Children, p 158). Previously unimmunized family members and other household contacts should be immunized if a household member is found to be HBsAg positive. Positive HBsAg test results are nationally notifiable (see Appendix III, p 1033), and people with positive HBsAg test results should be referred for medical management to reduce their risk of complications from chronic HBV infection and to reduce risk of transmission.

Inmates in Juvenile Detention and Other Correctional Facilities. Unimmunized or underimmunized people in juvenile and adult correctional facilities should be immunized. If the length of stay is not sufficient to complete the immunization series, the series should be initiated, and follow-up mechanisms with a health care facility should be established to ensure completion of the series.

International Travelers. People traveling to areas where the prevalence of chronic HBV infection is 2% or greater (see Fig 3.2, p 383) should be immunized. Ideally, HepB vaccination should be administered ≥6 months before travel so that a 3-dose regimen can be completed (see Pre-Exposure Universal Immunization of Infants, Children, and Adolescents, p 390). If fewer than 4 months are available before departure, the alternative 4-dose schedule of 0, 1, 2, and 12 months, licensed for one vaccine (see Table 3.20, p 388), might provide opportunity for more rapid development of protection. Individual health care providers may choose to use an accelerated schedule (eg, doses at days 0, 7, and 21–30, with a booster at 12 months) for travelers who will depart before an approved immunization schedule can be completed. People who receive immunization on an accelerated schedule that is not licensed by the FDA also should receive a dose at 12 months after initiation of the series to promote long-term immunity. For people 18 years and older, the 2-dose regimen of Heplisav-B can be completed in 1 month and offers greater flexibility before travel.

Postimmunization Testing for Anti-HBs. Routine postimmunization testing for anti-HBs is not necessary after routine vaccination of healthy people but is recommended 1 to 2 months after the final vaccine dose for the following specific groups: (1) hemodialysis patients (and other people who might require outpatient hemodialysis); (2) people with HIV infection; (3) other immunocompromised patients (eg, hematopoietic stem-cell transplant recipients or people receiving chemotherapy); (4) people at occupational risk of exposure from percutaneous injuries or mucosal or nonintact skin exposures (eg, certain health care and public safety workers); (5) sexual partners of HBsAg-positive people, and (6) infants born to HBsAg-positive women and infants born to women whose HBsAg status remains unknown (testing should consist of HBsAg and anti—HBs).

Management of Nonresponders. Vaccine recipients who do not develop a serum anti-HBs response ($\geq$10 mIU/mL) after a primary vaccine series should be tested for HBsAg to rule out the possibility of a chronic infection as an explanation of failure to respond to the vaccine. If the HBsAg test result is negative, a single dose of HepB vaccine can be administered followed by testing for anti-HBs in 1 to 2 months. If anti-HBs is $\geq$10 mIU/mL, no further testing is required. If anti-HBs is <10 mIU/mL, additional doses should be administered to complete the second vaccine series, with testing for anti-HBs 1 to 2 months after the last dose. For the 3-dose vaccine series using Engerix-B or Recombivax HB, this would require 2 additional doses of vaccine, and for the 2-dose series using Heplisav-B (licensed only in adults), this would require 1 additional dose. For very recently vaccinated HCP with anti-HBs <10 mIU/mL, in whom the low antibody concentration is more likely to reflect a failure to respond rather than waning antibody concentration, it may be more practical to revaccinate with an entire second series (3 doses of Engerix-B or Recombivax HB; 2 doses of Heplisav-B) followed by anti-HBs testing 1 to 2 months after the last dose. Heplisav-B may be used for revaccination following an initial HepB vaccine series that consisted of doses from a different manufacturer. A vaccine nonresponder is defined as a person with anti-HBs <10 mIU/mL after $\geq$6 doses of HepB vaccine.

Care of Exposed People (Postexposure Immunoprophylaxis).

Household Contacts and Sexual Partners of HBsAg-Positive People. Household and sexual contacts of HBsAg-positive people (with acute or chronic HBV infection) identified through prenatal screening, blood donor screening, or diagnostic or other serologic testing should be screened for HBV infection with anti-HBc, anti-HBs, and HBsAg tests. Unvaccinated and uninfected people should be immunized. The first dose of vaccine should be administered after the blood for serologic tests is obtained while waiting for the results. People with chronic HBV should be referred for medical evaluation to prevent complications of the infection.

Prophylaxis with HBIG for other unimmunized household contacts of HBsAg-positive people is not indicated unless they have a discrete, identifiable exposure to the index patient (see next paragraph).

Postexposure Prophylaxis for People With Discrete Identifiable Exposures to Blood or Body Fluids. Management of people with a discrete, identifiable percutaneous (eg, needle stick, laceration, bite or nonintact skin), mucosal (eg, ocular or mucous membrane), or sexual exposure to blood or body fluids includes consideration of whether the HBsAg status

Table 3.22. Guidelines for Postexposure Prophylaxis[a] of People with Nonoccupational Exposures[b] to Blood or Body Fluids That Contain Blood, by Exposure Type and Vaccination Status

Exposure	Treatment Unvaccinated Person[c]	Previously Vaccinated Person[d]
HBsAg-positive source		
Household member	Consider testing if significant exposure; if negative administer hepatitis B vaccine series	Ensure completion of vaccine series
Percutaneous (eg, bite or needlestick) or mucosal exposure to HBsAg-positive blood or body fluids	Administer hepatitis B vaccine series and hepatitis B immune globulin (HBIG)	Administer hepatitis B vaccine booster dose
Sexual or needle-sharing contact of an HBsAg-positive person	Administer hepatitis B vaccine series and HBIG	Administer hepatitis B vaccine booster dose
Victim of sexual assault/abuse by a perpetrator who is HBsAg positive	Administer hepatitis B vaccine series and HBIG	Administer hepatitis B vaccine booster dose
Source with unknown HBsAg status		
Victim of sexual assault/abuse by a perpetrator with unknown HBsAg status	Administer hepatitis B vaccine series	No treatment
Percutaneous (eg, bite or needlestick) or mucosal exposure to potentially infectious blood or body fluids from a source with unknown HBsAg status	Administer hepatitis B vaccine series	No treatment
Sex or needle-sharing contact of person with unknown HBsAg status	Administer hepatitis B vaccine series	No treatment

HBsAg indicates hepatitis B surface antigen.

[a] When indicated, immunoprophylaxis should be initiated as soon as possible, preferably within 24 hours. Studies are limited on the maximum interval after exposure during which postexposure prophylaxis is effective, but the interval is unlikely to exceed 7 days for percutaneous exposures or 14 days for sexual exposures. The hepatitis B vaccine series should be completed.

[b] These guidelines apply to nonoccupational exposures. Guidelines for occupational exposures can be found in Schillie S, Murphy TV, Sawyer M, et al. CDC guidance for evaluating health-care personnel for hepatitis B virus protection and for administering post exposure management. *MMWR Recomm Rep.* 2013;62(RR-10):1–19.

[c] A person who is in the process of being vaccinated but who has not completed the vaccine series should complete the series and receive treatment as indicated.

[d] A person who has written documentation of a complete hepatitis B vaccine series and who did not receive postvaccination testing.

Source: Schillie S, Vellozzi C, Reingold A, et al. Prevention of hepatitis B virus infection in the United States: recommendations of the Advisory Committee on Immunization Practices. *MMWR Recomm Rep.* 2018;67(1):1–31.

of the person who was the source of exposure and the hepatitis B immunization and response status of the exposed person are known (also see Table 3.22). If possible, a blood specimen from the person who was the source of the exposure should be tested for HBsAg, and appropriate prophylaxis should be administered according to the hepatitis B immunization status and anti-HBs response status (if known) of the exposed person (see Table 3.22). Detailed guidelines for management of health care personnel and other people exposed to blood that is or might be HBsAg positive is provided in the recommendations of the Advisory Committee on Immunization Practices of the Centers for Disease Control and Prevention.[1]

Child Care.

Children who are HBsAg positive and who have no behavioral or medical risk factors, such as unusually aggressive behavior (eg, frequent biting), generalized dermatitis, or a bleeding problem, should be admitted to child care without restrictions. Under these circumstances, the risk of HBV transmission in child care settings is negligible, and routine screening for HBsAg is not warranted. Admission of HBsAg-positive children with behavioral or medical risk factors should be assessed on an individual basis by the child's physician, in consultation with the child care staff. A susceptible child who bites another child or adult who is HBsAg-positive should initiate or complete the hepatitis B vaccine series; HBIG is not recommended in this circumstance (see Bite Wounds, p 169).

Hepatitis C

CLINICAL MANIFESTATIONS: Signs and symptoms of hepatitis C virus (HCV) infection are indistinguishable from those of hepatitis A or hepatitis B virus infections. Acute disease tends to be mild and insidious in onset, and most infections are asymptomatic. Jaundice occurs in less than 20% of patients with HCV infection, and abnormalities in serum alanine aminotransferase concentrations generally are less pronounced than in patients with hepatitis B virus infection. Persistent infection with HCV occurs in up to 80% of infected children, even in the absence of biochemical evidence of liver disease. In general, higher rates of spontaneous viral clearance have been observed in children with perinatal infection, with roughly 20% clearing virus by 2 years of age. Most children with chronic infection are asymptomatic. Liver failure secondary to HCV infection is one of the leading indications for liver transplantation among adults in the United States. Limited data indicate that cirrhosis and hepatocellular carcinoma occur less commonly in children than in adults.

ETIOLOGY: HCV is a small, single-stranded, positive-sense RNA virus and is a member of the family *Flaviviridae* in the genus *Hepacivirus*. At least 7 HCV genotypes exist with more than 50 subtypes. Distribution of genotypes and subtypes varies by geographic location, with genotype 1a being the most common in the United States.

EPIDEMIOLOGY: Prevalence of HCV infection in the general population of the United States is estimated at 1.0%, equating to an estimated 2.7 (2.0–2.8) million people in the United States with chronic HCV infection. Incidence of HCV infection decreased markedly in the United States in all age groups from the 1990s to reach its lowest incidence

---

[1]Schillie S, Murphy TV, Sawyer M, et al. CDC guidance for evaluating health-care personnel for hepatitis B virus protection and for administering post exposure management. *MMWR Recomm Rep.* 2013;62(RR-10):1–19

in 2006–2010. After 2010, there was an increase in reported cases of acute HCV in the United States, largely related to injection drug use, with the highest incidence in people 20 through 29 years of age (**www.cdc.gov/hepatitis/statistics/SurveillanceRpts. htm**). Worldwide, the prevalence of chronic HCV infection is highest in eastern Europe, central Asia, northern Africa, and the Middle East.

HCV is transmitted primarily through percutaneous (parenteral) exposures to infectious blood that can result from injection drug use, needlestick injuries, and inadequate infection control in health care settings. The most common risk factors for adults are injection drug use and male-to-male sexual contact. The most common route of infection for children is maternal-fetal transmission. The current risk of HCV infection after blood transfusion in the United States is estimated to be less than 1 per 2 million units transfused because of exclusion of high-risk donors and of HCV-positive units after antibody testing as well as screening of pools of blood units by nucleic acid amplification tests (NAATs). All intravenous and intramuscular Immune Globulin and plasma products now available commercially in the United States undergo an inactivation procedure for HCV or are documented to be HCV RNA negative before release.

Approximately 60% of acute HCV cases reported to public health authorities are in people who acknowledge they inject drugs and that they have shared needles or injection paraphernalia. Data from recent multicenter, population-based cohort studies indicate that approximately one third of people who inject drugs 18 to 30 years of age are infected with HCV. People with sporadic percutaneous exposures, such as health care professionals, may be infected; per exposure risk of HCV transmission from needlestick is estimated at 0.1%. Health care-associated outbreaks have been documented, especially in nonhospital settings with inadequate infection control and injection safety procedures. Prevalence of HCV is higher among people with frequent direct percutaneous exposures, such as patients receiving hemodialysis (7%).

Sexual transmission of HCV between monogamous heterosexual partners is extremely rare. Transmission can occur in male-to-male sexual contact, especially in association with sexual practices that result in mucosal trauma, presence of concurrent anogenital ulcerative disease, human immunodeficiency virus (HIV)-positive serostatus, or sex while using methamphetamines. HCV has been identified in semen, rectal fluids, and the genital tracts of women, especially in those coinfected with HCV and HIV.

Transmission among family contacts could occur from direct or inapparent percutaneous or mucosal exposure to blood, but this is extremely uncommon.

Seroprevalence among pregnant women in the United States is estimated at 1% to 2% but is higher in some areas. Risk of perinatal transmission averages 5% to 6%, and transmission is associated with presence of HCV viremia at or near the time of delivery. The exact timing of HCV transmission from mother to infant is not established. Recent recommendations from the Centers for Disease Control and Prevention (CDC) and the US Preventive Services Task Force suggest that all pregnant women should be tested for HCV with each pregnancy. Factors that increase risk of perinatal transmission include internal fetal monitoring, vaginal lacerations, and prolonged rupture of membranes (>6 hours). Method of delivery has no effect on perinatal infection risk. Antibody to HCV (anti-HCV) and HCV RNA have been detected in colostrum, but risk of HCV transmission is similar in breastfed and formula-fed infants. Maternal coinfection with HIV is associated with increased risk of perinatal transmission of HCV (twofold greater). Early and sustained control of HIV viremia with antiretroviral therapy (ART) may reduce risk of HCV transmission to infants.

All people with HCV RNA in their blood are considered to be infectious.

The **incubation period** for HCV infection averages 6 to 7 weeks, with a range of 2 weeks to 6 months. The time from exposure to development of viremia generally is 2 to 3 weeks.

DIAGNOSTIC TESTS[1]**:** Diagnostic assays for the detection of anti-HCV antibody are available in various formats, which include enzyme immunoassays (EIA), chemiluminescent immunoassays (CIA), and immunochromatographic or rapid tests. NAATs for both qualitative and quantitative detection of HCV RNA are used for detection of current HCV infection and for monitoring response to antiviral therapy. Screening for HCV infection usually is accomplished by serologic testing for anti-HCV with reflex testing of positive or equivocal HCV antibody test results with NAAT testing to diagnose current infection. Third-generation anti-HCV assays cleared by the US Food and Drug Administration (FDA) are at least 97% sensitive and more than 99% specific. Anti-HCV antibodies can be detected approximately 8 to 11 weeks after exposure. Within 15 weeks after exposure and within 5 to 6 weeks after onset of hepatitis, 80% of patients will have positive test results for anti-HCV antibody. Among infants born to anti-HCV–positive mothers, passively acquired maternal antibody may persist for up to 18 months. In clinical settings where exposure to HCV is considered likely, testing for HCV RNA by NAAT should be performed regardless of the anti-HCV result.

FDA-licensed diagnostic NAATs for detection of HCV RNA are available commercially and recommended in the 2013 CDC HCV testing algorithm as reflex testing for patients with anti-HCV positive test results. HCV RNA can be detected in serum or plasma within 1 to 2 weeks after exposure to the virus and weeks before onset of liver enzyme abnormalities or appearance of anti-HCV antibody. Assays for detection of HCV RNA are used commonly in clinical practice to: (1) detect HCV infection after needlestick or transfusion and before seroconversion; (2) identify active infection in anti-HCV–positive patients; (3) identify infection in infants early in life (ie, perinatal transmission) when maternal antibody interferes with ability to detect antibody produced by the infant; (4) identify HCV infection in severely immunocompromised or hemodialysis patients in whom antibody test results may be falsely negative; and (5) monitor patients receiving antiviral therapy. False-positive and false-negative results of NAATs can occur from improper handling, storage, and contamination of test specimens. Highly sensitive quantitative assays for measuring the concentration of HCV RNA largely have replaced qualitative assays. HCV genotyping is still needed for determining which direct-acting antiviral (DAA) agents should be used in individual patients. With the availability of pan-genotypic DAAs, genotype testing may become less relevant.

Because infants exposed to HCV perinatally have a low risk of HCV acquisition, usually do not exhibit symptoms for years, and there are no antiviral therapies available in the first 3 years of life, testing for HCV infection usually relies on serologic testing at 18 months of age. Liver enzyme testing can be performed at approximately 6-month intervals to detect the rare perinatally HCV-infected infant who has significant liver injury before 18 months of age. When there is concern about follow-up of a perinatally

---

[1]Centers for Disease Control and Prevention. Testing for HCV Infection: an update of guidance for clinicians and laboratorians. *MMWR Morb Mortal Wkly Rep.* 2013;62(18):362-365

HCV-exposed infant until 18 months of age, in situations where a family is not willing to wait until 18 months of age to determine the child's HCV infection status, or if antiviral therapy becomes available to younger infants, NAAT for HCV RNA detection can be performed between 2 and 6 months of age. Regardless of NAAT test result, serologic testing also should be performed at 18 months of age for more definitive diagnosis.

TREATMENT: Children with a diagnosis of HCV infection should be referred to a pediatric infectious diseases specialist or gastroenterologist for clinical monitoring and consideration for treatment. A number of highly effective interferon-free DAA drug regimens have been approved by the FDA, an increasing number of which are now approved in children as young as 3 years (see Non-HIV Antiviral Drugs, p 930). All HCV-infected children 3 years or older should be treated with FDA age-approved antiviral medications. Because this is a rapidly changing field, the American Association for the Study of Liver Disease and the Infectious Diseases Society of America are continually updating recommended antiviral drug treatment for adults (**www.hcvguidelines.org**) and children (**www. hcvguidelines.org/unique-populations/children**).

Management of Chronic HCV Infection. Because of the very high rate of severe hepatitis in patients with HCV-associated chronic liver disease, all patients with chronic HCV infection should be immunized against hepatitis A and hepatitis B. Risk of liver-related morbidity and mortality, including cirrhosis and primary hepatocellular carcinoma, increases with advancing age in individuals with chronic HCV infection. Among children, progression of liver disease appears to be accelerated when comorbid conditions, including HIV, childhood cancer, iron overload, or thalassemia, are present. Pediatricians should be alert for conditions that may worsen liver disease in patients with HCV infection, such as concomitant infections, alcohol abuse, and concomitant use of prescription and nonprescription drugs, such as acetaminophen, some antiretroviral agents, and herbal medications. Children with chronic infection should be followed closely, including sequential monitoring of serum alanine aminotransferase concentrations, because of the potential for chronic liver disease. Evidence-based, consensus recommendations from the Infectious Diseases Society of America, the American Association for the Study of Liver Diseases, and the International Antiviral Society–USA for screening, treatment, and management of patients with HCV, including children and pregnant women, can be found online (**www.hcvguidelines.org**).

ISOLATION OF THE HOSPITALIZED PATIENT: Standard precautions are recommended.

CONTROL MEASURES:

Care of Exposed People.

Immunoprophylaxis. Use of Immune Globulin for postexposure prophylaxis against HCV infection is not recommended based on lack of clinical efficacy in humans and data from animal studies. Potential donors of immune globulin are screened for antibody to HCV and excluded from donation if positive, so Immune Globulin preparations are devoid of anti-HCV antibody.

Breastfeeding. Transmission of HCV by breastfeeding has not been documented. According to current guidelines of the US Public Health Service, maternal HCV infection is not a contraindication to breastfeeding. Mothers who are HCV infected and choose to breastfeed should interrupt breastfeeding temporarily if their nipples are bleeding or cracked and can consider expressing and discarding their milk until the nipples are healed. Once the nipples no longer are cracked or bleeding, HCV-infected mothers may resume breastfeeding.

Child Care. Exclusion of children with HCV infection from out-of-home child care is not indicated.

Serologic Testing for HCV Infection.

Universal Testing Recommendations.

- Individuals 18 years or older should be tested at least once in their lifetime, except in settings where the prevalence of HCV infection is <0.1%, in which case testing is not recommended.
- Pregnant women (during each pregnancy), except in settings where prevalence of HCV infection is <0.1%.

People Who Have Risk Factors for HCV Infection.

In addition to the universal testing recommendations above, HCV testing is recommended for anyone at increased risk for HCV infection and other populations, including[1,2,3,4]:

- Children born to HCV-positive mothers;
- People who have ever injected drugs, including those who injected only once many years ago;
- Recipients of clotting factor concentrates made before 1987;
- Recipients of blood transfusions or solid organ transplants before July 1992;
- Patients who have ever received long-term hemodialysis treatment;
- People with known exposures to HCV, such as
  - ◆ Health care workers after needlesticks involving HCV-positive blood;
  - ◆ Recipients of blood or organs from a donor who later tested HCV-positive;
- All people with HIV infection (at least yearly);
- Patients with signs or symptoms of liver disease (eg, abnormal liver enzyme test results);
- Incarcerated people; and
- People who use intranasal illicit drugs or received tattoos from unregulated settings; and
- Any person who requests hepatitis C testing, regardless of disclosure of risk, because many people might be reluctant to disclose stigmatizing risks.

Pregnant Women. Pregnant women should be tested for HCV infection during each pregnancy, except in settings where prevalence of HCV infection is <0.1%.

Children Born to Women With HCV Infection. Children born to HCV-infected women should be tested for HCV infection, because 5% to 6% of these children will acquire the infection.

---

[1]Centers for Disease Control and Prevention. Recommendations for the identification of chronic hepatitis C virus infection among persons born during 1945–1965. *MMWR Recomm Rep.* 2012;61(RR–4):1-32

[2]Centers for Disease Control and Prevention. Guidelines for prevention and treatment of opportunistic infections in HIV-infected adults and adolescents: recommendations from CDC, the National Institutes of Health, and the HIV Medicine Association of the Infectious Diseases Society of America. *MMWR Recomm Rep.* 2009;58(RR–4):1-207

[3]Panel on Opportunistic Infections in HIV-Exposed and HIV-Infected Children. Guidelines for the Prevention and Treatment of Opportunistic Infections in HIV-Exposed and HIV-Infected Children. Department of Health and Human Services. Available at: **https://clinicalinfo.hiv.gov/sites/default/files/inline-files/oi_guidelines_pediatrics.pdf**

[4]Moorman AC, de Perio MA, Goldschmidt R, et al. Testing and clinical management of health care personnel potentially exposed to hepatitis C virus—CDC guidance, United States, 2020. *MMWR Recomm Rep.* 2020;69(RR-6):1-8

Adoptees. See Medical Evaluation for Infectious Diseases for Internationally Adopted, Refugee, and Immigrant Children (p 158) for specific situations when serologic testing is warranted.

Counseling of Patients With HCV Infection. All people with HCV infection should be considered infectious, should be informed of the possibility of transmission to others, and should refrain from donating blood, organs, tissues, or semen and from sharing toothbrushes and razors.

Infected people should be counseled to avoid hepatotoxic agents, including medications, and should be informed of the risks of excessive alcohol ingestion. All patients with chronic HCV infection should be immunized against hepatitis A and hepatitis B.

Changes in sexual practices of infected people with a long-term, monogamous partner are not recommended, although these couples should be informed of possible risks and use of precautions to prevent transmission. People with multiple sexual partners should be advised to decrease number of partners and to use condoms to prevent transmission. No data exist to support counseling a woman against pregnancy. Currently, HCV antiviral therapy is not recommended during pregnancy.

The CDC Division of Viral Hepatitis maintains a website (**www.cdc.gov/hepatitis/HCV**) with information on hepatitis for health care professionals and the public, including specific information for people who have received blood transfusions before 1992. Information also can be obtained from the National Institutes of Health Web site (**www.niddk.nih.gov/health-information/liver-disease/viral-hepatitis/hepatitis-c**).

Hepatitis D

CLINICAL MANIFESTATIONS: Hepatitis D virus (HDV) causes infection only in people with acute or chronic hepatitis B virus (HBV) infection. HDV requires hepatitis B surface antigen (HBsAg) for virion assembly and secretion. The importance of HDV infection lies in its ability to convert an asymptomatic or mild chronic HBV infection into more severe or rapidly progressive disease. HDV infection can be acquired either simultaneously with HBV infection (coinfection) or subsequent to HBV infection among people already positive for HBsAg (superinfection). Coinfection is indistinguishable from acute hepatitis B and is usually transient and self-limited, whereas superinfection often results in chronic illness. Acute infection with HDV usually causes an illness indistinguishable from other viral hepatitis infections, except that the likelihood of fulminant hepatitis can be as high as 5%.

ETIOLOGY: Hepatitis delta virus is the only species in the *Deltavirus* genus and possesses the smallest genome of any human pathogen. HDV has a circular, negative sense ssRNA genome and approximately 70 copies of hepatitis delta antigen, all of which is coated with HBsAg.

EPIDEMIOLOGY: HDV infection is present worldwide, in all age groups. Over the past 20 years, HDV prevalence has varied geographically, with decreases in some regions attributable to long-standing hepatitis B vaccination programs and increases in others related to changing migration patterns. HDV remains a significant health problem in resource-limited countries. At least 8 genotypes of HDV have been described, each with a typical geographic pattern, with genotype 1 being found worldwide. Acquisition of HDV is by parenteral transmission from infected blood or body fluids such as through injection drug use or sexual contact. Transmission from mother to newborn infant is uncommon.

Intrafamilial spread can occur among people with chronic HBV infection. High-prevalence areas include parts of Eastern Europe, South America, Africa, Central Asia, and the Middle East, although considerable heterogeneity exists within specific countries. HDV infection is found in the United States most commonly in people who use injection drugs and people who have emigrated from areas with endemic HDV infection.

The **incubation period** for HDV superinfection is approximately 2 to 8 weeks. When HBV and HDV viruses infect simultaneously, the incubation period is similar to that of HBV (45 to 160 days; average 90 days).

DIAGNOSTIC TESTS: People with chronic HBV infection are at risk of HDV superinfection. Because of the dependence of HDV on HBV, the diagnosis of hepatitis D cannot be made in the absence of markers of HBV infection. Testing should be considered for patients with unusually severe or protracted hepatitis and for hepatitis B surface antigen (HBsAg)-positive patients with specific risk factors, such as emigration from a region with endemic infection (such as Eastern European countries, Mediterranean countries, and countries in Central America), injection drug use, men who have sex with men, coinfection with hepatitis C virus (HCV) or human immunodeficiency virus (HIV), or high-risk sexual practices. Testing for immunoglobulin G antibodies against HDV (IgG anti-HDV) using a commercially available test can be performed as an initial screening test. Anti-HDV becomes detectable several weeks after illness onset. In a person with anti-HDV, absence of IgM hepatitis B core antibody (IgM anti-HBc), which is indicative of chronic HBV infection, suggests that the person has both chronic HBV infection and superinfection with HDV. Because IgG anti-HDV is detectable during acute, chronic, and resolved phases of infection, testing for HDV RNA testing is required for diagnosing current HDV infection and for monitoring antiviral therapy. Patients with circulating HDV RNA should be staged for severity of liver disease, have surveillance for development of hepatocellular carcinoma, and be considered for treatment. Tests for IgM anti-HDV and hepatitis D antigen are of lesser utility because of low sensitivity and specificity.

TREATMENT: HDV has proven difficult to treat, and there are no approved therapies. Data suggest pegylated interferon-alfa may result in up to 40% of patients having a sustained response to treatment. Clinical trials suggest at least a year of therapy may be associated with sustained responses, and longer courses may be warranted if the patient is able to tolerate therapy. Novel therapies under investigation in adults include viral entry inhibitors, assembly inhibitors, and HBsAg secretion inhibitors. Liver transplantation in individuals with liver failure attributable to coinfections of HBV and HDV has been reported.

ISOLATION OF THE HOSPITALIZED PATIENT: Standard precautions are recommended.

CONTROL MEASURES: The same control and preventive measures used for HBV infection are indicated. Because HDV cannot be transmitted in the absence of HBV infection, HBV immunization protects against HDV infection. People with chronic HBV infection should take extreme care to avoid exposure to HDV.

Hepatitis E

CLINICAL MANIFESTATIONS: Hepatitis E virus (HEV) infection can be asymptomatic or can cause an acute illness with symptoms including jaundice, malaise, anorexia, fever, abdominal pain, and arthralgia. Disease is more common among young adults than among children and is more severe in pregnant women, in whom mortality rates can reach 10% to 25% if infection occurs during the third trimester. Chronic HEV infection is rare and, to date, has only been reported in more developed countries, mostly among organ transplant recipients with immunosuppression. Approximately 60% of recipients of solid organ transplants fail to clear the virus and develop chronic hepatitis, and 10% will develop cirrhosis.

ETIOLOGY: HEV is a spherical, nonenveloped, positive-sense, single-stranded RNA virus. HEV is classified in the genus *Orthohepevirus* of the family *Hepeviridae*. *Orthohepevirus* A comprises 8 genotypes (based on phylogenetic analyses); these may infect humans (HEV-1, -2, -3, -4, and -7), pigs (HEV-3 and -4), rabbits (HEV-3), wild boars (HEV-3, -4, -5, and -6), mongooses (HEV-3), deer (HEV-3), yaks (HEV-4), and camels (HEV-7 and -8). There is also a report of human infection caused by *Orthohepevirus* C, which is usually found in rats and ferrets.

EPIDEMIOLOGY: An estimated 20 million HEV infections occur each year worldwide, resulting in 3.4 million cases of acute hepatitis. A recent WHO estimate suggested that there were 44 000 deaths attributable to hepatitis E in 2015. Almost all HEV infections occur in resource-limited countries, where ingestion of fecally contaminated water is the most common route of HEV transmission, and large waterborne outbreaks occur frequently. HEV infection has been reported throughout the world, including Africa and Asia. Foodborne infection has occurred sporadically in developed countries following consumption of uncooked or undercooked pork or deer meat or sausage as well as from shellfish. Person-to-person transmission appears to be much less efficient than with hepatitis A virus but occurs sporadically and in outbreak settings. Mother-to-infant transmission of HEV, mainly HEV-1, occurs frequently and accounts for substantial fetal loss and perinatal mortality, but its contribution to overall disease burden appears to be small. It is unclear whether breastfeeding is a potential route of HEV transmission; there is sufficient concern to discourage breastfeeding among confirmed HEV-infected mothers until further data are available.

HEV also is transmitted through blood and blood product transfusion. Transfusion-transmitted hepatitis E occurs primarily in countries with endemic disease and also is reported in areas without endemic infection. Serologic studies have demonstrated that approximately 6% of the population of the United States has immunoglobulin (Ig) G antibodies against HEV, but symptomatic HEV infection in the United States is uncommon and generally occurs in people who acquire HEV-1 infection while traveling in countries with endemic HEV infection. A number of people without a travel history have been diagnosed with acute hepatitis E, and evidence for the infection should be sought in patients with acute hepatitis of unknown etiology. Hepatitis E may masquerade as drug-induced liver injury.

The **incubation period** is 2 to 10 weeks.

DIAGNOSTIC TESTS: HEV infection should be considered in any person with symptoms of viral hepatitis who has traveled to or from a region with endemic hepatitis E or from a region where an outbreak has been identified and who tests negative for serologic markers of hepatitis A, B, C, and other hepatotropic viruses. Testing for anti-HEV IgM and IgG is available through some research and commercial reference laboratories. Because anti-HEV assays are not approved by the US Food and Drug Administration and their performance characteristics are not well defined, results should be interpreted with caution, particularly in cases lacking a discrete onset of illness associated with jaundice or with no recent history of travel to a country with endemic HEV transmission. Definitive diagnosis can be made by demonstrating viral RNA in serum or stool samples by means of reverse transcriptase-polymerase chain reaction assay, which is available at a limited number of commercial laboratories and with prior approval through the Centers for Disease Control and Prevention. Because virus circulates in the body for a relatively short period, the inability to detect HEV in serum or stool does not eliminate the possibility that the person was infected with HEV.

TREATMENT: Management is supportive. Some case reports and case series have indicated that reduction of immunosuppression and/or use of antiviral drugs, such as ribavirin, with or without interferon-alpha, may result in viral clearance in immunocompromised patients with chronic hepatitis E, but no randomized controlled clinical trials have been performed.

ISOLATION OF THE HOSPITALIZED PATIENT: In addition to standard precautions, contact precautions are recommended for diapered and incontinent patients for the duration of illness.

CONTROL MEASURES: Provision of safe water and improved hygiene practices are the most effective prevention measures. A safe and effective recombinant HEV vaccine has been approved for use by the Chinese Food and Drug Administration but is not approved for use in the United States. In 2015, the World Health Organization published a position paper on hepatitis E vaccine development (**www.who.int/wer/2015/wer9018. pdf?ua=1**) in which it noted that immunogenicity and safety of the vaccine have not been established in people younger than 16 years or in pregnant women.

Herpes Simplex

CLINICAL MANIFESTATIONS:

Neonatal. In newborn infants, herpes simplex virus (HSV) infection can manifest as: (1) disseminated disease involving multiple organs, most prominently liver and lungs, and in 60% to 75% of cases also involving the central nervous system (CNS); (2) localized CNS disease, with or without skin, eye, or mouth involvement (CNS disease); or (3) disease localized to the skin, eyes, and/or mouth (SEM disease). Approximately 25% of cases of neonatal HSV manifest as disseminated disease, 30% manifest as CNS disease, and 45% manifest as SEM disease. Both HSV type 1 (HSV-1) and type 2 (HSV-2) can cause any of these manifestations of neonatal HSV disease. In the absence of skin lesions, the diagnosis of neonatal HSV infection is challenging and requires a high index of suspicion. More than 80% of neonates with SEM disease have skin vesicles; those without vesicles have infection limited to the eyes and/or oral mucosa. Approximately two thirds of neonates with disseminated or CNS disease have skin lesions, but these lesions may not be present at the time of onset of symptoms. Disseminated infection should be considered in neonates with sepsis syndrome with negative bacteriologic culture results, severe liver dysfunction, consumptive coagulopathy, or suspected viral pneumonia, especially hemorrhagic pneumonia. HSV should be considered as a causative agent in neonates with fever (especially within the first 3 weeks of life), a vesicular rash, or abnormal cerebrospinal fluid (CSF) findings (especially in the presence of seizures or during a time of year when enteroviruses are not circulating in the community). Although asymptomatic HSV infection is common in older children, it rarely, if ever, occurs in neonates. Recurrent skin lesions are common in surviving infants, occurring in approximately 50% of survivors, often within 1 to 2 weeks of completing the initial treatment course of parenteral acyclovir.

Initial signs of HSV infection can occur anytime between birth and approximately 6 weeks of age, although almost all infected infants develop clinical disease within the first month of life. Infants with disseminated disease and SEM disease have an earlier age of onset, typically presenting between the first and second weeks of life; infants with CNS disease usually present with illness between the second and third weeks of life.

Children Beyond the Neonatal Period and Adolescents. Most primary HSV childhood infections beyond the neonatal period are asymptomatic. Gingivostomatitis, which is the most common clinical manifestation of HSV during childhood, is almost exclusively caused by HSV-1 and is characterized by fever, irritability, tender submandibular adenopathy, and an ulcerative enanthem involving the gingiva and mucous membranes of the mouth, often with perioral vesicular lesions.

Genital herpes is characterized by vesicular or ulcerative lesions of the male or female genitalia, perineum, or perianal areas. Until the last 2 decades, genital herpes most often was caused by HSV-2, but likely because of an increase in oral sexual practices by adolescents and young adults, HSV-1 now accounts for more than half of all cases in the United States. Most cases of primary genital herpes infection in males and females are asymptomatic, so they are not recognized by the infected person or diagnosed by a health care professional.

In immunocompromised patients, severe local lesions and, less commonly, disseminated HSV infection with generalized vesicular skin lesions and visceral involvement can occur.

After primary infection, HSV persists for life in a latent form. Reactivation of latent virus most commonly is asymptomatic. When symptomatic, recurrent HSV-1 herpes labialis manifests as single or grouped vesicles in the perioral region, usually on the vermilion border of the lips (typically called "cold sores" or "fever blisters"). Symptomatic recurrent genital herpes manifests as vesicular lesions on the penis, scrotum, vulva, cervix, buttocks, perianal areas, thighs, or back. Among immunocompromised patients, genital HSV-2 recurrences are more frequent and of longer duration. Recurrences may be heralded by a prodrome of burning or itching at the site of an incipient recurrence, identification of which can be useful in instituting early antiviral therapy.

Ocular manifestations of HSV include conjunctivitis and keratitis that can result from primary or recurrent HSV infection. In addition, HSV can cause acute retinal necrosis and uveitis.

Eczema herpeticum can develop in patients with atopic dermatitis who are infected with HSV and can be difficult to distinguish from poorly controlled atopic dermatitis. Examination may reveal skin with punched-out erosions, hemorrhagic crusts, and/or vesicular lesions. Pustular lesions attributable to bacterial superinfection also may occur. Herpetic whitlow consists of single or multiple vesicular lesions on the distal parts of fingers. Wrestlers can develop herpes gladiatorum if they become infected with HSV-1. HSV infection can be a precipitating factor of other cutaneous manifestations, such as erythema multiforme. Recurrent erythema multiforme often is caused by symptomatic or asymptomatic HSV recurrences.

HSV encephalitis (HSE) occurs in children beyond the neonatal period, in adolescents, and in adults and can result from primary or recurrent HSV-1 infection. One fifth of HSE cases occur in the pediatric age group. Symptoms and signs usually include fever, alterations in the state of consciousness, personality changes, seizures, and focal neurologic findings. Encephalitis commonly has an acute onset with a fulminant course, leading to coma and death in untreated patients. HSE usually involves the temporal lobe, and magnetic resonance imaging is the most sensitive imaging modality to detect this. CSF pleocytosis with a predominance of lymphocytes is typical. Historically, erythrocytes in the CSF were considered suggestive of HSE, but with earlier diagnosis (prior to development of a hemorrhagic encephalitis), this finding is rare today.

HSV infection also can manifest as mild, self-limited aseptic meningitis, usually associated with genital HSV-2 infection. Unusual CNS manifestations of HSV include Bell's palsy, atypical pain syndromes, trigeminal neuralgia, ascending myelitis, transverse myelitis, postinfectious encephalomyelitis, and recurrent (Mollaret) meningitis.

ETIOLOGY: HSVs are large, enveloped, double-stranded DNA viruses. They are members of the family *Herpesviridae* and, along with varicella-zoster virus (human herpesvirus 3), are the subfamily *Alphaherpesviridae*. Two distinct HSV types exist: HSV-1 and HSV-2. Infections with HSV-1 traditionally involve the face and skin above the waist; however, an increasing number of genital herpes cases are attributable to HSV-1. Infections with HSV-2 usually involve the genitalia and skin below the waist in sexually active adolescents and adults. Both HSV-1 and HSV-2 cause herpetic disease in neonates. HSV-1 and HSV-2 establish latency following primary infection, with periodic reactivation to cause recurrent symptomatic disease or asymptomatic viral shedding. Genital HSV-2 infection is more likely to recur than is genital HSV-1 infection.

EPIDEMIOLOGY: HSV infections can be transmitted from people who are symptomatic or asymptomatic with primary or recurrent infections.

Neonatal. The incidence of neonatal HSV infection in the United States has increased over the past 2 decades to approximately 1 in 2000 live births. HSV is transmitted to a neonate most often during birth through an infected maternal genital tract but can be caused by an ascending infection through ruptured or apparently intact amniotic membranes. Other less common sources of neonatal infection include postnatal transmission from a parent, sibling, or other caregiver, most often from a nongenital infection (eg, mouth or hands), transmission from the mouth of a religious circumciser ("mohel") to the infant penis during ritual Jewish circumcisions that include direct orogenital suction (metzitzah b'peh), and intrauterine infection causing congenital malformations.

The risk of transmission to a neonate born to a mother who acquires primary genital HSV infection near the time of delivery is estimated to be 25% to 60%. In contrast, the risk to a neonate born to a mother shedding HSV as a result of reactivation of infection acquired during the first half of pregnancy or earlier is less than 2%. More than three quarters of infants who contract HSV infection are born to women with no history or clinical findings suggestive of genital HSV infection during or preceding pregnancy. Therefore, a lack of history of maternal genital HSV infection does not preclude a diagnosis of neonatal HSV disease.

Children Beyond the Neonatal Period and Adolescents. Patients with primary gingivostomatitis or genital herpes usually shed virus for at least 1 week and occasionally for several weeks. Patients with symptomatic recurrences shed virus for a shorter period, typically

3 to 4 days. Intermittent asymptomatic reactivation of oral and genital herpes is common and likely occurs throughout the remainder of a person's life. The greatest concentration of virus is shed during symptomatic primary infections and the lowest during asymptomatic reactivation.

Several single gene defects have been reported that predispose to HSE. The ones characterized so far are mainly involved in the toll-like receptor 3 (TLR3) pathway, including deficiencies of TLR3 itself or in downstream signal transduction pathways (UNC93B1, TRIF/TICAM1, TRAF, TBK1) or deficiencies in innate/type 1 interferon pathways (IFN-alpha/-beta, IFN-lamba, STAT1, IRF3).

The **incubation period** for HSV infection occurring beyond the neonatal period ranges from 2 days to 2 weeks.

DIAGNOSTIC TESTS: HSV grows readily in traditional cell culture. Special transport media are available that allow transport to local or regional laboratories for culture. Cytopathogenic effects typical of HSV infection usually are observed 1 to 3 days after inoculation. Methods of culture confirmation include fluorescent antibody staining, enzyme immunoassays (EIAs), and monolayer culture with typing. Cultures that remain negative by day 5 likely will remain negative. A viral isolate by culture is required if antiviral susceptibility studies are to be performed.

Polymerase chain reaction (PCR) assay usually can detect HSV DNA in CSF from neonates with CNS infection (neonatal HSV CNS disease) and from older children and adults with HSE and is the diagnostic method of choice for CNS HSV involvement. PCR assay of CSF can yield negative results in cases of HSE, especially early in the disease course. In difficult cases in which HSV central nervous system disease is expected but repeated CSF PCR assay results are negative, histologic examination and viral culture of a brain tissue biopsy specimen is the most definitive method of confirming the diagnosis of HSE. Detection of intrathecal antibody against HSV also can assist in the diagnosis. Viral cultures of CSF from a patient with HSE usually are negative.

For diagnosis of neonatal HSV infection, all of the following specimens should be obtained for each patient: (1) swab specimens from the conjunctivae, mouth, nasopharynx, and anus ("surface specimens") for HSV culture (if available) or PCR assay (can use a separate swab for each site, or a single swab starting with the conjunctivae); (2) specimens of skin vesicles for HSV culture (if available) or PCR assay; (3) CSF sample for HSV PCR assay; (4) whole blood sample for HSV PCR assay; and (5) whole blood sample for measuring alanine aminotransferase (ALT). The performance characteristics of PCR assay on skin and mucosal specimens from neonates has not been studied. Positive cultures obtained from any of the surface sites more than 12 to 24 hours after birth indicate viral replication and are, therefore, suggestive of infant infection, and therefore risk of progression to neonatal HSV disease, rather than merely contamination after intrapartum exposure. As with any PCR assay, false-negative and false-positive results can occur. Any of the 3 manifestations of neonatal HSV disease (disseminated, CNS, SEM) can have associated viremia, so a positive whole blood PCR assay result does not define an infant as having disseminated HSV and, therefore, should not be used to determine extent of disease and duration of treatment. Likewise, no data exist to support use of serial blood PCR assays to monitor response to therapy. Rapid diagnostic techniques are available, such as direct fluorescent antibody staining of vesicle scrapings or EIA detection of HSV antigens. These techniques are as specific but less sensitive than culture.

HSV PCR assay and cell culture are the preferred tests for detecting HSV in genital lesions. The sensitivity of viral culture is low, especially for recurrent lesions, and declines rapidly as lesions begin to heal. PCR assays for HSV DNA are more sensitive and increasingly are used in many settings. Failure to detect HSV in genital lesions by culture or PCR assay does not rule out HSV infection, because viral shedding is intermittent.

Type-specific antibodies to HSV develop during the first several weeks after infection and persist indefinitely. Approximately 20% of HSV-2 first episode patients seroconvert by 10 days, and the median time to seroconversion is 21 days with a type-specific enzyme-linked immunosorbent assay (ELISA); more than 95% of people seroconvert by 12 weeks following infection. Although type-specific HSV-2 antibody usually indicates previous anogenital infection, the presence of HSV-1 antibody does not distinguish anogenital from orolabial infection reliably because a substantial proportion of initial genital infections and virtually all initial orolabial infections are caused by HSV-1. Serologic testing is not useful in neonates. IgM testing for HSV-1 or HSV-2 is not useful because of the lack of a reliable commercially available IgM assay.

TREATMENT: For recommended antiviral dosages and duration of therapy with systemically administered acyclovir, valacyclovir, and famciclovir for different HSV infections, see Non-HIV Antiviral Drugs (p 930). In pediatric patients who cannot swallow large pills, instructions for preparing a compounded liquid suspension of valacyclovir with a 28-day refrigerated shelf-life are provided in the drug's package insert.

Neonatal. Parenteral acyclovir is the treatment for neonatal HSV infections. The dosage of acyclovir is 60 mg/kg per day in 3 divided doses (20 mg/kg/dose), administered intravenously for 14 days in SEM disease and for a minimum of 21 days in CNS disease or disseminated disease. All infants with CNS involvement should have a repeat lumbar puncture performed near the end of therapy to document that the CSF is negative for HSV DNA on PCR assay; in the unlikely event that the PCR result remains positive near the end of a 21-day treatment course, intravenous acyclovir should be administered for another week, with repeat CSF PCR assay performed near the end of the extended treatment period and another week of parenteral therapy if it remains positive. Parenteral antiviral therapy should not be stopped until the CSF PCR result for HSV DNA is negative. Consultation with a pediatric infectious diseases specialist is warranted in these cases.

Infants surviving neonatal HSV disease of any classification (disseminated, CNS, or SEM) should receive oral acyclovir suppression at 300 mg/m^2/dose, administered 3 times daily for 6 months after the completion of parenteral therapy for acute disease; the dose should be adjusted monthly to account for growth. Absolute neutrophil counts should be assessed at 2 and 4 weeks after initiating suppressive acyclovir therapy and then monthly during the treatment period. Longer durations or higher doses of antiviral suppression do not further improve neurodevelopmental outcomes. Valacyclovir has not been studied for longer than 5 days in young infants, so it should not be used routinely for antiviral suppression in this age group.

All infants with neonatal HSV disease, regardless of disease classification, should have an ophthalmologic examination and neuroimaging to establish baseline brain anatomy; magnetic resonance imaging is the most sensitive imaging modality but may require sedation, so computed tomography or ultrasonography of the head are acceptable alternatives. Topical ophthalmic drug (1% trifluridine or 0.15% ganciclovir), in addition to parenteral antiviral therapy, may be indicated in infants with ocular involvement attributable to HSV infection, including a positive virologic test result from a conjunctival swab sample, and an ophthalmologist should be involved in the management and treatment of acute neonatal ocular HSV disease. The older topical antiviral agents vidarabine and iododeoxyuridine no longer are available in the United States.

Genital Infection.

Primary. Oral acyclovir therapy shortens the duration of illness and viral shedding. Valacyclovir and famciclovir are not more effective than acyclovir but offer the advantage of less frequent dosing. Intravenous acyclovir is indicated for patients with a severe or complicated primary infection that requires hospitalization. Treatment of primary herpetic lesions does not affect the subsequent frequency or severity of recurrences. Antiviral drug dosages for primary genital HSV infection are found on p 930 in Table 4.10, Non-HIV Antiviral Drugs.

Recurrent. Antiviral therapy for recurrent genital herpes can be administered either episodically to ameliorate or shorten the duration of lesions or continuously as suppressive therapy to decrease the frequency of recurrences. Many patients benefit from antiviral therapy, and treatment options should be discussed with patients with recurrent disease. Acyclovir, valacyclovir, and famciclovir have been approved for suppression of genital herpes in immunocompetent adults. Acyclovir and valacyclovir are most commonly used in pregnant women with first-episode genital herpes or severe recurrent herpes, and acyclovir should be administered intravenously to pregnant women with severe HSV infection. Antiviral drug dosages for episodic and suppressive treatment of recurrent genital HSV infection are found on p 930 in Table 4.10, Non-HIV Antiviral Drugs.

Mucocutaneous.

Immunocompromised Hosts. Intravenous acyclovir is effective for treatment of mucocutaneous HSV infections. Acyclovir-resistant strains of HSV have been isolated from immunocompromised people receiving prolonged treatment with acyclovir. Foscarnet is the drug of choice for acyclovir-resistant HSV isolates.

Immunocompetent Hosts. Limited data are available on effects of acyclovir on the course of primary or recurrent nongenital mucocutaneous HSV infections in immunocompetent hosts. Therapeutic benefit has been noted in a limited number of children with primary gingivostomatitis treated with oral acyclovir. A small therapeutic benefit of oral acyclovir therapy has been demonstrated among adults with recurrent herpes labialis. Famciclovir or valacyclovir also can be considered. Antiviral drug dosages for episodic and suppressive treatment of recurrent orolabial HSV infection are found on p 932, 935, and 945 in Table 4.10, Non-HIV Antiviral Drugs.

Other HSV Infections.

Central Nervous System. Patients with HSE should be treated for 21 days with intravenous acyclovir. Use of concomitant corticosteroids has not been adequately studied in people and is not routinely recommended.

Ocular. Treatment of eye lesions should be undertaken in consultation with an ophthalmologist. Several topical drugs, such as 1% trifluridine and 0.15% ganciclovir, have proven efficacy for superficial keratitis. Topical corticosteroids administered without concomitant antiviral therapy are contraindicated in suspected HSV conjunctivitis; however, ophthalmologists may choose to use corticosteroids in conjunction with antiviral drugs to treat locally invasive infections. For children with recurrent ocular lesions, oral suppressive therapy with acyclovir may be of benefit and may be indicated for months or even years.

ISOLATION OF THE HOSPITALIZED PATIENT: In addition to standard precautions, the following recommendations should be followed.

Neonates With HSV Infection. Neonates with HSV infection should be hospitalized and managed with contact precautions if mucocutaneous lesions are present.

Neonates Exposed to HSV During Delivery. Infants born to women with active genital HSV lesions should be managed with contact precautions during the incubation period. The risk of HSV infection in infants born to mothers with a history of recurrent genital herpes who have no genital lesions at delivery is low, so special precautions are not necessary. Specific management options for neonates born to women with active genital HSV lesions are detailed in "Prevention of Neonatal Infection."

Postpartum Women With HSV Infection. Women with active HSV lesions should be instructed about the importance of careful hand hygiene before and after caring for their infants. A mother with herpes labialis or stomatitis should wear a disposable surgical mask when touching the newborn infant until the lesions have crusted. The mother should not kiss or nuzzle the newborn until lesions have cleared. Herpetic lesions on other skin sites should be covered.

Breastfeeding is acceptable if no lesions are present on the breasts and if active lesions elsewhere on the mother are covered (see Breastfeeding and Human Milk, p 107).

Children With Mucocutaneous HSV Infection. Contact precautions are recommended for patients with severe mucocutaneous HSV infection. Patients with localized recurrent lesions should be managed with standard precautions.

Patients With HSV Infection of the CNS. Standard precautions are recommended for patients with infection limited to the CNS.

CONTROL MEASURES:

Prevention of Neonatal Infection.

During Pregnancy. The American College of Obstetricians and Gynecologists recommends that women with active recurrent genital herpes be offered suppressive antiviral therapy at or beyond 36 weeks of gestation. However, cases of neonatal HSV disease have occurred among infants born to women who received such antiviral prophylaxis.

Care of Newborn Infants Whose Mothers Have Active Genital Lesions at Delivery. The risk of transmitting HSV to the newborn infant during delivery is influenced directly by the mother's classification of HSV infection (Table 3.23); women with primary genital HSV infections who are shedding HSV at delivery are 10 to 30 times more likely to transmit the virus to their newborn infants, compared with women with a recurrent genital infection. With the commercial availability of serologic tests that can reliably distinguish type-specific HSV antibodies, the means to further refine management of asymptomatic neonates delivered to women with active genital HSV lesions now is possible. The American Academy of Pediatrics developed algorithms (Fig 3.6 and 3.7) addressing evaluation and management of asymptomatic neonates following vaginal or cesarean delivery to women with active genital HSV lesions.[1] The algorithms are intended to outline one approach to the management of these neonates and may not be feasible in settings with limited access to PCR assays for HSV DNA or to type-specific serologic tests. If, at any point during the evaluation outlined in the evaluation algorithm (Fig 3.6), an infant develops symptoms that

---

[1]Kimberlin DW, Baley J; American Academy of Pediatrics, Committee on Infectious Diseases. Guidance on management of asymptomatic neonates born to women with active genital herpes lesions. *Pediatrics.* 2013;131(2):e635-e646

Table 3.23. Maternal Infection Classification by Genital HSV Viral Type and Maternal Type-Specific Serologic Test Results[a]

Classification of Maternal Infection	PCR/Culture From Genital Lesion	Maternal HSV-1 and HSV-2 IgG Type-Specific Antibody Status
Documented first-episode primary infection	Positive, either virus	Both negative
Documented first-episode nonprimary infection	Positive for HSV-1	Positive for HSV-2 AND negative for HSV-1
	Positive for HSV-2	Positive for HSV-1 AND negative for HSV-2
Assumed first-episode (primary or nonprimary) infection	Positive for HSV-1 OR HSV-2	Not available
	Negative OR not available[b]	Negative for HSV-1 and/or HSV-2, OR not available
Recurrent infection	Positive for HSV-1	Positive for HSV-1
	Positive for HSV-2	Positive for HSV-2

HSV indicates herpes simplex virus; PCR, polymerase chain reaction (assay); IgG, immunoglobulin G.
[a]To be used for women without a clinical history of genital herpes.
[b]When a genital lesion is strongly suspicious for HSV, clinical judgment should supersede the virologic test results for the conservative purposes of this neonatal management algorithm. Conversely, if, in retrospect, the genital lesion was not likely to be caused by HSV and the PCR assay result/culture is negative, departure from the evaluation and management in this conservative algorithm may be warranted.

could indicate neonatal HSV disease (eg, fever, hypothermia, lethargy, irritability, vesicular rash, seizures, etc), a full diagnostic evaluation should be undertaken and intravenous acyclovir therapy should be initiated. In applying this algorithm, obstetric and pediatric providers will need to work closely with their diagnostic laboratories to ensure that serologic and virologic testing is available and turnaround times are acceptable. In situations in which this is not possible, the approach detailed in the algorithm will have limited, and perhaps no, applicability.

Care of Newborn Infants Whose Mothers Have a History of Genital Herpes But No Active Genital Lesions at Delivery. An infant whose mother has a history of genital herpes but no genital lesions at delivery should be observed for signs of infection (eg, vesicular lesions of the skin, respiratory distress, seizures, or signs of sepsis) but should not have specimens for surface cultures for HSV obtained at 12 to 24 hours of life and should not receive empiric parenteral acyclovir. Education of parents and caregivers about the signs and symptoms of neonatal HSV infection during the first 6 weeks of life is prudent.

Infected Health Care Professionals. Health care professionals with cold sores who have contact with infants should cover and not touch their lesions and should comply with hand hygiene policies. Transmission of HSV infection from health care professionals with genital lesions is not likely as long as they comply with hand hygiene policies. Health care professionals with an active herpetic whitlow should not have responsibility for direct care of neonates or immunocompromised patients and should wear gloves and use hand hygiene during direct care of other patients.

FIG 3.6. ALGORITHM FOR THE <u>EVALUATION</u> OF ASYMPTOMATIC NEONATES FOLLOWING VAGINAL OR CESAREAN DELIVERY TO WOMEN WITH ACTIVE GENITAL HERPES LESIONS

FIG 3.7. ALGORITHM FOR THE <u>TREATMENT</u> OF ASYMPTOMATIC NEONATES FOLLOWING VAGINAL OR CESAREAN DELIVERY TO WOMEN WITH ACTIVE GENITAL HERPES LESIONS

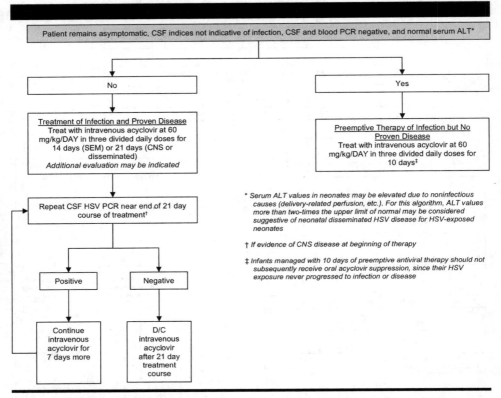

Adapted from Kimberlin DW, Baley J; American Academy of Pediatrics, Committee on Infectious Diseases. Guidance on management of asymptomatic neonates born to women with active genital herpes lesions. *Pediatrics.* 2013;131(2):e635-e646

Infected Household, Family, and Other Close Contacts of Newborn Infants. Household members with herpetic skin or mouth lesions (eg, stomatitis, herpes labialis, or herpetic whitlow) should be counseled about the risk of transmission and should avoid contact of their lesions with neonates by taking the same measures as recommended for infected health care professionals, as well as avoiding kissing and nuzzling the infant while they have active lip/mouth lesions or touching the neonate while they have a herpetic whitlow.

Care of People With Extensive Dermatitis. Patients with dermatitis should not be kissed by people with cold sores or touched by people with herpetic whitlow.

Care of Children With Mucocutaneous Infections Who Attend Child Care or School. Oral HSV infections are common among children who attend child care or school. Most of these infections are asymptomatic, with shedding of virus in saliva occurring in the absence of clinical disease. Only children with HSV gingivostomatitis (ie, primary infection) who do not have control of oral secretions should be excluded from child care. Exclusion of children with cold sores (ie, recurrent infection) from child care or school is not indicated. HSV lesions on other parts of the body should be covered with clothing or a bandage, if practical, for children attending school or day care. Additional control measures include avoiding the sharing of respiratory secretions through contact with objects and washing and sanitizing mouthed toys, bottle nipples, and utensils that have come in contact with saliva.

HSV Infections Among Wrestlers and Rugby Players.[1] HSV-1 has been identified as a cause of outbreak of skin infections among wrestlers (herpes gladiatorum) and rugby players (herpes rugbiorum) on numerous occasions, affecting up to 2.6% of high school and 7.6% of college wrestlers in the United States. During outbreaks, up to 34% of all high school wrestlers have been documented to be infected. The primary risk factor is direct skin-to-skin exposure to opponents with cutaneous lesions.

Three to 8 days of exclusion from competition of infected athletes with primary outbreaks of herpes gladiatorum and herpes rugbiorum will contain more than 90% of outbreaks. Valacyclovir (500 mg, once daily for 7 days), when given within 24 hours of symptoms onset, has been shown to shorten the duration of time until HSV PCR clearance from lesions of adolescent and adult wrestlers with recurrent herpes gladiatorum. Wrestlers receiving valacyclovir should be advised about the importance of good hydration to minimize the likelihood of nephrotoxicity. Efforts to reduce transmission should include (1) examination of wrestlers and rugby players for vesicular or ulcerative lesions on exposed areas of their bodies and around their mouths or eyes before practice or competition by a person familiar with the appearance of mucocutaneous infections (including HSV, herpes zoster, and impetigo); (2) excluding athletes with these lesions from competition until all lesions are fully crusted or production of a physician's written statement indicating that their condition is noninfectious; and (3) cleaning of wrestling mats with a freshly prepared solution of household bleach (one quarter cup of bleach in 1 gallon of water), applied for a minimum contact time of 15 seconds at least daily, and preferably, between matches. Athletes with a history of *recurrent* herpes gladiatorum, herpes rugbiorum, or herpes labialis should be considered for suppressive antiviral therapy, again with cautionary guidance about the importance of maintaining good hydration to avoid the likelihood of nephrotoxicity.

Histoplasmosis

CLINICAL MANIFESTATIONS: *Histoplasma capsulatum* causes symptoms in fewer than 5% of infected people. Clinical manifestations are classified according to site (pulmonary or disseminated), duration (acute, subacute, or chronic), and pattern (primary or reactivation) of infection. Most symptomatic patients have acute pulmonary histoplasmosis, a brief, self-limited illness characterized by fever, chills, nonproductive cough, and malaise. Radiographic findings may consist of hilar or mediastinal adenopathy, or diffuse interstitial or reticulonodular pulmonary infiltrates. Most patients recover without treatment 2 to 3 weeks after onset of symptoms.

Exposure to a large inoculum of conidia can cause severe pulmonary infection associated with high fevers, hypoxemia, diffuse reticulonodular infiltrates, and acute respiratory distress syndrome (ARDS). Mediastinal involvement, a rare complication of pulmonary histoplasmosis, includes mediastinal lymphadenitis, which can cause airway encroachment in young children. Inflammatory syndromes (pericarditis and rheumatologic

---

[1]Davies HD, Jackson MA; American Academy of Pediatrics, Committee on Infectious Diseases. Infectious Diseases Associated With Organized Sports and Outbreak Control. *Pediatrics*. 2017;140(4):e20172477

syndromes) can develop; erythema nodosum can occur in adolescents and adults. Primary cutaneous infections after trauma are rare, and chronic cavitary pulmonary histoplasmosis is extremely rare in children.

Progressive disseminated histoplasmosis (PDH) may occur in otherwise healthy infants and children younger than 2 years or in older children with primary or acquired cellular immune dysfunction. It can be a rapidly progressive illness following acute infection or can be a more chronic, slowly progressive disease. Early manifestations of PDH in children include prolonged fever, failure to thrive, and hepatosplenomegaly; if untreated, malnutrition, diffuse adenopathy, pneumonitis, mucosal ulceration, pancytopenia, disseminated intravascular coagulopathy, and gastrointestinal tract bleeding can ensue. PDH in adults occurs most often in people with underlying immune deficiency (eg, human immunodeficiency virus/acquired immunodeficiency syndrome, solid organ transplant, hematologic malignancy, and biologic response modifiers including tumor necrosis factor antagonists). Central nervous system involvement occurs in 5% to 25% of patients with chronic progressive disease. Chronic PDH generally occurs in adults with immune suppression and is characterized by prolonged fever, night sweats, weight loss, and fatigue; signs include hepatosplenomegaly, mucosal ulcerations, adrenal insufficiency, and pancytopenia. Clinicians should be alert to the risk of disseminated endemic mycoses in patients receiving tumor necrosis factor-alpha antagonists and disease-modifying antirheumatic drugs.

ETIOLOGY: *Histoplasma* strains, which may be classified into at least 7 distinct clades, are thermally dimorphic, endemic fungi that grow in the environment as a spore-bearing mold but convert to the yeast phase at 37°C.

EPIDEMIOLOGY: *H capsulatum* is encountered in most parts of the world (including Africa, the Americas, Asia, and Europe) and is highly endemic in the central and eastern United States, particularly the Mississippi, Ohio, and Missouri River valleys; Central America; the northernmost part of South America; and Argentina. *H capsulatum* var *duboisii* is found only in central and western Africa.

Infection is acquired following inhalation of conidia that are aerosolized by disturbance of soil, especially when contaminated with bat guano or bird droppings. Infections occur sporadically or rarely in point-source epidemics after exposure to activities that disturb contaminated sites. In regions with endemic disease, recreational activities, such as playing in hollow trees and caving, and occupational activities, such as construction, excavation, demolition, farming, and cleaning of contaminated buildings, have been associated with outbreaks. Person-to-person transmission may occur via transplantation of infected organs, vertical transmission, and possibly through exposure to cutaneous lesions. Prior infection confers partial immunity; reinfection can occur but may require a larger inoculum.

The **incubation period** is variable but usually is 1 to 3 weeks.

DIAGNOSTIC TESTS: Detection of *H capsulatum* polysaccharide antigen in serum, urine, bronchoalveolar lavage fluid, or cerebrospinal fluid using a quantitative enzyme immunoassay is the preferred method of testing. Antigen detection is most sensitive for progressive disseminated infections. Combining both urine and serum antigen testing increases the likelihood of antigen detection. Results often are transiently positive early in the course of acute, self-limited pulmonary infections. A negative test result does not exclude infection. If the result initially is positive, the antigen test also is useful for monitoring treatment response and, thereafter, identifying relapse or reinfection. Cross-reactions may occur in patients with dimorphic fungal diseases (eg, blastomycosis, coccidioidomycosis, paracoccidioidomycosis, sporotrichosis, *Emergomyces africanus* disease, and talaromycosis [formerly penicillosis]); clinical and epidemiologic distinctions aid in differentiating these entities.

Antibody detection testing is available and is most useful in patients with subacute or chronic pulmonary disease and central nervous system involvement. Complement fixation and immunodiffusion are available. A fourfold increase in mycelial-phase complement fixation titers or a single titer of ≥1:32 in either test is strong presumptive evidence of active or recent infection in patients exposed to or residing within endemic regions. Cross-reacting antibodies can result most commonly from *Blastomyces* and *Coccidioides* species. The immunodiffusion test is a qualitative method that is more specific, but slightly less sensitive, than the complement fixation test. It detects the H and M glycoproteins of *H capsulatum* found in histoplasmin. The M band develops with acute infection, generally by 6 weeks after infection, is often present in chronic forms of histoplasmosis, and persists for months to years after the infection has resolved. The H band is much less common; is rarely, if ever, found without an M band; and is indicative of chronic or severe acute forms of histoplasmosis. The immunodiffusion assay is approximately 80% sensitive but is more specific than the complement fixation assay. It commonly is used in conjunction with the complement fixation test.

Culture is the definitive method of diagnosis. *H capsulatum* organisms from bone marrow, blood, sputum, and tissue specimens grow in the mycelia (mold) phase on standard mycologic media, including Sabouraud dextrose or potato dextrose agar incubated at 25°C to 30°C in 1 to 6 weeks. The yeast phase of the organism can be recovered on primary culture using enriched media, such as brain-heart infusion agar with blood (BHIB) incubated at 35°C to 37°C. Mycelial-phase organisms in culture can be confirmed as *H capsulatum* by conversion to yeast-phase organisms by repeated passage on BHIB at 35°C to 37°C. The lysis-centrifugation method is preferred for blood and bone marrow cultures. A DNA probe for *H capsulatum* permits rapid identification of cultured isolates. Care should be taken in working with the organism in the laboratory, because mold-phase growth may release large numbers of infectious microconidia into the air.

Demonstration of typical intracellular yeast forms by examination with Wright or Giemsa stains of blood, bone marrow, or bronchoalveolar lavage specimens strongly supports the diagnosis of histoplasmosis when clinical, epidemiologic, and other laboratory studies are compatible.

TREATMENT: Immunocompetent children with uncomplicated or mild-to-moderate acute pulmonary histoplasmosis may not require antifungal therapy, because infection usually is self-limited. If the patient does not improve within 4 weeks, itraconazole should be given for 6 to 12 weeks.

Treatment is imperative for all forms of disseminated histoplasmosis, which can be either an acute (rapid onset and progression, usually in an immunocompromised patient) or chronic (slower evolution, usually in an immunocompetent patient) illness. Treatment with a lipid formulation of amphotericin B is recommended for severe acute pulmonary infection (see Table 4.7, p 909). Methylprednisolone during the first 1 to 2 weeks of therapy may be considered if severe respiratory complications develop but should be used only in conjunction with antifungals.

After clinical improvement occurs in 1 to 2 weeks, itraconazole is recommended for an additional 12 weeks. Itraconazole is preferred over other mold-active azoles by most experts; when used in adults, itraconazole is more effective, has fewer adverse effects, and is less likely to induce resistance than is fluconazole. Serum trough concentrations of itraconazole should be 1 to 2 µg /mL. Concentrations should be checked after several days of therapy to ensure adequate drug exposure. When measured by high-pressure liquid chromatography, both itraconazole and its bioactive hydroxy-itraconazole metabolite are reported, the sum of which should be considered in assessing drug levels.

All patients with chronic pulmonary histoplasmosis (eg, progressive cavitation of the lungs) should be treated. Mild to moderate cases should be treated with itraconazole for 1 to 2 years. Severe cases should be treated initially with a lipid formulation amphotericin B followed by itraconazole for the same duration.

Mediastinal and inflammatory manifestations of infection generally do not need to be treated with antifungal agents. Mediastinal adenitis that causes obstruction of a bronchus, the esophagus, or another mediastinal structure may improve with a brief course of corticosteroids. In these instances, itraconazole should be used concurrently and continued for 6 to 12 weeks thereafter. Dense fibrosis of mediastinal structures without an associated granulomatous inflammatory component does not respond to antifungal therapy, and surgical intervention may be necessary for severe cases. Pericarditis and rheumatologic syndromes may respond to treatment with nonsteroidal anti-inflammatory agents (indomethacin).

For treatment of moderately severe to severe progressive disseminated histoplasmosis (PDH) in an infant or child, a lipid formulation of amphotericin B is the drug of choice and usually is given for a minimum of 2 weeks. When the child has demonstrated substantial clinical improvement and a decline in the serum concentration of *Histoplasma* antigen, oral itraconazole is administered for a total of at least 12 months. Lifelong suppressive therapy with itraconazole may be required for patients with primary immunodeficiency syndromes, acquired immunodeficiency that cannot be reversed, or patients who relapse despite appropriate therapy. For those with mild to moderate PDH, itraconazole for at least 12 months is recommended. After completion of treatment for PDH, urine antigen concentrations should be monitored for 12 months. Stable, low, and decreasing concentrations that are unaccompanied by signs of active infection may not necessarily require prolongation or resumption of treatment.

ISOLATION OF THE HOSPITALIZED PATIENT: Standard precautions are recommended.

CONTROL MEASURES: Histoplasmosis is a reportable disease in some states and countries. Investigation for a common source of infection is indicated in outbreaks. Exposure to soil and dust from areas with significant accumulations of bird and bat droppings should be avoided, especially by immunocompromised individuals, including those receiving tumor necrosis factor inhibitors or disease-modifying antirheumatic drugs. If exposure is unavoidable, it should be minimized through use of respiratory protection (eg, N95 respirator), gloves, and disposable clothing. Although an N95 respirator is adequate in most circumstances, in environments with extremely high inoculum, powered air purifying respirators (PAPRs) with high-efficiency particulate air (HEPA) filters are recommended.

Areas suspected of being contaminated with *Histoplasma* species should be remediated. Old or abandoned structures likely to have been contaminated with bird or bat droppings should be saturated with water to reduce aerosolization of spores during demolition. Guidelines for preventing histoplasmosis have been designed for health and safety professionals, environmental consultants, and people supervising workers involved in activities in which contaminated materials are disturbed. Additional information about these guidelines is available from the National Institute for Occupational Safety and Health (NIOSH; publication No. 2005-109, available from Publications Dissemination, 4676 Columbia Parkway, Cincinnati, OH 45226-1998; telephone 800-356-4674) and the NIOSH website (**www.cdc.gov/niosh/docs/2005-109/pdfs/2005-109.pdf**).

Hookworm Infections
(*Ancylostoma duodenale* and *Necator americanus*)

CLINICAL MANIFESTATIONS: Patients with hookworm infection often are asymptomatic. The most common clinical manifestation is iron deficiency resulting from direct blood loss at the site where adult worms attach to the mucosa of the small intestine. Chronic hookworm infection is a common cause of moderate and severe hypochromic, microcytic anemia in people living in resource-limited tropical countries, and heavy infection can cause hypoproteinemia with edema. Chronic hookworm infection in children may lead to physical growth delay, deficits in cognition, and developmental delay. Transmission occurs when larvae in contaminated soil penetrate the skin, frequently through the feet. A stinging or burning sensation may occur, followed by pruritus and a papulovesicular rash ("ground itch"), persisting for 1 to 2 weeks. Pneumonitis associated with migrating larvae (Löffler-like syndrome) is uncommon and usually mild, except in heavy infections. Colicky abdominal pain, nausea, diarrhea, and marked eosinophilia may develop 4 to 6 weeks after exposure. Blood loss secondary to hookworm infection develops 10 to 12 weeks after initial infection, and symptoms related to serious iron-deficiency anemia can develop in long-standing moderate or heavy hookworm infections. Pharyngeal itching, hoarseness, nausea, and vomiting also may develop after ingestion of infectious *Ancylostoma duodenale* larvae.

ETIOLOGY: *Necator americanus* is the major cause of hookworm infection worldwide, although *A duodenale* also is an important hookworm in some regions. *Ancylostoma ceylanicum*, a zoonotic (eg, dogs and cats) hookworm, increasingly is being identified as a major cause of hookworm infections in humans, particularly in Asia. Mixed infections can occur. Each of these roundworms (nematodes) has a similar life cycle, with the exception of *A ceylanicum*. Other animal hookworm species (*Ancylostoma braziliense, Ancylostoma caninum, Uncinaria stenocephala*) cause cutaneous larva migrans when filariform larvae penetrate the skin and migrate in the upper dermis, causing an intensely pruritic track, although they do not usually develop further or cause systemic infection (an exception is *A caninum* which may rarely migrate to the intestine and cause eosinophilic enteritis).

EPIDEMIOLOGY: Hookworm is the second most common human helminthic infection following ascariasis. It has worldwide distribution but is most prominent in rural, tropical, and subtropical areas where soil is conducive to organism development and where contamination with human feces is common. *N americanus* is predominant in the Western hemisphere, sub-Saharan Africa, Southeast Asia, and a number of Pacific islands. *A duodenale* is the predominant species in the Mediterranean region, northern Asia, and selected foci of South America. *A ceylanicum* is found in Asia, Australia, some Pacific islands, South Africa, and Madagascar. Larvae and eggs survive in loose, sandy, moist, shady, well-aerated, warm soil (optimal temperature 23°C–33°C [73°F–91°F]). Hookworm eggs from stool hatch in soil in 1 to 2 days as rhabditiform larvae. These larvae develop into infective filariform larvae in soil within 5 to 7 days and can survive for 3 to 4 weeks. Percutaneous infection occurs after exposure to infectious larvae. *A duodenale* transmission can occur by ingestion and possibly through human milk. Untreated infected patients can harbor worms for 5 years or longer.

The **incubation period** from exposure to development of noncutaneous symptoms is 4 to 12 weeks. Eggs appear in feces approximately 5 to 8 weeks from the time of infection.

DIAGNOSTIC TESTS: Microscopic demonstration of hookworm eggs in feces is diagnostic. A direct stool smear with saline solution or potassium iodide saturated with iodine is adequate for diagnosis of heavy hookworm infection; light infections require concentration techniques. Quantification techniques (eg, Kato-Katz, Beaver direct smear, or Stoll egg-counting techniques) to determine the clinical significance of infection and the response to treatment may be available from state or reference laboratories. Stool microscopy is not very sensitive and multiple samples may be needed to detect infection; some experts recommend examining at least 3 consecutive samples using concentration techniques when index of suspicion of infection is high. Stool polymerase chain reaction is emerging as a sensitive and specific diagnostic technique, although it is not yet widely available. Cutaneous larva migrans attributable to transient cutaneous infection with dog or cat hookworms is diagnosed clinically.

TREATMENT: Albendazole and mebendazole are recommended and pyrantel pamoate is an effective alternative in the treatment of hookworm infection; only mebendazole is approved by the FDA for this indication (see Drugs for Parasitic Infections, p 949). Albendazole should be taken with food; a fatty meal increases oral bioavailability. Pyrantel pamoate suspension can be mixed with milk or fruit juice. Studies in children as young as 1 year of age suggest that albendazole can be administered safely to this population. Retreatment is indicated for persistent or recurrent infection. Nutritional supplementation, including iron, is important when addressing associated iron deficiency anemia. Severely affected children may require blood transfusion.

ISOLATION OF THE HOSPITALIZED PATIENT: Standard precautions are recommended. Direct person-to-person transmission does not occur.

CONTROL MEASURES: Sanitary disposal of feces to prevent contamination of soil is necessary in areas with endemic infection. Treatment of all known infected people and screening of high-risk groups (ie, children and agricultural workers) in areas with endemic infection can help decrease environmental contamination. Wearing shoes protects against hookworm infection; infection risk remains if other body surfaces are in contact with the soil. Periodic deworming treatments targeting preschool-aged and school-aged children have been advocated to prevent morbidity associated with heavy intestinal helminth infections. Certain populations immigrating to the United States (eg, refugees) receive presumptive albendazole treatment for soil-transmitted helminths, including hookworm, before departure for the United States.

Human Herpesvirus 6 (Including Roseola) and 7

CLINICAL MANIFESTATIONS: Human herpesvirus 6 and 7 comprise 3 distinct viral species, HHV-6B, HHV-6A, and HHV-7. Although many infections are asymptomatic, clinical manifestations of primary infection with human herpesvirus 6B (HHV-6B) include roseola (exanthem subitum) in approximately 20% of infected children as well as a nonspecific febrile illness without rash or localizing signs. Acute HHV-6B infection may be accompanied by cervical and characteristic postoccipital lymphadenopathy, gastrointestinal tract or respiratory tract signs, and inflamed tympanic membranes. Fever may be high (temperature >39.5°C [103.0°F]) and persist for 3 to 7 days. Approximately 20% of all emergency department visits for febrile children 6 through 12 months of age are attributable to HHV-6B. Roseola is distinguished by an erythematous maculopapular rash that typically appears once fever resolves and can last hours to days. Febrile seizures, sometimes leading to status epilepticus, are the most common complication and reason for hospitalization among children with primary HHV-6B infection. Approximately 10% to 15% of children with primary HHV-6B infection develop febrile seizures, predominantly between the ages of 6 and 18 months. Other reported neurologic manifestations include a bulging fontanelle and encephalopathy or encephalitis, the latter more commonly noted in infants in Japan than in the United States or Europe. Hepatitis has been reported as a rare manifestation of primary HHV-6B infection. Congenital infection with HHV-6B and HHV-6A, which occurs in approximately 1% of newborn infants, has not been linked to any clinical disease. In contrast to HHV-6B, primary infection with HHV-6A has not been associated with any recognized disease.

The clinical manifestations occurring with human herpesvirus 7 (HHV-7) infection are less clear than with HHV-6B. Most primary infections with HHV-7 presumably are asymptomatic or mild and not distinctive. Some initial infections can present as typical roseola and may account for second or recurrent cases of roseola. Febrile illnesses associated with seizures also have been documented to occur during primary HHV-7 infection.

Following infection, HHV-6B, HHV-6A, and HHV-7 remain in a latent state and may reactivate. The clinical circumstances and manifestations of reactivation in healthy people are unclear. Illness associated with HHV-6B reactivation has been described primarily among recipients of solid organ and hematopoietic stem cell transplants. Clinical findings associated with HHV-6B reactivation in solid organ and hematopoietic stem cell transplants include fever, rash, hepatitis, bone marrow suppression, acute graft-versus-host disease, graft rejection, pneumonia, delirium, and encephalitis. The best characterized of these is post-transplantation acute limbic encephalitis, a specific syndrome associated with HHV-6B reactivation in the central nervous system characterized by anterograde amnesia, seizures, insomnia, confusion, and the syndrome of inappropriate antidiuretic hormone secretion. Patients undergoing cord blood transplantation are at an increased risk of developing post-transplantation acute limbic encephalitis, with significant morbidity and mortality attributed to this complication. A few cases of central nervous system symptoms have been reported in association with HHV-7 reactivation in immunocompromised hosts, but clinical findings generally have been reported much less frequently with HHV-7 than with HHV-6B reactivation.

ETIOLOGY: HHV-6B, HHV-6A, and HHV-7 are lymphotropic viruses that are closely related members of the *Herpesviridae* family, subfamily *Betaherpesvirinae*. As betaherpesviruses, HHV-6B, HHV-6A, and HHV-7 are most closely related to cytomegalovirus. As with all human herpesviruses, they establish lifelong latency after initial acquisition. In 2012, HHV-6A and HHV-6B were recognized as distinct species rather than as variants of the same species. This increased the number of known human herpesviruses to 9.

EPIDEMIOLOGY: HHV-6B and HHV-7 cause ubiquitous infections in children worldwide. Humans are the only known natural host. Nearly all children acquire HHV-6B infection within the first 2 years of life, probably resulting from asymptomatic shedding of infectious virus in upper respiratory secretions of a healthy family member or other close contact. Virus-specific maternal antibody, which is present uniformly in the sera of infants at birth, provides transient partial protection. As maternal antibody concentration decreases during the first year of life, the infection rate increases rapidly, peaking between 6 and 24 months of age. During the acute phase of primary infection, HHV-6B and HHV-7 can be isolated from peripheral blood mononuclear cells and HHV-7 from saliva of some children. Viral DNA subsequently may be detected throughout life by polymerase chain reaction (PCR) assay in multiple body sites, including blood mononuclear cells, salivary glands, lung, skin, and the central nervous system. Infections occur throughout the year without a seasonal pattern. Secondary cases rarely are identified. Occasional outbreaks of roseola have been reported.

Several genetic mutations have been associated with severe central nervous system disease during primary HHV-6B infection. These include RandBP2, POLG, and carnitine palmitoyl-transferase 2 gene mutations.

Congenital infection occurs in approximately 1% of newborn infants, as determined by the presence of HHV-6A or HHV-6 B DNA in cord blood. Most congenital infections appear to result from the germline passage of maternal or paternal chromosomally integrated HHV-6 (ciHHV-6), a unique mechanism of transmission of human viral congenital infection. Transplacental HHV-6 infection also may occur from reinfection or reactivation of maternal HHV-6 infection or possibly from reactivated maternal ciHHV-6. HHV-6 has not been identified in human milk. Congenital infection typically is asymptomatic, and the clinical implications of ciHHV-6 are not fully known. However, reactivation of ciHHV-6 in severely immunocompromised hosts is possible and can be associated with disease.

HHV-7 infection usually occurs later in childhood than HHV-6B infection. By adulthood, the seroprevalence of HHV-7 is approximately 85%. Infectious HHV-7 is present in more than 75% of saliva specimens obtained from healthy adults. Acquisition of virus via infected respiratory tract secretions of healthy contacts is the probable mode of transmission of HHV-7 to young children. HHV-7 DNA has been detected in human milk, peripheral blood mononuclear cells, cervical secretions, and other body sites. Congenital HHV-7 infection has not been demonstrated.

The mean **incubation period** for HHV-6B is 9 to 10 days. For HHV-7, the **incubation period** is not known.

DIAGNOSTIC TESTS: Multiple assays for detection of HHV-6 and HHV-7 have been developed; some are available commercially, but because laboratory diagnosis of HHV-6 or HHV-7 usually does not influence clinical management (infections among the severely immunocompromised are an exception), these tests have limited utility in clinical practice.

Reference laboratories offer diagnostic testing for HHV-6B, HHV-6A, and HHV-7 infections by detection of viral DNA in blood, cerebrospinal fluid (CSF), other body fluids, or tissue specimens. However, detection of HHV-6A, HHV-6B, or HHV-7 DNA by PCR assay might not differentiate between new infection, persistence of virus from past infection, or chromosomal integration of HHV-6. At least one multiplexed PCR diagnostic panel designed to detect agents of meningitis and encephalitis in CSF cleared by the US Food and Drug Administration contains HHV-6 as one of its target pathogens; however, given the prevalence of ciHHV-6 (1%), which would yield a positive CSF PCR result, a positive test result should be interpreted with caution if there are no other findings to suggest encephalitis. Quantitative PCR assay has been used for monitoring the effectiveness of antiviral treatment in immunocompromised patients with viral reactivation.

Chromosomal integration of HHV-6 is supported by consistently positive PCR test results for HHV-6 DNA in whole blood, tissue, or other fluids, often with high viral loads (eg, 1×10^6 copies in whole blood, which with a normal white blood cell count is approximately 1 copy of HHV-6 DNA per cell). Droplet digital PCR or quantitative comparison of viral DNA copies to human cell number copies in whole blood samples may also be used to identify ciHHV-6. ciHHV-6 can be suggested by testing whole blood from both parents to see if one of them has a high viral load and confirmed by detection of HHV-6 DNA in hair follicles in research settings.

Serologic tests including immunofluorescent antibody assay, virus neutralization, immunoblot, and enzyme immunoassay (EIA) are often difficult to interpret. A four-fold increase in serum antibody concentration alone does not necessarily indicate new infection, because an increase in titer may occur with reactivation and in association with other infections, especially other betaherpesvirus infections. However, documented seroconversion is considered evidence of recent primary infection in infants and young children, and serologic tests may be useful for epidemiologic studies. Detection of specific immunoglobulin (Ig) M antibody is not reliable for diagnosing new infection, because IgM antibodies to HHV-6 and HHV-7 are not always detectable in children with primary infection and also may be present in asymptomatic previously infected people. These antibody assays do not differentiate HHV-6A from HHV-6B infections. In addition, the diagnosis of primary HHV-7 infection in children with previous HHV-6B infection is confounded by concurrent increase in HHV-6 antibody titer from antigenic cross-reactivity or from reactivation of HHV-6B by a new HHV-7 infection. Detection of low-avidity HHV-6 or HHV-7 antibody with subsequent maturation to high-avidity antibody has been used in such situations to identify recent primary infection.

TREATMENT: Management is supportive. The use of ganciclovir (and, therefore, valganciclovir) or foscarnet may be beneficial for immunocompromised patients with HHV-6 or HHV-7 disease and is recommended for treatment of HHV-6 encephalitis in hematopoietic stem cell and solid organ transplant patients. Antiviral resistance may occur. Routine monitoring of HHV-6 and HHV-7 DNA levels in blood during transplantation is not recommended. HHV-6 and HHV-7 have been reported as associated with various additional clinical syndromes in immunocompetent hosts, including multiple sclerosis, drug hypersensitivity, and uterine infection leading to infertility. None of these associations are generally accepted as etiological, and treatment of HHV-6 or HHV-7 in association with these syndromes is not recommended.

ISOLATION OF THE HOSPITALIZED PATIENT: Standard precautions are recommended.

CONTROL MEASURES: None.

Human Herpesvirus 8

CLINICAL MANIFESTATIONS: Human herpesvirus (HHV-8), also known as Kaposi sarcoma-associated herpesvirus (KSHV), is the cause of Kaposi sarcoma (KS), primary effusion lymphoma, multicentric Castleman disease (MCD), and the Kaposi sarcoma herpesvirus-associated inflammatory cytokine syndrome (KICS). HHV-8 also is a potential trigger of hemophagocytic lymphohistiocytosis (HLH). In regions with endemic HHV-8, a nonspecific primary infection syndrome in immunocompetent children consists of fever and a maculopapular rash, often accompanied by upper respiratory tract symptoms. Primary infection among immunocompromised people tends to present with more severe manifestations including pancytopenia, fever, rash, lymphadenopathy, splenomegaly, diarrhea, arthralgia, disseminated disease, and/or KS. In parts of Africa where HHV-8 is endemic, KS is a frequent, aggressive malignancy among children both with and without human immunodeficiency virus (HIV) infection. Clinical presentations can vary, but younger children most often present with prominent (>2 cm), firm, non-tender lymphadenopathy, associated cytopenias (significant anemia and thrombocytopenia), and frequently without the characteristic cutaneous lesions or "woody" edema more commonly seen in adults. In the United States, KS is rare in children and occurs primarily in adults with poorly controlled HIV infection. Immune reconstitution inflammatory syndrome (IRIS)-KS can occur, most notably among HIV-positive children adopted from HHV-8 endemic countries. Among solid organ and less often bone marrow transplant recipients, KS is an important cause of cancer-related deaths. Primary effusion lymphoma is rare among children. MCD has been described in immunosuppressed and immunocompetent children, but the proportion of cases attributable to infection with HHV-8 is unknown.

ETIOLOGY: HHV-8 is a member of the family *Herpesviridae*, the *Gammaherpesvirinae* subfamily, and the *Rhadinovirus* genus, and is a DNA virus closely related to Epstein-Barr virus and to herpesvirus saimiri of monkeys.

EPIDEMIOLOGY: In areas of Africa, the Amazon basin, the Mediterranean, and the Middle East with endemic HHV-8, seroprevalence ranges from approximately 30% to 80%. Low rates of seroprevalence, generally less than 5%, have been reported in the United States, Northern and Central Europe, and most areas of Asia. Higher rates, however, occur in specific geographic regions, among adolescents and adults with or at high risk of acquiring HIV infection, injection drug users, and children adopted from endemic regions including some Eastern European countries.

Acquisition of HHV-8 in areas with endemic infection frequently occurs before puberty, likely by exposure to saliva of close contacts, especially mothers and siblings. Virus is shed frequently in saliva of infected people and becomes latent for life in peripheral blood mononuclear cells and lymphoid tissue. In areas where infection is not endemic, sexual transmission appears to be the major route of infection, especially among men who have sex with men. Studies from areas with endemic infection have suggested transmission may occur by blood transfusion, but in the United States, evidence for this is lacking. Transplantation of infected donor organs has been documented to result in HHV-8 infection in the recipient. HHV-8 DNA has been detected in blood drawn at birth from infants born to HHV-8 seropositive mothers, but vertical transmission seems to be rare. Viral DNA has also been detected in human milk, but transmission via human milk is yet to be proven.

The **incubation period** of HHV-8 is unknown.

DIAGNOSTIC TESTS: Nucleic acid amplification testing and serologic assays for HHV-8 are available. Polymerase chain reaction (PCR) tests may be used on peripheral blood, fluid from body cavity effusions, and tissue biopsy specimens. When KS is suspected, biopsy with histologic confirmation is the gold standard. Detection of HHV-8 in peripheral blood specimens by PCR assay also has been used to identify exacerbations of other HHV-8-associated diseases, primarily MCD and KICS (especially at high copy number in these 2 diseases); however, HHV-8 DNA can be detected in the peripheral blood of asymptomatically infected people and conversely HHV-8 infected people may not have active viremia.

Currently available serologic assays measuring antibodies to HHV-8 include immuno-fluorescence antibody (IFA) assay, enzyme immunoassays (EIAs), and Western blot assays using recombinant HHV-8 proteins. These serologic assays detect both latent and lytic infection, but each has challenges with accuracy or convenience, with resulting limitations on their use in the diagnosis and management of acute clinical disease.

TREATMENT: Epidemic KS (KS in HIV-positive children) should be treated with both HIV antiretroviral therapy plus chemotherapy based on clinical staging. Retrospective cohort studies and in vitro assays suggest that antiretroviral therapy may inhibit HHV-8 replication. For clinically significant disease with tissue or fluid (primary effusion lymphoma) burden, the most widely used treatment modality is chemotherapy. Treatment of transplant KS may benefit from reduction in immunosuppressive therapy and use of sirolimus in lieu of tacrolimus as the suppressive agent.

Several antiviral agents have in vitro activity against HHV-8. Ganciclovir has been shown to inhibit HHV-8 replication in the only randomized trial of an antiviral drug for this infection. Case reports document an effect of ganciclovir, valganciclovir, ganciclovir combined with zidovudine, cidofovir, and foscarnet. Valacyclovir and famciclovir more modestly reduce HHV-8 replication. Antiviral therapy may play a more significant role in the treatment of diseases associated with active, lytic HHV-8 replication, specifically MCD and KICS, but this remains to be well established.

ISOLATION OF THE HOSPITALIZED PATIENT: Standard precautions are recommended.

CONTROL MEASURES: Although there are no standard guidelines on preventing HHV-8 transmission, avoidance of behavioral practices that lead to exposure to saliva might be effective.

Human Immunodeficiency Virus Infection[1]

CLINICAL MANIFESTATIONS: Human immunodeficiency virus (HIV) infection results in a wide array of clinical manifestations. HIV type 1 (HIV-1) is much more common in the United States than HIV type 2 (HIV-2). Unless otherwise specified, this chapter addresses HIV-1 infection. Acquired immunodeficiency syndrome (AIDS) is the name given to an advanced stage of HIV infection based on specific criteria for children, adolescents, and adults established by the Centers for Disease Control and Prevention (CDC).

Acute retroviral syndrome develops in 50% to 90% of adolescents and adults within the first few weeks after they become infected with HIV and is characterized by nonspecific mononucleosis-like symptoms, including fever, malaise, lymphadenopathy, and skin rash.

Clinical manifestations of untreated pediatric HIV infection include unexplained fevers, generalized lymphadenopathy, hepatomegaly, splenomegaly, failure to thrive, persistent oral and diaper candidiasis, recurrent diarrhea, parotitis, hepatitis, central nervous system (CNS) disease (eg, encephalopathy, hyperreflexia, hypertonia, floppiness,

---

[1]For a complete listing of current policy statements from the American Academy of Pediatrics regarding human immunodeficiency virus and acquired immunodeficiency syndrome, see **https://pediatrics.aappublications.org/hiv%3Aaids_sub.**

developmental delay), lymphoid interstitial pneumonia, recurrent invasive bacterial infections, and opportunistic infections (OIs) (eg, viral, parasitic, and fungal).[1]

In the era of antiretroviral therapy (ART), there has been a substantial decrease in frequency of all OIs. In the pre-ART era, the most common OIs observed among children in the United States were infections caused by invasive encapsulated bacteria, *Pneumocystis jirovecii* (previously called *Pneumocystis carinii*, hence the still-used acronym PCP for *Pneumocystis carinii* pneumonia), varicella-zoster virus, cytomegalovirus, herpes simplex virus, *Mycobacterium avium* complex, *Cryptococcus neoformans*, and *Candida* species. Less commonly observed opportunistic pathogens included Epstein-Barr virus (EBV), *Mycobacterium tuberculosis*, *Cryptosporidium* species, *Cystoisospora* (formerly *Isospora*) species, other enteric pathogens, *Aspergillus* species, and *Toxoplasma gondii*.

Immune reconstitution inflammatory syndrome (IRIS) is a paradoxical clinical deterioration often seen in severely immunosuppressed individuals that occurs shortly after the initiation of ART. Local and/or systemic symptoms develop secondary to an inflammatory response as cell-mediated immunity is restored. IRIS is observed in patients with previous infections with mycobacteria (including *Mycobacterium tuberculosis*), bacille Calmette-Guérin (BCG) vaccine, herpesviruses, and fungi (including *Cryptococcus* species).

Malignant neoplasms in children with HIV infection are relatively uncommon, but leiomyosarcomas and non-Hodgkin B-cell lymphomas of the Burkitt type (including those in the CNS) occur more commonly in children with HIV infection than in immunocompetent children. Kaposi sarcoma, caused by human herpesvirus 8, is rare in children in the United States but has been documented in HIV-infected children who have emigrated from sub-Saharan African countries. The incidence of malignant neoplasms in HIV-infected children has decreased during the ART era.

ETIOLOGY: HIV-1 and HIV-2 are cytopathic lentiviruses *(genus Lentivirus)* belonging to the family *Retroviridae*. Three distinct genetic groups of HIV exist: M (major), O (outlier), and N (new). Group M viruses are the most prevalent worldwide and comprise 8 genetic subtypes, or clades, known as A through K, each of which has a distinct geographic distribution.

HIV-2, the second AIDS-causing virus, is found predominantly in West Africa. HIV-2 has a milder disease course with a longer time to development of AIDS than HIV-1. Accurate diagnosis of HIV-2 is important clinically, because HIV-2 is intrinsically resistant to nonnucleoside reverse transcriptase inhibitors (NNRTIs) and the fusion inhibitor enfuvirtide.

EPIDEMIOLOGY: Humans are the only known reservoir for HIV-1 and HIV-2. Latent virus persists in peripheral blood mononuclear cells and in cells of the brain, bone marrow, and genital tract even when plasma viral load is undetectable. Only blood, semen, cervicovaginal secretions, and human milk have been implicated in transmission of infection.

Established modes of HIV transmission include: (1) sexual contact (vaginal, anal, or orogenital); (2) percutaneous blood exposure (from contaminated needles or other sharp materials); (3) mucous membrane exposure to contaminated blood or other body fluids; (4) mother-to-child transmission (MTCT) during prepartum, intrapartum, and

---

[1]Panel on Opportunistic Infections in HIV-Exposed and HIV-Infected Children. Guidelines for the Prevention and Treatment of Opportunistic Infections in HIV-Exposed and HIV-Infected Children. Department of Health and Human Services. Available at: **https://clinicalinfo.hiv.gov/sites/default/files/inline-files/oi_guidelines_pediatrics.pdf**

postpartum periods, including breastfeeding postnatally; and (5) transfusion with contaminated blood products. Cases of HIV transmission from HIV-infected caregivers to children through feeding blood-tinged premasticated food and from contact of nonintact skin with blood-containing body fluids have been reported in the United States. As a result of highly effective screening assays and protocols, transfusion of blood, blood components, and clotting factors has virtually been eliminated as a cause of HIV transmission in the United States since 1985. Since the mid-1990s, the number of reported pediatric AIDS cases has decreased significantly, primarily because of prevention of MTCT of HIV and the widespread availability of ART for children with HIV.

In the absence of breastfeeding, the risk of HIV infection for infants born to untreated women living with HIV (WLHIV) in the United States is approximately 25%, with most transmission occurring near the time of delivery. Maternal viral load is the critical determinant affecting the likelihood of MTCT of HIV, although transmission has been observed across the entire range of maternal viral loads. Current US guidelines recommend cesarean section before labor and before rupture of membranes at 38 completed weeks of gestation for WLHIV with viral load ≥1000 copies/mL (irrespective of antiretroviral [ARV] use in pregnancy) and for women with unknown viral load near the time of delivery (**https://clinicalinfo.hiv.gov/en/guidelines/perinatal/ whats-new-guidelines**).

The rate of acquisition of HIV infection among infants has decreased significantly in the United States. The rate of new HIV infections among adolescents and young adults aged 13 to 24 years overall also is decreasing but is increasing for young men who have sex with men in this age group. HIV infection in adolescents occurs disproportionately among youth of minority race or ethnicity and is attributable primarily to sexual exposure.

INCUBATION PERIOD: The usual age of onset of symptoms is approximately 12 to 18 months of age[1] for untreated infants and children in the United States who acquire HIV infection through MTCT. However, some HIV-infected children become ill in the first few months of life, whereas others remain relatively asymptomatic for more than 5 years and, rarely, until early adolescence.

Acute retroviral syndrome occurring in adolescents and adults following HIV acquisition occurs 7 to 14 days following viral acquisition and lasts for 5 to 7 days. Only a minority of patients are ill enough to seek medical care with acute retroviral syndrome, although more may recall a prior viral illness when queried later.

DIAGNOSTIC TESTS:

Serologic Assays. Immunoassays are used widely as the initial test for serum HIV antibody or for p24 antigen (see below) and HIV antibody. Serologic assays that are cleared by the US Food and Drug Administration (FDA) for the diagnosis of HIV include:

- Antigen/antibody combination immunoassays (fourth-generation tests) that detect HIV-1/HIV-2 antibodies as well as HIV-1 p24 antigen (see below): recommended for initial testing
- HIV-1/HIV-2 immunoassays that detect IgM (third-generation antibody tests): alternative for initial testing

---

[1] Centers for Disease Control and Prevention. HIV Surveillance Report, 2017; Vol 29. Atlanta, GA: Centers for Disease Control and Prevention; November 2018. Available at: **www.cdc.gov/hiv/pdf/library/reports/ surveillance/cdc-hiv-surveillance-report-2017-vol-29.pdf**

- HIV-1/HIV-2 antibody differentiation immunoassay that differentiates HIV-1 antibodies from HIV-2 antibodies (HIV-1/HIV-2 test): recommended for supplemental confirmatory testing
- HIV-1 Western blot and HIV-1 indirect immunofluorescent antibody assays (first-generation tests): alternative for supplemental confirmatory testing
- HIV-1 and HIV-2 antibodies (separate results for each) as well as p24 antigen (fifth-generation test): FDA cleared for initial HIV screening but not as a confirmatory test.

The 2018 CDC HIV laboratory testing algorithm (**https://stacks.cdc.gov/view/cdc/50872**) recommends an initial FDA-approved HIV-1/HIV-2 antigen/antibody combination immunoassay (fourth-generation assay). Specimens with a reactive antigen/antibody immunoassay result should be tested with an FDA-approved HIV-1/HIV-2 antibody differentiation immunoassay. Specimens that are reactive on the initial antigen/antibody immunoassay and nonreactive or indeterminate on the HIV-1/HIV-2 antibody differentiation immunoassay should be tested with an FDA-approved HIV-1 nucleic acid amplification test (NAAT). If acute HIV infection or end-stage AIDS is suspected, virologic testing may be indicated because of false-negative antibody assay results in these populations.

Nucleic Acid Amplification Tests. Plasma HIV DNA or RNA assays have been used to diagnose HIV infection. The DNA polymerase chain reaction (PCR) assays can detect 1 to 10 DNA copies of proviral DNA in peripheral blood mononuclear cells and are used qualitatively to diagnose HIV infection. An RNA qualitative assay that can detect 100 RNA copies per mL also is cleared by the FDA for diagnosis, using transcription mediated amplification (TMA). Quantitative RNA PCR (viral load) assays cleared by the FDA provide results that serve as a predictor of disease progression and are useful in monitoring changes in viral load during treatment with ART.

HIV-2 Detection. Most HIV immunoassays currently approved by FDA detect but do not routinely differentiate between HIV-1 and HIV-2 antibodies. It is important to notify the laboratory when ordering serologic tests for a patient in whom HIV-2 infection is a possibility so that FDA-approved HIV-1/HIV-2 antibody differentiation immunoassays can be used. NAATs approved by the FDA for detection and quantitation of viral load are specific to HIV-1 and do not detect HIV-2.

Diagnosis of Perinatally and Postnatally Acquired Infection. Because children born to HIV-infected mothers passively acquire maternal antibodies, antibody assays are not informative for the diagnosis of infection in children younger than 18 months unless assay results are negative. Therefore, laboratory diagnosis of HIV infection during the first 18 months of life is based on HIV NAATs (Table 3.24). In children 18 to 24 months and older, HIV antibody assays can be used for diagnosis. Despite a median age of seroreversion of 13.9 months, 14% of infants remain seropositive after 18 months, 4.3% remain seropositive after 21 months, and 1.2% remain seropositive after 24 months.

HIV-1 RNA or DNA NAATs for diagnosis of infection in infants are equally recommended in current diagnostic guidelines (**https://clinicalinfo.hiv.gov/en/guidelines/perinatal/whats-new-guidelines**). Because DNA PCR detects proviral DNA in cells while HIV RNA tests measure viral RNA in plasma, there is the potential for DNA testing to be more sensitive in infants with very low viral loads. However, studies have shown that RNA and DNA NAATs for the diagnosis of HIV-1 infection of infants produce comparable results, leading to the current recommendation that either assay can be used in this setting. HIV-1 RNA assays will identify 25% to 58% of infected infants in the first week of life, 89% by 1 month of age, and 90% to 100% by 2 to 3 months of age.

Table 3.24. Laboratory Diagnosis of HIV Infection[a]

Test	Comment
HIV DNA PCR or RNA PCR	Preferred tests to diagnose HIV infection in infants and children younger than 18–24 months; highly sensitive and specific by 2 weeks of age and available; DNA test performed on peripheral blood mononuclear cells; RNA test performed on plasma.
HIV p24 Ag	Less sensitive, false-positive results during first month of life, variable results; not recommended.
ICD p24 Ag	Negative test result does not rule out infection; not recommended.
HIV culture	Expensive, not readily available, requires up to 4 weeks for results; not recommended.

Ag indicates antigen; HIV, human immunodeficiency virus; ICD, immune complex dissociated; PCR, polymerase chain reaction.

[a]Adapted from Read JS; American Academy of Pediatrics, Committee on Pediatric AIDS. Diagnosis of HIV-1 infection in children younger than 18 months in the United States, *Pediatrics*. 2007;120(6):e1547–e1562 (Reaffirmed April 2010). Available at: **http://pediatrics.aappublications.org/cgi/content/full/120/6/e1547**

An HIV RNA assay result with only a low-level viral copy number in an HIV-exposed infant may indicate a false-positive result.

In HIV-exposed infants, diagnostic testing with HIV DNA or RNA assays is recommended at 14 to 21 days of age and, if results are negative, again at 1 to 2 months of age and at 4 to 6 months of age (Fig 3.8). An infant is considered infected if 2 samples from 2 different time points have positive test results by DNA or RNA NAAT. For infants at higher risk of perinatal HIV transmission, additional virologic diagnostic testing is recommended at birth and at 8 to 10 weeks of life (which is 2 to 4 weeks after cessation of antiretroviral prophylaxis) (Fig 3.8). If testing is performed shortly after birth, umbilical cord blood should not be used because of possible contamination with maternal blood. HIV-infected infants should promptly be transitioned from neonatal ARV prophylaxis to ART treatment.

In HIV-exposed children with 2 negative HIV DNA or RNA assay results, many clinicians will confirm the absence of antibody (ie, loss of passively acquired maternal antibody, or "seroreversion") to HIV on testing at 18 through 24 months of age. Some clinicians have a slightly more stringent requirement that the 2 separate antibody-negative blood samples obtained after 6 months of age be drawn at least 1 month apart for a child to be considered HIV-uninfected.

Adolescents and HIV Testing. The American Academy of Pediatrics recommends that routine HIV screening be offered to all youth 15 years or older, at least once in health care settings. Following initial screening, youth at increased risk, including those who are sexually active, should be rescreened at least annually, potentially as frequently as every 3 to 6 months if at very high risk (males reporting male sexual contact, active injection drug users, transgender youth; having sexual partners who are HIV-infected, of both genders, or injection drug users; exchanging sex for drugs or money; or those who have had a diagnosis of or request testing for other STIs).[1] Use of any FDA-cleared HIV antibody

[1]Hsu KK, Rakhmanina NY; American Academy of Pediatrics, Committee on Pediatric AIDS. Clinical report: Adolescents and young adults: the pediatrician's role in HIV testing and pre- and post-exposure HIV prophylaxis. *Pediatrics*. 2021; In press

FIG 3.8. RECOMMENDED VIROLOGIC TESTING SCHEDULES FOR INFANTS EXPOSED TO HIV BY PERINATAL HIV TRANSMISSION RISK

NAT indicates nucleic acid amplification test (referred to as NAAT in this chapter).

Low Risk: Infants born to mothers who received standard antiretroviral therapy (ART) during pregnancy with sustained viral suppression (usually defined as confirmed HIV RNA level below the lower limits of detection of an ultrasensitive assay) and no concerns related to maternal adherence.

Higher Risk: Infants born to women living with HIV infection who did not receive prenatal care, did not receive antepartum or intrapartum antiretrovirals (ARVs), received intrapartum ARV drugs only, initiated ART late in pregnancy (late second or third trimester), were diagnosed with acute HIV infection during pregnancy, or had detectable HIV viral loads close to the time of delivery, including those who received combination ARV drugs and did not have sustained viral suppression.

*For higher-risk infants, additional virologic diagnostic testing should be considered at birth and 2 to 4 weeks after cessation of ARV prophylaxis (ie, at 8–10 weeks of life).

Reproduced with permission from Spach DH. Preventing Perinatal HIV Transmission. Seattle, WA: National HIV Curriculum, Infectious Diseases Education and Assessment, University of Washington. Available at: **www.hiv.uw.edu/go/prevention/preventing-perinatal-transmission/core-concept/all**

test is appropriate. For any positive test result, immediate referral to an HIV specialist is appropriate to confirm diagnosis and initiate management. HIV testing is recommended and should be routine for all patients in sexually transmitted infection (STI) clinics and those seeking treatment for STIs in other clinical settings.

Suspicion of acute retroviral syndrome should prompt urgent assessment with an antigen/antibody immunoassay or HIV RNA NAAT in conjunction with an antibody test. If the immunoassay result is negative or indeterminate, then testing for HIV RNA using a NAAT should follow. Clinicians should not assume that a laboratory report of a negative HIV antibody test result indicates that the necessary RNA screening for acute HIV infection has been conducted. HIV home-testing kits only detect HIV antibodies and, therefore, will not detect acute HIV infection.

TREATMENT:

Antiretroviral Therapy. Consultation with an expert in pediatric HIV infection is recommended in the care of HIV-infected infants, children, and adolescents. Current treatment recommendations for HIV-infected infants and children (**https://clinicalinfo.hiv.gov/en/guidelines/pediatric-arv/whats-new-guidelines**) as well as adolescents (**https://clinicalinfo.hiv.gov/en/guidelines/adult-and-adolescent-arv/whats-new-guidelines**) are available online. Whenever possible, enrollment of HIV-infected infants, children, and adolescents in clinical trials should be encouraged. Information about trials for HIV-infected infants, children, and adolescents can be obtained by contacting the AIDS Clinical Trials Information Service (**www.actis.org/**).

ART is indicated for HIV-infected pediatric patients and should be initiated as soon as possible after diagnosis of HIV infection is established. Initiation of treatment of adolescents generally follows guidelines for adults and is recommended strongly for all HIV-infected adolescents or adults regardless of CD4+ T-lymphocyte count, as long as medication readiness is apparent. In general, ART with at least 3 active drugs is recommended for all HIV-infected individuals requiring ARV therapy. ARV resistance testing (viral genotyping) is recommended before starting treatment. Sustained suppression of virus to undetectable levels is the desired goal. A change in ARV therapy should be considered if there is evidence of disease progression (virologic, immunologic, or clinical), toxicity of or intolerance to drugs, development of drug resistance, or availability of data suggesting the possibility of a superior regimen.

Opportunistic Infections. Guidelines for prevention and treatment of OIs in children (**https://clinicalinfo.hiv.gov/en/guidelines/pediatric-opportunistic-infection/whats-new**) and adolescents and adults (**https://clinicalinfo.hiv.gov/en/guidelines/adult-and-adolescent-opportunistic-infection/whats-new-guidelines**) provide indications for administration of drugs for infection with *P jirovecii*, *M avium* complex, cytomegalovirus, *T gondii*, and other organisms.

Immunization Recommendations. (also see Immunization in Special Clinical Circumstances, p 67, and Table 1.17, p 73).[1] All recommended childhood immunizations should be administered to HIV-exposed infants. If HIV infection is confirmed, guidelines for the HIV-infected child should be followed. Children and adolescents with HIV infection should be immunized as soon as is age appropriate with all inactivated vaccines. Inactivated influenza vaccine (IIV) should be administered annually according to the most current recommendations. The 3-dose series of human papillomavirus vaccine; tetanus toxoid, reduced diphtheria toxoid, and acellular pertussis (Tdap) vaccine; and meningococcal conjugate vaccine all are indicated in HIV-infected adolescents (**https://redbook.solutions.aap.org/SS/Immunization_Schedules.aspx**).

The live-virus measles-mumps-rubella (MMR) vaccine and monovalent varicella vaccine can be administered to asymptomatic HIV-infected children and adolescents without severe immunosuppression (that is, can be administered to children 1 through 13 years of age with a CD4+ T-lymphocyte percentage ≥15% and to adolescents ≥14 years with a CD4+ T-lymphocyte count ≥200 lymphocytes/mm³). Severely immunocompromised HIV-infected infants, children, adolescents, and young adults (eg, children 1 through 13 years of age with a CD4+ T-lymphocyte percentage <15% and adolescents ≥14 years with a CD4+ T-lymphocyte count <200 lymphocytes/mm³) should not receive measles virus-containing vaccine, because vaccine-related pneumonia has been reported. The quadrivalent measles-mumps-rubella-varicella (MMRV) vaccine should not be administered to any HIV-infected infant, regardless of degree of immunosuppression, because of lack of safety data in this population.

Rotavirus vaccine should be administered to HIV-exposed and HIV-infected infants irrespective of CD4+ T-lymphocyte percentage or count.

All HIV-infected children should receive a dose of 23-valent polysaccharide pneumococcal vaccine after turning 24 months of age, with a minimal interval of 8 weeks since the last pneumococcal conjugate vaccine.

HIV-infected children who are 5 years and older and have not received *Haemophilus influenzae* type b (Hib) vaccine should receive 1 dose of Hib vaccine (see Table 3.12, p 354).

---

[1]Rubin LG, Levin MJ, Ljungman P, et al. 2013 IDSA clinical practice guideline for vaccination of the immuno-compromised host. *Clin Infect Dis.* 2014;58(3):309-318

Infants and children with HIV infection 2 months of age or older should receive an age-appropriate series of the meningococcal ACWY conjugate vaccine (MenACWY) (see Meningococcal Infections, p 519).[1] The same vaccine product should be used for all doses. However, if the product used for previous doses is unknown or unavailable, the vaccination series may be completed with any age- and formulation-appropriate meningococcal ACWY conjugate vaccine. Although no data on interchangeability of meningococcal conjugate vaccines in HIV-infected people are available, limited data from a postlicensure study in healthy adolescents suggests safety and immunogenicity of MenACWY-CRM are not adversely affected by prior immunization with MenACWY-D. For HIV-infected children aged 2 through 23 months of age, only MenACWY-CRM (Menveo) should be used, because interference with the immune response to pneumococcal conjugate vaccine occurs with MenACWY-D (Menactra) and MenACWY-TT (MenQuadfi) is not licensed for use in children younger than 2 years.

Children Who Are HIV Uninfected Residing in the Household of an HIV-Infected Person. Members of households in which an adult or child has HIV infection can receive MMR vaccine, because these vaccine viruses are not transmitted from person to person. To decrease the risk of transmission of influenza to patients with symptomatic HIV infection, all household members 6 months or older should receive yearly influenza immunization (see Influenza, p 447). Immunization with varicella vaccine of siblings and susceptible adult caregivers of patients with HIV infection is encouraged to prevent acquisition of wild-type varicella-zoster virus infection, which can cause severe disease in immunocompromised hosts. Transmission of varicella vaccine virus from an immunocompetent host to a household contact is very uncommon.

Postexposure Passive Immunization of HIV-Infected Children.

Measles (see Measles, p 503).[2] HIV-infected children who are exposed to measles require prophylaxis on the basis of immune status and measles vaccine history. HIV-infected children who have serologic evidence of immunity or who received 2 doses of measles vaccine after initiation of ART with no to moderate immunosuppression should be considered immune and will not require any additional measures to prevent measles. Asymptomatic mildly or moderately immunocompromised HIV-infected people without evidence of immunity to measles should receive IGIM at a dose of 0.5 mL/kg (maximum 15 mL), regardless of immunization status. Severely immunocompromised patients (eg, HIV-infected people with CD4+ T-lymphocyte percentages <15% [all ages] or CD4+ T-lymphocyte counts <200/mm^3 [age >5 years], regardless of vaccination status, and those who have not received MMR vaccine since receiving ART) who are exposed to measles should receive Immune Globulin Intravenous (IGIV) prophylaxis, 400 mg/kg, after exposure to measles, because they may not be protected by the vaccine. Some experts would include all HIV-infected people, regardless of immunologic status or MMR vaccine history, as needing IGIV prophylaxis. HIV-infected children who have received IGIV within 3 weeks of exposure do not require additional passive immunization.

---

[1]Centers for Disease Control and Prevention. Recommendations for use of meningococcal conjugate vaccines in HIV-infected persons—Advisory Committee on Immunization Practices, 2016. *MMWR Morb Mortal Wkly Rep.* 2016;65(43):1189–1194

[2]Centers for Disease Control and Prevention. Prevention of measles, rubella, congenital rubella syndrome, and mumps, 2013 summary: recommendations of the Advisory Committee on Immunization Practices (ACIP). *MMWR Recomm Rep.* 2013;62(RR-4):1-34

Tetanus. HIV-infected children with severe immune suppression who sustain wounds classified as tetanus prone (see Tetanus, p 750, and Table 3.68, p 753) should receive Tetanus Immune Globulin regardless of immunization status.

Varicella. HIV-infected children without a history of previous varicella infection or who lack evidence of immunity to varicella should receive Varicella Zoster Immune Globulin, if available, ideally within 96 hours but potentially beneficial up to 10 days, after close contact with a person who has chickenpox or shingles (see Varicella-Zoster Infections, p 831). An alternative to Varicella-Zoster Immune Globulin for passive immunization is IGIV, 400 mg/kg, administered once within 10 days after exposure. Children who have received IGIV for other reasons within 3 weeks of exposure do not require additional passive immunization.

ISOLATION OF THE HOSPITALIZED PATIENT: Standard precautions should be followed by all health care professionals regardless of suspected or confirmed HIV infection status of the patient.

CONTROL MEASURES: HIV is a nationally notifiable disease in the United States.
Maternal ARV Therapy and MTCT Prophylaxis.

Management of Infected Mother. Pregnant WLHIV should receive ART regimens, both for treatment of HIV infection and for prevention of MTCT of HIV. Sustained virologic suppression is the goal both during pregnancy and following delivery. Detailed recommendations for use of ARVs in pregnant WLHIV can be found online (**https://clinicalinfo.hiv.gov/en/guidelines/perinatal/whats-new-guidelines**). Ideally, WLHIV initiating such a regimen during pregnancy should be tested for the presence of ARV resistance. However, initiation of ART should not be delayed pending results of resistance testing, especially if decisions are being made late in pregnancy. WLHIV with detectable or unknown HIV RNA near delivery should receive intravenous (IV) zidovudine during labor, regardless of antepartum regimen or mode of delivery; in situations in which IV administration is not possible, oral administration can be considered. A pregnant woman already receiving treatment that does not include zidovudine need not have her ARV regimen changed if her viral load is suppressed.

A slightly increased risk of neural tube defects was found in Botswana among women who initiated dolutegravir (a second-generation integrase inhibitor) before they became pregnant, compared with women who conceived on a regimen that did not contain dolutegravir. An increased risk of infant neural tube defects has not been found in women who initiate dolutegravir during pregnancy. Because updated data indicate that the increased risk of neural tube defects associated with the use of dolutegravir is small and because dolutegravir has the advantages of once-daily dosing and producing rapid, durable viral load suppression, dolutegravir is still recommended as a preferred ARV drug throughout pregnancy.

Management of Exposed Infant. The newborn infant should be bathed and cleaned of maternal secretions (especially bloody secretions) immediately after birth, and begin ARV prophylaxis as soon as possible, preferably within 6 to 12 hours. Management options for evaluation and prophylactic therapy of newborn infants in the United States at low risk and at higher risk of perinatal transmission are presented in Fig 3.9 and Fig 3.10, respectively. These figures are adapted from "Management of Infants Born to Women with HIV Infection," in "Recommendations for the Use of Antiretroviral Drugs in Pregnant Women with HIV Infection and Interventions to Reduce Perinatal HIV Transmission in the United States" (**https://clinicalinfo.hiv.gov/en/guidelines/perinatal/whats-new-guidelines**).

FIG 3.9. NEWBORN TESTING AND PROPHYLAXIS RECOMMENDATIONS FOLLOWING LOW-RISK PERINATAL HIV EXPOSURE*

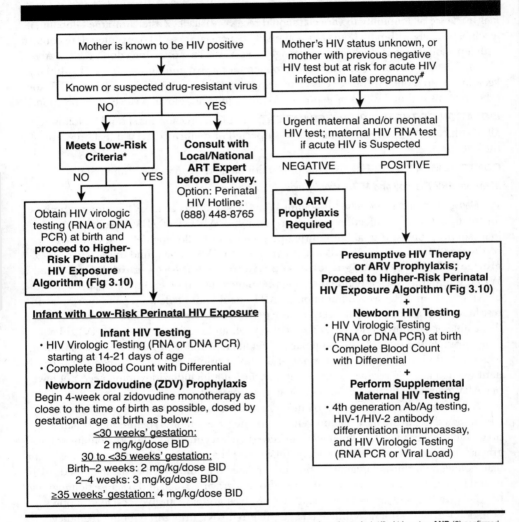

* Low-risk criteria: (1) mother with HIV who received ART throughout pregnancy or from the early 1st/2nd trimester; **AND** (2) confirmed maternal HIV RNA <50 copies/mL near delivery (within 4-6 weeks); **AND** (3) no concerns regarding ART adherence; **AND** (4) mother did not have primary or acute HIV infection during pregnancy.
# Mothers with previous negative HIV test at risk for seroconversion in late pregnancy are those with: documented STI, unprotected sex, partner with HIV, multiple partners, or IV drug use.
ART = Antiretroviral Therapy
Algorithm adapted by Paul Spearman, Rana Chakraborty and Athena Kourtis from Management of Infants Born to Women with HIV Infection, in Recommendations for the Use of Antiretroviral Drugs in Pregnant Women with HIV Infection and Interventions to Reduce Perinatal HIV Transmission in the United States, **clinicalinfo.hiv.gov**.

FIG 3.10. NEWBORN TESTING AND PROPHYLAXIS RECOMMENDATIONS FOLLOWING HIGHER-RISK PERINATAL HIV EXPOSURE*

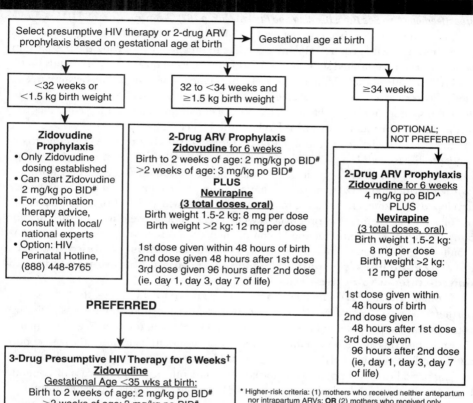

Select presumptive HIV therapy or 2-drug ARV prophylaxis based on gestational age at birth → Gestational age at birth

<32 weeks or <1.5 kg birth weight

Zidovudine Prophylaxis
- Only Zidovudine dosing established
- Can start Zidovudine 2 mg/kg po BID#
- For combination therapy advice, consult with local/national experts
- Option: HIV Perinatal Hotline, (888) 448-8765

32 to <34 weeks and ≥1.5 kg birth weight

2-Drug ARV Prophylaxis
Zidovudine for 6 weeks
Birth to 2 weeks of age: 2 mg/kg po BID#
>2 weeks of age: 3 mg/kg po BID#
PLUS
Nevirapine
(3 total doses, oral)
Birth weight 1.5-2 kg: 8 mg per dose
Birth weight >2 kg: 12 mg per dose

1st dose given within 48 hours of birth
2nd dose given 48 hours after 1st dose
3rd dose given 96 hours after 2nd dose
(ie, day 1, day 3, day 7 of life)

≥34 weeks

OPTIONAL; NOT PREFERRED

2-Drug ARV Prophylaxis
Zidovudine for 6 weeks
4 mg/kg po BID^
PLUS
Nevirapine
(3 total doses, oral)
Birth weight 1.5-2 kg: 8 mg per dose
Birth weight >2 kg: 12 mg per dose

1st dose given within 48 hours of birth
2nd dose given 48 hours after 1st dose
3rd dose given 96 hours after 2nd dose
(ie, day 1, day 3, day 7 of life)

PREFERRED

3-Drug Presumptive HIV Therapy for 6 Weeks†
Zidovudine
Gestational Age <35 wks at birth:
Birth to 2 weeks of age: 2 mg/kg po BID#
>2 weeks of age: 3 mg/kg po BID#
Gestational Age ≥35 weeks at birth:
4 mg/kg po BID#^

PLUS
Lamivudine (3TC)†
Birth to age 4 wks of age: 2 mg/kg/dose po BID
>4 wks of age: 4 mg/kg/dose po BID

PLUS EITHER
Nevirapine
Gestational Age ≥37 weeks
6 mg/kg/dose po BID^
Gestational Age 34–<37 weeks
Birth to 1 week of age: 4 mg/kg/dose po BID
>1 week of age: 6 mg/kg/dose po BID^

OR

Raltegravir§
Gestational Age ≥37 weeks
Birth to 1 week of age: 1.5 mg/kg/dose po QD
1 week to 4 weeks of age: 3 mg/kg/dose po BID
4 weeks to 6 weeks of age: 6 mg/kg/dose po BID

* Higher-risk criteria: (1) mothers who received neither antepartum nor intrapartum ARVs; **OR** (2) mothers who received only intrapartum ARVS; **OR** (3) mothers who received ante- and intrapartum ARVs but who do not have viral suppression (HIV RNA <50 copies/mL) near delivery, particularly if delivery was vaginal; **OR** (4) mothers with acute or primary HIV infection during pregnancy or breastfeeding, in which case the mother should discontinue breastfeeding.

For newborns who are unable to tolerate oral agents, the IV dose of zidovudine is 75% of the oral dose, while maintaining the same dosing interval.

† All infants at higher risk of perinatal HIV exposure should be tested by HIV RNA or DNA PCR at birth. If birth HIV virologic testing in newborn is negative, some experts would discontinue lamivudine and nevirapine after 2 weeks and complete 6 weeks of prophylaxis with zidovudine alone.

^ ARV doses (such as ZDV and nevirapine) may need to be changed and the ARV regimen may need to be optimized if the infant has confirmed HIV infection. See **clinicalinfo.hiv.gov** for full dosing guidelines for infants with confirmed HIV infection.

§ If the mother has taken raltegravir 2-24 hours prior to delivery, the neonate's first dose of raltegravir should be delayed until 24–48 hours after birth; additional ARV drugs should be started as soon as possible. Do not use raltegravir if gestational age <37 weeks.

Algorithm adapted by Paul Spearman, Rana Chakraborty and Athena Kourtis from Management of Infants Born to Women with HIV Infection, in Recommendations for the Use of Antiretroviral Drugs in Pregnant Women with HIV Infection and Interventions to Reduce Perinatal HIV Transmission in the United States, **clinicalinfo.hiv.gov**.

The newborn infant's physician should be informed of the mother's HIV infection status so appropriate care and follow-up of the infant can be accomplished. Whenever possible, an HIV-infected mother and her infant should be referred to a facility that provides HIV-related services for both women and children.

Breastfeeding (Also See Breastfeeding and Human Milk, p 107). Transmission of HIV by breastfeeding accounts for one third to one half of MTCT of HIV worldwide. It is more likely among mothers who acquire HIV infection late in pregnancy or during the postpartum period. In resource-limited settings, the World Health Organization recommends that WLHIV breastfeed their infants exclusively for the first 6 months of life, because infant morbidity associated with formula feeding is unacceptably high and safe alternatives to human milk may not be readily available. Replacement (formula) feeding continues to be recommended for infants born to WLWH in the United States.

Because of social and cultural reasons, a pregnant WLHIV may be pressured to or choose to breastfeed. It is critical that providers keep open channels of communication with a WLHIV. If, after counseling, a mother still chooses to breastfeed, it is important for the provider to be aware of this so that an appropriate plan of management can be developed, including encouraging maternal adherence with ARV during breastfeeding, use of ARVs in the infant as prophylaxis while breastfeeding, exclusive breastfeeding for 6 months followed by introduction of complementary foods, frequent maternal viral load monitoring, and frequent infant testing for HIV infection (**https://clinicalinfo.hiv. gov/en/guidelines/perinatal/counseling-and-managing-women-living-hiv-united-states-who-desire-breastfeed**).

Women who are HIV uninfected but who are known to have HIV-infected sexual partners or bisexual partners, or women who are active injection drug users, should be counseled about the potential risk of acquiring HIV infection themselves and of then transmitting HIV through human milk. Such women should be counseled to use condoms and to undergo frequent HIV testing (eg, monthly to every 3 months) during the breastfeeding period to detect potential maternal HIV seroconversion. In the case of condom breakage during sexual intercourse with the HIV-infected discordant partner, women should be counseled to undergo immediate HIV testing and to initiate HIV postexposure prophylaxis within 72 hours of the condom breakage. Breastfeeding women who are at continuing substantial risk for HIV infection could also be offered preexposure prophylaxis (PrEP), along with frequent clinical monitoring.

Premastication. Probable transmission of HIV by caregivers who premasticated food for infants has been described in the United States. The CDC recommends that HIV-infected caregivers be asked about whether they practice premastication and counseled not to premasticate food for infants.

HIV in the Athletic Setting. Athletes and staff of athletic programs can be exposed to blood during certain athletic activities. Recommendations have been developed by the AAP for prevention of transmission of HIV and other bloodborne pathogens in the athletic setting (see Children in Group Child Care and Schools, Bloodborne Infections, p 116).

Sexual Abuse. In cases of proven or suspected sexual abuse, the child should be tested with an HIV antibody test at the original assessment, with testing repeated at 6 weeks and 3 months (see Sexual Assault and Abuse in Children and Adolescents/Young Adults, p 150). Serologic evaluation for HIV infection of the perpetrator should be attempted as soon after the incident as possible. Counseling of the child and family needs to be provided (see Prophylaxis of Children and Adolescents After Sexual Victimization, p 155).

Prevention of HIV Transmission Through Sexual Activity. Abstinence from sexual activity is the only certain way to prevent sexual transmission of HIV. Safer sex practices, including use of condoms for all sexual encounters (vaginal, anal, and oral sex) can reduce HIV transmission significantly by reducing exposure to body fluids containing HIV. Suppressing HIV viral load to undetectable levels in the blood with ART regimens has resulted in decreases in transmission in discordant couples by as much as 96%.

Preexposure prophylaxis (PrEP) with antiretrovirals (tenofovir plus emtricitabine) reduces the risk of HIV acquisition from sex by 99% when taken consistently. Among people who inject drugs, PrEP reduces the risk of getting HIV by at least 74% when taken consistently. PrEP is much less effective if it is not taken consistently. Preexposure prophylaxis also is FDA approved for adolescents. The American Academy of Pediatrics recommends that youth at substantial risk for HIV acquisition be routinely offered HIV pre-exposure prophylaxis.[1] Detailed guidance is available from the CDC at **www.cdc.gov/hiv/risk/prep/index.html.** If advice is needed, clinicians may consult the National Clinicians Consultation Center PrEP Line at 1-855-448-7737 (9:00 am–8:00 pm Eastern Time).

ARV-based vaginal microbicides and ARV-coated vaginal rings have reduced HIV acquisition in uninfected women. Data from clinical trials conducted in African countries also provide evidence that medical male circumcision can reduce HIV acquisition in uninfected heterosexual males by 38% to 66% over 24 months.

Postexposure Prophylaxis for Possible Sexual or Other Nonoccupational Exposure to HIV. Decisions to provide ARVs after possible nonoccupational (ie, community) exposure to HIV must balance the potential benefits and risks. Decisions regarding the need for ARV prophylaxis in such instances are predicated on the probability that the source is infected or contaminated with HIV, the likelihood of transmission by the particular exposure, and the interval between exposure and initiation of therapy, balanced against expected adverse effects associated with the regimen.

The risk of transmission of HIV from a puncture wound attributable to a needle found in the community likely is lower than 0.3%, which is the estimated probability of HIV transmission from a puncture wound involving a known HIV-contaminated needle in a health care setting. The actual risks of HIV infection in an infant or child after a needlestick injury or sexual abuse are unknown, but to date there are no confirmed transmissions of HIV from accidental nonoccupational needlestick injuries (needles found in the community). The estimated risk of HIV transmission from receptive penile-anal sexual exposure is 138 per 10 000 exposures. The estimated risk per episode of receptive vaginal exposure is 8 per 10 000 exposures.

ARVs generally should not be used if the risk of transmission is low (eg, trivial needlestick injury with a drug needle from an unknown nonoccupational source) or if care is sought more than 72 hours after the reported exposure (see Injuries from Needles Discarded in the Community, p 166). The benefits of postexposure prophylaxis are greatest when risk of infection is high, intervention is prompt, and adherence is likely. Consultation with an experienced pediatric HIV health care professional is essential. Detailed guidelines for postexposure prophylaxis for children can be found at **https://stacks.cdc.gov/view/cdc/38856.** The American Academy of Pediatrics recommends that youth be offered HIV post-exposure prophylaxis following high-risk sexual exposures.[1]

---

[1] Hsu KK, Rakhmanina NY; American Academy of Pediatrics, Committee on Pediatric AIDS. Clinical report: Adolescents and young adults: the pediatrician's role in HIV testing and pre- and post-exposure HIV prophylaxis. *Pediatrics.* 2021; In press

Postexposure Prophylaxis for Occupational Exposure to HIV. Guidelines for use of occupational postexposure prophylaxis have been published by the CDC and should be started as soon as possible after the exposure but within 72 hours for maximal effectiveness (**https:// stacks.cdc.gov/view/cdc/38856**). In addition, the University of California, San Francisco maintains a Clinician Consultation Center at 1-888-448-4911 seven days a week between 9 am and 9 pm Eastern Time and can provide valuable support to providers.

Human Papillomaviruses

CLINICAL MANIFESTATIONS: Most human papillomavirus (HPV) infections are subclinical, and 90% resolve spontaneously within 2 years. However, persistent HPV infection can cause benign epithelial proliferation (warts) of the skin and mucous membranes as well as cancers of the lower anogenital tract and the oropharynx. HPVs can be grouped into cutaneous and mucosal types. The cutaneous types cause common skin warts, plantar warts, flat warts, and thread-like (filiform) warts. These cutaneous warts are benign. Certain mucosal types (low risk) are associated with warts or papillomas of mucous membranes, including the upper respiratory tract and anogenital, oral, nasal, and conjunctival areas. Other mucosal types (high risk) can cause precancers and cancers, including cervical, anogenital, and oropharyngeal cancers.

Warts are common, benign lesions, although they may be associated with significant clinical problems. Common **skin warts** are dome-shaped with conical projections that give the surface a rough appearance. Skin warts usually are painless and multiple, occurring commonly on the hands and around or under the nails. When small dermal vessels become thrombosed, black dots appear in the warts.

Plantar warts on the foot often are larger than warts at other sites and may not project through much of the skin surface. They can be painful when walking and are characterized by marked hyperkeratosis, sometimes with black dots.

Flat warts ("juvenile warts") commonly are found on the face and extremities of children and adolescents. Flat warts usually are small, multiple, and flat topped, seldom exhibit papillomatosis, and rarely cause pain. **Filiform warts** occur on the face and neck.

Anogenital warts, also called **condylomata acuminata,** are skin-colored warts with a papular, flat, or cauliflower-like surface that range in size from a few millimeters to several centimeters; these warts often occur in groups. In males, these warts may be found on the penis, scrotum, anal, or perianal area. In females, these lesions may occur on the vulvar, anal, or perianal areas and less commonly in the vagina or on the cervix. Warts usually are painless, although they may cause itching, burning, local pain, or bleeding.

Invasive cancers attributable to HPV include those of the cervix, vagina, vulva, penis, anus, and oropharynx (back of throat, base of tongue, and tonsils). Cervical cancer is the most common HPV-attributable cancer among females, and oropharyngeal cancer is the most common HPV-attributable cancer among males. Anogenital low-grade squamous intraepithelial lesions (LSILs) can result from persistent infection with low-risk or high-risk HPV types, whereas high-grade squamous intraepithelial lesions (HSILs) can result from persistent infection with high-risk HPV types. In the cervix, HSILs include cervical intraepithelial neoplasia (CIN) grades 2 or 3, and adenocarcinoma in situ (AIS), which are precancerous lesions. Intraepithelial lesions are detected through routine screening with cytologic testing (Papanicolaou [Pap] test); tissue biopsy is required to make the diagnosis of CIN.

Recurrent respiratory papillomatosis is a rare condition characterized by recurring papillomas in the larynx or other areas of the upper or lower respiratory tract. Age of onset can be in childhood or adulthood. Recurrent respiratory papillomatosis is referred to as juvenile onset RRP (JORRP) when it occurs before 12 years of age and as adult onset RRP (AORRP) in those 12 years and older. JORRP is believed to result most frequently from vertical transmission of HPV from a mother to her infant at the time of delivery. JORRP is diagnosed most commonly in children between 2 and 5 years of age, with manifestations of voice change (eg, hoarseness or abnormal cry), stridor, or respiratory distress. Respiratory papillomas can cause respiratory tract obstruction in young children, and repeated surgeries often are needed. Most cases of JORRP are caused by HPV 6 or 11. Less is known about AORRP.

Epidermodysplasia verruciformis is a rare, inherited disorder believed to be a consequence of a deficiency of cell-mediated immunity, resulting in an abnormal susceptibility to certain HPV types and manifesting as chronic cutaneous lesions and skin cancers. Lesions may resemble flat warts or pigmented plaques covering the torso and upper extremities. Most appear during the first decade of life, but malignant transformation, which occurs in 30% to 60% of affected people, usually is delayed until adulthood.

ETIOLOGY: HPVs are small, nonenveloped, double-stranded DNA viruses of the *Papillomaviridae* family, which can be grouped into a number of types based on DNA sequence variation. Different types display different specific tissue tropism. Types 6 and 11 cause anogenital warts (condylomata acuminata), recurrent respiratory papillomatosis, and conjunctival papillomas but rarely are found in cancer. High-risk HPV types can be detected in almost all cervical precancers and invasive cervical cancers. Approximately 50% of cervical cancers worldwide are attributable to HPV type 16; 70% are attributable to either type 16 or 18. The majority of other HPV-related cancers—anogenital cancers (vulvar, vaginal, penile, anal) and oropharyngeal cancers—also are attributable to HPV type 16. Infection with a high-risk HPV type is considered necessary but not sufficient to cause cancer. The vast majority of people with an HPV infection will not develop cancer. Risk of developing cancer precursors or cancers is greater in people with certain immunocompromising conditions, such as human immunodeficiency virus (HIV) infection or cellular immune deficiencies.

EPIDEMIOLOGY: Virtually all adults will be infected with some type of HPV during their lives. In the United States, HPV infection prevalence is 79 million, and annual incidence is 14 million infections.

Nongenital hand and foot warts occur commonly among school-aged children. Acquisition can occur through casual contact and is facilitated by minor skin trauma. Autoinoculation can result in spread of lesions. The intense and often widespread appearance of cutaneous warts in people with compromised cellular immunity (particularly those who have undergone transplantation or who have HIV infection) suggests that alterations in T-lymphocyte immunity may impair clearance of infection.

Genital HPV infections are transmitted by intimate skin-to-skin contact, for example through sexual intercourse or other close genital contact. In US females, the highest prevalence of infection is in 20- to 24-year-olds. Most infections are subclinical and clear spontaneously within 1 or 2 years. Cancer is an uncommon outcome of infection that generally requires decades of persistent infection with high-risk HPV types. There are more than 33 000 cases of HPV-attributable cancers annually in the United States.

HPV-attributable cervical cancer accounts for approximately one third of new HPV-attributable cancer cases and 4000 deaths annually in the United States. HPV-attributable oropharyngeal cancer accounts for more than one third of new HPV-attributable cancer cases per year. HPV is the cause of at least 90% of all cervical cancers, 70% of oropharyngeal cancers, and most vulvar, vaginal, penile, and anal cancers.

Rarely, HPV infection is transmitted to a child through the birth canal during delivery or transmitted from nongenital sites postnatally. When anogenital warts are diagnosed in a child, the possibility of sexual abuse must be considered while noting the possibility of vertical transmission to neonates (see STI Evaluation of Prepubertal Victims, p 152, and Table 2.5, p 151).

The **incubation period** for symptoms of HPV infection is estimated to range from 3 months to several years but most infections are asymptomatic. The period from infection to neoplastic changes is usually years to decades.

DIAGNOSTIC TESTS: Most cutaneous and anogenital warts can be diagnosed through clinical inspection. Serologic testing for HPV does not inform clinical decisions and is not commercially available. Routine cervical cancer screening guidelines have been established by multiple professional societies. These guidelines direct the age of initiation and interval at which screening with cytology (Pap testing) and/or HPV nucleic acid testing (primary screen or "cotesting") should be performed (see below). Criteria for screening abnormalities that require colposcopic evaluation and biopsy are also provided. Vulvar, vaginal, penile, and anal lesions may be identified using visual inspection, sometimes using magnification; in some cases, cytologic screening is used and suspicious lesions are biopsied, but there is no routine screening recommended for cancers at these sites. Many dentists screen for oral cancer but there is no widely accepted screening program. For all anogenital, oropharyngeal, and respiratory tract precancers and cancers, diagnosis is made histologically.

Although cytologic and histologic changes can be suggestive of HPV, these findings are not diagnostic of HPV. Documentation of HPV infection is based on detection of viral nucleic acid (DNA or RNA). Nucleic acid tests for high-risk HPV types may be used as a primary screen for cervical cancer in women starting at age 25 years, in combination with Pap testing in women 30 years or older and for triage of equivocal Pap test abnormalities (atypical squamous cells of undetermined significance [ASCUS]) in women 21 years or older. The benefit of HPV nucleic acid testing is that a negative test result for high-risk HPV types allows longer intervals (eg, 3–5 years) between routine screening.

A number of HPV DNA or mRNA detection and genotyping assays have been cleared for use in the United States by the US Food and Drug Administration (FDA). Liquid-based cytology collection and transport kits permit performance of Pap smear cytology and HPV detection and genotyping on the same specimen. There are differences in the appropriate clinical applications for each of these assays, including whether they can be used as an initial standalone test (ie, without cervical cytology) or in a primary screening algorithm; none is recommended for use in women younger than 21 years or for men.

TREATMENT[1]: There is no FDA approved treatment for HPV infection. Treatment may be directed toward lesions caused by HPV.

---

[1]Centers for Disease Control and Prevention. Sexually transmitted infections treatment guidelines, 2021. *MMWR Recomm Rep.* 2021; in press

Regression of **nongenital and genital warts** occurs in approximately 30% of cases within 6 months, even without treatment. Most methods of treatment of cutaneous warts use chemical or physical destruction of the infected epithelium, including cryotherapy with liquid nitrogen, laser or surgical removal of warts, application of salicylic acid products, or application of topical immune-modulating agents. Many agents used for treatment of warts have not been tested for safety and efficacy in children, and some are contraindicated in pregnancy.

Daily treatment with tretinoin has been useful for widespread flat warts in children. Systemic treatments, including cimetidine, have been used for refractory warts with variable success. Treatments for genital warts are characterized as patient-applied or provider administered. Interventions include ablational/excisional treatments, topical antiproliferative medications, or immune-modulating medications. Oral warts can be removed through cryotherapy, electrocautery, or surgical excision. Although most forms of therapy are successful for initial removal of warts, treatment may not eradicate HPV infection from the surrounding tissue. Recurrences are common and may be attributable to reactivation rather than reinfection.

Cancer precursor lesions that are identified in the cervix (eg, HSILs, AIS) or elsewhere in the genital tract may require excision or destruction. Treatment of cervical lesions can cause substantial economic, emotional, and reproductive adverse effects, including higher risk of preterm birth and perinatal mortality. Management of invasive cervical and other anogenital and oropharyngeal cancers requires a specialist and should be conducted according to current guidelines.

Respiratory papillomatosis is difficult to treat and is best managed by an experienced otolaryngologist. Local recurrence is common, and repeated surgical debulking procedures are often necessary to relieve airway obstruction. Extension or dissemination of respiratory papillomas from the larynx into the trachea, bronchi, or lung parenchyma happens rarely but results in increased morbidity and mortality; malignant transformation occurs rarely. Intralesional interferon, oral indole-3-carbinole, systemic bevacizumab, photodynamic therapy, intralesional cidofovir, and HPV vaccination have been used as investigational treatments; however, efficacy with any of these is unproven.

ISOLATION OF THE HOSPITALIZED PATIENT: Standard precautions are recommended.

CONTROL MEASURES AND CARE OF EXPOSED PEOPLE: Sexual abuse should be considered if anogenital warts are found in a child. When anogenital warts are found in a child who is prepubertal, clinicians should refer patients to a child abuse management pediatrician for an abuse evaluation (see STI Evaluation of Prepubertal Victims, p 152, and Table 2.5, p 151). Suspected child sexual abuse should be reported to the appropriate local agency.

Most cancer-causing HPV infections can be prevented by vaccination (see below). Delaying sexual debut and minimizing the lifetime number of sex partners are other modes of reducing risk of HPV infection. Consistent and correct use of latex condoms may reduce the risk of anogenital HPV infection when infected areas are covered or protected by the condom. The degree and duration of contagiousness in patients with a history of genital HPV infection is unknown. People with genital warts should refrain from sex with new partners while warts are present, and should inform their current sex partners, who also may benefit from a clinical evaluation for anogenital warts or other sexually transmitted infections.

Although respiratory papillomatosis is believed to be caused by transmission of HPV types 6 and 11 during passage through the birth canal, this condition has occurred in infants born by cesarean delivery. Because the preventive value of cesarean delivery is unknown, it should not be performed solely to prevent transmission of HPV to the newborn infant.

Cervical Cancer Screening. Women who have received HPV vaccine should continue to have regular cervical cancer screening. HPV vaccines do not provide protection against all HPV types associated with development of cervical cancer and do not alter the course of infections existing before vaccination. Several professional organizations offer guidance on cervical cancer screening, including the American College of Obstetricians and Gynecologists (**www.acog.org**), the American Cancer Society (**www.cancer.org**), and the US Preventive Services Task Force (**www.uspreventiveservicestaskforce.org**). These organizations recommend that Pap testing begin at 21 years of age for all healthy women, regardless of sexual history. Female adolescents with a recent diagnosis of HIV infection should undergo cervical Pap test screening at the time of diagnosis and again in the next 6 to 12 months (**https://clinicalinfo.hiv.gov/en/guidelines**). Sexually active female adolescents who have had an organ transplant or are receiving long-term corticosteroid therapy also should undergo similar cervical Pap test screening.

HPV Vaccines. Three HPV vaccines have been licensed by the FDA for use in the United States but only one, a 9-valent vaccine, is currently on the market in the United States. A quadrivalent vaccine (4vHPV [types 6, 11, 16, and 18], Gardasil) was licensed by the FDA in 2006. A bivalent vaccine (2vHPV [types 16 and 18], Cervarix) was licensed in 2009. A 9-valent HPV vaccine (9vHPV [types 6, 11, 16, 18, 31, 33, 45, 52, and 58], Gardasil 9) was licensed by the FDA in 2014.

Immunogenicity. More than 97% of healthy vaccine recipients develop antibodies to HPV vaccine types after vaccination. Antibody titers are higher in adolescent females and males aged 9 through 15 years compared with females and males 16 through 26 years of age.

Antibody titers for all HPV vaccines decrease over time but plateau by 18 to 24 months after vaccination. Follow-up studies through 8 and 10 years after 4vHPV and 2vHPV vaccination, respectively, have shown no waning of protection. Studies of all 3 HPV vaccines have found that antibody titers after 2 doses administered 6 to 12 months apart to 9- through 14-year-olds are similar to 3 doses administered to women 16 through 26 years of age, the age group in which efficacy was demonstrated in clinical trials.

Efficacy. 4vHPV and 2vHPV have been shown to be highly effective in preventing cervical precancers related to HPV types 16 and 18 in clinical trials among females 15 through 26 years of age. 4vHPV has been shown to be highly effective in preventing genital warts related to HPV types 6 and 11 in clinical trials among females and males 16 through 26 years of age. 4vHPV also has been shown to be highly effective in preventing anal precancers in males 16 through 26 years of age. 9vHPV has been shown in a clinical trial among women 16 through 26 years of age to provide 97% protection against the additional 5 HPV types in the 9-valent product (31, 33, 45, 52, and 58) and to produce noninferior immunogenicity for the 4 HPV types in the quadrivalent product (6, 11, 16, and 18). Clinical trials of 2vHPV and 4vHPV in women older than age 26 years also have been conducted; efficacy has been demonstrated for a combined endpoint of vaccine-type infection and cervical precancers. HPV vaccines have not been proven to have a therapeutic effect on existing HPV infection or disease and do not offer protection against progression of infection to disease from HPV acquired before immunization. Therefore, HPV vaccines are most effective when administered before exposure to any of the HPV types included in the vaccine.

Assessment of the full impact of HPV vaccination on anogenital and oropharyngeal cancers may take decades, given the natural history of HPV-driven oncogenesis. Demonstrated impacts include significant reductions in early and intermediate HPV-related outcomes, including vaccine-type HPV prevalence, anogenital warts, and cervical precancers. Long-term follow-up studies are being conducted to determine the duration of efficacy for all HPV vaccines.

Vaccine Recommendations.[1,2] The American Academy of Pediatrics (AAP) and the Advisory Committee on Immunization Practices (ACIP) of the Centers for Disease Control and Prevention recommend routine HPV vaccination for females and males. The AAP recommends starting the series between 9 and 12 years, at an age that the provider deems optimal for acceptance and completion of the vaccination series. The ACIP recommends starting the series at age 11 or 12 years of age and states that vaccination can be administered starting at age 9 years. When HPV vaccine is begun at 9 or 10 years of age, other adolescent vaccines (eg, MenACWY and Tdap) still are recommended to be administered at 11 to 12 years of age.

Providers are encouraged to recommend use of HPV vaccine as they do all other routine childhood and adolescent vaccines. Research has demonstrated that parents are influenced by strong recommendations and personal testimonials from their child's pediatrician. Opportunities to prevent cancers and deaths are being missed by clinicians who describe HPV vaccine as a sexually transmitted infection vaccine rather than a cancer prevention vaccine or who fail to announce HPV vaccination as routinely recommended.

Catch-up HPV vaccination is recommended for all people through age 26 years who are not adequately vaccinated. Catch-up HPV vaccination is not recommended for all adults >26 years of age. Instead, shared clinical decision-making regarding HPV vaccination is recommended for some adults 27 through 45 years of age who are not adequately vaccinated.

Dosage and Administration. HPV vaccine is administered in either 2 or 3 doses of 0.5 mL, intramuscularly, preferably in a deltoid muscle.
- For people initiating vaccination before their 15th birthday, the recommended schedule is 2 doses of HPV vaccine, with the second dose administered 6 to 12 months after the first dose (minimum interval 5 months).
- For people initiating vaccination on or after their 15th birthday, the recommended schedule is 3 doses of HPV vaccine. In a 3-dose schedule, the second dose should be administered at least 1 to 2 months after the first dose (minimum interval 4 weeks), and the third dose should be administered 6 months after the first dose (minimum interval 5 months after first dose, and 12 weeks after second dose).
- People considered adequately vaccinated:
  - People who initiated vaccination before their 15th birthday and received 2 doses of any HPV vaccine (9vHPV, 4vHPV, or 2vHPV) at the recommended dosing schedule

[1]American Academy of Pediatrics, Committee on Infectious Diseases. HPV vaccine recommendations. *Pediatrics.* 2012;129(3):602–605

[2]Meites E, Szilagyi PG, Chesson HW, Unger ER, Romero JR, Markowitz LE. Human papillomavirus vaccination for adults: updated recommendations of the Advisory Committee on Immunization Practices. *MMWR Morb Mortal Wkly Rep.* 2019;68(32):698–702. DOI: **http://dx.doi.org/10.15585/mmwr.mm6832a3**

(0, 6–12 months), or 3 doses of any HPV vaccine at the recommended dosing schedule (0, 1–2, 6 months).

    ◆ People who initiated vaccination on or after their 15th birthday and received 3 doses of any HPV vaccine (9vHPV, 4vHPV, or 2vHPV) at the recommended dosing schedule (0, 1–2, 6 months). (Also see section on recommendations for special populations, below).

- If the vaccine schedule is interrupted, the vaccine series can be continued with the next recommended dose and does not need to be restarted.
- 9vHPV may be used to complete a series started with 4vHPV or 2vHPV.
- There is no recommendation regarding additional vaccination with 9vHPV for people who previously completed a 4vHPV or 2vHPV vaccination series.
- Evidence of past HPV exposure or current HPV infection or disease, such as abnormal Pap test results, cervical lesions, anogenital warts, or a positive HPV DNA test result, are not contraindications to HPV immunization. Males and females in the recommended age ranges still should receive HPV vaccine to protect against any HPV types not already acquired.
- HPV vaccines can be coadministered with any live or inactivated vaccine indicated at the same visit.

    Recommendations for Special Populations. HPV vaccines are not live vaccines. For people ages 9 through 26 years with immunocompromising conditions (including primary or secondary immunocompromising conditions that might reduce cell-mediated or humoral immunity, such as B-lymphocyte antibody deficiencies, T-lymphocyte complete or partial defects, HIV infection, malignant neoplasms, transplantation, autoimmune disease, or immunosuppressive therapy), a 3-dose schedule of HPV vaccine is recommended regardless of age at initiation. Immune response and vaccine efficacy in immunocompromised people might be less than that in immunocompetent people.

    For children with a history of sexual abuse or assault, the HPV vaccination series should be started at 9 years of age. Children who are victims of sexual abuse or assault are recognized to be at greater risk for subsequent high risk sexual behaviors at an earlier age than nonabused children; they also may be at higher risk of future victimization.

Vaccine Adverse Events, Precautions, and Contraindications. Studies of more than 15 000 people in clinical trials for each of the HPV vaccines have shown no serious safety concerns. In addition, more than 100 million doses of HPV vaccines have been distributed in the United States without evidence for serious safety concerns. Injection site discomfort or pain, redness, and swelling are the most commonly reported local adverse events. Systemic symptoms after HPV vaccine can include headache, fever, nausea, dizziness, and fatigue/malaise. Syncope (fainting) has been reported in adolescents after receipt of any vaccination, including HPV vaccine. Despite common misinformation disseminated mainly on the internet and through social media, HPV vaccine has not been associated with ovarian damage, infertility, or postural orthostatic tachycardia syndrome (POTS). HPV vaccines can be administered to people with minor acute illnesses.

- Immunization of people with moderate or severe acute illnesses should be deferred until after their condition improves.
- HPV vaccines are produced in yeast and are contraindicated in people with a history of immediate hypersensitivity to any vaccine component, including yeast.
- HPV vaccines are not recommended for use during pregnancy because of limited information about safety. The health care professional should inquire about pregnancy

in patients who are known to be sexually active, but a pregnancy test is not required before starting the HPV vaccination series. If a vaccine recipient becomes pregnant, subsequent doses should be postponed until she is no longer pregnant. If a dose has been administered inadvertently during pregnancy, no intervention is needed. Data to date show no evidence of adverse effect of any HPV vaccine on outcomes of pregnancy. Health care professionals can report inadvertent administrations of 9vHPV to pregnant women by calling the vaccine manufacturer at 1-800-986-8999.

- Vaccine providers, particularly when vaccinating adolescents, should observe patients (with patients seated or lying down) for 15 minutes after vaccination to decrease the risk for injury should they faint. If syncope develops, patients should be observed until symptoms resolve.
- HPV vaccines can be administered to lactating women.

Influenza

CLINICAL MANIFESTATIONS: Influenza illness typically begins with sudden onset of fever, often accompanied by nonproductive cough, chills or rigors, diffuse myalgia, headache, and malaise. Subsequently, respiratory tract symptoms, including sore throat, nasal congestion, rhinitis, and cough, become more prominent. Less commonly, abdominal pain, nausea, vomiting, and diarrhea are associated with influenza illness. In some children, influenza can appear as an upper respiratory tract illness or as a febrile illness with few respiratory tract symptoms. In infants, influenza can produce a nonspecific sepsis-like illness picture, and in infants and young children, influenza can cause otitis media, croup, pertussis like-illness, bronchiolitis, or pneumonia. Acute myositis secondary to influenza can present with calf tenderness and refusal to walk.

Although the majority of children with influenza recover fully after 3 to 7 days of illness, complications may occur, even in previously healthy children. Neurologic complications associated with influenza range from febrile seizures to severe encephalopathy and encephalitis with status epilepticus, resulting in neurologic sequelae or death. Reye syndrome, now a very rare condition, has been associated with influenza infection and the use of aspirin therapy during the illness. Children with influenza or suspected influenza should not be given aspirin, and children with diseases that necessitate long-term aspirin therapy or salicylate-containing medication, including juvenile idiopathic arthritis or Kawasaki disease, should be recognized as being at increased risk for complications from influenza. Death from influenza-associated myocarditis has been reported. Invasive secondary infections or coinfections with *Staphylococcus aureus* (including methicillin-resistant *S aureus* [MRSA]), *Streptococcus pneumoniae,* group A streptococcus, or other bacterial pathogens can result in severe disease and death.

ETIOLOGY: Influenza viruses are orthomyxoviruses of 3 genera or types (A, B, and C). Annual epidemics are caused by influenza virus types A and B, and both influenza A and B virus antigens are included in seasonal influenza vaccines. Type C influenza viruses can cause sporadic mild influenza-like illness in children. Type C antigens are not included in influenza vaccines. Influenza A viruses are subclassified into subtypes based on their surface antigens, hemagglutinin (HA) and neuraminidase (NA). Examples of these virus subtypes include H1N1 and H3N2 influenza A viruses. Specific antibodies to these various antigens, especially to hemagglutinin, are important determinants of immunity.

A minor antigenic variation that leads to changes in the HA or NA surface proteins of influenza A or B viruses is termed *antigenic drift*. Antigenic drift occurs continuously and results in new strains of influenza A and B viruses, resulting in seasonal epidemics.

A major antigenic variation that leads to new subtypes containing a unique HA and/or NA is termed *antigenic shift*. When the new virus subtype can infect humans and be transmitted efficiently from person to person in a sustained manner, this can lead to a pandemic because the human population has little or no preexisting immunity to the newly emerged influenza strain. Antigenic shift occurs only among influenza A viruses and has produced 4 influenza pandemics in the 20th and 21st centuries, the most recent in 2009. As with previous antigenic shifts, the 2009 pandemic influenza A (H1N1) viral strain subsequently replaced the previously circulating seasonal influenza A (H1N1) strain in the ensuing influenza seasons.

Humans of all ages may sporadically be infected with emerging influenza A viruses of swine or avian origin. Most notable among avian influenza viruses are A (H5N1), which emerged in 1997 in Hong Kong, and A (H7N9), first detected in 2013 in China, both of which have been associated with severe disease and high case-fatality rates. Since 2017, Asian (H7N9) is considered the influenza virus with the highest potential pandemic risk. Infection with a novel influenza A virus is a nationally notifiable disease and should be reported to the Centers for Disease Control and Prevention (CDC) through state health departments.

EPIDEMIOLOGY: Influenza is spread person to person, primarily through large-particle respiratory droplet transmission (eg, coughing or sneezing), which requires close proximity between the person who is the source and the person who is the recipient because droplets generally only travel short distances. Another mode of transmission comes from contact with influenza virus from droplet-contaminated hands or surfaces, where it can remain for up to 24 hours, with transfer from hands to mucosal surfaces of the face. Airborne transmission via small-particle aerosols in the vicinity of the infectious individual also may occur. Influenza is highly contagious. Patients may be infectious 24 hours before onset of symptoms. Viral shedding in nasal secretions usually peaks during the first 3 days of illness and ceases within 7 days but can be prolonged (10 days or longer) in young children and immunodeficient patients.

Influenza activity in the United States can occur anytime from October to May but most commonly peaks between December and February. Seasonal epidemics can last 8 to 12 weeks or longer. Circulation of 2 or 3 influenza virus strains in a community may be associated with a prolonged influenza season and may produce bimodal peaks in activity.

Seasonal influenza epidemics are associated with an estimated 9.3 to 45 million illnesses, 140 000 to 810 000 hospitalizations, and 12 000 to 61 000 respiratory and circulatory deaths annually in the United States. The CDC estimates that on average, 8% (range, 3%–11%) of the US population develops symptomatic influenza illness each season, depending on the circulating strains. During community outbreaks of influenza, the highest influenza incidence occurs among children, ranging from 10% to 40%, particularly school-aged children. Secondary spread to adults and other children within a family is common.

Hospitalization rates among children younger than 5 years are high and are similar to hospitalization rates among people 65 years and older. Although rates vary across studies (190–480 per 100 000 population) because of differences in methodology and severity of influenza seasons, children younger than 2 years consistently are at a substantially higher risk of hospitalization than are older children. Rates of hospitalization and morbidity attributable to complications, such as bronchitis and pneumonia, are greater in children with high-risk conditions, including chronic pulmonary diseases such as asthma, neurologic and neurodevelopmental disorders, hemodynamically significant cardiac disease, obesity, immunosuppression, metabolic diseases such as diabetes mellitus, and hemoglobinopathies such as sickle cell disease. However, 40% to 50% of all children hospitalized with influenza have no known underlying conditions, and almost half of children who die from influenza do not have an underlying high-risk condition. The number of reported annual influenza-related deaths among both chronically ill and previously healthy children usually ranges from 35 to 188, with higher numbers reported in some seasons. All influenza-associated pediatric deaths are nationally notifiable and must be reported to the CDC through state health departments.

Information about influenza surveillance is available through the CDC Voice Information System (influenza update, 888-232-3228) or through **www.cdc.gov/flu/**.

The **incubation period** usually is 1 to 4 days, with a mean of 2 days.

DIAGNOSTIC TESTS: Influenza testing should be performed when the results are anticipated to influence clinical management (eg, to inform the decision to initiate antiviral therapy or antibiotic agents, to pursue other diagnostic testing, or to implement infection prevention and control measures). The decision to test is related to the level local influenza activity, clinical suspicion for influenza, and the sensitivity and specificity of commercially available influenza tests (Table 3.25, p 450). These include rapid molecular assays for influenza RNA or nucleic acid detection, reverse transcriptase-polymerase chain reaction (RT-PCR) single-plex or multiplex assays, real time or other RNA-based assays, immunofluorescence assays (direct [DFA] or indirect [IFA] fluorescent antibody staining) for antigen detection, rapid influenza diagnostic tests (RIDTs) based on antigen detection, rapid cell culture (shell vial culture), and viral tissue cell culture (conventional) for virus isolation. The optimal choice of influenza test depends on the clinical setting.

The sensitivity and specificity of any influenza test varies by the type of test used, the time from illness onset to specimen collection, the quality of the specimen collected, the source of the specimen, and the handling and processing of the specimen, including the time from specimen collection to testing. To diagnose influenza in the outpatient or inpatient setting, testing should occur as soon after illness onset as possible, because the quantity of virus shed decreases rapidly as illness progresses. Nasopharyngeal swab specimens have the highest yield of upper respiratory tract specimens for detection of influenza viruses. Mid-turbinate nasal swab or wash specimens are also acceptable. Testing with combined nasal and throat swab specimens may increase the detection of influenza viruses over single specimens from either site (particularly over throat swab specimens alone). Using flocked swabs likely improves influenza virus detection over nonflocked swabs. For patients with respiratory failure receiving mechanical ventilation, including patients with negative influenza testing results on upper respiratory tract specimens, endotracheal aspirate or bronchoalveolar lavage (BAL) fluid specimens should be obtained. Nonrespiratory specimens such as blood, plasma, serum, cerebrospinal fluid, urine, and stool should not be used for routine diagnosis of influenza. Results of influenza testing should be properly interpreted in the context of clinical findings and local community influenza activity, because the prevalence of circulating influenza viruses influences the positive and negative predictive values of these influenza screening tests. False-positive

Table 3.25. Summary of Influenza Diagnostic Tests

Influenza Diagnostic Test	Method	Availability	Typical Processing Time	Sensitivity	Types Detected
Rapid influenza diagnostic tests (RIDTs)[a]	Antigen detection	Wide	<15 min	10%–70%	A and B
Rapid molecular assays[b]	RNA or nucleic acid detection	Wide	15–30 min	86%–100%	A and B
Nucleic acid amplification (RT-PCR and other molecular assays)[c]	RNA or nucleic acid detection	Limited	1–8 h	86%–100%	A and B
Direct and indirect Immunofluorescence antibody assays[c]	Antigen detection	Wide	1–4 h	70%–100%	A and B
Rapid cell culture (shell vials and cell mixtures)[c]	Virus isolation	Limited	1–3 days	100%	A and B
Tissue cell culture[c]	Virus isolation	Limited	3–10 days	100%	A and B

RT-PCR indicates reverse transcriptase-polymerase chain reaction. May be single-plex or multiplex, real time, and other RNA-based assays.
[a] Most rapid influenza diagnostic tests are Clinical Laboratory Improvement Amendments (CLIA) waived.
[b] Some rapid influenza molecular assays are CLIA waived, depending on the specimen.
[c] Not CLIA waived. Requires laboratory expertise.
Adapted from **www.cdc.gov/flu/professionals/diagnosis/index.htm.**

results are more likely to occur during periods of low influenza activity; false-negative results are more likely to occur during periods of peak influenza activity.

TREATMENT: In the United States, 3 classes of antiviral medications with different mechanisms of action currently are approved for treatment or prophylaxis of influenza infections. Two of these classes are used in clinical management of influenza disease: 3 drugs in the neuraminidase inhibitor class (oral oseltamivir, inhaled zanamivir, and intravenous peramivir) and 1 drug in the cap-dependent endonuclease inhibitor class (oral baloxavir marboxil). Guidance for use of these antiviral agents is summarized in Table 3.26 and at **www.aapredbook.org/flu** and **www.cdc.gov/flu/professionals/antivirals/index.htm.**

Oseltamivir remains the antiviral drug of choice for treatment of influenza A and B. The US Food and Drug Administration (FDA) has approved oseltamivir for influenza treatment in children as young as 2 weeks of age. Given available pharmacokinetic data and safety data, though, oseltamivir can be used to treat influenza in both term and preterm infants from birth, because benefits of therapy are likely to outweigh possible risks of treatment.

Inhaled zanamivir is an acceptable alternative for older children. Intravenous peramivir is approved for use in people 2 years and older. Oral baloxavir is approved for people

Table 3.26. Antiviral Drugs for Influenza[a]

Drug (Trade Name)	Virus	Administration	Treatment Indications	Chemoprophylaxis Indications	Adverse Effects
Oseltamivir (Tamiflu)	A and B	Oral twice daily for 5 days	Birth or older[b]	3 mo or older	Nausea, vomiting, headache; skin reactions
Zanamivir (Relenza)	A and B	Inhalation twice daily for 5 days	7 y or older	5 y or older	Bronchospasm, skin reactions
Peramivir (Rapivab)	A and B[c]	Intravenous as a single dose	2 y or older	Not recommended	Diarrhea, skin reactions
Baloxavir marboxil (Xofluxa)[d]	A and B	Oral as a single dose	12 y or older and weight ≥40 kg	Not recommended	Nausea, vomiting, diarrhea

[a] Recommended dosages for drugs approved for treatment and prophylaxis of influenza are provided in Table 4.10 (p 930). For current recommendations about treatment and chemoprophylaxis of influenza, including specific dosing information, see **www.aapredbook.org/flu** and **www.cdc.gov/flu/professionals/antivirals/index.htm.** Antiviral susceptibilities of viral strains are reported weekly at **www.cdc.gov/flu/weekly/fluactivitysurv.htm.**

[b] Approved by the FDA for children as young as 2 wk of age. Given available pharmacokinetic data and limited safety data, the AAP believes that oseltamivir can be used to treat influenza in both term and preterm infants from birth because benefits of therapy are likely to outweigh possible risks of treatment.

[c] Peramivir efficacy is based on clinical trials in which the predominant influenza virus type was influenza A; a limited number of subjects infected with influenza B virus were enrolled.

[d] Long-acting endonuclease inhibitor with different mechanism of action than neuraminidase inhibitors. Greater activity on influenza B reported compared with oseltamivir.

12 years and older. Recommended dosages for drugs approved for treatment and prophylaxis of influenza are provided in Table 4.10 (p 930).

Resistance to oseltamivir and zanamivir has been documented in less than 1% of the tested influenza viral samples during the past seasons. Decreased susceptibility to baloxavir has been reported in Japan, where use has been more common, and surveillance for resistance among circulating influenza viruses is ongoing in the United States. Each year, options for treatment or chemoprophylaxis of influenza in the United States will depend on influenza strain resistance patterns.

Regardless of influenza vaccination status, antiviral treatment should be offered as early as possible to the following individuals:

• Any hospitalized child with suspected or confirmed influenza disease, regardless of the duration of symptoms;

• Any child, inpatient or outpatient, with severe, complicated, or progressive illness attributable to influenza, regardless of the duration of symptoms or presence of high-risk conditions; and

• Children with influenza virus infection of any severity who are at high risk of complications of influenza, regardless of the duration of symptoms.

Antiviral treatment may be considered for the following individuals:

• Any previously healthy, symptomatic outpatient not at high risk for influenza complications in whom an influenza diagnosis is confirmed or suspected on the basis of clinical judgment, if treatment can be initiated within 48 hours of illness onset; and

- Children with suspected or confirmed influenza disease whose siblings or household contacts either are younger than 6 months or have a high-risk condition that predisposes them to complications of influenza.

Children with severe influenza should be evaluated carefully for possible coinfection with bacterial pathogens (eg, *S aureus* or *S pneumoniae*) that might require antimicrobial therapy.

The most common adverse effects of oseltamivir are nausea and vomiting. Postmarketing reports, almost exclusively from Japan, have noted self-injury and delirium with use of oseltamivir among pediatric patients, but other data suggest that these occurrences may have been related to influenza disease itself rather than antiviral therapy. An FDA review of controlled clinical trial data and ongoing surveillance did not establish a link between oseltamivir (or any influenza antiviral medication) and neurologic or psychiatric events. Zanamivir use has been associated with bronchospasm in some people and is not recommended for use in patients with underlying reactive airway disease. The most common adverse effects of baloxavir are nausea, vomiting, and diarrhea.

Control of fever with acetaminophen or another appropriate nonsalicylate-containing antipyretic agent may be important in some children, because fever and other symptoms of influenza could exacerbate underlying chronic conditions. Children and adolescents with influenza should not receive aspirin or any salicylate-containing products because of the potential risk of developing Reye syndrome.

ISOLATION OF THE HOSPITALIZED PATIENT: In addition to standard precautions, droplet precautions are recommended for children hospitalized with influenza or an influenza-like illness for the duration of illness.

CONTROL MEASURES:

Influenza Vaccines. All people 6 months and older should be vaccinated annually against influenza. Two types of influenza vaccines are available: inactivated influenza vaccines (IIVs), which contain no live virus and are given via intramuscular (IM) injection; and the live attenuated influenza vaccine (LAIV), which is given as a nasal spray. All influenza vaccines are formulated with the same viral strains. The influenza virus strains selected for inclusion in the seasonal vaccine may change yearly in anticipation of the predominant influenza strains expected to circulate in the northern hemisphere in the upcoming influenza season on the basis of influenza circulation in the southern hemisphere and/or in the northern hemisphere's prior season. All pediatric influenza vaccines available in the United States since the 2019–2020 season are quadrivalent, containing 2 influenza A strains and 2 influenza B strains. All licensed pediatric vaccines in the United States are manufactured using virus grown in eggs (egg-based), except for 1 inactivated cell-based vaccine. The age indication and dose varies among licensed influenza vaccines for children (see Fig 3.11). FDA approved formulations of licensed influenza vaccines are available with a standard volume of 0.5 mL per dose for children 6 through 36 months of age (see Table 3.27, p 454). The AAP has no preference for any type of vaccine (IIV or LAIV) or formulation over the other.

An adjuvanted, cell-based vaccine designed to protect against H5N1 in the event of a pandemic has been approved for children 6 months or older. Recommendations for its use would be made in the event that such a pandemic develops.

Immunogenicity and Dosing in Children. Children 9 years and older require only 1 dose of influenza vaccine annually, regardless of their influenza immunization history. Children

FIG 3.11. AVAILABLE INFLUENZA VACCINES IN THE UNITED STATES, BY FDA-LICENSED AGE INDICATION

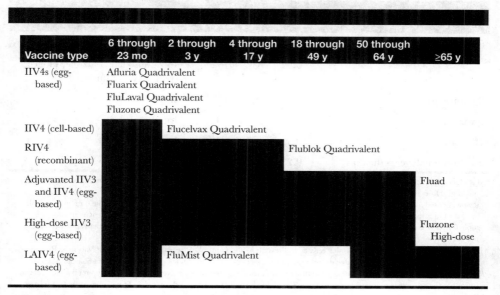

Vaccine type	6 through 23 mo	2 through 3 y	4 through 17 y	18 through 49 y	50 through 64 y	≥65 y
IIV4s (egg-based)	Afluria Quadrivalent Fluarix Quadrivalent FluLaval Quadrivalent Fluzone Quadrivalent					
IIV4 (cell-based)		Flucelvax Quadrivalent				
RIV4 (recombinant)				Flublok Quadrivalent		
Adjuvanted IIV3 and IIV4 (egg-based)						Fluad
High-dose IIV3 (egg-based)						Fluzone High-dose
LAIV4 (egg-based)		FluMist Quadrivalent				

6 months through 8 years of age who are receiving the influenza vaccine for the first time or who have received only 1 dose before the upcoming influenza season should receive 2 doses of influenza vaccine administered at least 4 weeks apart. For children requiring 2 doses, vaccination should not be delayed to obtain a specific product for either dose. Any available, age-appropriate vaccine can be used. Protection against disease is achieved 1 to 2 weeks after the second dose.

Children 6 through 35 months of age may receive either a 0.25-mL or 0.5-mL dose of any licensed, age-appropriate inactivated influenza vaccine available (see Table 3.27). No product is preferred over another for this age group. Children 36 months (3 years) and older should receive a 0.5-mL dose of any available, licensed, age appropriate inactivated vaccine (**https://redbook.solutions.aap.org/redbook.aspx**).[1]

Coadministration With Other Vaccines. Influenza vaccines can be administered simultaneously with other live and inactivated vaccines. Receipt of recommended childhood vaccines during a single visit has important benefits of protecting children against many infectious diseases and minimizing the number of visits that parents, caregivers, and children must make.

Recommendations for Influenza Immunization.[1,2] All people 6 months and older should receive influenza vaccine annually. Influenza vaccine should be administered before the start of

---

[1]American Academy of Pediatrics, Committee on Infectious Diseases. Recommendations for prevention and control of influenza in children, 2020–2021. *Pediatrics.* 2020;146(4):e2020024588

[2]Centers for Disease Control and Prevention. Prevention and control of seasonal influenza with vaccines: recommendations of the Advisory Committee on Immunization Practices (ACIP)—United States, 2017–2018 influenza season. *MMWR Recomm Rep.* 2017;66(RR-2):1–20 (for updates, see **www.cdc.gov/flu**)

Table 3.27. Schedule for Influenza Vaccine Dosing by Age[a]

Age	Dose, mL[b]	No. of Doses	Route[c]
6 through 35 mo	0.25	1–2[d]	Intramuscular (Afluria)
	0.5	1–2[d]	Intramuscular (Fluzone, Fluarix, FluLaval, Afluria)
3 y through 8 y	0.5	1–2[d]	Intramuscular
9 y through 17 y	0.5	1	Intramuscular
18 y or older	0.5	1	Intramuscular
2 y through 49 years (healthy)	0.2	1–2[d]	Intranasal[e]

[a] Manufacturers include Sanofi Pasteur (Fluzone Quadrivalent, split-virus vaccines licensed for people 6 months or older, Fluzone High-Dose, trivalent split virus vaccine licensed for people 65 years and older, and Flublok Quadrivalent, recombinant vaccine licensed for people 18 years or older), Seqirus (Afluria Quadrivalent, split virus vaccine for people 6 months and older; Flucelvax Quadrivalent cell-based vaccine licensed for people 2 years and older, and Fluad adjuvanted trivalent vaccine for people 65 years and older), GlaxoSmithKline Biologicals (Fluarix Quadrivalent and FluLaval Quadrivalent split-virus vaccines licensed for people 6 months or older).

[b] From: Grohskopf LA, Alyanak E, Broder KR, et al. Prevention and Control of Seasonal Influenza with Vaccines: Recommendations of the Advisory Committee on Immunization Practices — United States, 2020–21 Influenza Season. *MMWR Recomm Rep*. 2020;69(RR-8):1–24. Dosages are those recommended in recent years. Refer to the product circular each year to ensure that the appropriate dosage is given for each available formulation. **www.cdc.gov/flu/professionals/vaccines. htm.**

[c] For adults and older children, the recommended site of immunization is the deltoid muscle. For infants and young children, the preferred site is the anterolateral aspect of the thigh.

[d] Two doses administered at least 4 weeks apart are recommended for children younger than 9 years who are receiving influenza vaccine for the first time.

[e] Manufacturer: AstraZeneca (Flumist Quadrivalent, live attenuated influenza vaccine licensed for otherwise healthy persons 2–49 years of age).

influenza season, preferably by end of October, or at the time specified in the annual recommendations of the ACIP (**www.cdc.gov/flu/**). Providers should continue to offer vaccine until the vaccine expiration date (typically June 30, marking the end of the influenza season), because influenza circulation is unpredictable. Particular efforts should be on the vaccination of all children and adolescents with factors associated with an elevated risk of complications from influenza, including the following:

- Age <5 years, and especially <2 years, regardless of the presence of underlying medical conditions.
- Chronic pulmonary disease (including asthma and cystic fibrosis), hemodynamically significant cardiovascular disease (except hypertension alone), or renal, hepatic, hematologic (including sickle cell disease and other hemoglobinopathies), or metabolic disorders (including diabetes mellitus).
- Immunosuppression attributable to any cause, including that caused by medications (see Special Considerations, p 455) or by HIV infection (see Human Immunodeficiency Virus Infection, p 427).
- Neurologic and neurodevelopment conditions (including disorders of the brain, spinal cord, peripheral nerve, and muscle such as cerebral palsy, epilepsy, stroke, intellectual disability, moderate-to-severe developmental delay, muscular dystrophy, or spinal cord injury).

- Conditions that compromise respiratory function or handling of secretions (including tracheostomy and mechanical ventilation).
- Women who are pregnant or postpartum during the influenza season.
- Receipt of long-term aspirin therapy or salicylate containing medications (including those with Kawasaki disease and rheumatologic conditions) because of increased risk of Reye syndrome.
- American Indian/Alaska Native people.
- Extreme obesity.

Special Considerations. In children receiving immunosuppressive chemotherapy, influenza immunization may result in a less robust response than in immunocompetent children. The optimal time to immunize children with malignant neoplasms who must undergo chemotherapy is more than 3 weeks after chemotherapy has been discontinued, when the peripheral granulocyte and lymphocyte counts are greater than $1000/\mu L$ ($1.0 \times 10^9/L$). Children who no longer are receiving chemotherapy generally have adequate rates of seroconversion.

Children with hemodynamically unstable cardiac disease are at high risk of complications of influenza. The immune response to and safety of IIV in these children are comparable to the immune response and safety in healthy children.

Corticosteroids administered daily for brief periods or every other day seem to have a minimal effect on antibody response to influenza vaccine. Prolonged administration of high doses of corticosteroids (ie, a dose of prednisone of either 2 mg/kg or greater or a total of 20 mg/day or greater for children who weigh 10 kg or more or an equivalent dose of other corticosteroids) may impair antibody response. Influenza immunization can be deferred temporarily during the time of receipt of high-dose corticosteroids, provided deferral does not compromise the likelihood of immunization before the start of influenza season (see Vaccine Administration, p 26).

Breastfeeding. Breastfeeding is not a contraindication for influenza immunization. Special effort should be made to vaccinate all women who are breastfeeding during the influenza season if they were not vaccinated during pregnancy.

Influenza Control in Peri- and Postpartum Settings. Strategies to decrease the likelihood of transmission from a mother to her newborn child during the birth hospitalization are provided at **www.cdc.gov/flu/professionals/infectioncontrol/peri-post-settings.htm.**

Close Contacts of High-Risk Patients. Immunization of everyone who is in close contact with children younger than 5 years or children with high-risk conditions (see Recommendations for Influenza Immunization, p 453) is an important strategy to ensure protection for these children who may not benefit from adequate protection from vaccination alone.

Health Care Personnel. The AAP supports mandatory annual immunization programs for HCP, because HCP frequently come into contact with patients at high risk of influenza illness in clinical settings.[1]

Reactions, Adverse Effects, and Contraindications. The most common reactions after IIV administration are local injection site pain and tenderness. Fever may occur within

[1]Bernstein HH; Starke JR; and the American Academy of Pediatrics, Committee on Infectious Diseases. Policy statement: influenza immunization for all health care personnel: keep it mandatory. *Pediatrics*. 2015;136(4):809-818

24 hours after immunization in approximately 10% to 35% of children younger than 2 years but rarely in older children and adults. Mild systemic symptoms, such as nausea, lethargy, headache, muscle aches, and chills, may occur after administration of IIV. LAIV may result in nasal congestion, rhinorrhea, and sore throat, as well as wheezing, particularly in younger children and those with underlying reactive airway disease. Anaphylaxis after receipt of any influenza vaccine is a contraindication to influenza vaccination. Children who have had an allergic reaction after a previous dose of any influenza vaccine should be evaluated by an allergist to determine whether or not future receipt of the vaccine is appropriate. Minor illnesses, with or without fever, are not contraindications to the use of influenza vaccines, including among children with mild upper respiratory infection symptoms or allergic rhinitis. In children with a moderate to severe febrile illness (eg, high fever, active infection, requiring hospitalization, etc), on the basis of the judgment of the clinician, vaccination should be deferred until resolution of the illness. Similarly, children with an amount of nasal congestion that would notably impede vaccine delivery into the nasopharyngeal mucosa should have LAIV vaccination deferred until resolution, or should receive IIV, because nasal congestion would not impact its delivery. LAIV is contraindicated in immunocompromised hosts and pregnant women, as well as in patients with asplenia or CNS anatomic barrier defects (eg, cochlear implant, congenital dysplasia of the inner ear, persistent CSF communication with naso-/oropharynx) (see Table 1.17, p 73).

Although most influenza vaccines are produced in eggs and contain measurable amounts of egg protein, they are well tolerated by recipients with egg allergy of any severity. Special precautions for egg-allergic recipients of IIV or LAIV are not warranted, as the rate of anaphylaxis after administration is no greater in egg-allergic than non–egg-allergic recipients or from other universally recommended vaccines. Patients who prefer to receive a non-egg-based vaccine may be vaccinated with an age-appropriate recombinant or cell-based product.

History of Guillain-Barré syndrome (GBS) following influenza vaccine is considered a precaution for the administration of influenza vaccines. Data on the risk of GBS following vaccination with seasonal influenza vaccine are variable and have been inconsistent across seasons. GBS is rare, especially in children, and there is a lack of evidence on risk of GBS following influenza vaccine in children. The decision not to immunize should be thoughtfully balanced against the potential morbidity and mortality associated with influenza for that individual.

Chemoprophylaxis. Chemoprophylaxis with influenza antivirals should not be considered a substitute for immunization. If not contraindicated, influenza vaccine always should be offered, even after influenza virus has begun circulating in the community. Providers should inform recipients of antiviral chemoprophylaxis that the risk of influenza is lowered but still remains while taking medication, and susceptibility to influenza returns when medication is discontinued. Chemoprophylaxis is not a contraindication to immunization with IIV, and does not interfere with the immune response to IIV. Chemoprophylaxis should not be administered in conjunction with LAIV immunization, as antivirals will interfere with LAIV. On the basis of drug half-lives, it is prudent to assume interference is possible during the following periods: (1) for oseltamivir and zanamivir, from 48 hours before to 2 weeks after LAIV; (2) for peramivir, from 5 days before to 2 weeks after LAIV; and (3) for baloxavir, from 17 days before to 2 weeks after LAIV.

Chemoprophylaxis is not recommended for infants younger than 3 months, unless the situation is judged critical, because of limited safety and efficacy data in this age group. For current recommendations about chemoprophylaxis against influenza, see **www.cdc. gov/flu/professionals/antivirals/index.htm** or **www.aapredbook.org/flu/**.

Kawasaki Disease

CLINICAL MANIFESTATIONS: Kawasaki disease is a vasculitis of medium-sized arteries, the diagnosis of which is made in patients with fever in addition to the presence of the following clinical criteria:

1. Bilateral injection of the bulbar conjunctivae with limbic sparing and without exudate;
2. Erythematous mouth and pharynx, strawberry tongue, and red, cracked lips;
3. A polymorphous, generalized, erythematous rash, often with accentuation in the groin, which can be morbilliform, maculopapular, scarlatiniform, or erythema multiforme-like;
4. Changes in the peripheral extremities consisting of erythema of the palms and soles and firm, sometimes painful, induration of the hands and feet, often with periungual desquamation usually beginning 10 to 14 days after fever onset;
5. Acute, nonsuppurative, usually unilateral, anterior cervical lymphadenopathy with at least 1 node ≥1.5 cm in diameter.

The diagnosis of classic (or complete) Kawasaki disease is based on the presence of ≥5 days of fever and ≥4 of the 5 principal features described. Clinicians should consider Kawasaki disease in their differential diagnosis before the fifth day of fever if several of the principal features are present without alternative explanation. Individual clinical manifestations may appear and self-resolve rather than all being present simultaneously. It is important to question about previous presence of relevant manifestations when a patient seeks medical attention for persistent fever.

The correct diagnosis sometimes is delayed in patients who seek medical attention because of fever and unilateral neck swelling, which mistakenly is thought to be attributable to bacterial lymph node or para- or retropharyngeal infection. A distinguishing clinical and imaging feature in these cases is that suppuration generally is not observed in Kawasaki disease. Concurrent viral upper respiratory infection sometimes is present in a patient with Kawasaki disease and, even if confirmed by virus detection, should not delay treatment of Kawasaki disease. (An exception is the patient with fever, exudative conjunctivitis, and exudative pharyngitis, in whom adenovirus is detected. In such cases, Kawasaki disease is considered extremely unlikely.)

The following mucocutaneous or laboratory findings should prompt a search for an alternative diagnosis to Kawasaki disease: bullous, vesicular, or petechial rash; oral ulcers; pharyngeal or conjunctival exudates; generalized lymphadenopathy or splenomegaly; or leukopenia or relative lymphocyte predominance. Prior infection with severe acute respiratory syndrome coronavirus 2 (SARS-CoV-2), the virus that causes COVID-19 and is the cause of the worldwide pandemic that began in early 2020, increases the likelihood of multisystem inflammatory syndrome in children (MIS-C) as the cause in a child presenting with symptoms suggestive of Kawasaki disease (see Coronaviruses, Including SARS-CoV-2 and MERS-CoV, p 280). Although features of MIS-C overlap with those of Kawasaki disease, MIS-C has a wider spectrum of symptoms. Patients with MIS-C are typically older than 7 years, of African or Hispanic origin, and show greater elevation of inflammatory markers. More than 80% of patients with MIS-C also present with an unusual cardiac injury shown by high concentrations of troponin and brain natriuretic peptide, whereas others develop arrhythmia, left ventricle dysfunction, and unusual coronary dilatation or aneurysms.

The diagnosis of incomplete Kawasaki disease should be considered in children with unexplained fever who lack all of the principal clinical criteria. Supportive laboratory and echocardiography data also are sought when considering the diagnosis of incomplete Kawasaki disease. In 2017, the American Heart Association (AHA) published updated guidelines for the diagnosis, treatment, and long-term management of Kawasaki disease.[1] An algorithm for diagnosis and treatment of suspected incomplete Kawasaki disease is provided in Fig 3.12. A high index of suspicion for Kawasaki disease should be maintained for infants, particularly those younger than 6 months, because compared with older children, infants have heightened risk of incomplete manifestations, delayed diagnosis, and development of coronary artery aneurysms. Kawasaki disease should be considered in infants younger than 12 months with prolonged unexplained fever, with or without aseptic meningitis, with evidence of systemic inflammation, even with fewer than 2 of the characteristic features of Kawasaki disease. Other presentations of Kawasaki disease include infants and children with a shock-like syndrome in whom an inciting infection is not confirmed and those with presumed bacterial cervical lymphadenitis or para- or retropharyngeal phlegmon that fail to respond to appropriate antibiotic therapy.

If coronary artery aneurysm or ectasia is evident (z score ≥ 2.5) in any patient evaluated for fever, a presumptive diagnosis of Kawasaki disease should be made. A normal early echocardiographic study is typical and does not exclude the diagnosis but may be useful in evaluation of patients with suspected incomplete Kawasaki disease. In one study, 80% of patients with Kawasaki disease who ultimately developed coronary artery disease had abnormalities (z score ≥ 2.5) on an echocardiogram obtained during the first 10 days of illness.

Other clinical features of Kawasaki disease include irritability, abdominal pain, diarrhea, and vomiting. Other examination and laboratory findings include urethritis with sterile pyuria (70% of cases), mild anterior uveitis (80%), mild elevation of serum hepatic aminotransferase concentrations (50%), arthralgia or arthritis (10%–20%), marked irritability with cerebrospinal fluid pleocytosis (40%), hydrops of the gallbladder (<10%), pericardial effusion of at least 1 mm (<5%), myocarditis manifesting as congestive heart failure (<5%), and cranial nerve palsy (<1%). Persistent resting tachycardia and a hyperdynamic precordium are common findings, and an S3 gallop can be present. Fine desquamation in the groin area can occur in the acute phase of disease (Fink sign).[1]

[1]McCrindle BW, Rowley AH, Newburger JW, et al; American Heart Association Rheumatic Fever, Endocarditis, and Kawasaki Disease Committee of the Council on Cardiovascular Disease in the Young; Council on Cardiovascular and Stroke Nursing; Council on Cardiovascular Surgery and Anesthesia; and Council on Epidemiology and Prevention. Diagnosis, treatment, and long-term management of Kawasaki disease: a scientific statement for health professionals from the American Heart Association. *Circulation*. Published online March 29, 2017; www.ahajournals.org/doi/full/10.1161/CIR.0000000000000484

FIG 3.12. EVALUATION OF SUSPECTED INCOMPLETE KAWASAKI DISEASE.[a]

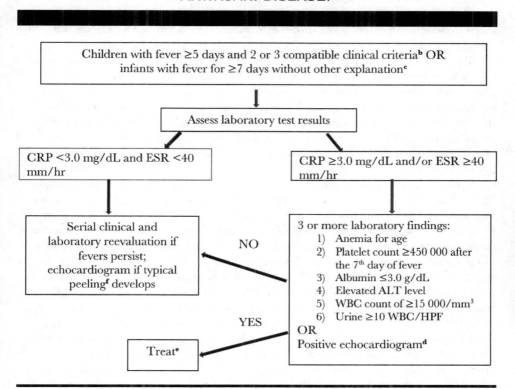

CRP indicates C-reactive protein; ESR, erythrocyte sedimentation rate; ALT, alanine aminotransferase; WBC, white blood cell; HPF, high-powered field.

[a]In the absence of a "gold standard" for diagnosis, this algorithm cannot be evidence based but rather represents the informed opinion of the expert committee. Consultation with an expert should be sought anytime assistance is needed.

[b]See text for clinical findings of Kawasaki disease.

[c]Infants ≤6 months of age are the most likely to develop prolonged fever without other clinical criteria for Kawasaki disease; these infants are at particularly high risk of developing coronary artery abnormalities.

[d]Echocardiography is considered positive for purposes of this algorithm if any of 3 conditions are met: z score of left anterior descending coronary artery or right coronary artery ≥2.5; coronary artery aneurysm is observed; or ≥3 other suggestive features exist, including decreased left ventricular function, mitral regurgitation, pericardial effusion, or z scores in left anterior descending coronary artery or right coronary artery of 2 to 2.5.

[e]Treatment should be given within 10 days of fever onset. See text for indications for treatment after the tenth day of fever.

[f]Typical peeling begins under the nail beds of fingers and toes.

Source: McCrindle BW, Rowley AH, Newburger JW, et al; American Heart Association Rheumatic Fever, Endocarditis, and Kawasaki Disease Committee of the Council on Cardiovascular Disease in the Young; Council on Cardiovascular and Stroke Nursing; Council on Cardiovascular Surgery and Anesthesia; and Council on Epidemiology and Prevention. Diagnosis, treatment, and long-term management of Kawasaki disease: a scientific statement for health professionals from the American Heart Association. *Circulation.* Published online March 29, 2017; **www.ahajournals.org/doi/full/10.1161/CIR.0000000000000484**

Inflammation or ulceration may be observed at the inoculation scar of previous bacille Calmette-Guérin immunization. Rarely, Kawasaki disease can present with acute shock; these children often have significant thrombocytopenia attributable to consumption coagulopathy, which also causes a low erythrocyte sedimentation rate (ESR). Group A streptococcal or *Staphylococcus aureus* toxic shock syndrome should be excluded in such cases.

The average duration of fever in untreated Kawasaki disease is 10 days; however, fever can last 2 weeks or longer. After fever resolves, patients can remain anorexic and/or irritable with decreased energy for 2 to 3 weeks. During this phase, branny desquamation of fingers, toes, hands, and feet may occur. Transverse lines across the nails (Beau lines) sometimes are noted month(s) later. Recurrent disease develops in approximately 1% to 2% of patients in the United States a median of 1.5 years after the index episode. The recurrence rate is 3.5% in Asian and Pacific Islander populations.

Coronary artery abnormalities are serious sequelae of Kawasaki disease, occurring in 20% to 25% of untreated children. Increased risk of developing coronary artery abnormalities is associated with male sex; age <12 months or >8 years; fever for more than 10 days; white blood cell count >15 000/mm^3; high relative neutrophil (>80%) and band count; low hemoglobin concentration (<10 g/dL); hypoalbuminemia, hyponatremia, or thrombocytopenia; and fever persisting or recurring >36 hours after completion of Immune Globulin Intravenous (IGIV) administration. Aneurysms of the coronary arteries most typically occur between 1 and 4 weeks after onset of illness; onset later than 6 weeks is extremely uncommon. Giant coronary artery aneurysms (internal diameter ≥8 mm) are highly predictive of long-term complications. Aneurysms occurring in other medium-sized arteries (eg, iliac, femoral, renal, and axillary vessels) are uncommon and generally do not occur in the absence of significant coronary abnormalities. In addition to coronary artery disease, carditis can involve the pericardium, myocardium, or endocardium, and mitral or aortic regurgitation or both can develop. Carditis generally resolves when fever resolves.

In children with only mild coronary artery dilation, coronary artery dimensions often return to baseline within 6 to 8 weeks after onset of disease. Approximately 50% of coronary aneurysms (but only a small proportion of giant aneurysms) regress by echocardiography to normal luminal size within 1 to 2 years, although this process can result in luminal stenosis or a poorly compliant, fibrotic vessel wall or both.

The current case-fatality rate for Kawasaki disease in the United States and Japan is less than 0.2%. The principal cause of death is myocardial infarction resulting from coronary artery occlusion attributable to thrombosis or progressive stenosis. The relative risk of mortality is highest within 6 weeks of onset of acute symptoms, but myocardial infarction and sudden death can occur months to years after the acute episode. There is no current evidence that the vasculitis of Kawasaki disease predisposes to premature atherosclerotic coronary artery disease.

ETIOLOGY: The etiology is unknown. Epidemiologic and clinical features suggest an infectious and/or an environmental cause or trigger in genetically susceptible individuals. The disease was first described in 1967 by Dr. Tomisaku Kawasaki in a landmark paper entitled "Acute Febrile Mucocutaneous Syndrome With Lymphoid Involvement With Specific Desquamation of the Fingers and Toes in Children" in the Japanese journal *Arerugi* ("Allergy"). This is now known universally as Kawasaki disease, although he did not use that term himself. Dr. Kawasaki died on June 5, 2020, at age 95.

EPIDEMIOLOGY: Peak age of occurrence in the United States is 6 to 24 months. Fifty percent of patients are younger than 2 years, and 80% are younger than 5 years; cases are uncommon in children older than 8 years, but rare cases have occurred even in adults. The prevalence of coronary artery abnormalities is higher if treatment (Immune Globulin Intravenous) is delayed beyond the 10th day of illness. The male-to-female ratio is approximately 1.5:1. In the United States, 4000 to 5500 cases are estimated to occur each year; the incidence is highest in children of Asian ancestry. Kawasaki disease first was described in Japan, where a pattern of endemic occurrence with superimposed epidemic outbreaks was recognized. More cases, including clusters, occur during winter and spring. Little evidence indicates person-to-person or common-source spread, although the incidence is tenfold higher in siblings of children with the disease than in the general population, and more than 50% of sibling cases occur within 10 days of the index case.

The **incubation period** is unknown.

DIAGNOSTIC TESTS: No specific diagnostic test is available. The diagnosis is established by fulfillment of the clinical criteria (see Clinical Manifestations, p 457) after consideration of other possible illnesses, such as staphylococcal or streptococcal toxin-mediated disease; drug reactions (eg, Stevens-Johnson syndrome); MIS-C; measles, adenovirus, Epstein-Barr virus, parvovirus B19, or enterovirus infections; rickettsial exanthems; leptospirosis; systemic-onset juvenile idiopathic arthritis; and reactive arthritis. The identification of a respiratory virus by molecular testing does not exclude the diagnosis of Kawasaki disease in infants and children who otherwise have met diagnostic criteria. A markedly increased ESR and/or serum C-reactive protein (CRP) concentration during the first 2 weeks of illness and an increased platelet count ($>450\,000/mm^3$) on days 10 to 21 of illness are almost universal laboratory features. ESR and platelet count usually are normal within 6 to 8 weeks; CRP concentration returns to normal much sooner.

TREATMENT: Management during the acute phase is directed at decreasing inflammation of the myocardium and coronary artery wall and providing supportive care. Therapy should be initiated as soon as the diagnosis is established or strongly suspected. Once the acute phase has subsided, therapy is directed at prevention of coronary artery thrombosis.

Primary Treatment

Immune Globulin Intravenous. A single dose of IGIV, 2 g/kg, administered over 10 to 12 hours, results in rapid resolution of fever and other clinical and laboratory indicators of acute inflammation in approximately 85% of patients and has been proven to reduce the risk of coronary artery aneurysms from 17% to 4% in children with a normal first echocardiogram. IGIV plus aspirin (see below) is the treatment of choice and should be initiated as soon as the diagnosis is established or strongly suspected and alternative diagnoses are unlikely, whether or not coronary artery abnormalities are detected. Despite prompt treatment with IGIV and aspirin, approximately 2% to 4% of patients develop coronary artery aneurysms even when treatment is initiated before the onset of coronary artery abnormalities.

Efficacy of therapy initiated later than the 10th day of illness or after detection of aneurysms has not been evaluated fully. However, therapy with IGIV and aspirin should be provided for patients in whom the diagnosis is made more than 10 days after the onset of fever (ie, the diagnosis was not made earlier) who have manifestations of continuing inflammation (ie, elevated ESR or CRP ≥3.0 mg/dL) plus either fever or coronary artery luminal dimension z score >2.5.

IGIV infusion reactions (fever, chills, hypotension) are not uncommon. Occasionally, Coombs-positive hemolytic anemia can complicate IGIV therapy, especially in individuals with AB blood type, and usually occurs within 5 to 10 days of infusion. Aseptic meningitis can result from IGIV therapy and resolves quickly without neurologic sequelae. IGIV infusion results in elevation of the ESR; therefore, ESR is not a useful test to monitor disease activity after infusion; CRP is not affected by IGIV administration and can be used.

Aspirin. Aspirin is used for its anti-inflammatory (high-dose) and antithrombotic (low-dose) activity, although aspirin alone does not decrease the risk of coronary artery abnormalities. Guidelines vary with regard to dose, with Japanese and Western European clinicians frequently using 30 to 50 mg/kg per day and US clinicians using 80 to 100 mg/kg per day in 4 divided doses when the diagnosis is made and concurrently with IGIV administration. There are no data to suggest that either aspirin dose is superior. Children with acute Kawasaki disease have decreased aspirin absorption and increased clearance and rarely achieve therapeutic serum concentrations. It generally is not necessary to monitor salicylate concentrations. High-dose aspirin therapy usually is given until the patient has been afebrile for 48 to 72 hours. Low-dose aspirin (3 to 5 mg/kg/day, in a single daily dose; maximum 81–325 mg/day) then is given until a follow-up echocardiogram at 6 to 8 weeks after onset of illness is normal or is continued indefinitely for children in whom coronary artery abnormalities are present. In general, ibuprofen should be avoided in children with coronary aneurysms taking aspirin, because ibuprofen and other nonsteroidal anti-inflammatory drugs with known or potential effects on the cyclooxygenase pathway interfere with the antiplatelet effect of ASA to prevent thrombosis. Because of the potential risk of Reye syndrome in patients with influenza or varicella receiving salicylates, parents of children receiving aspirin should be instructed to contact their child's physician promptly if the child develops symptoms of or is exposed to either of these diseases. The child and all household contacts older than 6 months should receive influenza vaccine according to seasonal recommendations. The inactivated injectable influenza vaccine (not live attenuated vaccine) should be used in the child receiving aspirin. Family members can receive either inactivated or live attenuated influenza vaccine; refer to the annual influenza policy statement from the American Academy of Pediatrics, which can be found at **https://redbook.solutions.aap.org/selfserve/sspage.aspx?selfservecontent id=influenza-resources**.

Adjunctive Therapies for Primary Treatment. The following are 2017 consensus recommendations of the AHA[1]: (1) single-dose pulse methylprednisolone should not be administered with IGIV as routine primary therapy for patients with Kawasaki disease; and (2) administration of a longer course of corticosteroids (eg, prednisolone, 2 mg/kg/day IV, divided every 8 hours until afebrile, then an oral corticosteroid until CRP normalizes, with subsequent tapering over 2–3 weeks) together with IGIV and aspirin may be considered for treatment of high-risk patients with acute Kawasaki disease, when such risk can be identified before initiation of treatment.

---

[1]For further information on the diagnosis and management of Kawasaki disease, see McCrindle BW, Rowley AH, Newburger JW, et al; American Heart Association Rheumatic Fever, Endocarditis, and Kawasaki Disease Committee of the Council on Cardiovascular Disease in the Young; Council on Cardiovascular and Stroke Nursing; Council on Cardiovascular Surgery and Anesthesia; and Council on Epidemiology and Prevention. Diagnosis, treatment, and long-term management of Kawasaki disease: a scientific statement for health professionals from the American Heart Association. *Circulation.* Published online March 29, 2017. Available at: **www.ahajournals.org/doi/full/10.1161/CIR.0000000000000484**

Management of IGIV Resistance and Retreatment. Approximately 30% of patients who receive IGIV, 2 g/kg, plus aspirin have fever within the first 36 hours after completing the IGIV infusion, which is not an indication of therapeutic failure. However, 10% to 20% of treated patients have recrudescent or persistent fever beyond 36 hours after completion of their IGIV infusion and are termed IGIV-resistant. In these situations, the diagnosis of Kawasaki disease should be reevaluated. If Kawasaki disease still is considered to be most likely, retreatment with IGIV, 2 g/kg, usually is given and high-dose aspirin is continued. Several small series and observational studies have described children with IGIV-resistant Kawasaki disease in whom administration of a single dose of infliximab or a variety of regimens of corticosteroids was associated with an improvement of symptoms, without adverse events. Evidence of alteration of coronary artery outcomes associated with different therapies is limited.

Management of patients with Kawasaki disease refractory to a second dose of IGIV, infliximab, or a course of corticosteroids has included use of cyclosporine, other immune modulating therapies, or plasma exchange but should be undertaken in consultation with an expert in KD.[1]

Cardiac Care.[1] Echocardiography should be performed at the time of suspected diagnosis and repeated at 2 weeks and 6 to 8 weeks after diagnosis in children with normal coronary arteries on initial evaluation. Coronary abnormalities warrant closer follow-up with echocardiography. Children at higher risk—for example, children with persistent or recrudescent fever after initial IGIV, baseline coronary artery abnormalities, or very young patients— may require more frequent echocardiograms to guide the need for additional therapies. Children should be assessed during this time for arrhythmias, congestive heart failure, and valvular regurgitation. The care of patients with significant cardiac abnormalities should involve a pediatric cardiologist experienced in management of patients with Kawasaki disease and in assessing echocardiographic studies of coronary arteries in children.

Long-term management of Kawasaki disease should be based on the extent of coronary artery involvement. In patients with persistent moderately large coronary artery aneurysms that are not large enough to warrant anticoagulation, clopidogrel (0.2–1 mg/kg/d) to antagonize adenosine diphosphate-mediated platelet activation in combination with prolonged low-dose aspirin are recommended.

Development of giant coronary artery aneurysms (luminal diameter ≥ 8 mm or larger in a child, but smaller diameter in an infant based on relative body surface area, z score ≥ 10) usually requires addition of anticoagulant therapy, such as warfarin or low-molecular weight heparin, to prevent thrombosis. The AHA has provided recommendations regarding criteria for systemic anticoagulation and frequency of echocardiography in those with coronary aneurysms.[2]

---

[1]For further information on the diagnosis and management of Kawasaki disease, see McCrindle BW, Rowley AH, Newburger JW, et al; American Heart Association Rheumatic Fever, Endocarditis, and Kawasaki Disease Committee of the Council on Cardiovascular Disease in the Young; Council on Cardiovascular and Stroke Nursing; Council on Cardiovascular Surgery and Anesthesia; and Council on Epidemiology and Prevention. Diagnosis, treatment, and long-term management of Kawasaki disease: a scientific statement for health professionals from the American Heart Association. *Circulation.* Published online March 29, 2017; **www.ahajournals.org/doi/full/10.1161/CIR.0000000000000484**

[2]Giglia TM, Massicotte MP, Tweddell JS, et al. Prevention and treatment of thrombosis in pediatric and congenital heart disease: a scientific statement from the American Heart Association. American Heart Association Congenital Heart Defects Committee of the Council on Cardiovascular Disease in the Young, Council on Cardiovascular and Stroke Nursing, Council on Epidemiology and Prevention, and Stroke Council. *Circulation.* 2013;128(24):2622-2703

Subsequent Immunization. Measles- and varicella-containing vaccines should be deferred until 11 months after receipt of IGIV, 2 g/kg, for treatment of Kawasaki disease because of possible interference with development of an adequate immune response (see Table 1.11, p 40). If the child's risk of exposure to measles or varicella within this period is high, the child should be immunized and then reimmunized at least 11 months after administration of IGIV. Live attenuated varicella-containing vaccines should be avoided during aspirin therapy because of a theoretical concern of Reye syndrome. If the child is receiving low-dose aspirin therapy and the risk of varicella exposure is high, or if aspirin therapy is prolonged beyond 11 months, benefits and theoretical risk of Reye syndrome should be discussed; usually, varicella vaccine is administered in this circumstance. The schedule for administration of inactivated childhood vaccines should not be interrupted.

ISOLATION OF THE HOSPITALIZED PATIENT: Standard precautions are indicated.

CONTROL MEASURES: None.

Kingella kingae Infections

CLINICAL MANIFESTATIONS: The most common infections attributable to *Kingella kingae* are pyogenic arthritis, osteomyelitis, and bacteremia. Other infections caused by *K kingae* include diskitis, endocarditis (*K kingae* belongs to the HACEK group of organisms), meningitis, ocular infections, and pneumonia. The vast majority of *K kingae* infections affect children between 6 and 48 months of age, with most cases occurring in children younger than 2 years.

    K kingae is a primary cause of skeletal infections in the first 4 years of life. *K kingae* pyogenic arthritis generally is monoarticular and most commonly involves the knee, hip, or ankle. *K kingae* osteomyelitis most often involves the femur or tibia. The organism also shows an unusual predilection for the small joints of the hand and foot. Compared with the clinical manifestations of pyogenic arthritis and osteomyelitis in immunocompetent children caused by other pathogens, skeletal infections caused by *K kingae* can be milder and evolution can be more insidious, resulting in a more subacute presentation in many cases. Evolution to chronicity or long-term sequelae are rare; however, Brodie abscesses of bone attributable to *K kingae* have been reported.

    K kingae bacteremia can occur in previously healthy young children and in children with preexisting chronic medical problems. Children with *K kingae* bacteremia present with fever and frequently have concurrent symptoms of respiratory or gastrointestinal tract disease.

ETIOLOGY: *K kingae* is a gram-negative, encapsulated organism that belongs to the *Neisseriaceae* family. It is a fastidious, facultative anaerobic, b-hemolytic, coccobacillus that appears as pairs or short chains with tapered ends. It often resists decolorization, sometimes resulting in misidentification as a gram-positive organism.

EPIDEMIOLOGY: The usual habitat of *K kingae* is the human posterior pharynx. The organism colonizes young children more frequently than older children or adults and can be transmitted among children in child care centers, occasionally causing clusters of cases. Infection may be associated with preceding or concomitant viral infections that cause hand, foot, and mouth disease, herpetic gingivostomatitis, or nonspecific upper respiratory tract infections.

    The **incubation period** relative to acquisition of colonization is not well defined.

DIAGNOSTIC TESTS: *K kingae* can be isolated from blood, synovial fluid, bone, cerebrospinal fluid, respiratory tract secretions, and other fluid or tissues. Patients with pyogenic arthritis or osteomyelitis attributable to *K kingae* often have negative blood cultures. Organisms grow best in aerobic conditions with enhanced carbon dioxide. *K kingae* is difficult to isolate on routinely used solid media. Therefore, synovial fluid and bone aspirates from patients with suspected *K kingae* infection should be inoculated on both solid media and into an aerobic blood culture vial and held for 5 to 7 days to maximize recovery. Once recovered in culture, standard biochemical tests readily identify the organism; alternatively, mass spectrometry of bacterial cellular components may be used for rapid identification. When available, conventional and real-time polymerase chain reaction (PCR) methods markedly improve detection of *K kingae* in young children with culture-negative skeletal infections. There currently are no PCR assays cleared by the US Food and Drug Administration for *K kingae*, and such tests are available only in specialty laboratories.

TREATMENT: *K kingae* usually is highly susceptible to penicillins and cephalosporins, but in vitro susceptibility to oxacillin is relatively reduced. Nearly all isolates are susceptible to aminoglycosides, macrolides, tetracyclines, and fluoroquinolones. Between 40% and 100% of isolates are resistant to clindamycin, and virtually all isolates are resistant to glycopeptide antibiotics (eg, vancomycin) and trimethoprim (although most strains are susceptible to trimethoprim-sulfamethoxazole). Occasional isolates in parts of the United States and other countries have demonstrated TEM-1 beta-lactamase production resulting in low-level resistance to penicillin and ampicillin. The TEM-1 beta-lactamase is susceptible to beta-lactamase inhibitors and lacks activity against second and third generation cephalosporins.

Ampicillin-sulbactam or a first- or second-generation cephalosporin is recommended for children with osteoarticular infections suspected to be attributable to *K kingae* (definitive therapy can be determined after beta-lactamase production of the isolate is known). For more invasive or severe infections (eg, endocarditis), treatment with a third-generation cephalosporin or, if beta-lactamase production has been ruled out, ampicillin plus an aminoglycoside should be considered.

ISOLATION OF THE HOSPITALIZED PATIENT: Standard precautions are recommended.

CONTROL MEASURES: None. Although small clusters of cases have been reported in child care facilities in multiple countries, antimicrobial prophylaxis in contacts of a case is not standard practice. Prophylactic therapy has been used in the setting of an outbreak, and public health advice should be sought if more than a single case is identified in young children with close contact.

Legionella pneumophila Infections

CLINICAL MANIFESTATIONS: Legionellosis is associated primarily with 2 clinically and epidemiologically distinct illnesses: Legionnaires' disease and Pontiac fever. **Legionnaires' disease** presents as pneumonia characterized by fever, cough with or without chest pain, and progressive respiratory distress. Legionnaires' disease can be associated with chills and rigors, headache, myalgia, and gastrointestinal tract, central nervous system, and renal manifestations. Overall (including adults) case fatality rate is approximately 10%. **Pontiac fever** is a milder febrile illness without pneumonia that is characterized by an abrupt onset of a self-limited, influenza-like illness (fever, myalgia, headache, weakness) resulting from the host inflammatory response to the bacterium.

Cervical lymphadenitis caused by *Legionella* species has been reported and may produce a syndrome clinically similar to nontuberculous mycobacterial infection. Other extrapulmonary infections including endocarditis, graft infections, joint infections, and wound infections also have been reported.

ETIOLOGY: *Legionella* species are fastidious, small, gram-negative, aerobic bacilli that grow on buffered charcoal yeast extract (BCYE) media. They constitute a single genus in the family *Legionellaceae*. At least 20 of the more than 60 known species have been implicated in human disease, but the most common species causing infections in the United States is *Legionella pneumophila*, with most isolates belonging to serogroup 1. Multiplication of *Legionella* organisms in water sources occurs optimally in temperatures between 25°C (77°F) and 42°C (108°F), although *Legionella* organisms have been recovered from water outside this temperature range.

EPIDEMIOLOGY: Legionnaires' disease is usually acquired through inhalation of aerosolized water containing *Legionella* species. Less frequently, transmission can occur via aspiration of *Legionella*-containing water. Only one case of possible person-to-person transmission has been reported. Outbreaks commonly are associated with buildings or structures that have complex water systems, like hotels and resorts, long-term care facilities, hospitals, and cruise ships. The most likely sources of infection include *Legionella*-containing water aerosolized from showerheads, cooling towers (parts of centralized air-conditioning systems for large buildings), hot tubs, decorative fountains, and humidifiers. Health care-associated infections can be related to contamination of the hot water supply. Legionnaires' disease should be considered in the differential diagnosis of patients who develop pneumonia during or after their hospitalization. Most cases of Legionnaires' disease are sporadic, although they may be connected with unrecognized outbreaks or clusters. Legionnaires' disease is more common among older individuals (50 years or older), males, smokers, and individuals with weakened immune systems, malignancy, or chronic disease. Infection in children is rare, with ≤1% cases of pneumonia caused by *Legionella* infection, and may be asymptomatic or mild and unrecognized. Severe disease has occurred in children with malignancy, severe combined immunodeficiency, chronic granulomatous disease, organ transplantation, end-stage renal disease, and underlying pulmonary disease and those treated with systemic corticosteroids or other immunosuppression. Health care-associated cases of *Legionella* infection in newborn infants, including severe and sometimes fatal cases, have been associated with a *Legionella*-containing water source (eg, humidifiers). Severe and fatal infections in neonates have occurred after birth in water (eg, utilizing a birthing pool or hot tub).

The **incubation period** for Legionnaires' disease most commonly is 2 to 10 days, with an average of 5 to 6 days but can rarely occur up to 26 days. For Pontiac fever, the **incubation period** generally is 1 to 3 days but can be as short as 4 hours.

DIAGNOSTIC TESTS: When a patient is suspected of having Legionnaires' disease, testing should include both culture of a lower respiratory tract specimen and urine antigen testing. Recovery of *Legionella* organisms from lower respiratory tract secretions, lung tissue, pleural fluid, or other normally sterile fluid specimens by using supplemented BCYE media provides definitive evidence of infection, but the sensitivity of culture is laboratory dependent. Specimens should be plated onto both supplemented, nonselective BCYE and selective BCYE containing appropriate antimicrobial agents and incubated at 35°C to 37°C for up to 14 days. Suspicious colonies commonly are identified by demonstrating growth dependence on L-cysteine followed by staining with specific fluorescein-labeled antibodies for *L pneumophila*. Culture is an important diagnostic tool, because it can detect all *Legionella* species and *L pneumophila* serogroups. Comparative genetic analysis of clinical and environmental isolates can be useful in outbreak investigations.

Detection of *Legionella* lipopolysaccharide antigen in urine by commercially available immunoassays is highly specific. This test detects only *L pneumophila* serogroup 1, and thus other testing methods are needed to detect other *L pneumophila* serogroups and other *Legionella* species. Urinary antigen test sensitivity is dependent on the assay method used and on the severity of disease.

Genus-specific polymerase chain reaction (PCR)-based assays have been developed that detect *Legionella* DNA in lower respiratory tract specimens and blood. There is a commercially available PCR assay, present in a multiplexed nucleic acid format for detection of *Legionella pneumophila* in lower respiratory tract specimens.

Direct detection of the bacterium in lower respiratory tract specimens by direct immunofluorescent assay is rarely performed, because the specificity is technician dependent and the sensitivity is lower than that for culture or urine immunoassay.

Detection of serum immunoglobulin (Ig) M antibodies is not useful for diagnosis, and the positive predictive value of a single IgG titer of ≥1:256 is low and does not provide definitive evidence of acute infection. A fourfold increase in *Legionella pneumophila*-specific IgG antibody titer, as measured by indirect immunofluorescent antibody (IFA), confirms a recent infection. This serologic result is not useful for treatment decisions however, because convalescent titers take 3 to 4 weeks to increase (and the increase may be delayed for 8 to 12 weeks). Antibodies to several gram-negative organisms, including *Pseudomonas* species, *Bacteroides fragilis*, and *Campylobacter jejuni*, can cause false-positive IFA test results.

Because *Legionella* species are relatively inert biochemically, biochemical test systems are not helpful to identify *Legionella* organisms in culture. However, mass spectrometry of cellular components can be used as a rapid identification method.

TREATMENT: Patients with Legionnaires' disease should receive antimicrobial agents. Intravenously administered azithromycin or levofloxacin (or another respiratory fluoroquinolone) is recommended. Once the patient is improved clinically, oral therapy can be substituted. Doxycycline is an alternative agent; however, *Legionella longbeachae* often is resistant (this species is common in some geographic areas such as Australia and New Zealand). Duration of therapy is 5 to 10 days for azithromycin and 14 to 21 days for other drugs, with the longer courses of therapy for patients who are immunocompromised or who have severe disease.

Antimicrobial treatment for patients with Pontiac fever is not recommended, because the disease results from host inflammation (not bacterial replication) and, thus, is self-limiting.

ISOLATION OF THE HOSPITALIZED PATIENT: Standard precautions are recommended.

CONTROL MEASURES: The most effective strategy for prevention of Legionnaires' disease in buildings with large or complex water systems is through the development and implementation of water management programs.[1] Water management programs identify

---

[1]American Society of Heating, Refrigerating and Air-Conditioning Engineers. Legionellosis: risk management for building water systems. ANSI/ASHRAE Standard 188–2018. Atlanta, GA: ASHRAE; 2018. Available at: **www.ashrae.org/technical-resources/bookstore/ansi-ashrae-standard-188-2018-legionellosis-risk-management-for-building-water-systems.**

hazardous conditions and implement steps to minimize the risk associated with *Legionella* and other waterborne pathogens in building water systems. Adequate levels of disinfectant should be maintained in all building water systems. Hospitals should maintain hot water at the highest temperature allowable by state regulations or codes, preferably stored at 60°C (140°F) or greater with a minimum return temperature of 51°C (124°F); precaution should be taken to avoid scalding. Cold water temperature should be maintained at less than 20°C (68°F) to minimize waterborne *Legionella* growth. Occurrence of even a single laboratory-confirmed health care-associated case of legionellosis warrants consideration of an epidemiologic and environmental investigation. Hospitals with transplantation programs (solid organ or hematopoietic stem cell) should maintain a high index of suspicion of legionellosis, use sterile water for the filling and terminal rinsing of nebulization devices, and consider performing periodic culturing for *Legionella* species in the potable water supply of the transplant unit. Some hospitals may choose to perform periodic, routine culturing of water samples from the hospital's potable water system to detect *Legionella* species.

For emergency disinfection, superheating (to 71°C–77°C [160°F–170°F] or greater) and/or shock chlorination or targeted use of point-of-use water filters can be used. Optional supplemental measures for long-term control of potable water supplies to prevent health care-associated cases include copper-silver ionization; addition of chlorine, monochloramine, or chlorine dioxide; and ultraviolet light.

Infection with *Legionella* species is a nationally notifiable disease in the United States.

Leishmaniasis

CLINICAL MANIFESTATIONS:

Cutaneous Leishmaniasis. After inoculation by the bite of an infected female phlebotomine sand fly (approximately 2–3 mm long), parasites proliferate locally in mononuclear phagocytes, leading to an erythematous papule, which typically enlarges slowly to become a nodule and then an ulcerative lesion with raised, indurated borders. Ulcerative lesions may become dry and crusted or may develop a moist granulating base with overlying exudate. Lesions can, however, persist as nodules, papules, or plaques and may be single or multiple. Lesions commonly appear on exposed areas of the body (eg, face and extremities) and may be accompanied by satellite lesions, sporotrichoid-like nodules, and regional adenopathy. Spontaneous resolution of lesions may take weeks to years—depending, in part, on the *Leishmania* species/strain—and usually results in a flat, atrophic scar.

Mucosal Leishmaniasis (Espundia). Mucosal leishmaniasis traditionally refers to a metastatic sequela of New World cutaneous infection resulting from dissemination of the parasite from the skin to the naso-oropharyngeal/laryngeal mucosa. This form of leishmaniasis typically is caused by species in the *Viannia* subgenus. (Mucosal involvement attributable to local extension of cutaneous facial lesions has a different pathophysiology.) Mucosal disease usually becomes evident clinically months to years after the original cutaneous lesions have healed, although mucosal and cutaneous lesions may be noted simultaneously, and some affected people have had subclinical cutaneous infection. Untreated mucosal leishmaniasis can progress to cause ulcerative destruction of the mucosa (eg, perforation of the nasal septum) and facial disfigurement.

Visceral Leishmaniasis (Kala-Azar). After cutaneous inoculation by an infected sand fly, the parasite spreads throughout the reticuloendothelial system (ie, within macrophages in spleen, liver, and bone marrow) leaving no or a minimal skin lesion at the bite site.

Clinical manifestations include fever, weight loss, hepatosplenomegaly, pancytopenia (anemia, leukopenia, and thrombocytopenia), hypoalbuminemia, and hypergammaglobulinemia. Hemophagocytic lymphohistiocytosis has been reported as a complication of visceral leishmaniasis. Peripheral lymphadenopathy is common in East Africa (eg, South Sudan). Some patients in South Asia (the Indian subcontinent) develop grayish discoloration of their skin; this manifestation gave rise to the Hindi term kala-azar ("black sickness"). Untreated, advanced cases of visceral leishmaniasis almost always are fatal, either directly from the disease or from complications, such as secondary bacterial infections or hemorrhage. Visceral infection can, alternatively, be asymptomatic or have few symptoms. Latent visceral infection can reactivate years to decades after exposure in people who become immunocompromised (eg, because of coinfection with human immunodeficiency virus [HIV] or immunosuppressive/immunomodulatory therapy). Some patients develop post-kala-azar dermal leishmaniasis during or after treatment of visceral leishmaniasis.

Post-Kala-Azar Dermal Leishmaniasis (PKDL). Post-kala-azar dermal leishmaniasis is a dermatosis that generally develops as a sequela after apparent successful cure from visceral leishmaniasis. In the Indian subcontinent variant, polymorphic lesions (coexistence of macules/patches along with papulonodules) are prevalent, whereas the Sudanese variant has papular or nodular lesions.

ETIOLOGY: In the human host, *Leishmania* species are obligate intracellular protozoan parasites of mononuclear phagocytes. Together with *Trypanosoma* species, they constitute the family *Trypanosomatidae*. Approximately 20 *Leishmania* species (in the *Leishmania* and *Viannia* subgenera) are known to infect humans. Cutaneous leishmaniasis typically is caused by Old World species *Leishmania tropica, Leishmania major,* and *Leishmania aethiopica* and by New World species *Leishmania mexicana, Leishmania amazonensis, Leishmania (Viannia) braziliensis, Leishmania (V) panamensis, Leishmania (V) guyanensis,* and *Leishmania (V) peruviana*. Mucosal leishmaniasis typically is caused by species in the *Viannia* subgenus (especially *L [V] braziliensis* but also *L [V] panamensis* and *L [V] guyanensis*). Most cases of visceral leishmaniasis are caused by *Leishmania donovani* or *Leishmania infantum (Leishmania chagasi* is synonymous). *L donovani* and *L infantum* also can cause cutaneous and mucosal leishmaniasis, although people with typical cutaneous leishmaniasis caused by these organisms rarely develop visceral leishmaniasis. Recently, emerging foci of both cutaneous and visceral infection with *Leishmania enriettii* complex have been reported from the Caribbean, Ghana, and Thailand. PKDL has been reported to be caused primarily by *L donovani,* both in the Indian subcontinent and Sudan.

EPIDEMIOLOGY: In most settings, leishmaniasis is a zoonosis, with mammalian reservoir hosts, such as rodents or dogs. Some transmission cycles are anthroponotic: infected humans are the primary or only reservoir hosts of *L donovani* in South Asia (potentially also in East Africa) and of *L tropica*. Congenital and parenteral (ie, shared needles, blood transfusion) transmission also have been reported.

Leishmaniasis has been endemic in more than 90 countries in the tropics, subtropics, and southern Europe. Visceral leishmaniasis (50 000–90 000 new cases annually) is found in focal areas in the Old World; in parts of Asia (particularly South, Southwest, and Central Asia), Africa (particularly East Africa), the Middle East, and southern Europe; and in the New World, particularly in Brazil. Most (>95%) of the world's cases of visceral leishmaniasis occur in 10 countries: Bangladesh, Brazil, China, Ethiopia, India, Kenya, Nepal, Somalia, South Sudan, and Sudan.

Cutaneous leishmaniasis is more common (0.6 to 1 million new cases annually). Approximately 90% of cutaneous leishmaniasis occurs in the Americas, the

Mediterranean basin, parts of the Middle East, and Central Asia. In 2017, 7 countries (Afghanistan, Algeria, Brazil, Colombia, Iran, Iraq, and Syria) accounted for 95% of new cases. Cutaneous leishmaniasis has been acquired in Texas and occasionally in Oklahoma. In general, the geographic distribution of leishmaniasis cases identified in the United States reflects immigration from and travel patterns to regions with endemic disease.

PKDL is confined mainly to 2 regions with endemic kala-azar: the Indian subcontinent (India, Nepal, Sri Lanka, and Bangladesh) and East Africa, mainly Sudan, although case reports have emanated from China, Iraq, and Iran. In the Indian subcontinent, transmission of VL is anthroponotic, whereas in Sudan it is zoonotic and anthroponotic; therefore, patients with PKDL are the proposed disease reservoir of VL in the Indian subcontinent. Young adults are more affected in the Indian subcontinent and children are more affected in Sudan.

Incubation periods for the various forms of leishmaniasis range from weeks to years. The primary skin lesions of cutaneous leishmaniasis typically appear within several weeks of exposure. The **incubation period** of visceral infection usually ranges from approximately 2 to 6 months. PKDL in Sudan develops within 6 months of treatment but in India can develop decades after cure of VL.

DIAGNOSTIC TESTS: Definitive diagnosis is made by detecting the parasite (amastigote stages) in infected tissue (eg, of aspirates, scrapings, touch preparations, or histologic sections) by light-microscopic examination of slides stained with Giemsa, hematoxylin, and eosin or other stains, by in vitro culture (available at reference laboratories), or increasingly by molecular methods (detection of parasite DNA by polymerase chain reaction [PCR] testing). The latter are reported to be more sensitive than microscopy or culture. The SMART-Leish PCR used by the US military leishmaniasis diagnostic laboratory is cleared by the US Food and Drug Administration (FDA) for use. In cutaneous and mucosal disease, tissue can be obtained by a 3-mm punch biopsy, lesion scrapings, or needle aspiration of the raised nonnecrotic edge (biopsy) or the ulcer base of the lesion. In visceral leishmaniasis, although the sensitivity is highest (approximately 95%) for splenic aspiration, the procedure can be associated with life-threatening hemorrhage; bone marrow aspiration is safer and generally preferred. Other potential sources of specimens include liver, lymph node, and in some patients (eg, those coinfected with HIV) whole blood or buffy coat. Identification of *Leishmania* species (eg, via isoenzyme analysis of cultured parasites or molecular approaches) may affect prognosis and influence treatment decisions. The Centers for Disease Control and Prevention (CDC) (**www.cdc.gov/ parasites/leishmaniasis**) can assist in all aspects of diagnostic testing. Serologic testing usually is not helpful in the evaluation of potential cases of cutaneous leishmaniasis but can provide supportive evidence for the diagnosis of visceral or mucosal leishmaniasis, particularly if the patient is immunocompetent. The rK39 immunochromatographic assay is FDA cleared for the presumptive diagnosis of visceral leishmaniasis and is commercially available.

TREATMENT: Guidelines published in 2016 from the Infectious Diseases Society of America and the American Society of Tropical Medicine and Hygiene provide a detailed approach to diagnosis and treatment.[1] Systemic antileishmanial treatment always is indicated for

---

[1]Aronson N, Herwaldt BL, Libman M, et al. Diagnosis and treatment of leishmaniasis: clinical practice guidelines by the Infectious Diseases Society of America (IDSA) and the American Society of Tropical Medicine and Hygiene (ASTMH). *Clin Infect Dis*. 2016;63(12):e202-e264

patients with visceral or mucosal leishmaniasis, whereas not all patients with cutaneous leishmaniasis need to be treated or require systemic therapy (see Drugs for Parasitic Infections, p 949, for specific treatment recommendations). Consultation with infectious disease or tropical medicine specialists and with staff of the CDC Division of Parasitic Diseases and Malaria is recommended (telephone: 404-718-4745; e-mail: **parasites@ cdc.gov**; CDC Emergency Operations Center [after business hours and on weekends]: 770-488-7100). The relative merits of various treatment approaches/regimens for an individual patient should be considered, taking into account that the therapeutic response may vary, not only for different *Leishmania* species but also for the same species in different geographic regions. Special considerations apply in the United States regarding the availability of particular medications. For example, the pentavalent antimonial compound, sodium stibogluconate, is not commercially available but can be obtained by US-licensed physicians through the CDC Drug Service (404-639-3670), under an investigational new drug (IND) protocol, for parenteral (intravenous or, less commonly, intramuscular) treatment of leishmaniasis. Liposomal amphotericin B is approved by the FDA for treatment of visceral leishmaniasis. The oral agent miltefosine is approved for treatment of cutaneous, mucosal, and visceral leishmaniasis; the FDA-approved indications are limited to infection caused by particular *Leishmania* species and to patients who are at least 12 years of age, weigh at least 30 kg (66 lb), and are not pregnant or breastfeeding during and for 5 months after the treatment course.

ISOLATION OF THE HOSPITALIZED PATIENT: Standard precautions are recommended.

CONTROL MEASURES: The best way for travelers to prevent leishmaniasis is by protecting themselves from sand fly bites. Vaccines and drugs for preventing infection are not available. To decrease the risk of being bitten, travelers should take the following measures:

- Stay in well-screened or air-conditioned areas when feasible. Avoid outdoor activities, especially from dusk to dawn, when sand flies generally are most active.
- When outside, wear long-sleeved shirts, long pants, and socks.
- Apply insect repellent on uncovered skin and under the ends of sleeves and pant legs. Follow instructions on the label of the repellent. The most effective repellents generally are those that contain the chemical N,N-diethyl-meta-toluamide (DEET) (see Prevention of Mosquitoborne and Tickborne Infections, p 175).
- Spray clothing items with a pyrethroid-containing insecticide several days before travel, and allow them to dry. The insecticide should be reapplied after every 5 washings. Permethrin should never be applied to skin.
- Spray living and sleeping areas with an insecticide.
- Use a bed net tucked under the mattress if not sleeping in an area that is well screened or air conditioned. If at all possible, a bed net that has been soaked in or sprayed with a pyrethroid-containing insecticide should be used; the insecticide will be effective for several months if the bed net is not washed. Because sand flies are much smaller than mosquitoes and can penetrate through smaller holes, fine-mesh netting, which may be uncomfortable in hot weather, is needed for an effective physical barrier against sand flies if the bed net is not impregnated.
- Purchase bed nets, repellents containing DEET, and permethrin before traveling.

Other considerations for prevention of leishmaniasis include early, effective treatment of infected persons, particularly those infected with anthroponotically transmitted parasites for which competent vectors exist; and treatment (to prevent potential congenital transmission) of pregnant women with visceral leishmaniasis. Leukoreduction filtering of blood products may decrease risk of acquiring visceral leishmaniasis through transfusion.

Leprosy

CLINICAL MANIFESTATIONS: Leprosy (Hansen's disease) is a curable infection primarily involving skin, peripheral nerves, and mucosa of the upper respiratory tract. The clinical forms of leprosy reflect the cellular immune response to *Mycobacterium leprae* and, in turn, the number, size, structure, and bacillary content of the lesions. The organism has unique tropism for peripheral nerves, and all forms of leprosy exhibit nerve involvement. Leprosy skin lesions are quite varied and may present as macular hypopigmented or erythematous anesthetic lesions, discolored patches, scaly plaques, sharply defined macules with central clearing, painless ulcers, or nodules. Leprosy lesions usually do not itch or hurt. They lack sensation to heat, touch, and pain but otherwise may be difficult to distinguish from other common maladies. There may be madarosis (loss of eyelashes or eyebrows). Although the nerve injury caused by leprosy is irreversible, early diagnosis and drug therapy can prevent those sequelae.

Leprosy manifests over a broad clinical and histopathologic spectrum. In the United States, the Ridley-Jopling scale is used to classify patients according to the histopathologic features of their lesions and organization of the underlying granuloma. The scale is as follows: (1) tuberculoid; (2) borderline tuberculoid; (3) mid-borderline; (4) borderline lepromatous; and (5) lepromatous. A simplified scheme introduced by the World Health Organization for circumstances in which pathologic examination and diagnosis is unavailable is based purely on clinical skin examination. This scheme classifies leprosy by the number of skin patches as either paucibacillary (1–5 lesions, usually tuberculoid or borderline tuberculoid) or multibacillary (>5 lesions, usually mid-borderline, borderline lepromatous, or lepromatous). Patients in the tuberculoid spectrum have active cell-mediated immunity with low antibody responses to *M leprae* and few well-defined lesions containing few bacilli. Lepromatous spectrum cases have high antibody responses with little cell-mediated immunity to *M leprae* and several somewhat diffuse lesions usually containing numerous bacilli.

Serious consequences of leprosy occur from immune reactions and nerve involvement with resulting anesthesia, which can lead to repeated unrecognized trauma, ulcerations, fractures, and even bone resorption. Leprosy is a leading cause of permanent physical disability among communicable diseases worldwide. Eye involvement can occur, especially corneal scarring, and patients should be examined by an ophthalmologist. A diagnosis of leprosy should be considered in any patient with a hypoesthetic or anesthetic skin rash or skin patches who has a history of residence in areas with endemic leprosy or who has had contact with armadillos.

Leprosy Reactions. Acute clinical exacerbations reflect abrupt changes in the immunologic balance. These reactions are especially common during initial years of treatment but can occur in the absence of therapy. Two major types of leprosy reactions (LRs) are observed. Type 1 (reversal reaction [LR-1]) is observed predominantly in borderline tuberculoid and borderline lepromatous leprosy and is the result of a sudden increase in effective cell-mediated immunity. Acute tenderness and swelling at the site of cutaneous and neural lesions with development of new lesions are major manifestations. Ulcerations can occur, but polymorphonuclear leukocytes are absent from the LR-1 lesion. Fever and systemic toxicity are uncommon. Type 2 (erythema nodosum leprosum [LR-2]) occurs in border-line and lepromatous forms as a systemic inflammatory response. Tender, red subcutane-ous papules or nodules resembling erythema nodosum can occur along with high fever, migrating polyarthralgia, painful swelling of lymph nodes and spleen, iridocyclitis, and rarely, nephritis.

ETIOLOGY: Leprosy is caused by *M leprae*, an obligate intracellular rod-shaped bacterium that can have variable findings on Gram stain and is weakly acid-fast on standard Ziehl-Neelsen staining but is best visualized using the Fite stain. *M leprae* has not been cultured successfully in vitro. *M leprae* is the only bacterium known to infect Schwann cells of peripheral nerves, and demonstration of acid-fast bacilli in peripheral nerves is pathogno-monic for leprosy. A newly described genomic variant, *Mycobacterium lepromatosis*, also has been implicated to cause leprosy, but the organism is not yet well characterized.

EPIDEMIOLOGY: Leprosy is considered a neglected tropical disease and is most prevalent in tropical and subtropical zones. It is not highly infectious. Several human genes have been identified that are associated with susceptibility to *M leprae* and a minority of people appear to be genetically susceptible to the infection. Accordingly, spouses of leprosy patients are not likely to develop leprosy, but biological parents, children, and siblings who are household contacts of untreated patients with leprosy are at some increased risk.

Transmission is believed to be most effective through long-term close contact with an infected individual and likely occurs through respiratory shedding of organisms. The 9-banded armadillo (*Dasypus novemcinctus*) is a recognized nonhuman reservoir of *M leprae*, and zoonotic transmission is reported in the southern United States. There are reports of *M leprae* infection among 9-banded armadillos as well as the 6-banded armadillo (*Euphractus sexcinctus*) in both Central and South America, mainly Argentina and Brazil. In addition, red squirrels (*Sciuris vulgarus*) in the British Isles may harbor *M leprae* and *M lepro-matosis*. People living with human immunodeficiency virus (HIV) infection do not appear to be at increased risk of becoming infected with *M leprae*. However, concomitant HIV infection and leprosy can lead to worsening of leprosy symptoms during HIV treatment and result in immune reconstitution inflammatory syndrome. Like many other chronic infectious diseases, onset of leprosy is associated increasingly with use of anti-inflamma-tory autoimmune therapies and immunologic senescence among elderly patients.

A total of 14 029 leprosy cases have been documented in the United States since 1894. There are approximately 6500 people with leprosy currently living in the United States, with 3500 under active medical management. The majority of leprosy cases reported in the United States occurred among residents of Texas, California, and Hawaii or among immigrants and other people who lived or worked in countries with endemic leprosy. More than 65% of the world's leprosy patients reside in South and Southeast Asia, primarily India. Other areas of high endemicity include Angola, Brazil, the Central African Republic, Democratic Republic of Congo, Madagascar, Mozambique, the Republic of the Marshall Islands, South Sudan, the Federated States of Micronesia, and the United Republic of Tanzania.

The **incubation period** usually is 3 to 5 years but may range from 1 to 20 years. The average age at onset varies according to endemicity within a population. All age groups are susceptible.

DIAGNOSTIC TESTS: There are no diagnostic tests or methods to detect subclinical lep-rosy. Histopathologic examination of a skin biopsy by an experienced pathologist is the best method of establishing the diagnosis and establishing classification of the disease. Formalin fixed or paraffin embedded biopsies can be sent to the National Hansen's Disease (Leprosy) Program (NHDP [800-642-2477; **www.hrsa.gov/hansens-disease/diagnosis/biopsy.html**]). Acid-fast bacilli may be found in slit smears or biopsy specimens of skin lesions from patients with lepromatous (multibacillary) forms of the disease but rarely are visualized from patients with the paucibacillary tuberculoid and indeterminate (first lesion with slightly diminished sensation) forms of disease. A polymerase chain reaction test for *M leprae* and *M lepromatosis* also is available at the NHDP, as are molecular tests for genetic mutations associated with drug resistance, and strain typing based on single nucleotide polymorphisms and other genomic elements. Tuberculin skin tests and interferon-gamma release assays are not used to diagnose leprosy.

TREATMENT: Leprosy is curable. Therapy for patients with leprosy should be undertaken in consultation with an expert in leprosy. The NHDP (800-642-2477) provides consultation on clinical and pathologic issues and information about local Hansen's disease clinics and clinicians who have experience with the disease. Prevention of permanent nerve damage and disability is an important goal of treatment and care and requires education and self-awareness of the patient. Combination antimicrobial multidrug therapy can be obtained free of charge from the NHDP in the United States and from the World Health Organization in other countries (**www.hrsa.gov/hansensdisease/diagnosis/recommendedtreatment.html**).

The infectivity of leprosy patients to others ceases within only a few days of initiating standard multidrug therapy. It is important to treat *M leprae* infections with more than 1 antimicrobial agent to minimize development of antimicrobial-resistant organisms. Adults are treated with dapsone, rifampin, and clofazimine. Regimens and doses for children are available and should be chosen with assistance from NHDP. Resistance to all 3 drugs has been documented but is extremely rare. Before beginning antimicrobial therapy, patients should be tested for glucose-6-phosphate dehydrogenase deficiency, have baseline complete blood cell counts and serum aminotransferase results documented, and be evaluated for any evidence of tuberculosis infection, especially if infected with HIV. This consideration is important to avoid monotherapy of active tuberculosis with rifampin while treating active leprosy.

Management of leprosy reactions is complex and expert guidance should be sought. Reactions should be treated aggressively to prevent peripheral nerve damage. Treatment with prednisone (1 mg/kg per day, orally) can be initiated for short-term management and rescue situations. Long-term use of prednisone should incorporate a sparing agent such as methotrexate. LR-2 may be treated with thalidomide (100–400 mg/day for 4 days). Thalidomide is used under strict supervision and is available through Celgene (**www.thalomidrems.com** or 888-423-5436). Thalidomide is not approved for use in children younger than 12 years. Most patients can be treated on an outpatient basis. Rehabilitative measures, including surgery and physical therapy, may be necessary for some patients.

All patients with leprosy should be educated about signs and symptoms of neuritis and cautioned to report them immediately so that corticosteroid therapy can be instituted. Patients should receive counseling because of the social and psychological effects of this disease.

Relapse of disease after completing multidrug therapy is rare (0.01%–0.14%); the presentation of new skin patches usually is attributable to a late type 1 reaction (LR-1).

When it does occur, relapse usually is attributable to reactivation of drug-susceptible organisms. People with relapses of disease require another course of multidrug therapy.

ISOLATION OF THE HOSPITALIZED PATIENT: Standard precautions are indicated; isolation is not required. Many patients suffer profound anxiety because of the stigma historically associated with leprosy.

CONTROL MEASURES: Leprosy is a reportable disease in the United States. Newly diagnosed cases should be reported to state public health authorities, the Centers for Disease Control and Prevention, and the NHDP. Household contacts should be examined initially, but long-term follow-up of asymptomatic contacts is not warranted. Chemoprophylaxis is not recommended.

There are no vaccines approved for use in the United States. A single bacille Calmette-Guérin (BCG) immunization is reported to be from 28% to 60% protective against leprosy, and BCG vaccine is used as an adjunct to drug therapy in Brazil. However, BCG vaccine administration also may precipitate leprosy among subclinically infected individuals incubating the infection. The effectiveness of combined drug and immunotherapy is unknown.

Leptospirosis

CLINICAL MANIFESTATIONS: Leptospirosis is an acute febrile disease with varied manifestations. The severity of disease ranges from asymptomatic or subclinical to a self-limited systemic febrile illness (approximately 90% of patients) to a life-threatening illness that can include jaundice, renal failure (oliguric or nonoliguric), myocarditis, hemorrhage (particularly pulmonary), aseptic meningitis, or refractory shock. Clinical presentation may be mono- or biphasic. Classically described biphasic leptospirosis has an acute septicemia phase usually lasting up to 1 week, during which time *Leptospira* organisms are present in blood, followed by a second immune-mediated phase that is less likely to respond to antimicrobial therapy. Regardless of its severity, the acute phase is characterized by nonspecific symptoms, including fever, chills, headache, myalgia, nausea, vomiting, or rash. Distinct clinical findings include notable conjunctival suffusion without purulent discharge (28%–99% of cases) and myalgia of the calf and lumbar regions (40%–97% of cases). Manifestations of the immune phase are more variable and milder than the initial illness. The hallmark of the immune phase is aseptic meningitis; uveitis is a late finding (4–8 months after the illness has begun). Supportive therapies are appropriate during this phase. Severe manifestations include jaundice and renal dysfunction (Weil syndrome), pulmonary hemorrhage, cardiac arrhythmias, and circulatory collapse. Abnormal potassium (high or low) and/or magnesium (low) levels may require aggressive management. The estimated case-fatality rate is 5% to 15% with severe illness, although it can increase to >50% in patients with pulmonary hemorrhage syndrome.

ETIOLOGY: Leptospirosis is caused by pathogenic spirochetes of the genus *Leptospira*. Leptospires are classified by species and subdivided into more than 300 antigenically defined serovars and grouped into serogroups on the basis of antigenic relatedness. Currently, the molecular classification divides the genus into 23 named pathogenic (n=10), intermediate (n=5) and saprophytic (nonpathogenic; n=8) genomospecies as determined by DNA-DNA hybridization, 16S ribosomal gene phylogenetic clustering, and whole genome sequencing. This newer nomenclature supersedes the former division of these organisms into 2 species: *Leptospira interrogans*, comprising all pathogenic strains, and *Leptospira biflexa*, comprising all saprophytic stains found in the environment. All leptospires are tightly coiled spirochetes, obligate aerobic, with an optimum growth temperature of 28°C to 30°C.

EPIDEMIOLOGY: Leptospirosis is among the most important zoonoses globally, affecting people in resource-rich and resource-limited countries in both urban and rural contexts. It has been estimated that more than 1 million people worldwide are infected annually (95% confidence interval [CI], 434 000–1 750 000), with approximately 58 900 deaths (95% CI, 23 800–95 900) occurring each year. The reservoirs for *Leptospira* species include a wide range of wild and domestic animals, including rodents, dogs, livestock (cattle, pigs), and horses that may shed organisms asymptomatically for years. *Leptospira* organisms excreted in animal urine may remain viable in moist soil or water for weeks to months in warm climates. Humans usually become infected via entry of leptospires through contact of mucosal surfaces (especially conjunctivae) or abraded skin with urine-contaminated environmental sources such as soil and water. Infection also may be acquired through direct contact with infected animals or their tissues, urine, or other body fluids. Epidemics are associated with seasonal flooding and natural disasters, including hurricanes and monsoons. Populations in regions of high endemicity in the tropics and subtropics likely encounter *Leptospira* organisms during routine activities of daily living. People predisposed by occupation include abattoir and sewer workers, miners, veterinarians, farmers, and military personnel. Recreational exposures and clusters of disease have been associated with adventure travel, sporting events including triathlons, and wading, swimming, or boating in contaminated water, particularly during flooding or following heavy rainfall. Common history includes head submersion in or swallowing water during such activities. Person-to-person transmission is not described convincingly.

The **incubation period** usually is 5 to 14 days, range 2 to 30 days.

DIAGNOSTIC TESTS: Clinical features and routine laboratory findings are not specific for leptospirosis; a high index of suspicion must be maintained for diagnosis. *Leptospira* organisms can be isolated from blood during the early septicemic phase (first week) of illness, from urine specimens starting approximately 1 week after symptom onset, and from cerebrospinal fluid when clinical signs of meningitis are present. Specialized culture media are required but are not available routinely in most clinical laboratories. *Leptospira* organisms can be subcultured to specific *Leptospira* semi-solid medium (ie, EMJH) from blood culture bottles used in automated systems within 1 week of inoculation. Isolation of the organism may be difficult, requiring incubation for up to 16 weeks, weekly darkfield microscopic examination, and avoidance of contamination. Sensitivity of culture for diagnosis is low. Isolated leptospires are identified either by serologic methods using agglutinating antisera or more recently by molecular methods.

Serum specimens always should be obtained to facilitate diagnosis, and paired acute and convalescent sera are recommended, ideally collected 10 to 14 days apart. Antibodies develop by 5 to 7 days after onset of illness, but increases in antibody titer may not be detected until more than 10 days after onset, especially if antimicrobial therapy is initiated early. Antibodies can be measured by commercially available immunoassays, most of which are based on sonicates of the saprophyte *L biflexa*. These assays have variable sensitivity according to regional differences of the various *Leptospira* species. In populations with high endemicity, background reactivity requires establishing regionally relevant diagnostic criteria and establishing diagnostic versus background titers. Antibody increases can be transient, delayed, or absent in some patients, which may be related to antibiotic use, bacterial virulence, immunogenetics of the individual, or other unknown factors. Microscopic agglutination, the gold standard serologic test, is performed only in reference laboratories and seroconversion demonstrated between acute and convalescent specimens is diagnostic.

Immunohistochemical and immunofluorescent techniques can detect leptospiral antigens in infected tissues. Polymerase chain reaction (PCR) assays for detection of *Leptospira* DNA in clinical specimens are available but are sensitive only in acute specimens and sometimes convalescent urine. *Leptospira* DNA can be detected in whole blood during the first 7 days of illness, with highest sensitivity between days 1 and 4; *Leptospira* DNA can be found after 7 days of illness in urine and may be detectable for weeks to months in the absence of antimicrobial treatment. *Leptospira* DNA also can be detected in CSF from symptomatic patients with clinical signs of meningitis.

TREATMENT: Antimicrobial therapy should be initiated as soon as possible after symptom onset. Intravenous penicillin is the drug of choice for patients with severe infection requiring hospitalization; penicillin has been shown to be effective in shortening duration of fever when given as late as 7 days into the course of illness. Penicillin G decreases the duration of systemic symptoms and persistence of associated laboratory abnormalities and may prevent development of leptospiruria. A Jarisch-Herxheimer reaction (an acute febrile reaction accompanied by headache, myalgia, and an aggravated clinical picture lasting less than 24 hours) can develop after initiation of penicillin therapy, as with other spirochetal infections. Parenteral cefotaxime, ceftriaxone, and doxycycline have been demonstrated in randomized clinical trials to be equal in efficacy to penicillin G for treatment of severe leptospirosis. For patients with mild disease, oral doxycycline has been shown to shorten the course of illness and decrease occurrence of leptospiruria; doxycycline can be used for short durations (ie, 21 days or less) without regard to patient age (see Tetracyclines, p 866). Ampicillin or amoxicillin also can be used to treat mild disease. Azithromycin has been demonstrated in a clinical trial to be as effective as doxycycline. Severe cases require appropriate supportive care, including fluid and electrolyte replacement. Patients with oliguric renal insufficiency require prompt dialysis, and those with pulmonary hemorrhage may require mechanical ventilation to improve clinical outcome.

ISOLATION OF THE HOSPITALIZED PATIENT: Standard precautions are recommended for patient care. Contact precautions are advised for contact with urine.

CONTROL MEASURES:

- Immunization of livestock, horses, and dogs can prevent clinical disease attributable to infecting serovars contained within the vaccine. Immunization may not prevent the shedding of leptospires in urine of animals and, thus, contamination of environments with which humans may come in contact.
- Rodent-control programs may be useful in areas with endemic infection.
- Swimming, immersion, and swallowing water should be avoided in bodies of potentially contaminated fresh water.
- Appropriate protective clothing, boots, and gloves should be worn by people with exposure to urine or potentially contaminated water or mud, such as during floods.
- Doxycycline, 200 mg, administered orally once a week to adults, may provide effective prophylaxis against clinical disease and could be considered for high-risk groups with short-term exposure, but infection may not be prevented, and adverse gastrointestinal tract events are common. Indications for prophylactic doxycycline use for children have not been established.

Listeria monocytogenes Infections
(Listeriosis)

CLINICAL MANIFESTATIONS: Listeriosis is a relatively uncommon but often severe invasive infection caused by *Listeria monocytogenes*. Transmission predominantly is foodborne, and illness, especially with severe manifestations, occurs most frequently among pregnant women and their fetuses or newborn infants, older adults, and people with impaired cell-mediated immunity resulting from underlying illness or treatment (eg, organ transplant, hematologic malignancy, immunosuppression resulting from therapy with corticosteroid or anti-tumor necrosis factor agents, or acquired immunodeficiency syndrome). Infections during pregnancy can result in spontaneous abortion, fetal death, preterm delivery, and neonatal illness or death. In pregnant women, infections can be asymptomatic or associated with a nonspecific febrile illness with myalgia, back pain, and occasionally gastrointestinal tract symptoms. Fetal infection generally results from transplacental transmission following maternal bacteremia. Additional mechanisms of infection in neonates with listeriosis are thought to include inhalation of infected amniotic fluid and infection ascending from maternal vaginal colonization. Approximately 65% of pregnant women with *Listeria* infection experience a prodromal illness before the diagnosis of listeriosis in their newborn infants. Amnionitis during labor, brown staining of amniotic fluid, or asymptomatic perinatal infection can occur.

Neonates can present with early- or late-onset disease. Preterm birth, pneumonia, and septicemia are common in early-onset disease (within the first week), with fatality rates of 14% to 56%. An erythematous rash with small, pale papules characterized histologically by granulomas, termed "granulomatosis infantisepticum," can occur in severe newborn infection. Late-onset infections occur at 8 to 30 days following term deliveries and usually result in meningitis with fatality rates of approximately 25%. Late-onset infection may result from acquisition of the organism during passage through the birth canal or, rarely, from environmental sources. Health care-associated nursery outbreaks have been reported.

Clinical features characteristic of invasive listeriosis outside the neonatal period or pregnancy are bacteremia and meningitis, with or without parenchymal brain involvement, and less commonly brain abscess or endocarditis. *L monocytogenes* also can cause rhombencephalitis (brain stem encephalitis) in otherwise healthy adolescents and young adults. Outbreaks of febrile gastroenteritis caused by food contaminated with a very large inoculum of *L monocytogenes* have been reported.

ETIOLOGY: *L monocytogenes* is a facultatively anaerobic, nonspore-forming, nonbranching, motile, gram-positive rod that multiplies intracellularly. It has been assigned to the family *Listeriaceae* along with 5 other traditional and several newly named species. The organism grows readily on blood agar and produces incomplete hemolysis. *L monocytogenes* serotypes 1/2a, 4b, and 1/2b grow well at refrigerator temperatures (4°C–10°C).

EPIDEMIOLOGY: *L monocytogenes* causes approximately 1000 cases of invasive disease annually in the United States, and approximately 15% of cases are associated with pregnancy. Pregnant women are 10 times more likely to be infected than other people. The mortality rate is 15% to 20%, with higher rates among older adults and the immunocompromised, including neonates. The saprophytic organism is distributed widely in the environment and is an important cause of illness in ruminants. Foodborne transmission causes outbreaks and sporadic infections in humans. Commonly incriminated foods include deli-style, ready-to-eat meats, particularly poultry; unpasteurized milk[1]; and soft cheeses, including Mexican-style cheese. Approximately 25% of global outbreaks are attributable to foods not traditionally associated as sources of *L monocytogenes*, such as ice cream and fresh and frozen fruits and vegetables. Listeriosis is a relatively rare foodborne illness (<1% of pathogens causing reported foodborne illness in the United States) but has the highest case-fatality rate among all foodborne pathogens and causes 20% of foodborne disease-related deaths.[2] The incidence of listeriosis decreased substantially in the United States during the 1990s, when regulatory agencies began enforcing rigorous screening guidelines for *L monocytogenes* in processed foods and better detection methods became available to identify contaminated foods. The prevalence of stool carriage of *L monocytogenes* among healthy, asymptomatic adults is estimated to be 1% to 5%.

The **incubation period** for invasive disease is longer for pregnancy-associated cases (2–4 weeks or occasionally longer) than for nonpregnancy-associated cases (1 to 14 days). The **incubation period** for self-limiting, febrile gastroenteritis following ingestion of a large inoculum is 24 hours; illness typically lasts 2 to 3 days.

DIAGNOSTIC TESTS: *L monocytogenes* can be recovered readily on blood agar from cultures of blood, cerebrospinal fluid (CSF), meconium, placental or fetal tissue specimens, amniotic fluid, and other infected tissue specimens, including joint, pleural, or peritoneal fluid. Attempts to recover the organism from clinical specimens from nonsterile body sites, including stool, should include the use of selective medium. Gram stain of meconium, placental tissue, biopsy specimens of the rash of early-onset infection, or CSF from an infected patient may demonstrate the organism. The organisms can be gram-variable and can resemble diphtheroids, cocci, or diplococci. Laboratory misidentification is not uncommon, and the isolation of a "diphtheroid" from blood or cerebrospinal fluid (CSF) should always alert one to the possibility that the organism is *L monocytogenes*.

A number of laboratory-derived polymerase chain reaction (PCR) assays have been described for detection of *L monocytogenes* in blood and CSF. At least 1 multiplexed PCR diagnostic panel designed to detect agents of meningitis and encephalitis in CSF cleared by the US Food and Drug Administration contains *L monocytogenes* as one of its target organisms; however, there are limited clinical data with the use of PCR for this purpose, and parallel culture of CSF also should be performed to allow for susceptibility testing and molecular characterization, especially for outbreak detection.

TREATMENT: No controlled trials have established the drug(s) of choice or duration of therapy for listeriosis. Combination therapy using ampicillin and a second agent in doses appropriate for meningitis is recommended for severe infections. An aminoglycoside, typically gentamicin, usually is used as the second agent in combination therapy. Use of an alternative second agent that is active intracellularly (eg, trimethoprim-sulfamethoxazole [contraindicated in infants younger than 2 months], fluoroquinolones, linezolid, or rifampin) is supported by case reports in adults. If alternatives to gentamicin are used, susceptibility should be confirmed because resistance to trimethoprim-sulfamethoxazole, fluoroquinolones, linezolid, or rifampin occasionally has been reported. In the penicillin-allergic patient, options include either penicillin desensitization or use of either

---

[1] American Academy of Pediatrics, Committee on Infectious Diseases and Committee on Nutrition. Consumption of raw or unpasteurized milk and milk products by pregnant women and children. *Pediatrics*. 2014;133(1):175-179 (Reaffirmed November 2019)

[2] **www.cdc.gov/foodnet/pdfs/FoodNet-Annual-Report-2015-508c.pdf**

trimethoprim-sulfamethoxazole or a fluoroquinolone, both of which have been used successfully as monotherapy for *Listeria* meningitis and in the setting of brain abscess. Treatment failures with vancomycin have been reported. Cephalosporins are not active against *L monocytogenes*.

For bacteremia without associated central nervous system infection, 14 days of treatment is recommended. For *L monocytogenes* meningitis, most experts recommend 3 to 4 weeks of treatment. Longer courses are necessary for patients with endocarditis or parenchymal brain infection (cerebritis, rhombencephalitis, brain abscess). Iron may enhance the pathogenicity of *L monocytogenes*; iron supplements should be withheld until treatment for listeriosis is complete. Diagnostic imaging of the brain near the end of the anticipated duration of therapy allows determination of parenchymal involvement of the brain and the need for prolonged therapy in neonates with complicated courses and in immunocompromised patients.

ISOLATION OF THE HOSPITALIZED PATIENT: Standard precautions are recommended.

CONTROL MEASURES:

- Antimicrobial therapy for infection diagnosed during pregnancy may prevent fetal or perinatal infection and its consequences.
- Neonatal listeriosis complicating successive pregnancies is virtually unknown, and intrapartum antimicrobial therapy is not recommended for mothers with a history of perinatal listeriosis.
- General and specific guidelines for preventing listeriosis from foodborne sources are provided in Table 3.28.

Table 3.28. Recommendations for Preventing Foodborne Listeriosis

General recommendations:
Washing and handling food
- **Rinse** raw produce, such as fruits and vegetables, thoroughly under running tap water before eating, cutting, or cooking. Even if the produce will be peeled, it should still be washed first.
- **Scrub** firm produce, such as melons and cucumbers, with a clean produce brush.
- **Dry** the produce with a clean cloth or paper towel.
- **Separate** uncooked meats and poultry from vegetables, cooked foods, and ready-to-eat foods.

Keep your kitchen and environment cleaner and safer
- Wash hands, knives, countertops, and cutting boards after handling and preparing uncooked foods.
- Be aware that *Listeria monocytogenes* can grow in foods in the refrigerator. Use an appliance thermometer, such as a refrigerator thermometer, to check the temperature inside your refrigerator. The refrigerator temperature should be 40°F or lower and the freezer temperature should be 0°F or lower.
- Clean up all spills in your refrigerator right away—especially juices from hot dog and lunch meat packages, raw meat, and raw poultry.
- Clean the inside walls and shelves of your refrigerator with hot water and liquid soap, then rinse.

Cook meat and poultry thoroughly
- Thoroughly cook raw food from animal sources, such as beef, pork, or poultry to a safe internal temperature. For a list of recommended temperatures for meat and poultry, visit the safe minimum cooking temperatures chart at **FoodSafety.gov (www.foodsafety.gov/keep/charts/mintemp.html)**.

Table 3.28. Recommendations for Preventing Foodborne Listeriosis, continued

Store foods safely

- Use precooked or ready-to-eat food as soon as you can. Do not store the product in the refrigerator beyond the use-by date; follow USDA refrigerator storage time guidelines:
  - o Hot dogs – store opened package no longer than 1 week and unopened package no longer than 2 weeks in the refrigerator.
  - o Luncheon and deli meat – store factory-sealed, unopened package no longer than 2 weeks. Store opened packages and meat sliced at a local deli no longer than 3 to 5 days in the refrigerator.
- Divide leftovers into shallow containers to promote rapid, even cooling. Cover with airtight lids or enclose in plastic wrap or aluminum foil. Use leftovers within 3 to 4 days.

Choose safer foods

- Do not drink raw (unpasteurized) milk[a] (**www.cdc.gov/foodsafety/rawmilk/raw-milk-index.html** and **http://pediatrics.aappublications.org/content/pediatrics/early/2013/12/10/peds.2013-3502.full.pdf**), and do not eat foods that have unpasteurized milk in them.
- Find more specific information about this topic on the CDC Listeriosis Prevention website (**www.cdc.gov/listeria/prevention.html**).

Recommendations for people at higher risk, such as pregnant women, people with weakened immune systems, and older adults, in addition to the recommendations listed above:

Meats

- Do not eat hot dogs, luncheon meats, cold cuts, other deli meats (eg, bologna), or fermented or dry sausages unless they are heated to an internal temperature of 165°F or until steaming hot just before serving.
- Avoid getting fluid from hot dog and lunch meat packages on other foods, utensils, and food preparation surfaces, and wash hands after handling hot dogs, luncheon meats, and deli meats.
- Pay attention to labels. Do not eat refrigerated pâté or meat spreads from a deli or meat counter or from the refrigerated section of a store. Foods that do not need refrigeration, like canned or shelf-stable pâté and meat spreads, are safe to eat. Refrigerate after opening.

Soft cheeses

- Do not eat soft cheese, such as feta, queso blanco, queso fresco, brie, Camembert, blue-veined, or panela (queso panela) unless it is labeled as "MADE WITH PASTEURIZED MILK."
- Be aware that Mexican-style cheeses made from pasteurized milk, such as queso fresco, have caused *Listeria* infections as they were presumably contaminated during cheese-making.

Seafood

- Do not eat refrigerated smoked seafood, unless it has been cooked (such as a casserole) or is a canned or shelf-stable product.
- Do not eat refrigerated smoked seafood, such as salmon, trout, whitefish, cod, tuna, and mackerel. These fish typically are found in the refrigerator section or sold at seafood and deli counters of grocery stores and delicatessens. Canned and shelf-stable tuna, salmon, and other fish products are not considered foods at risk of causing listeriosis.

Safety tips for eating melons

- Consumers and food preparers should wash their hands with warm water and soap for at least 20 seconds *before* and *after* handling any whole melon such as cantaloupe, watermelon, or honeydew.
- Scrub the surface of melons, such as cantaloupes, with a clean produce brush under running water and dry them with a clean cloth or paper towel before cutting. Be sure that your scrub brush is sanitized after each use to avoid transferring bacteria between melons.
- Promptly consume cut melon or refrigerate promptly. Keep your cut melon refrigerated at, or less than 40°F (32°F–34°F is best) for no more than 7 days.
- Discard cut melons left at room temperature for more than 4 hours.

[a] American Academy of Pediatrics, Committee on Infectious Diseases and Committee on Nutrition. Consumption of raw or unpasteurized milk and milk products by pregnant women and children. *Pediatrics*. 2014;133(1):175-179 (Reaffirmed November 2019)

- Trimethoprim-sulfamethoxazole, given as pneumocystis prophylaxis for those with acquired immunodeficiency syndrome, transplant recipients, or others on long-term, high-dose corticosteroids, effectively prevents listeriosis.
- Listeriosis is a nationally notifiable disease in the United States. Cases should be reported promptly to the state or local health department to facilitate early recognition and control of common-source outbreaks. Clinical isolates should be forwarded to a public health laboratory for genetic sequencing.

Lyme Disease[1]
(Lyme Borreliosis, *Borrelia burgdorferi* sensu lato Infection)

CLINICAL MANIFESTATIONS: Clinical manifestations of Lyme disease are divided into 3 stages: early localized, early disseminated, and late manifestations. Early localized disease is characterized by a distinctive lesion, erythema migrans (EM), at the site of a recent tick bite. Erythema migrans is by far the most common manifestation of Lyme disease in children. Erythema migrans appears days to weeks after a tick bite and begins as a red macule or papule that usually expands to form a large (often ≥5 cm in diameter) annular, erythematous lesion, sometimes with partial central clearing. The lesion typically is painless and nonpruritic. Localized erythema migrans can vary greatly in size and shape and can be confused with cellulitis; lesions may have a purplish discoloration or central vesicular or necrotic areas. A classic "bulls-eye" appearance with concentric rings appears in a minority of cases. Factors that distinguish erythema migrans from local allergic reaction to a tick bite include larger size, gradual expansion, less pruritus, and slower onset of EM. Constitutional symptoms, such as malaise, headache, mild neck stiffness, myalgia, and arthralgia, but not joint swelling or effusion, often accompany erythema migrans. Fever may be present but is not universal and generally is mild.

In early disseminated disease, multiple EM lesions may appear several weeks after an infective tick bite and consist of secondary annular, erythematous lesions similar to but usually smaller than the primary lesion. Other manifestations of early disseminated illness (which may occur with or without a skin lesion) are palsies of the cranial nerves (most commonly cranial nerve VII), lymphocytic meningitis (often associated with cranial neuropathy or papilledema), and radiculitis. Carditis usually manifests as various degrees of atrioventricular block and can be life threatening. Systemic symptoms, such as low-grade fever, arthralgia, myalgia, headache, and fatigue, may be present during the early disseminated stage.

Patients with early Lyme disease can be infected simultaneously with *Borrelia miyamotoi* and agents of babesiosis and anaplasmosis (see Babesiosis, p 217; *Ehrlichia, Anaplasma,* and Related Infections, p 308; and *Borrelia* Infections, p 235). These diagnoses should be suspected in patients who manifest high fever, have hematologic abnormalities consistent with these infections, or who do not respond as expected to therapy prescribed for Lyme disease, such as fever persisting for more than 1 day after starting treatment. Patients

[1]Lantos PM, Rumbaugh J, Bockenstedt LK, et al. Clinical practice guidelines by the Infectious Diseases Society of America (IDSA), American Academy of Neurology (AAN), and American College of Rheumatology (ACR): 2020 Guidelines for the prevention, diagnosis and treatment of Lyme disease. *Clin Infect Dis*. Published online November 30, 2020. Doi: **https://doi.org/10.1093/cid/ciaa1215.** The full guideline is available at: **www.idsociety.org/practice-guideline/lyme-disease/**

who contract Lyme disease may be coinfected with Powassan virus (deer tick virus) if bitten in the United States or with tickborne encephalitis virus if infection was acquired in Europe.

Late Lyme disease occurs in patients who are not treated at an earlier stage of illness and manifests in children most commonly as arthritis. Lyme arthritis is characterized by inflammatory arthritis that usually is mono- or oligoarticular and affects large joints, particularly the knees. Although arthralgia can be present at any stage of Lyme disease, Lyme arthritis has objective evidence of joint swelling and white blood cells in synovial fluid specimens. Most cases of arthritis occur without a history of earlier stages of illness (including erythema migrans) or prior treatment. Compared with pyogenic arthritis, Lyme arthritis tends to manifest with joint swelling/effusion out of proportion to pain or disability and with lower peripheral blood neutrophilia and erythrocyte sedimentation rate (ESR). The effusion may be episodic lasting weeks at a time and then resolve with later occurrence. Polyneuropathy, encephalopathy, and encephalitis are rare late manifestations. Children treated with antimicrobial agents in the early stage of disease rarely develop late manifestations.

Other rare clinical manifestations include ophthalmic conditions such as conjunctivitis, optic neuritis, keratitis, and uveitis.

Lyme disease is not thought to produce a congenital infection syndrome. No causal relationship between maternal Lyme disease and abnormalities of pregnancy or congenital disease caused by *Borrelia burgdorferi* sensu lato has been documented. No evidence exists that Lyme disease can be transmitted via human milk.

ETIOLOGY: In the United States, Lyme disease is caused by the spirochete *B burgdorferi* sensu stricto (hereafter referred to as *B burgdorferi*) and rarely by the recently discovered *Borrelia mayonii*. In Eurasia, *B burgdorferi*, *Borrelia afzelii*, and *Borrelia garinii* cause borreliosis. *Borrelia* species are members of the family *Spirochaetaceae*, which also includes *Treponema* species.

EPIDEMIOLOGY: In 2017, 29 513 confirmed cases of Lyme disease were reported in the United States, although the actual number of cases may be up to 10-fold greater because of underreporting. Lyme disease occurs primarily in 2 distinct geographic regions of the United States, with more than 80% of cases occurring in New England and the eastern Mid-Atlantic States, as far south as Virginia. The disease also occurs, but with lower frequency, in the upper Midwest, especially Wisconsin and Minnesota. The geographic range is not static and has expanded considerably in the eastern and Midwestern states since 2000. Transmission also occurs at a low level on the west coast, especially northern California. The occurrence of cases in the United States correlates with distribution and frequency of infected tick vectors—*Ixodes scapularis* in the east and Midwest and *Ixodes pacificus* in the west. In Southern states, *I scapularis* ticks are rarer than in the northeast; those ticks that are present do not feed commonly on competent reservoir mammals and are less likely to bite humans because of different questing habits. Cases reported from states without known endemic transmission may have been imported from endemic states or may be misdiagnoses resulting from false-positive serologic test results or results that are misinterpreted as positive. Late manifestations, such as arthritis, can occur months after exposure highlighting the importance of eliciting a travel history to areas with endemic transmission.

Most cases of early localized and early disseminated Lyme disease occur between April and October; approximately 50% occur during June and July. People of all ages can be affected, but incidence in the United States is highest among children 5 through 9 years of age and adults 55 through 69 years of age.

With lesion(s) similar to erythema migrans, "southern tick-associated rash illness" (STARI) has been reported mainly in south central and southeastern states without endemic *B burgdorferi* infection. The etiology is unknown. STARI results from the bite of the lone star tick, *Amblyomma americanum*, which is abundant in southern states and is biologically incapable of transmitting *B burgdorferi*. Patients with STARI may present with constitutional symptoms in addition to erythema migrans, but STARI has not been associated with any of the disseminated complications of Lyme disease. Appropriate treatment of STARI is unknown.

B mayonii is a newly described species identified in a small number of patients from the upper Midwest with symptoms similar to those of Lyme disease. Patients with *B mayonii* infection can be expected to test positive for Lyme disease using the 2-tier serologic testing described below, and therapy used for Lyme disease is effective against *B mayonii*.

Lyme disease also is endemic in eastern Canada, Europe, states of the former Soviet Union, China, Mongolia, and Japan. The primary tick vector in Europe is *Ixodes ricinus*, and the primary tick vector in Asia is *Ixodes persulcatus*. Clinical manifestations vary somewhat from those seen in the United States. European Lyme disease can cause the skin lesions borrelial lymphocytoma and acrodermatitis chronica atrophicans and is more likely to produce neurologic disease, whereas arthritis is uncommon. These differences are attributable to the different genospecies of *Borrelia* responsible for European Lyme disease.

The **incubation period** for US Lyme disease from tick bite to appearance of single or multiple erythema migrans lesions ranges from 3 to 32 days, with a median time of 11 days. Late manifestations such as arthritis can occur months after the tick bite in people who do not receive antimicrobial therapy.

DIAGNOSTIC TESTS: Diagnosis of Lyme disease rests first and foremost on the recognition of a consistent clinical illness in people who have had plausible geographic exposure. Early Lyme disease in patients with erythema migrans is diagnosed clinically on the basis of the characteristic appearance of this skin lesion. Although erythema migrans is not pathognomonic for Lyme disease, it is highly distinctive and characteristic. In areas with endemic Lyme disease, it is expected that the vast majority of erythema migrans occurring in the appropriate season is attributable to *B burgdorferi* infection. Sensitivity of serologic testing is low during early infection, and less than half of children with solitary EM lesions will be seropositive. Patients who seek medical attention with 1 or more lesions of EM and without extracutaneous manifestations should be treated based on a clinical diagnosis of Lyme disease without serologic testing.

There is a broad differential diagnosis for extracutaneous manifestations of Lyme disease. Diagnosis of extracutaneous Lyme disease, including late-stage disease, requires a typical clinical illness, plausible geographic exposure, and a positive serologic test result.

The standard testing method for Lyme disease is a 2-tier serologic algorithm. The initial screening test identifies antibodies to a whole-cell sonicate, to peptide antigen, or to recombinant antigens of *B burgdorferi* using an enzyme-linked immunosorbent assay (ELISA or EIA) or immunofluorescent antibody (IFA) test. It should be noted that clinical laboratories vary somewhat in their description of this test. It may be described as "Lyme

ELISA," "Lyme antibody screen," "total Lyme antibody," or "Lyme IgG/IgM." Many commercial laboratories offer EIA/IFA with reflex to Western immunoblot if the first-tier assay result is positive or equivocal. Although the initial EIA or IFA test result may be reported quantitatively, its sole importance is to categorize the result as negative, equivocal, or positive.

If the first-tier EIA result is negative, the patient is considered seronegative and no further testing is indicated. If the result is equivocal or positive, then a second-tier test is required to confirm the result. There are 2 options for second tier testing: (1) a western immunoblot, which is the standard 2-tiered testing algorithm; or (2) an EIA test that has been specifically cleared by FDA for use as a second-tier confirmatory test, which is the modified 2-tiered testing algorithm (**www.cdc.gov/mmwr/volumes/68/wr/ mm6832a4.htm?s_cid=mm6832a4_w**). Some assays marketed in the United States have reduced sensitivity for European strains of *B burgdorferi*. For patients potentially infected in Europe, check with the test provider or laboratory director to select tests that have been validated for this purpose.

Two-tier serologic testing increases test specificity. False-positive results are partly explained by antigenic components of *B burgdorferi* that are not specific to this species. Antibodies produced in response to other spirochetal infections, spirochetes in normal oral flora, other acute infections, and certain autoimmune diseases may be cross-reactive. In areas with endemic infection, previous subclinical infection with seroconversion may occur, and a seropositive patient's symptoms may be coincidental. Patients with active Lyme disease almost always have objective signs of infection (eg, erythema migrans, facial nerve palsy, arthritis). Nonspecific symptoms commonly accompany these specific signs but almost never are the only evidence of Lyme disease. Serologic testing for Lyme disease should not be performed for children without symptoms or signs suggestive of Lyme disease and plausible geographic exposure.

Western immunoblot testing should not be performed if the initial EIA or IFA test result is negative or without a prior EIA or IFA test, because specificity of immunoblot diminishes if the test is performed alone. The immunoblot assay tests for presence of antibodies to specific *B burgdorferi* antigens, including immunoglobulin (Ig) M antibodies to 3 spirochetal antigens (the 23/24, 39, and 41 kDa polypeptides) and IgG antibodies to 10 spirochetal antigens (the 18, 23/24, 28, 30, 39, 41, 45, 60, 66, and 93 kDa polypeptides). Although some clinical laboratories report presence of antibody to each of 13 bands, describing each band as positive or negative, a positive immunoblot result is defined as presence of at least 2 IgM bands or 5 IgG bands. Physicians must be careful not to misinterpret a positive band as a positive test result or interpret a result as positive despite presence of 4 or fewer IgG bands. It is noteworthy that IgG antibodies to flagella protein, the p41 band, are present in 30% to 50% of healthy people.

A positive IgM immunoblot result can be falsely positive. The IgM assay is useful only for patients in the first 4 weeks after symptom onset. The IgM immunoblot result should be disregarded (or, if possible, not ordered) in patients who have had symptoms for longer than 4 weeks, or symptoms consistent with late Lyme disease, because false-positive IgM assay results are common, and because most untreated patients with disseminated Lyme disease will have a positive IgG result by week 4 of symptoms.

Lyme disease test results for *B burgdorferi* in patients treated for syphilis or other spirochete diseases are difficult to interpret. Consultation with an infectious diseases specialist is recommended. Although immunodeficiency theoretically could affect serologic testing results, reports have described infected patients who produced anti-*B burgdorferi* antibodies and had positive test results despite various immunocompromising conditions.

No polymerase chain reaction (PCR) test for *B burgdorferi* currently is cleared by the FDA. PCR testing of joint fluid from a patient with Lyme arthritis often yields positive results and can be informative in establishing a diagnosis of Lyme arthritis. The role of a PCR assay on blood is not well established; test results usually are negative in early and late Lyme disease and is not recommended routinely. Yield of PCR testing on cerebrospinal fluid samples from patients with neuroborreliosis is too low to be useful in excluding this diagnosis.

Some patients treated with antimicrobial agents for early Lyme disease never develop detectable antibodies against *B burgdorferi;* they are cured and are not at risk of late disease. Development of antibodies in patients treated for early Lyme disease does not indicate lack of cure or presence of persistent infection. Ongoing infection without development of antibodies ("seronegative Lyme") has not been demonstrated. Most patients with early disseminated disease and virtually all patients with late disease have antibodies against *B burgdorferi.* Once such antibodies develop, they may persist for many years. Tests for antibodies should not be repeated or used to assess success of treatment.

A number of tests for Lyme disease have been found to be invalid on the basis of independent testing or to be too nonspecific to exclude false-positive results. These include urine tests for *B burgdorferi*, CD57 assay, novel culture techniques, and antibody panels that differ from those recommended as part of standardized 2-tier testing. Although these tests are commercially available from some clinical laboratories, they are not FDA cleared and are not appropriate diagnostic tests for Lyme disease.

Current evidence indicates that patients with *B mayonii* infection develop a serologic response similar to that of patients infected with *B burgdorferi*. Standardized 2-tier testing can be expected to have positive results in patients with *B mayonii* infection.

TREATMENT: Consensus practice guidelines for assessment, treatment, and prevention of Lyme disease have been published by the Infectious Diseases Society of America.[1] Care of children should follow recommendations in Table 3.29. Antimicrobial therapy for nonspecific symptoms or for asymptomatic seropositivity is not recommended. Antimicrobial agents administered for durations not specified in Table 3.29 are not recommended. Alternative diagnostic approaches or therapies without adequate validation studies and publication in peer-reviewed scientific literature are discouraged. Physicians have successfully treated patients with *B mayonii* infection with antimicrobial regimens used for Lyme disease.

Erythema Migrans (Single or Multiple). Doxycycline, amoxicillin, or cefuroxime can be used to treat children of any age who present with erythema migrans. Azithromycin generally is regarded as a second-line antimicrobial agent for erythema migrans in the United States, but further research on the efficacy of this agent is warranted. Selection of an oral antimicrobial agent for treatment of erythema migrans should be based on the following considerations: presence of neurologic disease (for which doxycycline is the drug of choice), drug allergy, adverse effects, frequency of administration (doxycycline and cefuroxime are administered twice a day, amoxicillin is administered 3 times a day), ability

---

[1]Lantos PM, Rumbaugh J, Bockenstedt LK, et al. Clinical practice guidelines by the Infectious Diseases Society of America (IDSA), American Academy of Neurology (AAN), and American College of Rheumatology (ACR): 2020 Guidelines for the prevention, diagnosis and treatment of Lyme disease. *Clin Infect Dis*. Published online November 30, 2020. Doi: **https://doi.org/10.1093/cid/ciaa1215.** The full guideline is available at: **www.idsociety.org/practice-guideline/lyme-disease/**

Table 3.29. Recommended Treatment of Lyme Disease in Children

Disease Category	Drug(s) and Dose
Erythema migrans (single or multiple) (any age)	Doxycycline, 4.4 mg/kg per day, orally, divided into 2 doses (maximum 200 mg/day) for 10 days **OR** Amoxicillin, 50 mg/kg per day, orally, divided into 3 doses (maximum 1.5 g/day) for 14 days **OR** Cefuroxime, 30 mg/kg per day, orally, in 2 divided doses (maximum 1 g/day) for 14 days **OR,** for a patient unable to take a beta-lactam or doxycycline, Azithromycin, 10 mg/kg/day, orally, once daily for 7 days
Isolated facial palsy	Doxycycline, 4.4 mg/kg per day, orally, divided into 2 doses (maximum 200 mg/day), for 14 days[a]
Arthritis	An oral agent as for early localized disease, for 28 days[b]
Persistent arthritis after first course of therapy	Retreat using an oral agent as for first-episode arthritis for 28 days[b] **OR** Ceftriaxone sodium, 50–75 mg/kg, IV, once a day (maximum 2 g/day) for 14–28 days
Atrioventricular heart block or carditis	An oral agent as for early localized disease, for 14 days (range 14–21 days) **OR** Ceftriaxone sodium, 50–75 mg/kg, IV, once a day (maximum 2 g/day) for 14 days (range 14–21 days for a hospitalized patient); oral therapy (using an agent as for early localized disease) can be substituted when the patient is stabilized or discharged, to complete the 14- to 21-day course
Meningitis	Doxycycline, 4.4 mg/kg per day, orally, divided into 1 or 2 doses (maximum 200 mg/day) for 14 days **OR** Ceftriaxone sodium, 50–75 mg/kg, IV, once a day (maximum 2 g/day) for 14 days

IV indicates intravenously.

[a] Corticosteroids should not be given. Use of amoxicillin for facial palsy in children has not been studied. Treatment has no effect on the resolution of facial nerve palsy; its purpose is to prevent late disease.

[b] There are limited safety data on the use of doxycycline for >21 days in children <8 years of age.

to minimize sun exposure (photosensitivity may be associated with doxycycline use), likelihood of coinfection with *Anaplasma phagocytophilum* or *Ehrlichia muris*-like agent (neither is sensitive to beta-lactam antimicrobial agents), and when *Staphylococcus aureus* cellulitis cannot be distinguished easily from erythema migrans (doxycycline is effective against most strains of methicillin-sensitive and methicillin-resistant *S aureus*). Erythema migrans should be treated orally for 10 days if doxycycline is used and for 14 days if amoxicillin or cefuroxime is used. Because STARI may be indistinguishable from early Lyme disease and questions remain about appropriate treatment, some physicians treat STARI with the same antimicrobial agents orally as for Lyme disease.

Treatment of erythema migrans results in resolution of the skin lesion within several days of initiating therapy and almost always prevents development of later stages of Lyme disease.

Early Disseminated Disease. Oral antimicrobial agents are appropriate and effective for most manifestations of disseminated Lyme disease. Doxycycline is preferred therapy for facial nerve palsy caused by *B burgdorferi* in children of any age. The purpose of therapy for cranial nerve palsies is to reduce the risk of late disease; treatment has no effect on resolution of the facial palsy. Amoxicillin has not been studied sufficiently for treatment of facial nerve palsies in young children to make a recommendation. Amoxicillin is unlikely to reach therapeutic levels in the central nervous system.

A growing body of evidence suggests that oral doxycycline is effective for treatment of Lyme meningitis and may be used as an alternative to hospitalization and parenteral ceftriaxone therapy in children well enough to be treated as outpatients. Lumbar puncture is indicated for a child with a stiff neck and other symptoms of meningitis in whom the possibility of a bacterial (nonspirochetal) meningitis cannot be ruled out. Neurologic disease is treated for 14 days.

Late Disseminated Disease. Children with Lyme arthritis are treated with oral antimicrobial agents for 28 days. Because of this duration, patients younger than 8 years should be treated with an oral agent other than doxycycline (eg, amoxicillin; see Table 3.29, footnote b). For patients 8 years and older, any of the oral options, including doxycycline, may be used (see Tetracyclines, p 866).

Management of patients with Lyme arthritis who have a partial response to therapy is uncertain. Consideration should be given to medication adherence, duration of symptoms before treatment, extent of synovial proliferation compared to joint swelling, cost, and patient preference. A second 28-day course of oral therapy is reasonable when synovial proliferation is modest compared with joint swelling or when the patient prefers a trial of oral therapy before considering intravenous treatment. Patients who demonstrate no or minimal response or who experience worsening of their arthritis can be treated with ceftriaxone parenterally for 14 to 28 days.

Approximately 10% to 15% of patients treated for Lyme arthritis will develop persistent synovitis that can last for months to years. Theories of pathophysiology include delayed resolution of inflammation because of slow clearance of nonviable bacteria following treatment versus an autoimmune mechanism. Misdiagnosis also should be considered (ie, Lyme antibodies in serum present from a previous infection or cross-reacting because of another disorder). Persisting synovitis following Lyme disease, termed "antibiotic-refractory Lyme arthritis," is a strongly HLA-associated phenomenon. Patients with persistent synovitis despite repeat treatment initially should be managed with nonsteroidal anti-inflammatory drugs. More severe cases should be referred to a rheumatologist who may treat the inflammation with an intra-articular steroid injection. Methotrexate has been used successfully in some cases. Arthroscopic synovectomy is required rarely for disabling or refractory cases.

Persistent Post-treatment Symptoms. Some patients have prolonged, persistent symptoms following standard treatment for Lyme disease. It is not clear whether this phenomenon is unique to Lyme disease or whether it is a more general occurrence during convalescence from other systemic illnesses. Persistent, treatment-refractory infection with *B burgdorferi* ("chronic Lyme disease") has not been substantiated scientifically. Patients with persistent symptoms following Lyme disease usually respond to symptomatic treatment and recover gradually.

Several double-blinded, randomized, placebo-controlled trials have found that retreatment with additional antimicrobial agents for patients with residual post-treatment Lyme disease subjective symptoms may be associated with harm and does not offer benefit.[1,2,3,4] Administration of additional antimicrobial agents to a patient with post-treatment Lyme disease symptoms following standard treatment for Lyme disease is strongly discouraged.

Retreatment is appropriate for subsequent acute infections caused by *B burgdorferi*.

Pregnancy. Tetracyclines are contraindicated in pregnancy. Doxycycline has not been studied adequately during pregnancy to make a recommendation regarding its use. Otherwise, therapy is the same as recommended for nonpregnant people.

ISOLATION OF THE HOSPITALIZED PATIENT: Standard precautions are recommended.

CONTROL MEASURES: Lyme disease is a nationally notifiable disease in the United States.

Ticks. See Prevention of Mosquitoborne and Tickborne Infections (p 175).

Chemoprophylaxis. In areas of high endemicity (the coastal northeast), where 30% to 50% of *I scapularis* ticks harbor *B burgdorferi*, the overall risk of Lyme disease following a recognized tick bite is no higher than 3%. After a high-risk deer tick bite, defined as an engorged tick that has fed for >72 hours, the risk of infection may be 25% in an area with hyperendemic disease. The risk is extremely low after brief attachment, defined as <36 hours (eg, a flat, nonengorged deer tick is found). Testing of the tick for spirochete infection has a poor predictive value and is not recommended.

Studies of doxycycline prophylaxis have been conducted in adults and older children (≥12 years). In areas of high risk, a single prophylactic 200-mg dose (or 4.4 mg/kg for children weighing less than 45 kg) of doxycycline can be used in children of any age to reduce risk of acquiring Lyme disease after the bite of an infected *I scapularis* tick. Benefits of prophylaxis may outweigh risks when the tick is engorged (ie, has been attached for at least 36 hours based on exposure history) and prophylaxis can be started within 72 hours of tick removal. Amoxicillin prophylaxis has not been studied sufficiently, but likely would require a longer course than doxycycline because of its shorter half-life and is not recommended. There are no clinical data to support antibiotic prophylaxis for anaplasmosis, ehrlichiosis, babesiosis or Rocky Mountain spotted fever.

Blood Donation. No documented cases of *B burgdorferi* transmission have occurred to date as a result of spirochete transmission via blood transfusion, but because spirochetemia occurs in early Lyme disease, patients with active disease should not donate blood. Patients who have been treated for Lyme disease can be considered for blood donation.

Vaccines. A Lyme disease vaccine was licensed by the FDA in 1998 for people 15 to 70 years of age but was withdrawn in 2002, principally because of poor sales and unsubstantiated public concerns about adverse effects. A phase I/II trial of a new vaccine performed in Europe found the vaccine to be immunogenic and without safety concerns.

[1]Feder HM, Johnson BJ, O'Connell S, et al; Ad Hoc International Lyme Disease Group. A critical appraisal of "chronic Lyme disease." *N Engl J Med.* 2007;357(14):1422–1430

[2]Lantos PM, Rumbaugh J, Bockenstedt LK, et al. Clinical practice guidelines by the Infectious Diseases Society of America (IDSA), American Academy of Neurology (AAN), and American College of Rheumatology (ACR): 2020 Guidelines for the prevention, diagnosis and treatment of Lyme disease. *Clin Infect Dis.* Published online November 30, 2020. Doi: **https://doi.org/10.1093/cid/ciaa1215.** The full guideline is available at: **www.idsociety.org/practice-guideline/lyme-disease/**

[3]Berende A, ter Hofstede HJ, Vos FJ, et al. Randomized trial of longer-term therapy for symptoms attributed to Lyme disease. *N Engl J Med.* 2016;374(13):1209–1220

[4]Marzec NS, Nelson C, Waldron PR, et al. Serious bacterial infections acquired during treatment of patients given a diagnosis of chronic Lyme disease—United States. *MMWR Morb Mortal Wkly Rep.* 2017;66(23):607–609

Lymphatic Filariasis
(Bancroftian, Malayan, and Timorian)

CLINICAL MANIFESTATIONS: Lymphatic filariasis (LF) is caused by infection with the filarial parasites *Wuchereria bancrofti, Brugia malayi*, or *Brugia timori*. Adult worms cause lymphatic dilatation and dysfunction, which result in abnormal lymph flow and eventually may lead to lymphedema in the legs, scrotal area (for *W bancrofti* only), and arms. Recurrent secondary bacterial infections hasten progression of lymphedema to the more severe form known as elephantiasis. Although the infection occurs commonly in young children living in areas with endemic LF, chronic manifestations of infection, such as hydrocele and lymphedema, occur infrequently in people younger than 20 years. Most filarial infections remain clinically asymptomatic, but even then, they commonly cause subclinical lymphatic dilatation and dysfunction. Lymphadenopathy, most frequently of the inguinal, crural, and axillary lymph nodes, is the most common clinical sign of lymphatic filariasis in children. There can be an acute inflammatory response that progresses from the lymph node distally (retrograde) along the affected lymphatic vessel, usually in the limbs. Accompanying systemic symptoms, such as headache or fever, generally are mild. In postpubertal males, adult *W bancrofti* organisms are found most commonly in the intrascrotal lymphatic vessels; thus, inflammation around dead or dying adult worms may present as funiculitis (inflammation of the spermatic cord), epididymitis, or orchitis. A tender granulomatous nodule may be palpable at the site of dying or dead adult worms. Chyluria can occur as a manifestation of bancroftian filariasis. Tropical pulmonary eosinophilia, characterized by cough, fever, wheezing, marked eosinophilia, and high serum immunoglobulin (Ig) E concentrations, is a rare manifestation of lymphatic filariasis.

ETIOLOGY: Filariasis is caused by 3 filarial nematodes in the family *Filaridae*: *W bancrofti, B malayi*, and *B timori*.

EPIDEMIOLOGY: The parasite is transmitted by the bite of infected mosquitoes of various genera, including *Culex, Aedes, Anopheles*, and *Mansonia. W bancrofti*, the most prevalent cause of lymphatic filariasis, is found in Haiti, the Dominican Republic, Guyana, northeast Brazil, sub-Saharan and North Africa, and Asia, extending from India through the Indonesian archipelago to the western Pacific islands. Humans are the only definitive host for the parasite. *B malayi* is found mostly in Southeast Asia and parts of India. *B timori* is restricted to certain islands at the eastern end of the Indonesian archipelago. Live adult worms release microfilariae into the bloodstream. Adult worms live for an average of 5 to 8 years, and reinfection is common. Microfilariae that can infect mosquitoes may be present in a patient's blood for decades, although individual microfilariae have a lifespan between 3 and 12 months. The adult worm is not transmissible from person to person or by blood transfusion; microfilariae can be transmitted by transfusion, but they do not develop into adult worms.

The **incubation period** is not well established; the period from acquisition to the appearance of microfilariae in blood can be 3 to 12 months, depending on the species of parasite.

DIAGNOSTIC TESTS: Diagnosis requires epidemiologic risk and consistent laboratory findings (identification of microfilariae or antibody). Microfilariae generally can be detected microscopically on blood smears obtained at night (10 pm–4 am), although variations in the periodicity of microfilaremia have been described depending on the parasite strain and the geographic location. Adult worms or microfilariae can be identified based on general morphology, size, and presence or absence of a sheath in Giemsa-stained fluid or tissue specimens obtained at biopsy. Serologic enzyme immunoassays are available, but interpretation of results is affected by cross-reactions of filarial antibodies with antibodies against other helminths. Determination of serum antifilarial IgG and IgG4 is available through the Laboratory of Parasitic Diseases at the National Institutes of Health (301-496-5398) or for antifilarial IgG4 through the Centers for Disease Control and Prevention (CDC [**www.dpd.cdc.gov/dpdx;** 404-718-4745; **parasites@cdc.gov**]). Assays for circulating filarial antigen of *W bancrofti* are available commercially but are not cleared for use by the US Food and Drug Administration (FDA), nor are they available in the United States. Polymerase chain reaction assays can detect parasite-specific DNA in fluids and tissues with high sensitivity and specificity, but none are FDA cleared. Ultrasonography can be used to visualize adult worms. Patients with lymphedema may no longer have microfilariae or antifilarial antibody present.

TREATMENT: The main goal of treatment of an infected person is to kill the adult worm. Diethylcarbamazine citrate (DEC), which is both microfilaricidal and active against the adult worm, is the drug of choice for lymphatic filariasis (see Drugs for Parasitic Infections, p 967). DEC is no longer sold in the United States but can be obtained from the CDC (404-718-4745; **parasites@cdc.gov;** or **www.cdc.gov/parasites/lymphaticfilariasis**). DEC is contraindicated in patients who may also have onchocerciasis or loiasis because of the possibility of exacerbation of skin or eye involvement or severe adverse effects. Treatment with DEC should be undertaken by a specialist with experience in treating lymphatic filariasis, because DEC therapy has been associated with life-threatening adverse events, including encephalopathy and renal failure in people with circulating *Loa loa* microfilariae concentrations >8000/mm^3. Ivermectin is effective against the microfilariae of *W bancrofti* and the 2 *Brugia* species but has no effect on the adult parasite. The safety of ivermectin in children weighing less than 15 kg and in pregnant women has not been established. Albendazole also has demonstrated macrofilaricidal activity. Studies in children as young as 1 year of age suggest that albendazole can be administered safely to this population. Two- or 3-drug combination therapies have been used in the Global Program for Elimination of Lymphatic Filariasis. Doxycycline, a drug that targets *Wolbachia* species, an intracellular rickettsial-like bacterial endosymbiont in adult worms, has been shown to be macrofilaricidal and has been used in combination with DEC.

Antifilarial chemotherapy has been shown to have limited efficacy for reversing or stabilizing lymphedema in its early forms. Doxycycline, in limited studies, has been shown to decrease the severity of lymphedema. Complex decongestive physiotherapy can be effective for treating lymphedema and requires strict attention to hygiene in the affected anatomical areas. Prompt identification and treatment of bacterial superinfections, particularly streptococcal and staphylococcal infections, and careful treatment of intertriginous and ungual fungal infections are important aspects of therapy for lymphedema. Surgery may be indicated for management of hydrocele. Chyluria originating in the bladder responds to fulguration; chyluria originating in the kidney is difficult to correct.

ISOLATION OF THE HOSPITALIZED PATIENT: Standard precautions are recommended.

CONTROL MEASURES: Annual mass drug administration of DEC and albendazole; albendazole and ivermectin; or ivermectin, DEC, and albendazole, to decrease or possibly eliminate transmission, has been instituted in selected settings. The use of insecticide-treated bed nets also has been shown to decrease transmission. No vaccine is available for lymphatic filariasis.

Lymphocytic Choriomeningitis Virus

CLINICAL MANIFESTATIONS: Child and adult infections with lymphocytic choriomeningitis virus (LCMV) are asymptomatic in approximately one third of cases. Symptomatic infection may result in a mild to severe illness, which can include fever, malaise, myalgia, retro-orbital headache, photophobia, anorexia, and nausea and vomiting. Sore throat, cough, arthralgia or arthritis, and orchitis also may occur. Initial symptoms may last from a few days to 3 weeks. Leukopenia, lymphopenia, thrombocytopenia, and elevation of lactate dehydrogenase and aspartate aminotransferase occur frequently. A biphasic febrile course is common; after a few days without symptoms, the second phase may occur in up to half of symptomatic patients, consisting of neurologic manifestations that vary from aseptic meningitis to severe encephalitis. Transverse myelitis, eighth nerve deafness, Guillain-Barré syndrome, and hydrocephalus also have been reported, but a causal link remains to be established. Extraneural disease has included reports of myocarditis and dermatitis. Rarely, LCMV has caused a disease resembling viral hemorrhagic syndrome. Transmission of LCMV through organ transplantation and infection in other immunocompromised populations can result in fatal disseminated infection with multiple organ failure.

Current prevalence and seasonality are not known, because diagnostic testing is not often performed. Recovery without sequelae is the usual outcome, but convalescence may take several weeks, with asthenia, poor cognitive function, headaches, and arthralgia. LCMV infection should be suspected in presence of: (1) aseptic meningitis or encephalitis, especially during periods of colder weather; (2) febrile illness, followed by brief remission, followed by onset of neurologic illness; and (3) cerebrospinal fluid (CSF) findings of lymphocytosis and hypoglycorrhachia.

Infection during pregnancy has been associated with spontaneous abortion. Congenital infection may cause severe abnormalities, including hydrocephalus, chorioretinitis, intracranial calcifications, microcephaly, and mental retardation. Congenital LCMV infection should be included in the differential diagnosis whenever intrauterine infections with toxoplasma, rubella, cytomegalovirus, herpes simplex virus, enterovirus, parechovirus, Zika virus, *Treponema pallidum*, or parvovirus B19 are being considered.

ETIOLOGY: LCMV is a single-stranded RNA virus that belongs to the family *Arenaviridae* (so named because of its appearance on electron microscopy, which resembles grains of sand). Other members of this family included in the genus *Mammarenaviruses* are Lassa virus and the New World *Arenaviruses* Junin, Machupo, Guanarito, Sabiá, and Chapare.

EPIDEMIOLOGY: LCMV is a chronic infection of common house mice, which often are infected asymptomatically and chronically shed virus in urine and other excretions. Congenital murine infection is common and results in a normal-appearing litter with chronic viremia and particularly high virus excretion. In addition, hamsters, laboratory mice, and guinea pigs can have chronic infection and can be sources of human infection. Humans are infected mostly by inhalation of aerosol generated by rodents shedding virus from the urine, feces, blood, or nasopharyngeal secretions. Other less likely routes of entry of infected secretions include conjunctival and other mucous membranes, ingestion, and cuts in the skin. The disease is observed more frequently in young adults. Human-to-human transmission has occurred during pregnancy from infected mothers to their fetus and through solid organ transplantation from an infected organ donor. Several such clusters of cases have been described following transplantation, and one case was traced to a pet hamster purchased by the donor. Laboratory-acquired LCMV infections have occurred, both through infected laboratory animals and contaminated tissue-culture stocks.

The **incubation period** usually is 6 to 13 days and occasionally is as long as 3 weeks.

DIAGNOSTIC TESTS: Patients with central nervous system disease have a mononuclear pleocytosis with 30 to 8000 cells in CSF. Hypoglycorrhachia, as well as mild increase in protein, may occur. LCMV usually can be isolated from CSF obtained during the acute phase of illness and, in severe disseminated infections, also from blood, urine, and nasopharyngeal secretion specimens. Reverse transcriptase-polymerase chain reaction assays available through reference or commercial laboratories can be used on serum during the acute stage and on CSF during the neurologic phase; however, none of these assays are cleared by the US Food and Drug Administration (FDA). Serum specimens from the acute and convalescent phases of illness can be tested for increases in antibody titers by enzyme immunoassays and neutralization tests. Demonstration of virus-specific immunoglobulin M antibodies in serum or CSF specimens is useful. In congenital infections, diagnosis usually is suspected when ocular or neurologic signs develop, and diagnosis usually is made by serologic testing. In immunosuppressed patients, seroconversion can take several weeks. Diagnosis can also be made by immunohistochemical assay of fixed tissues.

TREATMENT: Management is supportive. Limited data suggest a possible role for ribavirin in immunosuppressed patients infected with LCMV. However, ribavirin is not FDA approved for treatment of LCMV.

ISOLATION OF THE HOSPITALIZED PATIENT: Standard precautions are recommended.

CONTROL MEASURES: Infection can be controlled by preventing rodent infestation in animal and food storage areas. Because the virus is excreted for long periods of time by rodent hosts, attempts should be made to monitor laboratory and commercial colonies of mice and hamsters for infection. Pet rodents or wild mice in a patient's home should be considered likely sources of infection. Guidelines for minimizing risk of human LCMV infection associated with rodents are available[1] (also see Diseases Transmitted by Animals [Zoonoses], p 1048). Although the risk of LCMV infection from pet rodents is low, pregnant women should avoid exposure to wild or pet rodents and their aerosolized excreta. Pregnant women also should avoid working in the laboratory with LCMV.

Malaria

CLINICAL MANIFESTATIONS: The classic symptoms of malaria, which may be paroxysmal, are high fever with chills, rigor, sweats, and headache. Other manifestations can include nausea, vomiting, diarrhea, cough, tachypnea, arthralgia, myalgia, and abdominal and back pain. Anemia and thrombocytopenia are common. Hepatosplenomegaly frequently is present in infected children in areas with endemic malaria and may be present in adults and in people previously not infected with malaria. Severe disease

---

[1]Centers for Disease Control and Prevention. Update: interim guidance for minimizing risk for human lymphocytic choriomeningitis virus infection associated with pet rodents. *MMWR Morb Mortal Wkly Rep.* 2005;54(32):799–801

occurs more frequently in people without immunity acquired as a result of previous infection; young children; pregnant women, especially primigravidae; or in those who are immunocompromised.

Infection with *Plasmodium falciparum*, one of the 5 *Plasmodium* species that naturally infect humans, potentially is fatal and most commonly manifests as a nonspecific febrile illness often without localizing signs. Severe disease (which may occur with any of the infecting species but is most commonly caused by *P falciparum*) may manifest as one of the following clinical syndromes, all of which are medical emergencies and may be fatal unless treated:

- **Cerebral malaria,** characterized by altered mental status and manifesting with a range of neurologic signs and symptoms, including generalized seizures, signs of increased intracranial pressure (confusion and progression to stupor or coma), and death;
- **Severe anemia** attributable to dyserythropoiesis, high parasitemia and hemolysis, sequestration of infected erythrocytes to capillaries, coagulopathy, and hemolysis of infected erythrocytes associated with hypersplenism; late onset hemolytic anemia has been described following treatment of severe disease with artemisinin derivatives;
- **Hypoglycemia,** which can present with metabolic acidosis and hypotension associated with hyperparasitemia; it also can be a consequence of quinine or quinidine-induced hyperinsulinemia;
- **Renal failure** caused by acute tubular necrosis (rare in children younger than 8 years);
- **Respiratory failure,** without pulmonary edema;
- **Abnormal bleeding**, which can include hemoglobinuria and is attributable to thrombocytopenia, an exaggerated hemolytic response, or disseminated coagulopathy;
- **Jaundice**, secondary to hemolysis of infected blood cells, coagulopathy, and/or hepatic dysfunction;
- **Metabolic acidosis,** usually attributed to lactic acidosis, hypovolemia, liver dysfunction, and impaired renal function; or
- **Vascular collapse and shock** associated with hypothermia and adrenal insufficiency.

Syndromes primarily associated with *Plasmodium vivax* and *Plasmodium ovale* infection are as follows:

- **Anemia** attributable to acute parasitemia;
- **Hypersplenism** with danger of splenic rupture;
- **Thrombocytopenia** which may be severe with P vivax;
- **Relapse of infection,** for as long as 3 to 5 years after the primary infection, attributable to latent hepatic stages (hypnozoites); and
- **Severe, and even fatal, infection** with *P vivax*.

Syndromes associated with *Plasmodium malariae* infection include:

- **Chronic asymptomatic parasitemia**, which persists at undetectable levels for as long as decades after the primary infection; and
- **Nephrotic syndrome** resulting from deposition of immune complexes in the kidney.

Plasmodium knowlesi is a nonhuman primate malaria parasite that also can infect humans and has been misdiagnosed as *P malariae*, which causes more benign infection. Disease can be characterized by very rapid replication of the parasite and hyperparasitemia resulting in severe disease. *P knowlesi* infection should be treated aggressively, because hepatorenal failure and subsequent death have been documented.

Congenital malaria resulting from perinatal transmission occurs infrequently, with increased risk among primigravidae in areas with endemic infection. Most congenital cases have been caused by *P vivax* and *P falciparum; P malariae* and *P ovale* account for fewer than 20% of such cases. Manifestations can resemble those of neonatal sepsis, including fever and nonspecific symptoms of poor appetite, irritability, and lethargy.

ETIOLOGY: The genus *Plasmodium* includes species of intraerythrocytic parasites that infect a wide range of mammals, birds, and reptiles. The 5 species that infect humans are *P falciparum, P vivax, P ovale, P malariae,* and *P knowlesi*. Coinfection with multiple species has been documented.

EPIDEMIOLOGY: Malaria is endemic throughout the tropical areas of the world and is acquired primarily from the bite of the female *Anopheles* genus of mosquito. Half of the world's population lives in areas where transmission occurs. Worldwide, 219 million cases and 435 000 deaths were reported in 2017. Approximately 10% of these are cases of severe malaria, which have a significantly higher chance of death. Most deaths occur in children younger than 5 years. Infection by the malaria parasite poses substantial risks to pregnant women and their fetuses, especially primigravid women in areas with endemic infection, and may result in spontaneous abortion and stillbirth. Malaria also contributes to low birth weight in countries where *P falciparum* or *P vivax* is endemic.

Risk of malaria is highest, but variable, for travelers to sub-Saharan Africa, Papua New Guinea, the Solomon Islands, and Vanuatu; risk is intermediate on the Indian subcontinent and is low in most of Southeast Asia and Latin America. Potential for malaria reintroduction exists in areas where malaria has been eliminated. Climate change may also affect the geographic range of malaria. Health care professionals can check the Centers for Disease Control and Prevention (CDC) website for the most current information (**www.cdc.gov/malaria**) to determine malaria endemicity when providing pretravel malaria advice or evaluating a febrile returned traveler. Transmission is possible in more temperate climates, including areas of the United States where *Anopheles* mosquitoes are present.

Nearly all of the approximately 2078 annual reported cases in the United States in 2016 resulted from infection acquired outside the United States.[1] Uncommon modes of malaria transmission are congenital, through transfusions, or through the use of contaminated needles or syringes.

P vivax and *P falciparum* are the most prevalent species worldwide. *P vivax* malaria is prevalent on the Indian subcontinent and in Central America. *P falciparum* malaria is prevalent in Africa, Papua New Guinea, and on the island of Hispaniola (Haiti and the Dominican Republic). *P vivax* and *P falciparum* species are the most common malaria species in southern and Southeast Asia, Oceania, and South America. *P malariae,* although much less common, has a wide distribution. *P ovale* malaria occurs most frequently in West Africa but has been reported in other areas. Reported cases of human infections with *P knowlesi* have been from certain countries of Southeast Asia, specifically Borneo, Malaysia, Philippines, Thailand, Myanmar, Singapore, and Cambodia.

Relapses may occur in *P vivax* and *P ovale* infections because of a persistent hepatic (hypnozoite) stage of infection. Recrudescence of *P falciparum* and *P malariae* infection occurs when a persistent low-density parasitemia produces recurrence of symptoms of the disease, such as when incomplete treatment or drug resistance prevents elimination of the parasite. Asymptomatic parasitemia can occur in individuals with partial immunity.

Drug resistance in both *P falciparum* and *P vivax* has been evolving throughout areas with endemic malaria, generally proportional to the use of particular drugs in a

---

[1]Centers for Disease Control and Prevention. Malaria surveillance—United States, 2016. *MMWR Surveill Summ.* 2019;68(5):1-35

population. The spread of chloroquine-resistant *P falciparum* strains throughout the world dates back to the 1960s. Chloroquine-resistant *P vivax* has been reported in Indonesia, Papua New Guinea, the Solomon Islands, Myanmar, India, and Guyana. *P falciparum* resistance to sulfadoxine-pyrimethamine is distributed throughout Africa and other endemic regions as well. Mefloquine resistance has been documented in Myanmar (Burma), Lao People's Democratic Republic (Laos), Thailand, Cambodia, and Vietnam. Resistance to artemisinin compounds has been reported across the same region.

The **incubation period** (time to onset of malaria symptoms) in most cases ranges from as soon as 7 days after being bitten by an infected mosquito to about 30 days and is shortest for *P falciparum* and longest for *P malariae*. Antimalarial drugs discontinued before completing the recommended course of prophylaxis for *P falciparum* may delay symptoms for weeks to months; relapses of *P vivax* and *P ovale* may occur months after initial infection.

DIAGNOSTIC TESTS: Definitive parasitologic diagnosis historically has been based on identification of *Plasmodium* parasites microscopically on stained blood films. There is an increasing range of rapid diagnostic test methods available that detect specific malaria antigens in blood, one of which is approved by the US Food and Drug Administration (FDA) and is available for use by many hospitals and commercial laboratories. Rapid diagnostic testing is recommended to be conducted in parallel with routine microscopy to provide further information needed for patient treatment, such as the percentage of erythrocytes harboring parasites. Both positive and negative rapid diagnostic test results should be confirmed by microscopic examination, because low-level parasitemia may not be detected (ie, false-negative result), false-positive results occur, and mixed infections may not be detected accurately. Both thick and thin blood films should be examined. The thick film allows for concentration of the blood to find parasites that may be present at low density, whereas the thin film is most useful for species identification and determination of the density of red blood cells infected with parasites. If initial blood smears test negative for *Plasmodium* species but malaria remains a possibility, the smear should be repeated every 12 to 24 hours during a 72-hour period, ideally with at least 3 smears.

Confirmation and identification of the species of malaria parasites on the blood smear is essential in guiding therapy. Serologic testing generally is not helpful, except in epidemiologic surveys. Polymerase chain reaction (PCR) assay is available in reference laboratories and many state health departments, but same-day results may not be available to make treatment decisions. PCR is most useful to confirm species of malaria. Information about sensitivity of rapid diagnostic tests for the 3 less common species of malaria, *P ovale*, *P malariae*, and *P knowlesi*, is limited. Additional information about rapid diagnostic testing for malaria is available on the CDC website. Species confirmation and antimalarial drug resistance testing is available free of charge at the CDC for all cases of malaria diagnosed in the United States (**www.cdc.gov/malaria/diagnosis_treatment/index.html**).

TREATMENT: Choice of malaria treatment is based on the infecting species, possible drug resistance, and severity of disease. Selection of appropriate therapy is presented in Drugs for Parasitic Infections beginning on p 968. Severe malaria (largely a consideration for *P falciparum* infections) is defined as any one or more of the following: parasitemia greater than 5% of red blood cells infected, signs of central nervous system or other end-organ involvement, severe anemia requiring transfusion, shock, acidosis, abnormal bleeding, and/or hypoglycemia. Patients with severe malaria require intensive care and parenteral treatment with intravenous artesunate. Intravenous quinidine is no longer available in the United States. Sequential blood smears to determine percentage of erythrocytes infected with parasites may be monitored to assess therapeutic efficacy. A recent review of available literature suggests exchange transfusion for severe disease is not efficacious in patients with end-organ involvement.

For patients with severe malaria in the United States or patients with malaria who are unable to tolerate an oral medication despite attempts, intravenous artesunate is the treatment of choice. If commercially available intravenous artesunate is not available within 24 hours, intravenous artesunate is available through a CDC investigational new drug (IND) protocol. When the distribution of intravenous artesunate expands nationwide and is stocked in the states where the most cases of malaria are found (before the end of 2021), the CDC will discontinue its distribution of intravenous artesunate. Clinicians may contact the CDC Malaria Hotline (770-488-7788, Monday–Friday, 9:00 am–5:00 pm Eastern Time; or 770-488-7100 at all other times) for additional information and release of the drug under the conditions of the protocol.[1] Assistance with management of malaria is available 24 hours a day through the CDC Emergency Operations Center (770-488-7100). Additional information on artesunate and guidelines for the treatment of malaria are available on the CDC website (**www.cdc.gov/malaria/diagnosis_treatment/artesunate.html** and **www.cdc.gov/malaria/resources/pdf/Malaria_Treatment_Table.pdf**).

ISOLATION OF THE HOSPITALIZED PATIENT: Standard precautions are recommended.

CONTROL MEASURES: Malaria is a nationally notifiable disease in the United States. There is no licensed vaccine against malaria in the United States. Effective measures to reduce risk of acquiring malaria include control of *Anopheles* mosquito populations, protection against mosquito bites, treatment of infected people, and chemoprophylaxis of travelers to areas with endemic infection (see Table 3.30). Measures to prevent contact with mosquitoes, especially from dusk to dawn (because of the nocturnal biting habits of most female *Anopheles* mosquitoes), include use of bed nets impregnated with insecticide, mosquito repellents (see Prevention of Mosquitoborne and Tickborne Infections, p 175), and protective clothing. The most current information on country-specific malaria transmission, drug resistance, and resulting recommendations for travelers can be obtained by contacting the CDC (**www.cdc.gov/malaria** or the Malaria Hotline at 770-488-7788). *Chemoprophylaxis for Travelers to Areas With Endemic Malaria.[2]* Drugs for prevention of malaria currently available in the United States include chloroquine, mefloquine, doxycycline, atovaquone-proguanil, primaquine, and tafenoquine. Table 3.30 details use of these drugs for prophylaxis against malaria.

The appropriate chemoprophylactic regimen is determined by the traveler's risk of acquiring malaria in the area(s) to be visited and by local prevalence of drug resistance. The travel itinerary should be reviewed in detail and compared with information on where malaria transmission occurs within a given country to determine whether the traveler will be traveling in a part of the country where malaria occurs and if antimalarial

---

[1]Centers for Disease Control and Prevention. Notice to readers: new medication for severe malaria available under an investigational new drug protocol. *MMWR Morb Mortal Wkly Rep.* 2007;56(30):769–770

[2]For further information on prevention of malaria in travelers, see the biennial publication: *Health Information for International Travel.* (Centers for Disease Control and Prevention. CDC Yellow Book 2020: Health Information for International Travel. New York: Oxford University Press; 2020. Available at: **wwwnc.cdc.gov/travel/page/yellowbook-home**

Table 3.30. Drugs to Consider for Use in Children for Malaria Prophylaxis[a]

Locale	Drug	Dosing	Timing	Adverse Effects and Contraindications	Other Considerations
Only chloroquine-sensitive areas	Chloroquine or hydroxychloroquine	Chloroquine dose: 5 mg/kg base (8.3 mg/kg salt), orally, once weekly, up to maximum adult dose 300 mg base Hydroxychloroquine dose: 5 mg/kg base (6.5 mg/kg salt), orally, once weekly, up to maximum 310 mg base	Begin 1–2 weeks before travel and take weekly throughout and for 4 weeks after leaving area	Most common adverse effects: gastrointestinal tract disturbance, headache, dizziness, blurred vision, pruritus, insomnia Can exacerbate psoriasis	Take with meals
Only mefloquine-sensitive areas	Mefloquine	≤9 kg: 4.6 mg/kg base (5 mg/kg salt), once weekly >9–19 kg: 1/4 tablet, once weekly >19–30 kg: 1/2 tablet, once weekly >30–45 kg: 3/4 tablet, once weekly >45 kg: 1 tablet, once weekly Each tablet contains 228 mg base (250 mg salt)	Begin ≥2 wk before travel, then weekly on same day each wk throughout and for 4 wk after leaving area Initiating 2–3 wk before travel can help assess tolerability	Most common adverse effects: gastrointestinal tract disturbance, headache, insomnia, vivid dreams, visual disturbance, anxiety, dizziness CONTRAINDICATED in travelers with a known hypersensitivity to the drug, and in those with active or recent history depression, anxiety disorder, psychosis, schizophrenia, other major psychiatric disorder or seizures Do not use in those with cardiac conduction defects	Black box warning for neurologic (dizziness, vestibular problems, tinnitus) and psychiatric (anxiety, paranoia, depression, hallucinations) side effects that may occur at any time during drug use, and may last for months to years after the drug is stopped. Patients must be given copy of FDA medication guide May be given in all trimesters of pregnancy

Table 3.30. Drugs to Consider for Use in Children for Malaria Prophylaxis,[a] continued

Locale	Drug	Dosing	Timing	Adverse Effects and Contraindications	Other Considerations
All areas	Atovaquone-proguanil	Pediatric tablets, 62.5 mg atovaquone and 25 mg proguanil hydrochloride 5–8 kg: ½ tab >8–10 kg: ¾ tab >10–20 kg: 1 tab >20–30 kg: 2 tabs >30–40 kg: 3 tabs >40 kg: 1 adult tab (250 mg atovaquone/100 mg proguanil)	Start 1–2 days before travel, take daily throughout travel and for 7 days after leaving area	Most common adverse effects: abdominal pain, nausea, vomiting, headache Do not use in those with creatinine clearance <30 mL/min; not recommended for infants <5 kg, pregnant women, or women who are breastfeeding infants <5 kg	Take with meals Generally well tolerated Proguanil can increase warfarin effect; dosage adjustment may be needed

Table 3.30. Drugs to Consider for Use in Children for Malaria Prophylaxis,[a] continued

Locale	Drug	Dosing	Timing	Adverse Effects and Contraindications	Other Considerations
All areas	Doxycycline	2.2 mg/kg, up to maximum adult dose 100 mg/day	Start 1–2 days before travel, take daily throughout travel, and for 4 wk after leaving area	Most common adverse effects: photosensitivity, gastrointestinal disturbance	Take with meals
				Not recommended for pregnant women, or for children <8 y since duration of prophylaxis exceeds 21 days	Also active against rickettsiae and leptospirae (hikers, campers, fresh water swimmers)
			Licensed for use for 4 mo but may be safely given up to 2 y		Complete oral typhoid vaccine >72 h before starting doxycycline
Short-duration travel (<6 months) to all areas	Primaquine	0.5 mg/kg base (0.8 mg/kg salt) up to adult dose of 30 mg base (52.6 mg salt) daily	Start 1–2 days before travel, take daily throughout travel, and for 7 days after leaving area	CONTRAINDICATED in those with G6PD deficiency and pregnant women	Test for G6PD deficiency before prescribing
				Should not be given to lactating woman unless infant has normal G6PD level	Also used for presumptive therapy (ie, terminal prophylaxis) to decrease risk of P vivax or P ovale relapse

Table 3.30. Drugs to Consider for Use in Children for Malaria Prophylaxis,[a] continued

Locale	Drug	Dosing	Timing	Adverse Effects and Contraindications	Other Considerations
Short-duration travel (<6 months) to all areas	Tafenoquine	Loading dose: 200 mg once daily for 3 days before departure Maintenance regimen (while in malaria transmission area): 200 mg weekly Post-trip dose: 200 mg once, 7 days after the last weekly dose	Start 3 days before travel, weekly during the trip, and a single dose during the week after returning.	CONTRAINDICATED in those with G6PD deficiency and pregnant women Should not be given to lactating woman unless infant has normal G6PD level	Test for G6PD deficiency using a quantitative test before prescribing Approved for 18 years of age and older for prophylaxis (and for antirelapse therapy in people aged ≥16 years) Also used for presumptive therapy (ie, terminal prophylaxis) to decrease risk of *P vivax* or *P ovale* relapse (different formulation and dosing schedule)

G6PD indicates glucose-6-phosphate dehydrogenase.

[a] No drug is 100% effective; always combine chemoprophylaxis with personal protection measures.

drug resistance has been reported in that location (see the chapter "Yellow Fever and Malaria Information, by Country" in the CDC *Yellow Book* **[wwwnc.cdc.gov/travel/ yellowbook/2020/preparing-international-travelers/yellow-fever-vaccine- and-malaria-prophylaxis-information-by-country]**). Additional factors to consider are the patient's other medical conditions (including pregnancy), medications being taken (to assess potential drug interactions), cost of the medicines, and potential adverse effects. Indications for prophylaxis for children are identical to those for adults. Pediatric dosages should be calculated on the basis of the child's current weight, and children's dosages should never exceed adult dosages. Drugs used for malaria chemoprophylaxis generally are well tolerated, although adverse reactions can occur. Minor adverse reactions do not require stopping or adjusting drug dosage. Those who provide malaria chemoprophylaxis should provide travelers with information about management of mild adverse events and what to do in the event of serious adverse reactions.

Medications for chemoprophylaxis of malaria should not be obtained at overseas locations, as quality of these products is unknown. Travelers also should avoid medications and combinations that are commonly prescribed abroad but not recommended in the United States. Chemoprophylaxis should begin before arrival in the area with endemic malaria.

Prophylaxis During Pregnancy and Lactation. Malaria during pregnancy carries significant risks for both the mother and fetus. Malaria may increase risk of adverse outcomes in pregnancy, including abortion, preterm birth, and stillbirth. For these reasons and because no chemoprophylactic regimen is absolutely effective, women who are pregnant or likely to become pregnant should try to avoid travel to areas where they could contract malaria.

Women traveling to areas where chloroquine-resistant malaria has not been reported may take chloroquine prophylaxis. Harmful effects on the fetus have not been demonstrated when chloroquine is given in recommended doses for malaria prophylaxis. Pregnancy and lactation, therefore, are not contraindications for malaria prophylaxis with chloroquine.

The CDC recommends mefloquine chemoprophylaxis in all trimesters of pregnancy when exposure to chloroquine-resistant *P falciparum* is unavoidable. Lactating mothers of infants may use mefloquine, or for infants weighing more than 5 kg, atovaquone-proguanil for prophylaxis when exposure to chloroquine-resistant *P falciparum* is unavoidable. Primaquine and tafenoquine are contraindicated in pregnancy because of the unknown glucose-6-phosphate dehydrogenase (G6PD) status of the fetus.

Assessment for Malaria While Traveling. Travelers to areas with endemic malaria should seek medical attention immediately if they develop fever. Malaria treatment is most effective if begun early in the course of disease, and delay of appropriate treatment can have serious or even fatal consequences.

Travelers taking atovaquone-proguanil as their chemoprophylactic drug regimen should not take atovaquone-proguanil for treatment if they develop malaria and should use an appropriate alternative antimalarial regimen.

Travelers should be advised that any fever or influenza-like illness that develops within 3 months of departure from an area with endemic malaria requires immediate medical evaluation, including appropriate blood testing to rule out malaria.

Prevention of Relapses. There is no test to determine the potential for relapses of *P vivax* or *P ovale* infection. Antirelapse therapy can be provided along with treatment of symptomatic infection or after leaving an endemic area following a prolonged stay. Presumptive antirelapse therapy, also known as terminal prophylaxis, uses a medication toward the end of the exposure period or immediately thereafter to prevent relapses or delayed onset clinical presentations of malaria caused by hypnozoites. Primaquine and tafenoquine (in patients 16 years and older) both are approved for use to prevent relapses of *P vivax*. Both can be used to prevent *P ovale* relapse, but tafenoquine is not approved by the FDA for this use. Screening for G6PD deficiency using a quantitative test must be performed before using primaquine and tafenoquine, because both drugs can cause hemolysis in patients with G6PD deficiency.

Personal Protective Measures. All travelers to areas where malaria is endemic should be advised to use personal protective measures, including the following: (1) insecticide-impregnated mosquito nets while sleeping; (2) remaining in well-screened, or air-conditioned areas at dusk and at night; (3) protective clothing, preferably permethrin treated; and (4) mosquito repellents. Most repellents require frequent reapplications to be effective (see Prevention of Mosquitoborne and Tickborne Infections, p 175).

Measles

CLINICAL MANIFESTATIONS: Measles is an acute viral disease characterized by fever, cough, coryza, and conjunctivitis, followed by a maculopapular rash beginning on the face and spreading cephalocaudally and centrifugally. During the prodromal period, a pathognomonic enanthema (Koplik spots) may be present. Complications of measles, including otitis media, bronchopneumonia, laryngotracheobronchitis (croup), and diarrhea, occur commonly in young children and immunocompromised hosts. Acute encephalitis, which often results in permanent brain damage, occurs in approximately 1 of every 1000 cases. In the postelimination era in the United States, death, predominantly resulting from respiratory and neurologic complications, has occurred in 1 to 3 of every 1000 cases reported. Case-fatality rates are increased in children younger than 5 years, pregnant women, and immunocompromised children, including children with leukemia, human immunodeficiency virus (HIV) infection, and severe malnutrition (including vitamin A deficiency). Sometimes the characteristic rash does not develop in immunocompromised patients.

Measles inclusion body encephalitis (MIBE) is a rare manifestation of measles infection in immunocompromised individuals usually presenting within 1 year of measles infection. Disease onset is subacute with progressive neurologic dysfunction occurring over weeks to months. Subacute sclerosing panencephalitis (SSPE) is a rare degenerative central nervous system disease characterized by behavioral and intellectual deterioration and seizures that occurs 7 to 11 years after wild-type measles virus infection, occurring at a rate of 4 to 11 per 100 000 measles cases. Rates of SSPE as high as approximately 1:1000 measles case have been seen in some recent studies, with the highest rates in children infected before 2 years of age.

Several recent studies have documented that children who have had measles have long-term blunted immune responses to other pathogens and increased mortality attributable to the known effects of measles virus on lymphocytes. This effect is another reason why measles prevention is so important.

ETIOLOGY: Measles virus is an enveloped RNA virus with 1 serotype, classified as a member of the genus *Morbillivirus* in the *Paramyxoviridae* family.

EPIDEMIOLOGY: The only natural host of measles virus is humans. Measles virus is transmitted by direct contact with infectious droplets or, less commonly, by airborne spread. Measles is one of the most highly communicable of all infectious diseases; the attack rate in a susceptible individual exposed to measles is 90% in close-contact settings. Population immunity as high as 95% or greater is often needed to stop ongoing transmission. In temperate areas, the peak incidence of infection usually occurs during late winter and spring. In the prevaccine era, most cases of measles in the United States occurred in preschool- and young school-aged children, and few people remained susceptible by 20 years of age. Following implementation of routine childhood vaccination in the United States at age 12 to 15 months, measles occurred more often in infants younger than 1 year and in older adolescents and adults who had not been adequately vaccinated. Infant susceptibility occurs around the time when transplacentally acquired maternal antibodies are no longer present. The childhood and adolescent immunization program in the United States began with licensure of the measles vaccine in 1963 and has resulted in a greater than 99% decrease in the reported incidence of measles, with interruption of endemic disease transmission being declared in 2000.

From 1989 to 1991, the incidence of measles in the United States increased because of low immunization rates in preschool-aged children, especially in urban areas, and because of primary vaccine failures after 1 measles vaccine dose. Following improved coverage in preschool-aged children and implementation of a routine second dose of measles, mumps, and rubella (MMR) vaccine for children, the incidence of measles declined to extremely low levels (<1 case per 1 million population). Unfortunately, increasing numbers of cases and outbreaks of measles have occurred over the last decade. The majority of these cases are linked to importation of measles from countries where it is endemic, including countries in Western Europe, and subsequent spread among unimmunized individuals, including intentionally unimmunized children.

Progress continues toward global control and regional measles elimination, with an 80% drop in measles deaths worldwide between 2000 and 2017. By the end of 2018, 89% of children globally had received 1 dose of measles vaccine by their second birthday. All World Health Organization (WHO) regions have established goals to eliminate measles by 2020, including the adoption of a second dose of a measles-containing vaccine for all children.

Inadequate response to vaccine (ie, primary vaccine failure) occurs in as many as 7% of people who received a single dose of vaccine at 12 months or older. Most cases of measles in previously immunized children seem to be attributable to primary vaccine failures, but waning immunity after immunization (ie, secondary vaccine failure) may be a factor in some cases. Primary vaccine failure was the main reason a 2-dose vaccine schedule was recommended routinely for children and high-risk adults.

Patients infected with wild-type measles virus are contagious from 4 days before the rash through 4 days after appearance of the rash. Immunocompromised patients who may have prolonged excretion of the virus in respiratory tract secretions can be contagious for the duration of the illness. Patients with SSPE are not contagious.

The **incubation period** generally is 8 to 12 days from exposure to onset of prodromal symptoms. In family studies, the average interval between appearance of rash in the index case and subsequent cases is 14 days, with a range of 7 to 21 days. In SSPE, the mean **incubation period** of 84 cases reported between 1976 and 1983 was 10.8 years.

DIAGNOSTIC TESTS: Measles virus infection can be confirmed by: (1) detection of measles viral RNA by reverse transcriptase-polymerase chain reaction (RT-PCR); (2) detection of measles virus-specific immunoglobulin (Ig) M; (3) a fourfold increase in measles IgG antibody concentration in paired acute and convalescent serum specimens (collected at least 10 days apart); or (4) isolation of measles virus in cell culture. Detection of IgM in serum samples by enzyme immunoassay has been the preferred method for case confirmation; however, as the incidence of disease decreases, the positive predictive value of IgM detection decreases. For this reason, detection of viral RNA in blood; throat, nasal, and posterior nasopharyngeal swab specimens; bronchial lavage samples; or urine samples (respiratory samples are preferred specimens, and sampling more than 1 site may increase sensitivity) is playing an increasing role in case confirmation. A serum sample as well as a throat swab specimen should be obtained from any patient in whom measles is suspected. Additionally, it is ideal to obtain a urine sample because sampling from all 3 sites will increase the likelihood of establishing a diagnosis. Many state public health laboratories and the Measles Laboratory at the Centers for Disease Control and Prevention (CDC) can perform RT-PCR assays to detect measles RNA. Isolation of measles virus in cell culture is not recommended for routine case confirmation because isolation can take up to 2 weeks to complete.

The sensitivity of measles IgM assays varies by timing of specimen collection, immunization status of the patient, and the assay method itself. Up to 20% of assays for IgM may have a false-negative result in the first 72 hours after rash onset. If the measles IgM result is negative and the patient has a generalized rash lasting more than 72 hours the measles IgM test should be repeated. Measles IgM is detectable for at least 1 month after rash onset in unimmunized people but might be absent or present only transiently in people immunized with 1 or 2 vaccine doses. Therefore, a negative IgM test result should not be used to rule out the diagnosis in immunized people.

Detection of viral RNA by RT-PCR provides a rapid and sensitive method for case confirmation. It is important to collect samples for RNA detection as soon as possible after rash onset, because viral shedding declines with time after rash. Specimen timing and quality greatly influence the results of RT-PCR testing, so a negative result should not be the only criterion used to rule out a case of measles. Another advantage of collecting samples for molecular detection of the virus is that these samples can also be used to genotype the virus, which is important to determine patterns of importation and transmission.

In populations with high vaccine coverage, such as those in the United States, comprehensive serologic and virologic testing generally is not available locally and requires submitting specimens to state public health laboratories or the CDC. Individuals with a febrile rash illness who are seronegative for measles IgM and have negative RT-PCR assay results for measles should be tested for rubella using the same specimens.

TREATMENT: No specific antiviral therapy is available. Measles virus is susceptible in vitro to ribavirin, which has been given by the intravenous and aerosol routes to treat severely affected and immunocompromised children with measles. However, no controlled trials have been conducted, and ribavirin is not licensed by the US Food and Drug Administration for treatment of measles.

Vitamin A. The WHO currently recommends vitamin A for all children with measles, regardless of their country of residence, and many US experts concur for all children regardless of hospitalization status with measles in the United States. Vitamin A treatment of children with measles in resource-limited countries has been associated with decreased morbidity and mortality rates. Low serum concentrations of vitamin A also have been found in children in the United States, and children with more severe measles illness may have lower vitamin A concentrations. There is no need to measure vitamin A concentrations, though, because the result should not change management. Vitamin A for treatment of measles is administered once daily for 2 days (ie, immediately on diagnosis and repeated the next day), at the following doses:

- 200 000 IU (60 000 μg retinol activity equivalent [RAE]) for children 12 months or older;
- 100 000 IU (30 000 μg RAE) for infants 6 through 11 months of age; and
- 50 000 IU (15 000 μg RAE) for infants younger than 6 months.
- An additional (ie, a third) age-specific dose of vitamin A should be given 2 through 6 weeks later to children with clinical signs and symptoms of vitamin A deficiency.

ISOLATION OF THE HOSPITALIZED PATIENT: In addition to standard precautions, airborne transmission precautions are indicated for 4 days after the onset of rash in otherwise healthy children and for the duration of illness in immunocompromised patients. Exposed susceptible patients should be placed on airborne precautions from day 5 after first exposure until day 21 after last exposure.[1]

CONTROL MEASURES:

Evidence of Immunity to Measles.[2] Evidence of immunity to measles includes any of the following:

1. Documentation of age-appropriate vaccination with a live measles virus-containing vaccine:
   - Preschool-aged children: 1 dose administered after the first birthday;
   - School-aged children (grades K-12): 2 doses; the first dose administered after the first birthday and the second dose administered at least 28 days after the first dose;
2. Laboratory evidence of immunity;
3. Laboratory confirmation of disease; or
4. Born before 1957.

Care of Exposed People.

Table 3.31 and Table 3.32 summarize the use of vaccine and Immune Globulin (IG) for postexposure prophylaxis in people who are not immunocompromised or pregnant and people who are immunocompromised or pregnant, respectively.

Use of Vaccine. Available data suggest that measles vaccine, if administered within 72 hours of measles exposure to susceptible individuals, will provide protection or disease modification in some cases. Measles vaccine should be considered in all exposed individuals who are vaccine eligible and who have not been vaccinated or have received only 1 dose of vaccine (the second measles vaccine dose can be administered ≥28 days after the first measles vaccine dose). If the exposure does not result in infection, the vaccine should induce protection against subsequent measles exposures. Immunization is the intervention of choice for control of measles outbreaks in schools and child care centers and for

[1]Centers for Disease Control and Prevention. Immunization of health-care personnel: recommendations of the Advisory Committee on Immunization Practices (ACIP). *MMWR Recomm Rep.* 2011;60(RR-7):1-45

[2]Centers for Disease Control and Prevention. Prevention of measles, rubella, congenital rubella syndrome, and mumps, 2013 summary: recommendations of the Advisory Committee on Immunization Practices (ACIP). *MMWR Recomm Rep.* 2013;62(RR-4):1-34

Table 3.31. Post-exposure Prophylaxis (PEP) for Measles Exposures Who Are NOT Pregnant or Immunocompromised

Age Range	Measles Immune Status[a]	PEP Type Depending on Time After Initial Exposure		
		≤3 days (≤72 hours)	4–6 days	>6 days
All ages	Immune (IgG positive, 2 MMR vaccine doses, or born before 1957[b])	• PEP not indicated. Exposed person has documented immunity.		
<6 months	Non-immune (due to age)	• Give intramuscular immunoglobulin (IMIG).[c,d] • Home quarantine[e] for 28 days after last exposure.		• PEP not indicated (too late).[f] • Home quarantine[e] for 21 days after last exposure.
6–11 months	Non-immune (due to age)	• Give MMR vaccine (MMR vaccine preferred over IG). • No quarantine needed.[b]	• Give intramuscular immunoglobulin (IMIG).[c,d] • Home quarantine[e] for 28 days after last exposure.	• PEP not indicated (too late).[f] • Home quarantine[e] for 21 days after last exposure.
≥12 months	Non-immune (0 doses MMR vaccine or IgG negative)	• Give MMR vaccine. • No quarantine needed.[b]	• PEP not indicated (too late).[f] • Home quarantine[e] for 21 days after last exposure, then give MMR vaccine to protect from future exposures.	
≥12 months	1 dose of MMR vaccine[b]	• Give 2nd MMR vaccine dose if ≥28 days from last dose of live vaccine. • No quarantine needed.	Household member of a confirmed/suspected case • Obtain IgG titers to determine immunity. Home quarantine[e] while awaiting results; if IgG negative, quarantine for 21 days after last exposure (too late for PEP).[f] Not a household member of a confirmed/suspected case • Age 1–3 years: Less likely to get sick because has 1 dose of MMR. • Age ≥4 years: Less likely to get sick because has 1 dose of MMR, and give 2nd MMR to protect from future exposures.	

Table 3.31. Post-exposure Prophylaxis (PEP) for Measles Exposures Who Are NOT Pregnant or Immunocompromised, continued

Age Range	Measles Immune Status[a]	PEP Type Depending on Time After Initial Exposure		
		≤3 days (≤72 hours)	4–6 days	>6 days
Adults	Unknown measles immune status	• Give MMR vaccine. • No quarantine needed.[b]	<u>Household member of a confirmed/suspected case</u> • Obtain IgG titers to determine immunity. Home quarantine[e] while awaiting results; if IgG negative, quarantine for 21 days after last exposure (too late for PEP).[f] **Not** a household member of a confirmed/suspected case Does contact work in setting with children (daycare/school) or healthcare facility • <u>Yes</u>: Obtain titers to determine immunity. Home quarantine[e] while awaiting results; if IgG negative, quarantine for 21 days after last exposure (too late for PEP).[f] • <u>No</u>: Contact can reach out to their own provider to obtain measles IgG titers.[f]	

Reproduced with permission from New York City Department of Health: **https://www1.nyc.gov/assets/doh/downloads/pdf/imm/pep-measles-providers.pdf**

[a] All persons exposed to measles must be notified of their exposure, regardless of their evidence of immunity to measles.

[b] Birth before 1957 or 1 dose of MMR should not be considered sufficient for household members of confirmed measles cases or healthcare workers exposed to measles; without documented positive measles IgG titers or 2 MMR doses, consider them to have unknown immunity. Furlough non-immune healthcare workers for 21 days even if they get MMR PEP.

[c] For patients who receive IG, provide these instructions: **www1.nyc.gov/assets/doh/downloads/pdf/imm/stay-home-non-cases.pdf.**

[d] Dosing of intramuscular IG for infants aged <12 months is 0.5 mL/kg of body weight (max dose 15 mL). Administration of MMR or varicella vaccines must be delayed by 6 months after administration of intramuscular IG and by 8 months after intravenous IG.

[e] When instructing home quarantine, ensure that all household members of the exposed individual are immune to measles. IG prolongs the incubation period to 28 days.

[f] For patients who do not receive PEP, provide these instructions: **www1.nyc.gov/assets/doh/downloads/pdf/imm/stay-home-cases.pdf.**

Table 3.32. Post-exposure Prophylaxis (PEP) for Measles Exposures Who ARE Pregnant or Immunocompromised

Category	Age Range	Measles Immune Status[a]	PEP Type Depending on Time After Initial Exposure		
			≤3 days (≤72 hours)	4–6 days	>6 days
Severely Immuno-compromised[b]	<12 months	Will need IG regardless of measles immune status	• Give intramuscular immunoglobulin (IMIG)[c,d] • Home quarantine[e] for 28 days after last exposure		• PEP not indicated (too late)[f] • Home quarantine[e] for 21 days after last exposure
	≥12 months		• Give intravenous immunoglobulin (IVIG)[c,d] • Home quarantine[e] for 28 days after last exposure		
Pregnant	n/a	Immune (IgG positive or 2 MMR vaccine doses)	• PEP not indicated[f]		
		Non-immune (IgG negative)	• Give intravenous immunoglobulin (IVIG)[c,d] • Home quarantine[e] for 28 days after last exposure		• PEP not indicated (too late)[f] • Home quarantine[e] for 21 days after last exposure
		Unknown immunity	• Draw titers (measles IgG) STAT to determine immunity; proceed as above based on titer results		• PEP not indicated (too late)[f] • Home quarantine[e] for 21 days after last exposure

Reproduced with permission from New York City Department of Health: **https://www1.nyc.gov/assets/doh/downloads/pdf/imm/pep-measles-providers.pdf**

[a] All persons exposed to measles must be notified of their exposure, regardless of their evidence of immunity to measles.

[b] Management of immunocompromised persons can be challenging and may require individualized decisions with provider based on immunocompromising condition or medications.

Table 3.32. Post-exposure Prophylaxis (PEP) for Measles Exposures Who ARE Pregnant or Immunocompromised, continued

Severely immunocompromising conditions (per ACIP and IDSA)* include:

- Severe primary immunodeficiency;
- Bone marrow transplant until ≥12 months after finishing all immunosuppressive treatment and maybe longer in patients who have developed graft-versus-host disease;
- On treatment for acute lymphoblastic leukemia (ALL) within and until ≥6 months after completion of immunosuppressive chemotherapy;
- On cancer chemotherapy**
- Post solid organ transplantation**
- Receiving daily corticosteroid therapy with a dose ≥20 mg (or >2 mg/kg/day for patients who weigh <10 kg) of prednisone or equivalent for ≥14 days
- Receiving certain biologic immune modulators, such as tumor necrosis factor-alpha (TNF-α) blockers or rituximab**
- After hematopoietic stem cell transplant, duration of high-level immunosuppression is highly variable and depends on type of transplant (longer for allogenic than autologous), type of donor and stem cell source, and post-transplant complications such as graft-versus-host disease and their treatments**
- AIDS or HIV with severe immunosuppression defined as CD4 <15% (all ages) or CD4 count <200 lymphocytes/mm³ (age >5 years).

Low-level immunosuppression: In the absence of published guidance on exposed persons with low-level immunosuppression, consider assessing presumptive immunity to measles (measles IgG positive or 2 MMR vaccine doses) to determine if PEP is indicated. If not immune to measles, give PEP as MMR (if not contraindicated and within 72 hours of initial exposure). Consider intravenous IG[c] if MMR is contraindicated or if it is too late for MMR (day 4–6 after initial exposure) with home quarantine for 28 days after last exposure. If no PEP is given because it is too late, home quarantine for 21 days after last exposure.[e]

[c] For patients who receive IG, provide these instructions: **www1.nyc.gov/assets/doh/downloads/pdf/imm/stay-home-non-cases.pdf.**

[d] Dosing of intramuscular IG for infants aged <12 months: 0.5 mL/kg of body weight (max dose 15mL). Dosing of intravenous IG for pregnant women not immune to measles and immunocompromised persons: 400 mg/kg. MMR or varicella vaccine administration must be delayed by 6 months and 8 months after intramuscular and intravenous IG, respectively.

[e] When implementing home quarantine, ensure that all household members of the exposed individual are immune to measles. IG prolongs the incubation period to 28 days.

[f] For patients who do not receive PEP, provide these instructions: **www1.nyc.gov/assets/doh/downloads/pdf/imm/stay-home-cases.pdf.**

* References: Centers for Disease Control and Prevention. Prevention of measles, rubella, congenital rubella syndrome, and mumps, 2013. *MMWR Recomm Rep.* 2013;62(RR-4):1-34; and Rubin LG, Levin MJ, Ljungman P, et al. 2013 IDSA Clinical practice guideline for vaccination of the immunocompromised host. *Clin Infect Dis.* 2014;58(3):e44-e100

** Check guidance/discuss with treating provider as duration of immunosuppression during or following chemotherapy, transplants, or biologic immune modulators may vary.

vaccine-eligible people 12 months and older and has been used starting at 6 months of age with good efficacy in previous measles epidemics in the United States.

Use of Immune Globulin. IG can be administered either intramuscularly (IGIM) or intravenously (IGIV) within 6 days of exposure to prevent or modify measles in people who do not have evidence of measles immunity. Concentrations of measles antibodies in IGIM or IGIV products produced internationally may be different from those of products available in the United States. The recommended dose of IGIM is 0.50 mL/kg (the maximum dose by volume is 15 mL). IGIV is the recommended IG preparation for pregnant women without evidence of measles immunity and for severely immunocompromised hosts,[1] regardless of immunologic or vaccination status, including patients with severe primary immunodeficiency; patients who have received a hematopoietic stem cell transplant, until at least 12 months after finishing all immunosuppressive treatment or longer in patients who have developed graft-versus-host disease; patients undergoing treatment for acute lymphoblastic leukemia, within and until at least 6 months after completion of immunosuppressive chemotherapy; people who have received a solid organ transplant; people with human immunodeficiency virus (HIV) infection who have severe immunosuppression; and patients younger than 12 months whose mothers received biologic response modifiers during pregnancy. IGIV is recommended for these people, because they may be at higher risk of severe measles and complications, and people who weigh >30 kg will receive less than the recommended dose with IGIM preparations. IGIV is administered at a dose of 400 mg/kg. For patients who already are receiving IGIV at regularly scheduled intervals, the usual dose of 400 mg/kg should be adequate for measles prophylaxis after exposures occurring within 3 weeks of receiving IGIV. For people routinely receiving Immune Globulin Subcutaneous (IGSC) therapy, administration of at least 200 mg/kg for 2 consecutive weeks before measles exposure should be sufficient. IG is not indicated for household or other close contacts who have received 1 dose of vaccine at 12 months or older unless they are severely immunocompromised (as defined previously).

For children who receive IGIM for modification or prevention of measles after exposure, measles vaccine (if not contraindicated) should be administered 6 months after IGIM administration, provided the child is at least 12 months of age. Intervals vary between administration of IGIV or other biologic products and measles-containing vaccines (see Table 1.11, p 40).

HIV Infection.[1] HIV-infected children who are exposed to measles require prophylaxis on the basis of immune status and measles vaccine history. HIV-infected children who have serologic evidence of immunity or who received 2 doses of measles vaccine after initiation of combination antiretroviral therapy (ART) with no to moderate immunosuppression (see Human Immunodeficiency Virus Infection, p 427) should be considered immune and will not require any additional measures to prevent measles. Asymptomatic mildly or moderately immunocompromised HIV-infected people without evidence of immunity to measles should receive IGIM at a dose of 0.5 mL/kg (maximum 15 mL), regardless of immunization status. Severely immunocompromised patients (including HIV-infected people with CD4+ T-lymphocyte percentages <15% [all ages] or CD4+ T-lymphocyte

[1]Centers for Disease Control and Prevention. Prevention of measles, rubella, congenital rubella syndrome, and mumps, 2013 summary: recommendations of the Advisory Committee on Immunization Practices (ACIP). *MMWR Recomm Rep.* 2013;62(RR-4):1-34

counts <200/mm^3 [age >5 years], regardless of immunization status, and those who
have not received MMR vaccine since receiving ART) who are exposed to measles should
receive IGIV prophylaxis, 400 mg/kg, after exposure to measles, regardless of vaccination
status. Some experts would include all HIV-infected people, regardless of immunologic
status or MMR vaccine history, as needing IGIV prophylaxis. HIV-infected children
who have received IGIV within 3 weeks of exposure do not require additional passive
immunization.

Health Care Personnel. To decrease health care-associated infection, immunization programs should be established to ensure that all people who work or volunteer in health
care facilities (including students) have presumptive evidence of immunity to measles (see
Immunization in Health Care Personnel, p 92).

Measles Vaccine Recommendations. (see Table 3.33 for summary).

Use of MMR Vaccine. The only measles vaccine licensed in the United States is a live
further-attenuated strain prepared in chicken embryo cell culture. Measles vaccines
provided through the Expanded Programme on Immunization in resource-limited countries meet the WHO standards and usually are comparable with the vaccine available
in the United States. Measles vaccine is available in the United States as combination
formulations, which include MMR and measles, mumps, rubella, and varicella (MMRV)
vaccines. Single-antigen measles vaccine no longer is available in the United States.
Measles-containing vaccine in a dose of 0.5 mL is administered subcutaneously. Measles-
containing vaccines can be administered simultaneously with other immunizations in a
separate syringe at a separate site (see Simultaneous Administration of Multiple Vaccines,
p 36).

Serum measles antibodies develop in approximately 95% of children immunized
at 12 months of age and 98% of children immunized at 15 months of age. Protection
conferred by a single dose is durable in most people. A small proportion (5% or less)
of immunized people may lose protection after several years. For measles elimination,
2 doses of vaccine are required. More than 99% of people who receive 2 doses (separated
by at least 28 days, and the first dose administered on or after the first birthday) develop
serologic evidence of measles immunity. The second dose provides protection to those
failing to respond to their primary measles immunization and, therefore, is not a booster
dose. Immunization is not deleterious for people who already are immune. Immunized
people do not shed or transmit measles vaccine virus.

Improperly stored vaccine may fail to protect against measles. Since 1979, an
improved stabilizer has been added to the vaccine that makes it more resistant to heat
inactivation. For recommended storage of MMR and MMRV vaccines, see the manufacturers' package labels. MMRV vaccine must be stored frozen between −58°F and
+5°F.

Age of Routine Immunization. The first dose of MMR vaccine should be administered at
12 through 15 months of age. Delays in administering the first dose contributed to large
outbreaks in the United States from 1989 to 1991. The second dose is recommended routinely at school entry (ie, 4 through 6 years of age) but can be administered at an earlier
age (eg, during an outbreak or before international travel), provided the interval between
the first and second MMR doses is at least 28 days. Catch-up second-dose immunization should occur for all school-aged children (elementary, middle, high school) who have
received only 1 dose, including at the adolescent visit at 11 through 12 years of age and

Table 3.33. Recommendations for Measles Immunization[a]

Category	Recommendations
Unimmunized, no history of measles (12 through 15 mo of age)	MMR or MMRV vaccine is recommended at 12 through 15 mo of age; a second dose is recommended at least 28 days after the first dose (or 90 days for MMRV) and usually is administered at 4 through 6 y of age.
Children 6 through 11 mo of age in outbreak situations[b] or before international travel	Immunize with MMR vaccine, ideally at least 2 weeks prior to travel, but this dose is not considered valid, and 2 valid doses administered on or after the first birthday are required. MMRV should not be administered to children <12 mo of age.
Students in kindergarten, elementary, middle, and high school who have received 1 dose of measles vaccine at 12 mo of age or older	Administer the second dose.
Students in college and other postsecondary institutions who have received 1 dose of measles vaccine at 12 mo of age or older	Administer the second dose.
History of immunization before the first birthday	Dose not considered valid; immunize (2 doses).
History of receipt of inactivated measles vaccine or unknown type of vaccine, 1963–1967	Dose not considered valid; immunize (2 doses).
Further attenuated or unknown vaccine administered with IG	Dose not considered valid; immunize (2 doses).
Allergy to eggs	Immunize; no reactions likely (see text for details).
Neomycin allergy, nonanaphylactic	Immunize; no reactions likely (see text for details).
Severe hypersensitivity (anaphylaxis) to neomycin or gelatin	Avoid immunization.
Tuberculosis	Immunize (see Tuberculosis, p 786); if patient has untreated tuberculosis disease, start antituberculosis therapy before immunizing.
Measles exposure	Immunize or give IG, depending on circumstances (see Care of Exposed People, p 522, Table 3.31, and Table 3.32).
HIV infected	Immunize (2 doses) unless severely immunocompromised (see text, p 511); administration of IG if exposed to measles is based on degree of immunosuppression and measles vaccine history (see text, p 511).

Table 3.33. Recommendations for Measles Immunization,[a] continued

Category	Recommendations
Personal or family history of seizures	Immunize; advise parents of slightly increased risk of seizures.
Immunoglobulin or blood recipient	Immunize at the appropriate interval (see Table 1.11, p 40).

HIV indicates human immunodeficiency virus; IG, Immune Globulin; MMR, measles-mumps-rubella vaccine; MMRV, measles-mumps-rubella-varicella vaccine.

[a]See text for details and recommendations for use of MMRV vaccine.

[b]See Outbreak Control (p 518).

older. If a child receives a dose of measles vaccine before 12 months of age, this dose is not counted toward the required number of doses; the universally recommended 2 doses are still required in the United States beginning at 12 through 15 months of age and separated by at least 28 days.

Use of MMRV Vaccine.[1]

- MMRV vaccine is indicated for simultaneous immunization against measles, mumps, rubella, and varicella among children 12 months through 12 years of age; MMRV vaccine is not indicated for people outside this age group. See Varicella-Zoster Infections, p 831, for recommendations for use of MMRV vaccine for the first dose.
- Children with HIV infection also should not receive MMRV vaccine because of lack of safety data of the quadrivalent vaccine in children infected with HIV.
- MMRV vaccine may be administered with other vaccines recommended at 12 through 15 months of age and before or at 4 through 6 years of age (**https://redbook. solutions.aap.org/SS/Immunization_Schedules.aspx**).
- At least 28 days should elapse between a dose of measles-containing vaccine, such as MMR vaccine, and a dose of MMRV vaccine. However, the recommended minimal interval between MMRV vaccine doses is 90 days.

Colleges and Other Institutions for Education Beyond High School. Colleges and other educational institutions should require that all entering students have documentation of evidence of measles immunity (see Evidence of Immunity to Measles, p 506). Students without documentation of measles immunity should receive MMR vaccine on entry, followed by a second dose 28 days later, if not contraindicated.

Immunization During an Outbreak. During an outbreak, MMR vaccine should be offered to all people exposed or in the outbreak setting who lack evidence of measles immunity. During a community-wide outbreak that affects infants, MMR vaccine has been shown to be efficacious and may be recommended for infants 6 through 11 months of age (see Outbreak Control, p 518). Doses received prior to the first birthday do not count toward the recommended 2-dose series.

---

[1]Centers for Disease Control and Prevention. Use of combination measles, mumps, rubella, and varicella vaccine: recommendations of the Advisory Committee on Immunization Practices (ACIP). *MMWR Recomm Rep.* 2010;59(RR–3):1–12

International Travel. People traveling internationally (any country outside of the United States) should be immune to measles prior to travel. Infants 6 through 11 months of age should receive 1 dose of MMR vaccine at least 2 weeks before departure if possible, and then should receive a second dose of measles-containing vaccine at 12 through 15 months of age (at least 28 days after the initial measles immunization) and a third dose at 4 through 6 years of age. Children 12 months or older as well as adults who have received 1 dose and are traveling to areas where measles is endemic or epidemic should receive their second dose before departure, provided the interval between doses is 28 days or more.

International Adoptees. The US Department of State requires that internationally adopted children 10 years and older receive MMR vaccine before entry into the United States. Internationally adopted children who are younger than 10 years are exempt from Immigration and Nationality Act regulations pertaining to immunization of immigrants before arrival in the United States (see Children Who Received Immunizations Outside the United States or Whose Immunization Status is Unknown or Uncertain, p 96); adoptive parents are required to sign a waiver indicating their intention to comply with US immunization recommendations after their child's arrival in the United States.

Health Care Personnel.[1] Adequate presumptive evidence of immunity to measles for people who work in health care facilities is: (1) documented administration of 2 doses of live-virus measles vaccine with the first dose administered at ≥12 months of age and the second dose at least 28 days after the first; (2) laboratory evidence of immunity or laboratory confirmation of disease; or (3) birth before 1957. Birth before 1957 is not a guarantee of measles immunity, and therefore, facilities should consider vaccinating unimmunized personnel born before 1957 who lack laboratory evidence of immunity with 2 doses of MMR vaccine at the appropriate interval (see Immunization in Health Care Personnel, p 92). For recommendations during an outbreak, see Outbreak Control (p 518).

Adverse Events. A body temperature of 39.4°C (103°F) or higher develops in approximately 5% to 15% of vaccine recipients, usually between 6 and 12 days after receipt of MMR vaccine; fever generally lasts 1 to 2 days but may last as long as 5 days. Most people with fever do not have other symptoms. Transient rashes have been reported in approximately 5% of vaccine recipients. Recipients who develop fever and/or rash are not considered contagious. Febrile seizures 5 to 12 days after immunization occur in 1 in 3000 to 4000 people immunized with MMR vaccine. Transient thrombocytopenia occurs in 1 in 22 000 to 40 000 people after administration of measles-containing vaccines, specifically MMR (see Thrombocytopenia, p 516). There is no evidence that reimmunization increases the risk of adverse events in people already immune to these diseases. Data indicate that only people who are not immune to the viruses in MMR tend to have adverse effects. Thus, events following a second dose of MMR vaccine would be expected to be substantially lower than after a first dose because most people who received a first dose would be immune.

Rates of most local and systemic adverse events for children immunized with MMRV vaccine are comparable with rates for children immunized with MMR and varicella vaccines administered concomitantly. However, recipients of a first dose of MMRV vaccine have a greater rate of fever 102°F (38.9°C) or higher than do recipients of MMR and varicella administered concomitantly (22% vs 15%, respectively). Febrile seizures occur in

---

[1] Centers for Disease Control and Prevention. Immunization of health-care personnel: recommendations of the Advisory Committee on Immunization Practices (ACIP). *MMWR Recomm Rep.* 2011;60(RR–07):1–45

1 in 1100 to 1400 children immunized with a first dose of MMRV vaccine at 12 through 23 months of age and in 1 in 2500 to 3000 children immunized with a first dose of MMR and varicella vaccines administered separately at the same visit. The period of risk for febrile seizures is from 5 to 12 days following receipt of the vaccine. The benefit of using MMRV instead of MMR and monovalent varicella vaccines separately is that the quadrivalent product results in 1 fewer injection. Either MMRV or separate MMR and varicella vaccines are acceptable option for dose 1 at 12 through 15 months of age and pediatricians should discuss risks and benefits of the vaccine choices with the parents or caregivers. For the first dose of measles, mumps, rubella, and varicella vaccines at ages 48 months and older and for dose 2 at any age (15 months through 12 years), use of MMRV vaccine generally is preferred over separate injections of MMR and varicella vaccines to minimize the number of injections.

The reported frequency of central nervous system conditions, such as encephalitis and encephalopathy, after measles immunization is less than 1 per million doses administered in the United States. Because the incidence of encephalitis or encephalopathy after measles immunization in the United States is lower than the observed incidence of encephalitis of unknown cause, some or most of the rare reported severe neurologic disorders may be related temporally, rather than causally, to measles immunization. Multiple studies, as well as the National Academy of Medicine Vaccine Safety Review, refute a causal relationship between autism and MMR vaccine or between inflammatory bowel disease and MMR vaccine.

Precautions and Contraindications.

Febrile Illnesses. Children with minor illnesses, such as upper respiratory tract infections, may be immunized. Fever is not a contraindication to immunization. However, if other manifestations suggest a more serious illness, immunization should be deferred until the illness has resolved.

Allergic Reactions. Hypersensitivity reactions occur rarely and usually are minor, consisting of wheal-and-flare reactions or urticaria at the injection site. Reactions have been attributed to trace amounts of neomycin or gelatin or some other component in the vaccine formulation. Anaphylaxis is rare. Measles vaccine is produced in chicken embryo cell culture and does not contain significant amounts of egg white (ovalbumin) cross-reacting proteins. Children with egg allergy are at low risk of anaphylactic reactions to measles-containing vaccines (including MMR and MMRV). Skin testing of children for egg allergy is not predictive of reactions to MMR vaccine and is not recommended before administering MMR or other measles-containing vaccines. People with allergies to chickens or feathers are not at increased risk of reaction to the vaccine.

People who have had a significant hypersensitivity reaction after the first dose of measles-containing vaccine should: (1) be tested for measles immunity, and if immune, should not receive a second dose; or (2) receive evaluation and possible skin testing before receiving a second dose.

Thrombocytopenia. Rarely, MMR vaccine can be associated with thrombocytopenia within 2 months of immunization, with a temporal clustering 2 to 3 weeks after immunization. On the basis of case reports, the risk of vaccine-associated thrombocytopenia may be higher for people who previously experienced thrombocytopenia, especially if it occurred in temporal association with earlier MMR immunization. The decision to immunize these children should be based on assessment of immunity after the first dose and the benefits of protection against measles, mumps, and rubella in comparison with the risks of recurrence of thrombocytopenia after immunization. The risk of thrombocytopenia is higher after the first dose of vaccine than after the second dose. There have been no reported cases of thrombocytopenia associated with receipt of MMR vaccine that have resulted in hemorrhagic complications or death in otherwise healthy people.

Recent Administration of IG or Other Blood Products. IG preparations interfere with the serologic response to measles vaccine for variable periods, depending on the dose of IG administered. Suggested intervals between IG or blood-product administration and measles immunization are provided in Table 1.11 (p 40). If vaccine is administered at intervals shorter than those indicated, as may be warranted if the risk of exposure to measles is imminent, the child should be reimmunized at or after the appropriate interval for immunization (and at least 28 days after the earlier immunization) unless serologic testing indicates that measles-specific antibodies were produced.

MMR vaccine should be administered at least 2 weeks before planned administration of IG, blood transfusion, or other blood products because of the theoretical possibility that antibody will neutralize vaccine virus and interfere with successful immunization. If IG must be administered within 14 days after administration of MMR or MMRV, these vaccines should be administered again after the interval specified in Table 1.11 (p 40).

Tuberculosis. Tuberculin skin testing is not a prerequisite for measles immunization. Antituberculosis therapy should be initiated before administering MMR vaccine to people with untreated tuberculosis infection or disease. Tuberculin skin testing, if otherwise indicated, can be performed any time before or on the day of immunization. Otherwise, testing should be postponed for 4 to 6 weeks, because measles immunization temporarily may suppress tuberculin skin test reactivity. The effects of measles vaccination on interferon gamma release assay (IGRA) characteristics have not been determined; the same precautions as for tuberculin skin testing should be followed.

Altered Immunity. Immunocompromised patients with disorders associated with increased severity of viral infections should not receive live-virus measles vaccine (the exception is people with HIV infection, unless they have evidence of severe immunosuppression; see Immunization and Other Considerations in Immunocompromised Children, p 72, and HIV Infection, p 518). The risk of exposure to measles for immunocompromised patients can be decreased by immunizing their close susceptible contacts. Immunized people do not shed or transmit infectious measles vaccine virus. Management of immunodeficient and immunosuppressed patients exposed to measles can be facilitated by previous knowledge of their immune status. If possible, children should receive measles vaccine before initiating treatment with biological response modifiers, such as tumor necrosis factor antagonists, and before transplantation, ideally with 2 doses. Severely immunocompromised patients should receive IG after measles exposure regardless of immunologic or vaccination status (see Care of Exposed People, p 522, Table 3.31, and Table 3.32).

Corticosteroids. For patients who have received high doses of corticosteroids ($\geq$2 mg/kg of body weight or $\geq$20 mg/day of prednisone or its equivalent for people who weigh $\geq$10 kg) for 14 days or more and who otherwise are not immunocompromised, the recommended interval between stopping the corticosteroids and immunization is at least 4 weeks (see Immunization and Other Considerations in Immunocompromised Children, p 72). In general, inhaled steroids do not cause immunosuppression and are not a contraindication to measles immunization.

HIV Infection.[1] Measles immunization (administered as MMR vaccine) is recommended for all people ≥12 months of age with HIV infection who do not have evidence of measles immunity and who do not have evidence of severe immunosuppression, because measles can be severe and sometimes is fatal in patients with HIV infection (see Human Immunodeficiency Virus Infection, p 427). For vaccination purposes, severe immunosuppression is defined in children 1 through 13 years of age as a CD4+ T-lymphocyte percentage <15% and in adolescents ≥14 years as a CD4+ T-lymphocyte count <200 lymphocytes/mm^3. Severely immunocompromised HIV-infected infants, children, adolescents, and young adults should not receive measles virus-containing vaccine. MMRV vaccine should not be administered to any HIV-infected infant, regardless of degree of immunosuppression, because of lack of safety data in this population. The first dose of MMR vaccine should be administered at age 12 through 15 months and the second dose at age 4 through 6 years, or as early as 28 days after the first dose. Children, adolescents, and adults with newly diagnosed HIV infections and without evidence of measles immunity should complete a 2-dose schedule with MMR vaccine as soon as possible after diagnosis, unless they have evidence of severe immunosuppression. People with perinatally acquired HIV infection who were vaccinated against measles before initiation of ART should be considered unvaccinated and should be revaccinated with 2 doses of MMR vaccine once effective ART has been administered, unless they have other acceptable current evidence of measles immunity. All members of the household of an HIV-infected person who lack evidence of measles immunity should receive 2 doses of MMR. Because measles vaccine virus is not shed after immunization, HIV-infected people are not at risk of measles vaccine virus infection if household members are immunized.

Personal or Family History of Seizures. Children with a personal or family history of seizures should be immunized after parents or guardians are advised that the risk of seizures after measles immunization is increased slightly. Children receiving anticonvulsants should continue such therapy after measles immunization.

Pregnancy. A measles-containing vaccine should not be administered to women known to be pregnant. Women who receive MMR vaccine should not become pregnant for at least 28 days. This precaution is based on the theoretical risk of fetal infection, which applies to administration of any live-virus vaccine to women who might be pregnant or who might become pregnant shortly after immunization. No data from women who were inadvertently vaccinated while pregnant substantiate this theoretical risk. When immunizing adolescents and young adults against measles, recommended precautions include asking women if they are pregnant, excluding women who are, and explaining the theoretical risks to others. Pregnancy testing prior to immunization is not required.

Outbreak Control. Every suspected measles case should be reported immediately to the local health department, and every effort must be made to obtain laboratory evidence that would confirm that the illness is measles (including obtaining specimens for virus detection), especially if the illness may be the first case in the community. Subsequent prevention of spread of measles depends on prompt immunization of people at risk of exposure or people already exposed. People who have not been immunized, including those who have been exempted from measles immunization for medical reasons, should be excluded

[1]Rubin LG, Levin MJ, Ljungman P, et al. 2013 IDSA clinical practice guideline for vaccination of the immunocompromised host. *Clin Infect Dis.* 2014;58(3):309-318

from school, child care, and health care settings until at least 21 days after the onset of rash in the last case of measles.

Schools and Child Care Facilities. During measles outbreaks in child care facilities, schools, and colleges and other institutions of higher education, all students, their siblings, and personnel born in 1957 or after who cannot provide evidence of measles immunity should be immunized. People receiving their second dose, as well as unimmunized people receiving their first dose as part of the outbreak-control program, may be readmitted immediately to the school or child care facility.

Health Care Facilities. If an outbreak occurs in an area served by a hospital or within a hospital, all employees and volunteers who cannot provide evidence of immunity to measles should receive 2 doses of MMR vaccine. Because some health care personnel born before 1957 have acquired measles in health care facilities, immunization with 2 doses of MMR vaccine is recommended for health care personnel without serologic evidence of immunity in this age category during outbreaks. Serologic testing before immunization is not recommended during an outbreak because rapid immunization is required to halt disease transmission. Health care personnel without evidence of immunity who have been exposed should be relieved of direct patient contact from the fifth to the 21st day after exposure, regardless of whether they received vaccine or IG after the exposure. Health care personnel who become ill should be relieved of patient contact until 4 days after rash develops.

Meningococcal Infections

CLINICAL MANIFESTATIONS: Invasive meningococcal infection usually results in septicemia (35%–40% of cases), meningitis (~50% of cases), or both. Bacteremic pneumonia is less common (10% of cases). Rarely, young children have occult bacteremia. Onset of invasive infections can be insidious and nonspecific, but onset of septicemia (meningococcemia) typically is abrupt, with fever, chills, malaise, myalgia, limb pain, prostration, and a rash that initially can be macular or maculopapular but typically becomes petechial or purpuric within hours. A similar rash can occur with viral infections or with severe sepsis attributable to other bacterial pathogens. In fulminant cases, purpura, limb ischemia, coagulopathy, pulmonary edema, shock, coma, and death can ensue within hours despite appropriate management. Signs and symptoms of meningococcal meningitis are indistinguishable from those associated with pneumococcal meningitis. In severe and fatal cases of meningococcal meningitis, raised intracranial pressure is a predominant presenting feature. Invasive infections can be complicated by arthritis, myocarditis, pericarditis, and endophthalmitis. Noninvasive meningococcal infections, such as conjunctivitis and urethritis, also occur. The overall case-fatality rate for invasive meningococcal disease is 15% and is somewhat higher in late adolescence and in older adults. Clinical predictors of mortality include coma, hypotension, leukopenia, and thrombocytopenia. A self-limiting postinfectious inflammatory syndrome occurs in fewer than 10% of cases, begins a minimum 4 days after onset of meningococcal infection, and most commonly presents as fever and arthritis or vasculitis with less common manifestations including iritis, scleritis, conjunctivitis, pericarditis, and polyserositis.

Sequelae associated with meningococcal disease occur in up to 19% of survivors and include hearing loss, neurologic disability, digit or limb amputations, and skin scarring. In addition, patients may experience subtle long-term neurologic deficits, such as impaired school performance, behavioral problems, and attention deficit disorder.

ETIOLOGY: *Neisseria meningitidis* is a gram-negative diplococcus with 12 confirmed serogroups based on capsular type.

EPIDEMIOLOGY: *N meningitidis* disease rates are highest in infants <1 year of age, followed by children 1 year of age and adolescents and young adults 16 to 20 years of age. Household contacts of cases have 500 to 800 times the rate of disease for the general population. A predominance of US cases is observed in the winter, often noted 2 to 3 weeks following onset of influenza outbreaks, with peak of cases in January, February, and March. Patients with persistent complement-component deficiencies (eg, C3, C5–C9, properdin, or factor D or factor H deficiencies), with anatomic or functional asplenia or human immunodeficiency virus, or treated with eculizumab are at increased risk of invasive and recurrent meningococcal disease. Asymptomatic colonization of the upper respiratory tract is most common in older adolescents and young adults and is the reservoir from which the organism is spread. Transmission occurs from person to person through droplets from the respiratory tract and requires close contact. Patients should be considered capable of transmitting the organism for up to 24 hours after initiation of effective antimicrobial treatment.

Distribution of meningococcal serogroups in the United States has shifted in the past 2 decades. Serogroups B accounts for most cases currently, followed by serogroups C, W, and Y and nongroupable (nonencapsulated) meningococci. Serogroup distribution varies by age, location, and time. More than 85% of cases among adolescents and young adults are caused by serogroups B, C, Y, or W and, therefore, potentially are preventable with available vaccines. In infants and children younger than 60 months, approximately two thirds of cases are caused by serogroup B.

Since the early 2000s, annual incidence rates for invasive meningococcal disease have decreased, and during 2017, 350 cases occurred (incidence of 0.11 per 100 000 population) in the United States. The decrease in cases in the United States started before the 2005 introduction of ACWY meningococcal conjugate vaccine into the routine immunization schedule at age 11 through 12 years and the 2010 recommendation for a booster vaccine at age 16 years. Reasons for this decrease in incidence are postulated to be related to the increased use of influenza vaccine, reduction in the carriage rates, the use of meningococcal conjugate vaccines in preadolescents and adolescents, immunity of the population to circulating meningococcal strains unrelated to vaccination, and changes in behavioral risk factors (eg, decreases in smoking and exposure to secondhand smoke among adolescents and young adults).

Strains belonging to groups A, B, C, Y, W, and X are implicated most commonly in invasive disease worldwide. Serogroup A has historically been associated with epidemics outside the United States, primarily in sub-Saharan Africa. A serogroup A meningococcal conjugate vaccine was introduced in the "meningitis belt" of sub-Saharan Africa starting in December 2010, and its widespread use has been associated with a marked reduction in serogroup A disease rates; recent outbreaks in the meningitis belt have been associated with serogroups C, W, and X. In Europe, Australia, and South America, the incidence of meningococcal disease ranged from 0.3 to 2 cases per 100 000 population in recent years. Serogroups B, C, W, and Y are most commonly reported in these regions.

Most cases of meningococcal disease are sporadic, with fewer than 10% associated with outbreaks. Outbreaks occur in communities and institutions, including child care centers, schools, colleges, and military recruit camps. Multiple outbreaks of serogroup B meningococcal disease have occurred on college campuses, and outbreaks of serogroup

C meningococcal disease have been reported among men who have sex with men and among people experiencing homelessness.

The **incubation period** for invasive disease is 1 to 10 days, usually less than 4 days.

DIAGNOSTIC TESTS: Cultures of blood and cerebrospinal fluid (CSF) are indicated for patients with suspected invasive meningococcal disease. Cultures of a petechial or purpuric lesion scraping, synovial fluid, and other usually sterile body fluid specimens sometimes are positive. Specimens for culture should be plated onto both sheep blood and chocolate agar and incubated at 35°C to 37°C with 5% carbon dioxide in a moist atmosphere. The organism is readily identified with standard biochemical tests as well as by the newer method of mass spectrometry of bacterial cell components. A Gram stain of a petechial or purpuric scraping, CSF, or buffy coat smear of blood may reveal gram negative diplococci. Because *N meningitidis* can be a component of the nasopharyngeal flora, isolation of *N meningitidis* from this site is not helpful diagnostically. A serogroup-specific polymerase chain reaction (PCR) test to detect *N meningitidis* from clinical specimens is useful particularly in patients who receive antimicrobial therapy before cultures are obtained. In the United States, commercially available multiplex PCR assays have excellent sensitivity and specificity for detection of serogroups A, B, C, W, X, and Y. Antigen detection tests, primarily by latex agglutination, to detect select meningococcal polysaccharide types in CSF were developed more than 2 decades ago. These assays no longer are commonly used because of concerns about test sensitivity and specificity.

Surveillance case definitions for invasive meningococcal disease are provided in Table 3.34. Serologic typing and other characterization such as whole genome sequencing can be useful epidemiologic tools during a suspected outbreak to detect concordance among invasive strains.

TREATMENT: The priority in management of meningococcal disease is treatment of shock in meningococcemia and of raised intracranial pressure in severe meningitis. Empirical therapy for suspected meningococcal disease should include cefotaxime or ceftriaxone. Once the microbiologic diagnosis is established, treatment options include cefotaxime, ceftriaxone, penicillin G, or ampicillin. Five to 7 days of antimicrobial therapy is adequate. Because of recent detections of β-lactamase-producing organisms in the United States, meningococcal isolate susceptibility to penicillin should be determined before switching to penicillin or ampicillin.[1] Ceftriaxone clears nasopharyngeal carriage effectively after 1 dose. For patients with a life-threatening penicillin allergy characterized by anaphylaxis, meropenem can be used with caution as the rate of cross-reactivity in penicillin-allergic adults is very low. In meningococcemia, early and rapid fluid resuscitation and early use of inotropic and ventilatory support may reduce mortality. The postinfectious inflammatory syndromes associated with meningococcal disease often respond to nonsteroidal anti-inflammatory drugs. Treating physicians should consider evaluating for conditions that increase risk of disease, such as underlying complement component deficiencies. In some studies, underlying complement deficiency has been identified in up to 10% to 50% of patients with meningococcal disease, although no recent data are available on complement deficiency prevalence among US patients with meningococcal disease.

---

[1] McNamara LA, Potts C, Blain AE, et al. Detection of ciprofloxacin-resistant, β-lactamase–producing *Neisseria meningitidis* serogroup Y isolates—United States, 2019–2020. *MMWR Morb Mortal Wkly Rep.* 2020;69(24):735–739. DOI: **http://dx.doi.org/10.15585/mmwr.mm6924a2**

Table 3.34. Surveillance Case Definitions for Invasive Meningococcal Disease

Confirmed case

A clinically compatible case and isolation of *Neisseria meningitidis* from a usually sterile site, for example:

- Blood
- Cerebrospinal fluid (CSF)
- Synovial fluid
- Pleural fluid
- Pericardial fluid
- Isolation from skin scraping of petechial or purpuric lesions

OR

Detection of *N meningitidis*-specific nucleic acid in a specimen obtained from a normally sterile body site (eg, blood or CSF), using a validated polymerase chain reaction (PCR) assay

Probable case

A clinically compatible case with EITHER a positive result of antigen test OR immunohistochemistry of formalin-fixed tissue

Suspect case

- A clinically compatible case and gram-negative diplococci in any sterile fluid, such as CSF, synovial fluid, or scraping from a petechial or purpuric lesion
- Clinical purpura fulminans without a positive culture

ISOLATION OF THE HOSPITALIZED PATIENT: In addition to standard precautions, droplet precautions are recommended until 24 hours after initiation of effective antimicrobial therapy.

CONTROL MEASURES:

Care of Exposed People.

Postexposure Chemoprophylaxis. Regardless of immunization status, close contacts including household contacts of all people with invasive meningococcal disease (see Table 3.35), whether endemic or in an outbreak situation, are at high risk of infection and should promptly receive chemoprophylaxis. Chemoprophylaxis should be provided even if the close contact has received meningococcal vaccine. The decision to give chemoprophylaxis to other contacts is based on risk of contracting invasive disease related to specific exposure to the secretions from the infected patient. Throat and nasopharyngeal cultures are not recommended, because these cultures are of no value in deciding who should receive chemoprophylaxis.

Table 3.34 provides the surveillance case definition for invasive meningococcal disease. Table 3.35 provides prophylaxis recommendations for contacts of a person with invasive meningococcal disease, and Table 3.36 provides recommended prophylaxis regimens. Routine prophylaxis is not recommended for health care personnel unless they have had intimate exposure to respiratory tract secretions, such as occurs with unprotected mouth-to-mouth resuscitation, intubation, or suctioning before or less than 24 hours after antimicrobial therapy was initiated. Chemoprophylaxis ideally should be initiated within 24 hours after the index patient is identified; prophylaxis is not indicated more than 2 weeks after exposure. If antimicrobial agents other than ceftriaxone or cefotaxime (each of which will eradicate nasopharyngeal carriage) are used for treatment of invasive

Table 3.35. Disease Risk for Contacts of People With Invasive Meningococcal Disease

High risk: chemoprophylaxis recommended (close contacts)
- Household contact
- Child care or preschool contact at any time during 7 days before onset of illness
- Direct exposure to index patient's secretions through kissing or through sharing toothbrushes or eating utensils, markers of close social contact, at any time during 7 days before onset of illness
- Mouth-to-mouth resuscitation, unprotected contact during endotracheal intubation at any time from 7 days before onset of illness to 24 h after initiation of effective antimicrobial therapy
- Frequently slept in same dwelling as index patient during 7 days before onset of illness
- Passengers seated directly next to the index case during airline flights lasting more than 8 hours (gate to gate), or passengers seated within one seat in any direction from an index case on a flight of any duration if the index case was coughing or vomiting during the flight

Low risk: chemoprophylaxis not recommended
- Casual contact: no history of direct exposure to index patient's oral secretions (eg, school or work)
- Indirect contact: only contact is with a high-risk contact, no direct contact with the index patient
- Health care personnel without direct exposure to patient's oral secretions

In outbreak or cluster
- Chemoprophylaxis for people other than people at high risk (close contacts) should be administered only after consultation with local public health authorities

---

meningococcal disease, the child should receive chemoprophylaxis before hospital discharge to eradicate nasopharyngeal carriage of *N meningitidis*.

Ciprofloxacin-resistant strains of *N meningitidis* have been detected over the past 15 years.[1,2] If fluoroquinolone resistance has been identified in a community, ciprofloxacin should not be used for chemoprophylaxis. Prophylaxis failures and antimicrobial resistance among meningococcal isolates should be monitored to inform meningococcal prophylaxis recommendations.

Meningococcal Vaccines. In the United States, 3 meningococcal vaccines are licensed and available for use in children and adults against serogroups A, C, W, and Y (MenACWY), and 2 vaccines are licensed for people 10 through 25 years of age against serogroup B (MenB). All 3 MenACWY vaccines are protein conjugate vaccines, while the 2 MenB vaccines are protein-based vaccines using 2 different technologies. Tables 3.37 (p 526) and 3.38 (p 528) provide recommendations on meningococcal vaccines.

Serogroup A, C, W, and Y Vaccines. Meningococcal groups A, C, W, and Y polysaccharide diphtheria toxoid conjugate vaccine (MenACWY-D) (Menactra, Sanofi Pasteur) is licensed for use in people 9 months through 55 years of age. Meningococcal groups A, C, W, and Y oligosaccharide diphtheria CRM_{197} conjugate vaccine (MenACWY-CRM) (Menveo, GSK) is licensed for use in people 2 months through 55 years of age. Meningococcal groups A, C, W, and Y polysaccharide tetanus toxoid conjugate vaccine

---

[1]Centers for Disease Control and Prevention. Emergence of fluoroquinolone-resistant *Neisseria meningitidis*—Minnesota and North Dakota, 2007–2008. *MMWR Morb Mortal Wkly Rep.* 2008;57(7):173-175

[2]McNamara LA, Potts C, Blain AE, et al. Detection of ciprofloxacin-resistant, β-lactamase–producing Neisseria meningitidis serogroup Y isolates—United States, 2019–2020. *MMWR Morb Mortal Wkly Rep.* 2020;69(24):735–739. DOI: **http://dx.doi.org/10.15585/mmwr.mm6924a2**

Table 3.36. Recommended Chemoprophylaxis Regimens for High-Risk Contacts and People With Invasive Meningococcal Disease

Age of Infants, Children, and Adults	Dose	Duration	Efficacy, %	Cautions
Rifampin[a]				
<1 mo	5 mg/kg per dose, orally, every 12 h	2 days		Discussion with an expert for infants <1 mo
≥1 mo	10 mg/kg per dose (maximum 600 mg), orally, every 12 h	2 days	90–95	Can interfere with efficacy of oral contraceptives and some seizure and anticoagulant medications; can stain soft contact lenses
Ceftriaxone				
<15 y	125 mg, intramuscularly	Single dose	90–95	To decrease pain at injection site, dilute with 1% lidocaine
≥15 y	250 mg, intramuscularly	Single dose	90–95	To decrease pain at injection site, dilute with 1% lidocaine
Ciprofloxacin[a,b]				
≥1 mo	20 mg/kg (maximum 500 mg), orally	Single dose	90–95	
Azithromycin	10 mg/kg (maximum 500 mg)	Single dose	90	Not recommended routinely; equivalent to rifampin for eradication of *Neisseria meningitidis* from nasopharynx in one study of young adults

[a] Not recommended for use in pregnant women.

[b] Use only if fluoroquinolone-resistant strains of *N meningitidis* have not been identified in the community (McNamara LA, Potts C, Blain AE, et al. Detection of ciprofloxacin-resistant, β-lactamase–producing *Neisseria meningitidis* serogroup Y isolates—United States, 2019–2020. *MMWR Morb Mortal Wkly Rep*. 2020;69(24):735–739. DOI: **http://dx.doi.org/10.15585/mmwr.mm6924a2**).

(MenACWY-TT [MenQuadfi, Sanofi Pasteur]) is licensed for use in people 2 years and older. Each is administered intramuscularly as a 0.5-mL dose. Dosing during the primary series varies by product, age, and underlying risk for disease.

Recommendations for use of MenACWY conjugate vaccine are as follows[1] (Tables 3.37 and 3.38):

- Adolescents should be immunized routinely at the 11- through 12-year health care visit (see **https://redbook.solutions.aap.org/SS/Immunization_Schedules. aspx**), when immunization status and other preventive health services can be addressed (Table 3.37). A booster dose at 16 years of age is recommended for adolescents immunized at 11 through 12 years of age.
- Adolescents who receive their first dose at age 13 to 15 years should receive a booster dose at age 16 to 18 years; the booster dose can be administered at any time, as long as a minimum interval of 8 weeks between doses is maintained.
- Adolescents who receive a first dose after their 16th birthday do not need a booster dose unless they become at increased risk for meningococcal disease (Table 3.38).
- People 19 to 21 years of age who have not received a dose after their 16th birthday can receive a single MenACWY dose as part of catch-up vaccination.
- Routine childhood immunization with meningococcal conjugate vaccines is not recommended for children 2 months through 10 years of age because of the low proportion of infections that are preventable with vaccination; approximately two thirds of disease among children 59 months and younger is caused by serogroup B, and MenB vaccines are not approved for use in those ages in the United States.
- People at increased risk of invasive meningococcal disease (defined, by age, in the subgroup column of Table 3.38) should be immunized with a meningococcal conjugate vaccine beginning at 2 months of age. Table 3.38 also details dosing recommendations for each of the three MenACWY vaccines in these increased-risk populations.
- Because of the high risk for invasive pneumococcal disease, children with functional or anatomic asplenia or HIV infection should not be vaccinated with MenACWY-D before age 2 years to avoid interference with the immune response to the 13-valent pneumococcal conjugate vaccine (PCV13); only MenACWY-CRM (Menveo) should be used in this group (see Table 3.38). MenACWY-TT (MenQuadfi) should not be used in this situation because it is only approved in children ≥2 years of age.
- When MenACWY-D is administered 30 days after diphtheria and tetanus toxoids and acellular pertussis (DTaP) vaccine, it interferes with the immune response for all four meningococcal serogroups. Therefore, MenACWY-D should be administered either before or at the same time as DTaP. Alternatively, Menveo or MenQuadfi (if ≥2 years of age) may be administered.

Serogroup B Meningococcal Vaccines. MenB-FHbp (Trumenba, Pfizer) is based on a surface-exposed lipoprotein named factor H binding protein (FHbp). It can be administered as either a 2- or 3-dose series (0 and 6 months or 0, 1–2, and 6 months), depending on risk factors for disease and on outbreak conditions (see Tables 3.37 and 3.38).

MenB-4C (Bexsero, GSK) contains 4 antigenic components: 1 FHbp fusion protein, NadA, NHBA fusion protein, and outer membrane vesicle. It is administered as a 2-dose series (0, ≥1 month [see Tables 3.37 and 3.38]).

[1]Mbaeyi SA, Bozio CH, Duffy J, et al. Meningococcal vaccination: recommendations of the Advisory Committee on Immunization Practices, United States, 2020. *MMWR Recomm Rep.* 2020;69(RR-9):1–41. DOI: **http://dx.doi.org/10.15585/mmwr.rr6909a1**

Table 3.37. Recommended Meningococcal Vaccines for Immunocompetent Children and Adults

Age	Vaccine	Status
Meningococcal ACWY Vaccines		
2 mo through 10 y	MenACWY-D[a] (Menactra, Sanofi Pasteur) or MenACWY-CRM[b] (Menveo, GSK) or MenACWY-TT[c] (MenQuadfi, Sanofi Pasteur)	**Not routinely recommended;** see Table 3.38 (p 528) for recommendations for people at increased risk
11 through 21 y	MenACWY-D or MenACWY-CRM or MenACWY-TT	• 11 through 18 y of age, with first dose at age 11–12 y and booster dose at age 16 y (give booster only if first dose administered prior to 16th birthday) • 19 through 21 y of age, not routinely recommended but may be administered as catch-up immunization for those who have not received a dose after their 16th birthday
Meningococcal B Vaccines		
10 y through 15 y	MenB-FHbp[d] (Trumenba, Pfizer, Inc) or MenB-4C[e] (Bexsero, GSK)	**Not routinely recommended** see Table 3.38 (p 528) for recommendations for people at increased risk
16 y through 23 y	MenB-FHbp or MenB-4C	• Administer based on shared clinical decision-making (formerly called Category B) with preferred age of 16 y through 18 y and 2-dose series recommended • For MenB-4C (Bexsero), dose 1 administered initially, then followed by dose 2 administered ≥1 month later • For MenB-FHbp (Trumenba), dose 1 administered initially, then followed by dose 2 administered 6 months later; in setting of serogroup B meningococcal outbreak, a 3-dose vaccine series administered at 0, 1–2, and 6 months

Table 3.37. Recommended Meningococcal Vaccines for Immunocompetent Children and Adults, continued

Age	Vaccine	Status
	See Table 3.38 (p 528) for recommendations for people at increased risk	

[a] Licensed for people 9 months through 55 years of age but should not be used before 2 y of age in patients with asplenia or HIV to avoid interference with the immune response to the 13-valent pneumococcal conjugate vaccine (PCV13). In all patients (not just those with asplenia or HIV infection), administration of MenACWY-D 30 days after diphtheria and tetanus toxoids and acellular pertussis (DTaP) vaccine interferes with the immune response for all four meningococcal serogroups; therefore, MenACWY-D should be administered either before or at the same time as DTaP, or alternatively one of two other MenACWY vaccines could be used.

[b] Licensed for people 2 months through 55 years of age.

[c] Licensed for people 2 years of age and older.

[d] Licensed for people 10 years through 25 years of age.

[e] Licensed for people 10 years through 25 years of age.

Data on effectiveness against clinical disease endpoints and duration of protection for either vaccine in the age groups for which they are licensed in the United States are limited. Recommendations for use of a serogroup B meningococcal vaccine are as follows[1] (Tables 3.37 and 3.38):

- People 10 years and older at increased risk for meningococcal disease should receive a meningococcal serogroup B vaccine, using the same vaccine for all doses in the vaccination series (Table 3.38). Vaccination may further activate complement, and as a result, patients with complement-mediated diseases may experience increased symptoms of their underlying disease, such as hemolysis, following vaccination.

- A MenB vaccine series may be considered for people 16 through 23 years based on shared clinical decision-making (decided in the context of the provider patient relationship and joint decision-making) with a preferred age at vaccination of 16 through 18 years (Table 3.37). It may be administered with other vaccines at the same visit but at a different injection site.

Immunization During Eculizumab Therapy.[1] Use of complement inhibitors (eg, eculizumab [Soliris] and its long-acting derivative ravulizumab [Ultomiris] monoclonal antibody therapies that block C5) is associated with a substantially increased risk for meningococcal disease. Eculizumab use is associated with an approximately 2000-fold increased incidence of meningococcal disease. Eculizumab and ravulizumab recipients should receive both meningococcal ACWY and meningococcal B vaccines. Because these monoclonal antibodies inhibit terminal complement activation, patients receiving them are still at risk for invasive meningococcal disease even if they develop antibodies following vaccination. Providers therefore should also consider antimicrobial prophylaxis (usually penicillin prophylaxis) for the duration of eculizumab or ravulizumab treatment, and until immunocompetence is restored once the monoclonal antibody therapy is stopped, to potentially reduce the risk for meningococcal disease.

Reimmunization/Booster Doses. Children previously immunized with a meningococcal conjugate vaccine (ACWY or B) who are at ongoing increased risk for meningococcal disease should receive booster immunizations (see Table 3.38). If a child was vaccinated

[1] Mbaeyi SA, Bozio CH, Duffy J, et al. Meningococcal vaccination: recommendations of the Advisory Committee on Immunization Practices, United States, 2020. *MMWR Recomm Rep.* 2020;69(RR-9):1–41. DOI: **http://dx.doi.org/10.15585/mmwr.rr6909a1**

Table 3.38. Recommended Immunization Schedule and Intervals for People at Increased Risk of Invasive Meningococcal Disease[a]

Age	Subgroup	Primary Immunization	Booster Dose
Meningococcal ACWY Vaccines			
2 through 23 mo of age	Children who: • have persistent complement deficiencies • have functional or anatomic asplenia • have human immunodeficiency virus (HIV) infection • travel to or are residents of countries where meningococcal disease is hyperendemic or epidemic • are at risk during a community outbreak attributable to a vaccine serogroup	**MenACWY-CRM (Menveo):** 4 doses at 2, 4, 6, and 12 mo In children initiating vaccination at 7 through 23 mo of age, MenACWY-CRM is to be administered as a 2-dose series, with the second dose administered in the second year of life and at least 3 mo after the first dose **MenACWY-D (Menactra):** MenACWY-D SHOULD NOT BE USED before 2 y of age in children with asplenia or HIV to avoid interference with the immune response to the pneumococcal conjugate vaccine (PCV) series For children aged ≥9 mo who are at increased risk because of complement deficiency, travel or an outbreak, MenACWY-D can be administered as a 2-dose series at 9 and 12 months (3 months apart) **MenACWY-TT (MenQuadfi):** SHOULD NOT BE USED before 2 y of age because not approved in this age group	Person remains at increased risk and first dose received at age: • **2 mo through 6 y of age:** Should receive additional dose of MenACWY 3 y after primary immunization. Boosters should be repeated every 5 y.[b]

Table 3.38. Recommended Immunization Schedule and Intervals for People at Increased Risk of Invasive Meningococcal Disease,[a] continued

Age	Subgroup	Primary Immunization	Booster Dose
≥2 y[d]	People who: • have persistent complement deficiencies • have functional or anatomic asplenia • have HIV infection	2 doses of either **MenACWY-CRM** or **MenACWY-D**[c] or **MenACWY-TT**, 8–12 wk apart **MenACWY-D** (Menactra) may be used if at least 4 wk after completion of PCV doses	• **2 y through 6 y of age:** Should receive additional dose of MenACWY 3 y after primary immunization. Boosters should be repeated every 5 y.[b] • **≥7 y of age:** should receive an additional dose of MenACWY 5 y after primary immunization. Boosters should be repeated every 5 y.[b]
≥2 y[d]	People who: • are at risk during a community outbreak attributable to a vaccine serogroup • travel to or are residents of countries where meningococcal disease is hyperendemic or epidemic • are laboratory workers routinely exposed to isolates of *Neisseria meningitidis*	1 dose of **MenACWY-CRM** or **MenACWY-D**[c] or **MenACWY-TT**	

Table 3.38. Recommended Immunization Schedule and Intervals for People at Increased Risk of Invasive Meningococcal Disease,[a] continued

Age	Subgroup	Primary Immunization	Booster Dose
Meningococcal B Vaccines			
≥10 y[e]	People who: • have persistent complement deficiencies (including complement inhibitor use) • have functional or anatomic asplenia • are laboratory workers routinely exposed to isolates of *Neisseria meningitidis* • are at increased risk, as determined by public health officials, because of a serogroup B meningococcal disease outbreak	2-dose series of **MenB-4C**, ≥1 mo apart OR 3-dose series of **MenB-FHbp**, with 2nd and 3rd doses administered 1–2 and 6 mo after initial doses	For subgroup at increased risk: • Other than outbreak: booster[f] 1 year following completion of a MenB primary series followed by MenB booster every 2–3 years thereafter.[b] • For outbreak: booster[f] if it has been ≥1 year since completion of a MenB primary series (≥6 months interval might also be considered by public health officials).

[a]Includes children who have persistent complement deficiencies (eg, C3, C5-C9, properdin, or factor D or factor H or receiving eculizumab or ravulizumab) or anatomic or functional asplenia; travelers to or residents of countries in which meningococcal disease is hyperendemic or epidemic; and children who are part of a community outbreak of a vaccine-preventable serogroup.

[b]If person remains at increased risk of meningococcal disease.

[c]When MenACWY-D and DTaP are being administered to children 4 through 6 years of age, preference should be given to simultaneous administration of the 2 vaccines or administration of MenACWY-D before administration of DTaP, because administration of MenACWY-D 1 month after Daptacel has been shown to reduce meningococcal antibody response to MenACWY-D. Alternatively, one of two other MenACWY vaccines could be used.

[d]Meningococcal polysaccharide vaccine is no longer available in the United States.

[e]According to the Advisory Committee on Immunization Practices, people >25 years who are at increased risk for meningococcal B disease, can receive MenB vaccine (no preference for MenB vaccine, but same vaccine should be used for full series).

[f]The same MenB vaccine should be used for boosters as was used in the primary series.

with ACWY meningococcal vaccine because of an outbreak or travel at <10 years of age, he or she would still need the adolescent doses. For meningococcal B vaccine, the same meningococcal B vaccine product used in the primary series should be used for booster doses.

Immunization During Outbreaks. During an outbreak, additional cases can occur several weeks or more after onset of disease in the index case; therefore, meningococcal vaccine is recommended when an outbreak is caused by a serogroup prevented by a meningococcal vaccine. For control of meningococcal outbreaks caused by serogroups A, C, W, and Y, the preferred vaccine is a meningococcal conjugate ACWY conjugate vaccine that can be administered to individuals 2 months and older (see Tables 3.37 and 3.38). The CDC Advisory Committee on Immunization Practices (ACIP) has recommended that either of the 2 licensed serogroup B vaccines be used in people 10 years and older during a serogroup B meningococcal disease outbreak; the same vaccine product should be used for all doses.

Adverse Events. Common adverse events after quadrivalent meningococcal conjugate vaccines include pain, erythema, and swelling at the injection site; headache; fatigue; and irritability. Similar adverse effects are observed after MenB vaccines, although effects are more common and may be more severe, and often include myalgia. Syncope can occur after any vaccination and is most common among adolescents and young adults. Adolescents should be seated or lying down during vaccination. Remaining that way *for at least 15 minutes* after immunization could avert many syncopal episodes and secondary injuries. If syncope develops, patients should be observed until symptoms resolve.[1] Syncope following receipt of a vaccine is not a contraindication to subsequent doses.

Pregnant Women.[2] Pregnant and lactating women should receive MenACWY vaccine if indicated. Because limited data are available for MenB vaccination during pregnancy, vaccination with MenB should be deferred unless the woman is at increased risk and, after consultation with her health care provider, the benefits of vaccination are considered to outweigh the potential risks.

Reporting. All confirmed, suspected, and probable cases of invasive meningococcal disease (see Table 3.34) must be immediately reported to the appropriate public health department. Timely reporting can facilitate early administration of chemoprophylaxis to close contacts, recognition and containment of outbreaks, and characterization of isolates so that appropriate prevention recommendations can be implemented rapidly.

Counseling and Public Education. When a case of invasive meningococcal disease is detected, the physician should provide accurate and timely information about meningococcal disease and the risk of transmission to families and contacts of the infected person, provide or arrange for chemoprophylaxis, and contact the public health department. Some experts recommend that patients with invasive meningococcal disease be evaluated for a complement component deficiency; screening can be accomplished with inexpensive CH50 and AH50 testing. If a specific complement component deficiency is detected, patients should receive a MenACWY vaccine series if 2 months or older and a MenB series if 10 years or older. Patients and parents should be counseled about the risk of

[1]Centers for Disease Control and Prevention. Syncope after vaccination—United States, January 2005–July 2007. *MMWR Morb Mortal Wkly Rep.* 2008;57(17):457–460

[2]Mbaeyi SA, Bozio CH, Duffy J, et al. Meningococcal vaccination: recommendations of the Advisory Committee on Immunization Practices, United States, 2020. *MMWR Recomm Rep.* 2020;69(No. RR-9):1–41. DOI: **http://dx.doi.org/10.15585/mmwr.rr6909a1**

recurrent invasive meningococcal disease and the need for immediate medical evaluation when fever develops. Patients on eculizumab or ravulizumab or with other complement deficiencies should be counseled about the risk of invasive infection. Public health questions, such as whether a mass immunization program or an expanded chemoprophylaxis program is needed, should be referred to the local or state public health department. In appropriate situations, early provision of information in collaboration with the health department to schools or affected groups, and to the media may help minimize public anxiety and unrealistic or inappropriate demands for intervention.

Human Metapneumovirus

CLINICAL MANIFESTATIONS: Human metapneumovirus (hMPV) causes acute respiratory tract illness in people of all ages and is one of the leading causes of bronchiolitis in infants. In children, hMPV also causes pneumonia, asthma exacerbations, croup, upper respiratory tract infections (URIs), and acute otitis media; these may be accompanied by fever. As with other respiratory viral infections, secondary bacterial pneumonia can occur. hMPV is associated with acute exacerbations of chronic obstructive pulmonary disease (COPD) and pneumonia in adults. Otherwise healthy, young children infected with hMPV usually have mild or moderate respiratory symptoms, but some young children have severe disease requiring hospitalization. hMPV infection in immunocompromised people can result in severe disease, and fatalities have been reported in hematopoietic stem cell or lung transplant recipients. Preterm birth and underlying cardiopulmonary disease are risk factors for severe disease. Children with a history of birth at gestational age <32 weeks are at higher risk for hospitalization, suffer more severe disease, and require longer stays and more supplementary oxygen. Recurrent infections occur throughout life and, in previously healthy people, are usually mild or asymptomatic.

ETIOLOGY: hMPV is an enveloped single-stranded negative-sense RNA virus in the genus *Metapneumovirus* of the family *Pneumoviridae*. hMPV is divided into 2 major antigenic lineages further subdivided into 2 clades within each lineage (designated A1, A2, B1, and B2) based on sequence differences in the fusion (F) and attachment (G) surface glycoproteins. Viruses from these different clades cocirculate each year in varying proportions.

EPIDEMIOLOGY: Humans are the only source of infection. Spread occurs by direct or close contact with contaminated secretions. Health care-associated infections have been reported.

In temperate climates, hMPV circulation usually occurs during late winter and early spring, overlapping with parts of the respiratory syncytial virus (RSV) season, but typically peaks 1 to 2 months later than RSV. Sporadic infection may occur throughout the year. In otherwise healthy infants, the duration of viral shedding is 1 to 2 weeks. Prolonged shedding (weeks to months) has been reported in severely immunocompromised individuals.

Serologic studies suggest that nearly all children are infected at least once by 5 years of age. The incidence of hospitalizations attributable to hMPV is lower than that attributable to RSV but comparable to that of influenza and parainfluenza 3 in children younger than 5 years. Large studies have shown that hMPV is detected in 5% to 15% of children with medically attended lower respiratory tract illnesses. Overall annual rates of hospitalization associated with hMPV infection are highest in the first year of life but occur throughout childhood. In infants, the peak age of hospitalization is 6 to 12 months (compared with 2 to 3 months for RSV). Coinfection with other respiratory viruses occurs.

The **incubation period** is 3 to 7 days.

DIAGNOSTIC TESTS: Reverse transcriptase-polymerase chain reaction (RT-PCR) assays are the diagnostic method of choice for hMPV. Several RT-PCR assays for hMPV are available commercially and have been cleared for use by the US Food and Drug Administration. These include a test for hMPV alone and multiplexed tests for hMPV with other respiratory pathogens. hMPV is difficult to isolate in cell culture. Direct fluorescent antibody (DFA) testing for hMPV detection in respiratory specimens is available in some reference laboratories, with reported sensitivity of 85%. Serologies are only used in research settings.

TREATMENT: Treatment is supportive. In vitro studies and animal models have shown that ribavirin and some preparations of Immune Globulin Intravenous have activity against hMPV. There are anecdotal reports using these therapies in humans, but there are no controlled clinical data available to assess whether these have any therapeutic benefit, and their use is not routinely recommended. Antimicrobial agents are not indicated in the treatment of infants hospitalized with uncomplicated hMPV bronchiolitis or pneumonia unless evidence exists for the presence of a concurrent bacterial infection. Additional management recommendations for infants with bronchiolitis can be found in the bronchiolitis guidelines from the American Academy of Pediatrics.[1]

ISOLATION OF THE HOSPITALIZED PATIENT: In addition to standard precautions, contact precautions are recommended for the duration of hMPV-associated illness. Prolonged shedding of virus in respiratory tract secretions may occur, particularly in immunocompromised people, and the duration of contact precautions should be extended in these situations.

CONTROL MEASURES: Appropriate respiratory hygiene and cough etiquette should be followed. Control of health care-associated hMPV infection depends on adherence to contact precautions. Exposure to hMPV-infected people, including other patients, staff, and family members, may not be recognized, because illness may be mild.

Preventive measures include limiting exposure to settings where contact with hMPV may occur (eg, child care centers) and emphasizing hand hygiene in all settings, including the home, especially when contacts of high-risk children have respiratory tract infections.

Microsporidia Infections
(Microsporidiosis)

CLINICAL MANIFESTATIONS: Microsporidia infections can be asymptomatic; patients with symptomatic intestinal infection have watery, nonbloody diarrhea; nausea; and diffuse abdominal pain. Abdominal cramping can occur. Symptomatic intestinal infection, often protracted diarrhea, is most common in immunocompromised people, especially in organ transplant recipients and people who are infected with human immunodeficiency virus (HIV) with low CD4+ lymphocyte counts (<100 cells/μL). Complications include malnutrition, progressive weight loss, and failure to thrive. Different infecting microsporidia species may result in different clinical manifestations, including ocular, biliary cerebral, respiratory, muscle, and genitourinary involvement (see Table 3.39). Chronic infection in immunocompetent people is rare.

---

[1]American Academy of Pediatrics, Subcommittee on Diagnosis and Management of Bronchiolitis. Clinical practice guideline: the diagnosis, management, and prevention of bronchiolitis. *Pediatrics.* 2014;134(5):e1474-e1502

Table 3.39. Clinical Manifestations of Microsporidia Infections

Microsporidia species	Clinical Manifestation
Anncaliia algerae	Myositis, ocular infection, cellulitis myositis
Anncaliia connori	Disseminated disease
Anncaliia vesicularum	Myositis
Encephalitozoon cuniculi	Infection of the respiratory and genitourinary tract, disseminated infection
Encephalitozoon hellem	Ocular infection
Encephalitozoon intestinalis	Infection of the gastrointestinal tract causing diarrhea, and dissemination to ocular, genitourinary, and respiratory tracts
Enterocytozoon bieneusi	Diarrhea, acalculous cholecystitis
Microsporidium species *(M africanum* and *M ceylonensis)*	Ocular infection
Nosema species *(N ocularum)*	Ocular infection
Pleistophora species	Myositis
Trachipleistophora anthropophthera	Disseminated infection, encephalitis, ocular infection
Trachipleistophora hominis	myositis, sinusitis, encephalitis, ocular infection
Tubulinosema acridophagus	Disseminated infection, myositis
Vittaforma corneae	Ocular infection, urinary tract infection

Adapted from: Han B, Weiss LM. Microsporidia: obligate intracellular pathogens within the fungal kingdom. *Microbiol Spectr.* 2017;5(2). DOI: **10.1128/microbiolspec.FUNK-0018-2016**
See also: **www.cdc.gov/dpdx/microsporidiosis/**

ETIOLOGY: Microsporidia are obligate intracellular, spore-forming organisms classified as fungi. More than 1400 species belonging to about 200 genera have been identified with at least 15 reported in human infection (Table 3.39). *Enterocytozoon bieneusi* and *Encephalitozoon intestinalis* are the most commonly reported pathogens in humans and are most often associated with chronic diarrhea in HIV-infected people.

EPIDEMIOLOGY: Most microsporidia infections are transmitted by oral ingestion of spores. *Microsporidium* spores commonly are found in surface water, and strains responsible for human infection have been identified in municipal water supplies and ground water. Spores can survive for extended periods in the environment. Several studies indicate that waterborne transmission occurs. Donor-derived infections in organ transplant recipients have been documented. Person-to-person spread by the fecal-oral route also occurs. Spores also have been detected in other body fluids, but their role in transmission is unknown. Data suggest the possibility of zoonotic transmission.

The **incubation period** is unknown.

DIAGNOSTIC TESTS: Infection with gastrointestinal tract microsporidia can be documented by microscopic identification of spores in stool or biopsy specimens. The laboratory should be alerted and specific stains for microsporidia should be requested, because routine ova and parasite examination usually does not detect microsporidia spores. Microsporidia spores can be detected in formalin-fixed or unfixed stool, other fluid, or tissue specimens stained with a chromotrope-based stain (a modification of the trichrome stain) and examined by an experienced microscopist. Fluorescent techniques including calcofluor or Fungi-Fluor also can be used to detect organisms in stool or tissue sections. Identification and diagnostic confirmation of species requires transmission electron microscopy or molecular methods (polymerase chain reaction), which are available through the Centers for Disease Control and Prevention for some common species. Isolation of select microsporidia species has been accomplished using cell culture. The value of serologic testing, when available, has not been substantiated.

TREATMENT: Restoration of immune function is critical for control of microsporidia infection. Effective antiretroviral therapy is the primary initial treatment for these infections in people infected with HIV and can result in resolution of symptoms even without specific therapy against microsporidia. Albendazole is the drug of choice for infections caused by microsporidia other than *E bieneusi* and *Vittaforma corneae* infections, which may respond to fumagillin. Studies in children as young as 1 year of age suggest that albendazole can be administered safely to this population. Fumagillin for systemic use is not available in the United States; it is associated with bone marrow toxicity, and recurrence of diarrhea is common after therapy is discontinued. Limited data suggest that nitazoxanide may be effective for treatment of *E bieneusi* gastroenteritis. None of these therapies have been studied in children with microsporidia infection. Topical voriconazole (1%), as well as topical fluoroquinolones have been reported effective for treatment of microsporidial ocular infection, but more study is needed. Supportive care for malnutrition and dehydration may be necessary. Antimotility agents may be useful to control chronic diarrhea.

ISOLATION OF THE HOSPITALIZED PATIENT: In addition to standard precautions, contact precautions are recommended for diapered and incontinent children for the duration of illness.

CONTROL MEASURES: In HIV-infected and other immunocompromised people, attention to hand hygiene, drinking bottled or boiled water, and avoiding unpeeled fruits and vegetables may decrease exposure. No chemoprophylactic regimens are known to be effective in preventing microsporidiosis, although continuation of treatment regimens is recommended as secondary prophylaxis in HIV-infected individuals until immune reconstitution.

Molluscum Contagiosum

CLINICAL MANIFESTATIONS: Molluscum contagiosum is a benign viral infection of the skin with no systemic manifestations. It usually is characterized by 1 to 20 discrete, 2- to 5-mm-diameter, flesh-colored to translucent, dome-shaped papules, some with central umbilication. Lesions commonly occur on the trunk, face, and extremities but rarely are generalized. Molluscum contagiosum is a self-limited epidermal infection with individual lesions often spontaneously resolving in 6 to 12 months but some taking as long as 3 to 4 years to disappear completely. An eczematous reaction (molluscum dermatitis) encircling the lesions is common. People with atopic dermatitis and immunocompromising conditions, including human immunodeficiency virus infection and patients with congenital DOCK8 deficiency or CARD11 mutations, tend to have more widespread and prolonged eruptions, which often are recalcitrant to therapy.

ETIOLOGY: Molluscum contagiosum virus (MCV) is the sole member of the genus *Molluscipoxvirus*, family *Poxviridae*. DNA subtypes of MCV can be differentiated, but the specific subtype probably is insignificant in pathogenesis. Other poxviruses include the agents of smallpox, monkeypox, vaccinia, and cowpox.

EPIDEMIOLOGY: Humans are the only known source of the virus, which is spread by direct contact, scratching, shaving, sexual contact, or fomites. Vertical transmission has been linked with neonatal molluscum contagiosum infection. Lesions can be disseminated by autoinoculation. Infectivity generally is low, but occasional outbreaks may occur in facilities such as child care centers. The period of communicability is unknown.

The **incubation period** is generally between 2 and 7 weeks but may be as long as 6 months.

DIAGNOSTIC TESTS: The diagnosis usually can be made clinically from the characteristic appearance of umbilicated papules. Wright or Giemsa staining of cells expressed from the central core of a lesion reveals characteristic intracytoplasmic inclusions. Electron microscopic examination of these cells identifies typical poxvirus particles. The virus does not grow readily in culture. Serologic testing is not available routinely for clinical practice. If uncertainty persists in the differential diagnosis (eg, warts, trichoepithelioma, tuberous sclerosis), nucleic acid testing by polymerase chain reaction is available at certain reference centers. Adolescents and young adults with genital molluscum contagiosum should prompt a screening for other sexually transmitted diseases.

TREATMENT: There is no consensus on management of molluscum contagiosum in children and adolescents. Genital lesions in older patients should be treated to prevent spread to sexual contacts. Treatment of nongenital lesions is sometimes provided for cosmetic reasons. Lesions in healthy people typically are self-limited, so treatment may be unnecessary. However, therapy may be warranted to: (1) alleviate discomfort, including itching; (2) reduce autoinoculation; (3) limit transmission of the virus to close contacts; (4) reduce cosmetic concerns; and (5) prevent secondary infection.

Physical destruction of the lesions is the most rapid and effective means of curing molluscum contagiosum. Modalities available include curettage, cryodestruction with liquid nitrogen, electrodesiccation, and chemical agents designed to initiate a local inflammatory response (podophyllin, tretinoin, cantharidin, 25%–50% trichloroacetic acid, liquefied phenol, silver nitrate, tincture of iodine, or potassium hydroxide). Most data available for any of these modalities are anecdotal. Randomized trials generally are limited because of small sample sizes, and no therapies are approved by the US Food and Drug Administration. When treatment is desired, the most support exists for cryotherapy, curettage, or cantharidin. These treatments require an experienced provider, as they can result in postprocedural pain, irritation, dyspigmentation, and scarring. Because physical destruction of the lesions is painful, appropriate local anesthesia may be required, particularly in young children.

Cidofovir is a cytosine nucleotide analogue with in vitro activity against molluscum contagiosum; successful intravenous treatment of immunocompromised adults with severe involvement has been reported. However, use of cidofovir should be reserved for extreme cases because of potential carcinogenicity and known toxicities (neutropenia and potentially permanent nephrotoxicity) associated with systemic administration of cidofovir. Successful treatment using compounded formulations of topical cidofovir has been reported in both adult and pediatric cases, most of whom were immunocompromised.

Solitary genital lesions in children usually are not acquired by sexual transmission and do not necessarily denote sexual abuse, as other modes of direct contact with the virus, including autoinoculation, may result in genital infection.

ISOLATION OF THE HOSPITALIZED PATIENT: Standard precautions are recommended.

CONTROL MEASURES: No control measures are known for isolated cases. For outbreaks, which are common in the tropics, restricting direct person-to-person contact and sharing of potentially contaminated fomites, such as towels and bedding, may decrease spread. Molluscum contagiosum should not prevent a child from attending child care or school or from swimming in public pools. Covering lesions is not necessary for child care, but when possible, localized lesions not covered by clothing may be covered with a gas-permeable dressing followed by under wrap and tape when participating in sports activities.[1] When children will be entering swimming pools, a watertight bandage can be placed on visible lesions.

Moraxella catarrhalis Infections

CLINICAL MANIFESTATIONS: *Moraxella catarrhalis* is commonly implicated in acute otitis media (AOM), otitis media with effusion, and sinusitis. AOM caused by *M catarrhalis* occurs predominantly in younger infants and frequently is recovered from middle ear and sinuses as part of mixed infections. Since introduction of 13-valent pneumococcal conjugate vaccine (PCV13), *M catarrhalis* appears to be recovered in a greater proportion of children undergoing tympanocentesis; however, it is unclear whether this represents an increase in cases attributable to *M catarrhalis* or a decrease in pneumococcal disease. *M catarrhalis* can cause pneumonia with or without bacteremia in immunocompetent infants and young children but is more common in children with chronic lung disease or impaired host defenses, such as leukemia with neutropenia or congenital immunodeficiency. In immunocompromised children, often no focus of infection is identified. Other clinical manifestations include hypotension with or without a rash indistinguishable from that observed in meningococcemia, neonatal meningitis, and focal infections, such as preseptal cellulitis, bacterial tracheitis, urethritis, osteomyelitis, or septic arthritis. Rare manifestations include endocarditis, peritonitis, shunt-associated ventriculitis, meningitis, and mastoiditis. Health care-acquired *M catarrhalis* bacteremia has been reported in hospitalized children with transnasal devices (nasogastric tube, elemental diet tube, or nasotracheal tube); foci of infection in these cases have included pneumonia or bronchitis. Other health care-associated outbreaks of *M catarrhalis* have been described.

ETIOLOGY: *M catarrhalis* is a gram-negative aerobic diplococcus.

EPIDEMIOLOGY: *M catarrhalis* is part of the normal microbiota of the upper respiratory tract of humans. At least two thirds of children are colonized within the first year of life. The mode of transmission is presumed to be direct contact with contaminated respiratory tract secretions or droplet spread. Infection is most common in infants and young children but also occurs in immunocompromised people at all ages. The duration of carriage by children with infection or colonization and the period of communicability are unknown. Recent studies suggest early colonization with *M catarrhalis* is associated with a stable microbiome and low risk for recurrent respiratory tract infection.

---

[1] Davies HH, Jackson MA, Rice SG; American Academy of Pediatrics, Committee on Infectious Diseases. Infectious diseases associated with organized sports and outbreak control. *Pediatrics.* 2017;140(4):e20172477

DIAGNOSTIC TESTS: The organism can be isolated on blood or chocolate agar culture media after incubation in air or with increased carbon dioxide. On Gram stain, *Moraxella* species are short and plump gram-negative cocci, usually occurring in pairs or short chains, and are mostly catalase and cytochrome oxidase positive. Polymerase chain reaction tests for *M catarrhalis* have been developed but currently are used for research purposes only.

TREATMENT: Almost all strains of *Moraxella* species produce beta-lactamase and are resistant to amoxicillin, unlike other common pathogens causing acute otitis media. *M catarrhalis* are typically susceptible to ampicillin-sulbactam (and amoxicillin-clavulanate), second- or third-generation cephalosporins, trimethoprim sulfamethoxazole, macrolides, and fluoroquinolones. Empiric and definitive therapy will depend on the severity of illness and type of infection, immunocompetence of the patient, and susceptibility of the isolate. The organism is resistant to clindamycin, vancomycin, and oxacillin. Macrolide-resistant isolates have been reported from Asia; only rarely have resistant strains been identified in the United States or Western Europe.

ISOLATION OF THE HOSPITALIZED PATIENT: Standard precautions are recommended.

CONTROL MEASURES: None.

Mumps

CLINICAL MANIFESTATIONS: Mumps is a systemic disease characterized by swelling of one or more of the salivary glands, usually the parotid glands. Approximately one fifth of infections in unvaccinated people may be asymptomatic. The frequency of asymptomatic infection in vaccinated persons is unknown, but mumps symptoms are usually milder and complications less common among vaccinated people. Orchitis is the most frequently reported complication and occurs in approximately 30% of unvaccinated and 6% of vaccinated postpubertal men. Approximately half of patients with mumps orchitis develop testicular atrophy of affected testicles. More than 50% of people with mumps have cerebrospinal fluid pleocytosis, but fewer than 1% have symptoms of viral meningitis. Uncommon complications include oophoritis, pancreatitis, encephalitis, hearing loss (either transient or permanent), arthritis, thyroiditis, mastitis, glomerulonephritis, myocarditis, endocardial fibroelastosis, thrombocytopenia, cerebellar ataxia, and transverse myelitis. Emergence of contralateral parotitis within weeks to months after apparent recovery has been described. In the absence of an immunization program, mumps typically occurs during childhood. Infection in adults is more likely to result in complications. Although mumps virus can cross the placenta, no evidence exists that this transmission results in congenital malformation.

ETIOLOGY: Mumps is an enveloped RNA virus with 12 genotypes in the genus *Rubulavirus* in the family *Paramyxoviridae*. The genus also includes human parainfluenza virus types 2 and 4. Other common infectious causes of parotitis include Epstein-Barr virus, cytomegalovirus, parainfluenza virus types 1 and 3, influenza A virus, enteroviruses, lymphocytic choriomeningitis virus, human immunodeficiency virus (HIV), nontuberculous mycobacterium, and gram-positive and gram-negative bacteria.

EPIDEMIOLOGY: Mumps occurs worldwide, and humans are the only known natural hosts. The virus is spread by contact with infectious respiratory tract secretions and saliva. Mumps virus is the only known cause of epidemic parotitis. Historically, the peak incidence of mumps was between January and May and among children younger than 10 years. Mumps vaccine was licensed in the United States in 1967 and recommended for routine childhood immunization in 1977. After implementation of the 2-dose measles, mumps, and rubella vaccine (MMR) recommendation in 1989 for measles control in the United States, mumps further declined to extremely low levels, with an incidence of 0.1/100 000 by 1999. From 2000 to 2005, there were fewer than 300 reported cases per year. However, since then, there has been an increase in the number of reported mumps cases with peak years in 2006, 2016-2017 (more than 6000 cases each year), and 2019 (more than 3000 cases). The majority of cases during these peak years were among college-aged young adults and persons who previously received 2 doses of MMR vaccine.

The **incubation period** usually is 16 to 18 days, but cases may occur from 12 to 25 days after exposure. The period of maximum communicability begins several days before parotitis onset. The recommended isolation period is 5 days after onset of parotid swelling. However, virus has been detected in patients' saliva as early as 7 days before and until 9 days after onset of swelling. Mumps virus has been isolated from urine and seminal fluids up to 14 days after onset of parotitis.

DIAGNOSTIC TESTS: Unvaccinated and vaccinated people with parotitis, orchitis, or oophoritis without other apparent cause should undergo diagnostic testing to confirm mumps virus as the cause. Mumps can be confirmed by detection of mumps virus nucleic acid by quantitative reverse transcriptase-polymerase chain reaction (RT-qPCR) assay in buccal swab specimens (Stenson duct exudates), throat or oral swab specimens, urine, or cerebrospinal fluid. The parotid should be massaged for 30 seconds prior to buccal swab specimen collection. The mumps RT-qPCR test developed by the Centers for Disease Control and Prevention (CDC) and available at the CDC, many state public health departments, and the Vaccine Preventable Disease Reference Centers (VPD-RC) is sensitive and specific. Other RT-PCR assays for mumps may be available at clinical or commercial laboratories, but the performance measures of these tests are unknown. Mumps virus may be isolated in cell culture using a variety of cell types, using either standard or rapid isolation and identification techniques. However, RT-qPCR is the preferred test for confirmation of mumps infection. Failure to detect mumps virus RNA by RT-PCR in samples from a person with clinically compatible mumps symptoms does not rule out mumps as a diagnosis. Vaccinated individuals may shed virus for a shorter period and may shed smaller amounts of virus.

Testing for mumps-specific immunoglobulin (Ig) M antibody, IgG seroconversion, or a significant increase between acute and convalescent IgG antibody titer can also aid in the diagnosis of mumps, but these serologic assays do not confirm a diagnosis of mumps. In previously vaccinated patients who acquire mumps, IgM response may be transient, delayed, or not detected. Collection of serum 3 to 10 days after parotitis onset improves the ability to detect IgM. A negative IgM in a person with clinically compatible mumps symptoms does not rule out mumps as a diagnosis. In vaccinated patients, collection of acute and convalescent phase serum samples to demonstrate a fourfold increase in IgG titer is not recommended, because by the time of onset of symptoms, IgG titers may already be elevated such that detection of a fourfold increase in titer is not possible.

To distinguish wild-type mumps virus from vaccine virus in a person with clinically compatible mumps symptoms who was recently vaccinated, it is necessary to obtain a buccal/oral swab specimen for genotyping. Serologic tests cannot differentiate between an exposure to vaccine and an exposure to wild-type mumps virus.

TREATMENT: Management is supportive.

ISOLATION OF THE HOSPITALIZED PATIENT: In addition to standard precautions, droplet precautions are recommended until 5 days after onset of parotid swelling.

CONTROL MEASURES: Mumps is a nationally notifiable disease in the United States.

Evidence of Immunity to Mumps.[1] Presumptive evidence of immunity to mumps includes any of the following:

1. Documentation of age-appropriate vaccination with a live mumps virus-containing vaccine:
   - Preschool-aged children: 1 dose after their first birthday;
   - School-aged children (grades K–12) and adults at high risk (ie, health care personnel, international travelers, and students at postsecondary educational institutions): 2 doses after their first birthday, with the second dose administered at least 28 days after the first dose;
   - Adults not at high risk: 1 dose;
2. Laboratory evidence of immunity (note: although the presence of mumps-specific IgG is considered evidence of prior exposure to mumps vaccine or mumps virus and is considered evidence of immunity for most situations [eg, employment or school vaccine requirements], it does not necessarily predict protection against mumps disease);
3. Laboratory confirmation of disease; or
4. Born before 1957 (note: health care workers of any age are not considered immune unless they have had 2 immunizations separated by at least 28 days or have serologic evidence of immunity).

School and Child Care. Children and young adults should be excluded for 5 days from onset of parotid gland swelling. When determining means to control outbreaks, exclusion of students without evidence of immunity from affected schools and schools judged by local public health authorities to be at risk of transmission should be considered. If implemented, unimmunized students should be excluded until at least 26 days after onset of parotitis in the last person with mumps. Excluded students can be readmitted immediately after receipt of a dose of MMR vaccine.

Care of Exposed People. Mumps vaccine has not been demonstrated to be effective in preventing infection or decreasing the severity of infection if administered after exposure. However, people without evidence of immunity who are exposed to mumps still should receive MMR vaccine (or measles, mumps, rubella, and varicella vaccine [MMRV], if 12 months through 12 years of age), because immunization will provide protection against subsequent exposures. Immunization during the incubation period presents no increased risk of adverse events. Immune Globulin (IG) preparations are not effective as postexposure prophylaxis for mumps.

During an outbreak, all people should be brought up to date on age-appropriate vaccinations (1 dose or 2 doses, depending on age). Health care workers of any age are not considered immune unless they have had 2 immunizations separated by at least 28 days or have serologic evidence of immunity. Public health authorities might also recommend that people who belong to groups at increased risk for mumps receive an additional dose of MMR to improve protection against mumps disease and related complications (second

---

[1]Centers for Disease Control and Prevention. Prevention of measles, rubella, congenital rubella syndrome, and mumps, 2013 summary: recommendations of the Advisory Committee on Immunization Practices (ACIP). *MMWR Recomm Rep.* 2013;62(RR-4):1-34

dose for people previously vaccinated with 1 dose or a third dose for people previously vaccinated with 2 doses). People who have evidence of presumptive immunity other than documented 2 doses of MMR vaccine should also receive a dose if determined to be part of a group at increased risk. Public health authorities will communicate to providers which groups are at increased risk and should receive a dose. Active and passive surveillance have not identified any new or unexpected short-term safety concerns following receipt of a third dose of mumps-containing vaccine.

Mumps Vaccine. Live attenuated mumps vaccine containing the Jeryl-Lynn strain (genotype A) has been licensed in the United States since 1967. Vaccine is administered by subcutaneous injection of 0.5 mL of MMR vaccine (licensed for people 12 months or older) or MMRV vaccine (licensed for children 12 months through 12 years of age). Monovalent mumps vaccine no longer is available in the United States.

Vaccine Recommendations.
- The first dose of MMR or MMRV (see MMRV-specific recommendations in Varicella-Zoster Infections, p 831) should be administered routinely to children at 12 through 15 months of age, with a second dose of MMR or MMRV administered at 4 through 6 years of age. The second dose of MMR or MMRV may be administered before 4 years of age, provided at least 28 days have elapsed since the first dose. MMR or MMRV is not harmful if administered to a person already immune to one or more of the viruses from previous infection or immunization.
- People should be immunized unless they have evidence of mumps immunity (p 540). Adequate immunization is 2 doses of mumps-containing vaccine ($\geq$28 days apart) for school-aged children and adults at high risk (ie, health care personnel, students at postsecondary educational institutions, and international travelers). Because mumps is endemic throughout most of the world, unless they have evidence of immunity, people 12 months or older should be offered 2 doses of MMR vaccine before beginning travel. Children younger than 12 months need not receive mumps vaccine before travel, but they may receive it as MMR vaccine starting at 6 months of age if measles immunization is indicated. If a child receives a dose of mumps vaccine before 12 months of age, this dose is not counted toward the recommended number of doses, and 2 additional doses are recommended beginning at 12 through 15 months of age and separated by at least 28 days.
- During a mumps outbreak, people previously vaccinated with 2 doses who are identified by public health authorities as being part of a group or population at increased risk for acquiring mumps should receive a third dose of MMR vaccine (or MMRV if age appropriate). People who have evidence of presumptive immunity for mumps other than receipt of 2 doses also should receive a dose of MMR vaccine (or MMRV if age appropriate) if they are part of the group at increased risk. No additional dose is recommended for people who already received 3 or more doses before the outbreak.
- Health care personnel born before 1957 should receive 2 doses of MMR vaccine unless they have laboratory evidence of immunity or disease.
- A mumps-containing vaccine may be administered with other vaccines at different injection sites and with separate syringes (see Simultaneous Administration of Multiple Vaccines, p 36).
- Vaccine documentation is required in multiple states for attendance in lower and higher educational institutions and is an effective public health tool to maximize immunization rates.

Adverse Reactions. Adverse reactions associated with the mumps component of US-licensed MMR or MMRV vaccines are rare. Orchitis, parotitis, and low-grade fever may occur. Causality has not been established for temporally related reactions, including nerve deafness, aseptic meningitis, encephalitis, rash, pruritus, and purpura. Allergic reactions also are rare (see Measles, Precautions and Contraindications [p 516], and Rubella, Precautions and Contraindications [p 654]). Other reactions that occur after immunization with MMR or MMRV vaccine may be attributable to other components of the vaccines (see Adverse Event sections in Measles, p 515, Rubella, p 654, and Varicella-Zoster Infections, p 840, chapters).

A second dose of MMR or MMRV is not associated with an increased incidence of reactions relative to the first dose.

Precautions and Contraindications. See Measles, p 516, Rubella, p 654, and, if MMRV is used, Varicella-Zoster Infections, p 841.

Febrile Illness. Children with minor illnesses, such as upper respiratory tract infections, should be immunized. Fever is not a contraindication to immunization. However, if other manifestations suggest a more serious illness, the child should not be immunized until recovered.

Allergies. Hypersensitivity reactions occur rarely and usually are minor, consisting of wheal-and-flare reactions or urticaria at the injection site. Reactions have been attributed to trace amounts of neomycin or gelatin or some other component in the vaccine formulation.

Anaphylaxis is rare. MMR and MMRV are produced in chicken embryo cell culture and do not contain significant amounts of egg white (ovalbumin) cross-reacting proteins, so children with egg allergy are at low risk of anaphylactic reactions. Skin testing of children for egg allergy is not predictive of reactions to MMR or MMRV vaccine and, therefore, is not required before administering vaccine. People with allergies to chickens or feathers are not at increased risk of reaction to the vaccine. People who have experienced anaphylactic reactions to gelatin or topically or systemically administered neomycin should receive mumps vaccine only in settings where such reactions could be managed and after consultation with an allergist or immunologist. Most often, however, neomycin allergy manifests as contact dermatitis, which is not a contraindication to receiving mumps vaccine (see Measles, p 516).

Recent Administration of IG. Administration of MMR or MMRV vaccine should be delayed from 3 to 11 months following receipt of specific blood products or IG (see Table 1.11, p 40). MMR vaccine should be administered at least 2 weeks before planned administration of IG, blood transfusion, or other blood products because of the theoretical possibility that antibody will neutralize vaccine virus and interfere with successful immunization; if IG must be administered within 14 days after administration of MMR or MMRV, these vaccines should be readministered after the interval specified in Table 1.11 (p 40).

Altered Immunity. Patients with immunodeficiency diseases and those receiving immunosuppressive therapy or expected to receive such therapy within 4 weeks, including high doses of systemically administered corticosteroids, alkylating agents, antimetabolites, or radiation, or people who otherwise are immunocompromised should not receive live attenuated vaccines including MMR or MMRV (see Immunization and Other Considerations in Immunocompromised Children, p 72).

Exceptions are patients with human immunodeficiency virus (HIV) infection who are not severely immunocompromised. The live-virus MMR vaccine can be administered to asymptomatic HIV-infected children and adolescents without severe immunosuppression. For vaccination purposes, severe immunosuppression is defined in children 1 through 13 years of age as a CD4+ T-lymphocyte percentage <15% and in adolescents ≥14 years as a CD4+ T-lymphocyte count <200 lymphocytes/mm^3. Severely immunocompromised HIV-infected infants, children, adolescents, and young adults should not receive measles virus-containing vaccine. The quadrivalent MMRV vaccine should not be administered to any HIV-infected infant, regardless of degree of immunosuppression, because of lack of safety data in this population (see Human Immunodeficiency Virus Infection, p 427).

The risk of mumps exposure for patients with altered immunity can be decreased by immunizing their close susceptible (ie, household) contacts. Vaccine recipients cannot transmit mumps vaccine virus.

After cessation of immunosuppressive therapy, MMR immunization should be deferred for at least 3 months (with the exception of corticosteroid recipients [see next paragraph]). This interval is based on the assumptions that immunologic responsiveness will have been restored in 3 months and the underlying disease for which immunosuppressive therapy was given is in remission or under control. However, because the interval can vary with the intensity and type of immunosuppressive therapy, radiation therapy, underlying disease, and other factors, a definitive recommendation for an interval after cessation of immunosuppressive therapy when mumps vaccine (as MMR) can be administered safely and effectively often is not possible.

Corticosteroids. Children receiving ≥2 mg/kg per day of prednisone or its equivalent, or ≥20 mg/day if they weigh 10 kg or more, for 14 days or more and who otherwise are not immunocompromised should not receive live-virus vaccines until 4 weeks after discontinuation (see Immunization and Other Considerations in Immunocompromised Children, p 72).

Pregnancy. Conception should be avoided for 4 weeks after mumps immunization because of the theoretical risk associated with live-virus vaccine. Susceptible postpubertal females should not be immunized if they are known to be pregnant. However, mumps immunization during pregnancy has not been associated with congenital malformations (see Immunization in Pregnancy, p 69).

Mycoplasma pneumoniae and Other *Mycoplasma* Species Infections

CLINICAL MANIFESTATIONS: *Mycoplasma pneumoniae* is a frequent cause of upper and lower respiratory tract infections in children, including pharyngitis, acute bronchitis, and pneumonia. Acute otitis media is uncommon. Bullous myringitis, once considered pathognomonic for mycoplasma, now is known to occur with other pathogens as well. Sinusitis and croup are rare. Symptoms are variable and include cough, malaise, fever, and occasionally headache. Acute bronchitis and upper respiratory tract illness caused by *M pneumoniae* generally are mild and self-limited. Approximately 25% of infected school-aged children will develop pneumonia with cough and rales on physical examination within days after onset of constitutional symptoms. Cough, initially nonproductive, can become productive, persist for 3 to 4 weeks, and be accompanied by wheezing. Approximately 10% of children with *M pneumoniae* infection will exhibit a rash, which most often is maculopapular. Radiographic abnormalities are variable; bilateral diffuse infiltrates or focal abnormalities, such as consolidation, effusion, or hilar adenopathy, can occur.

Unusual manifestations include nervous system disease (eg, aseptic meningitis, encephalitis, acute disseminated encephalomyelitis, cerebellar ataxia, transverse myelitis, and peripheral neuropathy) as well as myocarditis, pericarditis, arthritis (particularly in immunocompromised hosts), erythema nodosum, polymorphous mucocutaneous eruptions (eg, Stevens-Johnson syndrome or *Mycoplasma*-induced rash and mucositis [MIRM] syndrome), hemolytic anemia, thrombocytopenic purpura, and hemophagocytic syndromes. Severe pneumonia with pleural effusion can occur, particularly in patients with sickle cell disease, Down syndrome, immunodeficiencies, and chronic cardiorespiratory disease. Acute chest syndrome and pneumonia have been associated with *M pneumoniae* in patients with sickle cell disease. Infection also has been associated with exacerbations of asthma.

Several other *Mycoplasma* species colonize mucosal surfaces of humans and can produce disease in children. *Mycoplasma hominis* infection has been reported in neonates and children (both immunocompetent and immunocompromised). Intra-abdominal abscess, septic arthritis, endocarditis, pneumonia, meningoencephalitis, brain abscess, and surgical wound infection have been reported to be attributable to *M hominis*. *Mycoplasma genitalium* is now the second most common cause of nongonococcal urethritis in sexually active adolescents and adults with a frequency only slightly lower than *Chlamydia trachomatis*.

ETIOLOGY: Mycoplasmas are pleomorphic bacteria that lack a cell wall. They are classified in the family *Mycoplasmataceae*, which includes the *Mycoplasma* and *Ureaplasma* genera.

EPIDEMIOLOGY: Mycoplasmas are ubiquitous in animals and plants, but *M pneumoniae* causes disease only in humans. *M pneumoniae* is transmissible by respiratory droplets during close contact with a symptomatic person. Outbreaks have been described in hospitals, military bases, colleges, and summer camps. Occasionally, *M pneumoniae* causes ventilator-associated pneumonia. *M pneumoniae* is a leading cause of pneumonia in school-aged children and young adults but is an infrequent cause of community-acquired pneumonia (CAP) in children younger than 5 years. In the United States, an estimated 2 million infections are caused by *M pneumoniae* each year. Overall, approximately 10% to 20% of cases of CAP in hospitalized patients are believed to be caused by *M pneumoniae*. Infections occur throughout the world, in any season, and in all geographic settings. In family studies, approximately 30% of household contacts develop pneumonia. Asymptomatic carriage after infection may occur for weeks to months. Immunity after infection is not long lasting.

The **incubation period** usually is 2 to 3 weeks (range, 1–4 weeks), which can contribute to lengthy outbreaks.

DIAGNOSTIC TESTS: Nucleic acid amplification tests (NAATs), including polymerase chain reaction (PCR) tests for *M pneumoniae*, are available commercially and increasingly are replacing other tests, because PCR tests performed on respiratory tract specimens (nasal wash, nasopharyngeal swab, oropharyngeal swab, sputum, and bronchoalveolar lavage fluid) are rapid, have sensitivity and specificity between 80% and 100%, and yield positive results earlier in the course of illness. Several assays are cleared by the US Food and Drug Administration (FDA) for diagnostic use, including an assay targeting *M pneumoniae* alone and multiplex assays that simultaneously target other respiratory pathogens as well. Identification of *M pneumoniae* by NAAT or culture in a patient with compatible clinical manifestations suggests causation. However, attributing a nonclassic clinical disorder to *M pneumoniae* is problematic, because the organism can colonize the respiratory tract for several weeks after acute infection (even after appropriate antimicrobial therapy) and has been detected by PCR in 17% to 25% of asymptomatic children 3 months to 16 years of age. PCR assay of body fluids for *M hominis* is available at reference laboratories and may be helpful diagnostically.

Serologic tests using immunofluorescence and enzyme immunoassays that detect *M pneumoniae*-specific immunoglobulin (Ig) M, IgA, and IgG antibodies are available commercially. IgM antibodies generally are not detectable within the first 7 days after onset of symptoms. Although the presence of IgM antibodies may indicate recent *M pneumoniae* infection, false-positive test results occur, and antibodies may persist in serum for several months or even years and thus may not indicate acute infection. IgM antibodies may not be elevated in older children and adults who have had recurrent *M pneumoniae* infection. Serologic diagnosis is best accomplished by demonstrating a fourfold or greater increase in IgG antibody titer between acute and convalescent serum specimens. Complement-fixation assay results should be interpreted cautiously, because the assay is both less sensitive and less specific than is immunofluorescent assay or enzyme immunoassay. Measurement of serum cold hemagglutinin titer has limited value, because titers of $\geq 1:64$ are present in only 50% to 75% of patients with pneumonia caused by *M pneumoniae*, and lower titers are nonspecifically present during respiratory viral infections.

Mycoplasma organisms are not visible by cell-wall specific stains (eg, Gram stain) using light microscopy. *M pneumoniae* and *M hominis* can be grown in special enriched broth and agar media such as SP4 or on commercially available mixed liquid broth/agar slant media. However, most clinical laboratories lack the capacity to perform culture isolation; culture and identification may take longer than 21 days. *M genitalium* can be cultured in only a handful of laboratories in the world, and serologic tests are not available, so at the present time, only nucleic acid-based tests are available for diagnosis. At least 1 test is currently cleared by the FDA and is also capable of assessing the presence of mutations associated with macrolide resistance.

The diagnosis of mycoplasma-associated central nervous system disease is challenging, both because disease may not be the result of direct invasion and because there is no reliable single test for cerebrospinal fluid to establish a diagnosis.

TREATMENT: Evidence of benefit of antimicrobial therapy for nonhospitalized children with lower respiratory tract disease attributable to *M pneumoniae* is limited. Some data suggest benefit of appropriate antimicrobial therapy in hospitalized children. Antimicrobial therapy is not recommended for preschool-aged children with CAP, because viral pathogens are responsible for the great majority of cases.[1] There is no evidence that treatment of other possible manifestations of *M pneumoniae* infection (eg, upper respiratory tract infection) with antimicrobial agents alters the course of illness. However, despite a paucity of studies, it is reasonable to treat severe extrapulmonary infections such as central nervous system disease or septic arthritis in an immunocompromised patient with an expectation that it may shorten the duration and severity of illness.

Because mycoplasmas lack a cell wall, they inherently are resistant to beta-lactam agents. Macrolides, including azithromycin, clarithromycin, and erythromycin, are the preferred antimicrobial agents for treatment of *Mycoplasma* pneumonia in school-aged children who have moderate to severe infection and those with underlying conditions,

[1]Bradley JS, Byington CL, Shah SS, et al. The management of community-acquired pneumonia in infants and children older than 3 months of age: clinical practice guidelines by the Pediatric Infectious Diseases Society and the Infectious Diseases Society of America. *Clin Infect Dis.* 2011;53(1):e25-e76

such as sickle cell disease.[1] Fluoroquinolones and doxycycline are the other 2 classes of antibiotics to which *M pneumoniae* is sensitive. Macrolide-resistant strains are increasingly common in the United States (currently between 5% and 15%). Treatment of hospitalized children with CAP attributable to a macrolide-resistant *M pneumoniae* using a fluoroquinolone has been shown in some studies to shorten the duration of fever and the length of hospitalization, but other studies find no difference. Most children with CAP attributable to *M pneumoniae* have a relatively mild, self-limited illness, but effective antibiotic therapy may be more important with more severe infections, particularly if coinfection is present. The usual course of antimicrobial therapy for pneumonia is 7 to 10 days, except for azithromycin, for which it usually is 5 days.

M hominis usually is resistant to erythromycin and azithromycin but is variably susceptible to clindamycin, tetracyclines, and fluoroquinolones. Like *M pneumoniae,* to which it is closely related, *M genitalium* is susceptible in vitro to macrolides, tetracyclines, and fluoroquinolones, but for unknown reasons, tetracyclines usually fail to exhibit clinical efficacy in the treatment of nongonococcal urethritis. Resistance to macrolides in *M genitalium* has been increasing worldwide and now may stand at greater than 40%. Unfortunately, fluoroquinolone resistance, which has not been observed in *M pneumoniae*, is also increasing in *M genitalium*, making its treatment increasingly problematic. The new pleuromutilin antibiotic lefamulin has good in vitro activity against *M genitalium* but has not been studied in children.

ISOLATION OF THE HOSPITALIZED PATIENT: In addition to standard precautions, droplet precautions are recommended for the duration of symptomatic illness with *M pneumoniae.*

CONTROL MEASURES FOR *M PNEUMONIAE* INFECTIONS: Hand hygiene decreases household transmission of respiratory pathogens and should be encouraged.

Tetracycline or azithromycin prophylaxis for close contacts has been shown to limit transmission in family and institutional outbreaks. However, antimicrobial prophylaxis for asymptomatic exposed contacts is not recommended routinely, because most secondary illnesses will be mild and self-limited. Prophylaxis with a macrolide or tetracycline can be considered for people at increased risk of severe illness with *M pneumoniae,* such as children with sickle cell disease who are close contacts of a person who is acutely ill with *M pneumoniae* infection.

Nocardiosis

CLINICAL MANIFESTATIONS: Immunocompetent children typically develop cutaneous or lymphocutaneous disease with pustular or ulcerative lesions following soil contamination of a skin injury. Deep-seated tissue infection may follow traumatic soil-contaminated wounds. Immunocompromised people may develop invasive disease (pulmonary disease, which may disseminate). At-risk people include those with chronic granulomatous disease, chronic obstructive pulmonary disease (COPD), human immunodeficiency virus (HIV) infection, disease requiring long-term systemic corticosteroid/immunosuppressive therapy, solid organ or bone marrow transplantation, autoimmune disease, or people having received tumor necrosis factor inhibitors. Pulmonary disease commonly manifests as rounded nodular infiltrates that can undergo cavitation; the infection may be acute,

[1]Bradley JS, Byington CL, Shah SS, et al. The management of community-acquired pneumonia in infants and children older than 3 months of age: clinical practice guidelines by the Pediatric Infectious Diseases Society and the Infectious Diseases Society of America. *Clin Infect Dis.* 2011;53(1):e25-e76

subacute, or chronic suppurative. The most common clinical symptoms include fever, cough, pleuritic chest pain, chills and headache. Nocardia has a propensity to spread hematogenously to the brain (single or multiple abscesses) from the lungs. The organism also may spread to the skin (pustules, pyoderma, abscesses, mycetoma), or occasionally to other organs. *Nocardia* organisms can be recovered from respiratory specimens of patients with cystic fibrosis, but the clinical significance of this pathogen in these patients is unclear.

ETIOLOGY: *Nocardia* are Gram-stain positive, aerobic, intracellular, nonmotile, filamentous bacteria in the order Actinomycetales. Cell walls of *Nocardia* organisms contain mycolic acid and thus may be described as "acid fast" or "partially acid fast" using the modified Kinyoun or Fite Faraco acid-fast staining and light microscopy.

EPIDEMIOLOGY: *Nocardia* species are ubiquitous environmental saprophytes, living in soil, organic matter, and fresh or sea water. Infections caused by *Nocardia* species typically are the result of environmental exposure through inhalation of soil or dust particles or through traumatic inoculation with a soil-contaminated object. The most prevalent species reported from human clinical sources in the United States are *Nocardia nova* complex, *Nocardia farcinica*, *Nocardia cyriacigeorgica*, and *Nocardia abscessus* complex. Primary cutaneous infection and mycetoma most often are associated with *Nocardia brasiliensis*. Other less common pathogenic species include *Nocardia brevicatena-paucivorans* complex, *Nocardia otitidiscaviarum* complex, *Nocardia pseudobrasiliensis*, *Nocardia transvalensis* complex, and *Nocardia veterana*.

Health care-associated person-to-person transmission has been reported rarely. Animal-to-human transmission is not known to occur.

The **incubation period** is unknown.

DIAGNOSTIC TESTS: Isolation of *Nocardia* species from clinical specimens can require extended incubation periods because of their slow growth. Specimens from sterile sites can be inoculated directly onto enriched solid media such as trypticase soy agar supplemented with 5% sheep blood, chocolate, brain-heart infusion, Sabouraud dextrose agars, and buffered charcoal yeast extract (BCYE) agar. Colonies look like white snowballs because of aerial hyphae. Specimens from nonsterile or contaminated sites, such as tissue or sputum, should be inoculated onto selective media, such as Thayer Martin or BCYE supplemented with vancomycin, with a minimum incubation of 3 weeks. Recovery of *Nocardia* species from tissue can be improved if the laboratory is requested to observe cultures for up to 4 weeks in an appropriate liquid medium at optimal growth temperature (between 25°C and 35°C for most species). Stained smears of sputum, body fluids, or pus demonstrating beaded, branching rods that stain weakly gram-positive and partially acid-fast 086_06] by the modified Kinyoun method suggest the diagnosis. The Brown-Brenn tissue Gram stain method and Grocott-Gomori methenamine silver stains are recommended to demonstrate microorganisms in tissue specimens.

Accurate identification of *Nocardia* isolates paired with antimicrobial susceptibility testing greatly enhances selection of appropriate antimicrobial therapy, thereby increasing the likelihood of favorable patient care outcomes. Because of variability of phenotypic traits and difficulty growing organisms on commercial biochemical testing media, accurate identification is accomplished through molecular methods. Matrix-assisted laser desorption/ionization-time of flight (MALDI-TOF) mass spectrometry has become an established method to identify the *Nocardia* isolate down to the species level. Other complementary methods include 16S rRNA gene sequence analysis of full length or nearly full-length (~1440 bp) sequences, and whole genome analysis. Serologic tests for *Nocardia* species are not useful except for an ELISA test used to determine the presence of anti-bodies to *N brasiliensis* mycetoma.

Some experts recommend cerebrospinal fluid examination and/or neuroimaging in patients with pulmonary disease, even with a nonfocal neurologic examination, given the propensity of these organisms to infect the central nervous system.

TREATMENT: Rapid and accurate identification of *Nocardia* isolates and antimicrobial susceptibility testing are essential tools for successful treatment of nocardiosis. *Nocardia* species possess intrinsic resistance to multiple drugs. Antimicrobial susceptibility testing recommended by the Clinical and Laboratory Standards Institute (CLSI) is complex and generally requires a specialty or reference laboratory. Such testing should guide therapy and is recommended for all strains from patients with invasive disease, when patients are unable to tolerate a sulfonamide, or for patients in whom sulfonamide therapy fails.

Trimethoprim-sulfamethoxazole (TMP/SMX) or a sulfonamide alone (eg, sulfisoxa-zole or sulfamethoxazole) are the drugs of choice for mild infections. Certain *Nocardia* species including *N farcinica*, *N nova*, and *N otitidiscaviarum*, may demonstrate intrinsic resis-tance to TMP/SMX. If infection does not respond to TMP/SMX, a fluoroquinolone or a carbapenem may be considered, though most *Nocardia* species are resistant to ertape-nem. Linezolid has excellent activity against all *Nocardia* species but is not recommended for long-term administration because of hematologic and neurologic toxicity. Other agents with specific *Nocardia* coverage include clarithromycin *(N nova)* and amoxicillin-clavulanate *(N brasiliensis* and *N abscessus* complex). Pediatric data are lacking for many of these agents in treatment of nocardiosis. Immunocompetent patients with lymphocutane-ous disease usually respond after 6 to 12 weeks of monotherapy.

Combination drug therapy is recommended for patients with serious disease (pul-monary infection, disseminated disease, central nervous system involvement) and for infection in immunocompromised hosts. Initial combination treatment should include TMP/SMX, amikacin, and a carbapenem-cilastatin (resistance noted for some strains of *N brasiliensis*) or linezolid until susceptibilities are available. Ceftriaxone or cefotaxime are alternative agents, but resistance is noted for many strains of *N farcinica*, *N transvalensis* complex, and *N otitidiscaviarum* complex. Immunocompromised patients and patients with serious disease should be treated for 6 to 12 months and for at least 3 months after appar-ent cure because of the propensity for relapse. Patients living with HIV may need even longer therapy, and suppressive therapy should be considered for life. Patients with central nervous system disease should be monitored with serial neuroimaging studies.

Drainage of abscesses is beneficial, and removal of infected foreign bodies (eg, central venous catheters) is recommended.

ISOLATION OF THE HOSPITALIZED PATIENT: Standard precautions are recommended.

CONTROL MEASURES: People with weakened immune systems should be advised to cover their skin when working with soil. TMP/SMX administered 3 times per week for prophylaxis against *Pneumocystis jirovecii* generally is ineffective in preventing nocardiosis.

Norovirus and Sapovirus Infections

CLINICAL MANIFESTATIONS: Abrupt onset of vomiting and/or watery diarrhea, accom-panied by abdominal cramps and nausea, are characteristic of norovirus and sapovirus gastroenteritis. Symptoms typically last from 24 to 72 hours. However, more prolonged courses of illness can occur, particularly among elderly people, young children, and hospitalized patients. Norovirus illness also is recognized as one of the possible causes of chronic gastroenteritis in immunocompromised patients. Systemic manifestations, including fever, myalgia, malaise, anorexia, and headache, may accompany gastrointestinal tract symptoms.

ETIOLOGY: *Norovirus* and *Sapovirus* are genera in the family *Caliciviridae* and are 23- to 40-nm, nonenveloped, single-stranded RNA viruses. Noroviruses are genetically diverse, with viruses from genogroups (G) I and GII causing most of the infections in humans. GII genotype 4 viruses have been causing >50% of all outbreaks globally over the past 15 years. Sapovirus genogroups I, II, IV, and V cause acute gastroenteritis with symptoms indistinguishable to norovirus in humans. At least 17 different sapovirus genotypes have been recognized.

EPIDEMIOLOGY: Norovirus causes an estimated 1 in 15 US residents to become ill each year as well as 56 000 to 71 000 hospitalizations and 570 to 800 deaths annually, predominantly among young children and the elderly. As a result of the success of rotavirus vaccines, noroviruses have become the predominant cause of medically attended acute gastroenteritis in the United States, causing both sporadic cases and outbreaks. Outbreaks of sapovirus infection are relatively rare, but its prevalence in children younger than 5 years ranges from 3% to 17%.

Outbreaks with high attack rates tend to occur in semi-closed populations, such as long-term care facilities, schools, child care centers, and cruise ships. Transmission is via the fecal-oral or vomitus-oral routes, either directly person to person or indirectly by ingesting contaminated food or water, or by touching surfaces contaminated with the virus and then touching the mouth. Common-source outbreaks have been described after ingestion of ice, shellfish, and a variety of ready-to-eat foods, including salads, berries, and bakery products, usually contaminated by infected food handlers. Transmission via vomitus has been documented, and exposure to contaminated surfaces and aerosolized vomitus has been implicated in some outbreaks. Asymptomatic shedding of norovirus is common across all age groups, with the highest prevalence in children.

Most norovirus strains bind to histo-blood group antigens, which are expressed on intestinal epithelial cells and are genetically regulated by the fucosyltransferase 2 (FUT2) gene. Individuals with a functional FUT2 gene are referred to as "secretors" whereas nonsecretors have a single point mutation in FUT2 making them nonsusceptible to most norovirus infections.

The **incubation period** for both norovirus and sapovirus is 12 to 48 hours. Viral shedding may start before onset of symptoms, peaks several days after exposure, and in some cases, may persist for 4 weeks or more. Prolonged shedding (>6 months) has been reported in immunocompromised hosts. Infection occurs year-round but is more common during the colder months of the year.

DIAGNOSTIC TESTS: Molecular diagnostic methods, such as real-time quantitative reverse transcriptase polymerase chain reaction (RT-qPCR) are the most sensitive assays to detect norovirus and sapovirus. Several multiplex nucleic acid-based assays for the detection of gastrointestinal pathogens are cleared by the US Food and Drug Administration, with the majority including norovirus testing and some including sapovirus. In children, interpretation of test results may be complicated by coinfection with other enteric pathogens.

State and local public health laboratories use RT-qPCR for detection of norovirus and sapovirus RNA in clinical specimens. Both norovirus and sapovirus can be genotyped by amplification of small regions of the capsid regions followed by sequencing and comparison with reference samples. Several online typing tools are available for typing the obtained sequences. Laboratory and epidemiologic support for investigation of suspected viral gastroenteritis outbreaks in the United States is available through local and state health departments.

TREATMENT: Supportive therapy includes oral or intravenous rehydration solutions to replace and maintain fluid and electrolyte balance.

ISOLATION OF THE HOSPITALIZED PATIENT: In addition to standard precautions, contact precautions are recommended for suspected cases of acute gastroenteritis attributable to norovirus infection until 48 hours after symptom resolution.

CONTROL MEASURES: Appropriate hand hygiene is the most important method to prevent norovirus and sapovirus infections and control transmission. Reducing these viruses present on hands is best accomplished by thorough handwashing with running water and plain or antiseptic soap. Washing hands with soap and water after contact with a patient with norovirus or sapovirus infection is more effective than using alcohol-based hand sanitizers for reducing transmission.

Several factors favor transmission of noroviruses, including low infectious dose, large numbers of virus particles excreted, prolonged shedding, and persistence of the virus in the environment. The risk of infection can be decreased by standard measures for control of vomiting and diarrhea, such as educating child care providers and food handlers about infection control, maintaining cleanliness of surfaces and food preparation areas, using appropriate disinfectants (principally sodium hypochlorite [chlorine bleach]), excluding caregivers or food handlers who are ill and for at least 2 days after symptoms stop, and exercising appropriate hand hygiene, as discussed previously. If a source of transmission can be identified (eg, contaminated food or water) during an outbreak, then specific interventions to interrupt transmission can be effective.

Infants and children should be excluded from child care centers until stools are contained in the diaper or when toilet-trained children no longer have accidents using the toilet and when stool frequency becomes no more than 2 stools above that child's normal frequency for the time the child is in the program, even if the stools remain loose.

Sporadic cases are not nationally notifiable, but outbreaks should be reported to local and state public health authorities as required and to the CDC via the National Outbreak Reporting System (NORS) (**www.cdc.gov/nors),** and laboratory test data including genotype information should be submitted to CaliciNet (**www.cdc. gov/norovirus/reporting/calicinet/index.html**). Guidance on norovirus is available on the CDC website (**www.cdc.gov/mmwr/pdf/rr/rr6003.pdf).** A toolkit designed to help health care professionals control and prevent norovirus gastroenteritis in health care settings also is available (**www.cdc.gov/hai/pdfs/ norovirus/229110-ANorovirusIntroLetter508.pdf).**

Onchocerciasis
(River Blindness, Filariasis)

CLINICAL MANIFESTATIONS: The disease involves skin, subcutaneous tissues, lymphatic vessels, and eyes. Subcutaneous, nontender nodules that can be up to several centimeters in diameter containing male and female worms develop 6 to 12 months after initial infection. In patients in Africa, nodules tend to be found on the lower torso, pelvis, and lower extremities, whereas in patients in Central and South America, the nodules more often are located on the upper body (the head and trunk) but also may occur on the extremities. After the worms mature, fertilized female worms produce prelarval stages called microfilariae that migrate to the dermis and may cause a papular dermatitis. Pruritus often is highly intense, resulting in patient-inflicted excoriations over the affected areas. After a period of years, skin can become lichenified and hypo- or hyperpigmented. Microfilariae may invade ocular structures, leading to inflammation of the cornea, iris, ciliary body, retina, choroid, and optic nerve. Loss of visual acuity and blindness can result over time if the disease is left untreated. Infection with *Onchocerca volvulus* has been associated with development of epilepsy.

ETIOLOGY: *O volvulus* is a filarial nematode.

EPIDEMIOLOGY: *O volvulus* has no significant animal or environmental reservoir. Humans are infected when infectious larvae are transmitted through the bites of *Simulium* species flies (black flies). Black flies breed in fast-flowing streams and rivers (hence, the colloquial name for the disease, "river blindness"). The disease occurs primarily in equatorial Africa, but small foci are found in Venezuela, Brazil, and Yemen. Prevalence is greatest among people who live near vector breeding sites. The infection is not transmissible by person-to-person contact, blood transfusion, or breast feeding; congenital transmission does not occur.

The **incubation period** from larval inoculation to microfilariae in the skin usually is 12 to 18 months but can be as long as 3 years.

DIAGNOSTIC TESTS: Direct microscopic examination of a 1- to 2-mm biopsy specimen of the epidermis and upper dermis (usually taken from the posterior iliac crest area), incubated in saline, can reveal emerging microfilariae. Microfilariae are not found in blood. Adult worms may be demonstrated in excised nodules that have been sectioned and stained. A slit-lamp examination of an involved eye may reveal motile microfilariae in the anterior chamber or "snowflake" corneal lesions. Eosinophilia is common. Specific serologic tests and polymerase chain reaction techniques for detection of microfilariae in skin are available in the United States in research and public health laboratories, including those of the National Institutes of Health and Centers for Disease Control and Prevention.

TREATMENT: Ivermectin and moxidectin, microfilaricidal agents, are available for treatment of onchocerciasis (see Drugs for Parasitic Infections, p 982). Moxidectin, approved by the US Food and Drug Administration in 2018 as a single oral dose for patients 12 years and older, showed superior efficacy to a single dose of ivermectin, but safety and efficacy of repeated doses have not been studied. Treatment decreases dermatitis and the risk of developing severe ocular disease but does not kill the adult worms (which can live for more than a decade) and, thus, is not curative. Oral ivermectin is given every 6 to 12 months until asymptomatic. The safety of ivermectin in children weighing less than 15 kg and in pregnant women has not been established. Adverse reactions to treatment are caused by death of microfilariae and can include rash, edema, fever, myalgia, and rarely, asthma exacerbation and hypotension. Such reactions are more common in people with higher skin loads of microfilaria and decrease with repeated treatment in the absence of re-exposure. Precautions to ivermectin/moxidectin treatment include pregnancy (class C drug), central nervous system disorders, and in co-infection with *Loa loa* (see Lymphatic

Filariasis, p 490). Treatment of patients with high levels of circulating *L loa* microfilare-mia rarely can result in fatal encephalopathy. Referral to a specialist familiar with treating these infections would be indicated for people coinfected with *O volvulus* and *L loa*. Ivermectin usually is compatible with breastfeeding. Because low levels of drug are found in human milk after maternal treatment, some experts recommend delaying maternal treatment until the infant is 7 days of age, but risk versus benefit should be considered.

A 6-week course of doxycycline can be used to kill adult worms through depletion of the endosymbiotic rickettsia-like bacteria *Wolbachia*, which appear to be required for survival of *O volvulus*. Doxycycline can be used for short durations (ie, 21 days or less) without regard to patient age, but for the longer treatment durations required for treatment of *O volvulus*, for whom the alternative treatment of ivermectin exists, doxycycline is not recommended for children younger than 8 years (see Tetracyclines, p 866). Doxycycline may be used for children 8 years or older and nonpregnant adults to obviate the need for years of ivermectin treatment. Doxycycline treatment may be initiated 1 week after treatment with ivermectin/moxidectin; for patients without symptoms, a 6-week course of doxycycline may be given, followed by a dose of ivermectin/moxidectin. There are no studies of the safety of simultaneous treatment.

The microfilaricide diethylcarbamazine (DEC) is contraindicated for the treatment of onchocerciasis because it may cause adverse ocular reactions. Nodules can be removed surgically, but not all nodules may be clinically detectable or surgically accessible.

ISOLATION OF THE HOSPITALIZED PATIENT: Standard precautions are recommended.

CONTROL MEASURES: Repellents and protective clothing (long sleeves and pants) can decrease exposure to bites from black flies, which bite by day. Treatment of vector breeding sites with larvicides is effective for controlling black fly populations. Vector control, however, largely has been supplanted by community-wide mass ivermectin administration programs. A highly successful global initiative being led by the World Health Organization has distributed hundreds of millions of ivermectin treatments (donated by the drug manufacturer for this purpose) in communities endemic for onchocerciasis. As a result of these programs, morbidity and transmission largely have been eliminated from the Americas (where most mass treatment programs now have halted) and markedly curtailed throughout Africa.

Paracoccidioidomycosis
(Formerly Known as South American Blastomycosis)

CLINICAL MANIFESTATIONS: Most disease occurs in adults (90%–95% of cases), in whom the site of initial infection is the lungs. Clinical patterns include subclinical infection or progressive disease that can be either acute-subacute (juvenile type) or chronic (adult type). Constitutional symptoms, such as fever, malaise, anorexia, and weight loss, are common in both adult and juvenile forms.

In the juvenile form, the initial pulmonary infection usually is asymptomatic, and manifestations are related to dissemination of infection to the reticuloendothelial system, resulting in enlarged lymph nodes and involvement of liver, spleen, and bone marrow. Skin lesions are observed regularly and are located typically on the face, neck, and trunk. Involvement of bones, joints, and mucous membranes is less common. Enlarged lymph nodes occasionally coalesce and form abscesses or fistulas. The chronic form of the illness can be localized to the lungs or can disseminate. Oral mucosal lesions are observed in half of the cases, and skin involvement is common but occurs in a smaller proportion than in patients with the acute-subacute form. Infection can be latent for years before causing illness.

ETIOLOGY: *Paracoccidioides brasiliensis* is a thermally dimorphic fungus with yeast and mycelia (mold) phases. *P brasiliensis* contains 4 different phylogenetic lineages (S1, PS2, PS3, and PS4). A new species, *Paracoccidioides lutzii*, also causes paracoccidioidomycosis.

EPIDEMIOLOGY: The infection occurs in Latin America, from Mexico to Argentina, with 80% of cases in Brazil. The natural reservoir is unknown although soil is suspected, and most disease is associated with agricultural work. The mode of transmission is unknown, but most likely occurs via inhalation of contaminated soil or dust; person-to-person transmission does not occur. The armadillo is a known reservoir of *P brasiliensis*.

The **incubation period** is highly variable, ranging from 1 month to decades. Cases have been diagnosed outside endemic regions, so prior residence in Latin America is important to determine.

DIAGNOSTIC TESTS: Diagnosis is confirmed by visualization of fungal elements. Round, multiple-budding yeast cells with a distinguishing pilot's wheel appearance can be seen in preparations of sputum, bronchoalveolar lavage specimens, scrapings from ulcers, and material from lesions or in tissue biopsy specimens. Specimens can be prepared with several procedures, including wet or KOH wet preparations, or histologic staining with hematoxylin and eosin, silver, or periodic-acid Schiff. The mycelia form of *P brasiliensis* can be cultured on most enriched media, including blood agar at 37°C and Mycosel or Sabouraud dextrose agar at 25°C to 30°C. Cultures should be held at least 6 weeks. Its appearance is not distinctive, and confirmation requires conversion to the yeast phase or DNA sequence determination. Complement fixation and immunodiffusion are available for antibody detection; semiquantitative immunodiffusion is the preferred test and is the most widely available test in endemic regions.

TREATMENT: Oral therapy with itraconazole is the treatment of choice for less severe or localized infection; oral solution is preferred to capsules. Voriconazole may be as effective as itraconazole but has not been studied as extensively. Isavuconazole has been efficacious in adults, but there are no pediatric data for paracoccidioidomycosis. See Table 4.8 (p 917) for dosing. Prolonged therapy for 9 to 18 months is necessary to minimize the relapse rate, and children with severe disease can require a longer course.

Trimethoprim-sulfamethoxazole orally is an inferior alternative, and treatment must be continued for 2 years or longer to lessen risk of relapse, which occurs in 10% to 15% of optimally treated patients. Ketoconazole and fluconazole generally are not recommended. Amphotericin B generally is given only for initial treatment of severe paracoccidioidomycosis for 2 to 4 weeks, with intravenous trimethoprim-sulfamethoxazole being another option. Children treated initially by the intravenous route can transition to orally administered therapy after clinical improvement has been observed, usually after 3 to 6 weeks.

Serial serologic testing by complement fixation or semi-quantitative immunodiffusion is useful for monitoring the response to therapy. The expected response is a progressive decline in titers after 1 to 3 months of treatment with stabilization at a low titer for years or even for life.

ISOLATION OF THE HOSPITALIZED PATIENT: Standard precautions are recommended.

CONTROL MEASURES: None.

Paragonimiasis

CLINICAL MANIFESTATIONS: There are 2 major forms of paragonimiasis. Primary pulmonary disease with or without extrapulmonary manifestations principally is attributable to *Paragonimus westermani, Paragonimus heterotremus, Paragonimus africanus, Paragonimus uterobilateralis,* and *Paragonimus kellicotti.* Extrapulmonary disease caused by aberrant migrating immature flukes, sometimes resulting in a visceral larva migrans syndrome similar to that caused by *Toxocara canis,* is attributable to other species of *Paragonimus,* most notably *Paragonimus skrjabini,* for which humans are accidental hosts.

Pulmonary infections are mostly asymptomatic or result in mild symptoms but may be associated with chronic cough and dyspnea, often of insidious onset. During worm migration in the lungs, migratory infiltrates may be noted on serial imaging. Heavy infestations cause paroxysms of coughing, which often produce blood-tinged sputum that is brown because of the presence of the pigmented *Paragonimus* eggs and hemosiderin. Hemoptysis can be severe. Eosinophilic pleural effusion, pneumothorax, bronchiectasis, and pulmonary fibrosis with clubbing can develop.

Extrapulmonary manifestations may involve the liver, spleen, abdominal cavity, intestinal wall, intra-abdominal lymph nodes, skin, or central nervous system, with meningo-encephalitis, seizures, and space-occupying tumors attributable to invasion of the brain by adult flukes. Cerebral paragonimiasis is the most common extrapulmonary manifestation and is more common in children. Extrapulmonary paragonimiasis also is associated with migratory subcutaneous nodules, which contain juvenile worms. Symptoms tend to subside after approximately 5 years but can persist for as many as 20 years.

ETIOLOGY: Paragonimiasis is caused by the lung fluke (trematode, flat worm) *Paragonimus.* In Asia, classical paragonimiasis is caused by adult flukes and eggs of *P westermani* and *P heterotremus.* In Africa, the adult flukes and eggs of *P africanus* and *P uterobilateralis* produce the disease. *P kellicotti* is the endemic species in North America, where it parasitizes mink, opossums, and other animals, and can cause infection in humans.

The adult flukes of *P westermani* are up to 12 mm long and 7 mm wide and occur throughout Asia. A triploid parthenogenetic form of *P westermani,* which is larger, produces more eggs, and elicits greater disease, has been described in Japan, Korea, Taiwan, and parts of eastern China. *P heterotremus* occurs in Southeast Asia and adjacent parts of China.

Extrapulmonary paragonimiasis (ie, visceral larva migrans syndrome) can be caused by larval stages of *P skrjabini* and *P miyazakii.* The worms rarely mature in infected human tissues. *P skrjabini* occurs in China, whereas *P miyazakii* occurs in Japan. *P mexicanus* and *P ecuadoriensis* occur in Mexico, Costa Rica, Ecuador, and Peru.

EPIDEMIOLOGY: Transmission occurs when raw or undercooked freshwater crabs or crayfish, including pickled and soy sauce-marinated products, containing larvae (metacercariae) are ingested. Numerous cases of *P kellicotti* infection have occurred when people have ingested uncooked or undercooked crayfish while canoeing or camping in the Midwestern United States. In North America, disease also has been caused by *P westermani* present in imported crab. A less common mode of transmission that also may occur is human infection through ingestion of meat from a paratenic host, most commonly ingestion of raw pork, usually from wild pigs, containing the juvenile stages of *Paragonimus* species (described as occurring in Japan). Humans are accidental ("dead-end") hosts for *P skrjabini* and *P miyazakii* in visceral larva migrans. These flukes cannot mature in humans and do not produce eggs. *Paragonimus* species also infect a variety of other mammals, such as canids, mustelids, felids, and rodents, which serve as animal reservoir hosts.

The **incubation period** is variable. Egg production begins by approximately 8 weeks after ingestion of *P westermani* metacercariae.

DIAGNOSIS: Paragonimiasis should be considered in patients with unexplained fever, cough, eosinophilia, and pleural effusion or other chest radiographic abnormalities who have eaten raw or undercooked crayfish. Microscopic examination of stool, sputum, pleural fluid, cerebrospinal fluid, and other tissue specimens may reveal operculate eggs. A Western blot serologic antibody test based on *P westermani* antigen, available at the Centers for Disease Control and Prevention (CDC), is sensitive and specific; antibody concentrations detected by immunoblot decrease slowly after the infection is cured by treatment. Charcot-Leyden crystals and eosinophils in sputum are useful diagnostic elements. Peripheral blood eosinophilia also is characteristic. Chest radiographs may appear normal or may resemble radiographs from patients with tuberculosis or malignancy.

TREATMENT: Praziquantel in a 2-day course is the treatment of choice (see Drugs for Parasitic Infections, p 949) and is associated with high cure rates, as demonstrated by disappearance of egg production and resolution of radiographic lesions in the lungs. The drug also is effective for some extrapulmonary manifestations. An alternative drug for patients unable to take praziquantel (eg, because of previous allergic reaction) is triclabendazole, given in 1 or 2 doses. Triclabendazole is a narrow-spectrum anthelmintic with activity against *Fasciola* and *Paragonimus*. In February 2019, the US Food and Drug Administration (FDA) approved triclabendazole for the treatment of human fascioliasis; it is not approved by the FDA for paragonimiasis. A short course of steroids may be beneficial in addition to the praziquantel, for patients with central nervous system paragonimiasis, to reduce the inflammatory response associated with dying flukes. Other supportive care, including anti-epileptics and shunt placement, may be needed.

ISOLATION OF THE HOSPITALIZED PATIENT: Standard precautions are recommended.

CONTROL MEASURES: Crabs and crayfish should be cooked for several minutes to at least 145°F [63°C]. Meat from wild pigs should be cooked to an internal temperature of at least 160°F [71°C] before eating. Control of animal reservoirs is not possible.

Parainfluenza Viral Infections

CLINICAL MANIFESTATIONS: Parainfluenza viruses (PIVs) are the major cause of laryngotracheobronchitis (croup) and may cause bronchiolitis and pneumonia as well as upper respiratory tract infection.[1] PIV type 1 (PIV1) and, to a lesser extent, PIV type 2 (PIV2) are the most common pathogens associated with croup. PIV type 3 (PIV3) most commonly is associated with bronchiolitis and pneumonia in infants and young children. Infections with PIV type 4 (PIV4) are less well characterized but have been associated with both upper and lower respiratory tract infections. Longitudinal studies have demonstrated that upper respiratory infections caused by viruses, including PIVs, can be associated with acute otitis media, which is frequently a mixed viral-bacterial infection. Rarely, PIVs have been isolated from patients with parotitis, myopericarditis, aseptic meningitis,

---

[1]American Academy of Pediatrics, Subcommittee on Diagnosis and Management of Bronchiolitis. Clinical practice guideline: the diagnosis, management, and prevention of bronchiolitis. *Pediatrics.* 2014;134(5):e1474-e1502

encephalitis, febrile seizures, and Guillain-Barré syndrome. PIV infections can exacerbate symptoms of chronic lung disease and asthma in children and adults. In children with immunodeficiency and recipients of hematopoietic stem cell transplants, PIVs, most commonly PIV3, can cause refractory infections with persistent shedding, severe pneumonia with viral dissemination, and even fatal disease. PIV infections do not confer complete protective immunity; therefore, reinfections can occur with all serotypes and at any age, but reinfections usually are mild and limited to the upper respiratory tract.

ETIOLOGY: PIVs are enveloped single-stranded negative-sense RNA viruses classified in the family *Paramyxoviridae.* Four antigenically distinct types—1, 2, 3, and 4 (with 2 subtypes, 4A and 4B)—that infect humans have been identified. PIV1 and PIV3 are in the genus *Respirovirus* and PIV2 and PIV4 are classified in the genus *Rubulavirus.*

EPIDEMIOLOGY: PIVs are transmitted from person to person by direct contact with contaminated nasopharyngeal secretions through large respiratory tract droplets and fomites. PIV infections can be sporadic or associated with outbreaks of acute respiratory tract disease. Seasonal patterns of infection are distinct, predictable, and cyclic in temperate regions. Different serotypes have distinct epidemiologic patterns. PIV1 tends to produce outbreaks of respiratory tract illness, usually croup, in the autumn of every other year. A major increase in the number of cases of croup in the autumn usually indicates a PIV1 outbreak. PIV2 also can cause outbreaks of respiratory tract illness in the autumn, but PIV2 outbreaks tend to be less severe, irregular, and less common. PIV3 is endemic and usually is prominent during spring and summer in temperate climates but often continues into autumn, especially in years when autumn outbreaks of PIV1 or PIV2 are absent. PIV4 seasonal patterns are not as well characterized, but studies have shown that infections with PIV4 had year-round prevalence with peaks during the fall and winter.

The age of primary infection varies with serotype. Primary infection with all types usually occurs by 5 years of age. Infection with PIV3 more often occurs in infants and is a frequent cause of bronchiolitis and pneumonia in this age group. By 12 months of age, 50% of infants have acquired PIV3 infection. Infections with PIV1 and, to a lesser extent, PIV2 are more likely to occur between 1 and 5 years of age. Acquisition of PIV4 also occurs more often during preschool years.

Immunocompetent children with primary PIV infection may shed virus for up to 1 week before onset of clinical symptoms and for 1 to 3 weeks after symptoms have disappeared, depending on serotype. Severe lower respiratory tract disease with prolonged shedding of the virus can occur in immunocompromised individuals. In these patients, infection may disseminate.

The **incubation period** ranges from 2 to 6 days.

DIAGNOSTIC TESTS: Reverse transcriptase-polymerase chain reaction (RT-PCR) assays are the preferred diagnostic method for detection and differentiation of PIVs and have become the standard method in clinical practice. PIVs are included in many multiplex PCR-based respiratory pathogen panels, although PIV4 is less commonly included. PIVs may be isolated from nasopharyngeal secretions in cell culture, usually within 4 to 7 days of culture inoculation. Serologic diagnosis, made by a significant increase in antibody titer between acute and convalescent serum specimens, is less useful because results are delayed and infection may not always be accompanied by a significant homotypic antibody response.

TREATMENT: Specific antiviral therapy is not available. Racemic epinephrine aerosol commonly is given to severely affected hospitalized patients with laryngotracheobronchitis (croup) to decrease airway obstruction. Parenteral, oral, and nebulized corticosteroids have been demonstrated to lessen the severity and duration of symptoms and hospitalization in patients with moderate to severe laryngotracheobronchitis. Oral steroids also are effective for outpatients with less severe croup. Management otherwise is supportive.

Antimicrobial agents should be reserved for documented secondary bacterial infections. Use of ribavirin (usually inhaled), with or without concomitant administration of Immune Globulin Intravenous (IGIV), has been reported anecdotally in immunocompromised patients with severe pneumonia; however, controlled studies are lacking and this use is not routinely recommended.

ISOLATION OF THE HOSPITALIZED PATIENT: In addition to standard precautions, contact precautions are recommended for hospitalized infants and young children diagnosed with PIV for the duration of illness. Before a specific pathogen has been identified, contact and droplet precautions are required if influenza virus or adenovirus infections are considered. In immunocompromised patients, the duration of contact precautions should be extended because of possible prolonged shedding.

CONTROL MEASURES: Appropriate respiratory hygiene and cough etiquette should be followed. Exposure to PIV-infected people, including other patients, staff, and family members, may not be recognized, because illness may be mild. Additional infection control measures should be considered in certain settings (eg, child care centers, nursing homes) when respiratory infections have been identified.

Parasitic Diseases

Parasites are among the most common causes of morbidity and mortality in various and diverse geographic locations worldwide. Outside the tropics and subtropics, parasitic diseases are common among travelers, immigrants, and immunocompromised people. Toxocariasis occurs in the United States, most commonly in the South. Malaria infections in the United States occur among people who have traveled to regions with ongoing malaria transmission, and the diagnosis should be considered when evaluating fever in a returned traveler. Certain parasitic infections have long latency periods and the diseases they cause, such as Chagas disease, neurocysticercosis, schistosomiasis, and strongyloidiasis, are encountered in immigrants from regions with endemic infection. Clinicians need to be aware of where these infections may be acquired, their clinical presentations, methods of diagnosis, and how to prevent infection. A number of human parasitic infections are discussed in individual chapters in Section 3; diseases are arranged alphabetically. Table 3.40 provides details on some infrequently encountered parasitic diseases not discussed elsewhere.

Consultation and assistance in diagnosis and management of parasitic diseases are available from the Centers for Disease Control and Prevention (CDC), state health departments, and university departments or hospitals that have divisions of travel medicine, tropical medicine, infectious diseases, international or global health, and public health.

Drugs for Parasitic Infections can be found beginning on p 949 and are compiled from recommendations on the CDC website and other sources. Treatment recommendations may vary based on expert opinion, and because a number of commonly used drugs

Table 3.40. Selected Parasitic Diseases Not Covered Elsewhere[a]

Disease and/or Agent	Where Infection May Be Acquired	Definitive Host	Intermediate Host	Modes of Human Infection	Diagnostic Laboratory Tests in Humans	Parasitic Form Causing Human Disease	Common Manifestations in Humans
Angiostrongylus cantonensis (neurotropic disease)	Widespread in the tropics, particularly Pacific Islands and Southeast Asia, Central and South America, the Caribbean, and the United States	Rats	Snails and slugs	Eating improperly cooked infected mollusks or food contaminated by mollusk secretions containing larvae; possibly other modes	Eosinophils in CSF; rarely, identification of larvae in CSF; serologic testing or CSF PCR not available commercially	Larval worms	Eosinophilic meningitis, peripheral eosinophilia
Angiostrongylus costaricensis (gastrointestinal tract disease)	Central and South America	Rodents	Snails and slugs	Eating improperly cooked infected mollusks or food contaminated by mollusk secretions containing larvae	Identification of larvae and eggs in tissue; serologic testing not commercially available	Larval worms	Abdominal pain, nausea, vomiting, diarrhea (may mimic appendicitis) eosinophilia

Table 3.40. Selected Parasitic Diseases Not Covered Elsewhere,[a] continued

Disease and/or Agent	Where Infection May Be Acquired	Definitive Host	Intermediate Host	Modes of Human Infection	Diagnostic Laboratory Tests in Humans	Parasitic Form Causing Human Disease	Common Manifestations in Humans
Anisakiasis	Cosmopolitan, most common where eating raw fish is practiced	Marine mammal	Certain salt-water fish, squid, and octopus	Eating raw or undercooked infected marine fish or squid or octopus	Identification of recovered larvae on endoscopy or within tissue biopsies; serologic testing available	Larval worms	Abdominal pain, nausea, vomiting, diarrhea
Capillariasis–intestinal disease (*Capillaria philippinensis*)	Philippines, Thailand	Humans, fish-eating birds	Fish	Ingestion of uncooked infected fish	Eggs and parasite in feces or biopsies of small intestine	Larvae and mature worms	Abdominal pain, diarrhea, vomiting, weight loss
Clonorchis sinensis, Opisthorchis viverrini, Opisthorchis felineus (liver flukes)	East Asia, Eastern Europe, Russian Federation	Humans, cats, dogs, other mammals	Certain freshwater snails	Eating raw or undercooked infected freshwater fish, crabs, crayfish	Eggs in stool or duodenal fluid Serologic testing not commercially available	Larvae and mature flukes	Abdominal pain; hepatobiliary disease; cholangiocarcinoma

Table 3.40. Selected Parasitic Diseases Not Covered Elsewhere,[a] continued

Disease and/or Agent	Where Infection May Be Acquired	Definitive Host	Intermediate Host	Modes of Human Infection	Diagnostic Laboratory Tests in Humans	Parasitic Form Causing Human Disease	Common Manifestations in Humans
Dracunculiasis (*Dracunculus medinensis*) (guinea worm)	Foci in Africa; global eradication nearly achieved, with only 54 human cases worldwide in 2019	Humans	Crustacea (copepods)	Drinking water infested with infected copepods	Identification of emerging or adult worm in subcutaneous tissues; serology available but not necessary	Adult female worms	Emerging roundworm; inflammatory response; systemic and local blister or ulcer in skin
Fascioliasis (liver flukes; *Fasciola hepatica*)	Worldwide; predominantly in the tropics	Sheep and cattle most important; other ruminants	Snails	Eating raw freshwater plants (eg, watercress) or drinking water contaminated with larvae	Identifying eggs in stool, duodenal fluid, or bile; serologic testing; examination of surgical specimens	Larvae and mature flukes	Abdominal pain nausea, vomiting; hepatobiliary disease
Fasciolopsiasis (intestinal flukes; *Fasciolopsis buski*)	East Asia	Humans, pigs, dogs	Certain freshwater snails, plants	Eating uncooked infected plants	Eggs or worm in feces or duodenal fluid; serologic testing not commercially available	Larvae and mature flukes	Diarrhea, constipation, vomiting, anorexia, edema of face and legs, ascites

CSF, cerebrospinal fluid; PCR, polymerase chain reaction.

[a] For recommended drug treatment, see Drugs for Parasitic Infections (p 949).

do not have approved indications for a specific parasitic infection or a particular age group. Specific expertise or multiple sources should be consulted especially when there is a lack of familiarity with the parasite or the drugs recommended for treatment. The CDC distributes several drugs that are not available commercially in the United States for treatment of parasitic diseases. To request these drugs, a physician must contact the CDC Parasitic Diseases Inquiries office (see Appendix I, Directory of Resources, p 1027; 404-718-4745; email: **parasites@cdc.gov**). Consultation with a medical officer from the CDC is required before a drug is released for a patient. For drugs and consultation regarding malaria, a separate CDC hotline is available (770-488-7788).

Parechovirus Infections

CLINICAL MANIFESTATIONS: Parechoviruses (PeVs) primarily cause disease in young infants and present in a similar manner to enterovirus, disseminated herpes simplex virus, or bacterial infections, with a febrile illness, exanthem (maculopapular and/or generalized erythema or erythroderma, often with palmar and plantar erythema and at times in a distribution limited to the hands and feet), sepsis-like syndrome (frequently with leukopenia), and/or central nervous system manifestations. The latter includes meningitis (typically with little or no pleocytosis), encephalitis, seizures, and apnea, often with brain imaging abnormalities primarily affecting white matter; long-term neurodevelopmental sequelae may occur. Infections (particularly with PeV-A3) may be severe, with manifestations that include sepsis, hepatitis and coagulopathy, myocarditis, pneumonia, and/or meningoencephalitis, with long-term sequelae or death. PeV infections in older infants and toddlers have been associated with generally mild upper and lower respiratory tract disease and gastroenteritis (although causation has not been established consistently) and a variety of other less common manifestations, including acute flaccid paralysis, acute disseminated encephalomyelitis, myalgia and myositis, herpangina, hand-foot-and-mouth disease, sudden infant death syndrome, and hemophagocytic lymphohistiocytosis.

ETIOLOGY: PeVs are a group of small, nonenveloped, single-stranded, positive-sense RNA viruses in the family *Picornaviridae*. The *Parechovirus* genus consists of 4 species, *Parechovirus* A through D. *Parechovirus* A (formerly named Human *Parechovirus*) includes at least 19 PeV types (designated 1–19) and is the only species known to cause human disease. PeV-A1 and PeV-A2 previously were classified as echoviruses 22 and 23, respectively. PeV-A1 and PeV-A3 have been implicated in disease most frequently.

EPIDEMIOLOGY: Humans are the primary reservoir for PeVs, although zoonotic infection in a number of animals hosts has been demonstrated for different PeV species. PeV-A infections have been reported worldwide. Seroepidemiologic studies suggest that PeV-A infections occur commonly during early childhood. In some studies, most school-aged children have serologic evidence of prior infection, but seroprevalence appears to vary by geographic region and specific PeV-A type. Overall, PeV-A1 and PeV-A3 infections are most commonly reported in childhood and tend to infect children up to several years of age. PeV infections frequently are asymptomatic. Symptomatic infection is most frequent in children younger than 2 years, with the most severe disease occurring in infants (especially younger than 6 months of age with PeV-A3) and young children. Disease infrequently occurs in older children and adults.

Transmission appears to occur via the fecal-oral and respiratory routes, from symptomatic or asymptomatic individuals. On the basis of reports of very early onset neonatal disease, in utero transmission also may occur. Certain PeV-A types may circulate throughout the year, while infections by other types (eg, PeV-A3) occur more commonly during summer and fall months, with cyclic peaks described. Multiple PeV-A types may circulate in a community during the same time period, and community outbreaks have been described. Epidemiologic observations suggest household transmission, and health care-associated transmission in neonatal and pediatric hospital units has also been observed. Virus is shed from the upper respiratory tract for 1 to 3 weeks and in stool for less than 2 weeks to as long as 6 months. Shedding may occur in the absence of illness.

The **incubation period** for PeV infections has not been defined.

DIAGNOSTIC TESTS: Reverse transcriptase-polymerase chain reaction (RT-PCR) assays that detect PeVs, available at the Centers for Disease Control and Prevention and select reference and hospital-based laboratories, represent the best diagnostic modality currently available. Some of the assays may not detect all PeV-A types. Enterovirus RT-PCR assays will not detect PeVs (and vice versa). PeVs can be detected by RT-PCR in stool, throat swab specimens, nasopharyngeal aspirates, tracheal secretions, blood, and cerebrospinal fluid. Multiplex PCR assays designed to detect a number of bacterial and viral agents of meningitis and encephalitis, including PeVs, in cerebrospinal fluid are available. Clinical data on the use of these assays are limited. As with the enteroviruses, the PeVs can be shed from the respiratory and gastrointestinal tract for prolonged periods, so detection at these sites does not necessarily represent a current disease attributable to PeVs. Viral culture can be used, but recovery in culture is less sensitive than RT-PCR assay, viral culture requires multiple cell lines, recovery may take several days to weeks, and some types do not grow well in culture. The PeV type can be identified by partial or complete capsid sequencing of amplified nucleic acid. Serologic assays have been developed for research but are not available commercially for diagnostic purposes.

TREATMENT: No specific therapy is available for PeV infections. Immune Globulin Intravenous (IGIV) has been used in some published case reports of neonates with severe PeV infections.

ISOLATION OF THE HOSPITALIZED PATIENT: In addition to standard precautions, contact precautions are appropriate for infants and young children for the duration of PeV illness. Cohorting of infected neonates may be effective in controlling hospital nursery outbreaks.

CONTROL MEASURES: Hand hygiene and environmental cleaning are important in decreasing spread of PeVs within families and institutions.

Parvovirus B19
(Erythema Infectiosum, Fifth Disease)

CLINICAL MANIFESTATIONS: Infection with parvovirus B19 is clinically recognized most often as erythema infectiosum (EI), or fifth disease, which is characterized by a distinctive rash that may be preceded by mild systemic symptoms, including fever in 15% to 30% of patients. The facial rash can be intensely red with a "slapped cheek" appearance that often is accompanied by circumoral pallor. A symmetric, macular, lace-like, and often pruritic rash occurs on the trunk, moving peripherally to involve the arms, buttocks, and thighs. The rash can fluctuate in intensity and can recur with environmental changes, such as temperature and exposure to sunlight, for weeks to months. A brief, mild, non-specific illness consisting of fever, malaise, myalgia, and headache often precedes the

Table 3.41. Clinical Manifestations of Parvovirus B19 Infection

Conditions	Usual Hosts
Erythema infectiosum (EI, fifth disease)	Immunocompetent children
Polyarthropathy syndrome	Immunocompetent adults (more common in women)
Chronic anemia/pure red cell aplasia	Immunocompromised hosts
Transient aplastic crisis	People with hemolytic anemia (ie, sickle cell disease)
Hydrops fetalis/congenital anemia	Fetus (first 20 weeks of pregnancy)
Petechial, papular-purpuric gloves-and-socks syndrome (PPGSS)	Immunocompetent children and young adults

characteristic exanthem by approximately 7 to 10 days. Arthralgia and arthritis occur in fewer than 10% of infected children but commonly occur among adults, especially women. Knees are involved most commonly in children, but a symmetric polyarthropathy of knees, fingers, and other joints is common in adults.

Parvovirus B19 can cause asymptomatic or subclinical infections. Other manifestations (Table 3.41) include a mild respiratory tract illness with no rash, a rash atypical for EI that may be rubelliform or petechial, papular-purpuric gloves-and-socks syndrome (PPGSS; painful and pruritic papules, petechiae, and purpura of hands and feet, often with fever and an enanthem), polyarthropathy syndrome (arthralgia and arthritis in adults in the absence of other manifestations of EI), chronic erythroid hypoplasia with severe anemia in immunodeficient patients (eg, patients with human immunodeficiency virus [HIV] infection, patients receiving immune-suppressive therapy), and transient aplastic crisis lasting 7 to 10 days in patients with hemolytic anemias (eg, sickle cell disease and autoimmune hemolytic anemia). For children with other conditions associated with low hemoglobin concentrations, including hemorrhage and severe anemia, parvovirus B19 infection usually will not result in aplastic crisis but might result in prolongation of recovery from the anemia. Patients with transient aplastic crisis may have a prodromal illness with fever, malaise, and myalgia, but rash usually is absent. In addition, parvovirus B19 infection sometimes has been associated with decreases in numbers of platelets, lymphocytes, and neutrophils. In rare cases, parvovirus B19 infection has been associated with acute hepatitis, myocarditis, encephalopathies, and hemophagocytic lymphohistiocytosis in children and young adults. Parvovirus B19 infection occurring during pregnancy can cause fetal hydrops, intrauterine growth restriction, isolated pleural and pericardial effusions, and death, but the virus is not a proven cause of congenital anomalies. The risk of fetal death is between 2% and 6% when infection occurs during pregnancy. The greatest risk appears to occur during the first half of pregnancy.

ETIOLOGY: Parvovirus B19 is a small, nonenveloped, single-stranded DNA virus in the family *Parvoviridae*, genus *Erythroparvovirus*. Three distinct genotypes of the virus have been described, but there is no evidence of differences of virologic or disease characteristics among the genotypes. Parvovirus B19 replicates in human erythrocyte precursors, which accounts for some of the clinical manifestations following infection. Parvovirus B19-associated red blood cell aplasia is related to caspase-mediated apoptosis of erythrocyte precursors.

EPIDEMIOLOGY: Parvovirus B19 is distributed worldwide and is a common cause of infection in humans, who are the only known hosts. Modes of transmission include contact with respiratory tract secretions, percutaneous exposure to blood or blood products, and vertical transmission from mother to fetus. Parvovirus B19 infections are ubiquitous, and cases of EI can occur sporadically or in outbreaks in schools during late winter and early spring. Secondary spread among susceptible household members is common, with infection occurring in approximately 50% of susceptible contacts in some studies. The transmission rate in schools is lower, but infection can be an occupational risk for school and child care personnel, with approximately 20% of susceptible contacts becoming infected. In young children, antibody seroprevalence generally is 5% to 10%. In most communities, approximately 50% of young adults and often more than 90% of elderly people are seropositive.

The **incubation period** from acquisition of parvovirus B19 to onset of initial symptoms (rash or symptoms of aplastic crisis) is between 4 and 14 days but can be as long as 21 days. Timing of the presence of high-titer parvovirus B19 DNA in serum and respiratory tract secretions indicates that people with EI are infectious before rash onset and are unlikely to be infectious after onset of the rash and/or joint symptoms. In contrast, patients with aplastic crises are contagious from before the onset of symptoms through at least the week after onset. Symptoms of PPGSS can occur in association with viremia and before development of antibody response, and affected patients should be considered infectious.

DIAGNOSTIC TESTS: In the immunocompetent host, detection of serum parvovirus B19-specific immunoglobulin (Ig) M antibodies is the preferred diagnostic test for an acute or recent parvovirus B19-associated rash illness. A positive IgM test result indicates that infection probably occurred within the previous 2 to 3 months. Based on immunoassay results, IgM antibodies may be detected in 90% or more of patients at the time of the EI rash and by the third day of illness in patients with transient aplastic crisis. Serum IgG antibodies appear by approximately day 2 of EI and persist for life; therefore, presence of parvovirus B19 IgG is not necessarily indicative of acute infection. These assays are available through commercial laboratories and some state public health department laboratories. However, their sensitivity and specificity may vary, particularly for IgM.

Serum IgM and IgG assays are not reliable in immunocompromised patients. The optimal method for detecting transient aplastic crisis or chronic infection in the immunocompromised patient is demonstration of high titer of viral DNA by polymerase chain reaction (PCR) assays. Such patients generally have >10^6 parvovirus B19 DNA copies/mL of plasma. Currently, there are no PCR assays cleared by the US Food and Drug Administration for the qualitative or quantitative detection of parvovirus B19 DNA, but such assays are available through select commercial and reference laboratories and sometimes in larger hospital-based laboratories. With the availability of a World Health Organization (WHO) nucleic acid standard for parvovirus B19 DNA, assay results can be reported in international units per mL (IU/mL) to allow for comparison across assays. False-negative results can occur with PCR assays that do not detect all 3 genotypes. Because parvovirus B19 DNA can be detected at low levels by PCR assay in serum for months and even years after the acute viremic phase, detection does not necessarily indicate acute infection. Low levels of parvovirus B19 DNA also can be detected by PCR in tissues (skin, heart, liver, bone marrow), independent of active disease. Qualitative PCR may be used on amniotic fluid as an aid to diagnosis of hydrops fetalis. Parvovirus B19 cannot be propagated in standard cell culture.

TREATMENT: For most patients, only supportive care is indicated. Patients with aplastic crisis may require transfusions of blood products. Immune Globulin Intravenous (IGIV) therapy often is effective and should be used for the treatment of parvovirus B19 infection in immunodeficient patients. The optimal dosing regimen and duration of treatment have not been established. Reduction of immune suppression also should be attempted, if possible. There are no approved specific antivirals for the treatment of parvovirus B19. Some cases of parvovirus B19 infection in pregnancy concurrent with hydrops fetalis have been treated successfully with intrauterine blood transfusions of the fetus.

ISOLATION OF THE HOSPITALIZED PATIENT: In addition to standard precautions, droplet precautions are recommended for hospitalized children with aplastic crises, children with PPGSS, or immunosuppressed patients with chronic infection and anemia for the duration of hospitalization. For patients with transient aplastic or erythrocyte crisis, these precautions should be maintained for 7 days or until the reticulocyte count has recovered from suppression to at least 2%. Neonates who had hydrops attributable to parvovirus B19 in utero do not require isolation if the hydrops is resolved at the time of birth. Pregnant health care workers should be informed of the potential risks to their fetus from parvovirus B19 infections and about preventive measures that may decrease these risks (eg, attention to strict infection control procedures).

CONTROL MEASURES:

• Women who are exposed to children at home or at work (eg, teachers or child care providers) are at increased risk of infection with parvovirus B19. However, in view of the high prevalence of parvovirus B19 infection, the low incidence of adverse effects on the fetus, and the fact that avoidance of child care or classroom teaching can decrease but not eliminate the risk of exposure, routine exclusion of pregnant women from the workplace where EI is occurring is not recommended. Women of childbearing age who are concerned can undergo serologic testing for IgG antibody to parvovirus B19 to determine their susceptibility to infection.

• Pregnant women who discover that they have been in contact with children who were in the incubation period of EI or with children who were in aplastic crisis should have the relatively low potential risk of infection explained to them. The American College of Obstetricians and Gynecologists recommends that pregnant women exposed to parvovirus B19 should have serologic testing performed to determine susceptibility and possible evidence of acute parvovirus B19 infection.[1] Pregnant women with evidence of acute parvovirus B19 infection should be monitored closely (eg, serial ultrasonographic examinations) by their obstetric provider. In pregnant women with suspected or proven intrauterine parvovirus B19 infection, amniotic fluid and fetal tissues should be considered infectious, and contact precautions should be used in addition to standard precautions if exposure is likely.

---

[1]American College of Obstetricians and Gynecologists. Cytomegalovirus, parvovirus B19, varicella zoster, and toxoplasmosis in pregnancy. Practice Bulletin No. 151. *Obstet Gynecol.* 2015;125(6):1510–1525

- Children with EI may attend child care or school, because they no longer are contagious once the rash appears.
- Transmission of parvovirus B19 is likely to be decreased through use of routine infection control practices, including hand hygiene.
- The FDA has issued guidance for nucleic acid amplification testing to reduce the possible risk of parvovirus B19 transmission by plasma-derived products (**www.fda.gov/ ucm/groups/fdagov-public/@fdagov-bio-gen/documents/document/ ucm078510.pdf**). The goal is to identify and prevent the use of plasma-derived products containing high levels of virus. Parvovirus B19 viral loads in manufacturing pools should not exceed 10^4 IU/mL.

Pasteurella Infections

CLINICAL MANIFESTATIONS: The most common manifestation is cellulitis at the site of a bite or scratch of a cat, dog, or other domestic or wild animal. Cellulitis typically develops within 24 hours of the injury and includes swelling, erythema, tenderness, and serosanguinous to purulent drainage at the wound site. Regional lymphadenopathy, chills, and fever can occur. The most frequent local complications are abscesses and tenosynovitis, but septic arthritis and osteomyelitis also occur. Other less common manifestations that are not always associated with an animal bite include septicemia, central nervous system infections (meningitis is the most common; however, brain abscess and subdural empyema have been observed), ocular infections (eg, conjunctivitis, corneal ulcer, endophthalmitis), endocarditis, respiratory tract infections (eg, pneumonia, pulmonary abscesses, pleural empyema, epiglottitis), appendicitis, hepatic abscess, peritonitis, and urinary tract infection. People with liver disease, solid organ transplant, or underlying host defense abnormalities are predisposed to bacteremia with *Pasteurella multocida*.

ETIOLOGY: The genus *Pasteurella* is one of 4 genera of human pathogens classified in the family *Pasteurellaceae;* the other genera are *Actinobacillus, Aggregatibacter,* and *Haemophilus.* Members of the genus *Pasteurella* are nonmotile, facultatively anaerobic, mostly catalase and oxidase positive, gram-negative coccobacilli that are primarily respiratory tract colonizers and pathogens in animals. The most common human pathogen is *Pasteurella multocida.* Most human infections are caused by the following species or subspecies: *P multocida* subspecies *multocida* (causing more than 50% of infections), *P multocida* subspecies *septica, Pasteurella canis, Pasteurella stomatis,* and *Pasteurella dagmatis.*

EPIDEMIOLOGY: *Pasteurella* species have a worldwide distribution. They colonize the upper respiratory tract of 70% to 90% of cats, 25% to 50% of dogs, and many other wild and domestic animals. Transmission most frequently occurs from the bite or scratch or licking of a previous wound by a cat or dog. Infected cat bite wounds contain *Pasteurella* species more often than do dog bite wounds. Rarely, respiratory tract spread occurs from animals to humans, and in a significant proportion of cases, no animal exposure can be identified. Human-to-human transmission has been documented vertically from mother to neonate, horizontally from colonized humans, and by contaminated blood products.

The **incubation period** usually is less than 24 hours.

DIAGNOSTIC TESTS: The isolation of *Pasteurella* species from a normally sterile body site (eg, blood, joint fluid, cerebrospinal fluid, pleural fluid, or suppurative lymph nodes) establishes the diagnosis of systemic infection. Recovery of the organism from a superficial site, such as drainage from a skin lesion subsequent to an animal bite, must be interpreted in the context of other potential pathogens isolated, and mixed infection may occur. *Pasteurella* species are somewhat fastidious but may be cultured on several media generally used in clinical laboratories, including tryptic soybean digest agar with 5% sheep blood and chocolate agars, at 35°C to 37°C without increased carbon dioxide concentration. Although they resemble several other organisms morphologically, laboratory identification to the genus level generally is not difficult, although species and subspecies differentiation is more challenging. Newer laboratory methods, including polymerase chain reaction (PCR) amplification of the 16S rRNA gene followed by sequencing and identification of cellular components by matrix-assisted laser desorption/ionization-time of flight (MALDI-TOF) mass spectroscopy, have significantly improved specific identification.

TREATMENT: The drug of choice is penicillin. Penicillin resistance is rare, but beta-lactamase–producing strains have been recovered. Other oral agents that usually are effective include ampicillin, amoxicillin, amoxicillin/clavulanate, cefuroxime, cefixime, cefpodoxime, doxycycline, and fluoroquinolones. Parenteral third-generation cephalosporins, including ceftriaxone and cefotaxime, demonstrate excellent in vitro activity. Oral and parenteral antistaphylococcal penicillins and first-generation cephalosporins including cephalexin are not as active and are not recommended for treatment. *Pasteurella* species usually are resistant to vancomycin, clindamycin, and erythromycin. For patients who are allergic to beta-lactam agents, azithromycin, trimethoprim-sulfamethoxazole, and the fluoroquinolones are alternative choices, but clinical experience with these agents is limited. For suspected polymicrobial infected bite wounds, oral amoxicillin-clavulanate or, for severe infection, intravenous ampicillin-sulbactam or piperacillin-tazobactam can be given. The duration of therapy usually is 7 to 10 days for local infections and 10 to 14 days for more severe infections. Antimicrobial therapy should be continued for 4 to 6 weeks for bone and joint infections. Wound drainage or débridement may be necessary.

ISOLATION OF THE HOSPITALIZED PATIENT: Standard precautions are recommended.

CONTROL MEASURES: Limiting contact with wild animals and education about appropriate contact with domestic animals can help to prevent *Pasteurella* infections (see Bite Wounds, p 169). Wounds from animal bites and scratches should be irrigated, cleansed, and débrided promptly. Following a bite wound, antimicrobial prophylaxis for selected children, depending on host factors and the type of animal bite wound, should be initiated according to the recommendations in Table 2.9, p 171, and the risk of rabies exposure and tetanus immunization status should be assessed.

Pediculosis Capitis[1]
(Head Lice)

CLINICAL MANIFESTATIONS: Itching is the most common symptom of head lice infestation, but many children are asymptomatic. Adult lice (2–3 mm long, tan to grayish-white, with claws on all 6 legs) or eggs (match hair color) and nits (empty egg casings, white) are found on the hair and are most readily apparent behind the ears and near the nape of the neck. Excoriations and crusting caused by secondary bacterial infection may occur and often are associated with regional lymphadenopathy. Head lice usually deposit their eggs on a hair shaft 1 to 2 mm from the scalp. Because hair grows at a rate of approximately

---

[1]Devore CD, Schutze GE; American Academy of Pediatrics, Committee on School Health and Committee on Infectious Diseases. Clinical report: head lice. *Pediatrics.* 2015;135(5):e1355-e1365

1 cm per month, duration of infestation can be estimated by the distance of the nit from the scalp.

ETIOLOGY: *Pediculus humanus capitis* is the head louse. Both nymphs and adult lice feed on human blood.

EPIDEMIOLOGY: Head lice infestation in the United States is most common in children attending child care, preschool, and elementary school and is not a sign of poor hygiene. All socioeconomic groups are affected. Head lice infestation is not influenced by hair length, hair texture, or frequency of shampooing or brushing. Head lice are not a health hazard and are not responsible for spread of any disease. Transmission occurs mainly by direct head-to-head contact with hair of infested people. Transmission by contact with personal belongings, such as combs, hair brushes, sporting gear, and hats, is uncommon. Head lice survive <1 day at room temperature away from the scalp, and their eggs generally become nonviable within a week and cannot hatch at a lower ambient temperature than that near the scalp.

The **incubation period** from the laying of eggs to hatching of the first nymph usually is about 1 week (range 6 to 9 days). Lice mature to the adult stage approximately 7 days later. Adult females then may lay eggs, but these will develop only if the female has mated.

DIAGNOSTIC TESTS: Identification of eggs, nymphs, and adult lice with the naked eye is possible; diagnosis can be confirmed by using a hand lens, dermatoscope (epiluminescence microscope), or traditional microscope. Nymphal and adult lice shun light and move rapidly to conceal themselves. Wetting the hair with water, oil, or a conditioner to "slow down" the movement of the lice and using a fine-tooth comb may improve ability to diagnose infestation and shorten inspection time. It is important to differentiate nits from dandruff, hair casts (a layer of follicular cells that slide easily off the hair shaft), plugs of desquamated cells, external hair debris, and fungal infections of the scalp. Finding nits attached firmly within ¼ inch of the base of the hair shaft suggests that a person has had infestation, but because nits remain affixed firmly to hair even after hatching or when dead, their mere presence (particularly >1 cm from the scalp) is not a conclusive sign of an active infestation.

TREATMENT: Treatment is recommended for people who have an active infestation. A number of effective pediculicidal agents are available to treat head lice infestation (see Drugs for Parasitic Infections, p 965, and Table 3.42). Costs and recommended age ranges vary by product (see Table 3.42). Safety is a major concern with pediculicides, because lice infestation itself presents minimal risk to the host. Pediculicides should be used only as directed and with care and only when there is concern for active infestation. Instructions on proper use of any product should be explained carefully. Extra amounts should not be used, and multiple products should not be used concurrently. If medication gets into a child's eyes, it should be flushed out immediately with water. Skin exposure to pediculicide should be limited. Hair should be rinsed over a sink rather than during a shower or bath after topical pediculicide application, and warm rather than hot water used to minimize skin absorption attributable to vasodilatation. Therapy can be initiated with over-the-counter 1% permethrin lotion or with pyrethrin combined with piperonyl butoxide, both of which have good safety profiles. Resistance to these compounds has been documented in the United States, and clinical resistance may vary by region. Information about these agents and others are listed below and in Table 3.42 and in Drugs for Parasitic Infections (p 965). Drugs vary in their residual activity and no

Table 3.42. Pediculicides for the Treatment of Head Lice

Product	Brand Name	Recommended Age Range	Retreatment Interval (If Needed)	Availability	Cost Estimate[a]
Permethrin 1% lotion	Multiple products	≥2 mo	9–10 days	Over the counter	$
Pyrethrins + piperonyl butoxide Shampoo	Example: Rid	≥24 mo	9–10 days	Over the counter	$
Malathion 0.5%	Ovide	≥2 y (safety not established for ages 2-6 years)	7–9 days if live lice are seen after initial dose	Prescription	$$$$
Spinosad 0.9% suspension	Natroba	≥6 mo	7 days if live lice are seen after initial dose	Prescription	$$$$
Abametapir 0.74% lotion	Xeglyze	≥6 mo	Single use	Prescription	$$$$
Ivermectin 0.5% lotion	Sklice	≥6 mo	Single use	Over the counter	$$$$
Ivermectin (oral)	Stromectol	Any age, if weight ≥15 kg	9–10 days	Prescription	$$$$

[a]$ = ≤$25; $$ = $26–$99; $$$ = $100–$199; $$$$ = $200–$299.

treatment is 100% ovicidal. Retreatment may be needed after eggs present at the time of initial treatment have hatched but before new eggs are produced; retreatment intervals vary by product. Data are lacking to determine whether heat therapy or suffocation of lice by application of occlusive agents, such as petroleum jelly, olive oil, butter, or fat-containing mayonnaise, are effective methods of treatment.

- **Permethrin (1%) lotion.** Permethrin is available without a prescription in a 1% lotion. Infested hair and scalp are washed first with a nonconditioning shampoo and towel-dried. Permethrin then is applied to the scalp and entire length of wet hair, left for 10 minutes, and then rinsed off with water. Permethrin has a low potential for toxic effects and can be highly effective. Although residual permethrin is designed to kill emerging nymphs, many experts advise a second treatment 9 to 10 days after the first treatment, especially if hair is washed within a week after the first treatment or if live lice are seen.

- **Pyrethrin-based shampoo products.** Pyrethrins are natural extracts from the chrysanthemum flower, formulated with piperonyl butoxide, and are available without a prescription as shampoos or mousse preparations. The product is applied to dry hair in sufficient amounts to saturate the scalp and entire length of the hair, left for 10 minutes, and then rinsed off with water. Pyrethrins have no residual activity; repeat application 9 to 10 days after the first application is necessary to kill newly hatched lice. Pyrethrins are contraindicated in people who are allergic to chrysanthemums or ragweed.

- **Malathion (0.5%) lotion.** This organophosphate pesticide, which is both pediculicidal and partially ovicidal, is available only by prescription as a lotion. Malathion lotion is applied to dry hair in sufficient amounts to saturate the scalp and entire length of the hair, left to dry naturally, and then removed 8 to 12 hours later by washing and rinsing the hair. The product can be reapplied 7 to 9 days later only if live lice are still seen. The high alcohol content of the lotion makes it highly flammable; therefore, the lotion or lotion-coated hair during treatment should not be exposed to lighted cigarettes (no smoking around the individual during hair treatment), open flames, or electric heat sources such as hair dryers or curling irons. Malathion lotion should not be used in children younger than 2 years, and safety and effectiveness have not been assessed by the US Food and Drug Administration (FDA) in children younger than 6 years.
- **Spinosad (0.9%) suspension.** Spinosad is a novel neurotoxin derived from *Saccharopolyspora spinosa*. Spinosad suspension contains benzyl alcohol and is pediculicidal. The suspension is applied to dry hair in sufficient amounts to saturate the scalp and entire length of the hair, left for 10 minutes, and then rinsed off with water. A second treatment is applied at 7 days if live lice still are seen. This product should not be used in infants younger than 6 months because systemic absorption may lead to benzyl alcohol toxicity.
- **Abametapir (0.74%) lotion.** Abametapir inhibits metalloproteinases, which have a role in physiological processes critical to egg development and survival of lice. Abametapir lotion contains benzyl alcohol and is ovicidal. Abametapir lotion is applied to dry hair in sufficient amounts to thoroughly coat the hair and scalp, left on for 10 minutes, and then rinsed off with warm water. Treatment involves a single application. This product should not be used in infants younger than 6 months, because systemic absorption may lead to benzyl alcohol toxicity.
- **Ivermectin (0.5%) lotion.** Ivermectin interferes with the function of invertebrate nerve and muscle cells and is used widely as an anthelmintic agent. Ivermectin lotion is not ovicidal, but appears to prevent newly hatched lice (nymphs) from surviving. The lotion is applied to dry hair in sufficient amounts to saturate the scalp and entire length of the hair, left for 10 minutes, and then rinsed off with water. It is effective in most patients when given as a single application on dry hair without nit combing and may be used in children 6 months of age and older.
- **Oral ivermectin.** Ivermectin may be effective against head lice if sufficient concentration is present in the blood at the time a louse feeds. It has been given as a single oral dose of 200 µg/kg or 400 µg/kg, with a second dose given after 9 to 10 days. Fewer failures occur at the 400-µg/kg dose compared with the lower dose. Ivermectin should not be used in children weighing less than 15 kg because it blocks essential neural transmission if it crosses the blood-brain barrier and young children may be at higher risk of this adverse drug reaction.
- Lindane, although FDA approved for treatment of head lice, no longer is recommended by the American Academy of Pediatrics because of toxicity.

Detection of living lice on scalp inspection 24 hours or more after treatment suggests incorrect use of pediculicide, hatching of lice after treatment, reinfestation, or resistance to therapy, because pediculicides kill lice shortly after application. After excluding incorrect use, retreatment with a different pediculicide followed by a second application (with the exception of single-use topical ivermectin) at the intervals specified above and in Drugs for Parasitic Infections (p 965) is recommended in such situations.

Itching or mild burning of the scalp caused by inflammation of the skin in response to topical therapeutic agents can persist for many days after lice are killed; this is not a reason for retreatment. Topical corticosteroid and oral antihistamine agents may be beneficial for relieving these signs and symptoms.

Manual removal of nits after successful treatment with a pediculicide is helpful to decrease diagnostic confusion and to decrease the small risk of self-reinfestation and social stigmatization. Fine-toothed nit combs designed for this purpose are available, although the type of comb is less important than the actual action of combing. Other products, such as vinegar, should not be used to help remove nits, because these may interfere with effectiveness of the pediculicide.

ISOLATION OF THE HOSPITALIZED PATIENT: Standard precautions plus contact precautions are recommended until the patient has been treated with an appropriate pediculicide.

CONTROL MEASURES: Household and other close contacts should be examined and treated if infested. Bedmates of infested people should be treated prophylactically at the same time as the infested household members and contacts, even if bedmates do not have identifiable live lice. Prophylactic treatment of other noninfested people is not recommended. Children should not be excluded or sent home early from school because of head lice, because head lice have a low contagion within classrooms (see Table 2.3, p 128). Parents of children with infestation (ie, at least 1 live, crawling louse) should be notified and informed that their child should be treated. The presence of nits alone does not justify treatment.

"No-nit" policies requiring that children be free of nits before they return to a child care facility or school should be discouraged. Nits farther from the scalp are easier to discover but are of no consequence. Routine classroom or schoolwide screening for lice is discouraged, because it is not an accurate or cost-effective way of lowering the incidence of head lice in the school setting. Parents who are educated on the diagnosis of lice infestation may screen their own children's heads for lice regularly and if the child is symptomatic.

Supplemental measures generally are not required to eliminate an infestation. Head lice rarely are transferred via fomites from shared headgear, clothing, combs, or bedding. Special handling of such items, therefore, is not likely to be useful; protective headgear should not be refused because of fear of head lice. If desired, hats, bedding, clothing, and towels worn or used by the infested person in the 2-day period just before treatment is started can be machine-washed and dried using the hot water and hot air cycles, respectively, because lice and eggs are killed by exposure for 5 minutes to temperatures greater than 130°F. Clothing and items that are not washable can be dry cleaned or sealed in a plastic bag and stored for 2 weeks. Brushes and combs can be soaked in hot water (at least 130°F) for 5 to 10 minutes. Vacuuming furniture and floors can remove an infested person's hairs that might have viable eggs attached. Pediculicide spray is not necessary and should not be used. Treatment of dogs, cats, or other pets is not indicated, because they do not play a role in transmission of human head lice.

Pediculosis Corporis
(Body Lice)

CLINICAL MANIFESTATIONS: Patients affected with pediculosis corporis characteristically come to medical attention because of intense itching, particularly at night. Bites manifest as small erythematous macules, papules, and excoriations, primarily on the trunk. In heavily bitten areas, typically around the mid-section of the body (waist, groin, upper thighs), the skin can become thickened and discolored. Secondary bacterial infection of the skin (pyoderma) caused by scratching is common.

ETIOLOGY: *Pediculus humanus corporis* (or *humanus*) is the body louse. Both nymphs and adult lice feed on human blood.

EPIDEMIOLOGY: Body lice generally are restricted to people living in crowded conditions without access to regular bathing (at least weekly) or changes of clean clothing (refugees, victims of war or natural disasters, homeless people). Under these conditions, body lice can spread rapidly through direct contact or contact with contaminated clothing or bedding. Body lice live in clothes or bedding used by infested people, lay their eggs on or near the seams of clothing, and only move to the skin to feed. Body lice cannot survive away from a blood source for longer than approximately 5 to 7 days at room temperature. In contrast with head and pubic lice, body lice are well-recognized vectors of disease (eg, epidemic typhus, trench fever, epidemic relapsing fever, and bacillary angiomatosis).

The **incubation period** from laying eggs to hatching of the first nymph is approximately 1 to 2 weeks, depending on ambient temperature. Lice mature and are capable of reproducing 9 to 19 days after hatching, depending on whether infested clothing is removed for sleeping.

DIAGNOSTIC TESTS: Seams of clothing should be examined for eggs (nits), nymphs, and adult lice (2–4 mm) if body louse infestation is suspected. Nits and lice may be seen with the naked eye; diagnosis can be confirmed by using a hand lens, dermatoscope (epiluminescence microscope), or a traditional microscope. Adult and nymphal body lice seldom are seen on the body, because they generally are sequestered in clothing.

TREATMENT: Treatment consists of improving hygiene, including bathing and regular (at least weekly) changes to clean clothes and bedding. Infested materials can be discarded or decontaminated by machine-washed and dried using the hot water and hot air cycles, respectively, by dry cleaning, by sealing in a plastic bag and stored for 2 weeks or by pressing with a hot iron. Temperatures exceeding 130°F for 5 minutes are lethal to lice and eggs. Pediculicides for patients usually are not necessary if materials are laundered sufficiently hot at least weekly. People with abundant body hair may require full-body treatment with a pediculicide, because lice and eggs may occasionally adhere to body hair. Guidance for the choice of pediculicide (if desired for treatment) is the same as for head lice (see Pediculosis Capitis, p 567; and Drugs for Parasitic Infections, p 965).

ISOLATION OF THE HOSPITALIZED PATIENT: In addition to standard precautions, contact precautions are recommended and should continue until the patient's clothing and bedding have been cleaned effectively.

CONTROL MEASURES: The most important factor in the control of body lice infestation is the ability to change and wash clothing. Close contacts should be examined and treated appropriately. Fumigation or dusting with chemical insecticides sometimes is necessary to control and prevent certain diseases (epidemic typhus) that are spread by body lice.

Pediculosis Pubis
(Pubic Lice, Crab Lice)

CLINICAL MANIFESTATIONS: Pruritus of the anogenital area is a common symptom in pubic lice infestations ("crabs" or "phthiriasis"). Adult lice (1–2 mm long and flattened, tan to grayish-white with 4 of its 6 legs terminating in crab-like claws) or eggs (match hair color) and nits (empty egg casings, white) are found on hair, particularly near the hair-skin junction. The parasite most frequently is found in the pubic region, but infestation can involve other coarse body hair, including the eyelashes, eyebrows, beard, axilla, legs, perianal area, and rarely, the scalp. A characteristic sign of heavy pubic lice infestation is the presence of bluish or slate-colored macules (maculae ceruleae) on the chest, abdomen, or thighs.

ETIOLOGY: *Pthirus pubis* is the pubic or crab louse. Both nymphs and adult lice feed on human blood. Pubic lice are not a health hazard and are not responsible for the spread of any disease.

EPIDEMIOLOGY: Pubic lice infestations are more prevalent in teenagers and young adults and usually are spread through sexual contact. Transmission by contact with contaminated items, such as bed linens, towels, or shared clothing, can occur. Pubic lice on the eyelashes or eyebrows of children (likely the only areas of coarse hair) may be evidence of sexual abuse. People with pubic lice infestation should be examined for the presence of other sexually transmitted infections. Animals do not get or spread pubic lice.

The **incubation period** from the laying of eggs to the hatching of the first nymph is 6 to 10 days. Adult lice become capable of reproducing 2 to 3 weeks after hatching. Adult pubic lice can survive away from a host for up to 48 hours, and their eggs can remain viable for up to 10 days under suitable environmental conditions.

DIAGNOSTIC TESTS: Identification of eggs (nits), nymphs, and lice with the naked eye is possible, although it can be difficult to detect lice unless they have had a recent blood meal. The diagnosis can be confirmed by using a hand lens, traditional microscope, or dermatoscope (epiluminescence microscope) to examine hair shafts. Pubic lice may be difficult to find because of low numbers, and they do not crawl as quickly as head and body lice. If crawling lice are not seen, finding nits in the pubic area strongly suggests infestation and should lead to treatment.

TREATMENT[1]: All areas of the body with coarse hair should be examined for evidence of pubic lice infestation. Lice and their eggs can be removed manually, or the hairs can be shaved to eliminate infestation immediately (though topical pediculicides should still be used even when the affected area is shaved). Caution should be used when inspecting, removing, or treating lice on or near the eyelashes. Recommended therapies include either permethrin 1% cream rinse (applied to affected areas and washed off after 10 minutes) or pyrethrins with piperonyl butoxide (applied to the affected area and washed off after 10 minutes). Reported resistance to permethrin and pyrethrins has been increasing and is widespread. Evaluation should be performed after 1 week if symptoms persist. Retreatment might be necessary if lice are found or if eggs are observed at the hair-skin junction. If no clinical response is achieved to one of the recommended regimens, treatment with malathion (0.5% lotion applied to affected areas and washed off after 8–12 hours) or oral ivermectin (250 µg/kg orally, repeated in 7–14 days) is recommended.

Infested people should be examined for other sexually transmitted infections (see Sexually Transmitted Infections in Adolescents and Children, p 148). Pubic lice on the eyelashes or eyebrows of children should prompt evaluation for sexual abuse (see Sexual Assault and Abuse in Children and Adolescents/Young Adults, p 150).

ISOLATION OF THE HOSPITALIZED PATIENT: In addition to standard precautions, contact precautions are recommended until the patient has been treated with an appropriate pediculicide.

---

[1]Centers for Disease Control and Prevention. Sexually transmitted infections treatment guidelines, 2021. *MMWR Recomm Rep.* 2021; in press

CONTROL MEASURES: Lice are highly contagious; thus, all sexual contacts within the previous month should be treated. Patients should be advised to avoid sexual contact until they and their sex partners have been treated successfully, bedding and clothing have been decontaminated, and reevaluation has been performed to rule out persistent infestation. Bedding, towels, and clothing can be decontaminated by machine washing and drying using the hot water and hot air cycles, respectively, because lice and eggs are killed by exposure for 5 minutes at temperatures greater than 130°F. Clothing and items that are not washable can be dry cleaned or sealed in a plastic bag and stored for 2 weeks.

Pelvic Inflammatory Disease

CLINICAL MANIFESTATIONS: Pelvic inflammatory disease (PID) comprises a spectrum of inflammatory disorders of the female upper genital tract, including any combination of endometritis, parametritis, salpingitis, oophoritis, tubo-ovarian abscess, and pelvic peritonitis. Acute PID is difficult to diagnose because of the wide variation in symptoms and signs. Symptoms of acute PID include unilateral or bilateral lower abdominal or pelvic pain, fever, vomiting, abnormal vaginal discharge, irregular vaginal bleeding, and pain with intercourse. The severity of symptoms varies widely and may range from indolent to severe. Patients occasionally present with right upper quadrant abdominal pain resulting from peritoneal adhesions related to perihepatitis (Fitz-Hugh-Curtis syndrome). Many episodes of PID go undiagnosed and untreated because the patient and/or health care professional fails to recognize the implications of mild or nonspecific symptoms and signs. Subclinical PID is defined as inflammation of the upper reproductive tract in the absence of signs and symptoms of acute PID, and there is a growing body of evidence that this represents a large proportion of all PID cases. In both clinically apparent and subclinical PID, inflammation occurs within the reproductive tract that scars or damages the fallopian tubes or surrounding structures. Clinicians need to maintain a high degree of suspicion for PID when a woman of reproductive age presents with mild or nonspecific findings, particularly in a young female who might provide an incomplete or inaccurate sexual history.

Examination findings vary but may include oral temperature >101°F (>38.3°C), lower abdominal tenderness with or without peritoneal signs, abnormal cervical or vaginal discharge, tenderness with lateral motion of the cervix, uterine tenderness, unilateral or bilateral adnexal tenderness, and adnexal fullness. Pyuria (presence of white blood cells [WBCs] on urine microscopy), abundant WBCs on saline microscopy of vaginal fluid, an elevated erythrocyte sedimentation rate, elevated C-reactive protein, and/or an adnexal mass demonstrated by abdominal or transvaginal ultrasonography are findings that support a diagnosis of PID.

Complications of PID include perihepatitis (Fitz-Hugh-Curtis syndrome) and tubo-ovarian abscess/complex formation. Long-term sequelae include tubal scarring that can cause infertility in an estimated 10% to 20% of affected females, ectopic pregnancy in an estimated 9%, and chronic pelvic pain in an estimated 18%. Factors that may increase the likelihood of infertility are delay in diagnosis or delay in initiation of antimicrobial therapy, younger age at time of infection, chlamydial infection, recurrent PID, and PID determined to be severe by laparoscopic examination.

Any prepubertal female with PID needs to be assessed for sexual abuse (see Sexual Assault and Abuse in Children and Adolescents/Young Adults, p 150). Mandatory reporters should follow their state's regulations for reporting.

ETIOLOGY: *Neisseria gonorrhoeae* and *Chlamydia trachomatis* are the pathogens most commonly associated with PID, although in recent studies less than half of PID cases have evidence of these bacterial pathogens. A number of organisms other than *N gonorrhoeae* and *C trachomatis* have been isolated from upper genital tract cultures of females with PID, including anaerobes (such as *Prevotella* species), *Gardnerella vaginalis*, *Haemophilus influenzae*, *Streptococcus agalactiae*, enteric gram-negative rods, cytomegalovirus, *Mycoplasma hominis*, and *Ureaplasma urealyticum*. Therefore, PID is managed as a polymicrobial infection. In more than half of cases, however, no organism is identified from routine lower genital tract swab specimens (ie, endocervical or vaginal swab specimens). *Mycoplasma genitalium* also has been implicated in the etiology of PID in some studies, although the natural history of *M genitalium* in females remains unclear. PID may also be secondary to other causes of peritonitis, such as ruptured appendicitis.

EPIDEMIOLOGY: Although many of the issues pertaining to high-risk sexual behavior and acquisition of sexually transmitted infections (STIs) are common to both adolescents and adults, they often are intensified among adolescents because of both behavioral and biological predispositions. Adolescents and young women can be at higher risk of STIs and PID because of behavioral factors such as inconsistent barrier contraceptive use, douching, greater number of current and lifetime sexual partners, and use of alcohol and other substances that may impair judgment while engaging in sexual activity. Use of condoms may reduce the risk of PID. Adolescent and young adult females also have an increased biologic susceptibility to STIs. Cervical ectopy increases risk of chlamydia and gonorrhea infection by exposing columnar epithelium to a potential infectious inoculum.

An **incubation period** for PID is undefined.

DIAGNOSTIC TESTS[1]: Centers for Disease Control and Prevention (CDC) criteria for clinical diagnosis and presumptive treatment of PID are presented in Table 3.43. Acute PID is difficult to diagnose because of its wide variation in symptoms and signs. Many women with PID have subtle or nonspecific symptoms or are asymptomatic, and a diagnosis of PID usually is based on imprecise clinical findings. A clinical diagnosis of symptomatic PID has a positive predictive value for salpingitis of 65% to 90% compared with laparoscopy. No single historical, physical, or laboratory finding is both sensitive and specific for the diagnosis of acute PID. Because of the difficulty of diagnosis and the potential for damage to the reproductive health of women, health care providers should maintain a low threshold for the clinical diagnosis of PID.

A cervical or vaginal swab specimen should be obtained from all patients with suspected PID to perform a nucleic acid amplification test (NAAT) for *C trachomatis* and *N gonorrhoeae*. A swab specimen for culture of *N gonorrhoeae* may be collected from the cervix or vagina to allow susceptibility testing to be performed. The most specific criteria for diagnosing PID include endometrial biopsy with histopathologic evidence of endometritis; transvaginal ultrasonography or magnetic resonance imaging techniques showing thickened, fluid-filled tubes with or without free pelvic fluid or tubo-ovarian complex or

---

[1]Centers for Disease Control and Prevention. Sexually transmitted infections treatment guidelines, 2021. *MMWR Recomm Rep.* 2021; in press

Table 3.43. Criteria for Clinical Diagnosis and Presumptive Treatment of Pelvic Inflammatory Disease (PID)[a]

Minimum Criteria

Presumptive treatment for PID should be initiated in sexually active young women and other women at risk for STIs if they are experiencing pelvic or lower abdominal pain, if no cause for the illness other than PID can be identified, and if one or more of the following **minimum clinical criteria** are present on pelvic examination:

- Cervical motion tenderness

or

- Uterine tenderness

or

- Adnexal tenderness

One or more of the following **additional criteria** can be used to enhance the specificity of the minimum clinical criteria and support a diagnosis of PID:

- Oral temperature >101°F (>38.3°C);
- Abnormal cervical mucopurulent discharge or cervical friability;
- Presence of abundant numbers of WBC on saline microscopy of vaginal fluid;
- Elevated erythrocyte sedimentation rate;
- Elevated C-reactive protein; and
- Laboratory documentation of cervical infection with *N gonorrhoeae* or *C trachomatis*.

Most women with PID have either mucopurulent cervical discharge or evidence of WBCs on a microscopic evaluation of a saline preparation of vaginal fluid (ie, wet prep). If the cervical discharge appears normal and no WBCs are observed on the wet prep of vaginal fluid, the diagnosis of PID is unlikely, and alternative causes of pain should be considered. A wet prep of vaginal fluid also can detect the presence of concomitant infections (eg, bacterial vaginosis and trichomoniasis).

[a] Adapted from Centers for Disease Control and Prevention. Sexually transmitted infections treatment guidelines, 2021. *MMWR Recomm Rep.* 2021; in press

Doppler ultrasonography suggesting pelvic infection (eg, tubal hyperemia); or laparoscopic findings consistent with PID. A diagnostic evaluation that includes some of these more extensive procedures might be warranted in some cases. Endometrial biopsy is warranted in women undergoing laparoscopy who do not have visual evidence of salpingitis, because endometritis is the only sign of PID for some women.

In addition to determining whether WBCs are present in cervicovaginal secretions, a wet mount will assist in the diagnosis or exclusion of the commonly associated trichomonas or bacterial vaginosis. Serologic testing for human immunodeficiency virus (HIV) and syphilis also should be performed. The possibility of coexisting early pregnancy must always be assessed in patients who are being evaluated for PID.

TREATMENT[1]: A sexually active adolescent or young adult female with lower abdominal pain who exhibits uterine, adnexal, or cervical motion tenderness on bimanual

[1] Centers for Disease Control and Prevention. Sexually transmitted infections treatment guidelines, 2021. *MMWR Recomm Rep.* 2021; in press

examination should be treated for PID if no other cause is identified. To minimize risks of progressive infection and subsequent infertility, treatment should be initiated at the time of clinical diagnosis, and therapy should be completed, regardless of the STI test results.

Among females with mild to moderate PID, there is no difference in clinical course, recurrent PID, chronic pelvic pain, or infertility rates between females hospitalized and those treated on an outpatient basis for PID. The decision to hospitalize adolescent or young adult females with acute PID should be based on the provider's judgment and whether the patient meets any of the following suggested criteria:
- Surgical emergencies (eg, appendicitis) cannot be excluded;
- Tubo-ovarian abscess;
- Pregnancy;
- Severe illness, nausea and vomiting, or high fever;
- Unable to follow or tolerate an outpatient oral regimen;
- No clinical response to oral antimicrobial therapy.

Whether treated on an inpatient or outpatient basis, the antimicrobial regimen chosen should provide empiric, broad-spectrum coverage directed against the most common causative agents, including *N gonorrhoeae* and *C trachomatis*, even if these pathogens are not identified in lower genital tract specimens. If the *N gonorrhoeae* culture is positive, antimicrobial susceptibility testing should guide subsequent therapy. If the isolate is determined to be quinolone-resistant *N gonorrhoeae* or if antimicrobial susceptibility cannot be assessed (eg, if only NAAT testing is available), consultation with an infectious-disease specialist is recommended.

Table 4.4 (p 898) lists the parenteral regimens recommended by the CDC for treatment of hospitalized patients, and the intramuscular/oral regimens recommended for the treatment of patients in the outpatient setting. For management of women hospitalized and managed initially with the parenteral therapy options listed in Table 4.4, clinical experience should guide decisions regarding transition to oral therapy, which usually can be initiated within 24 to 48 hours of clinical improvement. In women with tubo-ovarian abscesses, at least 24 hours of inpatient observation is recommended.

Intramuscular/oral therapy (Table 4.4, p 898) can be considered for women with mild-to-moderately severe acute PID who can be managed in the outpatient setting from the outset, because the clinical outcomes among women treated with these regimens are similar to those treated with intravenous therapy. Women who do not respond to intramuscular/oral therapy within 72 hours should be reevaluated to confirm the diagnosis and be administered intravenous therapy. Women should demonstrate clinical improvement (eg, defervescence; reduction in direct or rebound abdominal tenderness; and reduction in uterine, adnexal, cervical motion tenderness) within 3 days after initiation of therapy. If no clinical improvement has occurred within 72 hours after outpatient intramuscular/oral therapy, hospitalization, assessment of the antimicrobial regimen, and additional diagnostics (including consideration of diagnostic laparoscopy for alternative diagnoses) are recommended.

If an adolescent or young woman with an intrauterine device (IUD) receives a diagnosis of PID, the IUD does not need to be removed. However, the patient should have close clinical follow-up and if there is no clinical improvement 48 to 72 hours after treatment initiation, removal of the IUD may be considered.

ISOLATION OF THE HOSPITALIZED PATIENT: Standard precautions are recommended.

CONTROL MEASURES[1,2]:

- All women who have received a diagnosis of chlamydial or gonococcal PID should be retested 3 months after treatment, regardless of whether their sex partners were treated. If retesting at 3 months is not possible, these women should be retested whenever they next present for medical care in the 12 months following treatment.
- Men who have had sexual contact with a woman with PID during the 60 days preceding her onset of symptoms should be evaluated, tested, and presumptively treated for chlamydia and gonorrhea, regardless of the etiology of PID or pathogens isolated from the woman. If a woman's last sexual intercourse was >60 days before onset of symptoms or diagnosis, the most recent sex partner should be treated.
- To minimize disease transmission, women should be instructed to abstain from sexual intercourse until therapy is completed, symptoms have resolved, and sex partners have been adequately treated.
- The patient and her partner(s) should be encouraged to use condoms consistently and correctly.
- The patient should be screened for other STIs, including HIV.
- Unimmunized or incompletely immunized patients should complete the immunization series for human papillomavirus and hepatitis B **(https://redbook.solutions.aap.org/SS/Immunization_Schedules.aspx).**
- The diagnosis of PID provides an opportunity to educate the adolescent about prevention of STIs, including abstinence, consistent use of barrier methods of protection, immunization, and the importance of receiving periodic screening for STIs.

Pertussis (Whooping Cough)

CLINICAL MANIFESTATIONS: Pertussis begins with mild upper respiratory tract symptoms similar to the common cold (catarrhal stage) and progresses to cough, usually paroxysms of cough (paroxysmal stage), characterized by inspiratory whoop (gasping) after repeated cough on the same breath, which commonly is followed by vomiting. Fever is absent or minimal. Symptoms wane gradually over weeks to months (convalescent stage). Cough illness in immunized children and adults can range from typical to very mild. The duration of classic pertussis is 6 to 10 weeks. Complications among adolescents and adults include syncope, weight loss, sleep disturbance, incontinence, rib fractures, and pneumonia; among adults, complications may increase with age. Pertussis is most severe when it occurs during the first 6 months of life, particularly in preterm and unimmunized infants. Disease in infants younger than 6 months can be atypical with a short catarrhal stage, followed by gagging, gasping, bradycardia, or apnea as prominent early manifestations; absence of whoop; and prolonged convalescence. Sudden unexpected death can be caused by pertussis. Complications among infants include pneumonia, pulmonary hypertension, and severe coughing spells with associated conjunctival bleeding, hernia, and hypoxia. Seizures (0.9%), encephalopathy (less than 0.5%), apnea, and death can occur in infants with pertussis. Approximately half of infants with pertussis in the United States are hospitalized. Case-fatality rates are approximately 1.6% in infants younger than

---

[1]Centers for Disease Control and Prevention. Recommendations for partner services programs for HIV infection, syphilis, gonorrhea, and chlamydial infection. *MMWR Recomm Rep.* 2008;57(RR-9):1–63

[2]Centers for Disease Control and Prevention. Sexually transmitted infections treatment guidelines, 2021. *MMWR Recomm Rep.* 2021; in press

2 months and less than 1.2% in infants 2 through 11 months of age. Maternal immunization during pregnancy and an infant's receipt of at least some doses of pertussis vaccine reduce morbidity and mortality in young infants.

ETIOLOGY: Pertussis is caused by a fastidious, gram-negative, pleomorphic bacillus, *Bordetella pertussis*. Other *Bordetella* species can cause sporadic prolonged cough illness in people, including *Bordetella parapertussis*, *Bordetella bronchiseptica* (the cause of canine kennel cough), and *Bordetella holmesii*.

EPIDEMIOLOGY: Humans are the only known hosts of *B pertussis*. Transmission occurs by close contact with infected individuals via large respiratory droplets generated by coughing or sneezing. Cases occur year-round, typically with a late summer-autumn peak. Neither infection nor immunization provides lifelong immunity. Waning immunity, particularly when acellular pertussis vaccine is used for the entire immunization series, is predominantly responsible for increased cases reported in school-aged children, adolescents, and adults. Additionally, waning maternal immunity of mothers who have not received Tdap vaccine during that pregnancy results in low concentrations of transplacentally transmitted antibody and an increased risk of pertussis in very young infants. Pertussis incidence is cyclic and in the United States and has increased between 2000 and 2016. Pertussis is highly contagious. As many as 80% of susceptible household contacts of symptomatic infant cases are infected with *B pertussis*, with symptoms in these contacts varying from mild to classic pertussis. Siblings and adults with cough illness are important sources of pertussis infection for young infants. Infected people are most contagious during the catarrhal stage through the third week after onset of paroxysms or until 5 days after the start of effective antimicrobial treatment. Factors affecting the length of communicability include age, immunization status or previous infection, and receipt of appropriate antimicrobial therapy.

The **incubation period** is 7 to 10 days, with a range of 5 to 21 days.

DIAGNOSTIC TESTS: Culture previously was considered the "gold standard" for laboratory diagnosis of pertussis but is not optimally sensitive and has largely been replaced by nucleic acid amplification tests (NAATs). Culture requires collection of an appropriate nasopharyngeal swab specimen, obtained either by aspiration or with polyester or flocked rayon swabs or calcium alginate swabs. Specimens must not be allowed to dry during prompt transport to the laboratory. Culture results can be negative if taken from a previously immunized person, if antimicrobial therapy has been started, if more than 2 weeks has elapsed since cough onset, or if the specimen is not collected or handled appropriately.

NAATs cleared by the US Food and Drug Administration (FDA), including polymerase chain reaction (PCR) assays, are commercially available as standalone tests or as multiplex assays and are the most commonly used laboratory method for detection of *B pertussis* because of greater sensitivity and more rapid turnaround time. The PCR test requires collection of an adequate nasopharyngeal specimen using a Dacron swab or nasopharyngeal wash or aspirate. Calcium alginate swabs can be inhibitory to PCR and should not be used. The PCR test has optimal sensitivity during the first 3 weeks of cough and is unlikely to be useful if antimicrobial therapy has been given for more than 5 days. The Centers for Disease Control and Prevention (CDC) has released a "best practices" document to guide pertussis PCR assays (**www.cdc.gov/pertussis/clinical/diagnostic-testing/diagnosis-pcr-bestpractices.html**) as well as a video demonstrating optimal specimen collection. PCR assays for pertussis are not standardized and assays vary in their diagnostic utility. Most PCR assays target only a multicopy insertion gene sequence (IS 481) found in *B pertussis* as well as the less commonly encountered *B holmesii* and some strains of *B bronchiseptica*. Multiple DNA target sequences are required to distinguish among clinically relevant *Bordetella* species.

Serologic tests for pertussis infection may be helpful for diagnosis, especially late in illness, but are not commonly used. The CDC and FDA have developed a pertussis antibody test that has been used by many state public health laboratories during outbreaks; however, no commercial kit is cleared by the FDA for diagnostic use. In the absence of recent immunization, an elevated serum immunoglobulin (Ig) G antibody to pertussis toxin (PT) present 2 to 8 weeks after onset of cough is suggestive of recent *B pertussis* infection. For single serum specimens, an IgG anti-PT value of approximately 100 IU/mL or greater (using standard reference sera as a comparator) has been recommended. Positive paired serologic results based on the World Health Organization pertussis case definition may also be considered diagnostic. IgA and IgM assays lack adequate sensitivity and specificity and should not be used for the diagnosis of pertussis. Direct fluorescent antibody (DFA) testing is not recommended.

An increased white blood cell count attributable to absolute lymphocytosis is suggestive of pertussis in infants and young children but often is absent in older people with pertussis and may be only mildly abnormal in some infants. A markedly elevated white blood cell count is associated with a poor prognosis in young infants.

TREATMENT: Antimicrobial therapy administered during the catarrhal stage may ameliorate the disease. Antimicrobial therapy is indicated before test results are received if the clinical history is strongly suggestive of pertussis or the patient is at high risk of severe or complicated disease (eg, is an infant). A 5-day course of azithromycin is the appropriate first-line choice for treatment and for postexposure prophylaxis (PEP [see Table 3.44, p 581]). After the paroxysmal cough is established, antimicrobial agents have no discernible effect on the course of illness but are recommended to limit spread of organisms to others. Resistance of *B pertussis* to macrolide antimicrobial agents has been reported but rarely in the United States. Penicillins and first- and second-generation cephalosporins are not effective against *B pertussis*.

Orally administered erythromycin and, to a lesser degree, azithromycin, when given in the first 6 weeks of life, are associated with increased risk of infantile hypertrophic pyloric stenosis (IHPS), but azithromycin remains the drug of choice for treatment or prophylaxis of pertussis in very young infants. Cases of IHPS in young infants who have been treated with a macrolide antibiotic should be reported to MedWatch (see MedWatch, p 1004).

Trimethoprim-sulfamethoxazole is an alternative for patients older than 2 months who cannot tolerate macrolides or who are infected with a macrolide-resistant strain, but studies evaluating trimethoprim-sulfamethoxazole as treatment for pertussis are limited.

Young infants are at increased risk of respiratory failure attributable to apnea or secondary bacterial pneumonia and are at risk of cardiopulmonary failure and death from severe pulmonary hypertension. Illness characteristics that would suggest the need for hospitalization of infants with pertussis include respiratory distress, inability to feed, cyanosis or apnea, and seizures. Some experts believe that age <4 months is itself an indication for hospitalization in infants with pertussis or suspected pertussis infection. Hospitalized young infants with pertussis should be managed in a setting/facility where these complications can be recognized and managed urgently. Exchange transfusions or leukopheresis

Table 3.44. Recommended Antimicrobial Therapy and Postexposure Prophylaxis for Pertussis in Infants, Children, Adolescents, and Adults[a]

| Age | Recommended Drugs | | | Alternative |
	Azithromycin	Erythromycin	Clarithromycin	TMP-SMX
Younger than 1 mo	10 mg/kg/day as a single dose daily for 5 days[b,c]	40 mg/kg/day in 4 divided doses for 14 days	Not recommended	Contraindicated at younger than 2 mo
1 through 5 mo	10 mg/kg/day as a single dose daily for 5 days[b]	40 mg/kg/day in 4 divided doses for 14 days	15 mg/kg/day in 2 divided doses for 7 days	2 mo or older: TMP, 8 mg/kg/day; SMX, 40 mg/kg/day in 2 doses for 14 days
6 mo or older and children	10 mg/kg as a single dose on day 1 (maximum 500 mg), then 5 mg/kg/day as a single dose on days 2 through 5 (maximum 250 mg/day)[b,d]	40 mg/kg/day in 4 divided doses for 7–14 days (maximum 2 g/day)	15 mg/kg/day in 2 divided doses for 7 days (maximum 1 g/day)	2 mo or older: TMP, 8 mg/kg/day; SMX, 40 mg/kg/day in 2 doses for 14 days
Adolescents and adults	500 mg as a single dose on day 1, then 250 mg as a single dose on days 2 through 5[b,d]	2 g/day in 4 divided doses for 7–14 days	1 g/day in 2 divided doses for 7 days	TMP, 320 mg/day; SMX, 1600 mg/day in 2 divided doses for 14 days

SMX indicates sulfamethoxazole; TMP, trimethoprim.

[a]Centers for Disease Control and Prevention. Recommended antimicrobial agents for the treatment and postexposure prophylaxis of pertussis: 2005 CDC guidelines. *MMWR Recomm Rep.* 2005;54(RR-14):1–16

[b]Azithromycin should be used with caution in people with prolonged QT interval and certain proarrhythmic conditions.

[c]Preferred macrolide for this age because of risk of idiopathic hypertrophic pyloric stenosis associated with erythromycin.

[d]A 3-day course of azithromycin for PEP or treatment has not been validated and is not recommended.

have been reported to be life-saving in infants with progressive pulmonary hypertension and markedly elevated lymphocyte counts.

Because data on the clinical effectiveness of antibiotic treatment on *B parapertussis* are limited, treatment decisions should be based on clinical judgment, with particular attention toward special populations that may be at increased risk for severe *B parapertussis* disease, including infants, elderly, and immunocompromised people. Limited available data suggest that *B parapertussis* is less susceptible to antimicrobial agents than *B pertussis*, although some studies indicate that macrolides, trimethoprim-sulfamethoxazole, and ciprofloxacin generally have activity against *B parapertussis*. *B bronchiseptica* has intrinsic resistance to macrolide antibiotics.

ISOLATION OF THE HOSPITALIZED PATIENT: In addition to standard precautions, droplet precautions are recommended for 21 days from onset of cough if appropriate antimicrobial therapy is not administered or for 5 days after initiation of effective therapy.

CONTROL MEASURES: Pertussis is a nationally notifiable disease in the United States. *Care of Exposed People.* Individuals in all settings who have been in close contact with a person infected with pertussis should be monitored closely for respiratory tract symptoms for 21 days after last contact with the infected person. Close contacts with cough should be evaluated. People in child care settings (both care takers and children), schools (both teachers and students), and health care settings with confirmed pertussis should be excluded from daycare, school, or work until completion of 5 days of the recommended course of antimicrobial therapy. Untreated individuals should be excluded until 21 days have elapsed from cough onset.

Household and Other Close Contacts. Close contacts who are unimmunized or underimmunized should have pertussis immunization initiated or continued as soon as possible using age-appropriate products according to the recommended schedule; this includes off-label use of tetanus toxoid, reduced-content diphtheria toxoid, and acellular pertussis vaccine (Tdap) in children 7 through 9 years of age who did not complete the diphtheria and tetanus toxoids and acellular pertussis vaccine (DTaP) series (see Table 3.45).

PEP is recommended for all household contacts of the index case and other close contacts, including children in child care, regardless of immunization status. (**www.cdc. gov/pertussis/outbreaks/pep.html).** When considering a nonhousehold contact with an uncertain amount of exposure, PEP should be administered if the contact personally is at high risk or lives in a household with a person at high risk of severe pertussis (eg, young infant, pregnant woman, person who has contact with infants). If 21 days have elapsed since onset of cough in the index case, PEP has limited value but may be considered for households with high-risk contacts. The agents, doses, and duration of PEP are the same as for treatment of pertussis (see Table 3.44, p 581). Prophylaxis for people exposed to *B parapertussis* is not recommended.

Child Care. Pertussis vaccine and chemoprophylaxis should be administered as recommended for household and other close contacts. In the setting of known pertussis exposure, children and child care providers who are symptomatic should be excluded pending physician evaluation.

Schools. Use of PEP for large groups of students usually is not recommended, especially in the setting of widespread community transmission, but exceptions for specific individuals can be considered. This occurs when close contact simulates household exposure or when pertussis in the exposed person may result in severe medical consequences. Public health officials should be consulted for recommendations to control pertussis transmission in schools. The immunization status of close contacts should be reviewed, and appropriate vaccines administered when indicated. Parents and teachers should be notified about possible exposures to pertussis. Exclusion of exposed people with cough illness within 21 days of last exposure should be considered pending evaluation by a physician.

Health Care Settings.[1] Health care facilities should maximize efforts to immunize all health care personnel (HCP) with Tdap. All HCP should observe droplet precautions when examining a patient with pertussis. People exposed to a patient with pertussis should be evaluated by infection control personnel for postexposure management and follow-up.

---

[1]Centers for Disease Control and Prevention. Immunization of health-care personnel. Recommendations of the Advisory Committee on Immunization Practices (ACIP). *MMWR Recomm Rep.* 2011;60(RR-07):1–45

Table 3.45. Composition and Recommended Use of Vaccines With Tetanus Toxoid, Diphtheria Toxoid, and Acellular Pertussis Components Licensed and Available in the United States[a]

Pharmaceutical	Manufacturer	Recommended Use
DTaP (Infanrix)	GlaxoSmithKline Biologicals	**All 5 doses,** children 6 wk through 6 y of age.
DTaP (Daptacel)	Sanofi Pasteur	**All 5 doses,** children 6 wk through 6 y of age.
DTaP-hepatitis B-IPV (Pediarix)	GlaxoSmithKline Biologicals	**First 3 doses, children 6 wk through 6 y of age; usual use** at 2, 4, and 6 months of age; then 2 doses of DTaP are needed to complete the 5-dose series before 7 y of age.
DTaP-IPV/Hib (Pentacel)	Sanofi Pasteur	**First 4 doses, children 6 wk through 4 y of age; usual use** at 2, 4, 6, and 15 through 18 mo of age; then 1 dose of DTaP is needed to complete the 5-dose series before 7 y of age.
DTaP-IPV-hepatitis B-Hib (Vaxelis)	Merck/Sanofi Pasteur	**First 3 doses, children 6 wk through 4 y of age: usual use** at 2, 4, and 6 months of age; then 2 doses of DTaP are needed to complete the 5-dose series before 7 y of age.
DTaP-IPV (Kinrix)	GlaxoSmithKline Biologicals	**Booster dose** for **fifth dose** of DTaP and **fourth dose** of IPV at 4 through 6 y of age.
DTaP-IPV (Quadracel)	Sanofi Pasteur	**Booster dose** for **fifth dose** of DTaP and **fourth dose** of IPV at 4 through 6 y of age.
Tdap (Boostrix)	GlaxoSmithKline Biologicals	**Single dose** at 11 through 12 y of age. Can be used in place of Td.
Tdap (Adacel)	Sanofi Pasteur	**Single dose** at 11 through 12 y of age. Can be used in place of Td.

DTaP indicates pediatric formulation of diphtheria and tetanus toxoids and acellular pertussis vaccines; FHA, filamentous hemagglutinin; Hib, *Haemophilus influenzae* type b vaccine; IPV, inactivated poliovirus; PT, pertussis toxoid; Td, tetanus and reduced diphtheria toxoids (for children 7 years of age or older and adults); Tdap, adolescent/adult formulation of tetanus toxoid, reduced diphtheria toxoid, and acellular pertussis vaccine.

[a]DTaP recommended schedule is 2, 4, 6, and 15 through 18 months and 4 through 6 years of age. The fourth dose can be administered as early as 12 months of age, provided 6 months have elapsed since the third dose was administered. The fifth dose is not necessary if the fourth dose was administered on or after the fourth birthday. Refer to manufacturers' product information for comprehensive product information regarding indications and use of the vaccines listed.

Data on the need for PEP in Tdap-immunized HCP are inconclusive. Some immunized HCP still are at risk of *B pertussis* infection.

Recommendations of the CDC are as follows:

- PEP is recommended for all HCP (even if immunized with Tdap) who have been exposed to pertussis and are likely to expose patients at risk of severe pertussis (eg, hospitalized neonates and pregnant women). Other exposed HCP either should receive

PEP or should be monitored daily for 21 days after exposure and treated at the onset of signs and symptoms of pertussis.

- Other people (patients, caregivers) defined as close contacts or high-risk contacts of a patient or HCP with pertussis should receive chemoprophylaxis (and immunization when indicated), as recommended for household contacts (see Table 3.44, p 581).

- HCP with symptoms of pertussis (or HCP with any respiratory illness within 21 days of exposure to pertussis who did not receive PEP) should be excluded from work for at least the first 5 days of the recommended antimicrobial therapy. HCP with symptoms of pertussis who do not accept antimicrobial therapy should be excluded from work for 21 days from onset of cough. Use of a respiratory mask is not sufficient protection during this time.

Immunization.

Vaccine Products. Acellular-component pertussis vaccines (DTaP) replaced previously used diphtheria, tetanus, and whole-cell pertussis vaccine (DTwP or DTP) exclusively in 1997; see Table 3.45 (p 583) for products. All pertussis vaccines in the United States are combined with diphtheria and tetanus toxoids; none contains thimerosal as a preservative. DTaP products may be formulated as combination vaccines that contain other vaccine components. Adolescent and adult formulations, known as Tdap vaccines, contain reduced quantities of diphtheria toxoid and some pertussis antigens compared with DTaP.

Dose and Route. Each 0.5-mL dose of DTaP or Tdap is administered intramuscularly. Use of a decreased volume of individual doses of pertussis vaccines or multiple doses of decreased-volume (fractional) doses is not recommended.

Interchangeability of Acellular Pertussis Vaccines. Insufficient data exist on the safety, immunogenicity, and efficacy of DTaP vaccines from different manufacturers when administered interchangeably for the primary series in infants. In circumstances in which the type of DTaP product(s) received previously is unknown or the previously administered product(s) is not readily available, any DTaP vaccine licensed for use in the primary series may be used. There is no need to match Tdap vaccine manufacturer with DTaP vaccine manufacturer used for earlier doses.

Recommendations for Routine Childhood Immunization With DTaP. Five doses of pertussis-containing vaccine are recommended prior to entering school. The first dose of DTaP may be administered as early as 6 weeks of age, followed by 2 additional doses at intervals of approximately 2 months. The fourth dose of DTaP is recommended at 15 through 18 months of age, and the fifth dose of DTaP is administered at 4 through 6 years of age. The fourth dose can be administered as early as 12 months of age, provided 6 months have elapsed since the third dose was administered. If the fourth dose of pertussis vaccine is delayed until after the fourth birthday, the fifth dose is not recommended.

Other recommendations are as follows:

- Simultaneous administration of DTaP and all other recommended vaccines is acceptable. Vaccines should not be mixed in the same syringe unless the specific combination is licensed by the FDA (see Simultaneous Administration of Multiple Vaccines, p 36, and *Haemophilus influenzae* Infections, p 345).

- Inadvertent administration of Tdap instead of DTaP to a child younger than 7 years as either dose 1, 2, or 3 of DTaP does not count as a valid dose; DTaP should be administered as soon as is feasible.

- Inadvertent administration of Tdap instead of DTaP to a child younger than 7 years of age as either dose 4 or 5 can be counted as valid for DTaP dose 4 or 5.

- During a pertussis outbreak in the community, public health authorities may recommend starting DTaP immunization as early as 6 weeks of age, with doses 2 and 3 in the primary series administered at intervals as short as 4 weeks.
- Children younger than 7 years who have begun but not completed their primary immunization schedule with DTwP outside the United States should receive DTaP to complete the pertussis immunization schedule.
- DTaP is not licensed or recommended for people 7 years or older.

Combined Vaccines. Several pertussis-containing combination vaccines are licensed for use (see Table 3.45, p 583) and may be used when feasible and when any components are indicated and none is contraindicated.

Recommendations for Scheduling Pertussis Immunization for Children Younger Than 7 Years in Special Circumstances.

- For children who have received fewer than the recommended number of doses of pertussis vaccine but who have received the recommended number of diphtheria and tetanus toxoid (DT) vaccine doses for their age, DTaP should be administered to complete the recommended pertussis immunization schedule.
- The total number of doses of diphtheria and tetanus toxoids (as DT, DTaP, or DTwP) should not exceed 6 before the seventh birthday.
- Although *B pertussis* infection confers protection against recurrent infection, the duration of protection is unknown. Age-appropriate DTaP dose(s) or a Tdap dose should be administered to complete the standard or catch-up immunization series on schedule in people who have had pertussis infection. No interval between disease and immunization is needed.

Adverse Events After DTaP Immunization in Children Younger Than 7 Years.

- **Local and febrile reactions.** Reactions to DTaP can occur within several hours of immunization and subside spontaneously within 48 hours without sequelae. Most commonly, these include redness, swelling, induration, and tenderness at the injection site as well as drowsiness. Less common reactions include irritability, anorexia, vomiting, crying, and slight to moderate fever.
- **Limb swelling** involving the entire thigh or upper arm has been reported in 2% to 3% of vaccine recipients after administration of the fourth and fifth doses of DTaP. Although thigh swelling may interfere with walking, most children have no limitation of activity; the condition resolves spontaneously and has no sequelae. Entire limb swelling is not a contraindication to further DTaP, Tdap, or Td immunization.
- A review by the National Academy of Medicine (NAM) based on case-series reports found evidence of a rare yet likely causal relationship between receipt of tetanus toxoid-containing vaccines and **brachial neuritis**. However, the frequency of this event has not been determined. Brachial neuritis is listed in the Vaccine Injury Table maintained as part of the National Vaccine Injury Compensation Program.
- **Other reactions.** Severe anaphylactic reactions are rare after pertussis immunization. Transient urticarial rashes that occur occasionally after pertussis immunization, unless appearing immediately (ie, within minutes), are unlikely to be anaphylactic (IgE mediated) in origin.
- **Seizures.** In contrast to DTwP, no increased risk of seizures has been observed after DTaP administration. A small increased risk for febrile seizures after DTaP when administered simultaneously with inactivated influenza vaccine was observed in a study by the CDC Vaccine Safety Datalink project. However, neither the CDC

Advisory Committee on Immunization Practices (ACIP) nor the American Academy of Pediatrics recommends administering vaccines on separate days.

- **Hypotonic-hyporesponsive episode.** Hypotonic-hyporesponsive episodes (HHE) (also termed "collapse" or "shock-like state") occur significantly less often after immunization with DTaP than previously shown with DTwP and are not a contraindication to subsequent dose(s).

Contraindications and Precautions to DTaP Immunization.

Contraindications to DTaP and Tdap:

- **Severe allergic reaction (eg, anaphylaxis)** to a dose of DTaP or Tdap or to a vaccine component (DT or Td) is a contraindication to DTaP, Tdap, DT, or Td. Because of the importance of tetanus vaccination, people who experience anaphylactic reactions should be referred to an allergist to determine whether they have a specific allergy to tetanus toxoid and can be desensitized to tetanus toxoid.
- **Encephalopathy (eg, coma, decreased level of consciousness, or prolonged seizures) not attributable to another identifiable cause** within 7 days after administration of a previous dose of diphtheria and tetanus toxoids and pertussis vaccine (DTwP, DTaP, or Tdap) is a contraindication to the pertussis component.

Precautions to DTaP and Tdap:

- **Guillain-Barré syndrome** within 6 weeks after a previous dose of tetanus toxoid-containing vaccine is a **precaution** to further doses of DTaP, Tdap, DT, or Td.
- Moderate or severe acute illness with or without a fever is a reason to defer administration of any vaccine until the person has recovered.
- **Evolving neurologic disorder** generally is a reason to defer DTaP or Tdap immunization temporarily to reduce confusion about reason(s) for a change in the clinical course. If deferred in the first year of life, DT should not be administered, because in the United States, the risk of acquiring diphtheria or tetanus by children younger than 1 year is remote. The decision to administer DTaP should be revisited, and if deferral is chosen after 1 year of age, DT immunization should be completed according to the recommended schedule (see Diphtheria, p 304, and/or Tetanus, p 750).

Recommendations for Routine Adolescent Immunization with Tdap.[1,2] Adolescents 11 years and older should receive a single dose of Tdap instead of Td for booster immunization against tetanus, diphtheria, and pertussis. The preferred age for Tdap immunizations is 11 through 12 years of age.

- Adolescents who received Td but not Tdap should receive a single dose of Tdap to provide protection against pertussis regardless of time since receipt of Td.
- Simultaneous administration of Tdap and all other recommended vaccines is recommended when feasible.
- Inadvertent administration of DTaP instead of Tdap in people 7 years and older is counted as a valid dose of Tdap.

[1]Centers for Disease Control and Prevention. Prevention of pertussis, tetanus, and diphtheria with vaccines in the United States: recommendations of the Advisory Committee on Immunization Practices, 2018. *MMWR Morb Mortal Wkly Rep.* 2018;67(2):1-44

[2]Havers FP, Moro PL, Hunter P, Hariri S, Bernstein H. Use of tetanus toxoid, reduced diphtheria toxoid, and acellular pertussis vaccines: updated recommendations of the Advisory Committee on Immunization Practices—United States, 2019. *MMWR Morb Mortal Wkly Rep.* 2020;69(3):77–83. DOI: **http://dx.doi.org/10.15585/mmwr.mm6903a5**

Recommendations for Scheduling Tdap in Children 7 Years and Older Who Did Not Complete Recommended DTaP Doses Before 7 Years of Age.[1]

- Children 7 through 10 years of age who have not completed their immunization schedule with DTaP before 7 years of age or who have an unknown vaccine history should receive at least one dose of Tdap. If further dose(s) of tetanus and diphtheria toxoids are needed in a catch-up schedule, either Td or Tdap can be used. The preferred schedule is Tdap followed by Td or Tdap at 2 months and 6 to 12 months (if needed).
- Children 7 through 9 years of age who receive Tdap or DTaP for any reason should receive the adolescent Tdap booster at 11 through 12 years of age.
- A Tdap or DTaP dose received by a 10 year-old for any reason can count as the adolescent Tdap booster dose.

Recommendations for Adolescent and Adult Immunization With Tdap in Special Situations.[1] Despite the burden of pertussis in the community, a decision analysis conducted by the CDC concluded that a routine second dose would have a limited effect on overall disease rates. However, repeat doses of Tdap are generally well tolerated, and either Td or a Tdap can be used regardless of prior receipt of Tdap for catchup immunization of individuals 7 years and older, for the routine decennial tetanus-diphtheria booster, and for wound prophylaxis when indicated.

Special situations for use of Tdap, or repeated use of Tdap off label, are provided in the following sections.

Use of Tdap in Pregnancy.[2] Providers of prenatal care should implement a Tdap immunization program for all pregnant women. In order to protect infants, who have a high risk for severe or fatal pertussis, the ACIP recommends that a dose of Tdap be administered during **each** pregnancy, irrespective of the mother's prior history of receiving Tdap or having had pertussis. Maternal immunization leads to transplacental transfer of antibody that may partially protect the infant. Tdap may be administered at any time during pregnancy, but current evidence suggests that immunization early in the interval between 27 and 36 weeks of gestation will maximize passive antibody transfer to the infant. For women not previously vaccinated with Tdap and in whom Tdap was not administered during pregnancy, Tdap should be administered immediately postpartum. Postpartum Tdap is not recommended for women who previously received Tdap at any time.

Protection of Young Infants: The Cocoon Strategy. Tdap vaccination during each pregnancy is the preferred strategy for protecting young infants from pertussis in the early months of life. In addition, the American Academy of Pediatrics, CDC, American College of Obstetricians and Gynecologists, and American Academy of Family Physicians recommend the "cocoon" strategy to help protect infants from pertussis by immunizing those around them. This strategy may offer indirect protection by decreasing their likelihood

[1]Havers FP, Moro PL, Hunter P, Hariri S, Bernstein H. Use of tetanus toxoid, reduced diphtheria toxoid, and acellular pertussis vaccines: updated recommendations of the Advisory Committee on Immunization Practices—United States, 2019. *MMWR Morb Mortal Wkly Rep.* 2020;69(3):77–83. DOI: **http://dx.doi. org/10.15585/mmwr.mm6903a5**

[2]Centers for Disease Control and Prevention. Prevention of pertussis, tetanus, and diphtheria with vaccines in the United States: recommendations of the Advisory Committee on Immunization Practices, 2018. *MMWR Morb Mortal Wkly Rep.* 2018;67(2):1-44

of acquisition and subsequent development of clinical pertussis. Immunizing parents or other adult family contacts in the pediatric office setting could increase immunization coverage for this population.[1]

- Underimmunized children younger than 7 years should receive DTaP, and underimmunized children 7 years and older should receive Tdap (see previous discussion).
- All adolescents and adults should have received a single dose of Tdap, ideally at least 2 weeks before beginning close contact with the infant. There is no minimum interval required between Tdap and prior Td.
- Cough illness in contacts of neonates should be investigated and managed promptly, with consideration given for azithromycin prophylaxis for the neonate if pertussis contact is likely (see Control Measures).

Special Situations.

- **Wound management.**[2] A tetanus toxoid–containing vaccine is indicated for wound management when >5 years have passed since the last tetanus toxoid–containing vaccine dose. If a tetanus toxoid–containing vaccine is indicated for persons aged ≥11 years, Tdap is preferred for persons who have not previously received Tdap or whose Tdap history is unknown. If a tetanus toxoid–containing vaccine is indicated for a pregnant woman, Tdap should be used. For nonpregnant persons with documentation of previous Tdap vaccination, either Td or Tdap may be used if a tetanus toxoid–containing vaccine is indicated.
- **Pregnant women for whom tetanus booster is due.** If Td booster immunization is indicated during pregnancy (ie, more than 10 years since previous Td), Tdap should be administered, preferably between weeks 27 and 36 of gestation.
- **Pregnant women with unknown or incomplete tetanus vaccination.** To ensure protection against maternal and neonatal tetanus, pregnant women who never have been immunized against tetanus should receive 3 doses of Td-containing vaccines during pregnancy. The recommended schedule is 0, 4 weeks, and 6 to 12 months, and at least 1 Tdap dose should be used in this series, preferably between 27 and 36 weeks of gestation; either Td or Tdap can be used to complete the series.

Health Care Professionals. The CDC recommends a single dose of Tdap as soon as is feasible for HCP of any age who previously have not received Tdap. There is no minimum interval suggested or required between Tdap and prior Td.

In certain cases (eg, documented transmission in the health care setting), revaccination of HCP with Tdap may be considered (**www.cdc.gov/vaccines/vpd/pertussis/tdap-revac-hcp.html**). In such a case, Tdap is not a substitute for infection prevention and control measures, including postexposure antimicrobial prophylaxis for exposed HCP. If implemented, HCP who work with infants or pregnant women should be prioritized for revaccination.

---

[1]Lessin HR; Edwards KM; American Academy of Pediatrics, Committee on Practice and Ambulatory Medicine, Committee on Infectious Diseases. Immunizing parents and other close family contacts in the pediatric office setting. *Pediatrics*. 2012;129(2):e247-e253

[2]Havers FP, Moro PL, Hunter P, Hariri S, Bernstein H. Use of tetanus toxoid, reduced diphtheria toxoid, and acellular pertussis vaccines: updated recommendations of the Advisory Committee on Immunization Practices—United States, 2019. *MMWR Morb Mortal Wkly Rep*. 2020;69(3):77–83. DOI: **http://dx.doi.org/10.15585/mmwr.mm6903a5**

Hospitals and ambulatory care facilities should provide Tdap for HCP and maximize immunization rates (eg, education about the benefits of immunization or mandatory requirement, convenient access, and provision of Tdap at no charge).

Recommendations for Adult Immunization With Tdap. The CDC recommends administration of a single dose of Tdap universally for adults of any age who previously have not received Tdap, with no minimum interval required between Tdap and prior dose of Td.

Adverse Events After Administration of Tdap. Local adverse events after administration of Tdap in adolescents and adults are common but usually are mild. Systemic adverse events also are common but usually are mild (eg, any fever, 3%–14%; any headache, 40%–44%; tiredness, 27%–37%). Postmarketing data suggest that these events occur at approximately the same rate and severity as following receipt of Td.

Contraindications, Precautions, and Deferral of Use of Tdap in Adolescents and Adults. Anaphylaxis that occurred after any component of the vaccine is a **contraindication** to Tdap (see Tetanus, p 750, for additional recommendations regarding tetanus immunization). In **latex-allergic** individuals, package inserts should be consulted regarding latex content.

History of **Guillain-Barré syndrome** within 6 weeks of a dose of a tetanus toxoid vaccine is a **precaution** to Tdap immunization. If the decision is made to continue tetanus toxoid immunization, Tdap is preferred if indicated. A history of severe **Arthus hypersensitivity reaction** after a previous dose of a tetanus or diphtheria toxoid-containing vaccine administered less than 10 years previously should lead to **deferral** of Tdap or Td immunization for 10 years after administration of the tetanus or diphtheria toxoid-containing vaccine.

Pinworm Infection
(Enterobius vermicularis)

CLINICAL MANIFESTATIONS: Pinworm infection (enterobiasis) commonly is asymptomatic but may cause pruritus ani and, rarely, pruritus vulvae. Pruritus ani can be severe enough to cause sleep disturbance. Bacterial superinfections can result from scratching and excoriation of the irritated area. Pinworms have been found in the lumen of the appendix, and in some cases, these intraluminal parasites have been associated with signs of acute appendicitis, but they have also been observed in histologically normal appendices removed for incidental reasons. Urethritis, vaginitis, salpingitis, or pelvic peritonitis may occur from aberrant migration of an adult worm from the perineum. Eosinophilic enterocolitis has been reported, although peripheral eosinophilia generally is not seen. Clinical findings such as grinding of teeth at night, weight loss, and enuresis, have been attributed to pinworm infections, but proof of a causal relationship has not been established.

ETIOLOGY: *Enterobius vermicularis* is a nematode or roundworm.

EPIDEMIOLOGY: Enterobiasis occurs worldwide and commonly clusters within families. Prevalence rates are higher in preschool- and school-aged children, in primary caregivers of infected children, and in institutionalized people. An estimated 40 million people in the United States have been infected with pinworms, with a prevalence of 20% to 30% in some age groups and communities.

Initial infection occurs by ingestion of contaminated food, or contact with hands, clothing, bedding, or other items contaminated with eggs. Alternative modes of transmission include person-to-person or sexual transmission. Eggs hatch and release larvae in the small intestine, and adult worms then locate themselves usually in the cecum, appendix, and ascending colon. Adult males die soon after copulating. Gravid females migrate, usually at night while the host is resting, to the perianal area to deposit eggs containing larvae, which mature in 6 to 8 hours. Females have an overall lifespan of up to 100 days. Adult females and eggs may induce intense perianal pruritus, leading to an autoinfection cycle during which the area is scratched and eggs are lodged on the hands and under the fingernails and are ingested when hands are put in the mouth. A person remains infectious as long as female nematodes are discharging eggs on perianal skin. Eggs may remain infective in an indoor environment for up to 2 weeks. Humans are the only known natural hosts. Pets are not reservoirs of infection.

The **incubation period** from ingestion of an egg until an adult gravid female migrates to the perianal region is 2 to 6 weeks or longer.

DIAGNOSTIC TESTS: Diagnosis is established via the classic cellulose tape test ("Scotch tape test") or with a commercially available pinworm paddle test, which is a clear plastic paddle coated with an adhesive surface on one side that is pressed on both sides of the perianal region during the night or at the time of waking and before bathing. The tape or paddle is then pressed on a slide and eggs can be visualized by microscopy. Eggs are 50 to 60 by 20 to 30 microns and flattened on one side, giving them a "bean-shaped" appearance. Testing on 3 different days will increase the sensitivity from around 50% for a single test to approximately 90%. Adult females, which are white and measure 8 to 13 mm, also can be seen in the perineal region. Stool examination is not helpful, because worms or eggs are found infrequently in the stool. Neither peripheral eosinophilia nor elevated immunoglobulin E concentrations are typical because of low invasiveness and, if present, should not be attributed to pinworm infection.

TREATMENT: Several drugs will treat pinworms (see Drugs for Parasitic Infections, p 949), including over-the-counter pyrantel pamoate and prescription mebendazole and albendazole. Mebendazole and albendazole are significantly more costly than pyrantel pamoate in the United States. Albendazole currently is not approved by the US Food and Drug Administration for treatment of pinworms. Each medication is recommended to be given in a single dose and repeated in 2 weeks, because these drugs are not completely effective against the egg or developing larvae stages. For children younger than 2 years, in whom experience with these three drugs is limited and use is off-label, risks and benefits should be considered before drug administration. Ivermectin has been evaluated and is partially effective; the safety of ivermectin in children weighing less than 15 kg and in pregnant women has not been established. Because reinfection is common even when effective therapy is given, treatment of the entire household as a group should be considered. Repeated infections should be treated by the same method as the first infection. Vaginitis is self-limited and does not require separate treatment. "Pulse" treatment with a single dose of mebendazole every 14 days for a period of 16 weeks has been used in refractory cases with multiple recurrences. Alternative diagnoses in cases being attributed to recurrent pinworm infections can include *Dipylidium caninum*, which is diagnosed by stool ova and parasite analysis and treated with praziquantel (see Other Tapeworm Infections [Including Hydatid Disease], p 747, and Table 4.11, p 957), as well as delusional parasitosis.

ISOLATION OF THE HOSPITALIZED PATIENT: Standard precautions are indicated.

CONTROL MEASURES: Control is difficult in child care centers and schools, because the rate of reinfection is high. In institutions, mass and simultaneous treatment, repeated in 2 weeks, can be successful. Hygienic measures, such as bathing in the morning to remove eggs, frequent hand hygiene, and clipping of fingernails, all are helpful for decreasing the risk of autoinfection and continued transmission. Bed linens and underclothing of infected children should be handled carefully, should not be shaken (to avoid scattering eggs), and should be laundered promptly.

Pityriasis Versicolor
(Formerly Tinea Versicolor)

CLINICAL MANIFESTATIONS: Pityriasis versicolor (formerly tinea versicolor) is a common and benign superficial infection of the skin, classically manifesting on the upper trunk and neck. Most patients are asymptomatic, although some may complain of pruritus. In infants and children, the infection is likely to involve the face, particularly the temples. Infection can include other areas, including the scalp, genital area, and thighs. Symmetrical involvement with ovoid discrete or coalescent lesions of varying size is typical; these macules or patches vary in color, even in the same person. White, pink, tan, or brown coloration is often surmounted by faint dusty scales. Lesions fail to tan during the summer and are relatively darker than the surrounding skin during the winter, hence the term versicolor. The differential diagnosis includes pityriasis alba, vitiligo, seborrheic dermatitis, pityriasis rosea, pityriasis lichenoides, progressive macular hypopigmentation, and dyschromatosis universalis hereditaria. Folliculitis also can occur, particularly in immunocompromised patients. Invasive infections can occur in neonates, particularly those receiving total parenteral nutrition with lipids.

ETIOLOGY: The cause of pityriasis versicolor is a number of species of the *Malassezia furfur* complex, a group of lipid-dependent yeasts that exist on healthy skin in yeast phase and cause clinical lesions only when substantial growth of hyphae occurs. Moisture, heat, and the presence of lipid-containing sebaceous secretions encourage rapid overgrowth of hyphae.

EPIDEMIOLOGY: Pityriasis versicolor can occur in any climate or age group but tends to favor adolescents and young adults. Living in hot and humid climates, sweating excessively, or a weakened immune system allows the fungus to flourish. Pityriasis versicolor is not contagious.

The **incubation period** is unknown.

DIAGNOSTIC TESTS: The presence of symmetrically distributed faintly scaling macules and patches of varying color concentrated on the upper back and chest is close to diagnostic. The "evoked scale" sign is when the clinician uses thumb and forefinger to stretch the skin, eliciting a visible white patch of scale overlying the affected area, which is still visible when the affected area is released. Another technique to evoke scales is scraping the involved skin with a scalpel blade or glass microscope slide, again yielding a pale and fuzzy scale that is confined to the lesion. Involved areas fluoresce yellow-green under Wood lamp evaluation. Potassium hydroxide wet mount prep of scraped scales reveals the classic "spaghetti and meatballs" short hyphae and clusters of yeast forms. Because this yeast is a common inhabitant of the skin, fungal culture from the skin surface is nondiagnostic. To grow the fungus in the laboratory, samples from pustules (if folliculitis is present) or sterile sites should be placed in media enriched with olive oil or another long-chain fatty acid.

TREATMENT: Multiple topical and systemic agents are efficacious, and recommendations vary substantially depending on expert opinion. For uncomplicated cases, most experts recommend initiating therapy with topical agents. The most cost-effective treatments are selenium sulfide shampoo/lotion and clotrimazole cream. Selenium sulfide shampoo is used for 3 to 7 days; application is once daily for 5 to 10 minutes, followed by rinsing. Topical azole therapy (eg, clotrimazole cream) is applied twice daily for 2 to 3 weeks. Adherence with these agents may be low because of unpleasant adverse effects (the shampoo has a sulfur-like odor) or duration and anatomic extent of required therapy. Other effective topical agents include ketoconazole, ciclopirox, econazole, oxiconazole, and off-label bifonazole, miconazole, econazole, oxiconazole, clotrimazole, terbinafine, and ciclopirox, as well as zinc pyrithione shampoo. Shampoos are easier to disperse, particularly on wet skin, than topical creams, and may increase compliance. Treatment response is measured by resolution of scale and/or disappearance of "spaghetti and meatball" microscopic findings. Restoration of normal pigmentation may take months after successful treatment.

Recurrence following discontinuation of therapy may approach 60% to 80%, and preventive treatments sometimes are used to decrease recurrences. Off-label regimens to decrease recurrence include use of the aforementioned shampoos/lotions on a weekly or monthly basis.

Systemic therapy is reserved for resistant infection or extensive involvement. Medications, including fluconazole, itraconazole, and pramiconazole, are not approved by the US Food and Drug Administration (FDA) for pityriasis versicolor. Fluconazole (preferred) can be administered at 300 mg weekly for 2 to 4 weeks or itraconazole 200 mg daily for 1 week. Although oral agents may be easier to use than topical agents, they are not necessarily more effective and have possible serious adverse effects. Drug interactions can occur when using oral drugs, and monitoring for liver toxicity must be considered in patients receiving systemic therapy, particularly if they receive multiple courses. Although ketoconazole can effectively treat pityriasis versicolor, the FDA reaffirmed in 2016 that it strongly discourages use of systemic ketoconazole for uncomplicated skin and nail infections due to significant risks of liver toxicity, adrenal insufficiency, and interactions with multiple medications which have resulted in at least one fatality. In several studies, topical therapy has appeared to be equivalent or superior to systemic therapy.

ISOLATION OF THE HOSPITALIZED PATIENT: Standard precautions are recommended.

CONTROL MEASURES: The organism that causes pityriasis versicolor is commensal and resides on normal skin.

Plague

CLINICAL MANIFESTATIONS: Naturally acquired plague most commonly manifests in the primary **bubonic form,** with fever and a painful swollen regional lymph node (bubo). Buboes develop most commonly in the inguinal region but also occur in axillary or cervical areas. Less commonly, plague manifests in the primary **septicemic form** without localizing signs (fever, hypotension, purpuric skin lesions, intravascular coagulopathy, organ failure) or as primary **pneumonic plague** (cough, fever, dyspnea, and hemoptysis) and rarely as **meningitic, pharyngeal, cutaneous, ocular,** or **gastrointestinal plague.** Occasionally, patients have symptoms of mild lymphadenitis or prominent gastrointestinal tract symptoms, which may obscure the correct diagnosis. Secondary septicemic, pneumonic, or other forms of plague can occur via hematogenous dissemination of bacteria. Untreated, plague often progresses to overwhelming sepsis and death. Plague has been referred to as the Black Death because of the tissue necrosis that it induces.

ETIOLOGY: Plague is caused by *Yersinia pestis,* a pleomorphic, bipolar-staining (with Giemsa, Wright, and Wayson stains), facultative intracellular gram-negative coccobacillus. *Y pestis* is a member of the *Enterobacteriaceae* family, along with more common *Yersinia* species and other enteric bacteria.

EPIDEMIOLOGY: Plague is a zoonotic infection primarily maintained in rodents and their fleas. Humans are incidental hosts who develop bubonic or primary septicemic manifestations, typically through the bite of infected rodent fleas or through direct contact with tissues of infected animals. Primary pneumonic plague is acquired by inhalation of respiratory tract droplets from a human or animal with pneumonic plague. Only the pneumonic form has been shown to be transmitted from person to person. Plague occurs worldwide with enzootic foci in parts of Asia, Africa, and the Americas. Most human plague cases are reported from rural, underdeveloped areas and mainly occur as isolated cases or in small, focal clusters. In the United States, plague is endemic in western states, with most cases reported from New Mexico, Colorado, Arizona, and California.[1] Cases of plague in states without endemic plague have been identified in travelers returning from these states.

Y pestis has also been identified as a potential bioterrorism agent, through widespread dispersal of an aerosolized form. Such an event would have potential for a large number of pneumonic plague cases.

The **incubation period** is 2 to 8 days for bubonic plague and 1 to 6 days for primary pneumonic plague.

DIAGNOSTIC TESTS: Diagnosis of plague usually is confirmed by culture of *Y pestis* from blood, bubo aspirate, sputum, or another clinical specimen. The organism is slow growing but not fastidious and can be isolated on sheep blood and chocolate agars with typical "fried-egg" colonies appearing after 48 to 72 hours of incubation. *Y pestis* has a bipolar (safety-pin) appearance when stained with Wright-Giemsa or Wayson stains. A positive direct fluorescent antibody test result for the presence of *Y pestis* in direct smears or cultures of blood, bubo aspirate, sputum, or another clinical specimen provides presumptive evidence of *Y pestis* infection. Automated, commercially available biochemical identification systems are not recommended, because they can misidentify *Y pestis.* Identification of suspected isolates of *Y pestis* should be based on guidelines recommended for "sentinel level" clinical microbiology laboratories using preliminary characterization tests, followed by definitive identification performed at the state or federal public health laboratory. Polymerase chain reaction assay and immunohistochemical staining for rapid diagnosis of *Y pestis* are available in some reference or public health laboratories.

A single positive serologic test result from a passive hemagglutination assay or enzyme immunoassay provides presumptive evidence of infection. Seroconversion, defined as a fourfold increase in antibody titer between serum specimens obtained 4 to 6 weeks apart, also confirms the diagnosis of plague.

In the United States, *Y pestis* is classified as a select agent, and the possession and transport of the organism requires adherence to strict federal guidelines. Laboratory-acquired cases, including fatal cases, have been reported. Clinical laboratories must handle a suspected or confirmed isolate using at least biosafety level 2 guidelines with

---

[1]Kwit N, Nelson C, Kugeler K, et al. Human plague—United States, 2015. *MMWR Morb Mortal Wkly Rep.* 2015;64(33):918-919

particular attention to preventing aerosolization of the organism. Isolates suspected as Y pestis should be reported immediately to the state health department.

TREATMENT: After obtaining diagnostic specimens, appropriate antibiotic therapy should be started immediately for any patient suspected of having plague. Pediatric treatment recommendations[1] are as follows:

- For naturally acquired primary bubonic or pharyngeal plague without signs of secondary pneumonic or septicemic plague and for early/mild primary pneumonic or septicemic plague, monotherapy with gentamicin, streptomycin, ciprofloxacin, or levofloxacin is recommended.
- Doxycycline also is a first-line option for treatment of naturally acquired bubonic or pharyngeal plague but is second-line therapy for naturally acquired pneumonic plague.
- Dual therapy with 2 distinct antimicrobial classes is recommended for initial treatment of patients with naturally acquired primary bubonic disease with large buboes or with naturally acquired moderate-severe septicemic or pneumonic plague. The recommended drugs are those listed in the first bullet.
- Alternative antibiotics for pneumonic, septicemic, bubonic, or pharyngeal plague are listed in the CDC plague document.
- For naturally acquired plague meningitis, chloramphenicol should be added to the patient's existing treatment regimen. If chloramphenicol is not available, moxifloxacin or levofloxacin should be added to the treatment regimen.
- For bioterrorism-related plague, dual therapy with 2 distinct classes of antimicrobials should be used for all patients until sensitivity patterns are known.

Neonates of pregnant women with plague at or around the time of delivery should be treated if they are symptomatic, using the antibiotic selections in the first 3 bullets. If the neonate is asymptomatic but the mother is untreated or has only recently begun treatment, the infant should receive antimicrobial prophylaxis, with the same antibiotic choices as those listed in Care of Exposed People. If the neonate is asymptomatic and the mother has been sufficiently treated and is improving, observation of the infant is acceptable.

The duration of antimicrobial treatment is 10 to 14 days; treatment duration can be extended for patients with ongoing fever or other concerning signs or symptoms. Drainage of abscessed buboes may be necessary; drainage material is considered infectious.

ISOLATION OF THE HOSPITALIZED PATIENT: For patients with bubonic or septicemic plague, standard precautions are recommended. For patients with suspected pneumonic plague, respiratory droplet precautions should be initiated immediately and continued for 48 hours after initiation of effective antimicrobial treatment.

CONTROL MEASURES:

Care of Exposed People. All people with exposure to a known or suspected plague source, such as Y pestis-infected fleas or infectious tissues, in the previous 6 days, should be offered antimicrobial prophylaxis or be cautioned to report fever greater than 38.3°C (101.0°F) or other illness to their physician. People with close exposure (less than 2 meters) to a patient with pneumonic plague and who are within the incubation period should receive antimicrobial prophylaxis, but isolation of asymptomatic people is not recommended. Pneumonic transmission typically occurs in the end stage of disease in patients with hemoptysis, thereby placing caregivers and health care professionals at higher risk. For children, including those younger

---

[1]Nelson CA, Meaney-Delman D, Fleck-Derderian S, Cooley KM, Yu PA, Mead P. Antimicrobial treatment and prophylaxis of plague: recommendations for naturally acquired infections and bioterrorism response. *MMWR Morb Mortal Wkly Rep.* 2021; in press

than 8 years, doxycycline, levofloxacin, or ciprofloxacin is recommended (see Tetracyclines, p 866, and Fluoroquinolones, p 864). The benefits of prophylactic therapy should be weighed against the risks. Prophylaxis is administered for 7 days and in the usual therapeutic doses.

Breastfeeding. There are no reports of suspected *Y pestis* transmission from mother to child through human milk. The risk of *Y pestis* transmission through human milk is believed to be low. Mothers with bubonic or septicemic plague and mothers taking antimicrobial prophylaxis after exposure to *Y pestis* can continue to breastfeed their infants if able. A mother with pneumonic plague may continue to breastfeed, as able, if she is receiving antimicrobial treatment and her infant is receiving antimicrobial treatment or postexposure prophylaxis for *Y pestis*. Because of the risk of person-to-person transmission of pneumonic plague, a mother with primary or secondary pneumonic plague whose infant is not receiving antimicrobial treatment or prophylaxis should avoid direct breastfeeding until she has received antimicrobial treatment for ≥48 hours and demonstrated clinical improvement. The mother's expressed milk may be given to the infant.

Other Measures. State public health authorities should be notified immediately of any suspected cases of human plague. People living in areas with endemic plague should be informed about the importance of eliminating sources of rodent food and harborage near residences, the role of dogs and cats in bringing plague-infected rodent fleas into peridomestic environments, the need for flea control and confinement of pets, and the importance of avoiding contact with sick and dead animals. Other preventive measures include surveillance of rodent populations and use of rodent control measures and insecticides by health authorities when surveillance indicates the occurrence of plague epizootics. For additional information on laboratory safety see CDC Biosafety in Microbiological and Biomedical Laboratories manual (**www.cdc.gov/biosafety/publications/bmbl5/**).

Vaccine. There is no vaccine currently licensed for use in the United States. New vaccines based on recombinant capsular subunit protein F1 and the low-calcium response V antigen (LcrV) are under evaluation.

Pneumocystis jirovecii Infections

CLINICAL MANIFESTATIONS: Symptomatic infection with *Pneumocystis jirovecii* is extremely rare in healthy people. However, in immunocompromised infants and children, *P jirovecii* causes a respiratory illness characterized by dyspnea, tachypnea, significant hypoxemia, nonproductive cough, chills, fatigue, and fever. The intensity of these signs and symptoms may vary, and in some immunocompromised children and adults, the onset may be acute and fulminant. Most children with *Pneumocystis* pneumonia are significantly hypoxic. Chest radiographs often show bilateral diffuse interstitial or alveolar disease but may appear normal in early disease. Atypical radiographic findings may include lobar, miliary, cavitary, and nodular lesions. The mortality rate in immunocompromised patients ranges from 5% to 40% in treated patients and approaches 100% without therapy.

ETIOLOGY: Nomenclature for *Pneumocystis* species has evolved. Human *Pneumocystis* is called *Pneumocystis jirovecii*, although the familiar acronym PCP (originally *Pneumocystis carinii* pneumonia) still is used commonly among clinicians. *P jirovecii* is an atypical fungus (based on DNA sequence analysis) with several morphologic and biologic similarities to protozoa, including susceptibility to a number of antiprotozoal agents but resistance to most antifungal agents. In addition, the organism exists as 2 distinct morphologic forms: the 5- to 7-μm-diameter cysts, which contain up to 8 intracystic bodies or sporozoites, and the smaller, 1- to 5-μm-diameter trophozoite or trophic form.

EPIDEMIOLOGY: *Pneumocystis* species are ubiquitous in mammals worldwide and have a tropism for respiratory tract epithelium. Asymptomatic or mild human infection occurs early in life, with more than 85% of healthy children showing seropositivity by 20 months of age. Animal models and studies of patients with acquired immunodeficiency syndrome (AIDS) do not support the existence of latency, and suggest that disease after the second year of life is likely reinfection.

The single most important factor in susceptibility to PCP is the status of cell-mediated immunity of the host, reflected by a marked decrease in percentage and numbers CD4+ T-lymphocytes, or a decrease in CD4+ T-lymphocyte function. In resource-limited countries and in times of famine, *Pneumocystis* pneumonia (also referred to as PCP, maintaining the same acronym as previously was used for the organism) can occur in epidemics, primarily affecting malnourished infants and children. In industrialized countries, PCP occurs almost entirely in immunocompromised people with deficient cell-mediated immunity, particularly people with human immunodeficiency virus (HIV) infection, recipients of immunosuppressive therapy after solid organ and hematopoietic stem cell transplantation, people undergoing treatment for hematologic malignancy, and children with primary immunodeficiency syndromes. Although onset of disease can occur at any age, PCP most commonly occurs in HIV-infected children in the first year of life, with peak incidence at 3 through 6 months of age. In patients with cancer, the disease can occur during remission or relapse of the malignancy.

The incidence of PCP has dramatically decreased in the United States as a result of combination antiretroviral therapy for people with HIV and the general adoption of recommendations for prophylaxis. Despite this decrease, it is still one of the leading opportunistic infections among people with HIV infection, particularly those not aware of their infection and not receiving antiretroviral therapy.

Animal studies have demonstrated animal-to-animal transmission by the airborne route; human-to-human transmission has been suggested by molecular epidemiology and global clustering of PCP cases in several studies. Outbreaks in hospitals have been reported. Vertical transmission has been postulated but never proven. The period of communicability is unknown.

The **incubation period** is unknown, but outbreaks of PCP in transplant recipients have demonstrated a median of 53 days from exposure to clinically apparent infection.

DIAGNOSTIC TESTS: A definitive diagnosis of PCP is made by visualization of organisms (*Pneumocystis* cysts) in lung tissue or respiratory tract secretion specimens. Bronchoscopy with bronchoalveolar lavage (BAL) is the diagnostic procedure of choice for most infants and children. Methenamine silver stain, toluidine blue stain, and fluorescently conjugated monoclonal antibody are useful tools for identifying the thick-walled cysts of *P jirovecii*. Sporozoites (within cysts) and trophozoites are identified with Giemsa or modified Wright-Giemsa stain. The sensitivity of all microscopy-based methods depends on the skill of the laboratory technician.

Polymerase chain reaction (PCR) assays to diagnose PCP are becoming more widely available. They are highly sensitive with a variety of specimen types from the respiratory tract, including nasopharyngeal aspirates. However, there are currently no US Food and Drug Administration (FDA)-cleared PCR tests for *P jirovecii*. Because highly sensitive PCR assays may detect colonization with these organisms, results from such assays must be interpreted in the context of clinical presentation.

Limited data suggest that serum 1,3-β-D-glucan (BG) assay, which is available as an FDA-cleared test in the United States for invasive fungal infections, may be a potential marker for *Pneumocystis* infection. This compound is a component of the cell wall of the cyst stage of the organism and may be found in high concentrations in serum of patients infected with *P jirovecii*; however, most other fungi also secrete the compound during infection, so correlation with clinical presentation is imperative.

TREATMENT[1]: The drug of choice is trimethoprim-sulfamethoxazole (TMP-SMX), usually administered intravenously. Oral therapy should be reserved for patients with mild disease who do not have malabsorption or diarrhea and for patients with a favorable clinical response to initial intravenous therapy. See Table 4.3 (p 882) for dosages. Duration of therapy is 21 days. The rate of adverse reactions to TMP-SMX (eg, rash, neutropenia, anemia, thrombocytopenia, renal toxicity, hepatitis, nausea, vomiting, and diarrhea) is higher in HIV-infected children than in non–HIV-infected patients. It is not necessary to discontinue therapy for mild adverse reactions (eg, vomiting). At least half of patients with more severe reactions that include rash require interruption of therapy. Desensitization to TMP-SMX may be considered after the acute reaction has abated.

Pentamidine, administered intravenously, is an alternative drug for treatment of *Pneumocystis* infection in children and adults who cannot tolerate TMP-SMX or who have severe disease and have not responded to TMP-SMX after 5 to 7 days of therapy. The therapeutic efficacy of intravenous pentamidine in adults with PCP is similar to that of TMP-SMX. Pentamidine is associated with a high incidence of adverse reactions, including renal toxicity, pancreatitis, diabetes mellitus, electrolyte abnormalities, hypoglycemia, hyperglycemia, hypotension, cardiac arrhythmias, fever, and neutropenia. Aerosolized pentamidine should not be used for treatment, because its efficacy is limited.

Atovaquone is approved for oral treatment of mild to moderate PCP in adults who are intolerant of TMP-SMX. Experience with use of atovaquone in children is limited, although a study comparing the efficacy of bacterial prophylaxis of atovaquone-azithromycin versus TMP-SMX noted that prevention of PCP was equivalent between the 2 drug regimens. Adverse reactions to atovaquone are limited to rash, nausea, and diarrhea.

Other potentially useful drugs for mild to moderate PCP in adults include clindamycin with primaquine (adverse reactions are rash, nausea, and diarrhea), dapsone with trimethoprim (associated with neutropenia, anemia, thrombocytopenia, methemoglobinemia, rash, and aminotransferase elevation), and trimetrexate with leucovorin. Experience with the use of these combinations in children is limited.

On the basis of studies in both adults and children, a course of corticosteroids is recommended in patients with moderate to severe PCP (as defined by an arterial oxygen pressure [PaO_2] of less than 70 mm Hg in room air or an arterial-alveolar gradient $\geq$35 mm Hg), starting within 72 hours of diagnosis. The recommended scheduled dosing of oral prednisone during treatment is presented in Table 3.46.

Coinfection with other organisms, such as cytomegalovirus or *Streptococcus pneumoniae*, has been reported in HIV-infected children. Children with dual infections may have more severe disease.

Chemoprophylaxis. Chemoprophylaxis is highly effective in preventing PCP among high-risk groups. Prophylaxis against a first episode of PCP is indicated for many patients with significant immunosuppression, including people with HIV infection (see Table 3.47 and Human Immunodeficiency Virus Infection, p 427) and people with primary or acquired cell-mediated immunodeficiency.

---

[1]Panel on Opportunistic Infections in HIV-Exposed and HIV-Infected Children. Guidelines for the Prevention and Treatment of Opportunistic Infections in HIV-Exposed and HIV-Infected Children. Department of Health and Human Services. Available at: **https://clinicalinfo.hiv.gov/sites/default/files/inline-files/oi_guidelines_pediatrics.pdf**

Table 3.46. Dosing of Oral Prednisone in the Treatment of *Pneumocystis* pneumonia[a]

Age	Days 1–5	Days 6–10	Days 11–21
<13 y	1 mg/kg/dose, twice daily	0.5 mg/kg/dose, twice daily	0.5 mg/kg/dose daily
≥13 y	40 mg, twice daily	40 mg daily	20 mg daily

[a] The maximum doses should not exceed the dose for children older than 13 years.

The recommended drug regimen for PCP prophylaxis for all immunocompromised patients is TMP-SMX. Acceptable dosing intervals and schedules are presented in Table 3.48. For patients who cannot tolerate TMP-SMX, alternative oral choices include atovaquone or dapsone. Atovaquone is effective and safe but expensive. Dapsone is effective and inexpensive but associated with more serious adverse effects than atovaquone. Aerosolized pentamidine is recommended for children who cannot tolerate TMP-SMX, atovaquone, or dapsone and are old enough to use a Respirgard II nebulizer. Intravenous pentamidine has been used but generally is not recommended for prophylaxis. Other drug combinations with potential for prophylaxis include pyrimethamine plus dapsone plus leucovorin or pyrimethamine-sulfadoxine. Experience with these drugs in adults and children for this indication is limited. These agents should be considered only in situations in which recommended regimens are not tolerated or cannot be used for other reasons.

In HIV-infected children, risk of PCP is associated with age-specific CD4+ T-lymphocyte cell counts and percentages that define severe immunosuppression (Immune Category 3). Because CD4+ T-lymphocyte counts and percentages can decline rapidly in HIV-infected infants, prophylaxis for PCP is recommended for all infants born to HIV-infected women in resource-limited settings beginning at 4 to 6 weeks of age and continuing until 12 months of age unless a diagnosis of HIV has been excluded presumptively or definitively, in which case prophylaxis should be discontinued (see Table 3.48). Children who are HIV infected or whose HIV status is indeterminate should continue prophylaxis throughout the first year of life. In the United States, in HIV-exposed infants who are deemed low risk for HIV seroconversion, PCP prophylaxis is not indicated unless there is evidence of HIV transmission in the infant.

For HIV-infected children aged 12 months or older, initiation and discontinuation of PCP prophylaxis is detailed in Table 3.47. In patients with AIDS, prophylaxis should be initiated at the end of therapy for acute infection. In most cases, secondary prophylaxis can be discontinued using the same criteria as for primary prophylaxis (see Table 3.47). Prophylaxis should be continued at least through 12 months of life for HIV-infected infants or lifelong if CD4+ T-lymphocyte counts or percentages do not exceed the thresholds shown in Table 3.47 in response to antiretroviral therapy.

Prophylaxis for PCP is recommended for children who have received hematopoietic stem cell transplants (HSCTs)[1] or solid organ transplants; children with hematologic malignancies (eg, leukemia or lymphoma) and some nonhematologic malignancies;

[1] Center for International Blood and Marrow Research; National Marrow Donor program; European Blood and Marrow Transplant Group; American Society of Blood and Marrow Transplantation; Canadian Blood and Marrow Transplant Group; Infectious Diseases Society of America; Society for Healthcare Epidemiology of America; Association of Medical Microbiology and Infectious Disease Canada; Centers for Disease Control and Prevention. Guidelines for preventing infectious complications among hematopoietic cell transplant recipients: a global perspective. *Biol Blood Marrow Transplant.* 2009;15(10):1143-1238

Table 3.47. Recommendations for *Pneumocystis jirovecii* Pneumonia (PCP) Prophylaxis for Human Immunodeficiency Virus (HIV)-Exposed Infants and Children, by Age and HIV Infection Status[a]

Age and HIV Infection Status	Initiation of PCP prophylaxis[b]	Discontinuation of PCP prophylaxis[b]
Birth through 4 to 6 wk of age, HIV exposed or HIV infected	No prophylaxis	Not applicable
4 to 6 wk through 12 mo of age		
HIV infected or indeterminate	Prophylaxis	Throughout first year of life
HIV infection presumptively or definitively excluded[c]	No prophylaxis	Not applicable
1 through 5 y of age, HIV infected	Prophylaxis if: CD4+ T-lymphocyte count is less than 500 cells/µL or percentage is less than 15%[d]	Discontinue if combination antiretroviral therapy administered for >6 months, and the following have been sustained for >3 consecutive months: CD4+ T-lymphocyte count 500 cells/µL or greater or percentage is 15% or greater
6 y of age or older, HIV infected	Prophylaxis if: CD4+ T-lymphocyte count is less than 200 cells/µL or percentage is less than 15%[d]	Discontinue if combination antiretroviral therapy administered for >6 months, and the following have been sustained for >3 consecutive months: CD4+ T-lymphocyte count 200 cells/ µL or greater or percentage is 15% or greater

[a] Panel on Opportunistic Infections in HIV-Exposed and HIV-Infected Children. Guidelines for the Prevention and Treatment of Opportunistic Infections in HIV-Exposed and HIV-Infected Children. Department of Health and Human Services. Available at: **https://clinicalinfo.hiv.gov/sites/default/files/inline-files/oi_guidelines_pediatrics.pdf.**

[b] Children who have had PCP should receive lifelong ("secondary") PCP prophylaxis unless/until their CD4+ T-lymphocyte cell counts and percentages achieve and maintain designated age-specific values greater than those indicative of severe immunosuppression (Immune Category 3) for at least 6 months (see Human Immunodeficiency Virus Infection, p 427).

[c] See Human Immunodeficiency Virus Infection, p 427.

[d] Prophylaxis should be considered on a case-by-case basis for children who might otherwise be at risk of PCP, such as children with rapidly declining CD4+ T-lymphocyte counts or percentages or children with Clinical Category C status of HIV infection.

Table 3.48. Drug Regimens for *Pneumocystis jirovecii* Pneumonia Prophylaxis for Children 4 Weeks and Older[a]

Recommended daily dose:

Trimethoprim-sulfamethoxazole (trimethoprim, 5–10 mg/kg per day; and sulfamethoxazole, 25–50 mg/kg per day, orally). The total daily dose should not exceed 320 mg TMP and 1600 mg SMX.

Acceptable dosing intervals and schedules:

- In divided doses twice daily, given 3 days per week on consecutive days or on alternate days
- In divided doses twice daily, given 2 days per week on consecutive days or on alternate days
- Total dose once daily, given 7 days per week

Alternative regimens if trimethoprim-sulfamethoxazole is not tolerated:

- **Atovaquone**
  - **children 1 through 3 mo of age and older than 24 mo through 12 y of age:** 30 mg/kg (maximum 1500 mg), orally, once a day
  - **children 4 through 24 mo of age:** 45 mg/kg (maximum 1500 mg), orally, once a day
  - **children older than 12 y:** 1500 mg, orally, once a day
- **Dapsone (children 1 mo or older)**
  2 mg/kg (maximum 100 mg), orally, once a day or 4 mg/kg (maximum 200 mg), orally, every week
- **Aerosolized pentamidine (children 5 y or older)**
  300 mg, inhaled monthly via Respirgard II nebulizer

[a]Panel on Opportunistic Infections in HIV-Exposed and HIV-Infected Children. Guidelines for the Prevention and Treatment of Opportunistic Infections in HIV-Exposed and HIV-Infected Children. Department of Health and Human Services. Available at **https://clinicalinfo.hiv.gov/sites/default/files/inline-files/oi_guidelines_pediatrics.pdf**

children with severe cell-mediated immunodeficiency, including children who received adrenocorticotropic hormone for treatment of infantile spasms; and children who otherwise are immunocompromised and who have had a previous episode of PCP. For this diverse group of immunocompromised hosts, the risk of PCP varies with duration and intensity of chemotherapy, with other immunosuppressive therapies, with coinfection with immunosuppressive viruses (eg, cytomegalovirus), and local epidemiologic rates of PCP. Guidelines for allogeneic HSCT recipients recommend that PCP prophylaxis be initiated at engraftment (or before engraftment, if engraftment is delayed) and administered for at least 6 months in autologous HSCT patients and for at least 1 year in allogeneic transplant recipients, especially matched unrelated or haploidentical transplants who may receive in vivo T-lymphocyte depletion with antithymocyte globulin (ATG) or Campath. It should be continued in all children receiving ongoing or intensified immunosuppressive therapy (eg, prednisone or cyclosporine) or in children with chronic graft-versus-host disease. Guidelines for PCP prophylaxis for solid organ transplant recipients are less definitive. In general, PCP prophylaxis is recommended for all solid organ transplant recipients for at least 6 to 12 months posttransplant, although longer durations should be considered. For lung and small bowel transplant recipients, as well as any transplant patient with a history of prior PCP infection or chronic CMV disease, lifelong prophylaxis may be indicated.

ISOLATION OF THE HOSPITALIZED PATIENT: Standard precautions are recommended. Some experts recommend that because of the theoretical risk for transmission, patients with PCP should not share a room with other immunocompromised patients, especially patients who are not receiving PCP prophylaxis. Data are insufficient to support this recommendation as standard practice.

CONTROL MEASURES: Appropriate therapy for infected patients and prophylaxis in immunocompromised patients are the only available means of control. Detailed guidelines for children, adolescents, and adults infected with HIV have been issued by the Department of Health and Human Services.[1,2]

Poliovirus Infections

CLINICAL MANIFESTATIONS: Approximately 70% of poliovirus infections in susceptible children are asymptomatic. Nonspecific illness with low-grade fever and sore throat (minor illness) occurs in approximately 25% of infected people, and viral meningitis (nonparalytic polio), sometimes accompanied by paresthesias, occurs in 1% to 5% of patients a few days after the minor illness has resolved. Rapid onset of asymmetric acute flaccid paralysis with areflexia of the involved limb (paralytic poliomyelitis) occurs in fewer than 1% of infections, with residual paresis in approximately two thirds of patients. Classical paralytic polio begins with a minor illness characterized by fever, sore throat, headache, nausea, constipation, and/or malaise for several days, followed by a symptom-free period of 1 to 3 days. Rapid onset of paralysis then follows. Typically, paralysis is asymmetric and affects the proximal muscles more than the distal muscles. Cranial nerve involvement (bulbar poliomyelitis) and paralysis of the diaphragm and intercostal muscles may lead to impaired respiration requiring assisted ventilation. Sensation usually is intact. The cerebrospinal fluid (CSF) profile is characteristic of viral meningitis, with mild pleocytosis and lymphocytic predominance.

Adults who contracted paralytic poliomyelitis during childhood may develop the noninfectious postpolio syndrome 15 to 40 years later, characterized by slow and irreversible exacerbation of weakness in the muscle groups affected during the original infection. Muscle and joint pain also are common manifestations. The estimated incidence of postpolio syndrome in poliomyelitis survivors is 25% to 40%.

ETIOLOGY: Polioviruses are classified as members of the family *Picornaviridae*, genus *Enterovirus*, in the species enterovirus C, and include 3 serotypes. They are nonenveloped, positive-sense, single-stranded RNA viruses that are highly stable in a liquid environment. Acute paralytic disease may be caused by naturally occurring (wild) polioviruses, and rarely by oral poliovirus (OPV) vaccine viruses. OPV-associated cases of vaccine-associated paralytic poliomyelitis (VAPP) may occur in vaccine recipients or their close contacts, or may be associated with circulating vaccine-derived polioviruses (cVDPVs) that have acquired virulence properties that are indistinguishable from naturally occurring polioviruses as a result of sustained person-to-person transmission in the absence of adequate population immunity. People with primary (but not acquired) B-lymphocyte immunodeficiencies are at increased risk both of VAPP and of persistent infection (immunodeficiency-associated vaccine-derived polioviruses, or iVDPVs) from vaccine virus.

[1]Panel on Opportunistic Infections in HIV-Exposed and HIV-Infected Children. Guidelines for the Prevention and Treatment of Opportunistic Infections in HIV-Exposed and HIV-Infected Children. Department of Health and Human Services. Available at: **https://clinicalinfo.hiv.gov/sites/default/files/inline-files/oi_guidelines_pediatrics.pdf**

[2]Panel on Opportunistic Infections in Adults and Adolescents with HIV. Guidelines for the Prevention and Treatment of Opportunistic Infections in Adults and Adolescents with HIV: Recommendations from the Centers for Disease Control and Prevention, the National Institutes of Health, and the HIV Medicine Association of the Infectious Diseases Society of America. Available at: **https://clinicalinfo.hiv.gov/sites/default/files/guidelines/documents/Adult_OI.pdf**

With continuing progress toward polio eradication, more global cases of paralytic disease are now caused by vaccine-related viruses (VAPP and cVDPV) than by wild polioviruses.

EPIDEMIOLOGY: Humans are the only natural reservoir for poliovirus. Spread is by contact with feces and/or respiratory secretions. Infection is more common in infants and young children and occurs at an earlier age among children living in poor hygienic conditions. In temperate climates, poliovirus infections are most common during summer and autumn; in the tropics, the seasonal pattern is less pronounced.

The last cases of poliomyelitis attributable to indigenously acquired, naturally occurring wild poliovirus in the United States were reported in 1979. Except for very rare imported cases, all poliomyelitis cases acquired in the United States have been attributable to VAPP, which, until 1998, occurred in an average of 6 to 8 people annually. Fewer VAPP cases were reported in 1998 and 1999, after a shift in US immunization policy in 1997 from use of OPV to a sequential inactivated poliovirus (IPV) vaccine/OPV schedule. Implementation of an all-IPV vaccine schedule in 2000 halted the occurrence of VAPP cases in the United States.

The risk of contact in the United States with imported wild polioviruses and cVDPV viruses has decreased in parallel with the success of the global eradication program. Of the 3 poliovirus serotypes, type 2 wild poliovirus was declared eradicated in 2015 with the last naturally occurring case detected in 1999 in India, and type 3 wild poliovirus was declared eradicated in October 2019 with the last naturally occurring case having occurred in Nigeria in 2012. Type 1 poliovirus now accounts for all polio cases attributable to wild poliovirus. Because the only source of disease from type 2 poliovirus is now related only to vaccine use, there was a global switch from trivalent OPV (tOPV) to bivalent OPV (bOPV) in April 2016, thus ending all routine immunization with live type 2 poliovirus-containing oral vaccines. Concurrent recommendations were made for all countries to provide at least one dose of IPV to all vaccinees. Similarly, following this vaccine change, the only remaining risk of type 2 infection would come from continued transmission of type 2 OPV viruses administered before the switch, long-term iVDPV type 2 excretors, and breach of containment at facilities maintaining type 2 polioviruses (both wild type and OPV strains). For this reason, containment of all type 2 poliovirus infectious and potentially infectious materials into accredited essential facilities has been initiated globally.

On August 25, 2020, the World Health Organization (WHO) African Region was certified as wild poliovirus free after 4 years without a case. With this historic milestone, 5 of the 6 WHO regions, representing more than 90% of the world's population, are now free of the wild poliovirus, moving the world closer to achieving global polio eradication.

Communicability of poliovirus is greatest shortly before and after onset of clinical illness, when the virus is present in the throat and excreted in high concentrations in feces. Virus persists in the throat for approximately 1 to 2 weeks after onset of illness and is excreted in feces for an average of 3 to 6 weeks. In recipients of OPV, virus also persists in the throat for 1 to 2 weeks and is excreted in feces for several weeks, although in rare cases, excretion for more than 2 months can occur. Immunocompromised patients with significant primary B-lymphocyte immune deficiencies have excreted iVDPV for periods of more than 30 years.

The **incubation period of nonparalytic poliomyelitis** is 3 to 6 days. For the onset of poliomyelitis, the **incubation period to paralysis** usually is 7 to 21 days (range, 3–35 days).

DIAGNOSTIC TESTS: Poliovirus can be detected in specimens from the pharynx and feces, less commonly from urine, and rarely from CSF by isolation in cell culture or polymerase chain reaction (PCR). The relatively low sensitivity of isolation in cell culture from CSF is likely attributable to low viral load. Fecal material and pharyngeal swab specimens are most likely to yield virus in cell culture.

The diagnostic test of choice for confirming poliovirus disease is viral culture of stool specimens and throat swab specimens obtained as early in the course of illness as possible. There currently are nucleic acid amplification tests for enteroviruses from CSF and at least several multiplexed assays that detect enteroviruses, in addition to a number of other bacterial and viral agents. Such commonly used molecular tests for enteroviruses will detect poliovirus but will not differentiate poliovirus from other enteroviruses and, therefore, are insufficient to demonstrate that poliovirus is the etiology of disease. In these situations, additional virus testing will be necessary to confirm the diagnosis of poliovirus-related disease. Interpretation of acute and convalescent serologic test results can be difficult because of high levels of population immunity.

Real-time reverse transcriptase (RT)-PCR assays generally have sensitivity that is nearly comparable to or better than cell culture and may be more likely to identify polioviruses in CSF. Two or more stool and throat swab specimens for enterovirus isolation or detection by RT-PCR should be obtained at least 24 hours apart from patients with suspected paralytic poliomyelitis as early in the course of illness as possible, ideally within 14 days of onset of symptoms. Poliovirus may be excreted intermittently, and a single negative test result does not rule out infection.

Molecular methods have replaced neutralization for identification and typing to differentiate wild type from vaccine derived virus strains.

Because OPV no longer is available in the United States, the chance of exposure to vaccine-type polioviruses has become remote. Therefore, if a poliovirus is isolated in the United States, the isolate should be reported immediately to the state health department and sent to the Centers for Disease Control and Prevention (CDC) through the state health department for further testing. Paralytic poliomyelitis and detection of polioviruses are nationally reportable conditions.

TREATMENT: Management is supportive.

ISOLATION OF THE HOSPITALIZED PATIENT: In addition to standard precautions, contact precautions are indicated for infants and young children for the duration of hospitalization.

CONTROL MEASURES:

Immunization of Infants and Children.

Vaccines. Only IPV is available in the United States. IPV contains the 3 serotypes, which are grown in Vero cells or human diploid cells and inactivated with formaldehyde. IPV also is available in combination with other childhood vaccines (see Table 1.10, p 37). As of May 16, 2016, bivalent live attenuated oral poliovirus vaccine (bOPV), which contains types 1 and 3 poliovirus serotypes, is now the primary vaccine used in low- and middle-income countries. bOPV is produced in monkey kidney cells or human diploid cells.

Immunogenicity and Efficacy. Both IPV and OPV, in their recommended schedules, are highly immunogenic and effective in preventing poliomyelitis. Administration of IPV results in seroconversion in 95% or more of vaccine recipients to each of the 3 serotypes after 2 doses and results in seroconversion in 99% to 100% of recipients after 3 doses. Immunity probably is lifelong. Following exposure to live polioviruses, most

IPV-immunized children will excrete virus from stool but not from the oropharynx. Stool excretion quantities and duration are modestly reduced compared with shedding from unimmunized people. Immunization with 3 or more doses of OPV induces excellent serum antibody responses and substantial intestinal immunity against poliovirus reinfection. A 3-dose series of OPV, as formerly used in the United States, results in sustained, probably lifelong immunity. After 3 doses of OPV, seroconversion rates are lower in some low income countries, because of chronic enteropathy and interference by other enteric pathogens with the replication of the OPV vaccine strains.

Administration With Other Vaccines. Either IPV or OPV may be administered concurrently with other routinely recommended childhood vaccines (see Simultaneous Administration of Multiple Vaccines, p 36). For administration of combination vaccines containing IPV (see Table 1.10, p 37) with other vaccines and interchangeability of the combined vaccine with other vaccine products, see Pertussis (p 578), Hepatitis B (p 381), *Haemophilus influenzae* Infections (p 345), and *Streptococcus pneumoniae* (Pneumococcal) Infections (p 717).

Adverse Reactions. Most adverse reactions to IPV are mild and self-limited (eg, injection site pain and fever). Serious reactions to IPV are rare. Because IPV may contain trace amounts of streptomycin, neomycin, and polymyxin B, allergic reactions are possible in recipients with hypersensitivity to one or more of these antimicrobial agents. Allergic reactions to other ingredients or components of IPV are also possible.

OPV can cause VAPP. Before exclusive use of IPV in the United States beginning in 2000, the overall risk of VAPP associated with OPV was approximately 1 case per 2.4 million doses of OPV distributed. The rate of VAPP following the first dose, including vaccine recipient and contact cases, was approximately 1 case per 750 000 doses.

Schedule.[1] Four doses of IPV are recommended for routine immunization of all infants and children in the United States.

Refugee and Immigrant Children. Refugee and immigrant children should meet recommendations of the Advisory Committee on Immunization Practices of the CDC for poliovirus vaccination, which include protection against all 3 poliovirus types by age-appropriate vaccination. For children incompletely immunized with tOPV (trivalent oral polio vaccine), the series should be completed with IPV according to the catch-up schedule outlined below. In the absence of adequate written vaccination records, vaccination or revaccination in accordance with the age appropriate IPV schedule for the United States is recommended. Serologic testing to assess immunity no longer is available.[2]

- The first 2 doses of the 4-dose IPV series should be administered at 2-month intervals beginning at 2 months of age (minimum age, 6 weeks), and a third dose is recommended at 6 through 18 months of age. Doses may be administered at 4-week intervals when accelerated protection is indicated.
- Administration of the third dose at 6 months of age has the potential advantage of enhancing the likelihood of completion of the primary series and does not compromise seroconversion.
- A fourth and final dose in the series should be administered at 4 years or older and at a minimum interval of 6 months from the third dose.

[1]Centers for Disease Control and Prevention. Updated recommendations of the Advisory Committee on Immunization Practices (ACIP) regarding routine poliovirus vaccination. *MMWR Morb Mortal Wkly Rep.* 2009;58(30):829-830

[2]Marin M, Patel M, Oberste S, Pallansch MA. Guidance for assessment of poliovirus vaccination status and vaccination of children who have received poliovirus vaccine outside the United States. *MMWR Morb Mortal Wkly Rep.* 2017;66(1):23-25

- The final dose in the IPV series at 4 years or older should be administered regardless of the number of previous doses; a fourth dose is not necessary if the third dose was administered at 4 years or older and a minimum of 6 months after the second dose.
- When IPV is administered in combination with other vaccines at 2, 4, 6, and 12 through 15 months of age, it is necessary to administer a fifth and final dose of IPV at 4 years or older. The minimum interval from dose 4 to dose 5 should be at least 6 months.
- If a child misses an IPV dose at 4 through 6 years of age, the child should receive a booster dose as soon as feasible.

OPV remains the vaccine of choice for global eradication, although the Strategic Advisory Group of Experts (SAGE) on Immunization of the World Health Organization (WHO) has recommended that all countries currently using bOPV introduce at least 1 dose of IPV into their routine immunization schedules to mitigate the risk of VDPV type 2 poliomyelitis.[1]

Children Incompletely Immunized. Children who have not received the recommended doses of poliovirus vaccines on schedule should receive sufficient doses of IPV to complete the immunization series for their age (**http://aapredbook.aappublications.org/site/resources/izschedules.xhtml**).

Vaccine Recommendations for Adults. Most adults residing in the United States are presumed to be immune to poliovirus from previous immunization and have only a small risk of exposure to wild poliovirus in the United States. For those traveling to areas where poliovirus infection occurs, immunization or booster should be provided as per CDC guidance (**wwwnc.cdc.gov/travel/yellowbook/2018/infectious-diseases-related-to-travel/poliomyelitis**). Countries are considered to have active poliovirus circulation if they have ongoing endemic circulation, active outbreaks, or environmental evidence of active circulation with either wild polioviruses or VDPVs.

For unimmunized adults traveling to poliovirus-affected areas, primary immunization with IPV is recommended. Adults without documentation of vaccination history should be considered unimmunized. Two doses of IPV should be administered at intervals of 1 to 2 months (4–8 weeks); a third dose is administered 6 to 12 months after the second dose. If time does not allow 3 doses of IPV to be administered according to the recommended schedule before protection is required, the following alternatives are recommended:

- If protection is not needed until 8 weeks or more, 3 doses of IPV should be administered at least 4 weeks apart (eg, at weeks 0, 4, and 8).
- If protection is not needed for 4 to 8 weeks, 2 doses of IPV should be administered at least 4 weeks apart (eg, at weeks 0 and 4).
- If protection is needed in fewer than 4 weeks, a single dose of IPV should be administered.

The remaining doses of IPV to complete the primary immunization schedule should be administered subsequently at the recommended intervals if the person remains at an increased risk.

Recommendations in other circumstances are as follows:

- **Incompletely immunized adults.** Adults who previously received less than a full primary series of OPV or IPV should receive the remaining required doses of IPV,

---

[1] Orenstein WA, Seib KG; American Academy of Pediatrics, Committee on Infectious Diseases. Eradicating polio: how the world's pediatricians can help stop this crippling illness forever. *Pediatrics.* 2015;135(1):196-202

a minimum of 4 weeks since the last dose and the type of vaccine that was received previously.

- **Adults who are at an increased risk of exposure to wild or vaccine-derived polioviruses and who previously completed primary immunization with OPV or IPV.** These adults can receive a single dose of IPV. Available data do not indicate the need for more than a single lifetime booster dose with IPV.

Travelers also may be affected by WHO and CDC polio vaccination recommendations for people residing for 4 or more consecutive weeks in countries with ongoing poliovirus transmission and who are traveling to polio-free countries.[1]

- All residents and long-term visitors (defined as a duration of more than 4 weeks) should receive an additional dose of IPV between 4 weeks and 12 months before international travel and have the dose documented.
- Residents and long-term visitors who currently are in those countries who must travel with fewer than 4 weeks' notice and have not been vaccinated with OPV or IPV within the previous 4 weeks to 12 months should receive a dose at least by the time of departure.

The list of countries affected by this new recommendation can be found online (**http://polioeradication.org/polio-today/polio-now/public-health-emergency -status/**).

Precautions and Contraindications to Immunization.

Immunocompromised People. Immunocompromised patients, including people with human immunodeficiency virus (HIV) infection; combined immunodeficiency; abnormalities of immunoglobulin synthesis (ie, antibody deficiency syndromes); or leukemia, lymphoma, or generalized malignant neoplasm or people receiving immunosuppressive therapy with pharmacologic agents (see Immunization and Other Considerations in Immunocompromised Children, p 72) or radiation therapy should receive IPV. OPV should not be used. The immune response to IPV in immunocompromised patients may vary based on their level of immunosuppression.

Household Contacts of Immunocompromised People or People With Altered Immune States, Immunosuppression Attributable to Therapy for Other Disease, or Known HIV Infection. IPV is recommended for these people, and OPV should not be used. If OPV inadvertently is introduced into a household of an immunocompromised or HIV-infected person, close contact between the patient and the OPV recipient should be minimized for approximately 4 to 6 weeks after immunization. Household members should be counseled on practices that will minimize exposure of the immunocompromised or HIV-infected person to excreted poliovirus vaccine. These practices include exercising hand hygiene after contact with the child by all and avoiding diaper changing by the immunosuppressed person.

Pregnancy. If a woman is at increased risk of exposure and protection against polioviruses is needed, IPV is recommended. There is no evidence that IPV is unsafe in pregnant women or their developing fetuses.

Hypersensitivity or Anaphylactic Reactions to IPV Vaccine or Antimicrobial Agents Contained in IPV. IPV is contraindicated for people who have experienced an anaphylactic reaction after a previous dose of IPV attributable to any component of the vaccine.

Breastfeeding. Breastfeeding and mild diarrhea are not contraindications to IPV or OPV administration.

---

[1]Centers for Disease Control and Prevention. Interim CDC guidance for polio vaccination for travel to and from countries affected by wild poliovirus. *MMWR Morb Mortal Wkly Rep.* 2014;63(27):591-594

Reporting of Adverse Events After Immunization. Any case of VAPP should be reported to the Vaccine Adverse Event Reporting System (VAERS). This and other reporting requirements for adverse events following IPV and OPV are listed in the VAERS Table of Reportable Events (**https://vaers.hhs.gov/docs/VAERS_Table_of_Reportable_Events_Following_Vaccination.pdf**). In addition, reporting is encouraged for any clinically significant adverse event following a vaccination, even if uncertainty exist as to whether a vaccine caused the event (see Vaccine Adverse Event Reporting System [VAERS], p 46).

Case Reporting and Investigation. A suspected case of poliomyelitis or a nonparalytic poliovirus infection, regardless of whether the virus is suspected to be wild poliovirus or VDPV, should be considered a **public health emergency** and reported immediately to the state health department; this results in an immediate epidemiologic investigation. Poliomyelitis should be considered in the differential diagnosis of all cases of acute flaccid paralysis, including Guillain-Barré syndrome, transverse myelitis, and acute flaccid myelitis (acute neurologic illness associated with limb weakness in children, which is associated with enterovirus D-68 and less commonly enterovirus A71; see Enterovirus [Nonpoliovirus], p 315).[1] If the course is compatible clinically with poliomyelitis, specimens should be obtained for virologic studies (see Diagnostic Tests, p 603). If evidence implicates wild poliovirus or a VDPV infection, an intensive investigation will be conducted, and a public health decision will be made about the need for supplementary immunizations, choice of vaccine, and other actions. Because the vast majority of people who transmit poliovirus either are clinically asymptomatic or have a minor illness, the source person who transmitted virus to the patient with paralytic polio may be very difficult to identify (eg, there may be no known contact with someone who traveled to an area with endemic or epidemic polio). Therefore, pediatricians should be guided by the clinical presentation in deciding whether a child with acute paralysis might have polio and might warrant reporting the suspected case to public health authorities.

Polyomaviruses (BK, JC, and Other Polyomaviruses)

CLINICAL MANIFESTATIONS: BK virus (BKV) infection and JC virus (JCV) infection in humans usually occur in childhood and seemingly result in lifelong persistence. More than 80% of adults are seropositive for BKV. Primary infection with BKV in immunocompetent children generally is asymptomatic, although it may result in mild upper respiratory tract symptoms. BKV is more likely to cause disease in immunocompromised people, including hemorrhagic cystitis in hematopoietic stem cell transplant recipients, and interstitial nephritis and ureteral stenosis in renal transplant recipients. The primary symptom of BKV-associated hemorrhagic cystitis among immunocompromised children is painful hematuria; blood clots in the urine and secondary obstructive nephropathy also can occur. BKV-associated nephropathy occurs in 3% to 8% of renal transplant recipients and less frequently in other solid organ transplant recipients. BKV-associated nephropathy should be suspected in any renal transplant recipient with allograft dysfunction. More than half of renal allograft patients with BKV-associated nephropathy may experience allograft loss.

---

[1]Centers for Disease Control and Prevention. Acute neurologic illness of unknown etiology in children— Colorado, August–September 2014. *MMWR Morb Mortal Wkly.* 2014;63(40):901-902

JCV is the cause of progressive multifocal leukoencephalopathy (PML), a demyelinating disease of the central nervous system that occurs in severely immunocompromised patients, including patients with acquired immunodeficiency syndrome (AIDS), patients receiving intensive chemotherapy, hematopoietic stem cell or solid organ transplant recipients, and patients receiving various monoclonal antibody therapies for treatment of autoimmune, oncologic, and neurologic diseases. PML, the only known disease caused by JCV, occurs in approximately 3% to 5% of untreated adults with AIDS but is rare in children with AIDS. Symptoms include cognitive disturbance, hemiparesis, ataxia, cranial nerve dysfunction, and aphasia. Lytic infection of oligodendrocytes by JCV is the primary mechanism of pathogenesis for PML. In the absence of restored T-lymphocyte function, PML almost always is fatal. PML is an AIDS-defining illness in human immunodeficiency virus (HIV)-infected people.[1] Approximately 50% to 60% of adults are infected by JCV, with infections being acquired during adolescence and early adulthood.

To date, 14 polyomaviruses have been detected in humans, but only a few have been associated with disease, including BK and JC viruses. The Merkel cell polyomavirus (MCPyV) has been detected in >80% of Merkel cell carcinomas, which are rare neuroendocrine tumors of the skin. The trichodysplasia spinulosa-associated polyomavirus (TSPyV) has been identified in tissue from patients with trichodysplasia spinulosa, a rare follicular disease of immunocompromised patients that primarily affects the face. The KI polyomavirus (KIPyV) and WU polyomavirus (WUPyV) have been identified in respiratory tract secretions, primarily in association with known pathogenic viruses of the respiratory tract. Human polyomaviruses 6 and 7 (HPyV6 and HPyV7) have been detected as asymptomatic inhabitants of human skin. Human polyomavirus 9 (HPyV9) has been detected in the serum of some renal transplant recipients. The natural history, prevalence, and pathogenic potential of these recently discovered human polyomaviruses have not yet been established.

ETIOLOGY: Polyomaviruses are members of the family *Polyomaviridae.* BKV, JCV, WUPyV, and KIPyV are members of the genus *Betapolyomavirus;* MCPyV, TSPyV, HPyV9, HPyV12, and New Jersey polyomavirus are members of the genus *Alphapolyomavirus;* HPyV6, HPyV7, Malawi polyomavirus, and St. Louis polyomavirus are members of the genus *Deltapolyomavirus.* They are nonenveloped viruses with a circular double-stranded DNA genome with icosahedral symmetry of the capsid ranging 40 to 50 nm in diameter. One of the biological characteristics of the polyomaviruses is the maintenance of a chronic viral infection in their host with few or no symptoms. Symptomatic disease caused by human polyomavirus infections occurs almost exclusively in immunosuppressed people.

EPIDEMIOLOGY: Humans are the only known natural hosts for BKV and JCV. The mode of transmission of BKV and JCV is uncertain, but the respiratory route and the oral route by water or food have been postulated. BKV and JCV are ubiquitous in the human population, with BKV infection occurring in early childhood and JCV infection occurring primarily in adolescence and adulthood. BKV persists in the kidney and gastrointestinal tract of healthy subjects, with urinary excretion occurring in 3% to 5% of healthy adults.

---

[1]Panel on Opportunistic Infections in HIV-Exposed and HIV-Infected Children. Guidelines for the Prevention and Treatment of Opportunistic Infections in HIV-Exposed and HIV-Infected Children. Department of Health and Human Services. Available at: **https://clinicalinfo.hiv.gov/sites/default/files/inline-files/oi_guidelines_pediatrics.pdf**

JCV persists in the kidney, gastrointestinal tract, and brain of healthy people. The prevalence of urinary excretion of JCV increases with age.

DIAGNOSTIC TESTS: Detection of BKV T-antigen by immunohistochemical analysis of renal biopsy material is the gold standard for diagnosis of BKV-associated nephropathy, but nucleic acid-based polymerase chain reaction (PCR) assays are the most sensitive tools for rapid viral screening for polyomaviruses and quantification of viral load. Prospective monitoring of BK viral load in plasma using PCR commonly is used after renal transplantation to monitor for BKV-associated nephropathy. Detection of BKV nucleic acid in plasma by PCR assay is associated with an increased risk of BKV-associated nephropathy, especially when BKV viral loads exceed 10 000 genomes/mL, but detection of BKV in urine of renal transplant recipients is common and does not predict BKV disease after renal transplantation. Both BKV and JCV can be propagated in cell culture, but culture plays no role in the laboratory diagnosis of infection attributable to these agents. Antibody assays commonly are used to detect the presence of specific antibodies against individual viruses.

The diagnosis of BKV-associated hemorrhagic cystitis is made clinically when other causes of urinary tract bleeding are excluded. Among hematopoietic stem cell transplant recipients, detection of BKV by PCR in urine is common (more than 50%), but BKV-associated hemorrhagic cystitis is much less common (10%–15%). Prolonged urinary shedding of BKV and detection of BKV in plasma after hematopoietic stem cell transplantation has been associated with increased risk of developing BKV-associated hemorrhagic cystitis. Urine cytologic testing may suggest urinary shedding of BKV on the basis of presence of decoy cells, which resemble renal carcinoma cells, but decoy cells do not have high sensitivity or specificity for BKV disease.

A confirmed diagnosis of PML attributable to JCV requires a compatible clinical syndrome and magnetic resonance imaging or computed tomographic findings showing lesions in the brain white matter coupled with brain biopsy findings. JCV can be demonstrated by in situ hybridization, electron microscopy, or immunohistochemistry of brain biopsy or autopsy material. There are no FDA-cleared nucleic acid amplification tests (NAATs) for detection of JCV. Diagnosis of PML can be facilitated when JCV DNA is detected in cerebrospinal fluid by a NAAT, which may obviate the need for a brain biopsy. Early in the course of PML, false-negative PCR assay results have been reported, so repeat testing is warranted when clinical suspicion of PML is high. Measurement of JCV DNA concentrations in cerebrospinal fluid samples may be a useful marker for managing PML in patients with AIDS who are receiving combination antiretroviral therapy.

TREATMENT: Multiple studies evaluating treatment options (eg, cidofovir, leflunomide, adoptive cellular immunotherapy) are ongoing (**www.clinicaltrials.gov**). Fluoroquinolones or Immune Globulin Intravenous (IGIV) provide little to no benefit in the treatment of BKV-associated nephropathy. Judicious reduction of immune suppression has been shown to prevent development of BKV-associated nephropathy without increasing the risk of rejection in renal transplant patients with BKV plasma viral loads greater than 10 000 genomes/mL.

Most patients with BKV-hemorrhagic cystitis after hematopoietic stem cell transplantation require only supportive care, because restoration of immune function by stem cell engraftment ultimately will control BKV replication. In severe cases, surgical intervention may be required to stop bladder hemorrhage. Parenteral and/or intravesicular cidofovir have been used for treatment, but data from prospective, controlled studies on its efficacy and safety are lacking. Use of systemic cidofovir must be balanced against its high risk of nephrotoxicity. Adoptive transfer of BKV-specific T lymphocytes has been used with varying success at some transplant centers.

Restoration of immune function (eg, combination antiretroviral therapy for patients with AIDS) is necessary for survival of patients with PML. Cidofovir has not been shown to be effective for treatment of PML. For patients with monoclonal antibody-associated PML, plasmapheresis and/or immune stimulatory agents (eg, granulocyte colony-stimulating factor) may be useful to improve outcomes.

ISOLATION OF THE HOSPITALIZED PATIENT: Standard precautions are recommended.

CONTROL MEASURES: None.

Prion Diseases: Transmissible Spongiform Encephalopathies

CLINICAL MANIFESTATIONS: Prion diseases, or transmissible spongiform encephalopathies (TSEs), constitute a group of rare, rapidly progressive, universally fatal, transmissible neurodegenerative diseases of humans and animals characterized by neuronal degeneration, reactive gliosis, and, most often, by spongiform degeneration in the cerebral cortical, subcortical, and cerebellar gray matter. Those findings are accompanied by accumulation of an abnormal misfolded, partially protease-resistant "prion" (proteinaceous infectious) protein. The normal protease-sensitive isomer of the protein is called "cellular" prion protein or PrP^C. The protease-resistant prion protein is variably called PrP^{res}, scrapie prion protein (PrP^{sc}, named for the first known prion disease affecting sheep), or as suggested by the World Health Organization, TSE-associated PrP (PrP^{TSE}). PrP^{TSE} distributes widely, albeit unevenly, throughout the central nervous system, sometimes forming plaques of varying morphologies.

Human prion diseases include several sporadic, familial, and acquired diseases: Creutzfeldt-Jakob disease (CJD), Gerstmann-Sträussler-Scheinker disease, fatal familial insomnia and sporadic fatal insomnia, kuru, and variant CJD (vCJD, caused by the agent of bovine spongiform encephalopathy [BSE], commonly called "mad cow" disease). Classic CJD can be sporadic (approximately 85% of cases), familial (approximately 15% of cases), or iatrogenic (fewer than 1% of cases). Sporadic CJD most commonly is a disease of older adults (median age of death in the United States, 68 years) but has also been described in adolescents and young adults. Iatrogenic CJD has been acquired through intramuscular injection of contaminated cadaveric pituitary hormones (growth hormone and human gonadotropin), dura mater allografts, corneal transplantation, contaminated instruments used in neurosurgery, and electroencephalographic probe electrodes. In 1996, an outbreak of a new variant of CJD (vCJD) was linked to consumption of beef from BSE-infected cattle in the United Kingdom and France, with index cases occurring in teenagers. Since the end of 2003, 4 presumptive cases of transfusion-transmitted vCJD have been reported: 3 clinical cases as well as 1 asymptomatic case in which PrP^{TSE} was detected in the spleen and lymph nodes but not brain tissues. A fifth possible iatrogenic vCJD infection was reported in the United Kingdom, affecting a hemophiliac patient, also asymptomatic, who had PrP^{TSE} in the spleen; preclinical vCJD was attributed to treatment with plasma-derived coagulation factor fractionated in the United Kingdom; the plasma product implicated in transmitting vCJD was never marketed in the United States.

The best-known prion diseases affecting animals include scrapie of sheep and goats, BSE, and a chronic wasting disease (CWD) of North American deer, elk, and moose (**www.cdc.gov/prions/index.html**). CWD recently was detected in reindeer and moose (European elk) in Norway, Sweden, and Finland. Except for vCJD, no human prion disease has yet been attributed convincingly to infection with an agent of animal origin.

CJD most typically manifests as a rapidly progressive neurologic disease with escalating defects in memory, personality, and other higher cortical functions. At presentation, approximately one third of patients have cerebellar dysfunction, including ataxia, incoordination, and dysarthria. Iatrogenic CJD also may manifest as dementia with cerebellar signs. Myoclonus develops in at least 80% of affected patients at some point in the course of disease. Death usually occurs in weeks to months (median, 4–5 months); only 10% to 15% of patients with sporadic CJD survive for more than 1 year.

vCJD is distinguished from classic CJD by younger age of onset (median age at death around 28 years), early "psychiatric" manifestations, and other features such as painful sensations in the limbs, delayed onset of overt neurologic signs, relative absence of diagnostic electroencephalographic changes, and a more prolonged duration of illness (median, 13–14 months). In vCJD, but not in classic CJD, a high proportion of people exhibit high signal abnormalities on T2-weighted brain magnetic resonance imaging in the pulvinar region of the posterior thalamus (known as the "pulvinar sign"). In vCJD, the neuropathologic examination reveals highly reproducible pathology with spongiform vacuolation and numerous "florid" plaques (compact flower-like amyloid plaques surrounded by vacuoles) and exceptionally striking punctate deposition of PrP^{TSE} in the basal ganglia. In addition, PrP^{TSE} is detectable by immunohistochemistry in the tonsils, appendix, spleen, and lymph nodes of patients with vCJD.

ETIOLOGY: The proteinaceous infectious particle (or prion), widely believed to cause human and animal prion diseases, consists of PrP^{TSE}, the misfolded form of PrP^C, a ubiquitous normal sialoglycoprotein of unknown function found on the surfaces of neurons and many other cells of humans and animals. It has been postulated by some authorities that sporadic CJD and atypical forms of BSE may result from a spontaneous structural change of host-encoded PrP^C into the self-replicating pathogenic PrP^{TSE} form. Prion propagation is proposed to occur by a "recruitment" reaction in which abnormal PrP^{TSE} serves as a template to convert PrP^C molecules into misfolded PrP^{TSE} molecules that precipitate in saline-detergent solutions, resist digestion with some proteolytic enzymes, and have a high potential to aggregate. Experimental efforts to confirm this hypothesis have yielded inconsistent results.

EPIDEMIOLOGY: Classic sporadic CJD is rare, occurring in the United States at a rate of approximately 1 to 1.5 cases per million people annually. Lifetime risk of CJD probably exceeds 1 in 10 000 people. Onset of disease peaks in the 60- through 74-year age group. Case-control studies of sporadic CJD have identified no consistent environmental risk factor. No increase in cases of sporadic CJD has been observed in people previously transfused with blood or blood components or injected with human plasma derivatives. Rate of sporadic CJD is not increased in patients with several diseases treated by repeated blood transfusions (eg, thalassemia and sickle cell disease) or in patients with hemophilia treated with human plasma derivatives. The American Red Cross traced a number of recipients of blood transfusions from donors later diagnosed with sporadic CJD; no cases of CJD were identified in recipients, some of whom survived for many years. Taken together, this information suggests that any risk of transfusion-transmitted classic sporadic CJD must be very low and appropriately regarded as theoretical. Except in families with familial forms of the disease, CJD has not been reported in progeny of mothers who died with CJD. Familial forms of prion diseases are expressed as autosomal dominant disorders with variable penetrance associated with a variety of mutations of the PrP-encoding gene (*PRNP*) located on chromosome 20. On average, familial CJD begins approximately 10 years earlier than does sporadic CJD, but age at onset varies widely, even for members of the same family harboring identical mutations.

As of May 2019 (**www.cjd.ed.ac.uk/surveillance**), the total number of vCJD cases reported was 178 patients in the United Kingdom, 28 in France, 5 in Spain, 4 in Ireland, 4 in the United States, 3 in the Netherlands, 3 in Italy, 2 in Portugal, 2 in Canada, and 1 each in Taiwan, Japan, and Saudi Arabia. Two of the 4 patients in the United States, 2 of the 4 in Ireland, and 1 each of the patients in France, Canada, and Taiwan are believed to have acquired vCJD during residence in the United Kingdom. A study using statistical analysis of probability density of exposure to BSE concluded that 2 vCJD patients in the United States and another in Canada probably were infected during childhood residence in the Kingdom of Saudi Arabia. On the basis of animal inoculation studies, comparative PrP immunoblotting, and epidemiologic investigations, almost all cases of vCJD are believed to have resulted from exposure to tissues from cattle infected with BSE. Authorities suspect that the Japanese patient was infected during a short visit of 24 days to the United Kingdom in 1990, 12 years before onset of vCJD. Most patients with vCJD were younger than 30 years at onset, and several were adolescents. Median age at death of the 175 primary vCJD cases was 27 years. The ages at death of the 3 iatrogenic vCJD transfusion-transmitted cases were 32, 69, and 75 years; they developed typical vCJD 6.3 to 8.5 years after transfusions with nonleukoreduced red blood cells from apparently healthy individuals who donated the blood 1.4 to 3.5 years before onset of vCJD, demonstrating that blood contained the infectious agent during a substantial part of the asymptomatic incubation period. One patient with hemophilia, also showing no clinical signs of prion disease, probably was infected through injections of human plasma-derived clotting factors.

The **incubation periods** for iatrogenic classic CJD vary by route of exposure and range from about 14 months to at least 42 years. No transfusion-transmitted cases of classic CJD have been recognized.

DIAGNOSTIC TESTS: The diagnosis of human prion diseases can be made with certainty only by neuropathologic examination of affected brain tissue, usually obtained at autopsy. Immunodetection methods for PrP such as immunohistochemistry with sections and Western blot with saline-detergent extracts can be used to test brain tissues. Electroencephalography (EEG), magnetic resonance imaging (MRI), and cerebrospinal fluid (CSF) testing can be used to diagnose prion disease in living patients. In most patients with classic CJD, characteristic 1-cycle to 2-cycles per second triphasic sharp-wave discharges on EEG tracing indicate CJD. The likelihood of finding this abnormality is enhanced by serial EEG recordings. Validated assays that detect 2 protein markers, 14-3-3 and tau, in CSF showed 83% to 90% sensitivity and 78% specificity. These proteins, sometimes detected in other neurologic diseases, are surrogate nonspecific markers found in CSF, probably as a result of the death of neurons. No validated blood test is available. Recent promising developments exploit the in vivo prion replication process to amplify and detect even minute amounts of prions in biological samples. One such technique, real-time quaking-induced conversion (RT-QuIC), has been applied successfully in the clinical diagnosis of CJD in CSF samples with high specificity and sensitivity. RT-QuIC also has been applied to diagnose CJD in olfactory epithelium brushings and, with additional validation, may be used in clinical settings.[1] RT-QuIC has not yet been applied successfully to blood samples. Some success has been reported with blood samples tested using another PrP^{TSE} amplification technique, called protein misfolding cyclic amplification (PMCA).[2] These are currently "research-use-only" tests not marketed for human diagnosis. Any person bearing a pathogenic mutation of the *PRNP* gene (not a normal polymorphism) with progressive neurologic signs suggestive of a TSE can be presumed to have a prion disease. Because no unique nucleic acid has been detected in prions causing TSEs, nucleic acid amplification studies such as polymerase chain reaction tests are not possible. Brain biopsies for patients with possible CJD should be considered only when other potentially treatable diseases remain in the differential diagnosis. Complete postmortem examination of the brain is encouraged to confirm the clinical diagnosis of prion disease, to detect emerging forms of CJD, such as vCJD, and to survey for potential zoonotic transmission of chronic wasting disease. State-of-the-art diagnostic testing, including assays of 14-3-3 and tau and RT-QuIC in CSF, *PRNP* gene sequencing, histopathology and Western blot analysis of brain to identify and characterize PrP^{TSE}, as well as expert neuropathologic consultation, are offered by the National Prion Disease Pathology Surveillance Center (telephone, 216-368-0587; **www.cjdsurveillance.com**). Clinical specimens that may contain prions, particularly specimens with substantial amounts of infectivity, including brain, spinal cord, and CSF, should be handled with extreme caution. Amounts of infectivity can be significantly but not completely inactivated by physical or chemical means commonly used in the laboratory. Potentially contaminated laboratory waste should be steam autoclaved, when possible, at 134°C, and then sent to incineration as medical-pathological waste.

TREATMENT: No treatment has stopped or slowed the progressive neurodegeneration in prion diseases. Experimental treatments are being studied. Supportive therapy aids in managing dementia, spasticity, rigidity, and seizures occurring during the course of illness. Compassionate counseling and emotional support should be offered to families of affected people. Skilled genetic counseling is indicated for familial disease, taking into account that penetrance has been variable in some kindreds in which people with a *PRNP* mutation survived to an advanced age without developing neurodegenerative disease. A family support and patient advocacy group, the CJD Foundation (telephone 800-659-1991; **www.cjdfoundation.org**), offers helpful information and advice together with information for professionals.

ISOLATION OF THE HOSPITALIZED PATIENT: Standard precautions are recommended. Available evidence indicates that even prolonged intimate contact with CJD patients has not transmitted disease. Tissues containing high levels of infectivity (eg, brains, eyes, spinal cords of affected people) and instruments in contact with those tissues are considered biohazards; incineration, prolonged autoclaving at high temperature and pressure

[1] Orrú CD, Bongianni M, Tonoli G, et al. A test for Creutzfeldt-Jakob disease using nasal brushings [erratum in: *N Engl J Med*. 2014;371(19):1852]. *N Engl J Med*. 2014;371(6):519-295

[2] Kramm C, Pritzkow S, Lyon A, Nichols T, Morales R, Soto C. Detection of prions in blood of cervids at the asymptomatic stage of chronic wasting disease. *Sci Rep* 2017;7(1):17241

after thorough cleaning, and, especially, exposure to a solution of 1 N or greater sodium hydroxide for 1 hour has been reported to decrease markedly or eliminate infectivity of contaminated surgical instruments. Work surfaces can be decontaminated effectively by exposure to 5.25% or stronger sodium hypochlorite (NaOCl, undiluted household chlorine bleach), but many surgical instruments corrode when exposed to NaOCl. The Centers for Disease Control and Prevention (CDC) offers advice for dealing with CJD patients (**www.cdc.gov/prions/index.html**) and recommendations for CJD infection control. Information on distribution of infectivity in various tissues and specific decontamination protocols are available online (**www.cdc.gov/prions/cjd/infection-control.html** and **www.who.int/csr/resources/publications/bse/WHO_CDS_CSR_APH_2000_3/en/**). Person-to-person transmission of classic sporadic CJD by blood, milk, saliva, urine, or feces has not been reported. Body fluids should be handled using standard infection control procedures. Universal blood precautions, routinely recommended for all patients, should be sufficient to prevent bloodborne transmission of TSEs.

CONTROL MEASURES: Immunization against prion diseases is not available, and no protective immune response to infection has been demonstrated. Iatrogenic transmission of CJD through cadaveric pituitary hormones has been obviated by use of recombinant products. Recognition that CJD had been spread by transplantation of infected dura mater allografts and corneal transplantation led to improved sourcing of those materials. After reports of transfusion-transmitted vCJD in the United Kingdom, blood establishments implemented more stringent blood and plasma donor selection criteria and improved collection protocols. Health care professionals should follow their state's prion disease reporting requirements and indicate CJD or other prion disease diagnoses appropriately on death certificates; the CDC uses mortality data from the United States to help monitor prion diseases. In addition, any suspected or confirmed diagnosis of a prion disease of special public health concern (eg, any suspected iatrogenic TSE, vCJD, or human TSE with onset before age of 55 years) should be reported promptly to the appropriate state or local health departments and to the CDC (telephone, 404-639-3091 or 404-639-4435; **www.cdc.gov/prions/cjd/index.html**). Current precautionary policies of the US Food and Drug Administration to reduce the risk of transmitting CJD by human blood or blood products are available online (**www.fda.gov/downloads/biologicsbloodvaccines/guidancecomplianceregulatoryinformation/guidances/blood/ucm307137.pdf**). General information about BSE and CWD is available from the US Food and Drug Administration (**www.fda.gov/AnimalVeterinary/ResourcesforYou/AnimalHealthLiteracy/ucm136222.htm**), from the US Department of Agriculture (**www.fsis.usda.gov/wps/portal/fsis/topics/food-safety-education/get-answers/food-safety-fact-sheets/production-and-inspection/bovine-spongiform-encephalopathy-bse/bse-resources**), from the CDC (**www.cdc.gov/prions/bse/index.html**), and from the World Organization for Animal Health (**www.oie.int/en/animal-health-in-the-world/bse-portal/**).

Pseudomonas aeruginosa Infections

CLINICAL MANIFESTATIONS: *Pseudomonas aeruginosa* causes a variety of localized and systemic infections including otitis externa, mastoiditis, folliculitis, cellulitis, ecthyma gangrenosum, wound infection, ocular infection, pneumonia, osteomyelitis, bacteremia, endocarditis, meningitis, and urinary tract infection. It is a common cause of health care-associated infections (particularly in the presence of invasive devices), infections in immunocompromised children, pulmonary infections in children with cystic fibrosis, and infections in children with burns. *Pseudomonas* ophthalmia occurs predominantly in preterm infants and presents with eyelid edema and erythema, purulent discharge, and pannus formation. It can progress to corneal perforation, endophthalmitis, sepsis, and meningitis.

ETIOLOGY: *P aeruginosa* is an aerobic, gram-negative, nonfermenting bacillus that is commonly found in the environment. The organism has a number of virulence factors, including the ability to form biofilms. *P aeruginosa* can convert to a mucoid phenotype, particularly in the setting of prolonged colonization, such as in individuals with cystic fibrosis.

EPIDEMIOLOGY: *P aeruginosa* is an opportunistic pathogen, causing infections in immunocompromised hosts (particularly those with neutropenia or poor granulocyte function), those with indwelling devices, burns, or cystic fibrosis. Children with cystic fibrosis commonly develop chronic endobronchial infection with *P aeruginosa*, which is often associated with a more rapid decline in pulmonary function. Children with cystic fibrosis can share epidemic strains of *P aeruginosa*. Hospital-acquired *P aeruginosa* infections include ventilator-associated pneumonia, catheter-associated urinary tract infections, and surgical site infections. Community-associated infections include "hot tub" folliculitis, otitis externa after swimming in fresh water, osteomyelitis after a puncture wound (particularly through a sneaker), and endocarditis in people who inject drugs. It is a common cause of "contact lens" keratitis. Auricular chondritis has occurred after upper ear piercing. Outbreaks of infection have occurred as a result of contaminated bronchoscopes.

P aeruginosa has intrinsic resistance to a variety of antibiotics and circulating strains are often multidrug resistant. Resistance may emerge during therapy. Production of beta-lactamases, loss of outer membrane proteins, and multidrug efflux pumps are common. Carbapenemase-producing strains (most commonly IMP and VIM) have occurred in the United States in recent years.

The **incubation period** is variable depending on the host and site of colonization/infection. Incubation period for folliculitis following immersion in a whirlpool is a few hours to several days after exposure.

DIAGNOSTIC TESTS: Diagnosis is established by growth of *P aeruginosa*. Isolates may be identified by traditional biochemical tests, by a variety of commercially available biochemical test systems, by mass spectrometry of bacterial cell components, or by molecular methods.

TREATMENT:

- Empiric combination therapy from different antimicrobial classes (eg, adding a fluoroquinolone or an aminoglycoside to an antipseudomonal β-lactam) may be indicated in severe sepsis, in patients with neutropenia, in patients who recently received broad-spectrum β-lactams, or in settings where antibiotic resistance is high to increase the probability of covering the infecting organism prior to knowing its identification and susceptibility.
- Cultures and susceptibilities should be sent prior to initiation of empiric therapy and therapy adjusted as per susceptibility data. In most patients, therapy can be simplified to a single active agent; there are no data to support continuation of combination

therapy for an isolate susceptible to an appropriate antipseudomonal drug (see below). When the clinical course is complicated or when there is multidrug resistance, it is recommended that an infectious disease expert assist in the management, particularly in the setting of carbapenem resistance.

- An important component of treatment is source control (ie, removal of catheters and devices, drainage of abscesses).
- Antimicrobial agents that have activity against *P aeruginosa* include piperacillin-tazobactam, ceftazidime, cefepime, aztreonam, ciprofloxacin, levofloxacin, meropenem, and imipenem/cilastatin (see Tables of Antibacterial Drugs, p 876); however, susceptibility patterns vary regionally. Aminoglycosides are often used as adjunctive therapy (but not as monotherapy beyond urinary tract infections). Polymyxins (ie, colistin and polymyxin B) can be considered in the setting of highly resistant organisms but should not be used as first-line treatments if newer agents (eg, imipenem/cilastatin-relebactam, ceftazidime-avibactam, or ceftolozane-tazobactam) are available because of their generally lower efficacy and higher adverse event rates compared with these newer agents.
- Management of children with cystic fibrosis should occur in conjunction with an expert in cystic fibrosis. Treatment for pulmonary exacerbation often includes 2 antipseudomonal agents in patients known to be chronically infected with *P aeruginosa*. The Cystic Fibrosis Foundation recommends early eradication of *P aeruginosa* with inhaled tobramycin (300 mg twice daily for 28 days). Once *P aeruginosa* becomes established, it can persist for years. Chronic suppressive treatment with inhaled antibiotics can decrease the bacterial burden. Inhaled antibiotics are generally not indicated for pulmonary exacerbations.
- Management of *Pseudomonas* neonatal ophthalmia urgently requires a combination of systemic and topical therapy, because systemic antibiotics alone have poor penetration in the anterior chamber of the eye. The diagnosis should be suspected when gram-stained specimens of exudate contain gram-negative bacilli, and should be confirmed by culture. Ophthalmology consultation is recommended.
- Duration of therapy is based on clinical and bacteriologic response of the patient and the site(s) of infection. Most bloodstream infections, ventilator-associated pneumonias, and urinary tract infections can be treated with 7 to 14 days of antibiotic therapy.

ISOLATION OF THE HOSPITALIZED PATIENT: Standard precautions for routine patients are recommended. For carbapenemase-producing organisms, contact precautions are indicated.[1] The Cystic Fibrosis Foundation recommends implementation of contact precautions in addition to standard precautions for care of all patients with cystic fibrosis in inpatient or ambulatory care settings, regardless of respiratory tract cultures.

CONTROL MEASURES: The Cystic Fibrosis Foundation recommends that all cystic fibrosis care centers limit contact between patients. This includes inpatient, outpatient, and social settings. When in a health care setting, patients with cystic fibrosis should wear a mask while outside of a clinic examination room or a hospital room. Education of patients and families about hand hygiene and appropriate personal hygiene is recommended.

---

[1]Centers for Disease Control and Prevention. Facility Guidance for Control of Carbapenem Resistant Enterobacteriaceae (CRE) November 2015 Update. Available at: **www.cdc.gov/hai/pdfs/cre/CRE-guidance-508.pdf**

Q Fever (*Coxiella burnetii* Infection)

CLINICAL MANIFESTATIONS: Approximately half of acute Q fever infections result in symptoms. Acute and persistent (chronic) forms of the disease exist and both can present as fever of unknown origin. Acute Q fever in children is typically characterized by abrupt onset of fever, and is often accompanied by chills, headache, weakness, cough, and other nonspecific systemic symptoms. Illness typically is self-limited, although a relapsing febrile illness lasting for several months has been documented in children. Gastrointestinal tract symptoms, such as diarrhea, vomiting, abdominal pain, and anorexia, are reported in 50% to 80% of children. Rash has been observed in some patients with Q fever. Q fever pneumonia usually manifests with a mild cough and shortness of breath but can progress to respiratory distress. Chest radiographic patterns are variable. In immunocompromised patients, a nodular pattern accompanied by a halo of ground-glass opacification and vessel connection, or findings suggestive of a necrotizing process, may be seen. More severe manifestations of acute Q fever are rare but include hepatitis, hemolytic-uremic syndrome, myocarditis, pericarditis, cerebellitis, encephalitis, meningitis, hemophagocytosis, lymphadenitis, cholecystitis, and rhabdomyolysis. The presence of anticardiolipin antibodies during acute Q fever has been associated with severe complications in adults. There appears to be a small link between Q fever and subsequent development of lymphoma in adulthood because of the risk factor of lymphadenitis. Persistent, localized (chronic) Q fever in children is rare but can present as blood culture-negative endocarditis, vascular infection, chronic relapsing or multifocal osteomyelitis, or chronic hepatitis. Osteomyelitis is a common presentation of persistent, localized Q fever in children. Children who are immunocompromised or have underlying valvular heart disease may be at higher risk of persistent, localized Q fever.

ETIOLOGY: *Coxiella burnetii,* the cause of Q fever, previously was considered to be a rickettsial organism but is a gram-negative intracellular bacterium that belongs to the order *Legionellales,* family *Coxiellaceae.* It shares many features, including relatedness of several virulence genes, with *Legionella pneumophila.* The infectious form of *C burnetii* is highly resistant to heat, desiccation, and disinfectant chemicals and can persist for long periods of time in the environment. *C burnetii* is classified as a category B bioterrorism agent by the Centers for Disease Control and Prevention (CDC).

EPIDEMIOLOGY: Q fever is a zoonotic infection that has been reported worldwide, including in every state in the United States. The "Q" comes from "query" fever, the name of the disease until its etiologic agent was identified in the 1930s. *C burnetii* infection usually is asymptomatic in animals. Many different species can be infected, although cattle, sheep, and goats are the primary reservoirs for human infection. Tick vectors may be important for maintaining animal and bird reservoirs but are not believed to be important in transmission to humans. Humans most often acquire infection by inhalation of fine-particle aerosols of *C burnetii* generated from birthing fluids or other excreta of infected animals or through inhalation of dust contaminated by these materials. Infection can occur by exposure to contaminated materials, such as wool, straw, bedding, or laundry. Windborne particles containing infectious organisms can travel prolonged distances, contributing to sporadic cases for which no apparent animal contact can be demonstrated. Unpasteurized dairy products also can contain the organism. Seasonal trends occur in farming areas with predictable frequency, and the disease often coincides with the livestock birthing season in spring.

The **incubation period** is 14 to 22 days, with a range from 9 to 39 days, depending on the inoculum size. Persistent, localized (chronic) Q fever can develop months to years after initial infection.

DIAGNOSTIC TESTS: Serologic evidence of a fourfold increase in phase II immunoglobulin (Ig) G via immunofluorescent assay (IFA) tests between paired sera taken 3 to 6 weeks apart is the most commonly used method to diagnose acute Q fever. A single high serum phase II IgG titer (≥1:128) by IFA in the convalescent stage may be considered as evidence of probable infection. Confirmation of persistent (chronic) Q fever is based on an increasing phase I IgG titer (typically ≥1:1024) that often is higher than the phase II IgG titer *and* an identifiable nidus of infection (eg, endocarditis, vascular infection, osteomyelitis, chronic hepatitis). Polymerase chain reaction (PCR) testing on whole blood or serum may be useful in the first 2 weeks of symptom onset and before antimicrobial administration. Although a positive PCR assay result can confirm the diagnosis, a negative PCR test result will not rule out Q fever. PCR and serologic testing for *C burnetii* are available through state public health laboratories and from some commercial diagnostic laboratories. Detection of *C burnetii* in tissues (eg, heart valve) by immunohistochemistry or PCR assay can also confirm a diagnosis of chronic Q fever. However, PCR test results may be negative in up to 66% of patients with endocarditis attributable to Q fever. Isolation of *C burnetii* from blood or tissue can be performed only in special laboratories with biosafety level 3 facilities using tissue culture, embryonated eggs, or animal inoculation because of the potential hazard to laboratory workers.

TREATMENT: Acute Q fever generally is a self-limited illness, and many patients recover without antimicrobial therapy. However, early treatment is effective in shortening illness duration and symptom severity and should be initiated in all symptomatic patients. For symptomatic patients with suspected Q fever, immediate empiric therapy should be given, because laboratory results are often negative early in illness onset pending production of quantifiable antibody. Doxycycline administered for 14 days is the drug of choice for severe infections in patients and can be used for acute Q fever regardless of patient age (see Tetracyclines, p 866). Pregnant women and patients allergic to doxycycline can be treated with trimethoprim-sulfamethoxazole.

Persistent (chronic) Q fever is much more difficult to treat, and relapses can occur despite appropriate therapy, necessitating repeated courses of therapy. For Q fever endocarditis in adults, the recommended therapy is a combination of doxycycline and hydroxychloroquine for a minimum of 18 months. There are limited data available on effective treatment of chronic Q fever in children, but in some cases, surgical replacement of infected tissue and/or surgical débridement may be required.

ISOLATION OF THE HOSPITALIZED PATIENT: Standard precautions are recommended for routine care. Airborne precautions should be used for patients who are undergoing procedures that could cause aerosolization or for pregnant women with Q fever who are delivering.

CONTROL MEASURES: Strict adherence to proper hygiene when handling infected parturient animals or their excreta can help decrease the risk of infection in the farm setting, as can ensuring that people do not consume unpasteurized milk and milk products. Improved prescreening of animal herds used by research facilities may decrease the risk of infection. Biosafety level 2 practices and facilities are recommended for nonpropagative laboratory procedures involving *C burnetii* and biosafety level 3 practices for all propagative procedures, and necropsy of infected animals. Special safety practices are recommended during high-risk worker exposures in biomedical facilities that house sheep and goats. Vaccines for domestic animals and people working in high-risk occupations have been developed but are not licensed in the United States. A small number of high-risk children in Australia have safely received the vaccine. Q fever is a nationally reportable disease, and all human cases should be reported to the state health department. Additional information about Q fever, is available on the CDC website (**www.cdc.gov/qfever/index.html**).

Rabies

CLINICAL MANIFESTATIONS: Infection with rabies virus and other lyssaviruses characteristically produces an acute illness with rapidly progressive central nervous system manifestations, including anxiety, radicular pain, dysesthesia or pruritus, hydrophobia, and dysautonomia. Some patients may have paralysis. Illness almost invariably progresses to death. The differential diagnosis of acute encephalitic illnesses of unknown cause or with features of Guillain-Barré syndrome should include rabies.

ETIOLOGY: Rabies virus is a single-stranded RNA virus classified in the *Rhabdoviridae* family, *Lyssavirus* genus. The genus *Lyssavirus* currently contains 14 species divided into 3 phylogroups.

EPIDEMIOLOGY: Understanding the epidemiology of rabies has been aided by viral variant identification using monoclonal antibodies and nucleotide sequencing. In the United States, human cases have decreased steadily since the 1950s, reflecting widespread immunization of dogs and the availability of effective prophylaxis after exposure to a rabid animal. From 2000 through 2017, 34 of 49 cases of human rabies reported in the United States were acquired indigenously. Among the 34 indigenously acquired cases, all but 5 were associated with bats. Despite the large focus of rabies in raccoons in the eastern United States, only 3 human deaths have been attributed to the raccoon rabies virus variant. Historically, 2 cases of human rabies were attributable to probable aerosol exposure in laboratories, and 2 unusual cases have been attributed to possible airborne exposures in caves inhabited by millions of bats, although alternative infection routes cannot be discounted. Transmission also has occurred by transplantation of organs, corneas, and other tissues from patients dying of undiagnosed rabies. Person-to-person transmission by bite has not been documented in the United States, although the virus has been isolated from saliva of infected patients.

Wildlife rabies perpetuates throughout all of the 50 United States except Hawaii, which remains "rabies free." Wildlife, including bats, raccoons, skunks, foxes, coyotes, bobcats, and mongoose, are the most important potential sources of infection for humans and domestic animals in the United States and its territories. Rabies in small rodents (squirrels, hamsters, guinea pigs, gerbils, chipmunks, rats, and mice) and lagomorphs (rabbits, pikas, and hares) is rare. Rabies may occur in woodchucks or other large rodents in areas where raccoon rabies is common. The virus is present in saliva and is transmitted by bites or, rarely, by contamination of mucosa or skin lesions by saliva or other potentially infectious material (eg, neural tissue). Worldwide, most rabies cases in humans result from dog bites in areas where canine rabies is enzootic (**www.who.int/rabies/Presence_dog_transmitted_human_Rabies_2014.png?ua=1**). Most rabid dogs, cats, and ferrets shed virus for a few days before there are obvious signs of illness. No case of human rabies in the United States has been attributed to a dog, cat, or ferret that has remained healthy throughout the standard 10-day period of confinement after an exposure.

The **incubation period** in humans averages 1 to 3 months but ranges from days to years.

DIAGNOSTIC TESTS: Infection in animals can be diagnosed by demonstration of the presence of rabies virus antigen in brain tissue using a direct fluorescent antibody (DFA) test. Suspected rabid animals should be euthanized in a manner that preserves brain tissue for appropriate laboratory diagnosis. Virus can be isolated in suckling mice or in tissue culture from saliva, brain, and other specimens and can be detected by identification of viral antigens by immunofluorescence or immunoperoxidase staining or nucleotide sequences by reverse transcriptase-polymerase chain reaction (RT-PCR) in affected tissues. Diagnosis in suspected human cases can be made postmortem by either immunofluorescent or immunohistochemical examination of brain tissue or by detection of viral nucleotide sequences; RT-PCR at the Centers for Disease Control and Prevention (CDC) currently is performed together with DFA while RT-PCR assays are being fully validated for this purpose. Antemortem diagnosis can be made by DFA testing on skin biopsy specimens from the nape of the neck, by isolation of the virus from saliva, by detection of antibody in serum (neutralization or indirect fluorescent antibody methods generally are used) in unvaccinated people and in cerebrospinal fluid (CSF) in all infected people, and by detection of viral nucleotide sequences in saliva, skin, or other tissues. RT-PCR assay plays a greater role in the diagnosis of rabies in such antemortem specimens in the absence of a brain biopsy specimen. No single test is sufficiently sensitive because of the unique nature of rabies pathobiology. State or local health departments should be consulted before submission of specimens to the CDC. Consultation with public health authorities facilitates cases inconsistent with rabies to be identified before specimens are collected and enables appropriate collection and transport of materials to be arranged when rabies testing is indicated. Step-by-step instructions can be found at **www.cdc. gov/rabies/resources/specimen-submission-guidelines.html.**

TREATMENT: There is no specific treatment. Once symptoms have developed, neither rabies vaccine nor Rabies Immune Globulin (RIG) improves the prognosis. A combination of sedation and intensive medical intervention may be valuable adjunctive therapy.[1] Details of one management protocol used can be found at **www.mcw.edu/rabies.** Eleven people have survived rabies in association with incomplete rabies vaccine schedules. Eight people who had not received rabies postexposure prophylaxis survived rabies. Approximately half of survivors have normal cognition.

ISOLATION OF THE HOSPITALIZED PATIENT: Standard precautions are recommended, including face mask, eye protection, gown, and gloves for procedures and patient care activities that could generate splashes or sprays or when contact with potentially infectious fluids is anticipated. If the patient has bitten another person or potentially infectious material from the patient has contaminated an open wound or mucous membrane, the involved area should be washed thoroughly with soap and water, and risk assessment should be completed to determine whether postexposure prophylaxis should be administered (see Care of Exposed People, p 623).

---

[1]Centers for Disease Control and Prevention. Recovery of a patient from clinical rabies—California, 2011. *MMWR Morb Mortal Wkly Rep.* 2012;61(4):61-65

CONTROL MEASURES: In the United States, animal rabies is common. Education of children to avoid contact with stray or wild animals is of primary importance. Inadvertent contact of family members and pets with potentially rabid animals, such as raccoons, foxes, coyotes, and skunks, may be decreased by securing garbage and pet food outdoors to decrease attraction of domestic and wild animals. Similarly, chimneys and other potential entrances for wildlife, including bats, should be identified and covered. Bats should be excluded from human living quarters. International travelers to areas with enzootic canine rabies should be warned to avoid exposure to stray dogs, and if traveling to an area with enzootic infection where immediate access to medical care or availability of biologic agents is limited, preexposure prophylaxis is indicated.

Exposure Risk and Decisions to Administer Prophylaxis. Exposure to rabies results from a break in the skin caused by the teeth of a rabid animal or by contamination of scratches, abrasions, or mucous membranes with saliva or other potentially infectious material, such as neural tissue, from a rabid animal. The decision to immunize a potentially exposed person should be made in consultation with the state or local health department, which can provide information on risk of rabies in a particular area for each species of animal and in accordance with the guidance in Table 3.49. Consultation with experts at the CDC may be helpful to guide decisions on prophylaxis (**www.cdc.gov/rabies/resources/ contacts.html**).

In the United States and Puerto Rico, all mammals are believed to be susceptible, but bats, raccoons, skunks, foxes, coyotes, and mongooses are reservoir species more likely to be infected than are other animals.[1] According to the CDC, all bites by such wildlife must be considered a possible exposure to the rabies virus. Postexposure prophylaxis should be initiated as soon as possible following exposure to these animals unless the animal has already been tested and determined not to be rabid. If postexposure prophylaxis has been initiated and subsequent testing shows that the exposing animal was not rabid, postexposure prophylaxis can be discontinued. Cattle, dogs, cats, ferrets, and other animals occasionally are infected. Bites of small rodents (such as squirrels, hamsters, guinea pigs, gerbils, chipmunks, mice, and rats) and lagomorphs (rabbits, hares, and pikas) rarely require prophylaxis, because these animals almost never are found to be infected with rabies and have not been known to transmit rabies to humans. Additional factors must be considered when deciding whether immunoprophylaxis is indicated. An unprovoked attack may be more suggestive of a rabid animal than a bite that occurs during attempts to feed or handle an animal. Properly immunized dogs, cats, and ferrets have only a minimal chance of developing rabies. However, in rare instances, rabies has developed in properly immunized animals.

Postexposure prophylaxis for rabies is recommended for all people bitten by domestic animals that are suspected to be rabid, or by bats or wild animals unless laboratory tests prove that the animal does not have rabies. The CDC Advisory Committee on Immunization Practices (ACIP) recommends dogs, cats, and ferrets be observed for 10 days if healthy and available to observe.[2] If the animal shows clinical signs of rabies, the exposed person can begin prophylaxis. Postexposure prophylaxis also is recommended for people who report an open wound, scratch, or mucous membrane that has been

---

[1] Centers for Disease Control and Prevention. Human rabies—Puerto Rico, 2015. *MMWR Morb Mortal Wkly Rep.* 2017;65(52):1474-1476

[2] Centers for Disease Control and Prevention. Human rabies prevention: United States, 2008. Recommendations of the Advisory Committee on Immunization Practices. *MMWR Recomm Rep.* 2008;57(RR-3):1-28

Table 3.49. Rabies Postexposure Prophylaxis Guide

Animal Type	Evaluation and Disposition of Animal	Postexposure Prophylaxis Recommendations
Dogs, cats, and ferrets	Healthy and available for 10 days of observation	Prophylaxis only if animal develops signs of rabies[b]
	Rabid or suspected of being rabid[a]	Immediate immunization and RIG[c]
	Unknown (escaped)	Consult public health officials for advice
Bats, skunks, raccoons, coyotes, foxes, mongooses, and most other carnivores; woodchucks	Regarded as rabid unless geographic area is known to be free of rabies or until animal proven negative by laboratory tests[a]	Immediate immunization and RIG[c]
Livestock, rodents, and lagomorphs (rabbits, hares, and pikas)	Consider individually	Consult public health officials; bites of squirrels, hamsters, guinea pigs, gerbils, chipmunks, rats, mice and other rodents, rabbits, hares, and pikas almost never require rabies postexposure prophylaxis

RIG indicates Rabies Immune Globulin.

[a] The animal should be euthanized and tested as soon as possible. Holding for observation is not recommended. Immunization is discontinued if immunofluorescent test result for the animal is negative.

[b] During the 10-day observation period, at the first sign of rabies in the biting dog, cat, or ferret, prophylaxis of the exposed person with RIG (human) and vaccine should be initiated. The animal should be euthanized immediately and tested.

[c] See text.

contaminated with saliva or other potentially infectious material (eg, brain tissue) from a rabid animal. The injury inflicted by a bat bite or scratch may be small and not readily evident, or the circumstances of contact with a bat may preclude accurate recall (eg, a bat in a room of a deeply sleeping or medicated person or a previously unattended child, especially an infant or toddler who cannot reliably communicate about a potential bite). Hence, postexposure prophylaxis may be indicated, following proper risk assessment, for situations in which a bat physically is present in the same room if a bite or mucous membrane exposure cannot reliably be excluded, unless prompt testing of the bat has excluded rabies virus infection. Prophylaxis should be initiated as soon as possible after bites by known or suspected rabid animals.

Risk Assessments for Contacts of Humans With Rabies. Risk assessment for the administration of postexposure prophylaxis is recommended for people who report a possibly infectious exposure (eg, bite, scratch, or open wound or mucous membrane contaminated with saliva or other infectious material, such as tears, CSF, or brain tissue) to a human with rabies. Rabies virus transmission after exposure to a human with rabies has not been documented convincingly in the United States, except after tissue or organ transplantation from donors who died of unsuspected rabies encephalitis. Casual contact with an infected person (eg, by touching a patient) or contact with noninfectious fluids or tissues (eg, blood or feces) alone does not constitute an exposure and is not an indication for prophylaxis. Administration of postexposure prophylaxis to hospital contacts of patients with rabies is required only in situations in which potentially infectious material (such as saliva, CSF, or brain tissue) comes into direct contact with broken skin or mucous membranes. It is expected that in cases in which people are using appropriate protective equipment, there will likely be no risk of exposure.

Handling of Animals Suspected of Having Rabies. A dog, cat, bat, or ferret that is suspected of having rabies and has bitten a human should be captured, confined, euthanized, and tested. Alternatively, if the dog, cat, or ferret appears healthy, it can be observed by a veterinarian for 10 days by order of public health authorities. If signs of rabies develop, the animal should be euthanized in a manner to allow its head to be removed and shipped to a qualified laboratory for examination. Instructions for packing can be found at **www. cdc.gov/rabies/resources/specimen-submission-guidelines.html**; freshly frozen and shipped with dry ice is preferred to refrigerated specimens.

Other biting animals that may have exposed a person to rabies virus should be reported immediately to the state or local health department. Management of animals depends on the species, the circumstances of the bite, and the epidemiology of rabies in the area. Previous immunization of an animal may not preclude the necessity for euthanasia and testing. Because clinical manifestations of rabies in a wild animal cannot be interpreted reliably, a wild mammal suspected of having rabies should be euthanized at once, and its brain should be examined for evidence of rabies virus infection. The exposed person need not receive prophylaxis if the result of rapid examination of the brain by DFA testing is negative for rabies virus infection.

Care of Exposed People.

Local Wound Care. The immediate objective of postexposure prophylaxis is to prevent virus from entering neural tissue. Prompt and thorough local treatment of all lesions is essential, because virus may remain localized to the area of the bite for a variable time. All wounds should be flushed thoroughly and cleaned with soap and water. Quaternary ammonium compounds (such as benzalkonium chloride) no longer are considered superior to soap. The need for tetanus prophylaxis and measures to control bacterial infection should be considered. The wound can be loosely sutured but only after Rabies Immune Globulin (RIG) is administered. For severe facial wounds, which often also are infected with bacteria, better cosmesis results from single sutures, widely placed, several hours after local instillation of RIG, followed by plastic surgery days later.

Prophylaxis (see Table 3.49, p 622). After wound care is completed, concurrent use of passive (RIG) and active (rabies vaccine) immunization is optimal, with the exceptions of people who previously have received complete vaccination regimens (pre- or postexposure) with a cell culture vaccine or people who have been vaccinated with other types of rabies vaccines and have previously had a documented rabies virus-neutralizing antibody titer; these people should receive only vaccine. Prophylaxis should begin as soon as possible after exposure, ideally within 24 hours. Although not ideal, a delay of several days or more may not compromise effectiveness, and prophylaxis should be initiated if reasonably indicated, regardless of the interval between exposure and initiation of therapy. In the United States, only human RIG is available for passive immunization. Licensed cell culture rabies vaccine should be used for active immunization. Physicians can obtain expert counsel from their state or local health departments when uncertain about administering these products.

Table 3.50. US Food and Drug Administration-Licensed Rabies Vaccines[a] and Rabies Immune Globulin Products

Category	Product	Manufacturer	Dose and Route of Administration
Human rabies vaccine	Human diploid cell vaccine (HDCV) (Imovax Rabies)	Sanofi Pasteur	1 mL, IM
	Purified chicken embryo cell vaccine (PCECV) (RabAvert)	Novartis Vaccines and Diagnostics	1 mL, IM
Rabies Immune Globulin	Imogam Rabies-HT	Sanofi Pasteur	20 IU/kg, infiltrate around wound[b]
	HyperRab S/D	Grifols USA	20 IU/kg, infiltrate around wound[b]
	Kedrab	Kedrion Biopharma	20 IU/kg, infiltrate around wound[b]

IM indicates intramuscular.
[a] Rabies vaccine adsorbed (RVA) is licensed in the United States but no longer is distributed in the United States.
[b] Any remaining volume should be administered intramuscularly.

Active Immunization (Postexposure). Human diploid cell vaccine (HDCV) and purified chicken embryo cell vaccine (PCECV) are licensed in the United States (see Table 3.50). For a previously unvaccinated immunocompetent person, a 1.0-mL dose of vaccine is injected intramuscularly in the deltoid area (the anterolateral aspect of the thigh is used for infants and young children) on the first day of postexposure prophylaxis (day 0), and repeated doses are administered on days 3, 7, and 14 after the first dose, for a total of 4 doses,[1] with 1 dose of RIG (based on body weight) administered on day 0. For a person with altered immunocompetence, postexposure prophylaxis should include a 5-dose vaccination regimen (ie, 1 dose of vaccine on days 0, 3, 7, 14, and 28), with 1 dose of RIG on day 0. Serologic testing to document seroconversion after administration of a rabies vaccine series usually is not necessary except for recipients who may be immunocompromised or for people with deviations from the recommended vaccination schedule. Immune response should be assessed by performing neutralizing antibody testing 7 to 14 days after administration of the final dose in the series. Ideally, a vaccination series should be initiated and completed with 1 vaccine product unless serious adverse reactions occur. Clinical studies evaluating efficacy or frequency of adverse reactions when the series is completed with a second product have not been conducted.

---

[1] Centers for Disease Control and Prevention. Use of a reduced (4-dose) vaccine schedule for postexposure prophylaxis to prevent human rabies: recommendations of the Advisory Committee on Immunization Practices. *MMWR Recomm Rep.* 2010;59(RR–02):1–9

Care should be taken to ensure that the vaccine is administered intramuscularly. Vaccines licensed in the United States are not approved for intradermal administration in the postexposure setting, although the World Health Organization (WHO) has recommended postexposure intradermal regimens as an alternative to intramuscular administration for reasons of cost and availability, and these are used in some countries **(apps.who.int/iris/handle/10665/272364)**. Because virus-neutralizing antibody responses in adults who received vaccine in the gluteal area sometimes have been less than in those who received vaccine in the deltoid muscle, the deltoid site always should be used for rabies vaccine, except in infants and young children, in whom the anterolateral thigh is the appropriate site.

ADVERSE REACTIONS AND PRECAUTIONS WITH HDCV AND PCECV. Reactions are uncommon in children. In adults, mild local reactions, such as pain, erythema, and swelling or itching at the injection site, are reported in 15% to 25%, and mild systemic reactions, such as headache, nausea, abdominal pain, muscle aches, and dizziness, are reported in 10% to 20% of recipients. Immune complex-like reactions in people receiving booster doses of HDCV have been observed, possibly because of interaction between propiolactone contained in the vaccine and human albumin. The reaction, characterized by onset 2 to 21 days after inoculation, begins with generalized urticaria and can include arthralgia, arthritis, angioedema, nausea, vomiting, fever, and malaise. The reaction is not life threatening, occurs in as many as 6% of adults receiving booster doses as part of a preexposure immunization regimen, and is rare in people receiving primary immunization with HDCV. Similar allergic reactions with primary or booster doses have been reported with PCECV. If the patient has a serious allergic reaction to HDCV, PCECV may be administered according to the same schedule as HDCV, and vice-versa. If reactions following vaccine are mild, pretreatment with antihistamines just before the next vaccination can be considered. All suspected serious, systemic, paralytic, or anaphylactic reactions to rabies vaccine should be reported immediately to the Vaccine Adverse Events Reporting System (see p 46).

Although the safety of rabies vaccine during pregnancy has not been studied specifically in the United States, pregnancy is not a contraindication to use of vaccine or RIG after exposure.

NERVE TISSUE VACCINES. Inactivated nerve tissue vaccines are not licensed in the United States and are not recommended by the WHO but still are used in some areas of the world. These preparations induce neuroparalytic reactions in 1 in 2000 to 1 in 8000 recipients. Vaccination with nerve tissue vaccine should be discontinued if meningeal or neuroparalytic reactions develop. Corticosteroids should be used only for life-threatening reactions, because they increase the risk of rabies in experimentally inoculated animals.

Passive Immunization. Human RIG should be used concomitantly with the first dose of vaccine for postexposure prophylaxis to bridge the time between possible infection and antibody production induced by the vaccine (see Table 3.50, p 624). If vaccine is not available immediately, RIG should be administered alone, and vaccination should be started as soon as possible. If RIG is not available immediately, vaccine should be administered, and RIG should be administered subsequently if obtained within 7 days after initiating vaccination. If administration of both vaccine and RIG is delayed, both should be used regardless of the interval between exposure and treatment, within reason.

The recommended dose of RIG is 20 IU/kg. RIG should never be administered in the same syringe as vaccine. As much of the RIG dose as is safely possible should be used to infiltrate the wound(s), if present. The remainder is administered intramuscularly into muscle that is not the same one where rabies vaccine was administered. In cases of multiple severe wounds in which RIG is insufficient for infiltration, dilution in saline solution to an adequate volume (twofold or threefold) has been recommended to ensure that all wound areas receive infiltrate. Since 2018, a concentrated RIG product, HyperRab, has been licensed for use in the United States. For children with small muscle mass, it may be necessary to administer RIG at multiple sites. Passive antibody can in some cases inhibit the response to rabies vaccines; therefore, the recommended dose should not be exceeded. Hypersensitivity reactions to RIG are rare.

Purified equine RIG containing rabies antibodies may be available outside the United States and generally is accompanied by a low rate of serum sickness (less than 1%). Equine RIG is administered at a dose of 40 IU/kg.

MANAGEMENT OF POSTEXPOSURE PROPHYLAXIS IN PREVIOUSLY IMMUNIZED PEOPLE. Administration of RIG is not recommended for people who are considered "previously vaccinated." A previously vaccinated person is defined as someone who has received one of the recommended pre- or postexposure regimens of HDCV, PCECV, or rabies vaccine adsorbed (the latter is a vaccine no longer available in the United States). Also acceptable is receipt of another vaccine along with a documented rabies virus neutralizing titer. Such individuals should receive two 1.0-mL booster doses of HDCV or PCECV; the first dose ideally is administered as soon as possible after exposure, and the second dose is administered 3 days later.

Preexposure Control Measures, Including Vaccination. The relatively low frequency of reactions to HDCV and PCECV has made provision of preexposure vaccination practical for people in high-risk groups, including veterinarians, animal handlers, certain laboratory workers, and people moving or traveling to areas where canine rabies is common. Others, such as spelunkers (cavers) or animal rehabilitators, who may have frequent exposures to bats and other wildlife, also should be considered for preexposure prophylaxis.

HDCV and PCECV are licensed in the United States for intramuscular administration. The preexposure prophylaxis schedule is three 1-mL intramuscular injections each, administered on days 0, 7, and 21 or 28. This series of immunizations has resulted in development of rabies virus-neutralizing antibodies in all immunocompetent people properly immunized. Therefore, routine serologic testing for antibody after primary immunization is not indicated unless the person is immunosuppressed.

Serum antibodies usually persist for very long periods of time after the primary series is administered intramuscularly. Preexposure booster immunization with 1.0 mL of HDCV or PCEC intramuscularly will produce an effective anamnestic response in most healthy individuals. The ACIP recommends rabies virus-neutralizing antibody titers should be determined at 6-month intervals for people at continuous risk of infection (eg, rabies research laboratory workers, rabies biologics production workers). Titers should be determined approximately every 2 years for people with risk of frequent exposure (eg, rabies diagnostic laboratory workers, spelunkers/cavers, veterinarians and staff, animal-control and wildlife workers in areas with enzootic rabies, and all people who frequently handle bats or other wildlife animals). A single booster dose of vaccine should be administered only as appropriate to maintain adequate antibody concentrations for these populations. The CDC currently specifies complete viral neutralization at a serum dilution of 1:5 (approximately 0.1 IU/mL or greater) by the rapid fluorescent-focus inhibition test as evidence of an adequate immune response; the WHO specifies a neutralizing antibody titer of 0.5 IU/mL or greater as acceptable. Most people, such as travelers to areas where canine rabies is common, do not need serologic testing and follow-up. If they received preexposure immunization at any time prior to the time they are exposed, then they should receive booster doses of vaccine at days 0 and 3 as postexposure prophylaxis (see "Management of Postexposure Prophylaxis in Previously Immunized People," above).

Public Health. A variety of approved public health measures, including vaccination of dogs, cats, and ferrets and management of the stray dog population and selected wildlife, are used to control rabies in animals.[1] In regions where oral vaccination of wildlife with recombinant rabies vaccine is undertaken, the prevalence of rabies among foxes, coyotes, and raccoons may be decreased. Unvaccinated dogs, cats, ferrets, or other pets bitten by a known rabid animal should be euthanized immediately. If the owner is unwilling to allow the animal to be euthanized, the animal should be placed in strict isolation for 6 months and immunized, at the latest, 1 month before release. If the exposed animal has been immunized within 1 to 3 years, depending on the vaccine administered and local regulations, the animal should be revaccinated and observed for 45 days.

Case Reporting. All suspected human cases of rabies should be reported promptly to state or local health departments.

Rat-Bite Fever

CLINICAL MANIFESTATIONS: Rat-bite fever is caused by *Streptobacillus moniliformis* or *Spirillum minus. S moniliformis* infection (streptobacillary fever or Haverhill fever) is characterized by relapsing fever, rash, and migratory polyarthritis. There is an abrupt onset of fever, chills, muscle pain, vomiting, headache, and rarely (unlike *S minus*) lymphadenopathy. A maculopapular, purpuric, or petechial rash develops, predominantly on the peripheral extremities including the palms and soles, typically within a few days of fever onset. The skin lesions may become purpuric or confluent and may desquamate. The bite site usually heals promptly and exhibits no or minimal inflammation. Nonsuppurative migratory polyarthritis or arthralgia follows in approximately 50% of patients. Symptoms of untreated infection may resolve within 2 weeks, but fever occasionally can relapse for weeks or months, and infection can lead to serious complications including soft tissue and solid-organ abscesses (brain, myocardium), septic arthritis, pneumonia, endocarditis, myocarditis, pericarditis, sepsis, and meningitis. The case-fatality rate is 7% to 13% in untreated patients, and fatal cases have been reported in children.

With *S minus* infection ("sodoku"), a period of initial apparent healing at the site of the bite usually is followed by fever and ulceration, discoloration, swelling, and pain at the site (about 1 to 4 weeks later), regional lymphangitis and lymphadenopathy, and a distinctive rash of red or purple plaques. Arthritis is rare.

ETIOLOGY: The causes of rat-bite fever are *S moniliformis*, a microaerophilic, facultatively anaerobic, gram-negative, pleomorphic bacillus, and *S minus*, a small, gram-negative, spiral-shaped bacterium with bipolar flagellar tufts.

---

[1]National Association of State Public Health Veterinarians Inc. Compendium of animal rabies prevention and control, 2011. *MMWR Recomm Rep.* 2011;60(RR-6):1-15

EPIDEMIOLOGY: Rat-bite fever is a zoonotic illness. The natural habitat of *S moniliformis* and *S minus* is the oropharynx and nasopharynx of rodents. *S moniliformis* is transmitted by bites or scratches from or exposure to oral secretions of infected rats (eg, kissing pet rodents), other rodents (eg, mice, gerbils, squirrels, weasels), and rodent-eating animals, including cats and dogs. Infection via contact with contaminated fomites (eg, rat cage) has been reported rarely. Haverhill fever refers to infection after ingestion of unpasteurized milk, water, or food contaminated with urine containing *S moniliformis* and may be associated with an outbreak of disease. *S minus* is transmitted by bites of rats and mice. *S moniliformis* infection accounts for almost all cases of rat-bite fever in the United States; *S minus* infections occur primarily in Asia.

The **incubation period** for *S moniliformis* usually is less than 7 days but can range from 3 days to 3 weeks; for *S minus*, the **incubation period** is 7 to 21 days.

DIAGNOSTIC TESTS: *S moniliformis* is a fastidious, slow-growing organism isolated from blood, synovial fluid, abscesses, or aspirates from the bite lesion. Growth is best in bacteriologic media enriched with blood (15% rabbit blood seems optimal), serum, and ascitic fluid; cultures should be kept in 5% to 10% carbon dioxide atmosphere at 37°C. The laboratory should be alerted that *S moniliformis* is suspected and to hold the culture for at least 1 week. A nucleic acid amplification-based assay may be available in research laboratories. The use of 16S ribosomal RNA gene sequencing and matrix-assisted laser desorption/ionization-time of flight (MALDI-TOF) mass spectrometry improve the diagnostic sensitivity and specificity of culture-based practices.

S minus has not been recovered on artificial media but can be visualized by darkfield microscopy in wet mounts of blood, exudate of a lesion, and lymph nodes. Blood specimens also should be viewed with Giemsa or Wright stain.

TREATMENT: Penicillin G procaine administered intramuscularly or penicillin G administered intravenously for 7 to 10 days is the treatment for rat-bite fever caused by either agent; currently in the United States and other countries, intravenous administration is the more acceptable route. Initial intravenous penicillin G therapy for 5 to 7 days followed by oral penicillin V for 7 days also has been successful. Limited experience exists for ampicillin, cefuroxime, ceftriaxone, and cefotaxime. Doxycycline or streptomycin can be substituted when a patient has a serious allergy to penicillin or while awaiting laboratory results when rickettsial infections (eg, Rocky Mountain spotted fever) are also among the differential diagnoses. Patients with endocarditis should receive intravenous high-dose penicillin G for at least 4 weeks. The addition of streptomycin or gentamicin for initial therapy may be useful in severe infections including endocarditis.

ISOLATION OF THE HOSPITALIZED PATIENT: Standard precautions are recommended.

CONTROL MEASURES: Exposed people should be observed for symptoms. Rat control is important in the control of disease. People with frequent rodent exposure should wear gloves and avoid hand-to-mouth contact during animal handling. Regular hand hygiene should be practiced, and surfaces that the rodent contacted should be disinfected.

Respiratory Syncytial Virus

CLINICAL MANIFESTATIONS: Respiratory syncytial virus (RSV) causes acute respiratory tract infections in people of all ages and is one of the most common diseases of early childhood. Most infants infected with RSV experience upper respiratory tract symptoms, and 20% to 30% develop lower respiratory tract disease (eg, bronchiolitis and/or pneumonia) with the first infection. Signs and symptoms of bronchiolitis typically begin with rhinitis and cough, which may progress to increased respiratory effort with tachypnea, wheezing, rales, crackles, intercostal and/or subcostal retractions, grunting, and nasal flaring. Fever may, but does not always, occur. Infection with RSV during the first few weeks of life, particularly among preterm infants, may present with more general symptoms such as lethargy, irritability, and poor feeding, accompanied with minimal respiratory tract symptoms. However, these infants are at risk of developing apnea, even in the absence of other respiratory symptoms.

Most previously healthy infants who develop RSV bronchiolitis do not require hospitalization, and most who are hospitalized improve with supportive care and are discharged after 2 or 3 days. However, approximately 1% to 3% of all children in the first 12 months of life will be hospitalized because of severe RSV lower respiratory tract disease, with the highest rate of RSV hospitalizations occurring in the first 6 months of life. Factors that increase the risk of severe RSV lower respiratory tract illness include prematurity, especially infants born before 29 weeks of gestation; chronic lung disease of prematurity (CLD [formerly called bronchopulmonary dysplasia]); certain types of hemodynamically significant congenital heart disease (CHD), especially conditions associated with pulmonary hypertension; certain immunodeficiency states; and neurologic and neuromuscular conditions. Identified risk factors with a more limited correlation with disease severity include low birth weight, maternal smoking during pregnancy, exposure to secondhand smoke in the household, family history of atopy, lack of breastfeeding, and household crowding. Mortality is rare when supportive care is available.

The association between RSV infection early in life and subsequent asthma remains incompletely understood. Infants who experience severe lower respiratory tract disease (eg, bronchiolitis or pneumonia) from RSV have an increased risk of developing asthma later in life. This association also is seen with other respiratory viral infections, particularly those caused by rhinoviruses. The unresolved question is whether the association between severe infection and reactive airway disease is causal and attributable to direct damage caused by viral replication and the host's response. Alternatively, the association may reflect a common genotype, indicating the same anatomic or immunologic abnormalities that predispose to asthma also predispose to severe viral lower respiratory tract disease. Results from 2 randomized, placebo-controlled trials demonstrate that providing RSV immunoprophylaxis to term and preterm infants had no measurable effect on medically attended wheezing, physician-diagnosed asthma, or lung function at 3 to 6 years of age.

Almost all children are infected by RSV at least once by 24 months of age, and reinfection throughout life is common. Subsequent infections are usually less severe than a primary infection. Particularly among otherwise healthy older children and adults, recurrent RSV infection manifests as mild upper respiratory tract illness and seldom involves the lower respiratory tract. However, serious disease involving the lower respiratory tract may develop in older children and adults, especially in immunocompromised people and frail, elderly people, particularly those with cardiopulmonary comorbidities.

ETIOLOGY: RSV is an enveloped, nonsegmented, negative-strand RNA virus of the genus *Orthopneumovirus* of the family *Pneumoviridae*. Human RSV exists as 2 antigenic subgroups, A and B, and often these cocirculate during the same RSV season. A consistent correlation between RSV subgroup and disease severity is unclear. The RSV envelope contains 3 surface glycoproteins: glycoprotein G, fusion protein F, and a small hydrophobic protein

(SH). Antibodies directed against F and G are protective and are neutralizing antibodies. G protein is involved in viral attachment to the cell and assists in the ability of the virus to evade host immunity. F protein enables viral penetration of the epithelial cell once viral attachment occurs. In contrast to G protein, F protein is conserved, making it an attractive target for vaccine and monoclonal antibody development.

EPIDEMIOLOGY: Humans are the only source of infection. RSV usually is transmitted by direct or close contact with contaminated secretions, which may occur from exposure to large-particle droplets at short distances (typically <6 feet) or by self-inoculation after touching contaminated surfaces or fomites. Viable RSV can persist on environmental surfaces for several hours and for 30 minutes or more on hands.

RSV occurs in annual epidemics generally beginning in fall and continuing through early spring in temperate climates. Spread among households and people in child care facilities, including adults, is common. Spread can also occur in the health care setting. The usual period of viral shedding is 3 to 8 days, but it may be longer, especially in young infants and immunosuppressed children, in whom shedding may continue for 3 to 4 weeks or longer.

The **incubation period** ranges from 2 to 8 days; 4 to 6 days is most common.

DIAGNOSTIC TESTS: For many years, laboratory diagnosis of RSV respiratory tract disease required viral isolation in cell culture. Although cell culture still is used, this approach requires a specialized laboratory and several days of incubation before characteristic cytopathic changes (syncytia formation) are observed. Centrifugation-enhanced, shell vial techniques shorten the time to results to 24 to 48 hours. Rapid diagnostic assays, including direct fluorescent antibody (DFA) assays and enzyme or chromatographic immunoassays, are available for detection of viral antigen in nasopharyngeal specimens and are reliable in infants and young children. Sensitivity in older children and adults is lower, because less virus is shed in the upper airways. As with all antigen detection assays, the predictive value is high during the peak season, but false-positive test results are more likely to occur when the incidence of disease is low, such as in the summer in temperate areas.

Molecular diagnostic tests using reverse transcriptase-polymerase chain reaction (RT-PCR) assays have largely replaced both culture and antigen detection assays. Some commercially available assays are designed as multiplex assays to facilitate testing for multiple respiratory viruses from a single nasopharyngeal specimen. Some complex multiplex tests can distinguish between RSV A and B subgroups. Using RT-PCR assays, as many as 30% of symptomatic children will demonstrate the presence of a viral coinfection with 2 or more viruses. Whether symptomatic children who are coinfected with more than one virus experience more severe or even less severe disease is not clear.

Testing for seroconversion with acute and convalescent serum specimens is rarely performed for the purposes of diagnosing RSV infection and may not be reliable in infants because the immune response to RSV infection may be limited.

In most outpatient settings for children with bronchiolitis, routine specific respiratory viral testing has little effect on management and is not recommended.[1] Among hospitalized children with bronchiolitis, testing for viral etiology is not routinely recommended.

---

[1]Ralston SL, Lieberthal AS, Meissner HC, et al. Clinical practice guideline: the diagnosis, management, and prevention of bronchiolitis. *Pediatrics.* 2014;134(5):e1474-e1502

However, if patient cohorting is necessary, identification of the specific viral etiology of a respiratory infection will aid hospital infection prevention efforts.

TREATMENT[1]: No available treatment shortens the course of bronchiolitis or hastens the resolution of symptoms. Management of young children hospitalized with bronchiolitis is supportive and should include hydration, careful assessment of respiratory status, and suction of the upper airway, as necessary. Supplemental oxygen is recommended only when oxyhemoglobin saturation persistently decreases below 90% in a previously healthy infant. Nasal continuous positive airway pressure and heliox have been used for respiratory support in hospitalized infants with bronchiolitis. Only limited data are available on the effectiveness of these therapies in bronchiolitis specifically caused by RSV. Because these therapies, as well as intubation and ventilation, typically are used in severely or critically ill infants with bronchiolitis, they should be used only in consultation with a critical care or pulmonary specialist.

Early studies with aerosolized ribavirin therapy demonstrated a small increase in oxygen saturation in small clinical trials; however, a decrease in the need for mechanical ventilation or a decrease in the length of stay was not shown. Because of limited evidence for a clinically relevant benefit, potential toxic effects, and high cost, routine use of aerosolized ribavirin is not recommended.

Alpha- and Beta-Adrenergic Agents. Beta-adrenergic agents are not recommended for care of wheezing associated with RSV bronchiolitis, and a trial of albuterol no longer is included as a recommended option in the management of RSV bronchiolitis.[1] Evidence does not support the use of nebulized epinephrine in children hospitalized with bronchiolitis. Insufficient data are available to recommend routine use of epinephrine for outpatient management of children with bronchiolitis.[2]

Glucocorticoid Therapy. Controlled clinical trials among children with bronchiolitis have demonstrated that corticosteroids do not reduce hospital admissions and do not reduce length of stay for inpatients. Corticosteroid treatment should not be used for infants and children with RSV bronchiolitis.

Antimicrobial Therapy. Antimicrobial therapy is not indicated for infants with RSV bronchiolitis or pneumonia unless there is evidence of concurrent bacterial infection. A young child with a distinct viral lower respiratory tract infection (bronchiolitis) has a low risk (<1%) of bacterial infection of the CSF or blood. Bacterial lung infections and bacteremia are uncommon in this setting. Acute otitis media (AOM) caused by RSV or bacterial superinfection may occur in infants with RSV bronchiolitis. Oral antimicrobial therapy for treatment of otitis media may be considered if bulging of the tympanic membrane is present.[2]

PREVENTION OF RSV INFECTIONS: Palivizumab is a humanized monoclonal immunoglobulin (Ig) G1K antibody produced by recombinant DNA technology. The antibody is directed against a conserved epitope of an antigenic site of the fusion protein (F), which resides on the viral surface and prevents the conformational change that is necessary for fusion of the viral RSV envelope with the plasma membrane of the respiratory epithelial cell. Without fusion, the virus is unable to enter the cell and unable to replicate.

---

[1]Ralston SL, Lieberthal AL, Meissner HC, et al. Clinical practice guideline: the diagnosis, management, and prevention of bronchiolitis. *Pediatrics.* 2014;134(5):e1474-e1502

[2]Lieberthal AS, Carroll AE, Chonmaitree T, et al. Clinical practice guideline: the diagnosis and management of acute otitis media. *Pediatrics.* 2013;131(3):e964-e999

Palivizumab may be considered to reduce the risk of RSV-associated hospitalizations in carefully selected children at significantly increased risk of severe disease. Palivizumab is administered intramuscularly at a dose of 15 mg/kg, once every 30 days. Children who qualify for palivizumab prophylaxis should receive the first dose at the onset of the RSV season. A patient with a history of a severe allergic reaction following a dose of palivizumab should not receive additional doses.

Palivizumab is not effective in treatment of RSV disease and is not approved or recommended for this indication.

Cost Considerations. Results of cost-effectiveness analyses of palivizumab prophylaxis depend on several assumptions, including baseline RSV hospitalization rates among different groups of high-risk children, the reduction in RSV hospitalization rates among recipients of prophylaxis in different risk groups, the cost of hospitalization (amount saved by avoiding hospitalization), the threshold criteria for hospitalization of a child with bronchiolitis (which differs among countries and providers), the number of monthly doses administered, the weight of an infant who receives prophylaxis, variation in the severity of the RSV season, and the acquisition cost and administration fee of palivizumab. Cost analyses conducted by independent investigators consistently demonstrate the cost of palivizumab prophylaxis exceeds the economic benefit from the small number of hospitalizations avoided, even among infants at highest risk.

Initiation and Termination of Immunoprophylaxis. During the 3 RSV seasons from July 2014 to June 2017, the Centers for Disease Control and Prevention reported the median peak of RSV activity occurred in early February (with median onset mid-October and median offset mid-May). Data regarding RSV circulation are obtained from 10 different US Department of Health and Human Services regions within the United States and are reported separately for Florida because patterns of RSV circulation there can be different from regional and national patterns. During these 3 years, the season onset ranged from early September to early December, demonstrating that determination of onset of the RSV season should be based on local activity. Season onset can be determined in real time by identifying the first week of 2 consecutive weeks that RSV RT-PCR test positivity is 3% or greater or antigen detection positivity is 10% or greater. Because 5 monthly doses of palivizumab at 15 mg/kg/dose will provide more than 6 months of serum palivizumab concentrations above the threshold for protection for most infants, administration of more than 5 monthly doses is not recommended within the continental United States. For qualifying infants born during the RSV season, fewer than 5 doses will be needed to provide protection until the RSV season ends in their region (maximum of 5 doses).

A small number of sporadic RSV hospitalizations will occur before or after the main season in many areas of the United States, but the greatest benefit from prophylaxis is derived during the peak of the season and not when the incidence of RSV hospitalization is low.

Timing of Prophylaxis for American Indian/Alaska Native Infants. Rates of RSV hospitalization are three- to fivefold higher for American Indian/Alaska Native infants in rural Alaska (particularly the Yukon Kuskokwim Delta region) and southwest Indian Health System regions than for other US infants of similar ages. RSV hospitalization rates for American Indian/Alaska Native infants in these areas are related in part to household crowding and lack of plumbing (Alaska) and are similar to medically high-risk infants in the overall US population. On the basis of the epidemiology of RSV in Alaska and Navajo/White Mountain Apache populations, particularly in remote regions where the cost of emergency air transport may alter a cost analysis, the selection of infants eligible for prophylaxis may differ from the remainder of the United States. Because of unique seasonality of RSV in Alaska, clinicians may wish to use RSV laboratory surveillance data generated by the state of Alaska to assist in determining onset and end of the RSV season for appropriate timing of palivizumab administration.

Limited information is available concerning the burden of RSV disease for other American Indian populations. However, local assessment of the cost-benefit, as occurs for Alaska Native and Navajo/White Mountain Apache populations, may be prudent for other American Indian populations. If local data support a high burden of RSV disease in select American Indian populations, selection of infants eligible for prophylaxis may differ from the remainder of the United States for infants for their first RSV season.

Eligibility Criteria for Prophylaxis of High-Risk Infants and Young Children.[1,2]

- **Preterm infants with CLD:**
  - Prophylaxis may be considered during the first RSV season for preterm infants who develop CLD of prematurity, defined as gestational age <32 weeks, 0 days, and a history of a requirement for >21% oxygen for at least the first 28 days after birth.
  - During the second RSV season for that child, consideration of palivizumab prophylaxis is recommended only for those who satisfy this definition of CLD of prematurity and continue to require medical support (chronic corticosteroid therapy, diuretic therapy, or supplemental oxygen) during the 6-month period before the start of the second RSV season.
  - For infants with CLD who do not continue to require medical support during the second RSV season, prophylaxis is not recommended.
- **Infants with CHD:**
  - Children with hemodynamically significant CHD who are most likely to benefit from immunoprophylaxis during their first RSV season include infants with acyanotic heart disease who are receiving medication to control congestive heart failure and will require cardiac surgical procedures and infants with moderate to severe pulmonary hypertension.
  - Decisions regarding palivizumab prophylaxis for infants with cyanotic heart defects for their first season of RSV may be made in consultation with a pediatric cardiologist, as the benefit of prophylaxis in infants with cyanotic heart disease is unknown.
  - The following groups of infants with CHD are <u>not</u> at increased risk of RSV infection and generally should not receive immunoprophylaxis:
    - Infants and children with hemodynamically insignificant heart disease (eg, secundum atrial septal defect, small ventricular septal defect, pulmonic stenosis, uncomplicated aortic stenosis, mild coarctation of the aorta, and patent ductus arteriosus);
    - Infants with lesions adequately corrected by surgery, unless they continue to require medication for congestive heart failure;

---

[1] American Academy of Pediatrics, Committee on Infectious Diseases, Bronchiolitis Guideline Committee. Technical report: updated guidance for palivizumab prophylaxis among infants and young children at increased risk of hospitalization for respiratory syncytial virus infection. *Pediatrics.* 2014;134(2):e620-e638

[2] American Academy of Pediatrics, Committee on Infectious Diseases, Bronchiolitis Guideline Committee. Policy statement: updated guidance for palivizumab prophylaxis among infants and young children at increased risk of hospitalization for respiratory syncytial virus infection. *Pediatrics.* 2014;134(2):415-420

  — Infants with mild cardiomyopathy who are not receiving medical therapy for the condition; and
  — Children in the second year of life.
- Because a mean decrease in palivizumab serum concentration of 58% was observed after surgical procedures that involve cardiopulmonary bypass, for children who are receiving prophylaxis and who continue to require prophylaxis following a surgical procedure, a postoperative dose of palivizumab (15 mg/kg) should be considered after cardiac bypass or at the conclusion of extracorporeal membrane oxygenation (ECMO) for infants and children younger than 2 years.
- Children younger than 2 years who undergo cardiac transplantation during the RSV season may be considered for palivizumab prophylaxis.

- **Preterm infants without CLD or CHD:**
  - Palivizumab prophylaxis may be considered for preterm infants born before 29 weeks, 0 days gestation who are younger than 12 months at the start of the RSV season.
  - For infants born during the RSV season, fewer than 5 monthly doses will be needed.
  - Available data for infants born at 29 weeks, 0 days gestation or later do not identify a gestational age cutoff for which the benefits of prophylaxis are clear. For this reason, otherwise healthy infants born at 29 weeks, 0 days gestation or later are not recommended to receive palivizumab prophylaxis. Infants born at 29 weeks, 0 days gestation or later may qualify to receive prophylaxis on the basis of CHD, CLD, or another condition.
  - Palivizumab prophylaxis is not recommended during the second RSV season on the basis of a history of prematurity alone, regardless of the degree of prematurity.

- **Children with anatomic pulmonary abnormalities or neuromuscular disorder:**
  - No prospective studies or population-based data are available to define the risk of RSV hospitalization in children with pulmonary abnormalities or neuromuscular disease. Infants with neuromuscular disease or a congenital anomaly that impairs the ability to clear secretions from the upper airway because of ineffective cough are at risk of a prolonged hospitalization related to lower respiratory tract infection and, therefore, may be considered for prophylaxis during their first RSV season.

- **Immunocompromised children:**
  - No population-based data are available on the incidence of RSV hospitalization in children who undergo hematopoietic stem cell transplantation. An increased risk of complications after RSV infection among pediatric liver transplant recipients was reported in a review of the national transplantation database. Data on the incidence of RSV hospitalizations among other solid organ transplant recipients are not readily available. Severe and even fatal disease attributable to RSV is recognized in children receiving chemotherapy or who are immunocompromised because of other conditions including hematopoietic or solid organ transplantation but the efficacy of prophylaxis in this cohort is not known. Prophylaxis may be considered for children younger than 24 months who will be profoundly immunocompromised during the RSV season.

- **Children with Down syndrome:**
  - Limited data suggest an increased risk of RSV-related hospitalization among children with Down syndrome.

- Data are insufficient to justify a recommendation for routine use of prophylaxis in children with Down syndrome unless qualifying heart disease, CLD, airway clearance issues, or prematurity (<29 weeks, 0 days gestation) is present.
- **Children with cystic fibrosis:**
  - Routine use of palivizumab prophylaxis in patients with cystic fibrosis, including neonates diagnosed with cystic fibrosis by newborn screening, should not be used, unless other indications are present.
  - An infant with cystic fibrosis with clinical evidence of CLD and/or nutritional compromise may be considered for prophylaxis for the first RSV season.
  - Continued use of palivizumab prophylaxis for the second RSV season may be considered for infants with manifestations of severe lung disease (previous hospitalization for pulmonary exacerbation in the first year or abnormalities on chest radiography or chest computed tomography that persist when stable) or weight-for-length less than the 10th percentile.
- **Preventive measures for all high-risk infants:**
  - Infants, especially those at high risk, never should be exposed to tobacco smoke. Tobacco smoke exposure is a known risk factor for many adverse health-related outcomes, and studies have shown increased severity of RSV infection in hospitalized children exposed to secondhand smoke. In addition, smoke exposure may increase the risk of developing wheezing after RSV infection. Families with infants, especially with infants who are at increased risk of RSV disease, should be advised to control exposure to tobacco smoke, and referrals for smoking cessation are appropriate.
  - In contrast to the well-documented beneficial effect of breastfeeding against many viral illnesses, existing data are conflicting regarding the specific protective effect of breastfeeding against RSV infection. Breastfeeding should be encouraged for all infants in accordance with recommendations of the American Academy of Pediatrics.
  - High-risk infants should be kept away from crowds and from situations in which exposure to infected people cannot be controlled. Participation in group child care should be restricted during the RSV season for high-risk infants whenever feasible.
  - Parents should be instructed on the importance of careful hand hygiene.
- **Special situations:**
  - Discontinuation of palivizumab prophylaxis among children who experience breakthrough RSV infection:
    - If any infant or young child receiving monthly palivizumab prophylaxis experiences a breakthrough RSV infection, monthly prophylaxis should be discontinued because of the extremely low likelihood of an RSV hospitalization following a second infection in the same season (<0.5%).
  - Prevention of health care-associated RSV disease:
    - No rigorous data exist to support palivizumab use in controlling outbreaks of health care-associated disease, and palivizumab use is not recommended for this purpose. Strict adherence to infection control practices is the basis for reducing health care-associated RSV disease.
    - Infants in a neonatal unit who qualify for prophylaxis because of CLD, prematurity, or CHD may receive the first dose 48 to 72 hours before discharge to home or promptly after discharge.

ISOLATION OF THE HOSPITALIZED PATIENT: Although RSV may be transmitted by the droplet route, direct contact with infected respiratory secretions is the most important determinant of transmission and consistent adherence to contact precautions in addition to standard precautions prevents transmission in health care settings. These precautions are recommended for the duration of illness for infants, and young children. In immunocompromised patients, the duration of contact precautions should be extended because of prolonged shedding. Even though droplet precautions are not recommended for RSV, protection for the eyes, nose, and mouth by using a mask and goggles, or face shield alone, is necessary when it is likely that there will be a splash or spray of any respiratory secretions or other body fluids, as defined in standard precautions. In addition, patients with RSV infection should be placed in single rooms or cohorted.

CONTROL MEASURES: The control of health care-associated RSV transmission is complicated by the continuing risk of introduction through infected patients, staff, and visitors. During the peak of the RSV season, many infants and children hospitalized with respiratory tract symptoms will be infected with RSV and should be cared for with contact and standard precautions (see Isolation of the Hospitalized Patient, discussed previously). A variety of measures have been demonstrated to reduce the risk of health care-associated transmission, including: (1) cohorting of symptomatic patients and staff; (2) excluding visitors with current or recent respiratory tract infections from health care settings; (3) excluding staff with respiratory tract illness or RSV infection from caring for high risk patients; (4) using gowns and gloves and possibly goggles or masks for protecting health care personnel; (5) emphasizing hand hygiene before and after direct contact with patients, after contact with inanimate objects in the direct vicinity of patients because of the likelihood of skin contamination from contact with respiratory secretions (alcohol-based gels and antibacterial hand soaps rapidly inactivate RSV), and after glove removal; and (6) limiting young children visiting during the RSV season.

A critical aspect of RSV prevention among high-risk infants is education of parents and other caregivers about the importance of decreasing exposure to and transmission of RSV. Preventive measures include limiting, where feasible, exposure to contagious settings (eg, child care centers); emphasis on hand hygiene in all settings, including the home, especially during periods when contacts of high-risk children have respiratory tract infections; and limiting exposure to secondhand smoke.

Rhinovirus Infections

CLINICAL MANIFESTATIONS: Rhinoviruses are the most frequent cause of the common cold, or rhinosinusitis. Typical clinical manifestations include sore throat, nasal congestion, and nasal discharge that initially is watery and clear but often becomes mucopurulent and viscous after a few days. Malaise, headache, myalgia, low-grade fever, cough, and sneezing may occur. Symptoms typically peak in severity after 2 to 3 days and have a median duration of 7 days but may persist for more than 10 days in approximately 25% of illnesses. Rhinoviruses also cause otitis media and lower respiratory tract infections (eg, bronchiolitis, pneumonia), particularly in infants, and are associated with approximately 60% to 70% of acute exacerbations of asthma in school-aged children.

ETIOLOGY: Rhinoviruses (RVs) are small, nonenveloped, single, positive-stranded RNA viruses classified into 3 species (RV-A, RV-B, and RV-C) in the family *Picornaviridae*, genus *Enterovirus*. More than 160 rhinovirus types have been identified by immunologic and molecular methods. Infection confers type-specific immunity, but protection is temporary.

EPIDEMIOLOGY: Rhinovirus infection is ubiquitous in human populations. Children have an average of 2 rhinovirus infections each year, and 93% of adults experience at least 1 rhinovirus infection annually. Rhinoviruses cause approximately two thirds of cases of the common cold and, thus, are responsible for more episodes of human illness than any other infectious agent. They can cause sinusitis and otitis media, either as the sole pathogen or with secondary bacterial infections. Rhinovirus infections are a major viral cause of exacerbations of asthma, cystic fibrosis, and chronic obstructive pulmonary disease and have been detected in the lower respiratory tract infections in patients of all ages hospitalized with wheezing or pneumonia.

Person-to-person transmission occurs predominantly by self-inoculation by contaminated secretions on hands or by large-particle aerosol spread. Infections occur throughout the year, but peak activity occurs during autumn and spring. Multiple types circulate simultaneously, and the prevalent types circulating in a given population change from season to season. Viral shedding in nasopharyngeal secretions is most abundant during the first 2 to 3 days of infection and usually ceases by 7 to 10 days. Viral RNA may be detectable in nasal secretions by molecular testing for as long as 30 days, although low amounts of virus detected by PCR in an asymptomatic person are unlikely to result in transmission.

The **incubation period** usually is 2 to 3 days.

DIAGNOSTIC TESTS: Rhinovirus infection is diagnosed by detection of virus in respiratory secretions, although a specific viral diagnosis generally is not useful clinically in terms of patient management. Because of the lack of common group antigen among the various types, antigen detection is not practical for clinical diagnosis. If a specific viral diagnosis is necessary, reverse transcriptase-polymerase chain reaction (RT-PCR) assays are the preferred method to identify rhinovirus infections, with several commercial assays cleared by the US Food and Drug Administration. Most of these assays are designed as multiplexed tests that detect a wide variety of viral and, in some cases, bacterial respiratory pathogens. In general, these assays cannot clearly distinguish rhinoviruses from enteroviruses because of the genetic similarity of the 2 groups. Given the prevalence of rhinovirus infection and the occurrence of shedding following infection, rhinovirus detection, even in symptomatic patients, may not be causal. Serologic diagnosis of rhinovirus infection is impractical because of the large number of antigenic types and the absence of a common antigen.

TREATMENT: Treatment is supportive. No specific antiviral therapy is currently available for treatment of rhinovirus infections. Antimicrobial agents should not be used for prevention of secondary bacterial infection, because their use may promote the emergence of resistant bacteria and subsequently complicate treatment for a bacterial infection, and because of the risk of antibiotic-associated side effects (eg, *Clostridioides difficile* disease; see Antimicrobial Resistance and Antimicrobial Stewardship: Appropriate and Judicious Use of Antimicrobial Agents, p 868).

ISOLATION OF THE HOSPITALIZED PATIENT: In addition to standard precautions, droplet precautions are recommended for symptomatic hospitalized infants and children for the duration of illness. Contact precautions should be added if copious moist secretions and close contact are likely to occur (eg, young infants). In symptomatic immunocompromised patients, the duration of contact precautions should be extended because of possible prolonged shedding.

CONTROL MEASURES: Appropriate respiratory hygiene and cough etiquette should be followed. Routine hand washing and alcohol-based hand sanitizers are effective for removal of rhinovirus from the hands.

Rickettsial Diseases

Rickettsial diseases comprise infections caused by bacterial species of the genera *Rickettsia* (endemic and epidemic typhus and spotted fever group rickettsioses), *Orientia* (scrub typhus), *Ehrlichia* (ehrlichiosis), *Anaplasma* (anaplasmosis), *Neoehrlichia*, and *Neorickettsia*. The genus *Rickettsia* is further divided into 4 groups on the basis of serologic and genomic analysis: typhus group, spotted fever group, ancestral group, and transitional group.

CLINICAL MANIFESTATIONS: Early signs and symptoms can be nonspecific and often mimic viral illness. Rickettsial infections have many features in common. Fever, rash (especially in spotted fever and typhus group rickettsiae), headache, myalgia, and respiratory symptoms are prominent features. The classic rash of Rocky Mountain spotted fever (RMSF) may not appear until 3 to 5 days after onset of symptoms, and approximately 10% of patients do not develop an identifiable rash. One or more inoculation eschars occur with many rickettsial diseases, especially most spotted fever group rickettsioses, rickettsialpox, and scrub typhus. Systemic endothelial damage of small blood vessels resulting in increased vascular permeability is the hallmark pathologic feature of most severe spotted fever and typhus group rickettsial infections. Some rickettsial diseases, particularly RMSF and Mediterranean spotted fever, can rapidly become life threatening. Risk factors for severe disease include glucose-6-phosphate dehydrogenase deficiency, male gender, and antecedent exposure to sulfonamides.

Immunity against reinfection by the same agent after natural infection is not well studied, but some anecdotal information suggests that prior infection confers immunity for at least 1 year. Documented reinfections with *Rickettsia* and *Ehrlichia* species have been described only rarely.

ETIOLOGY: Rickettsiae are small, coccobacillary gram-negative bacteria that are obligate intracellular pathogens and cannot be grown in cell-free media. *Orientia* and *Rickettsia* organisms reside free within the cytoplasm and *Anaplasmataceae* organisms reside in phagosomes. Currently recognized rickettsial pathogens of humans include more than 20 species of *Rickettsia*, 5 species of *Ehrlichia*, 2 species each of *Orientia* and *Anaplasma*, and *Neorickettsia sennetsu*. Tickborne neoehrlichiosis caused by *Candidatus Neoehrlichia mikurensis*, which features rodents as the primary host, is an emerging disease in Asia and Europe.

EPIDEMIOLOGY: Rickettsial diseases have various hematophagous arthropod vectors that include ticks, fleas, mites, and lice. Except for *Rickettsia prowazekii*, the cause of epidemic typhus, humans are incidental hosts for rickettsial pathogens. Rickettsial life cycles typically involve one or more arthropod species as well as various mammalian reservoirs or amplifying hosts, and transmission to humans occurs during environmental or occupational exposures to infected arthropods. Geographic and seasonal occurrences of each rickettsial disease are related directly to distributions and life cycles of the specific vector.

Incubation periods vary according to organism (see disease-specific chapters in Section 3).

Other Global Rickettsial Spotted Fever Infections. A number of other epidemiologically distinct fleaborne and tickborne spotted fever infections caused by rickettsiae have been recognized (also see **www.cdc.gov/otherspottedfever/**). These diseases may affect people living in, traveling to, or returning from areas where these agents are endemic. These infections have clinical and pathologic features that vary widely in severity. Many present with an eschar at the site of the tick bite and without rash. Information about spotted fevers occurring outside the United States can be found at **www.cdc.gov/ otherspottedfever/imported/index.html.** Causative agents of spotted fevers in the United States and of other rickettsial diseases most important for travelers include the following:

- *Rickettsia africae*, the causative agent of African tick bite fever that is endemic in sub-Saharan Africa, Oceania, and some Caribbean islands.
- *Rickettsia akari*, the causative agent of rickettsialpox, which occurs sporadically throughout the United States but is often reported from the Northeast, particularly New York City.
- *Rickettsia conorii* and subspecies, the causative agents of Mediterranean spotted fever, India tick typhus, Israeli tick typhus, and Astrakhan spotted fever, that are endemic in southern Europe, Africa, the Middle East, and the Indian subcontinent.
- *Rickettsia parkeri*, a causative agent of eschar-associated infections in the Americas.
- *Rickettsia* species 364D causes eschar, headache, and fever in California (Pacific Coast tick fever).

DIAGNOSTIC TESTS: Group-specific antibodies are detectable in the serum of most patients by 7 to 10 days after onset of illness, but slower antibody responses may occur, particularly in some diseases of lesser severity such as African tick bite fever. The utility of serologic testing during the acute illness generally is of limited value, and a negative serologic test result during the initial stage of the illness should never be used to exclude a diagnosis of rickettsial disease. Serologic assays provide an excellent method of retrospective confirmation when paired serum samples collected during the illness and 2 to 6 weeks later are tested in tandem. The indirect immunofluorescence antibody assay is recommended in most circumstances but cannot determine the causative agent to the species level. Treatment early in the course of illness can blunt or delay serologic responses. Polymerase chain reaction (PCR) assays can detect rickettsiae in whole blood or tissues collected during the acute stage of illness and before administration of antimicrobial agents; availability of these tests often is limited to reference and research laboratories. Immunohistochemical staining and PCR testing of skin biopsy specimens from patients with rash or eschar lesions can help to diagnose rickettsial infections early in the course of disease. PCR assays and sequencing of DNA collected during acute infection provide more accurate identification of the etiologic agent than serologic testing.

TREATMENT: Prompt initiation of treatment is indicated for all patients in all age groups with presumptive evidence of any rickettsial disease, and is of paramount importance when there is clinical suspicion of a potentially life-threatening infection such as RMSF, ehrlichiosis, epidemic typhus, murine typhus, or scrub typhus. Treatment decisions should be made on the basis of clinical findings and epidemiologic data and never should be delayed until test results are known because confirmatory laboratory tests are rarely available early in the course of illness. Therapy is less effective in preventing complications when disease remains untreated into the second week of illness. For all ages, the drug of choice for all rickettsioses, including RMSF and ehrlichiosis, is doxycycline, and the treatment course generally is 7 to 14 days.

CONTROL MEASURES: Limiting exposures to ticks and tick bites is the primary means of prevention (see Prevention of Mosquitoborne and Tickborne Infections, p 175).

Several rickettsial diseases, including spotted fevers, ehrlichiosis, and anaplasmosis, are nationally notifiable diseases and should be reported to state and local health departments.

For more details, the following chapters in Section 3 on rickettsial diseases should be consulted:

- *Ehrlichia, Anaplasma*, and Related Infections, p 308 (or **www.cdc.gov/ehrlichiosis/**).
- Rickettsialpox, p 640.
- Rocky Mountain Spotted Fever, p 641 (or **www.cdc.gov/rmsf/**).
- Louseborne Typhus (Epidemic or Sylvatic Typhus), p 825.
- Murine Typhus (Endemic or Fleaborne Typhus), p 827.

Rickettsialpox

CLINICAL MANIFESTATIONS: Rickettsialpox is a febrile, eschar-associated illness characterized by generalized, relatively sparse, erythematous, papulovesicular eruptions on the trunk, face, extremities (less often on palms and soles), and oral mucous membranes. The rash develops 1 to 4 days after onset of fever and 3 to 10 days after appearance of an eschar at the site of the bite of an infected house mouse mite. Regional lymph nodes in the area of the inoculation eschar typically become enlarged. Without specific antimicrobial therapy, systemic disease lasts approximately 7 to 14 days; manifestations include fever, headache, malaise, and myalgia. Less frequent manifestations include anorexia, vomiting, conjunctivitis, hepatitis, nuchal rigidity, and photophobia. The disease is mild compared with Rocky Mountain spotted fever, and although no rickettsialpox-associated deaths have been described, disease occasionally is severe enough to warrant hospitalization.

ETIOLOGY: Rickettsialpox is caused by *Rickettsia akari*, a gram-negative intracellular bacillus now classified along with *Rickettsia felis* and *Rickettsia australis* within the transitional group, which has features of both the spotted fever and typhus groups.

EPIDEMIOLOGY: The natural host for *R akari* in the United States is *Mus musculus*, the common house mouse. The organism is transmitted by the house mouse mite, *Liponyssoides sanguineus*. Disease risk is heightened in areas infested with house mice. The disease can occur wherever the hosts, pathogens, and humans coexist, but most frequently is reported in large urban settings. In the United States, rickettsialpox has been described predominantly in northeastern metropolitan centers, especially in New York City. It has been confirmed in many other countries, including the Netherlands, Croatia, Ukraine, Turkey, Russia, South Korea, South Africa, and Mexico. All age groups can be affected. No seasonal pattern of disease occurs. The disease is not communicable but occurs occasionally among families or people cohabiting a house mouse mite-infested dwelling.

The **incubation period** is 6 to 15 days.

DIAGNOSTIC TESTS: *R akari* can be isolated in cell culture from blood and eschar biopsy specimens during the acute stage of disease, but culture is not attempted routinely. Because antigens of *R akari* have extensive cross-reactivity with antigens of *Rickettsia* *rickettsii* (the cause of Rocky Mountain spotted fever) and other spotted fever-group rickettsiae, an indirect immunofluorescence antibody assay for *R rickettsii* can be used to demonstrate a fourfold or greater change in antibody titers between acute and convalescent serum specimens taken 2 to 6 weeks apart. Use of *R akari* antigen is recommended for a more accurate serologic diagnosis but may be available only in specialized research laboratories. Immunoglobulin (Ig) M and IgG are detected 7 to 15 days after illness onset. Immunohistochemical testing of formalin-fixed, paraffin-embedded eschars or papulovesicle biopsy specimens can detect rickettsiae in the samples and are useful diagnostic techniques, but because of antigenic cross-reactivity these assays are not able to confirm the etiologic agent. A polymerase chain reaction assay for detection of rickettsial DNA with subsequent sequence identification can confirm *R akari* infection but currently is not cleared by the US Food and Drug Administration for use in the United States.

TREATMENT: Doxycycline is the drug of choice in all age groups. The minimum course of therapy is 5 days. Doxycycline shortens the course of disease, and symptoms typically resolve within 12 to 48 hours after initiation of therapy. Chloramphenicol is an alternative drug but carries a risk of serious adverse events and is not available as an oral formulation in the United States. Use of chloramphenicol should be considered only in rare cases, such as for patients with an absolute contraindication to receiving doxycycline, because rickettsialpox usually is mild and self-limited. Untreated rickettsialpox usually resolves within 2 weeks.

ISOLATION OF THE HOSPITALIZED PATIENT: Person-to-person spread of rickettsialpox has not been reported. Standard precautions are recommended.

CONTROL MEASURES: Application of residual acaricides can be used in heavily mite-infested environments to eliminate the vector. Rodent-control measures are important in limiting or eliminating spread of rickettsialpox but they should be conducted only in conjunction with acaricide application to ensure vector control. No specific management of exposed people is necessary.

Rocky Mountain Spotted Fever

CLINICAL MANIFESTATIONS: Rocky Mountain spotted fever (RMSF) is a systemic, small-vessel vasculitis that often involves a characteristic rash. High fever, myalgia, headache (less commonly reported in young children), nausea, vomiting, and malaise are typical presenting symptoms. Abdominal pain and diarrhea can be present and obscure the diagnosis. The rash usually begins within the first 2 to 4 days of symptoms; a faint maculopapular rash first appears on the wrists and ankles, and spreads centripetally to include the trunk. The rash associated with RMSF can also involve the palms and soles. Although development of a rash is a useful diagnostic sign, the early rash may be faint, and rash can be absent altogether in up to 10% of patients. As the rash progresses, it becomes petechial, which is reflective of the small-vessel vasculitis and indicative of progression to severe disease. Delayed onset or atypical appearance of the rash is a risk factor for misdiagnosis and poor outcome. Meningismus, altered mental status, and coma may occur. Children may experience peripheral or periorbital edema. Thrombocytopenia, elevated liver aminotransferases, and hyponatremia (serum sodium concentrations <130 mg/dL are observed in 20%–50% of cases) are the laboratory abnormalities seen most frequently and worsen as disease progresses. White blood cell count is often normal until later stages of disease, but leukopenia and anemia can occur. Patients treated early in the course of symptoms may have a mild illness, with fever resolving in the first 48 hours of treatment. If appropriate antimicrobial treatment is not initiated or is delayed past the fifth day of symptoms the illness can be severe, with prominent central nervous system, cardiac, pulmonary, gastrointestinal tract, and renal involvement; disseminated intravascular coagulation; necrosis of digits and gangrene; and shock leading to death. RMSF can progress rapidly, even in previously healthy people. Case-fatality rates of untreated RMSF range from 20% to 80%, with a median time to death of 8 days. Significant long-term sequelae can occur in patients with severe RMSF, even if treated with appropriate antibiotics; these include neurologic (paraparesis; hearing loss; peripheral neuropathy; bladder and bowel incontinence; developmental and language delays; and cerebellar, vestibular, and motor dysfunction) and non-neurologic (disability from limb or digit amputation) sequelae.

ETIOLOGY: *Rickettsia rickettsii*, an obligate, intracellular, gram-negative bacillus and a member of the spotted fever group of rickettsiae, is the causative agent. The primary targets of infection in mammalian hosts are endothelial cells lining the small blood vessels of all major tissues and organs. Diffuse small vessel vasculitis leads to poor perfusion, infarction, and increased permeability.

EPIDEMIOLOGY: The pathogen is transmitted to humans by the bite of a tick of the *Ixodidae* family (hard ticks). The principal recognized vectors of *R rickettsii* are *Dermacentor variabilis* (the American dog tick) in the eastern and central United States and *Dermacentor andersoni* (the Rocky Mountain wood tick) in the northern and western United States. Another emergent vector is *Rhipicephalus sanguineus* (the brown dog tick), which feeds on dogs and has been confirmed as a vector of *R rickettsii* in Arizona and Mexico and may play a role in other regions. Ticks and their small mammal hosts serve as reservoirs of the pathogen in nature. Other wild animals and dogs have been found with antibodies to *R rickettsii*, but their role as natural reservoirs is not clear. Dogs can experience clinical symptoms similar to those described in humans. People with occupational or recreational exposure to the tick vector (eg, pet owners, animal handlers, and people who spend more time outdoors) are at increased risk of exposure to the organism. People of all ages can be infected. The period of highest incidence in the United States is from April to September, although RMSF can occur year-round in certain areas with endemic disease. Laboratory-acquired infection is rare. Transmission has occurred on rare occasions by blood transfusion. RMSF is the most severe and frequently fatal rickettsial illness in the United States.

Current national surveillance collects data on spotted fever rickettsiosis (SFR), including RMSF. SFR are widespread in the United States, with most cases reported in the south Atlantic, southeastern, and south central states. The southwestern United States is reporting increasing amounts of SFR, which is largely believed to be RMSF. During 2016 to 2017, reported cases of SFR increased 46% from 4269 to 6248 cases. It is unknown how many of those cases are RMSF.

The **incubation period** is approximately 1 week (typical range, 3–12 days).

DIAGNOSTIC TESTS[1]: The diagnosis of RMSF must be made on the basis of clinical signs and symptoms and can be confirmed later using diagnostic tests. Treatment should

---

[1]Biggs HM, Behravesh CB, Bradley KK, et al. Diagnosis and management of tickborne rickettsial diseases: Rocky Mountain spotted fever and other spotted fever group rickettsioses, ehrlichioses, and anaplasmosis—United States. A practical guide for health care and public health professionals. *MMWR Recomm Rep.* 2016;65(RR-2):1–44. Available at: **www.cdc.gov/mmwr/volumes/65/rr/rr6502a1.htm**

never be delayed while awaiting laboratory confirmation or because of lack of history of tick bite: approximately half of RMSF cases do not report tick bite. The gold standard confirmatory test is indirect immunofluorescence antibody (IFA) to *R rickettsii* antigen. Both immunoglobulin (Ig) G and IgM antibodies begin to increase around 7 to 10 days after onset of symptoms; IgM is less specific, and IgG is the preferred test. Confirmation requires a fourfold or greater increase in antigen-specific IgG between acute (first 1–2 weeks of illness while symptomatic) and convalescent (2–4 weeks later) sera. An elevated acute titer may represent prior exposure rather than acute infection, and a negative serologic test in the acute phase does not rule out diagnosis of RMSF. Low-level elevated antibody titers can be an incidental finding in a significant proportion of the general population in some regions. Cross-reactivity may be observed between antibodies to other spotted fever group rickettsiae, including *Rickettsia parkeri* and *Rickettsia africae*. Enzyme-linked immunosorbent assays also can be used for assessing antibody presence in acute and convalescent sera but are less useful for quantifying changes in titer values.

RMSF may be diagnosed by detection of *R rickettsii* DNA in acute whole blood, tissue, and serum specimens by polymerase chain reaction (PCR) assay. *R rickettsii* typically does not circulate in large numbers in whole blood until advanced stages of disease; assays relying on detection of DNA may lack sensitivity, and a negative result does not rule out RMSF. Specimens used for PCR should be obtained before doxycycline administration when possible. Diagnosis may be confirmed by detection of rickettsial DNA in biopsy or autopsy specimens by PCR assay or immunohistochemical (IHC) visualization of rickettsiae in tissues.

R rickettsii also may be isolated from acute blood specimens or through tissue culture, but culture requires specialized procedures (not routine blood culture) and a laboratory with a minimum Biosafety Level 3 designation. Cell culture cultivation of the organism must be confirmed by molecular methods.

TREATMENT[1]: Doxycycline is the drug of choice for treatment of RMSF in patients of any age and should be started as soon as RMSF is suspected (see Tetracyclines, p 866). Physicians should treat empirically if RMSF is being considered and should not postpone treatment while awaiting laboratory confirmation. The doxycycline dose for RMSF is 2.2 mg/kg of body weight per dose, twice daily, orally or intravenously (maximum 100 mg per dose); the adult dose is 100 mg twice daily. Treatment is most effective if initiated in the first 5 days of symptoms, and treatment started after that time is less likely to prevent death or other adverse outcomes. Antimicrobial treatment should be continued until the patient has been afebrile for at least 3 days and has demonstrated clinical improvement; the usual duration of therapy is 5 to 7 days, but may be longer in severe cases. Use of antimicrobial agents other than doxycycline increases risk of mortality. Chloramphenicol can be found in some references as an alternative treatment; however, its use is associated with a higher risk of fatal outcome. Chloramphenicol carries a risk of serious adverse events and is not available as an oral formulation in the United States. In the case of severe doxycycline allergy, a specialist should be consulted to discuss risks, benefits, and alternatives. Experts at the United States Centers for Disease Control and

[1]Biggs HM, Behravesh CB, Bradley KK, et al. Diagnosis and management of tickborne rickettsial diseases: Rocky Mountain spotted fever and other spotted fever group rickettsioses, ehrlichioses, and anaplasmosis—United States. A practical guide for health care and public health professionals. *MMWR Recomm Rep.* 2016;65(RR-2):1–44. Available at: **www.cdc.gov/mmwr/volumes/65/rr/rr6502a1.htm**

Prevention (CDC) are available by telephone to consult with health care providers on a specific patient at 1-800-CDC-INFO (1-800-232-4636).

ISOLATION OF THE HOSPITALIZED PATIENT: Standard precautions are recommended.

CONTROL MEASURES: Limiting exposures to ticks and tick bites is the primary means of prevention (see Prevention of Mosquitoborne and Tickborne Infections, p 175). Prophylactic use of antimicrobial agents is not recommended to prevent RMSF, even in children with a documented tick bite but who are asymptomatic. No licensed *R rickettsii* vaccine is available in the United States. Additional information is available on the Centers for Disease Control and Prevention's Web site (**www.cdc.gov/rmsf/**).

Rotavirus Infections

CLINICAL MANIFESTATIONS: The clinical manifestations vary and depend on whether it is the first infection or reinfection. After 3 months of age, the first infection generally is the most severe. Infection begins with acute onset of vomiting followed 24 to 48 hours later by watery diarrhea; up to one third of patients will have high fevers. Symptoms usually last for 3 to 7 days but improve over time. In moderate to severe cases or with prolonged diarrhea, dehydration, electrolyte abnormalities, and acidosis may occur. In certain immunocompromised children, including children with congenital cellular immunodeficiencies or severe combined immunodeficiency (SCID) and children who are hematopoietic stem cell or solid organ transplant recipients, severe, prolonged, and sometimes fatal rotavirus diarrhea may occur. The presence of rotavirus RNA in cerebrospinal fluid (CSF) has been detected in children with rotavirus-associated seizures.

ETIOLOGY: Rotaviruses are segmented, nonenveloped, double-stranded RNA viruses belonging to the family *Reoviridae*, with at least 10 distinct groups (A through J). Group A viruses are the major causes of human disease, although rotaviruses of groups B and C have also been associated with acute gastroenteritis. A binomial genotyping system, Gx-P[x], based on the 2 outer capsid viral proteins, VP7 glycoprotein (G) and VP4 protease-cleaved protein (P), is being replaced with an 11-gene typing system where the notations Gx-P[x]-Ix-Rx-Cx-Mx-Ax-Nx-Tx-Ex-Hx indicate the genotypes of the 6 structural viral proteins (VP7, VP4, VP6, VP1, VP2, VP3) and the 6 nonstructural proteins (NSP1, NSP2, NSP3, NSP4, NSP5/6), respectively. Before introduction of the rotavirus vaccine, genotypes G1P[8], G2P[4], G3P[8], G4P[8], and G9P[8] were the most common genotypes circulating in the United States. However, since 2012, G12P[8] has been the most common genotype identified.

EPIDEMIOLOGY: Rotavirus is present in high titer in stools of infected patients several days before and may continue for at least 10 days after onset of clinical disease. A small inoculum (100 colony forming units/g) is needed for transmission, which occurs via the fecal-oral route. Rotavirus can remain viable for weeks to months on contaminated environmental surfaces and fomites (such as toys) which can also lead to transmission. Airborne droplet transmission has not been proven but may play a minor role in disease transmission. Spread within families and institutions is common. Rarely, common-source outbreaks from contaminated water or food have been reported.

In temperate climates, rotavirus disease is most prevalent during the cooler months. Before licensure of rotavirus vaccines in North America, the annual rotavirus epidemic usually started during the fall in Mexico and the southwest United States and moved eastward, reaching the northeast United States and Maritime Provinces by spring. Such a seasonal pattern of disease is less pronounced in tropical climates.

The epidemiology and burden of rotavirus disease in the United States has changed dramatically following the introduction of rotavirus vaccines in 2006 and 2008. Before widespread use of these vaccines, rotavirus was the most common cause of community acquired gastroenteritis and health care-associated diarrhea in young children. Since the introduction of rotavirus vaccines in the United States, a biennial pattern has emerged, with small, short seasons (median 9 weeks) beginning in late winter/early spring (eg, 2009, 2011, 2013, 2015, 2017), alternating with years with extremely low circulation (eg, 2008, 2010, 2012, 2014, 2016). Beginning in 2008, annual hospitalizations for rotavirus disease among US children younger than 5 years declined by approximately 75%, with an estimated 40 000 to 50 000 fewer rotavirus hospitalizations nationally each year. In case-control evaluations in the United States, the rotavirus vaccines (full series) have been found to be approximately 80% to 90% effective against rotavirus disease resulting in hospitalization. The vaccines also are highly effective in reducing emergency department visits for rotavirus disease. During a 4-year period after vaccine introduction, an estimated 177 000 hospitalizations, 242 000 emergency department visits, and 1.1 million outpatient visits for diarrhea were averted among US children younger than 5 years.

The **incubation period** for rotavirus is short, usually less than 48 hours.

DIAGNOSTIC TESTS: It is not possible to diagnose rotavirus infection by clinical presentation or nonspecific laboratory tests. Diagnostic enzyme immunoassays (EIAs) and rapid chromatographic immunoassays for group A rotavirus antigen detection in stool are available commercially. Given the marked reduction in rotavirus disease prevalence because of vaccine use, the positive predictive value of the immunoassays can be expected to be lower, and the negative predictive value to be higher, now compared with the prevaccine period. Polymerase chain reaction (PCR)-based multipathogen detection systems that test stool for a panel of viral, bacterial, and parasitic gastrointestinal tract pathogens, including rotavirus, are being increasingly used. Although the advantages of such PCR-based systems are increased sensitivity and the ability to test for multiple pathogens in a single sample, the probability of coincidental detection of rotaviruses or other potential pathogens that may not be causing current symptoms complicates test interpretation. The virus from approved rotavirus vaccines can be detected in stool for at least 10 days after immunization.

The following tests are available in some research and reference laboratories: electron microscopy, polyacrylamide gel electrophoresis (PAGE) of viral RNA with silver staining, and viral culture. However, these tests generally are not used for clinical diagnosis of rotavirus disease.

TREATMENT: No specific antiviral therapy is available. Oral or parenteral fluids and electrolytes are given to prevent or correct dehydration. Orally administered Human Immune Globulin, administered as an investigational therapy in immunocompromised patients with prolonged infection, has decreased viral shedding and shortened the duration of diarrhea.

ISOLATION OF THE HOSPITALIZED PATIENT: In addition to standard precautions, contact precautions are indicated for diapered or incontinent children for the duration of illness.

CONTROL MEASURES: Breastfeeding is associated with milder rotavirus disease and should be encouraged (see Breastfeeding and Human Milk, p 107).

Child Care. General measures for interrupting enteric transmission in child care centers are available (see Children in Group Child Care and Schools, p 116). Hand washing and cleaning surfaces with soap and water followed by disinfection is recommended. Bleach solutions or other products with confirmed virucidal activity against rotavirus can be used to inactivate rotavirus and may help prevent disease transmission resulting from contact with environmental surfaces (**www.cdc.gov/infectioncontrol/guidelines/disinfection/disinfection-methods/chemical.html**). Infants and children with rotavirus diarrhea should be excluded from child care centers until stools are contained in the diaper or when toilet-trained children no longer have accidents using the toilet and when stool frequency becomes no more than 2 stools above that child's normal frequency, even if the stools remain loose.

Vaccines. Two rotavirus vaccines are licensed for use among infants in the United States: a live, oral human-bovine reassortant pentavalent rotavirus (RV5 [RotaTeq, Merck & Co Inc]) vaccine, given as a 3-dose series and a live, oral human attenuated monovalent rotavirus (RV1 [Rotarix, GlaxoSmithKline]) vaccine, given as a 2-dose series. The products differ in composition and schedule of administration. The American Academy of Pediatrics and the Centers for Disease Control and Prevention do not express a preference for either vaccine.

In 2010, porcine circovirus or porcine circovirus DNA was detected in both rotavirus vaccines. There is no evidence that this virus is a safety risk or causes illness in humans.

Postmarketing surveillance data from the United States, Australia, Mexico, Canada, and Brazil indicate that there is a small risk of intussusception from the currently licensed rotavirus vaccines. In the United States, the data currently available suggest the attributable risk is between approximately 1 and 5 excess intussusception cases per 100 000 vaccinated infants. The risk appears to be primarily during the first week following the first or second dose; data from Australia suggest some risk may extend up to 21 days following the first dose. In the United States as well as other parts of the world, the benefits of rotavirus vaccination in preventing severe rotavirus disease outweigh the risk of intussusception. Parents should be informed of the risk, the early signs and symptoms of intussusception, and the need for prompt care if these develop.

Postmarketing strain surveillance in the United States and other countries has revealed that RV5 vaccine reassortant strains have been detected occasionally in stool samples of children with diarrhea. In some of the reports, the reassortant virus seemed to cause diarrheal illness. An RV1 vaccine wild-type reassortant strain has also been reported outside the United States.

Following are recommendations for use of the currently licensed rotavirus vaccines[1,2] (see Table 3.51):

- Infants in the United States should be immunized routinely with a licensed rotavirus vaccine.
- Immunization should not be initiated for infants 15 weeks, 0 days of age or older. For infants to whom the first dose of rotavirus vaccine is administered inadvertently at

---

[1] American Academy of Pediatrics, Committee on Infectious Diseases. Prevention of rotavirus disease: updated guidelines for use of rotavirus vaccine. *Pediatrics.* 2009;123(5):1412-1420

[2] Centers for Disease Control and Prevention. Prevention of rotavirus gastroenteritis among infants and children. Recommendations of the Advisory Committee on Immunization Practices (ACIP). *MMWR Recomm Rep.* 2009;58(RR-2):1–25

Table 3.51. Recommended Schedule for Administration of Rotavirus Vaccine

Recommendation	RV5 (RotaTeq)	RV1 (Rotarix)
Number of doses in series	3	2
Recommended ages for doses	2, 4, and 6 months of age	2 and 4 months of age
Minimum age for first dose	6 weeks of age	6 weeks of age
Maximum age for first dose	14 weeks, 6 days of age	14 weeks, 6 days of age
Minimum interval between doses	4 weeks	4 weeks
Maximum age for last dose	8 months, 0 days of age	8 months, 0 days of age

15 weeks, 0 days of age or older, the remainder of the rotavirus immunization series should be completed according to the schedule.
- The maximum age for the last dose of rotavirus vaccine is 8 months, 0 days.
- The rotavirus vaccine series should be completed with the same product whenever possible. However, immunization should not be deferred if the product used for previous doses is not available or is unknown. In this situation, the health care professional should continue or complete the series with the product available.
- If any dose in the series was RV5 vaccine or the product is unknown for any dose in the series, a total of 3 doses of rotavirus vaccine should be administered.
- Rotavirus vaccine can be administered concurrently with other childhood vaccines.
- Infants with transient, mild illness, with or without low-grade fever, may receive rotavirus vaccine.
- Preterm infants may be immunized if the infant is at least 6 weeks of postnatal age and is clinically stable. Preterm infants should be immunized on the same schedule and with the same precautions as recommended for full-term infants. Rotavirus vaccine virus is shed by some infants in the weeks after vaccination. There are limited published studies on the transmission of vaccine virus in hospital settings, including neonatal intensive care units that have not documented nosocomial transmission. Individual institutions may consider administering rotavirus vaccine at the recommended chronologic age to otherwise eligible infants during hospitalization, including in the neonatal intensive care unit. Otherwise, the first dose of vaccine should be administered at the time of discharge to eligible infants.
- Infants living in households with immunocompromised people can be immunized. Highly immunocompromised patients should avoid handling diapers of infants who have been vaccinated with rotavirus vaccine for 4 weeks after vaccination.
- Infants living in households with pregnant women should be immunized.
- Rotavirus vaccine should not be administered to infants who have a history of a severe allergic reaction (eg, anaphylaxis) after a previous dose of rotavirus vaccine or to a vaccine component.
- Known SCID or history of intussusception are contraindications for use of both rotavirus vaccines. Gastroenteritis, including severe diarrhea and prolonged shedding of vaccine virus, has been reported in infants who were administered live, oral rotavirus vaccines and later identified as having SCID.

- Consultation with experts should be sought prior to administering rotavirus vaccine in infants with altered immunocompetence other than SCID (eg, condition that affects the immune system, including cancer or treatment with drugs such as steroids, chemotherapy, or radiation); moderate to severe illness, including gastroenteritis and preexisting chronic intestinal tract disease.
- Infants exposed in utero to maternally administered biologic response modifiers (BRMs) can have detectable drug concentrations for many months following delivery, resulting in concern for immunosuppression among infants in the 12 months after the last maternal dose during pregnancy. Data are sparse on the safety of rotavirus vaccines in infants who were exposed to maternally administered BRMs in utero. Considering that rotavirus disease is rarely life threatening in the United States, rotavirus vaccines should be avoided in infants for the first 12 months after the last in utero exposure to most BRMs. Exceptions include certolizumab, which is not transferred across the placenta because of its structure as a pegylated Fab fragment, and likely infliximab, although the data are more sparse for it; rotavirus vaccination of infants can be considered when mothers received treatment during pregnancy with either of these BRMs (see Biologic Response-Modifying Drugs Used to Decrease Inflammation, p 82). As more data become available for the other BRMs, recommendations are likely to change, so consultation with a pediatric infectious diseases physician is recommended.
- Rotavirus vaccine should be administered to human immunodeficiency virus (HIV)-exposed and HIV-infected infants, irrespective of CD4+ T-lymphocyte percentage or count, according to the schedule for uninfected infants (see Human Immunodeficiency Virus Infection, p 168). Rotavirus vaccine may be indicated for infants with other acquired immunocompromising conditions if the potential benefit of protection outweighs the risk of adverse reaction.
- The tip caps of the prefilled oral applicators of the RV1 vaccine may contain natural rubber latex, so infants with a severe (anaphylactic) allergy to latex (eg, some patients with spina bifida or bladder extrophy) should preferentially receive RV5 vaccine, because dosing tubes of RV5 do not contain natural rubber latex.
- Rotavirus vaccine may be administered at any time before, concurrent with, or after administration of any blood product, including antibody-containing blood products.
- Breastfeeding infants should be immunized according to the same schedule as non-breastfed infants.
- If an infant regurgitates, spits out, or vomits during or after vaccine administration, the vaccine dose should not be repeated.
- If a recently immunized infant is hospitalized, standard precautions should be followed.
- Infants who have had rotavirus gastroenteritis before receiving the full series of rotavirus immunization should begin or complete the schedule following the standard age and interval recommendations.

Rubella

CLINICAL MANIFESTATIONS:

Postnatal Rubella. Many cases of postnatal rubella are subclinical, with 25% to 50% of adults being asymptomatic. Clinical disease usually is mild and characterized by a generalized erythematous maculopapular rash, lymphadenopathy, and slight fever. The rash starts on the face, becomes generalized in 24 hours, and lasts a median of 3 days. Lymphadenopathy, which may precede rash, often involves posterior auricular or suboccipital lymph nodes, can be generalized, and lasts between 5 and 8 days. In addition, conjunctivitis, cough, headache, coryza, and palatal enanthema may occur 1 to 5 days prior to the rash. Transient polyarthralgia and polyarthritis rarely occur in children but are common in adolescents and adults, especially among females. Encephalitis (1 in 6000 cases) and thrombocytopenia (1 in 3000 cases) are complications.

Congenital Rubella Syndrome. Maternal rubella during pregnancy can result in miscarriage, fetal death, or a constellation of congenital anomalies (congenital rubella syndrome [CRS]). The most commonly described anomalies/manifestations associated with CRS are ophthalmologic (cataracts, pigmentary retinopathy, microphthalmos, congenital glaucoma), cardiac (patent ductus arteriosus, peripheral pulmonary artery stenosis), auditory (sensorineural hearing impairment), or neurologic (behavioral disorders, meningoencephalitis, microcephaly, developmental disabilities). Neonatal manifestations of CRS include growth restriction, interstitial pneumonitis, radiolucent bone disease, hepatosplenomegaly, thrombocytopenia, and dermal erythropoiesis (so-called "blueberry muffin" lesions). Mild forms of the disease can be associated with few or no obvious clinical manifestations at birth. Congenital defects primarily occur in women infected during the first trimester. CRS is one of the few known causes of autism.

ETIOLOGY: Rubella virus is an enveloped, positive-stranded RNA virus classified as a *Rubivirus* in the *Togaviridae* family.

EPIDEMIOLOGY: Humans are the only natural host. Postnatal rubella is transmitted primarily through direct or droplet contact from nasopharyngeal secretions. The peak incidence of infection is during late winter and early spring. Immunity from wild-type or vaccine virus usually is lifelong, but reinfection on rare occasions has been demonstrated and rarely has resulted in CRS. Although volunteer studies have demonstrated rubella virus in nasopharyngeal secretions from 7 days before to a maximum of 14 days after onset of rash, the period of maximal communicability extends from a few days before to 7 days after onset of rash.

Rubella virus has been recovered in high titer from lens aspirates in children with congenital cataracts for several years, and a small proportion of infants with congenital rubella continue to shed virus in nasopharyngeal secretions and urine for 1 year or more, with transmission to susceptible contacts (see Isolation of the Hospitalized Patient and Control Measures). Rubella also has been associated with Fuchs heterochromic uveitis, sometimes decades after the initial infection.

Before widespread use of rubella vaccine, rubella was an epidemic disease, occurring in 6- to 9-year cycles, with most cases occurring in children. In the postvaccine era, most cases in the mid-1970s and 1980s occurred in young unimmunized adults in outbreaks on college campuses and in occupational settings. More recent outbreaks have occurred in people born outside the United States or among underimmunized populations. The incidence of rubella in the United States has decreased by more than 99% from the prevaccine era (see Table 1.1, p 2).

The United States was determined no longer to have endemic rubella in 2004, and from 2004 through 2017, 107 cases of rubella and 17 cases of CRS were reported in the United States; all of the cases were import associated or from unknown sources. A national serologic survey from 2009–2010 indicated that among children and adolescents

6 through 19 years of age, seroprevalence was >97%. Epidemiologic studies of rubella and CRS in the United States have identified that seronegativity is higher among people born outside the United States or from areas with poor vaccine coverage, and the risk of CRS is highest in infants of women born outside the United States.

In 2003, the Pan American Health Organization (PAHO) adopted a resolution calling for elimination of rubella and CRS in the Americas by the year 2010. The strategy consisted of achieving high levels of measles-rubella vaccination coverage in the routine immunization program and in the supplemental vaccination campaigns to rapidly reduce the number of people in the country susceptible to acute infection. This was accomplished while simultaneously strengthening epidemiologic surveillance to monitor impact. The last confirmed endemic rubella case in the Americas was diagnosed in Argentina in February 2009, and the last confirmed endemic CRS case was diagnosed in Brazil in August 2009. In April 2015, the PAHO International Expert Committee for Verification of Measles and Rubella Elimination verified that the region of the Americas had achieved the rubella and CRS elimination goals.

The average **incubation period** of rubella virus is 17 days, with a range of 12 to 23 days. People infected with rubella are most contagious when the rash is erupting.

DIAGNOSTIC TESTS:

Rubella. Detection of rubella-specific immunoglobulin (Ig) M antibody usually indicates recent postnatal infection, but both false-negative and false-positive results occur, requiring additional specialized testing in a reference laboratory. Most postnatal cases are IgM-positive by 5 days after symptom onset. For diagnosis of postnatally acquired rubella, a fourfold or greater increase in antibody titer between acute and convalescent periods or seroconversion between acute and convalescent IgG serum titers also indicate infection. Acute serum must be collected as close to rash onset as possible, preferably in the first 3 days after symptom onset.

Congenital Rubella Syndrome. CRS can be confirmed by detection of rubella-specific IgM antibody usually within the first 6 months of life. Congenital infection also can be confirmed by stable or increasing serum concentrations of rubella-specific IgG over the first 7 to 11 months of life. Diagnosis of congenital rubella infection in children older than 1 year is difficult because of routine vaccination with measles, mumps, and rubella (MMR) vaccine; serologic testing usually is not diagnostic, and viral isolation, although confirmatory, is possible in only the small proportion of congenitally infected children who are still shedding virus at this age.

The most commonly used methods of serologic screening for previous rubella infection are enzyme immunoassays (EIAs) and latex agglutination tests. Individual test interpretation is challenging. As a general rule, both IgM and IgG antibody testing should be performed for suspected cases of both congenital and postnatal rubella, because both results may aid diagnosis.

A false-positive IgM test result may be caused by a number of factors including rheumatoid factor, parvovirus IgM, and heterophile antibodies. The use of IgM-capture EIA may reduce the occurrence of false-positive IgM results. The presence of high-avidity IgG or a lack of increase in IgG titers can be useful in identifying false-positive rubella IgM results. Low-avidity IgG is associated with recent primary rubella infection, whereas high-avidity IgG is associated with past infection or reinfection or with previous vaccination. The avidity assay is not a routine test and should be performed at reference laboratories like the Centers for Disease Control and Prevention (CDC).

Rubella virus can be isolated most consistently from throat or nasal swab specimens (and less consistently urine) by inoculation of appropriate cell culture. Detection of rubella virus RNA by real time reverse transcriptase-polymerase chain reaction (RT-PCR) assay of a throat/nasal swab or urine specimen with subsequent genotyping of strains may be valuable for diagnosis and molecular epidemiology. RT-PCR assays generally are available in commercial and public health laboratories. In most postnatal cases, viral detection is possible by culture or RT-PCR assay on the day of symptom onset, and in most congenital cases viral detection is possible at birth and in some cases for up to 12 months. Laboratory personnel should be notified immediately that rubella is suspected, because specialized cell culture methods are required to isolate and identify the virus. Blood, urine, and cataract specimens also may yield virus, particularly in infants with congenital infection. With the successful elimination of indigenous rubella and CRS in the Western Hemisphere, molecular typing of viral isolates is critical in defining a source in outbreak scenarios as well as for sporadic cases.

TREATMENT: Management is supportive.

ISOLATION OF THE HOSPITALIZED PATIENT: In addition to standard precautions, for postnatal rubella droplet precautions are recommended for 7 days after onset of the rash. Contact isolation is indicated for children with proven or suspected congenital rubella until they are at least 1 year of age, unless rubella RT-PCR testing of 2 sets of clinical specimens (eg, throat/nasal swab and urine specimen) obtained 1 month apart after 3 months of age do not detect rubella virus RNA. In addition, droplet precautions can be considered if the infant has a respiratory illness or an aerosol generating procedure is being performed. Infection-control precautions should be considered in children with CRS up to 3 years of age who are hospitalized for congenital cataract extraction.

CONTROL MEASURES:

School and Child Care. Children with postnatal rubella should be excluded from school or child care for 7 days after onset of the rash. During an outbreak, children without evidence of immunity should be immunized or excluded for 21 days after onset of rash of the last case in the outbreak. Children with CRS should be considered contagious as indicated in the section above on Isolation of the Hospitalized Patients. When infants with CRS who are still potentially contagious are considered for placement in a group child care setting, public health authorities should be contacted for guidance. Caregivers of these infants should be made aware of the potential hazard of the infants to susceptible pregnant contacts. Rubella is an enveloped virus; alcohol-based hand rubs are generally effective against enveloped viruses. Surfaces and items contaminated with potentially infectious material should be disinfected. A 1% bleach solution or 70% ethanol are effective at inactivating rubella virus.

Surveillance for Congenital Infections. Accurate diagnosis and reporting of CRS are extremely important in assessing control of rubella. All birth defects in which rubella infection is suspected etiologically should be investigated thoroughly and reported to the CDC through local or state health departments.

Care of Exposed People. Evidence of rubella immunity consists of documented receipt of at least 1 dose of rubella-containing vaccine on or after the first birthday or serologic evidence of immunity. People born prior to 1957 can be considered immune. Documented evidence of rubella immunity is especially important for women who could become pregnant. Prenatal IgG serologic screening for rubella immunity should be performed for all pregnant women. Women who have rubella-specific antibody concentrations above the standard positive cutoff value for the assay can be considered to have adequate evidence of rubella immunity. Those without antibody concentrations above the standard positive cutoff or those with equivocal test results should receive rubella vaccine during the immediate postpartum period before discharge. Vaccinated women of childbearing age who have received 1 or 2 doses of rubella-containing vaccine and have rubella serum IgG concentrations that are not clearly positive should receive 1 additional dose of measles-mumps-rubella vaccine (maximum of 3 doses) and do not need to be retested thereafter for serologic evidence of rubella immunity.

When a pregnant woman is exposed to rubella, a blood specimen should be obtained as soon as possible and tested for rubella antibody (IgG and IgM). An aliquot of frozen serum should be stored for possible repeated testing at a later time. The presence of rubella-specific IgG antibody at the time of exposure indicates that the person most likely is immune. If antibody is not detectable, a second blood specimen should be obtained 2 to 3 weeks later and tested concurrently with the frozen first specimen. If the second test result is negative, another blood specimen should be obtained 6 weeks after the exposure and also tested concurrently with the frozen first specimen; a negative test result in both the second and third specimens indicates that infection has not occurred, and a positive test result in the second or third specimen but not the first (seroconversion) indicates recent infection.

Immune Globulin. Administration of Immune Globulin to susceptible people experimentally exposed to rubella virus can prevent clinical rubella. However, there have also been many reports of the failure of Immune Globulin to prevent the anomalies of congenital rubella. For this reason, the routine use of Immune Globulin Intramuscular for the prevention of rubella in an exposed pregnant patient is not recommended.

Vaccine. Live-virus rubella vaccine administered after exposure has not been demonstrated to prevent illness. Immunization of exposed nonpregnant people may be indicated, because if the exposure did not result in infection, then immunization will protect these people in the future. Immunization of a person who is incubating natural rubella or who already is immune is not associated with an increased risk of adverse effects.

Rubella Vaccine.[1] The live-virus rubella vaccine distributed in the United States is the RA 27/3 strain. Vaccine is administered by subcutaneous injection as a combination vaccine—either MMR or measles, mumps, rubella, and varicella (MMRV) vaccine. Vaccine can be administered simultaneously with other vaccines (see Simultaneous Administration of Multiple Vaccines, p 36). Serum antibody to rubella is induced in more than 95% of recipients after a single dose at 12 months or older. Clinical efficacy and challenge studies have demonstrated that 1 dose confers long-term immunity against clinical and asymptomatic infection in more than 90% of immunized people. However, both symptomatic (rare) and asymptomatic reinfection have occurred in immunized people.

Because of the 2-dose recommendations for measles- and mumps-containing vaccine (as MMR) and varicella vaccine (as MMRV), 2 doses of rubella vaccine are administered routinely. This provides an added safeguard against primary vaccine failures.

Vaccine Recommendations. At least 1 dose of live attenuated rubella-containing vaccine is recommended for people 12 months or older. In the United States, rubella vaccine

[1]Centers for Disease Control and Prevention. Prevention of measles, rubella, congenital rubella syndrome, and mumps, 2013 summary: recommendations of the Advisory Committee on Immunization Practices (ACIP). *MMWR Recomm Rep.* 2013;62(RR-4):1-34

is recommended to be administered in combination with measles and mumps vaccines (MMR) or in combination with measles, mumps, and varicella (MMRV) when a child is 12 through 15 months of age, with a second dose of MMR or MMRV at school entry at 4 through 6 years of age or sooner, according to recommendations for routine measles, mumps, rubella, and varicella immunization. People who have not received the dose at school entry should receive their second dose as soon as possible but optimally no later than 11 through 12 years of age (see Measles, p 503).

Special emphasis must continue to be placed on the immunization of at-risk postpubertal males and females, especially college students, military recruits, recent immigrants, health care professionals, teachers, and child care providers. People who were born in 1957 or after and who have not received at least 1 dose of vaccine or who have no serologic evidence of immunity to rubella are considered susceptible and should be immunized with MMR vaccine. Clinical diagnosis of infection is unreliable and should not be accepted as evidence of immunity.

Specific recommendations are as follows:

- Postpubertal females without documentation of presumptive evidence of rubella immunity should be immunized unless they are pregnant. Postpubertal females should be advised not to become pregnant for 28 days after receiving a rubella-containing vaccine (see Precautions and Contraindications, p 654, for further discussion). Routine serologic testing of nonpregnant postpubertal women before immunization is unnecessary and is a potential impediment to protection against rubella, because it requires 2 visits.
- During annual health care examinations, premarital and family planning visits, and visits to sexually transmitted infection clinics, postpubertal females should be assessed for rubella susceptibility and, if deemed susceptible, should be immunized with MMR vaccine.
- Routine prenatal IgG screening for rubella immunity should be performed. If a woman is found to be susceptible, rubella vaccine should be administered during the immediate postpartum period before discharge.
- People who have rubella-specific antibody concentrations above the standard positive cutoff value for the assay can be considered to have adequate evidence of rubella immunity. Except for women of childbearing age, people who have an equivocal serologic test result should be considered susceptible to rubella unless they have documented receipt of 1 dose of rubella-containing vaccine or subsequent serologic test results indicate rubella immunity. Vaccinated women of childbearing age who have received 1 or 2 doses of rubella-containing vaccine and have rubella serum IgG concentrations that are not clearly positive should receive 1 additional dose of MMR vaccine (maximum of 3 doses) and do not need to be retested thereafter for serologic evidence of rubella immunity.
- Breastfeeding is not a contraindication to postpartum immunization of the mother (for additional information, see Breastfeeding and Human Milk, p 107).
- All susceptible health care personnel who may be exposed to patients with rubella or who provide care for pregnant women, as well as people who work in educational institutions or provide child care, should be immunized to prevent infection for themselves and to prevent transmission of rubella to pregnant patients.[1]

---

[1]Centers for Disease Control and Prevention. Immunization of health-care personnel: recommendations of the Advisory Committee on Immunization Practices (ACIP). *MMWR Recomm Rep.* 2011;60(RR-7):1-45

Adverse Reactions.

- Of susceptible children who receive MMR or MMRV vaccines, fever develops in 5% to 15% from 6 to 12 days after immunization. Rash occurs in approximately 5% of immunized people. Mild lymphadenopathy occurs commonly. Febrile seizures occur slightly more frequently among children 12 through 23 months of age after administration of MMRV vaccine compared with MMR and varicella administered as separate injections during the same visit (see Measles, p 503).
- Joint pain, usually in small peripheral joints, has been reported in approximately 0.5% of young children following vaccination with a rubella-containing vaccine. Arthralgia and transient arthritis tend to be more common in susceptible postpubertal females, occurring in approximately 25% and 10%, respectively, of vaccine recipients. Joint involvement usually begins 7 to 21 days after immunization and generally is transient. The incidence of joint manifestations after immunization is lower than after natural infection at the corresponding age.
- Transient paresthesia and pain in the arms and legs have rarely been reported.
- Central nervous system manifestations have been reported, but no causal relationship with rubella vaccine has been established.
- Other reactions that occur after immunization with MMR or MMRV are associated with the measles, mumps, and varicella components of the vaccine (see Measles, p 503, Mumps, p 538, and Varicella-Zoster Infections, p 831).

Precautions and Contraindications.

- **Pregnancy.** Rubella vaccine should not be administered to pregnant women. If vaccine is administered to an unknowingly pregnant woman or the pregnancy occurs within 28 days of immunization, the patient should be counseled on the theoretical risks to the fetus. The theoretical maximum risk for CRS after vaccine administration is 0.2%, which is considerably lower than the risk with wild rubella virus or risk of non–CRS-induced congenital defects in pregnancy. Of the 2931 women immunized while pregnant who have been followed globally, 3.3% of offspring had subclinical infection, none had congenital defects, and 96.7% were not infected. In view of these observations, receipt of rubella vaccine during pregnancy is not an indication for termination of pregnancy.
- **Children of pregnant women.** Immunizing susceptible children whose mothers or other household contacts are pregnant does not cause a risk. Most immunized people intermittently shed small amounts of virus from the pharynx 7 to 28 days after immunization, but no evidence of transmission of the vaccine virus from immunized children has been found.
- **Febrile illness.** Children with minor illnesses, such as upper respiratory tract infection, may be immunized (see Vaccine Safety, p 42). Fever is not a contraindication to immunization. However, if other manifestations suggest a more serious illness, the child should not be immunized until recovery has occurred.
- **Recent administration of IG.** IG preparations interfere with immune response to measles vaccine and theoretically may interfere with the serologic response to rubella vaccine (see p 40). If rubella vaccine is indicated postpartum for a woman who has received anti-Rho (D) IG or blood products, suggested intervals are the same as used between IG administration and measles immunization (see Table 1.11, p 40).
- **Altered immunity.** Immunocompromised patients with disorders associated with increased severity of viral infections should not receive live-virus rubella vaccine (see

Immunization and Other Considerations in Immunocompromised Children, p 72). Exceptions are patients with human immunodeficiency virus (HIV) infection who are not severely immunocompromised; these patients may be immunized against rubella with MMR vaccine (see Human Immunodeficiency Virus Infection, p 427). If possible, children receiving biologic response modifiers, such as anti-tumor necrosis factor-alpha (see Biologic Response-Modifying Drugs Used to Decrease Inflammation, p 82), should be immunized before initiating treatment.

- **Household contacts of immunocompromised people.** The risk of rubella exposure for patients with altered immunity is decreased by immunizing susceptible contacts. Although small amounts of vaccine virus may be isolated from the pharynx, no evidence of transmission of rubella vaccine virus from immunized children to immunocompromised contacts has been found. Precautions and contraindications appropriate for the measles, mumps, and varicella components of MMR or MMRV vaccines also should be reviewed before administration (see Measles, p 503, Mumps, p 538, and Varicella-Zoster Infections, p 831).

Corticosteroids. For patients who have received high doses of corticosteroids (2 mg/kg or greater or more than 20 mg/day) for 14 days or more and who otherwise are not immunocompromised, the recommended interval between stopping the steroids and immunization is at least 4 weeks (see Immunization and Other Considerations in Immunocompromised Children, p 72) after steroids have been discontinued.

Tuberculosis. Tuberculin skin testing is not a prerequisite for MMR immunization. Antituberculosis therapy should be initiated before administering MMR vaccine to people with untreated tuberculosis infection or disease. Tuberculin skin testing, if otherwise indicated, can be performed on the day of immunization with MMR vaccine. Otherwise, tuberculin skin testing should be postponed for 4 to 6 weeks, because measles immunization temporarily may suppress tuberculin skin test reactivity.

Salmonella Infections

CLINICAL MANIFESTATIONS:

Nontyphoidal **Salmonella** *Infection.* Nontyphoidal *Salmonella* (NTS) infection is associated with a spectrum of illness ranging from asymptomatic gastrointestinal tract carriage to gastroenteritis, urinary tract infection, bacteremia, and focal infections, including meningitis, brain abscess, and osteomyelitis (to which people with sickle cell anemia are predisposed). The most common illness associated with NTS infection is gastroenteritis, with manifestations of diarrhea, abdominal cramps, and fever. The site of infection usually is the distal small intestine as well as the colon. Sustained or intermittent bacteremia can occur, and focal infections are recognized in up to 10% of patients with NTS bacteremia. In the United States, the incidence of invasive NTS is highest among infants. Certain NTS serovars (eg, Dublin, Choleraesuis), although rare, are more likely to result in invasive infection than gastroenteritis. Invasive NTS disease in infants and toddlers, manifesting as severe clinical illness and accompanied by high case fatality rates, is prevalent in many parts of sub-Saharan Africa. *Salmonella* Typhimurium, *Salmonella* Enteritidis, and *Salmonella* I:4,[5],12:i:- (and to a lesser extent *Salmonella* Dublin) are the most frequent NTS serovars isolated from blood and cerebrospinal fluid. Severe anemia, malaria, human immunodeficiency virus (HIV), and malnutrition are known risk factors that contribute to the high case fatality rate (10%–30%).

Enteric Fever. *Salmonella enterica* serovars Typhi, Paratyphi A, Paratyphi B, and Paratyphi C (which occurs rarely) can cause a protracted bacteremic illness referred to, respectively, as typhoid and paratyphoid fever and collectively as enteric fever. In older children, the onset of enteric fever typically is gradual, with manifestations such as fever, constitutional symptoms (eg, headache, malaise, anorexia, and lethargy), abdominal pain, hepatomegaly, splenomegaly, dactylitis, and rose spots (present in approximately 30% of patients). Change in mental status and shock may ensue. Myocarditis or endocarditis occur rarely. In infants and toddlers, invasive infection with enteric fever serovars can manifest as a mild, nondescript febrile illness accompanied by self-limited bacteremia or as an invasive infection in association with more severe clinical symptoms and signs, sustained bacteremia, and meningitis. Diarrhea (resembling pea soup) or constipation can be early features. Gastrointestinal tract bleeding occurs in approximately 10% of hospitalized adults and children with enteric fever. Relative bradycardia (pulse rate slower than would be expected for a given body temperature) has been considered a common feature of typhoid fever in adults but in children is neither a discriminating feature in the assessment of a febrile child from an area where enteric fever is endemic, nor a feature of the disease per se. The propensity to become a chronic *S* Typhi carrier (excretion longer than 1 year) following acute typhoid infection correlates with the prevalence of cholelithiasis, increases with age, and is greater in females than males. Chronic carriage in children is uncommon.

ETIOLOGY: *Salmonella* organisms are gram-negative bacilli that belong to the family *Enterobacteriaceae*. Current taxonomy recognizes 2 *Salmonella* species: *S enterica* with 6 subspecies and *S bongori*. *S enterica* subspecies enterica (also called subspecies I) is responsible for most infections in humans and other warm-blooded animals; the other *S enterica* subspecies and *S bongori* are usually isolated from cold-blooded animals. More than 2600 *Salmonella* serovars have been described. In 2016, the most commonly reported human isolates in the United States were *Salmonella* serovars Enteritidis, Newport, Typhimurium, Javiana, and I 4,[5],12:i:-; these 5 serovars accounted for approximately 45% of all *Salmonella* infections in the United States (**www.cdc.gov/nationalsurveillance/ pdfs/2016-Salmonella-report-508.pdf**). *S* Typhi belongs to O serogroup 9, along with many other common serovars including Enteritidis and Dublin. The relative prevalence of other serovars varies by country.

EPIDEMIOLOGY:

Nontyphoidal* Salmonella *infection. Every year, NTS organisms are among the most common causes of laboratory-confirmed cases of enteric disease reported to the US Foodborne Diseases Active Surveillance Network (**www.cdc.gov/foodnet**). The incidence of NTS infection is highest in children younger than 4 years. In the United States, rates of invasive infections and mortality are higher in infants, elderly people, and people with hemoglobinopathies (including sickle cell disease) and immunocompromising conditions (eg, malignant neoplasms, HIV infection). Most reported cases are sporadic, but widespread outbreaks, including health care-associated and institutional outbreaks, have been reported. The incidence of foodborne cases of NTS gastroenteritis has not changed in recent years (**www.cdc.gov/foodnet/reports/prelim-data-intro-2018.html**).

The principal reservoirs for NTS organisms include birds, mammals, reptiles, and amphibians. The major food vehicles of transmission to humans in industrialized countries include seeded vegetables and other produce, as well as food of animal origin (such as poultry, beef, eggs, and dairy products). Multiple other food vehicles (eg, peanut butter, frozen pot pies, powdered infant formula, cereal, and bakery products) have been implicated in outbreaks in the United States and Europe. Other modes of transmission include ingestion of contaminated water or close contact with infected animals, mainly poultry (eg, chicks, chickens, ducks), reptiles or amphibians (eg, pet turtles, iguanas, geckos, bearded dragons, lizards, snakes, frogs, toads, newts, salamanders), and rodents (eg, hamsters, mice, guinea pigs) or other mammals (eg, hedgehogs). Reptiles and amphibians that live in tanks or aquariums can contaminate the water with bacteria, which can spread to people. Small turtles with a shell length of less than 4 inches are a well-known source of *Salmonella* organisms. Because of this risk, the US Food and Drug Administration (FDA) has banned the interstate sale and distribution of these turtles since 1975. Animal-derived pet foods and treats have been linked to *Salmonella* infections as well, especially in young children.

A risk of transmission of infection to others persists for as long as an infected person sheds NTS organisms. Twelve weeks after infection with the most common NTS serovars, approximately 45% of children younger than 5 years shed organisms, compared with 5% of older children and adults; antimicrobial therapy can prolong shedding. Approximately 1% of adults continue to shed NTS organisms for more than 1 year.

Enteric Fever. Although typhoid fever (approximately 300–400 cases annually) and paratyphoid fever (approximately 100 cases annually) are uncommon in the United States, these infections are highly endemic in many resource-limited countries, particularly in Asia. Consequently, most typhoid fever infections in US residents are acquired during international travel. Unlike NTS serovars, the enteric fever serovars (*S* Typhi, *S* Paratyphi A, *S* Paratyphi B) are restricted to human hosts, in whom they cause both clinical and subclinical infections. Chronic human *S* Typhi carriers (mostly involving chronic infection of the gall bladder but occasionally involving infection of the urinary tract) constitute the long-term reservoir in areas with endemic infection. Infection with enteric fever serovars implies ingestion of a food or water vehicle contaminated by a chronic carrier or person with acute infection.

The **incubation period** for NTS gastroenteritis usually is 6 to 48 hours, but incubation periods of a week or more have been reported. For enteric fever, the **incubation period** usually is 7 to 14 days (range, 3–60 days).

DIAGNOSTIC TESTS: Isolation of *Salmonella* organisms from cultures of stool, blood, urine, bile (including duodenal fluid containing bile), and material from foci of infection is diagnostic. Gastroenteritis is diagnosed by stool culture or molecular testing; stool cultures should be obtained in all children with bloody diarrhea or unexplained persistent or severe diarrhea. Blood and stool cultures (positive in up to 30%) should be obtained for all children who present with unexplained fever after travel to resource poor countries. In addition, blood cultures should be considered for patients at risk of severe illness (eg, age <3 months, those who are immunocompromised or have hemolytic anemia) and in patients with evidence of disseminated infection, septicemia, or enteric fever. Optimum recovery of *Salmonella* from stool is achieved with the use of enrichment broth and multiple selective agar plate media. Definitive identification requires confirmation by phenotypic methods (biochemical profiling), molecular methods such as whole genome sequencing or polymerase chain reaction assays, or mass spectrometry of cellular components and O serogroup determination. Serovar determination is helpful from an epidemiologic perspective and is usually performed at public health laboratories.

Diagnostic tests to detect *Salmonella* antigens by enzyme immunoassay, latex agglutination, and monoclonal antibodies have been developed, as have commercial immunoassays that detect antibodies to antigens of enteric fever serovars. The latter tests are more important in areas of the world where typhoid fever is endemic.

Several multiplex polymerase chain reaction (PCR) platforms for detection of multiple viral, parasitic, and bacterial pathogens, including *Salmonella,* directly in stool have been cleared for diagnostic use by the US Food and Drug Administration (FDA). Laboratories should maintain culture capabilities for *Salmonella* species, because antimicrobial susceptibility testing requires an isolate. In addition, isolates are useful for state public health laboratories to conduct genomic characterization of strains for outbreak detection and investigation.

If enteric fever is suspected, multiple cultures may be needed to isolate the pathogen. Blood, bone marrow, or bile cultures are often diagnostic, because organisms often are absent from stool. The sensitivity of blood culture and bone marrow culture in children with enteric fever is approximately 60% and 90%, respectively. The combination of a single blood culture plus culture of bile (collected from a bile-stained duodenal string) is 90% sensitive in detecting *S* Typhi infection in children with clinical enteric fever. The CDC does not recommend using serologic tests, such as the Widal test, to diagnose acute typhoid because these tests are difficult to interpret in endemic populations and where previous *Salmonella* infection or vaccination may result in a false positive result. Isolate recovery remains important for guiding antimicrobial therapy for enteric fever. Serologic testing may be helpful in identification of chronic carriers in outbreak situations.

TREATMENT:

Nontyphoidal Salmonella *Infection.*

- Antimicrobial therapy usually is not indicated for patients with either asymptomatic infection or uncomplicated gastroenteritis caused by NTS serovars, because therapy does not shorten the duration of diarrheal disease, can prolong duration of fecal shedding, and increases symptomatic relapse rate. Antimicrobial therapy is recommended for gastroenteritis caused by NTS serovars in people at increased risk for invasive disease, including infants younger than 3 months and people with chronic gastrointestinal tract disease, malignant neoplasms, hemoglobinopathies, HIV infection, or other immunosuppressive illnesses or therapies. It should also be considered for those experiencing severe symptoms such as severe diarrhea or prolonged or high fever.
- If antimicrobial therapy is initiated in patients in the United States with presumed or proven NTS gastroenteritis, a blood and a stool culture should be obtained prior to antibiotic administration and an initial dose of ceftriaxone should be given. The patient who does not appear ill or have evidence of disseminated infection can be discharged with oral azithromycin pending blood culture results. Once susceptibilities are available, ampicillin or trimethoprim-sulfamethoxazole may be considered for susceptible strains. A fluoroquinolone is an alternative option. For those who appear ill or have evidence of disseminated infection, hospitalization is required.
- For bacteremia caused by NTS, disseminated disease (meningitis, osteoarticular infection, endocarditis) should be excluded. Blood cultures should be repeated until negative. Initial therapy with ceftriaxone should be given. Transition from intravenous ceftriaxone to oral azithromycin or a fluoroquinolone may be considered after the blood culture has cleared and focal disease has been excluded, for a total 7- to 10-day course.

Specific antimicrobial, route of administration, and duration of therapy will depend on antimicrobial susceptibilities, patient age and other host factors, and clinical response. Aminoglycosides are not recommended for the treatment of any invasive *Salmonella* infections (including those attributable to *S* Typhi) despite in vitro sensitivity of strains, because the clinical effectiveness is poor.

- For meningitis, the duration of treatment should be 4 weeks, and for osteomyelitis or other focal metastatic infections, a duration of 4 to 6 weeks is recommended. Evaluation for underlying immunodeficiency (eg, asplenia, HIV) should be considered.
- Antibiotic-resistant nontyphoidal *Salmonella* strains are increasing. Ciprofloxacin-nonsusceptible strains increased from 2% in 2009 to 8% in 2017 (**www.cdc.gov/ drugresistance/pdf/threats-report/2019-ar-threats-report-508.pdf**).

Enteric Fever.

- Travel history and regional antibiotic resistance patterns should be carefully considered when choosing empiric antibiotic therapy for enteric fever. Most typhoid fever infections diagnosed in the United States are fluoroquinolone nonsusceptible; therefore, clinicians should not use fluoroquinolones as empiric therapy, especially in returning travelers from South Asia.
- Since 2016, in Pakistan, there has been an ongoing large epidemic of extensively drug-resistant (XDR) *S* Typhi with resistance to ceftriaxone, ampicillin, ciprofloxacin, and trimethoprim-sulfamethoxazole (TMP-SMX); isolates are susceptible only to azithromycin and carbapenems.[1] More than 5000 cases of XDR *S* Typhi have been reported in Pakistan since the start of the outbreak, and multiple confirmed cases of XDR typhoid have been documented in travelers returning to the United States and the United Kingdom from Pakistan. Clinicians are advised to check for updates on the outbreak of XDR typhoid fever.
- For enteric fever caused by *S* Typhi that is known or likely to be multidrug resistant (but not XDR), empiric therapy with a parenteral third-generation cephalosporin or azithromycin should be initiated. Drugs of choice, route of administration, and duration of therapy are based on susceptibility of the organism (or inferred susceptibility if this is not available), severity and site of infection, host, and clinical response. The optimal duration of therapy is unclear and depends on the antibiotic used. Most experts would treat for at least 7 to 10 days for people with uncomplicated disease; if amoxicillin or TMP-SMX is considered on the basis of susceptibility testing, a 14-day course of therapy should be considered. Consultation with an expert in infectious diseases may be useful for management of severe and complicated cases.
- Relapse of typhoidal *Salmonella* infection can occur in up to 17% of patients within 4 weeks and is a particular risk for immunocompromised patients, who may require longer duration of treatment as well as retreatment. Relapse rates appear to be lower in those treated with azithromycin than with fluoroquinolones or ceftriaxone.
- The chronic carrier state may be eradicated by 4 weeks of oral therapy with ciprofloxacin or norfloxacin, which are antimicrobial agents that are highly concentrated in bile. High-dose parenteral ampicillin also can be used if 4 weeks of oral fluoroquinolone therapy is not well tolerated and if the strain is susceptible. Cholecystectomy followed

---

[1] François Watkins LK, Winstead A, Appiah GD, et al. Update on extensively drug-resistant *Salmonella* serotype Typhi infections among travelers to or from Pakistan and report of ceftriaxone-resistant *Salmonella* serotype Typhi infections among travelers to Iraq—United States, 2018–2019. *MMWR Morb Mortal Wkly Rep*. 2020;69(20):618–622. DOI: **http://dx.doi.org/10.15585/mmwr.mm6920a2external icon**

by another course of antimicrobial agents may be indicated in some adults if antimicrobial therapy alone fails.

- Corticosteroids may be beneficial in children with severe enteric fever, which is characterized by delirium, obtundation, stupor, coma, or shock. These drugs should be reserved for critically ill patients in whom relief of manifestations of toxemia may be lifesaving. The usual regimen is high-dose dexamethasone, administered intravenously at an initial dose of 3 mg/kg, followed by 1 mg/kg, every 6 hours, for a total course of 48 hours.

- For enteric fever caused by *S* Typhi acquired from overseas travel, a stool culture should be performed on all people who traveled with the index case(s). If results are positive, treatment should be initiated with azithromycin or a fluoroquinolone and the patient should be monitored for development of any symptoms. Asymptomatic people in the United States who had contact with the index case(s) but did not travel overseas with them, should be evaluated on a case by case basis to determine necessity for culture of stool samples.

ISOLATION OF THE HOSPITALIZED PATIENT: In addition to standard precautions, contact precautions should be used for diapered and incontinent children for the duration of illness. In children with enteric fever, precautions should be continued until culture results are negative for 3 consecutive stool specimens obtained at least 48 hours after cessation of antimicrobial therapy. For XDR typhoid, contact precautions should be used throughout hospital stay, as per guidelines for multidrug-resistant organisms.

CONTROL MEASURES: Important measures include proper food hygiene practices; treated water supplies; proper hand hygiene; adequate sanitation to dispose of human fecal waste; exclusion of infected people from handling food or providing health care; education on the risk of *Salmonella* infections from animal contact; prohibiting the sale of pet turtles; limiting exposure of children younger than 5 years and immunocompromised children to reptiles, amphibians, live poultry, and rodents at home, at school, and in child care and public settings (see Diseases Transmitted by Animals [Zoonoses], p 1048); reporting cases to appropriate health authorities; and investigating outbreaks. Eggs and other foods of animal origin should be cooked thoroughly. People should not eat raw eggs or foods containing raw eggs or consume unpasteurized milk or raw milk products.[1] Notification of public health authorities, sending isolates (or specimens), and determination of serovar are of primary importance in detection and investigation of outbreaks.

Child Care. Outbreaks of *Salmonella* illness in child care centers are rare. Specific strategies for controlling infection in out-of-home child care involve adherence to hygiene practices, including meticulous hand hygiene, and limiting exposure to certain animals. Animals at higher risk of causing salmonellosis, including reptiles, amphibians, and poultry, are not recommended in schools, child care settings, hospitals, or nursing homes (see Children in Group Child Care and Schools, p 116).

When NTS serovars are identified in a symptomatic child care attendee or staff member with enterocolitis, older children and staff members do not need to be excluded unless they are symptomatic. Stool cultures are not required for asymptomatic contacts.

---

[1]American Academy of Pediatrics, Committee on Infectious Diseases and Committee on Nutrition. Consumption of raw or unpasteurized milk and milk products by pregnant women and children. *Pediatrics.* 2014;133(1):175-179 (Reaffirmed November 2019)

Likewise, children or staff members with NTS enterocolitis do not require negative culture results from stool samples; children can return to child care facilities if stools are contained in the diaper or when toilet-trained children are continent and when stool frequency becomes no more than 2 stools above that child's normal frequency for the time the child is in the program, even if the stools remain loose (see Children in Group Child Care and Schools, p 116).

When *S* Typhi infection is identified in a child care staff member, local or state health departments should be consulted regarding regulations for length of exclusion and testing, which may vary by jurisdiction. In general, because infections with *S* Typhi or *S* Paratyphi A, *S* Paratyphi B, or *S* Paratyphi C are transmitted easily and can be severe, exclusion of an infected child is warranted at least until negative results for 3 stool samples obtained at least 48 hours after cessation of antimicrobial therapy for *S* Typhi or *S* Paratyphi (see Children in Group Child Care and Schools, p 116).

Typhoid Vaccine. Protection against *S* Typhi is enhanced by typhoid immunization, but currently licensed vaccines do not provide complete protection. Two typhoid vaccines are licensed for use in the United States (see Table 3.52), one for use in people 6 years and older and the other in people 2 years and older.

The demonstrated efficacy of the 2 vaccines licensed by the FDA ranges from 50% to 80%, but the duration of protection differs notably between the vaccines. Vaccine is selected on the basis of age of the child, need for booster doses, and possible contraindications (see Precautions and Contraindications, p 663) and reactions (see Adverse Events, p 662).

Recommended Use. In the United States, immunization is recommended only for the following people:

- **Travelers to areas where risk of exposure to *S* Typhi is recognized.** Risk is greatest for travelers to the Indian subcontinent, South and Southeast Asia, Latin America, the Caribbean, the Middle East, and Africa who may have prolonged exposure to contaminated food and drink. Such travelers need to be cautioned that typhoid vaccine is not a substitute for careful selection of food and drink (see **www.cdc.gov/travel**).
- **People with intimate exposure to a documented typhoid fever carrier,** as occurs with continued household contact.
- **Laboratory workers with frequent contact with *S* Typhi.**

Dosages. For primary immunization, the following dosage is recommended for each vaccine:

Table 3.52. Commercially Available Typhoid Vaccines in the United States

Typhoid Vaccine	Type	Route	Minimum Age of Receipt, y	No. of Doses[a]	Booster Frequency, y
Ty21a	Live attenuated	Oral	6	4	5
ViCPS	Polysaccharide	Intramuscular	2	1	2

ViCPS indicates Vi capsular polysaccharide vaccine.

[a] Primary immunization. For further information on dosage, schedules, and adverse events, see text.

- **Typhoid vaccine live oral Ty21a (Vivotif [Crucell Switzerland LTD).** Children (6 years and older) and adults should take 1 enteric-coated capsule every other day for a total of 4 capsules. Each capsule should be swallowed whole (not chewed) with liquid, no warmer than 37°C (98°F), approximately 1 hour before a meal. The capsules should be kept refrigerated, and all 4 doses must be taken to achieve maximal efficacy. Immunization should be completed at least 1 week before possible exposure. Note that in December 2020, the manufacturer of Ty21a temporarily stopped making and selling it; this vaccine may be in limited supply or unavailable.
- **Typhoid Vi polysaccharide vaccine (Typhim Vi [Sanofi Pasteur]).** Primary immunization of people 2 years and older with unconjugated Vi capsular polysaccharide (ViCPS) vaccine consists of one 0.5-mL (25-μg) dose administered intramuscularly. Vaccine should be administered at least 2 weeks before possible exposure.
- **Vi conjugate vaccine (not available in the United States).** A new typhoid conjugate vaccine that consists of the Vi capsular polysaccharide of *S* Typhi linked to tetanus toxoid protein is manufactured and licensed in India (Typbar-TCV, Bharat Biotech International, Hyderabad, India), has been prequalified by the World Health Organization (WHO). The vaccine has been recommended by the WHO Scientific Advisory Group of Experts for use in infants as young as 6 months of age, based on results of clinical trials establishing its tolerability and immunogenicity in children 6 through 23 months of age, as well as in older children and adults. The vaccine is administered as a single dose, provides greater protection against typhoid fever than the other available vaccines, and serum IgG Vi antibody appears to endure for several years among children living in areas with endemic infection. Typbar-TCV is not licensed in the United States. However, if families with children younger than 2 years of age are traveling to live in areas of South Asia where XDR *S* Typhi is circulating, parents of infants and toddlers can be advised to contact local pediatricians to have their young children vaccinated with this vaccine. It is widely available in India and available in Pakistan in parts of Sindh Province, the center of the XDR *S* Typhi outbreak.
- **Protection against *S* Paratyphi A and *S* Paratyphi B.** Neither Ty21a nor ViCPS vaccine provides reliable protection against *S* Paratyphi A. Results of 2 field trials suggest that Ty21a may provide partial cross-protection against *S* Paratyphi B.

Booster Doses. In circumstances of continued or repeated exposure to *S* Typhi, periodic reimmunization is recommended to maintain immunity.

Continued efficacy for 7 years after immunization with the oral Ty21a vaccine has been demonstrated; however, the manufacturer of oral Ty21a vaccine recommends reimmunization (completing the entire 4-dose series) every 5 years if continued or renewed exposure to *S* Typhi is expected.

ViCPS vaccine elicits a T-independent antigen response that does not create immunologic memory to allow boosting of serum Vi antibody titers following an initial immunization. The manufacturer of ViCPS vaccine recommends reimmunization every 2 years if continued or renewed exposure is expected.

Oral Ty21a (which does not express Vi antigen) and ViCPS (which protects by stimulating serum IgG Vi antibody) vaccines mediate protection by distinct mechanisms. No data have been reported concerning use of one vaccine administered after primary immunization with the other.

Adverse Events. The oral Ty21a vaccine is very well tolerated, but mild adverse reactions may occur; these include abdominal pain, nausea, diarrhea, vomiting, fever, headache, and rash or urticaria. Reported adverse reactions to ViCPS vaccine also are minimal and include fever, headache, malaise, myalgia, and local reaction of tenderness and pain, erythema, or induration of 1 cm or greater.

Precautions and Contraindications. A contraindication to administration of intramuscular ViCPS vaccine is a history of hypersensitivity to any component of the vaccine. No safety data have been reported for typhoid vaccines in pregnant women. The oral Ty21a vaccine is a live attenuated vaccine and should not be administered to immunocompromised people, including people known to be infected with HIV; to have a phagocytic cell defect; or to have chronic granulomatous disease;[1] the intramuscular ViCPS vaccine may be an alternative, although the expected immune response may not be achieved. The oral Ty21a vaccine should not be administered during acute febrile illness or gastrointestinal tract illness. Antimalarial drugs mefloquine and chloroquine and the combination antimalarials atovaquone/proguanil and pyrimethamine/sulfadoxine, at doses used for prophylaxis, can be administered with the Ty21a vaccine. The manufacturer advises that other antimalarial agents be administered at least 3 days after the last dose of Ty21a vaccine (**www.cdc.gov/mmwr/preview/mmwrhtml/mm6411a4.htm**). Antimicrobial agents should be avoided for 3 days before the first dose of oral Ty21a vaccine and 3 days after the last dose of Ty21a vaccine.

Scabies

CLINICAL MANIFESTATIONS: Scabies is characterized by an intensely pruritic, erythematous eruption that may include papules, nodules, vesicles, or bullae that is caused by burrowing of adult female mites in upper layers of the epidermis, creating serpiginous burrows. Itching is most intense at night. In older children and adults, the sites of predilection are interdigital folds, flexor aspects of wrists, extensor surfaces of elbows, anterior axillary folds, waistline, thighs, navel, genitalia, areolae, abdomen, intergluteal cleft, and buttocks. In children younger than 2 years, the eruption more often is vesicular and often occurs in areas usually spared in older children and adults, such as the scalp, face, neck, palms, and soles. The eruption is caused by a hypersensitivity reaction to proteins of the parasite.

Characteristic scabietic burrows appear as thin, gray or white, serpiginous, thread-like lines. Excoriations are common, and most burrows are obliterated by scratching before a patient seeks medical attention. Occasionally, 2- to 5-mm red-brown nodules are present, particularly on covered parts of the body, such as the genitalia, groin, and axilla. These scabies nodules are a granulomatous response to dead mite antigens and feces; the nodules can persist for weeks and even months after effective treatment. Cutaneous secondary bacterial infection is a frequent complication and usually is caused by *Streptococcus pyogenes* or *Staphylococcus aureus*. Studies have demonstrated a rare correlation between scabies and development of poststreptococcal glomerulonephritis.

Crusted (formerly called Norwegian) scabies is an uncommon clinical syndrome characterized by a large number of mites and widespread, crusted, hyperkeratotic lesions. Crusted scabies usually occurs in people with debilitating conditions, people with developmental disabilities, or people who are immunocompromised, including patients receiving biologic response modifiers. Crusted scabies also can occur in otherwise healthy children after long-term use of topical corticosteroid therapy.

---

[1]Rubin LG, Levin MJ, Ljungman P, et al. 2013 IDSA clinical practice guideline for vaccination of the immunocompromised host. *Clin Infect Dis.* 2014;58(3):e44-e100

Postscabietic pustulosis is a reactive phenomenon that may follow successful treatment of primary infestation with scabies. Affected infants and young children manifest episodic crops of sterile, pruritic papules, and pustules predominantly in an acral distribution, but lesions may extend to a lesser degree onto the torso.

ETIOLOGY: The mite *Sarcoptes scabiei* subspecies *hominis* is the cause of scabies. The adult female burrows in the stratum corneum of the skin and lays eggs. Larvae emerge from the eggs in 2 to 4 days and molt to nymphs and then to adults, which mate and produce new eggs. The entire cycle takes approximately 10 to 17 days. *S scabiei* subspecies *canis,* acquired from dogs with clinical mange, can cause a self-limited and mild infestation in humans, usually involving the area in direct contact with the infested animal.

EPIDEMIOLOGY: Humans are the source of infestation. Transmission usually occurs through prolonged close, personal contact. Even minimal contact with patients with crusted scabies or their immediate environment can result in transmission because of the large number of mites in exfoliating scales. Infestation acquired from dogs and other animals is uncommon, and these mites do not replicate in humans. Scabies of human origin can be transmitted as long as the patient remains infested and untreated, including during the interval before symptoms develop. Scabies is endemic in many countries and occurs worldwide sporadically and in epidemics, which may be cyclical in some settings. Scabies affects people from all socioeconomic levels without regard to age, gender, or standards of personal hygiene. Scabies in adults may be acquired sexually.[1]

The **incubation period** in people without previous exposure usually is 4 to 6 weeks. People who previously were infested are sensitized and develop symptoms 1 to 4 days after repeated infestation with the mite; these reinfestations usually are milder than the original episode.

DIAGNOSTIC TESTS: Diagnosis of scabies typically is made by clinical examination. Diagnosis can be confirmed by identification of the mite, mite eggs, or scybala (feces) from scrapings of papules or intact burrows, preferably from the terminal portion where the mite generally is found. Mineral oil, microscope immersion oil, or water applied to skin facilitates collection of scrapings. A broad-blade scalpel is used to scrape the burrow. Scrapings and oil can be placed on a slide under a glass coverslip and examined microscopically under low power. Adult female mites average 330 to 450 μm in length. Skin scrapings provide definitive evidence of infestation but have low sensitivity. Handheld dermoscopy (epiluminescence microscopy) has been used to identify in vivo the pigmented mite parts or air bubbles corresponding to infesting mites within the stratum corneum. Reflectance in vivo microscopy and polymerase chain reaction assays on swabbed skin material are promising techniques with improved sensitivity and specificity.

TREATMENT: Topical permethrin 5% cream or off-label use of oral ivermectin both are effective agents for treatment of scabies (see Drugs for Parasitic Infections, p 983). Most experts recommend starting with topical 5% permethrin cream as the drug of choice, particularly for infants (not approved for infants younger than 2 months), young children, and pregnant or nursing women. Permethrin cream should be removed by bathing after 8 to 14 hours. Children and adults with infestation should apply lotion or cream containing this scabicide over their entire body below the head. Permethrin kills the scabies mite and eggs. Two (or more) applications, each about a week apart, may be necessary to eliminate

[1] Centers for Disease Control and Prevention. Sexually transmitted infections treatment guidelines, 2021. *MMWR Recomm Rep.* 2021; in press

all mites. Because scabies can affect the face, scalp, and neck in infants and young children, treatment of the entire head, neck, and body in this age group is required. Special attention should be given to trimming fingernails and ensuring application of medication to these areas.

A Cochrane review found that oral ivermectin is as effective as topical permethrin for treating scabies. Because ivermectin is not ovicidal, it is given as 2 doses, 7 to 14 days apart. Ivermectin is not approved for treatment of scabies by the US Food and Drug Administration (FDA). Oral ivermectin should be considered for patients who have failed treatment or who cannot tolerate FDA-approved topical medications for the treatment of scabies. The safety of ivermectin in children weighing less than 15 kg and in pregnant women has not been established.

Alternative drugs include 10% crotamiton cream or lotion (not FDA approved for children) or 5% to 10% precipitated sulfur compounded into petrolatum. Lindane lotion generally should not be used for treatment of scabies because of safety concerns and availability of other treatments but may be used if all other medications cannot be tolerated or have failed.

Because scabietic lesions are the result of a hypersensitivity reaction to the mite, itching may not subside for several weeks despite successful treatment. The use of oral antihistamines and topical corticosteroids can help relieve this itching. Topical or systemic antimicrobial therapy is indicated for secondary bacterial infections of excoriated lesions.

ISOLATION OF THE HOSPITALIZED PATIENT: In addition to standard precautions, contact precautions are recommended until the patient has been treated with an appropriate scabicide.

CONTROL MEASURES:

- Most experts recommend prophylactic therapy for household members, particularly those who have had prolonged direct skin-to-skin contact. Manifestations of scabies infestation can appear as late as 2 months after exposure, during which time the mite can be transmitted. Household members should be treated at the same time to prevent reinfestation. Bedding and clothing worn next to the skin during the 3 days before initiation of therapy should be laundered in a washer with hot water and dried using a hot cycle. Mites do not survive more than 3 days without skin contact. Clothing that cannot be laundered should be removed from the patient and stored for several days to a week to avoid reinfestation.
- Children should be treated at the end of the program day and allowed to return to child care or school after the first course of treatment has been completed. Children should not be excluded or sent home early from school because of scabies (see Table 2.3, p 128).
- Epidemics and localized outbreaks may require stringent and consistent measures to treat contacts. Health care workers and other caregivers who have had prolonged skin-to-skin contact with patients with infestation may benefit from prophylactic treatment.
- Environmental disinfestation is unnecessary and unwarranted. Thorough vacuuming of environmental surfaces is recommended after use of a room by a patient with non-crusted scabies.
- People with crusted scabies and their close contacts must be treated promptly and aggressively to avoid outbreaks. Information about environmental disinfection for crusted scabies is available from the Centers for Disease Control and Prevention (**www. cdc.gov/parasites/scabies/health_professionals/crusted.html**).

Schistosomiasis

CLINICAL MANIFESTATIONS: Schistosomiasis (bilharzia) is established by skin penetration of infecting larvae (cercariae, shed by freshwater snails). Initial infections often are asymptomatic. Skin manifestations include pruritus at the penetration site a few hours after water exposure, followed in 5 to 14 days by an intermittent pruritic, sometimes papular, eruption. More intense papular eruptions may occur more quickly and last for 7 to 10 days after exposure in people sensitized previously. Cercarial dermatitis (swimmer's itch) also can be caused by larvae of schistosome parasites of birds or other wildlife. These larvae can penetrate human skin but eventually die in the dermis and do not cause systemic disease.

Parasites capable of causing intestinal and urogenital schistosomiasis enter the bloodstream after penetration of the skin, migrate through the lungs, and eventually mature into adult worms that reside in the venous plexus that drains the intestines or, in the case of *Schistosoma haematobium*, the urogenital tract. Four to 8 weeks after exposure, worms develop into adults and females begin egg deposition, which can lead to an acute serum sickness-like illness (Katayama syndrome) that manifests as fever, malaise, cough, rash, abdominal pain, hepatosplenomegaly, diarrhea, nausea, lymphadenopathy, and eosinophilia. This syndrome is most common among nonimmune hosts, such as travelers. Severity of symptoms associated with chronic infection is related to worm burden. People with low to moderate worm burdens may have only subclinical disease or relatively mild manifestations, such as growth stunting or anemia. Higher worm burdens are associated with a range of symptoms primarily caused by inflammation and local fibrosis triggered by the immune response to eggs produced by adult worms. Severe forms of chronic intestinal schistosomiasis (*Schistosoma mansoni* and *Schistosoma japonicum* infections) can result in hepatosplenomegaly, abdominal pain, bloody diarrhea, portal hypertension, ascites, esophageal varices, and hematemesis. Urogenital schistosomiasis (*S haematobium* infections) can result in the bladder becoming inflamed and fibrotic. Urinary tract symptoms and signs include dysuria, urgency, terminal microscopic and gross hematuria, secondary urinary tract infections, hydronephrosis, and nonspecific pelvic pain. *S haematobium* is associated with lesions of the lower genital tract (vulva, vagina, and cervix) in women, prostatitis and hematospermia in men, and certain forms of bladder cancer. Other organ systems can be involved—for example, eggs can embolize to the lungs, causing pulmonary hypertension. Less commonly, eggs can lodge in the central nervous system, causing severe neurologic complications.

ETIOLOGY: The trematodes (flukes) *S mansoni, S japonicum, Schistosoma mekongi, Schistosoma guineensis,* and *Schistosoma intercalatum* cause intestinal schistosomiasis, and *S haematobium* causes urogenital disease. All species have similar life cycles.

EPIDEMIOLOGY: Persistence of schistosomiasis depends on presence of an appropriate snail as an intermediate host. Eggs excreted in stool (*S mansoni, S japonicum, S mekongi, S intercalatum,* and *S guineensis*) or urine *(S haematobium)* into fresh water hatch into motile miracidia, which infect snails. After development and asexual replication in snails, cercariae emerge and penetrate the skin of humans in contact with water. In areas with endemic schistosomiasis, children are infected first when they accompany their mothers to lakes, ponds, and other open fresh water sources. School-aged children typically are the most heavily infected people in the community because of prolonged wading and swimming in infected waters. Children have greater susceptibility to infection than older people because of a lack of high preexisting immunity to these parasites and are important in maintaining transmission through behaviors such as uncontrolled defecation and urination. Animals play an important zoonotic role (as a source of eggs) in maintaining the life cycle of *S japonicum*. Infection is not transmissible by person-to-person contact or blood transfusion.

The distribution of schistosomiasis is focal and limited by the presence of appropriate snail vectors, infected human reservoirs, and fresh water sources. *S mansoni* occurs throughout tropical Africa, in parts of several Caribbean islands, and in areas of Venezuela, Brazil, Suriname, and the Arabian Peninsula. *S japonicum* is found in China, the Philippines, and Indonesia. *S haematobium* occurs in Africa and the Middle East; in 2014, local transmission was reported in Corsica. *S mekongi* is found in Cambodia and Laos. *S intercalatum* is found in Central Africa, and *S guineensis* in West Africa. Adult worms of *S mansoni* usually survive for 5 to 7 years but can live as long as 30 years in the human host. Schistosomiasis can be diagnosed in patients many years after they have left an area with endemic transmission. Immunity is incomplete, and reinfection occurs commonly. Swimmer's itch can occur in all regions of the world after exposure to fresh water, brackish water, or salt water.

The **incubation period** is variable but is approximately 4 to 6 weeks for *S japonicum*, 6 to 8 weeks for *S mansoni*, and 10 to 12 weeks for *S haematobium*.

DIAGNOSTIC TESTS: Eosinophilia is common and may be intense in Katayama syndrome (acute schistosomiasis). Infection with *S mansoni* and other intestinal species is diagnosed by microscopic examination of stool specimens to detect characteristic eggs containing fully differentiated larvae, but results may be negative if performed too early in the course of infection. In light infections, several stool specimens examined by a concentration technique may be needed before eggs are found, or eggs may be seen in a biopsy of the rectal mucosa. *S haematobium* is diagnosed by examining urine for eggs; filtration or centrifugation and examination of the urinary sediment is required for optimum sensitivity. Egg excretion in urine often peaks between noon and 3 pm. Biopsy of the bladder mucosa may be used to diagnose *S haematobium* infection. Urine reagent dipsticks commonly will be positive for blood. Serologic tests, available through the Centers for Disease Control and Prevention and some commercial laboratories, may be helpful for detecting light infections; results of these antibody-based tests remain positive for many years and are not useful in differentiating ongoing infection from past infection or reinfection. Serologic test results are negative during acute infection, turn positive 6 to 12 weeks or more after infection, and may be positive before eggs are detectable. Polymerase chain reaction and antigen tests for detection of schistosomes have been developed but are considered to be research tools at present.

Swimmer's itch, which is caused by the cercariae of certain schistosome species whose normal hosts are birds and nonhuman mammals, can be difficult to differentiate from other causes of dermatitis. A skin biopsy may demonstrate larvae, but their absence does not exclude the diagnosis. A history of exposure to water used by waterfowl may be helpful in making the diagnosis.

TREATMENT: The drug of choice for schistosomiasis caused by any species is praziquantel (see Drugs for Parasitic Infections, p 983). The alternative drug for *S mansoni* is oxamniquine, although this drug no longer is available in the United States. Optimal timing of treatment after known exposures is uncertain, but it is reasonable to give treatment with praziquantel within 6 to 8 weeks of exposure. Praziquantel does not kill developing worms so treatment administered early (eg, 4 to 8 weeks after exposure) should be repeated 2 to 4 weeks later to improve parasitologic cure. Initial management of acute schistosomiasis and neuroschistosomiasis includes reduction of inflammation with steroids, although optimal dose and duration are uncertain. Initial treatment with praziquantel may exacerbate symptoms. The optimal timing of adding praziquantel is unknown; treating with this drug when inflammation has subsided generally is favored. Swimmer's itch is a self-limited disease that may require symptomatic treatment of the rash. More intense reactions may require a course of oral corticosteroids.

ISOLATION OF THE HOSPITALIZED PATIENT: Standard precautions are recommended. Schistosomiasis cannot be transmitted from person to person or by the fecal-oral route.

CONTROL MEASURES: Elimination of the intermediate snail host is difficult to achieve in most areas. Mass or selective treatment of infected populations, sanitary disposal of human waste, water sanitation programs, and education about the source of infection are key elements of current control measures. Travelers to areas with endemic schistosomiasis should be advised to avoid any contact with freshwater streams, rivers, ponds, or lakes. Swimming and wading should occur only in chlorinated pools. Human schistosomiasis is not transmitted in sea water.

Shigella Infections

CLINICAL MANIFESTATIONS: *Shigella* species primarily infect the large intestine, causing clinical manifestations that range from watery or loose stools with minimal or no constitutional symptoms to more severe symptoms, including high fever, abdominal cramps or tenderness, tenesmus, and mucoid stools with or without blood. *Shigella dysenteriae* serotype 1 often causes a more severe illness than other *Shigella* species, with a higher risk of complications, including septicemia, pseudomembranous colitis, toxic megacolon, intestinal perforation, hemolysis, and hemolytic-uremic syndrome (HUS). Infection attributable to *S dysenteriae* serotype 1 has become rare in industrialized countries. Generalized seizures have been reported among young children with shigellosis attributable to any serotype; although the pathophysiology and incidence are poorly understood, such seizures usually are self-limited and usually are associated with high fever or electrolyte abnormalities. Septicemia is rare during the course of illness and is caused either by *Shigella* organisms or by other gut flora that gain access to the bloodstream through intestinal mucosa damaged during shigellosis. Septicemia occurs most often in neonates, malnourished children, and people with *S dysenteriae* serotype 1 infection but may occur in healthy children with non-*S dysenteriae* shigellosis. Reactive arthritis with possible extraarticular manifestations is a rare complication that can develop weeks or months after shigellosis, especially in patients expressing HLA-B27. Postinfectious irritable bowel syndrome can occur and last weeks to months.

ETIOLOGY: *Shigella* species are facultative aerobic, gram-negative bacilli in the family *Enterobacteriaceae*. Four species (with more than 40 serotypes) have been identified, with *Shigella sonnei* being most common in the United States. The other species are *Shigella flexneri*, *S dysenteriae*, and *Shigella boydii*. In resource-limited countries, especially in Africa and Asia, *S flexneri* predominates, and *S dysenteriae* serotype 1 often causes outbreaks. Shiga toxin, a potent cytotoxin produced by *S dysenteriae* serotype 1, enhances the virulence of this serotype at the colonic mucosa and can cause small blood vessel and renal damage, leading to HUS in some individuals. The Shiga toxin genes are phage-encoded and have been found in a small number of strains belonging to other *Shigella* species and serotypes, including *S flexneri* serotype 2a, *S dysenteriae* serotype 4, and *S sonnei*. HUS has been associated with an infection attributable to *S sonnei* in an adult, although the non-*S dysenteriae* species are not commonly associated with HUS.

EPIDEMIOLOGY: Humans are the natural host for *Shigella* organisms. Whereas the primary mode of transmission is the fecal-oral route, transmission also can occur via contact with a contaminated inanimate object, ingestion of contaminated food or water, or sexual contact. Houseflies and cockroaches also may be vectors through physical transport of infected feces. Ingestion of as few as 10 organisms, depending on the species, is sufficient for infection to occur. Prolonged organism survival in water (up to 6 months) and food (up to 30 days) can occur with *Shigella* species. Children 5 years or younger in child care settings and their caregivers and people living in crowded conditions are at increased risk of infection. Men who have sex with men also are at increased risk of shigellosis, including infections with multidrug-resistant strains. Infections attributable to *S flexneri*, *S boydii*, and *S dysenteriae* are slightly more common among adults than among children. Travel to resource-limited countries with inadequate sanitation can place travelers at risk of infection. Even without antimicrobial therapy, the carrier state usually ceases within 1 to 4 weeks after onset of illness; long-term carriage is uncommon and does not correlate with underlying intestinal dysfunction.

Antibiotic resistance is increasing among *Shigella* isolates. From 1999–2015, 59% of 7391 *Shigella* isolates in the United States were resistant to ampicillin, 43% were resistant to trimethoprim-sulfamethoxazole, 3% were resistant to amoxicillin-clavulanate, <1% were resistant to ciprofloxacin, and <0.3% were resistant to ceftriaxone. From 2011–2015, 6% of 2085 isolates demonstrated decreased susceptibility to azithromycin (**wwwn.cdc. gov/narmsnow**). By 2017, 10% of *Shigella* isolates were resistant to ciprofloxacin and 24% had decreased susceptibility to azithromycin (**www.cdc.gov/drugresistance/ pdf/threats-report/2019-ar-threats-report-508.pdf**). The Centers for Disease Control and Prevention (CDC) has been monitoring *Shigella* isolates that harbor one or more quinolone resistance mechanisms (ie, those with a minimum inhibitory concentration [MIC] of ≥ 0.12 µg/mL for ciprofloxacin) but that have in vitro susceptibility to fluoroquinolones (**https://emergency.cdc.gov/han/han00411.asp**). Additional data are needed to determine whether fluoroquinolone treatment outcomes and risk of illness transmission are affected in patients with such isolates. Data from the National Antimicrobial Resistance Monitoring System (NARMS) indicate that many *Shigella* isolates with a quinolone resistance mechanism are nonsusceptible or resistant to many other commonly used treatment agents, such as azithromycin, trimethoprim-sulfamethoxazole, amoxicillin-clavulanic acid, and ampicillin. In addition, clinical laboratories are often unable to perform azithromycin susceptibility testing for *Shigella* organisms, because breakpoints have not been established for azithromycin. In June 2018, the CDC requested that clinicians monitor and report possible clinical treatment failures when treating with fluoroquinolones or azithromycin to state or local health departments and that clinicians obtain an isolate for susceptibility testing and consider infectious disease consultation (**https://emergency.cdc.gov/han/han00411.asp**).

The **incubation period** varies from 1 to 7 days but typically is 1 to 3 days.

DIAGNOSTIC TESTS: Isolation of *Shigella* organisms from feces or rectal swab specimens containing feces is diagnostic; sensitivity is improved by testing stool as soon as possible after it is passed, along with the use of enrichment broth media and selective agar plate media. If specimens cannot be transported to the testing laboratory within 2 hours, they should be transferred to appropriate transport media (eg, Cary-Blair or similar media) and kept and transported at 4°C. Definitive identification of the organism requires both biochemical profiling and serogrouping to differentiate *Shigella* from *Escherichia* species. Identification by mass spectrometry of cellular components should not be used, because this method cannot distinguish between the 2 genera. The presence of fecal lactoferrin (or fecal leukocytes) demonstrated on a methylene-blue stained stool smear is fairly sensitive for the diagnosis of colitis but is not specific for shigellosis. Although bacteremia is rare, blood should be cultured in severely ill, immunocompromised, or malnourished children. Multiplex polymerase chain reaction (PCR) platforms for detection of multiple bacterial (including *Shigella*), viral, and parasitic pathogens have high sensitivity but PCR will not distinguish between viable and nonviable organisms. To guide treatment, if needed, and to enable surveillance and outbreak detection, stool cultures are recommended if shigellosis is diagnosed using multiplex PCR platforms or other nonculture-based diagnostic tests. Other tests for bacterial detection, including qualitative and quantitative PCR assays, are available in research laboratories and some clinical laboratories. Isolates of *Shigella* species (or clinical specimens from positive nonculture diagnostic tests, if reflex culturing is not possible) should be submitted as required to local or state public health laboratories.

TREATMENT:

- Although severe dehydration is rare with shigellosis, correction of fluid and electrolyte losses, preferably by oral rehydration solutions, is the mainstay of treatment.
- Most clinical infections with *S sonnei* are self-limited (48 to 72 hours), and mild episodes do not require antimicrobial therapy.
- Antimicrobial treatment is recommended for patients with severe disease or with underlying immunosuppressive conditions; in these patients, empiric therapy should be given while awaiting culture and susceptibility results. Available evidence suggests that antimicrobial therapy is somewhat effective in shortening duration of diarrhea and in hastening eradication of organisms from feces; however, whether antimicrobial treatment reduces transmission is unclear.
- Antimicrobial susceptibility testing of clinical isolates is indicated to guide therapy, because resistance to antimicrobial agents is common and increasing. *Shigella* strains with decreased susceptibility to azithromycin and resistance to ciprofloxacin have been reported in the United States. Ceftriaxone resistance has been reported recently, although it is still relatively uncommon in the United States. For cases in which antibiotic treatment is required, oral administration is recommended, except for seriously ill patients. First-line therapy should consist of one of the following antibiotics:
  - A fluoroquinolone (eg, ciprofloxacin) for 3 days. Fluoroquinolones should be avoided if the *Shigella* strain has an MIC of ≥0.12 µg/mL for ciprofloxacin, even if the laboratory indicates that the isolate is "susceptible," until more is known about the clinical outcomes of ciprofloxacin treatment when MICs are ≥0.12 µg/mL.
  - Azithromycin for 3 days. Clinical laboratories are often unable to perform azithromycin susceptibilities for *Shigella* species, because the clinical breakpoints have not been established.
  - Parenteral ceftriaxone for 2 to 5 days. Oral cephalosporins (eg, cefixime) are of unclear efficacy.

♦ For susceptible strains, oral ampicillin or trimethoprim-sulfamethoxazole for 5 days are alternative options; amoxicillin is not effective because of its rapid absorption from the gastrointestinal tract.

- Antidiarrheal compounds that inhibit intestinal peristalsis are contraindicated, because they can prolong the clinical and bacteriologic course of disease and can increase the rate of complications.
- Nutritional supplementation, including vitamin A (200 000 IU) and zinc (elemental Zn, orally daily for 10–14 days, 10 mg/day for newborn infants to 6 months of age, and 20 mg/day for those older than 6 months), can be given to hasten clinical resolution in geographic areas where children are at risk of malnutrition.

ISOLATION OF THE HOSPITALIZED PATIENT: In addition to standard precautions, contact precautions are indicated for the duration of illness.

CONTROL MEASURES:

Child Care Centers. General measures for interrupting enteric transmission in child care centers are recommended (see Children in Group Child Care and Schools, p 116). Meticulous hand hygiene is the single most important measure to decrease transmission. Waterless hand sanitizers may be effective as an adjunct to washing with soap and water when access to soap or clean water is limited. Eliminating access to shared water-play areas and contaminated diapers also can decrease infection rates. Child care staff members should follow all standard infection control recommendations, specifically enhancing hand hygiene and ensuring that those who change diapers are not responsible for food preparation.

When *Shigella* infection is identified in a child care attendee or staff member, stool specimens from symptomatic attendees and staff members should be obtained. The local health department should be notified to evaluate and manage potential outbreaks. Infected people should be excluded until the state or local health department has deemed it safe to return to work per state or local child care exclusion regulations. Following this, children can return to child care facilities if stools are contained in the diaper or when toilet-trained children are continent and when stool frequency becomes no more than 2 stools above that child's normal baseline for the time the child is in the program, even if the stools remain loose (see Table 2.3, p 128).

Institutional Outbreaks. The outbreaks that are most difficult to control are those that involve children not yet or only recently toilet-trained, adults who are unable to care for themselves (cognitively impaired people or skilled nursing facility residents), or an inadequate supply of chlorinated water. A strong emphasis on hand hygiene, a cohort system and appropriate antimicrobial therapy should be considered until stool cultures no longer yield *Shigella* species. In residential institutions, ill people and newly admitted and well individuals should be housed in separate areas.

General Control Measures. Strict attention to hand hygiene is essential to limit spread. Other important control measures include improved sanitation, appropriately chlorinating the water supply, proper cooking and storage of food, excluding infected people such as food handlers and child care providers, ensuring safe diapering practices, and measures to decrease contamination of food and surfaces by houseflies. People should refrain from recreational water venues (eg, swimming pools, water parks) while they have diarrhea, and those who are incontinent should continue to avoid recreational water activities for at least 1 additional week after symptoms resolve (check with local authorities on policies) (see Prevention of Illness Associated with Recreational Water Use, p 180). Sexually active people should avoid engaging in sexual activity for at least 1 week after resolution of diarrhea. Breastfeeding provides some protection for infants. Case reporting to appropriate health authorities (eg, hospital infection control personnel and public health departments) is essential and exclusion policies differ from state to state.

Smallpox (Variola)

The last naturally occurring case of smallpox occurred in Somalia in 1977, followed by 2 cases with 1 death in 1978 after a photographer was infected during a laboratory exposure and later transmitted smallpox to her mother in the United Kingdom. In 1980, the World Health Assembly declared that smallpox (variola virus) had been eradicated successfully worldwide, and no subsequent human cases have been confirmed. The United States discontinued routine childhood immunization against smallpox in 1972 and routine immunization of health care professionals in 1976. Immunization of US military personnel continued until 1990. Following eradication, 2 World Health Organization reference laboratories were authorized to maintain stocks of variola virus. As a result of terrorism events on September 11, 2001, and concern that the virus might be used as a weapon of bioterrorism, the smallpox immunization policy was revisited. In 2002, the United States resumed immunization of military personnel deployed to certain areas of the world and in 2003 initiated a civilian smallpox immunization program for first responders to facilitate preparedness and response to a possible smallpox bioterrorism event. Such a bioterrorism event has not occurred.

CLINICAL MANIFESTATIONS: People infected with variola major strains develop a severe prodromal illness characterized by high fever (102°F–104°F [38.9°C–40.0°C]) and constitutional symptoms, including malaise, severe headache, backache, abdominal pain, and prostration, lasting for 2 to 5 days. Infected children may suffer from vomiting and seizures during this prodromal period. Most patients with smallpox are severely ill and bedridden during the febrile prodrome. The prodromal period is followed by development of lesions on mucosa of the mouth or pharynx, which may not be noticed by the patient. This stage occurs less than 24 hours before onset of rash, which usually is the first recognized manifestation of smallpox. With onset of oral lesions, the patient becomes infectious and remains so until all skin crust lesions have separated. The rash typically begins on the face and rapidly progresses to involve the forearms, trunk, and legs, with the greatest concentration of lesions on the face and distal extremities. The majority of patients will have lesions on the palms and soles. With rash onset, fever decreases but does not resolve. Lesions begin as macules that progress to papules, followed by firm vesicles and then deep-seated, hard pustules described as "pearls of pus." Each stage lasts 1 to 2 days. By the sixth or seventh day of rash, lesions may begin to umbilicate or become confluent. Lesions increase in size for approximately 8 to 10 days, after which they begin to crust. Once all the crusts have separated, 3 to 4 weeks after the onset of rash, the patient no longer is infectious. Variola major in unimmunized people is associated with case fatality rates of approximately 30% during epidemics of smallpox. The mortality rate is highest in pregnant women, children younger than 1 year, and adults older than 40 years. The potential for improved outcomes because of modern supportive therapy is not known.

Variola minor strains cause a disease that is indistinguishable clinically from variola major, except that it causes less severe systemic symptoms and has more rapid rash evolution, reduced scarring, and fewer fatalities.

In addition to the typical presentation of smallpox (90% of cases or greater), there are 2 uncommon severe forms of variola major: hemorrhagic (characterized either by a hemorrhagic diathesis before onset of the typical smallpox rash [early hemorrhagic smallpox] or by hemorrhage into skin lesions and disseminated intravascular coagulation [late hemorrhagic smallpox]) and malignant or flat type (in which the skin lesions do not progress to the pustular stage but remain flat and soft). Each variant occurs in approximately 5% of cases and is associated with a 95% to 100% mortality rate. Pregnancy is a risk factor for hemorrhagic variola. Defects in cellular immunity may be responsible for flat type variola major, which is seen more commonly in children than adults.

Varicella (chickenpox) is the condition most likely to be mistaken for smallpox. Generally, children with varicella do not have a febrile prodrome, but adults may have a brief, mild prodrome. Although the 2 diseases are confused easily in the first few days of the rash, smallpox lesions develop into pustules that are firm and deeply embedded in the dermis, whereas varicella lesions develop into superficial vesicles. Because varicella erupts in crops of lesions that evolve quickly, lesions on any one part of the body will be in different stages of evolution (papules, vesicles, and crusts), whereas all smallpox lesions on any one part of the body are in the same stage of development. The rash distribution of the 2 diseases differs. Varicella most commonly starts on the trunk and moves peripherally with less involvement of the extremities as compared with the trunk (centripetal). Variola lesions can be found distributed on all parts of the body but are generally found in higher numbers on the face and extremities compared with the trunk (centrifugal). Monkeypox also could be mistaken for smallpox as it produces a clinically similar but milder illness. Prominent lymphadenopathy can be a distinguishing feature of monkeypox virus infection, and its diagnosis should only be considered in the United States in the appropriate epidemiologic setting, as discussed below.

ETIOLOGY: Variola, the virus that causes smallpox, is a member of the *Poxviridae* family (genus *Orthopoxvirus*). Other members of this genus that can infect humans include monkeypox virus, cowpox virus, vaccinia virus, and several putative novel species. Cowpox virus is believed to have been used by Benjamin Jesty in 1774 and by Edward Jenner in 1796 as material for the first smallpox vaccine. Later, cowpox virus was replaced with vaccinia virus.

EPIDEMIOLOGY: Humans are the only natural reservoir for variola virus (smallpox). Smallpox is spread most commonly by large respiratory droplets from the oropharynx of infected people, although rare transmission from aerosol spread has been reported. Infection from direct contact with lesion material or indirectly via fomites, such as clothing and bedding, also has been reported. Because most patients with smallpox are extremely ill and bedridden, spread generally is limited to household contacts, hospital workers, and other health care professionals. Secondary household attack rates for smallpox were considerably lower than for measles and similar to or lower than rates for varicella.

In 2003, an outbreak caused by monkeypox virus was linked to prairie dogs exposed to rodents imported from Ghana occurred in the United States. In 2017–2018, Nigeria reported the largest ever outbreak of monkeypox in West Africa with cases epidemiologically linked to Nigeria subsequently reported in the United Kingdom, Israel, and Singapore. Ongoing sporadic monkeypox cases within and linked to Nigeria continued to be reported through 2019. Novel putative orthopox species with clinical presentations similar to cowpox virus and vaccinia virus have been reported in Alaska and in the country of Georgia.

The **incubation period** for smallpox is 7 to 17 days (mean, 10–12 days).

DIAGNOSTIC TESTS: Variola virus can be detected in vesicular or pustular fluid by a number of different methods, including electron microscopy, immunohistochemistry, culture, or polymerase chain reaction (PCR) assay. Only PCR assay can diagnose infection with variola virus definitively; all other methods simply screen for orthopoxviruses. Screening is available through the US Laboratory Response Network, and state or local public health departments should be consulted. Final, confirmatory variola-specific laboratory testing is available only at the Centers for Disease Control and Prevention (CDC). Diagnostic work-up includes exclusion of varicella-zoster virus or other common conditions that cause a vesicular/pustular rash illness. An algorithm to guide evaluation is available at **www.cdc.gov/smallpox/clinicians/algorithm-protocol. html.** Caution is required when collecting specimens from patients in whom a diagnosis of smallpox is considered. Detailed guidelines for safe collection of specimens can be obtained through consultation with the CDC (**www.cdc.gov/smallpox/**; 770-488-7100).

TREATMENT: Tecovirimat (TPOXX or ST-246) was licensed by the US Food and Drug Administration (FDA) in July 2018 for the treatment of smallpox in people who weigh at least 13 kg. It has been shown to be active against monkeypox and rabbitpox in animal models, although effectiveness against variola in humans is unknown. It inhibits the function of an envelope protein required for extracellular transmission of virus. Cidofovir, a nucleotide analogue of cytosine, has demonstrated antiviral activity against certain orthopoxviruses in vitro and in animal models. Its effectiveness in treatment of variola in humans is unknown. Tecovirimat and cidofovir are included in the US Strategic National Stockpile that is managed by the US Department of Health and Human Services, Office of the Assistant Secretary for Preparedness and Response. Brincidofovir (a lipophilic derivative of cidofovir) is an investigational agent with broad-spectrum antiviral activity including against poxviruses in vitro and in animal studies.

ISOLATION OF THE HOSPITALIZED PATIENT: At the time of admission, a patient suspected of having smallpox should be placed in a private, airborne infection isolation room equipped with negative-pressure ventilation with high-efficiency particulate air filtration. Standard, contact, and airborne precautions should be implemented immediately, and hospital infection control personnel and the state (and/or local) health department should be alerted immediately.

CONTROL MEASURES:

Care of Exposed People. Cases of febrile rash illness for which smallpox is considered in the differential diagnosis should be reported immediately to state or local health departments.

Use of Vaccine. Postexposure immunization (within 3–4 days of exposure) provides some protection against disease and significant protection against a fatal outcome. Except for severely immunocompromised people who are not expected to benefit from live vaccinia vaccine, any person with a significant exposure to a patient with proven smallpox during the infectious stage of illness requires immunization as soon after exposure as possible ("ring vaccination").

Preexposure Immunization.

Smallpox Vaccine. ACAM2000 is a licensed live-virus vaccine to prevent smallpox. The lyophilized vaccine does not contain variola virus but rather the related vaccinia virus, different from the virus initially used for immunization by Jesty and Jenner. ACAM2000 is grown in tissue culture and elicits an immune response similar to Dryvax, a previously licensed vaccinia vaccine (no longer available) that was highly effective in preventing smallpox. Vaccine protection wanes with time but substantial protection has been observed up to 15 to 20 years after immunization. The Advisory Committee on Immunization Practices of the CDC recommends smallpox vaccination for select laboratory workers and health care personnel. The ACAM2000 package insert states that individuals at high risk of exposure, such as those handling variola virus in a laboratory, may be revaccinated every 3 years. ACAM2000 is not available for use in the general population and can only be administered by specially trained providers. In the absence of a smallpox outbreak, preexposure smallpox immunization is not recommended for children. Inadvertent transmission of the vaccine virus may occur from vaccine recipients to their household contacts. Children who are immunocompromised or have atopic skin disease are at increased risk of serious complications following contact transmission, including progressive vaccinia and eczema vaccinatum. Information on smallpox vaccine can be found on the CDC website (**www.cdc.gov/smallpox/clinicians/index.html**). Detailed information about contraindications to preexposure smallpox immunization and adverse reactions to vaccination can be found in the ACAM2000 package insert and medication guide (**www.fda.gov/BiologicsBloodVaccines/Vaccines/ApprovedProducts/ucm180810.htm**).

A live, nonreplicating vaccinia vaccine (Jynneos-BN) was approved by the FDA in 2019 for prevention of smallpox and monkeypox in people 18 years and older who are at high risk for smallpox or monkeypox. It is the only FDA-approved vaccine for monkeypox disease prevention. Two doses are administered 4 weeks apart. This vaccine is part of the National Strategic Stockpile and is intended for emergency use during a smallpox event in people who do not have a known smallpox exposure but are at high risk of smallpox and have a relative contraindication to ACAM2000 (including individuals with immunocompromising conditions, atopic skin disease, or allergy to a component of ACAM2000). An investigational vaccinia vaccine similar to ACAM2000 (APSV) is also part of the strategic national stockpile for emergency use during a smallpox event. Guidelines on the use of these vaccines in a smallpox event are available at **www.cdc.gov/mmwr/preview/mmwrhtml/rr6402a1.htm**.

Evaluation and Treatment of Complications of Smallpox Vaccine.

Vaccinia Immune Globulin (VIG) is licensed for certain complications of vaccination with replication competent vaccinia and has no role in treatment of smallpox (**www.cdc.gov/smallpox/clinicians/vaccine-medical-management6.html**). Tecovirimat and brincidofovir have been used for the treatment of disseminated vaccinia through individual patient expanded access requests. Physicians should consult with their state or local health departments for diagnosis and management of patients with complications of vaccinia vaccination. CDC medical staff can be reached through the CDC emergency operations center at 770-488-7100. The CDC smallpox vaccine adverse events clinical consultation team can discuss need for treatment with VIG or antivirals and arrange shipment when indicated. Physicians at military medical facilities (or physicians treating a US Department of Defense health care beneficiary) can call the Defense Health Agency's 24/7 Immunization Healthcare Support Center at 877-GETVACC (877-438-8222) and select option #1.

Sporotrichosis

CLINICAL MANIFESTATIONS: There are 3 **cutaneous** patterns described for sporotrichosis. The classic lymphocutaneous process with multiple nodules is seen more commonly
in adults. Inoculation occurs at a site of minor trauma, causing a painless papule that
enlarges slowly to become a firm, slightly tender subcutaneous nodule that can develop
a violaceous hue or ulcerate. Secondary lesions follow the same evolution and develop
along the lymphatic distribution proximal to the initial lesion. A localized cutaneous form
of sporotrichosis, also called fixed cutaneous form, is seen more commonly in children
and presents as a solitary crusted papule or papuloulcerative or nodular lesion in which
lymphatic spread is not observed. The extremities and face are the most common sites of
infection. A disseminated cutaneous form with multiple lesions is rare, usually occurring
in immunocompromised patients.

Extracutaneous sporotrichosis accounts for 20% of all cases and usually
occurs in the setting of unusual areas of trauma or in immunocompromised patients.
Osteoarticular infection results from hematogenous spread or local inoculation. The most
commonly affected joints are the knees, elbows, wrists, and ankles. Pulmonary sporotrichosis clinically resembles tuberculosis and occurs after inhalation or aspiration of aerosolized conidia. Disseminated disease generally occurs after hematogenous spread from
primary skin or lung infection. Disseminated sporotrichosis can involve multiple foci (eg,
eyes, pericardium, genitourinary tract, central nervous system) and occurs predominantly
in immunocompromised patients. Pulmonary and disseminated forms of sporotrichosis
are uncommon in children.

ETIOLOGY: *Sporothrix schenckii* is a thermally dimorphic fungus that grows as a mold or
mycelial form at room temperature and as a budding yeast at 35°C to 37°C and in host
tissues. *S schenckii* is a complex of at least 6 species. Within this complex, *S schenckii sensu
stricto* is responsible for most infections, followed by *Sporothrix globosa;* in South America,
Sporothrix brasiliensis is a major cause of infection.

EPIDEMIOLOGY: *S schenckii* is a ubiquitous organism that has worldwide distribution but
is most common in tropical and subtropical regions of Central and South America and
parts of North America and Asia. The fungus has been isolated from soil and plant material, including hay, straw, sphagnum moss, and decaying vegetation. Thorny plants such
as rose bushes and pine trees commonly are implicated, because pricks from their thorns
or needles inoculate the organism from the soil or moss around the bush or tree. Zoonotic
spread from cats infected with *S brasiliensis* is responsible for hyperendemic cutaneous sporotrichosis involving mostly women and children in Rio de Janeiro.

The **incubation period** is 7 to 30 days after cutaneous inoculation, but can be as
long as 6 months.

DIAGNOSTIC TESTS: Culture of *Sporothrix* species from a tissue, wound drainage, or sputum specimen is diagnostic. The mold phase of the organism can be isolated on a variety
of fungal media, including Sabouraud dextrose agar at 25°C to 30°C. Filamentous colonies generally appear within 1 week. Definitive identification requires conversion to the
yeast phase by subculture to enriched media, such as brain-heart infusion agar with 5%
blood and incubation at 35°C to 37°C. In some cases, repeated subcultures are required
for conversion. Culture of *Sporothrix* species from a blood specimen is definite evidence for
the disseminated form of infection associated with immunodeficiency. Histopathologic
examination of tissue may be helpful but often is not, because the organism is seldom

abundant, but may exclude clinically similar infections such as cutaneous leishmaniasis. Fungal stains including periodic acid-Schiff or Gomori methenamine silver to visualize the oval or cigar-shaped organism are required. Antibody tests that are offered by some reference laboratories have been useful in a few cases of extracutaneous sporotrichosis. Molecular testing on tissue samples is available only in a few reference laboratories and is not standardized.

TREATMENT[1]: Sporotrichosis usually does not resolve without treatment. Itraconazole is the drug of choice for children with lymphocutaneous and localized cutaneous disease; many experts prefer using the oral solution, which is taken on an empty stomach and appears to achieve better concentrations. See Recommended Doses of Parenteral and Oral Antifungal Drugs (p 913) for dosing. The duration of therapy is 2 to 4 weeks after all lesions have resolved, usually for a total duration of 3 to 6 months. Serum trough concentrations of itraconazole should be 1 to 2 µg/mL. Concentrations should be checked after several days of therapy to ensure adequate drug exposure. When measured by high-pressure liquid chromatography, both itraconazole and its bioactive hydroxy-itraconazole metabolite are reported, the sum of which should be considered in assessing drug levels. Saturated solution of potassium iodide (1 drop, 3 times daily, increasing as tolerated to a maximum of 1 drop/kg of body weight or 40 to 50 drops, 3 times daily, whichever is lowest) is an alternative therapy for nonsevere forms.

Amphotericin B is recommended as the initial therapy for visceral or disseminated sporotrichosis in children (see Recommended Doses of Parenteral and Oral Antifungal Drugs, p 913). After clinical response to amphotericin B therapy is documented, itraconazole can be substituted and should be continued for at least 12 months. Itraconazole may be required for lifelong therapy in children with human immunodeficiency virus infection. Pulmonary and disseminated infections respond less well than cutaneous infection, despite prolonged therapy.

ISOLATION OF THE HOSPITALIZED PATIENT: Standard precautions are indicated.

CONTROL MEASURES: Use of protective gloves and clothing for occupational and recreational activities that could lead to exposure to *S schenckii* can decrease risk of disease.

Staphylococcal Food Poisoning

CLINICAL MANIFESTATIONS: Staphylococcal foodborne illness is characterized by abrupt and sometimes violent onset of severe nausea, abdominal cramps, vomiting, and prostration, often accompanied by diarrhea. Low-grade fever or mild hypothermia can occur. The illness typically lasts no longer than 1 day, but symptoms are intense and can require hospitalization. The short incubation period, brevity of illness, and usual lack of fever help distinguish staphylococcal from other infectious causes of food poisoning, with the exception of the vomiting syndrome caused by *Bacillus cereus*. *Clostridium perfringens* food poisoning usually has a longer incubation period and chemical food poisoning usually has a shorter incubation period. Patients with foodborne *Salmonella*, *Campylobacter*, or *Shigella* infection are more likely to have fever and a longer incubation period (see Appendix VI, Clinical Syndromes Associated With Foodborne Diseases, p 1041).

---

[1]Kauffman CA, Bustamante B, Chapman SW, Pappas PG; Infectious Diseases Society of America. Clinical practice guidelines for the management of sporotrichosis: 2007 update by the Infectious Diseases Society of America. *Clin Infect Dis*. 2007;45(10):1255-1265

ETIOLOGY: Enterotoxins produced by strains of *Staphylococcus aureus* and, rarely, *Staphylococcus epidermidis* and *Staphylococcus intermedius* cause the symptoms of staphylococcal food poisoning.

EPIDEMIOLOGY: Illness is caused by ingestion of food containing heat-stable staphylococcal enterotoxins. The most commonly implicated foods are pork, beef, and chicken. Meats can be contaminated by staphylococci carried by animals. Foods may also be contaminated by enterotoxigenic strains of *S aureus* via contact with food handlers; approximately 25% of people are asymptomatically colonized with *S aureus*. When contaminated foods remain at room temperature for several hours, the toxin-producing staphylococcal organisms multiply and produce toxins that are heat-stable (ie, not inactivated by reheating). Much less commonly, the toxigenic staphylococci are of bovine origin (eg, from cows with mastitis) from contaminated milk or milk products, especially cheeses.

The **incubation period** ranges from 30 minutes to 8 hours after ingestion, typically 2 to 4 hours.

DIAGNOSTIC TESTS: In most cases, given the short duration of illness and rapid recovery with supportive care, diagnostic testing to confirm the diagnosis is not necessary. However, tests for enterotoxin are commercially available. In an outbreak, recovery of large numbers of staphylococci ($\geq 10^5$ *S aureus* per gram) from stool or vomitus or detection of enterotoxin in an implicated food can confirm the diagnosis, as can identification of the same subtype of *S aureus* from the stool or vomitus of 2 or more ill people. Guidance for confirming cases of staphylococcal food poisoning can be found online (**www.cdc. gov/foodsafety/outbreaks/investigating-outbreaks/confirming_diagnosis.html**). To aid in outbreak investigations, public health laboratories can determine whether strains are similar by molecular methods. Local public health authorities should be notified to help determine the source of the outbreak.

TREATMENT: Treatment is supportive. Antimicrobial agents are not indicated.

ISOLATION OF THE HOSPITALIZED PATIENT: Staphylococcal food poisoning is not spread from person to person. Standard precautions are recommended.

CONTROL MEASURES: Strict hand hygiene should be enforced for all food handlers. People with boils, abscesses, or other purulent lesions that could be from staphylococcal skin infection should be especially careful to wash hands thoroughly and use gloves or other protective equipment while handling food. Prepared foods should be refrigerated in wide, shallow containers within 2 hours after cooking (within 1 hour if the ambient temperature is higher than 90°F). Information on good food handling practices, including time and temperature recommendations for cooking, storage, and reheating, is available online (**www.foodsafety.gov**).

Staphylococcus aureus

CLINICAL MANIFESTATIONS: *Staphylococcus aureus* causes a variety of localized and invasive suppurative infections and 3 toxin-mediated syndromes: toxic shock syndrome, scalded skin syndrome, and food poisoning (see Staphylococcal Food Poisoning, p 677). Localized infections include cellulitis, skin and soft tissue abscesses, furuncles, carbuncles, pustulosis, impetigo (bullous and nonbullous), paronychia, mastitis, hordeola, omphalitis, sinusitis, orbital cellulitis/abscess, peritonsillar abscesses (Quinsy), parotitis, lymphadenitis, and wound infections. Bacteremia can be associated with focal complications including osteomyelitis; septic arthritis; endocarditis; pneumonia; pleural empyema; septic pulmonary emboli; pericarditis; soft tissue, muscle, or visceral abscesses; and septic thrombophlebitis of small and large vessels. In patients with neutropenia, ecthyma gangrenosum may occur. Primary *S aureus* pneumonia also can occur after aspiration of organisms from the upper respiratory tract and can occur in the context of concurrent or antecedent viral infections from the community (eg, influenza) or in ventilated patients. Meningitis may occur in preterm infants but otherwise is rare unless accompanied by an intradermal foreign body (eg, ventriculoperitoneal shunt) or a congenital or acquired defect in the dura. *S aureus* also causes infections with and without bacteremia associated with foreign bodies, including intravascular catheters or grafts, peritoneal catheters, cerebrospinal fluid shunts, spinal instrumentation or intramedullary rods, pressure equalization tubes, pacemakers and other intracardiac devices, vagal nerve stimulators, and prosthetic joints. *S aureus* infections can be fulminant. Certain chronic diseases, conditions, and events, such as diabetes mellitus, malignancy, prematurity, immunodeficiency, kidney disease, nutritional disorders, dialysis, surgery, and transplantation, increase the risk for severe *S aureus* infections. Metastatic foci and abscess formation need to be drained and foreign bodies should be removed when possible. Prolonged antimicrobial therapy often is necessary to achieve cure.

Staphylococcal toxic shock syndrome (TSS), a toxin-mediated disease, usually is caused by strains producing TSS toxin-1 or possibly other related staphylococcal enterotoxins. Characterized by acute onset of fever, generalized erythroderma, rapid-onset hypotension, and signs of multisystem organ involvement, including profuse watery diarrhea, vomiting, conjunctival injection, and severe myalgia (see Table 3.53, p 680, for clinical case definition). TSS can occur in menstruating females using tampons or following childbirth or abortion. TSS also can occur in males and females after surgical procedures, in association with cutaneous lesions, or without a readily identifiable focus of infection. Prevailing clones (eg, USA300) of methicillin-resistant *S aureus* (MRSA) rarely produce TSS toxin. People with TSS, especially menses-associated illness, are at risk of a recurrent episode.

Staphylococcal scalded skin syndrome (SSSS) is a toxin-mediated disease caused by circulation of exfoliative toxins A and B. The manifestations of SSSS are age related and include Ritter disease (generalized exfoliation) in the neonate, a tender scarlatiniform eruption and localized bullous impetigo in older children, or a combination of these with thick white/brown flaky desquamation of the entire skin, especially on the face and neck, in older infants and toddlers. The hallmark of SSSS is the toxin-mediated cleavage of the stratum granulosum layer of the epidermis (ie, Nikolsky sign). Proper pain management is a mainstay of therapy for SSSS. Healing occurs without scarring. Bacteremia is rare, but dehydration and superinfection can occur with extensive exfoliation.

ETIOLOGY: Staphylococci are catalase-positive, gram-positive cocci that appear microscopically as grape-like clusters. Staphylococci are ubiquitous and can survive extreme conditions of drying, heat, and low-oxygen and high-salt environments. *S aureus* has many surface proteins, including the microbial surface components recognizing adhesive matrix molecule (MSCRAMM) receptors, which allow the organism to bind to tissues and foreign bodies coated with fibronectin, fibrinogen, and collagen. This permits a low inoculum of organisms to adhere to sutures, catheters, prosthetic valves, and other devices.

Table 3.53. *Staphylococcus aureus* Toxic Shock Syndrome: Clinical Case Definition[a]

Clinical Findings
- Fever: temperature 38.9°C (102.0°F) or greater
- Rash: diffuse macular erythroderma
- Desquamation: 1–2 weeks after onset of rash, particularly on palms, soles, fingers, and toes
- Hypotension: systolic pressure 90 mm Hg or less for adults; lower than fifth percentile for age for children younger than 16 years
- Multisystem organ involvement: 3 or more of the following:
  1. Gastrointestinal tract: vomiting or diarrhea at onset of illness
  2. Muscular: severe myalgia or creatinine phosphokinase concentration greater than twice the upper limit of normal
  3. Mucous membrane: vaginal, oropharyngeal, or conjunctival hyperemia
  4. Renal: serum urea nitrogen or serum creatinine concentration greater than twice the upper limit of normal or urinary sediment with 5 white blood cells/high-power field or greater in the absence of urinary tract infection
  5. Hepatic: total bilirubin, aspartate aminotransferase, or alanine aminotransferase concentration greater than twice the upper limit of normal
  6. Hematologic: platelet count 100 000/mm^3 or less
  7. Central nervous system: disorientation or alterations in consciousness without focal neurologic signs when fever and hypotension are absent

Laboratory Criteria
- *Negative* results on the following tests, if obtained:
  1. Blood, throat, or cerebrospinal fluid cultures; blood culture rarely may be positive for *S aureus*
  2. Serologic tests for Rocky Mountain spotted fever, leptospirosis, or measles

Case Classification
- ***Probable:*** a case that meets the laboratory criteria and in which 4 of 5 clinical findings are present
- ***Confirmed:*** a case that meets laboratory criteria and all 5 of the clinical findings, including desquamation, unless the patient dies before desquamation occurs.

[a]Adapted from **wwwn.cdc.gov/nndss/conditions/toxic-shock-syndrome-other-than-streptococcal/case-definition/2011/**

EPIDEMIOLOGY: *S aureus* is the most common cause of skin and soft tissue infections and musculoskeletal infections in otherwise healthy children. *S aureus* colonizes the skin and mucous membranes of 30% to 50% of healthy adults and children. The anterior nares, throat, axilla, perineum, vagina, and rectum are usual sites of colonization. *S aureus* is second only to coagulase-negative staphylococci (CoNS) as a cause of health care-associated bacteremia, is one of the most common causes of health care-associated pneumonia in children, and is the most common pathogen responsible for surgical site infections. Patients with neutrophil dysfunction, such as those with chronic granulomatous disease (CGD), are also at risk for *S aureus* infections.

S aureus-mediated TSS was recognized in 1978 by Dr. Jim Todd, and many early cases were associated with tampon use. Although changes in tampon composition and use have resulted in a decreased proportion of cases associated with menses, menstrual and non-menstrual cases of TSS continue to occur and are reported with similar frequency. Risk factors for TSS include absence of antibody to TSS toxin-1 and focal *S aureus* infection with a TSS toxin-1–producing strain. TSS toxin-1–producing strains can be part of normal flora of the anterior nares or vagina, and colonization at these sites is believed to result in protective antibody in more than 90% of adults.

Transmission of S aureus. Rates of skin carriage of more than 50% occur in children with desquamating skin disorders or burns and in people with frequent needle use (eg, diabetes mellitus, hemodialysis, people who inject drugs, allergy shots). Although domestic animals can be colonized, data suggest that colonization is acquired from other humans. Hospitalized children who are colonized with MRSA on admission or acquire MRSA colonization in the hospital are at increased risk for subsequent MRSA infection compared with noncolonized children.

S aureus is transmitted most often by direct contact in community settings and indirectly from patient to patient via transiently colonized hands of health care professionals in health care settings. Health care professionals and family members who are colonized with S aureus in the nares or on skin also can serve as a reservoir for transmission. Contaminated environmental surfaces and objects also can play a role in transmission of S aureus. Although not transmitted by the droplet route routinely, S aureus can be dispersed into the air over short distances. Dissemination of S aureus from people with nasal carriage, including infants, is related to density of colonization, and increased dissemination occurs during viral upper respiratory tract infections. Maternal S aureus colonization at a variety of body sites has been associated with neonatal colonization.

Health Care-Associated MRSA. MRSA has been endemic in most US hospitals since the 1980s and in 2016 accounted for approximately 40% of health care-associated S aureus bloodstream infections in pediatric inpatients. Risk factors for health care-associated MRSA infections include hospitalization, surgery, dialysis, long-term care stay within the previous year, presence of an indwelling device, presence of wounds, and history of prior MRSA infection or colonization. The incidence of invasive health care-associated MRSA infections has decreased in many communities since the mid-2000s.

Health care-associated MRSA strains (ie, those that historically were responsible for most health care-associated MRSA infections) are usually multidrug resistant and predictably are susceptible only to vancomycin, ceftaroline, linezolid, daptomycin, and agents not approved by the US Food and Drug Administration (FDA) for use in children.

Community-Associated MRSA. Community-associated MRSA infections attributable to strains different from traditional health care-associated MRSA emerged in the 1990s. These strains most commonly cause skin and soft tissue abscesses, although they can also cause more severe infections. Clinical infections are more common in settings where there is crowding; frequent skin-to-skin contact; sharing of personal items, such as towels and clothing; and poor personal hygiene and among those with nonintact skin including body piercings. Outbreaks have been reported among athletic teams, in correctional facilities, and in military training facilities. Community-associated MRSA strains can also circulate in hospitals and cause health care-associated MRSA infections. Unlike health care-associated strains, community-associated MRSA strains are usually susceptible to a variety of non–beta-lactam antibiotics (eg, trimethoprim-sulfamethoxazole, clindamycin, tetracycline), in addition to the antibiotics listed above for health care-associated MRSA strains.

Vancomycin-Intermediately Susceptible S aureus. Vancomycin-intermediately susceptible S aureus (VISA) strains (minimum inhibitory concentration [MIC], 4–8 µg/mL) have been isolated from people (historically, dialysis patients) who have received multiple courses of vancomycin. Strains of MRSA can be heterogeneous for vancomycin resistance (see

Diagnostic Tests). Extensive vancomycin use allows VISA strains to develop during therapy. Control measures recommended by the Centers for Disease Control and Prevention (CDC) have included using proper methods to detect VISA, using appropriate infection-control measures, and adopting measures to ensure appropriate vancomycin use.

Vancomycin-Resistant S aureus. Vancomycin-resistant *S aureus* (VRSA) infections (MIC >8 µg/mL) are very rare, and in all confirmed cases, reported patients had underlying medical conditions, a history of MRSA infections, and prolonged exposure to vancomycin.

The **incubation period** is variable for staphylococcal disease. A long delay can occur between acquisition of the organism and onset of disease. For SSSS, the **incubation period** usually is 1 to 10 days; for postoperative TSS, the **incubation period** can be as short as 12 hours. Menses-related cases can develop at any time during menstruation.

DIAGNOSTIC TESTS: Gram stains of specimens from skin lesions or pyogenic foci showing gram-positive cocci in clusters can provide presumptive evidence of staphylococcal infection. Isolation of organisms from culture of otherwise sterile body fluid is the method for definitive diagnosis. Molecular assays have been approved by the FDA for detection of *S aureus* from blood cultures growing gram-positive organisms. These assays include nonamplified molecular assays, such as peptide nucleic acid fluorescent in situ hybridization (PNA-FISH) and Verigene (Luminex), as well as nucleic acid amplification tests, such as BD GenOhm Staph SR (BD Molecular Diagnostics), Xpert MRSA/SA BC (Cepheid), and the FilmArray Blood Culture Identification Panel (BCID) (Biofire). Matrix-assisted laser desorption/ionization-time of flight (MALDI-TOF) mass spectometry can rapidly identify *S aureus* colonies on culture plates or from growth in blood cultures. *S aureus* is almost never a contaminant when isolated from a blood culture.

S aureus-mediated TSS is a clinical diagnosis (Table 3.53); *S aureus* is isolated from blood cultures in fewer than 5% of patients with TSS. Specimens for culture should be obtained from an identified focus of infection, because these sites usually will yield the organism. Because approximately one third of isolates of *S aureus* from nonmenstrual cases produce toxins other than TSS toxin-1, and TSS toxin-1–producing organisms can be present as normal flora, TSS toxin-1 production by an isolate is not a useful diagnostic test.

Antimicrobial susceptibility testing should be performed for all *S aureus* specimens isolated from normally sterile sites. Laboratory practice includes routine screening (D-testing) to exclude inducible clindamycin resistance. Another phenomenon that has been described is heteroresistance to antibiotics, in which the heterogeneous or heterotypic strains appear susceptible by disk diffusion but contain resistant subpopulations that are only apparent when cultured with antibiotic-containing media. When these resistant subpopulations are cultured on antibiotic-free media, they can continue as stable resistant mutants or revert to susceptible strains (heterogeneous resistance). Bacteria expressing heteroresistance grow more slowly than the susceptible bacteria and can be missed at growth conditions greater than 35°C (95°F). The clinical significance of heteroresistance is not clear, but some have suggested that it could be a cause of some vancomycin treatment failures.

S aureus strain genotyping, in conjunction with epidemiologic information, can facilitate identification of the source, extent, and mechanism of transmission in an outbreak. A number of molecular typing methods are available for *S aureus*, including pulsed-field gel electrophoresis, spa typing, and whole genome sequencing. Choice of method should consider purpose of typing and available resources.

TREATMENT:

Skin and Soft Tissue Infection. Skin and soft tissue infections, such as diffuse impetigo or cellulitis attributable to methicillin-susceptible *S aureus* (MSSA), optimally are treated with oral penicillinase-resistant beta-lactam drugs, such as a first- or second-generation cephalosporin. For the penicillin-allergic patient and in cases in which MRSA is considered, trimethoprim-sulfamethoxazole, doxycycline, or clindamycin can be used if the isolate is susceptible. Topical mupirocin is recommended for localized impetigo.

The most frequent manifestation of community-associated MRSA infection is skin and soft tissue infection, which can range from mild to severe. Drainage is an important part of managing these types of infections. A randomized placebo-controlled study evaluating treatment strategies for uncomplicated skin infections included children with simple abscesses ≤3 cm (6–11 months of age), ≤4 cm (1–8 years of age), or ≤5 cm (>8 years of age) in diameter and found that drainage plus systemic oral therapy with either clindamycin or trimethoprim-sulfamethoxazole is associated with better outcomes compared with drainage alone. Applying mupirocin to the nares and bathing using chlorhexidine for 5 consecutive days for all family members have been associated with decreased recurrences. Studies in adults have reported success with a 7-day course of the combination of oral rifampin and doxycycline plus nasal mupirocin.

Invasive Staphylococcal Infections. Empiric therapy for suspected invasive staphylococcal infection, including pneumonia, osteoarticular infection, visceral abscesses, and foreign body-associated infection with bacteremia, is vancomycin plus a semisynthetic beta lactam (eg, nafcillin, oxacillin). Subsequent therapy should be based on antimicrobial susceptibility results. Serious MSSA infections require intravenous therapy with an antistaphylococcal beta-lactam antimicrobial agent, such as nafcillin, oxacillin, or cefazolin, because most *S aureus* strains produce beta-lactamase enzymes and are resistant to penicillin and ampicillin (see Table 3.54, p 684). The addition of rifampin may be considered for those with invasive disease associated with an indwelling foreign body, especially if removal of the infected implant or device is not feasible. Vancomycin is not recommended for treatment of serious MSSA infections (including endocarditis), because it is weakly bactericidal and outcomes are inferior with vancomycin compared with antistaphylococcal beta lactams. First- or second-generation cephalosporins (eg, cefazolin) or vancomycin are less effective than nafcillin or oxacillin for treatment of MSSA meningitis. Clindamycin is bacteriostatic and should not be used for treatment of primary bacteremia or endovascular infection.

Guidelines for management of serious skin/soft tissue infection, complicated pneumonia/empyema, central nervous system (CNS) infection, osteomyelitis, and endocarditis caused by MRSA are available (**www.idsociety.org/IDSA_Practice_Guidelines/**). For MRSA pneumonia complicating influenza in children, vancomycin monotherapy in the first 24 hours of treatment was associated with higher mortality compared with vancomycin combined with a second antibiotic (clindamycin, linezolid, or ceftaroline) in a retrospective, multicenter study. Thus, a combination of vancomycin plus one of these agents is recommended for empiric treatment of children with life-threatening pneumonia complicating influenza. Antibiotic therapy can be de-escalated to a single agent if there is clinical improvement and antibiotic susceptibility information to guide treatment.

Table 3.54. Parenteral Antimicrobial Agent(s) for Treatment of Bacteremia and Other Serious *Staphylococcus aureus* Infections

Antimicrobial Agents		Comments
I. Initial empiric therapy (organism of unknown susceptibility)		
Drugs of choice:	Vancomycin (15 mg/kg, every 6 h) + nafcillin or oxacillin[a,b]	For life–threatening infections (ie, septicemia, endocarditis, CNS infection); ceftaroline or linezolid are alternatives, but there are limited efficacy data in children
	Vancomycin (15 mg/kg, every 6–8 h)[b]	For non–life-threatening infection without signs of sepsis (eg, skin infection, cellulitis, osteomyelitis, pyarthrosis) when rates of MRSA colonization and infection in the community are substantial; ceftaroline or linezolid are alternatives
	Clindamycin	For non–life-threatening infection without signs of sepsis when rates of MRSA colonization and infection in the community are substantial and prevalence of clindamycin resistance is <15%
II. Methicillin-susceptible *S aureus* (MSSA)		
Drugs of choice:	Nafcillin or oxacillin[c]	
	Cefazolin	
Alternatives:	Clindamycin	Only for patients with a serious penicillin allergy and clindamycin-susceptible strain
	Vancomycin[b]	Only for patients with a serious penicillin and cephalosporin allergy
	Ampicillin + sulbactam	For patients with polymicrobial infections caused by susceptible isolates
III. Methicillin-resistant *S aureus* (MRSA; oxacillin MIC, 4 µg/mL or greater)		
A. Health care-associated (multidrug resistant)		
Drugs of choice:	Vancomycin ± gentamicin[b,c]	

Table 3.54. Parenteral Antimicrobial Agent(s) for Treatment of Bacteremia and Other Serious *Staphylococcus aureus* Infections, continued

	Antimicrobial Agents	Comments
Alternatives: susceptibility testing results available before alternative drugs are used	Trimethoprim-sulfamethoxazole	
	Ceftaroline[d]	
	Linezolid[d]	
	Daptomycin[d,e]	
B. Community-associated (not multidrug resistant)		
Drugs of choice:	Vancomycin ± gentamicin[b,c]	For life-threatening infections or endovascular infections including those complicated by venous thrombosis
	Clindamycin (if strain susceptible)	For pneumonia,[a] septic arthritis, osteomyelitis, skin or soft tissue infections
	Trimethoprim-sulfamethoxazole	For skin or soft tissue infections
	Doxycycline (if strain susceptible)	
Alternative:	Vancomycin[b]	For serious infections
	Linezolid	For serious infections caused by clindamycin resistant isolates in patients with renal dysfunction or those intolerant of vancomycin
IV. Vancomycin-intermediately susceptible *S aureus* (VISA; MIC, 4 to 16 μg/mL)[d]		
Drugs of choice:	Optimal therapy is not known	Dependent on in vitro susceptibility test results
	Linezolid[d]	
	Ceftaroline[d]	
	Daptomycin[e]	
	Quinupristin–dalfopristin[d]	
	Tigecycline[d]	

Table 3.54. Parenteral Antimicrobial Agent(s) for Treatment of Bacteremia and Other Serious *Staphylococcus aureus* Infections, continued

Antimicrobial Agents	Comments
Alternatives: Vancomycin[b] + linezolid ± gentamicin Vancomycin[b] + trimethoprim-sulfamethoxazole[e]	

CNS indicates central nervous system; MIC, minimum inhibitory concentration.

[a] For suspected MRSA pneumonia complicating influenza in critically ill children, add clindamycin, ceftaroline, or linezolid to vancomycin empiric treatment. Empiric selection of antibiotics is highly dependent on the local/regional susceptibility data.

[b] The area-under-the-curve to minimum inhibitory concentration (AUC/MIC) has been identified as the most appropriate pharmacokinetic/pharmacodynamic (PK/PD) target for vancomycin in adult patients with MRSA. Although there are limitations in prospective outcomes data in pediatric patients with serious MRSA infections, the most recent consensus guideline from the American Society of Health-System Pharmacists, the Infectious Diseases Society of America, the Pediatric Infectious Diseases Society, and the Society of Infectious Diseases Pharmacists recommends AUC guided therapeutic monitoring, preferably with Bayesian estimation, for all pediatric age groups receiving vancomycin.[f,g,h] This estimation accounts for developmental changes of vancomycin clearance from newborn to adolescent. Dosing in children should be designed to achieve an AUC of 400 to 600 μg-hour/L (assuming MIC of 1) and/or trough levels <15 μg/mL to minimize AKI risks. Bayesian estimation can be completed with 2 levels, with one level being recommended 1-2 hours after end of vancomycin infusion, and the second level being drawn 4 to 6 hours after end of infusion. Levels can be obtained as early as after the second dose. Software to assist with these calculations is available online and for purchase. It is recommended to avoid AUC >800 and troughs >15. Most children younger than 12 years will require higher doses to achieve optimal AUC/MIC compared with older children. Consultation with an infectious diseases specialist should be considered to determine which agent to use and duration of use.

[c] Gentamicin and rifampin for the first 2 weeks should be added for endocarditis of a prosthetic device. Addition of rifampin is recommended for other device-related infections (spinal instrumentation, prosthetic joint).

[d] Linezolid, ceftaroline, quinupristin-dalfopristin, and tigecycline are agents with activity *in vitro* and efficacy in adults with multidrug-resistant, gram-positive organisms, including *S aureus*. Because experience with these agents in children is limited, consultation with a specialist in infectious diseases should be considered before use. Further, tigecycline should not be used in children younger than 8 years if there are effective alternatives, because there may be reversible inhibition of bone growth and adverse effects on tooth development.

[e] Daptomycin is active in vitro against multidrug-resistant, gram-positive organisms, including *S aureus*. Daptomycin is approved by the US Food and Drug Administration only for treatment of complicated skin and skin structure infections and for *S aureus* bloodstream infections. Daptomycin is ineffective for treatment of pneumonia. Because experience with these agents in children is limited, consultation with a specialist in infectious diseases should be considered before use.

[f] Rybak MJ, Le J, Lodise TP, et al. Therapeutic monitoring of vancomycin for serious methicillin-resistant *Staphylococcus aureus* infections: a revised consensus guideline and review by the American Society of Health-System Pharmacists, the Infectious Diseases Society of America, the Pediatric Infectious Diseases Society, and the Society of Infectious Diseases Pharmacists. *Am J Health Syst Pharm*. Published online March 19, 2020. Available at: **https://doi.org/10.1093/ajhp/zxaa036**

[g] Rybak MJ, Le J, Lodise TP, et al. Executive summary: Therapeutic monitoring of vancomycin for serious methicillin-resistant *Staphylococcus aureus* infections: a revised consensus guideline and review by the American Society of Health-System Pharmacists, the Infectious Diseases Society of America, the Pediatric Infectious Diseases Society, and the Society of Infectious Diseases Pharmacists. *J Pediatr Infect Dis Soc*. 2020;9(3):281-284

[h] Heil EL, Claeys KC, Mynatt RP, et al. Making the change to area under the curve-based vancomycin dosing. *Am J Health Syst Pharm*. 2018;75(24):1986-1995. DOI: **https://doi.org/10.2146/ajhp180034**

VISA infection is rare in children. For seriously ill patients with a history of recurrent MRSA infections or for patients failing vancomycin therapy in whom VISA strains are a consideration, initial therapy could include linezolid or trimethoprim-sulfamethoxazole, with or without gentamicin. If antimicrobial susceptibility results document multidrug resistance, alternative agents, such as ceftaroline, daptomycin (except for pneumonia, for which daptomycin should not be used due to inhibition by pulmonary surfactant), tigecycline, or quinupristin-dalfopristin, could be considered. However, data are limited on the use of daptomycin, quinupristin-dalfopristin, and tigecycline in children, and consultation with a specialist in infectious diseases should be considered. In addition, in children younger than 8 years, there may be reversible inhibition of bone growth and adverse effects on tooth development with tigecycline use.

Duration of therapy for serious MSSA or MRSA infections depends on the site and severity of infection but usually is 4 weeks or more for endocarditis, osteomyelitis, necrotizing pneumonia, or disseminated infection, assuming a documented clinical and microbiologic response. In assessing whether modification of therapy is necessary, clinicians should consider whether the patient is improving clinically, should identify and drain sequestered foci of infection and remove foreign material (such as a central catheter) when possible, and for MRSA strains, should consider the vancomycin MIC and the achievable vancomycin exposure. The area-under-the-curve to minimum inhibitory concentration (AUC/MIC) has been identified as the most appropriate pharmacokinetic/pharmacodynamic (PK/PD) target for vancomycin in adult patients with MRSA. Although there are limitations in prospective outcomes data in pediatric patients with serious MRSA infections, the most recent consensus guideline from the American Society of Health-System Pharmacists, the Infectious Diseases Society of America, the Pediatric Infectious Diseases Society, and the Society of Infectious Diseases Pharmacists recommends AUC guided therapeutic monitoring, preferably with Bayesian estimation, for all pediatric age groups receiving vancomycin.[1,2,3] This estimation accounts for developmental changes of vancomycin clearance from newborn to adolescent. Dosing in children should be designed to achieve an AUC of 400 to 600 µg-hour/L (assuming MIC of 1) and/or trough levels <15 µg/mL to minimize AKI risks. Bayesian estimation can be completed with 2 levels, with one level being recommended 1 to 2 hours after end of vancomycin infusion and the second level being drawn 4 to 6 hours after end of infusion. Levels can be obtained as early as after the second dose. Software to assist with these calculations is available online and for purchase. It is recommended to avoid AUC >800 and troughs >15. Most children younger than 12 years will require higher doses to achieve optimal AUC/MIC compared with older children.

[1]Rybak MJ, Le J, Lodise TP, et al. Therapeutic monitoring of vancomycin for serious methicillin-resistant *Staphylococcus aureus* infections: a revised consensus guideline and review by the American Society of Health-System Pharmacists, the Infectious Diseases Society of America, the Pediatric Infectious Diseases Society, and the Society of Infectious Diseases Pharmacists. *Am J Health Syst Pharm.* Published online March 19, 2020. Available at: **https://doi.org/10.1093/ajhp/zxaa036**

[2]Rybak MJ, Le J, Lodise TP, et al. Executive summary: Therapeutic monitoring of vancomycin for serious methicillin-resistant *Staphylococcus aureus* infections: a revised consensus guideline and review by the American Society of Health-System Pharmacists, the Infectious Diseases Society of America, the Pediatric Infectious Diseases Society, and the Society of Infectious Diseases Pharmacists. *J Pediatr Infect Dis Soc.* 2020;9(3):281-284

[3]Heil EL, Claeys KC, Mynatt RP, et al. Making the change to area under the curve-based vancomycin dosing. *Am J Health Syst Pharm.* 2018;75(24):1986-1995. DOI: **https://doi.org/10.2146/ajhp180034**

Completion of the treatment course with an oral drug can be considered in children if an endovascular infection (ie, endocarditis or infected thrombus) or CNS infection is not a concern. For endovascular and CNS infections, parenteral therapy is recommended for the entire treatment course. Drainage of large abscesses, often more than once, and removal of foreign bodies are almost always required in addition to medical therapy. In some cases, multiple débridement procedures are necessary for children with complicated *S aureus* osteoarticular infection.

Duration of therapy for *S aureus* central line-associated bloodstream infections is controversial and depends on a number of factors—the type and location of the catheter, the site of infection (exit site vs tunnel vs line), the feasibility of using an alternative vascular access site at a later date, the presence or absence of a catheter-related thrombus, and host immunity. Infections are more difficult to treat when associated with a thrombus, thrombophlebitis, or intra-atrial thrombus, and a longer course is suggested if the patient is immunocompromised. Expert opinion differs on recommended treatment duration, but many suggest a minimum of 14 days provided there is no evidence of a metastatic focus and the patient responds to antimicrobial therapy with rapid sterilization of the blood cultures. If the patient needs a new central line, waiting 48 to 72 hours after bacteremia apparently has resolved before insertion is optimal. If a tunneled catheter is needed for ongoing care, treatment of the infection without removal of the catheter can be attempted but may not always be successful. Vegetations or a thrombus in the heart or great vessels always should be considered when a central line becomes infected and should be suspected more strongly if blood cultures remain positive for more than 2 days on appropriate antimicrobial therapy following removal of the central line or if there are other clinical manifestations associated with endocarditis. Transesophageal echocardiography is the most sensitive technique for identifying vegetations, but transthoracic echocardiography generally is adequate for children younger than 10 years and/or weighing <60 kg.

Management of* S aureus *Toxin-Mediated Diseases. The principles of therapy for TSS include aggressive fluid management (and vasoactive agents, as needed) to maintain adequate venous return and cardiac filling to prevent end organ damage, source control that includes prompt identification and removal of any indwelling foreign body (eg, tampon) or drainable focus, and anticipation and management of the commonly observed multiorgan complications of TSS (eg, acute respiratory distress syndrome, renal dysfunction). Initial antimicrobial therapy should include a parentally administered antistaphylococcal beta-lactam antimicrobial agent and a protein synthesis-inhibiting drug, such as clindamycin, at maximum dosages. Vancomycin should be added to the beta-lactam agent in regions where MRSA infections are common, although MRSA-associated TSS is rare in the United States (see Table 3.54, p 684). Empiric antibiotic therapy should be modified to targeted therapy once antibiotic susceptibilities are known. An active antimicrobial agent should be continued for 10 to 14 days. Administration of antimicrobial agents can be changed to the oral route once the patient is tolerating oral alimentation. The total duration of therapy is based on the usual duration of established foci of infection (eg, pneumonia, osteomyelitis). Immune Globulin Intravenous (IGIV) can be considered in patients with severe staphylococcal TSS unresponsive to other therapeutic measures, because IGIV may neutralize circulating toxin. Although data on the use of IGIV are not robust, it may be considered for critically ill children with shock that is unresponsive to fluid resuscitation, an undrainable focus of infection, or persistent oliguria with pulmonary edema. The optimal IGIV regimen is unknown, but 150 to 400 mg/kg per day for 5 days or a single dose of 1 to 2 g/kg has been used. SSSS in infants should be treated with a parenteral antistaphylococcal beta-lactam antimicrobial agent or clindamycin, depending on local susceptibility patterns and the severity of the disease. If MRSA is a consideration, vancomycin or clindamycin (depending on local susceptibility patterns) can be used. Transition to an oral agent is appropriate in nonneonates who have demonstrated excellent clinical response to parenteral therapy.

ISOLATION OF THE HOSPITALIZED PATIENT: Contact precautions should be added to standard precautions for patients with abscesses or draining wounds that cannot be covered, regardless of staphylococcal strain, and should be maintained until wound drainage ceases or can be contained by a dressing. Infants and young children with staphylococcal furunculosis and patients with SSSS should be placed on contact precautions for the duration of their illness. Although there has been debate about the practice, the CDC continues to recommend contact precautions for patients known to be infected or colonized with MRSA (**www.cdc.gov/hai/prevent/staph-prevention-strategies.html**).

To prevent transmission of VRSA, the CDC has issued specific infection control recommendations that should be followed (**www.cdc.gov/hai/pdfs/VRSA-Investigation-Guide-05_12_2015.pdf**).

CONTROL MEASURES: Measures to prevent and control *S aureus* infections can be considered separately for individual patients and for health care facilities.

Individual Patient. Community-associated *S aureus* infections in immunocompetent hosts are difficult to prevent in the absence of clearly apparent risk factors or an outbreak, because the organism is ubiquitous and there is no effective vaccine. Strategies focusing on hand hygiene, environmental disinfection, and wound care have been effective at limiting transmission of *S aureus* and preventing spread of infections in community settings. Specific strategies include appropriate wound care, minimizing skin trauma and keeping abrasions and cuts covered, optimizing hand hygiene and personal hygiene practices (eg, shower after activities involving skin-to-skin contact), avoiding sharing of personal items (eg, towels, razors, clothing), cleaning shared equipment between uses, and regular cleaning of frequently touched environmental surfaces. For patients who experience recurrent *S aureus* infections or who are predisposed to *S aureus* infections because of disorders of neutrophil function, chronic skin conditions, or obesity, a variety of techniques have been used to prevent infection, including scrupulous attention to skin hygiene, bleach baths, and the use of clothing and bed linens that minimize sweating, but none have shown definitive effectiveness in preventing recurrent infections with community-associated MRSA. Household contacts of people with *S aureus* infections generally do not need to be tested for colonization; however, for patients with multiple recurrent staphylococcal infections, decolonization of an entire household can be attempted, because household contacts and environmental sources play important roles in transmission of MRSA (see Eradication of Nasal Carriage, below).

Measures to prevent health care-associated *S aureus* infections in individual patients include strict adherence to recommended infection-control precautions and appropriate intraoperative antimicrobial prophylaxis, and in some circumstances, use of preoperative antimicrobial regimens to attempt to eradicate nasal carriage; use of chlorhexidine in certain patients also can be considered. Guidelines for prevention of surgical site infections can be found at **www.cdc.gov/infectioncontrol/guidelines/ssi/index.html**.

Child Care or School Settings. Children with *S aureus* colonization or infection should not be excluded routinely from child care or school settings. Children with draining or open abrasions or wounds should have these covered with a clean, dry dressing. Routine hand hygiene should be emphasized for personnel and children in these facilities.

General Measures. Published recommendations of the CDC Healthcare Infection Control Practices Advisory Committee (HICPAC)[1] for prevention of health care-associated pneumonia should be effective for decreasing the incidence of *S aureus* pneumonia. CDC/HICPAC guidelines for preventing intravascular catheter-related infections include careful preparation of the skin before surgery, including cleansing of skin before placement of intravascular catheters using barrier methods (**www.cdc.gov/infectioncontrol/guidelines/bsi/updates.html**). Meticulous surgical technique with minimal trauma to tissues, maintenance of good oxygenation, and minimal hematoma and dead space formation will minimize risk of surgical site infection. Appropriate hand hygiene, including before and after use of gloves, by health care professionals and strict adherence to contact precautions are of paramount importance.

Intraoperative Antimicrobial Prophylaxis. Most clean surgical procedures do not require antimicrobial prophylaxis because the risk of overall infection (most commonly caused by *S aureus*) is only 1% to 2%. However, antimicrobial prophylaxis is used in complicated surgeries such as organ transplantation, neurosurgical procedures, or insertion of a major prosthetic device, such as a ventriculoperitoneal shunt or a heart valve, or for a known MRSA carrier undergoing a major surgical procedure (see Antimicrobial Prophylaxis in Pediatric Surgical Patients, p 1010). If antimicrobial prophylaxis is used, the agent, usually cefazolin, is administered 30 to 60 minutes before the operation (vancomycin should be administered over a longer period, approximately 60–120 minutes before skin incision), and a total duration of therapy of less than 24 hours after surgery is recommended in most cases. Administering a single preoperative dose of vancomycin in addition to cefazolin is reasonable for patients known to be colonized with MRSA for whom antibiotic prophylaxis is indicated.

Eradication of Nasal Carriage. The combination of preoperative chlorhexidine baths and intranasal mupirocin has been demonstrated to be beneficial in reducing deep surgical site infections in adult MRSA carriers, but data are limited in children. Use of intermittent or continuous intranasal mupirocin for eradication of nasal carriage also has been shown to decrease the incidence of invasive *S aureus* infections in adult patients undergoing long-term hemodialysis or ambulatory peritoneal dialysis. However, long-lasting eradication of nasal carriage of *S aureus* is difficult, and the practice has not been widely adopted for outpatient dialysis because mupirocin-resistant strains can emerge with repeated or widespread use. Intranasal mupirocin treatment is not recommended for routine use but is considered for those with recurrent skin abscesses.

---

[1]Centers for Disease Control and Prevention. Guidelines for preventing health-care–associated pneumonia, 2003: recommendations of CDC and the Healthcare Infection Control Practices Advisory Committee. *MMWR Recomm Rep.* 2004;53(RR-3):1–36

Institutions. Measures to control spread of *S aureus* within health care facilities involve use and careful monitoring of adherence to HICPAC guidelines.[1,2,3] The CDC also recommends strategies for controlling spread of MRSA (**www.cdc.gov/drugresistance/index.html**). These strategies focus on administrative issues; engagement, education, and training of personnel; judicious use of antimicrobial agents; monitoring of prevalence trends over time; use of standard precautions for all patients; and use of contact precautions when appropriate. The CDC has also published a collection of strategies to prevent hospital-onset *S aureus* bloodstream infections (**www.cdc.gov/hai/prevent/staph-prevention-strategies.html**), which focuses on prevention of device and procedure-associated infections, source control strategies for high-risk patients during high-risk periods, interventions to prevent transmission of MRSA in acute care hospitals, and infrastructure needed for prevention. In addition to those contained in HICPAC guidelines for specific device or procedure associated infections, strategies also include intranasal antistaphylococcal antibiotic/antiseptic in conjunction with chlorhexidine wash or wipes before high-risk surgery (eg, cardiothoracic, orthopedic, neurologic, especially those with implantable devices). Some centers use chlorhexidine wash for patients being cared for in the pediatric intensive care unit (the package insert recommends using with care in infants younger than 2 months and preterm infants because of concerns about burns). When rates of endemicity are not decreasing despite adherence to the aforementioned measures, additional interventions, such as use of active surveillance cultures to identify colonized patients and to place them in contact precautions, may be warranted. Decolonization of a health care professional can be considered if the health care professional has been found to be a carrier of *S aureus* and has been epidemiologically linked as a likely source of ongoing transmission to patients. In this situation, attempts to eradicate carriage with topical nasal mupirocin therapy often are made. Both low-level (MIC 8–256 μg/mL) and high-level (MIC ≥512 μg/mL) resistance to mupirocin have been identified in *S aureus*, with high-level resistance associated with failure of decolonization.

Recommendations for investigation and control of VRSA have been published by the CDC (**www.cdc.gov/hai/pdfs/VRSA-Investigation-Guide-05_12_2015.pdf**). The CDC should be contacted for confirmatory testing if *S aureus* isolates with vancomycin MIC of ≥8 μg/mL are identified (generally, notification to the local or state health department should occur first; some initial testing can done at many state public health laboratories). Ongoing review and restriction of vancomycin use is critical in attempts to control the emergence of VISA and VRSA (see Antimicrobial Resistance and Antimicrobial Stewardship: Appropriate and Judicious Use of Antimicrobial Agents, p 868). To date, the use of catheters impregnated with various antimicrobial agents or

[1]Walters M, Lonsway D, Rasheed K, Albrecht V, McAllister S, Limbago B, Kallen A. *Investigation and Control of Vancomycin -Resistant Staphylococcus aureus: A Guide for Health Departments and Infection Control Personnel.* Atlanta, GA: Centers for Disease Control and Prevention; 2015. Available at: **www.cdc.gov/hai/pdfs/VRSA-Investigation-Guide-05_12_2015.pdf**

[2]Siegel JD, Rhinehart E, Jackson M, Chianello L, and the Healthcare Infection Control Practices Advisory Committee. *2007 Guideline for Isolation Precautions: Preventing Transmission of Infectious Agents in Healthcare Settings. Recommendations of the Healthcare Infection Control Practices Advisory Committee.* Atlanta, GA: Centers for Disease Control and Prevention; 2007. Available at: **www.cdc.gov/hicpac/2007IP/2007isolationPrecautions.html**

[3]Siegel JD, Rhinehart E, Jackwson M, Chiarello L; HICPAC. Management of multidrug-resistant organisms in healthcare settings, 2006. Atlanta, GA: Centers for Disease Control and Prevention, 2006. Available at: **www.cdc.gov/infectioncontrol/guidelines/mdro/index.html**

metals to prevent health care-associated infections has not been evaluated adequately in children.

Nurseries. Outbreaks of *S aureus* infections in newborn nurseries require unique measures of control. Hand hygiene should be emphasized to all personnel and visitors. Standard umbilical cord care currently does not include use of topical products (eg, chlorhexidine). Other measures recommended during outbreaks include reinforcement of hand hygiene, alleviating overcrowding and understaffing, surveillance of *S aureus* colonization of newborn infants at admission and periodically thereafter, use of contact precautions for colonized or infected infants, and cohorting of colonized or infected infants and their caregivers. During an outbreak, decolonization measures for infants can be considered, although this needs to be weighed against possible harms such as the risk of caustic cutaneous effects or of systemic absorption of products used for decolonization. In addition, the optimal regimen for decolonization of infants is not known. Decolonization of colonized health care professionals who are epidemiologically implicated in *S aureus* transmission can be attempted but may not be successful. The Centers for Disease Control and Prevention has issued guidance on the prevention and control of *S aureus* infections in newborn nurseries, which can be accessed at **www.cdc.gov/infectioncontrol/guidelines/NICU-saureus/**.

Coagulase-Negative Staphylococcal Infections

CLINICAL MANIFESTATIONS: Most coagulase-negative staphylococci (CoNS) isolates from patient specimens represent contamination of culture material (see Diagnostic Tests, p 693). Of the isolates that do not represent contamination, most come from infections associated with health care, such as patients with obvious disruptions of host defenses caused by surgery, medical device insertion, immunosuppression, or prematurity (eg, very low birth weight infants). CoNS are the most common cause of late-onset bacteremia and septicemia among preterm infants, typically infants weighing less than 1500 g at birth, and of episodes of health care-associated bacteremia in all age groups. CoNS are responsible for bacteremia in children with intravascular catheters, vascular grafts, intracardiac patches, prosthetic cardiac valves, or pacemaker wires. Infection may also be associated with other indwelling foreign bodies, including cerebrospinal fluid shunts, peritoneal catheters, spinal instrumentation, baclofen pumps, pacemakers, or prosthetic joints. Mediastinitis after open-heart surgery, endophthalmitis after intraocular trauma, and omphalitis and scalp abscesses in preterm neonates have been described. CoNS also can enter the bloodstream from the respiratory tract of mechanically ventilated preterm infants or from the gastrointestinal tract of infants with necrotizing enterocolitis. Some species of CoNS are associated with urinary tract infection, including *Staphylococcus saprophyticus* in adolescent females and young adult women, often after sexual intercourse, and *Staphylococcus epidermidis* and *Staphylococcus haemolyticus* in hospitalized patients with urinary tract catheters. *Staphylococcus lugdunensis* is particularly virulent and may cause infections resembling *Staphylococcus aureus*, including skin and soft tissue infection and bacteremia with or without endocarditis.

ETIOLOGY: There are more than 40 named coagulase-negative *Staphylococcus* species in the family; *Staphylococcus epidermidis*, *S haemolyticus*, *S saprophyticus*, *Staphylococcus schleiferi*, and *S lugdunensis* most often are associated with human infections. Many CoNS produce an exopolysaccharide slime biofilm that enables these organisms to bind to medical devices (eg, catheters) and makes them relatively inaccessible to host defenses and antimicrobial agents.

EPIDEMIOLOGY: CoNS are common inhabitants of the skin and mucous membranes. Virtually all neonates are colonized with CoNS at multiple sites by 2 to 4 days of age. The most frequently isolated CoNS organism is *S epidermidis,* which is found widely in most areas of skin. Different species colonize specific areas of the body. *S haemolyticus* is found on areas of skin with numerous apocrine glands, and *S lugdunensis* has a predilection for colonization of the inguinal and groin areas. Infants and children in intensive care units, including neonatal intensive care units, have the highest incidence of CoNS bloodstream infections. CoNS can be introduced at the time of medical device placement, through mucous membrane or skin breaks, through loss of bowel wall integrity (eg, necrotizing enterocolitis in very low birth weight neonates), or during catheter manipulation. Less often, health care professionals with environmental CoNS colonization on their hands transmit the organism.

The **incubation period** is variable for CoNS disease. A long delay can occur between acquisition of the organism and onset of disease.

DIAGNOSTICS TESTS: CoNS are readily isolated in culture using the same media and incubation conditions used for *S aureus*. Tests for coagulase by traditional methods or by latex agglutination are the same as are used for *S aureus*. CoNS isolated from a single blood culture commonly are classified as skin contaminants introduced into the blood culture bottle during venipuncture, and full identification and antimicrobial susceptibility testing are not performed by most clinical laboratories. Fluorescent in situ hybridization (FISH) probes or multiplex polymerase chain reaction (PCR) panel assays can rapidly differentiate CoNS and *S aureus* in positive blood cultures. In a very preterm neonate, an immunocompromised person, or a patient with an indwelling catheter or prosthetic device, repeated isolation of the same species of CoNS from blood cultures or another normally sterile body fluid suggests true infection. For central line-associated bloodstream infection, blood cultures drawn from the catheter generally become positive 2 or more hours before cultures from a peripheral blood vessel. This type of analysis requires that both a peripheral and line blood culture be performed at the same time using equal volumes of blood.

Criteria that suggest CoNS as bloodstream pathogens, rather than contaminants, include the following:

- Two or more positive blood cultures with the same *Staphylococcus* species from different collection sites;
- A positive culture from blood and from another sterile site (eg, cerebrospinal fluid, joint) with the same *Staphylococcus* species and identical antimicrobial susceptibility patterns for each isolate;
- Growth in a continuously monitored blood culture system within 15 hours of incubation;
- Clinical findings of infection;
- An intravascular catheter that has been in place for 3 days or more; and
- Similar or identical genotypes among all isolates.

TREATMENT: More than 90% of health care-associated CoNS strains are methicillin resistant. Methicillin-resistant strains are resistant to all beta-lactam drugs, including cephalosporins (except ceftaroline), and usually several other drug classes. Intravenous vancomycin is recommended for treatment of serious infections caused by CoNS strains resistant to beta-lactam antimicrobial agents. Ceftaroline, daptomycin, and linezolid are alternative agents when vancomycin cannot be used. An exception to this is *S lugdunensis*, which generally is methicillin susceptible. Treatment of infected foreign bodies often involves removal of the device, in addition to antibiotic therapy. Prolonged therapy is likely necessary when there is endocarditis or if the infected device (eg, spinal hardware) cannot be removed entirely. Antimicrobial lock therapy of tunneled central lines may result in a higher rate of catheter salvage in adults with CoNS infections, but experience with this approach is limited in children. If blood cultures remain positive for more than 3 to 5 days after initiation of appropriate antimicrobial therapy for CoNS or if the patient fails to improve, the central line should be removed, parenteral therapy should be continued, and the patient should be evaluated for metastatic foci of infection. If a central line is removed, there is no demonstrable thrombus, and bacteremia resolves promptly, a 5-day course of therapy is generally appropriate for CoNS infections in immunocompetent hosts. The exception is *S lugdunensis*, which should be managed similarly to *S aureus* catheter-related infections (see *Staphylococcus aureus*, p 678).

ISOLATION OF THE HOSPITALIZED PATIENT: Standard precautions are used.

CONTROL MEASURES: Prevention and control of CoNS infections involves prevention of intraoperative contamination by skin flora and sterile insertion of intravascular and intraperitoneal catheters and other prosthetic devices. Catheter-related bloodstream infections can be markedly reduced with a "bundled" prevention approach. Preoperative antibiotic administration lowers the incidence of infection after cardiac surgery and implantation of synthetic vascular grafts and prosthetic devices and often has been used at the time of cerebrospinal fluid shunt placement.

Group A Streptococcal Infections

CLINICAL MANIFESTATIONS: The most common group A streptococcal (GAS) infection is acute pharyngotonsillitis (pharyngitis), which manifests as sore throat with tonsillar inflammation and often tender anterior cervical lymphadenopathy, palatal petechiae, or a strawberry tongue. Purulent complications of pharyngitis include peritonsillar or retropharyngeal abscesses, suppurative cervical adenitis, and rarely, sinusitis and otitis media. Nonsuppurative complications include acute rheumatic fever (ARF) and acute glomerulonephritis (AGN). The goal of antimicrobial therapy for GAS pharyngitis is to reduce acute morbidity, suppurative and nonsuppurative (ARF) complications, and transmission to close contacts. Antimicrobial therapy to prevent AGN after pyoderma or pharyngitis is not effective.

Scarlet fever occurs most often with pharyngitis and, rarely, with pyoderma or an infected wound. Scarlet fever, which has re-emerged in the United Kingdom, China, and Hong Kong, involves a characteristic confluent erythematous sandpaper-like rash caused by one or more GAS erythrogenic exotoxins. Other than rash, the epidemiologic features, symptoms, signs, sequelae, and treatment of scarlet fever are the same as those of streptococcal pharyngitis.

Acute streptococcal pharyngitis is uncommon in children younger than 3 years. Instead, they may present with rhinitis and a protracted illness with moderate fever, irritability, and anorexia (streptococcal fever or streptococcosis). The second most common site of GAS infection is the skin. Streptococcal skin infections (eg, pyoderma or impetigo) can be followed by AGN, occasionally in epidemics. GAS skin infection has not been proven to lead to ARF.

Other GAS infections include erysipelas, cellulitis (including perianal), vaginitis, bacteremia, sepsis, pneumonia, endocarditis, pericarditis, septic arthritis, necrotizing fasciitis, purpura fulminans, osteomyelitis, myositis, puerperal sepsis, surgical wound infection, mastoiditis, and neonatal omphalitis. Invasive GAS infections often encompass bacteremia with or without a focus of infection and can present as streptococcal toxic shock syndrome (STSS), overwhelming sepsis, or necrotizing fasciitis (NF). Necrotizing fasciitis can follow minor or unrecognized trauma but uncommonly pharyngitis, often involves an extremity, and manifests as pain out of proportion to examination findings.

STSS is caused by infection of normally sterile body site(s) (blood, pleura, cerebrospinal fluid, etc) with a toxin-producing GAS strain, typically manifesting as a severe acute illness with fever, generalized erythroderma, rapid-onset hypotension, and signs of multiorgan involvement, including renal failure. Local soft tissue infection (eg, cellulitis, myositis, or NF) associated with severe, rapidly increasing pain is common, although STSS can occur without an identifiable focus of infection.

Rheumatic fever is a nonsuppurative sequela of GAS pharyngitis and is endemic in parts of Africa, Asia, and the Pacific, including the Australian and New Zealand indigenous populations. The United States, Canada, and most of Europe are considered ARF low-risk populations, although sporadic cases continue to occur.

An association between GAS infection and sudden onset of obsessive-compulsive behavior, tic disorders, or other unexplained acute neurologic changes—pediatric autoimmune neuropsychiatric disorders associated with streptococcal infections (PANDAS), as a subset of pediatric acute-onset neuropsychiatric syndrome (PANS)—has been proposed. Data for an association with GAS infection and either PANDAS or PANS rely on a number of small and as yet unduplicated studies. In the absence of acute clinical symptoms and signs of pharyngitis, GAS testing (by culture, antigen detection, or serology) is not recommended for such patients (see Indications for GAS Testing). There also is insufficient evidence to support antibiotic treatment or prophylaxis, Immune Globulin, or plasmapheresis for children suspected to have PANDAS or PANS. Management is best directed by specialists with experience with the presenting symptoms and signs, such as child psychiatrists, behavioral and developmental pediatricians, or child neurologists.

ETIOLOGY: More than 240 distinct serotypes or genotypes of group A streptococci *(Streptococcus pyogenes)* have been identified based on M-protein serotype or M-protein gene sequence *(emm* types). In general, *emm* typing is more discriminating than M-protein serotyping. Epidemiologic studies indicate an association between certain *emm* types (eg, types 1, 3, 5, 6, 14, 18, 19, and 24) and rheumatic fever, but a specific rheumatogenic factor remains unidentified. Several *emm* types (eg, types 2, 49, 55, 57, 59, 60, and 61) are more commonly associated with pyoderma and acute glomerulonephritis. Other serotypes (eg, types 1, 6, and 12) are associated with pharyngitis and acute glomerulonephritis. Although many M types can cause STSS, most cases are caused by *emm* 1 and *emm* 3 strains producing at least 1 pyrogenic exotoxin, most commonly streptococcal pyrogenic exotoxin A *(speA)*. These toxins are superantigens, stimulating production of tumor necrosis factor and other inflammatory mediators causing capillary leak and other physiologic changes including hypotension and multiorgan damage. In the United Kingdom, an increase in scarlet fever cases since 2016 has been associated with a new strain of *emm*1 (M1UK lineage).

EPIDEMIOLOGY: Pharyngitis usually results from contact with respiratory secretions of someone with GAS pharyngitis. Fomites and household pets, such as dogs, are not vectors. Pharyngitis and impetigo (and their nonsuppurative complications) can be associated with crowding, often present in socioeconomically disadvantaged populations. Close contact in schools, child care centers, contact sports (eg, wrestling), boarding schools, and military installations facilitates transmission. Rare foodborne outbreaks of pharyngitis are a consequence of human contamination of food with improper food preparation or refrigeration.

GAS pharyngitis occurs at all ages but is most common among school-aged children and adolescents, peaking at 7 to 8 years of age. GAS pharyngitis and pyoderma are substantially less common in adults than children.

Geographically, GAS pharyngitis and pyoderma are ubiquitous. Pyoderma is more common in tropical climates and warm seasons, in part because of antecedent insect bites and other minor skin trauma. Streptococcal pharyngitis is more common during late autumn, winter, and spring in temperate climates in part because of close contact in schools. Communicability of streptococcal pharyngitis peaks during acute infection and when untreated, gradually diminishes over a period of weeks.

Throat culture surveys of healthy asymptomatic children during the streptococcal season and during school outbreaks of pharyngitis yield GAS infection prevalence rates as high as 25%. GAS carriage can persist for many months, but the risk of transmission is low.

In streptococcal impetigo, the organism usually is acquired by direct contact from another person. GAS colonization of healthy skin usually precedes impetigo. Impetiginous lesions occur at the site of breaks in skin (eg, insect bites, burns, traumatic wounds, varicella lesions). After development of impetiginous lesions, the upper respiratory tract can become colonized with GAS organisms. Infection of surgical wounds and postpartum (puerperal) sepsis usually result from transmission through direct contact. Health care workers who are pharyngeal, anal, or vaginal GAS carriers and those with skin infection or skin colonization can transmit GAS infection to patients, particularly surgical and obstetrical patients, resulting in health care-associated outbreaks. Infections in neonates, uncommon in the United States but common in many developing countries, result from intrapartum or contact transmission; the latter infection can begin as omphalitis, cellulitis, or necrotizing fasciitis. In the United States, the incidence of invasive GAS infections is highest in infants and the elderly. Fatal cases in children are not common, but they can progress very rapidly (eg, overwhelming sepsis). Before varicella vaccine, varicella infection (chickenpox) was the most common predisposing factor for invasive GAS infection in children. Other risk factors include exposure to other children and household crowding. The portal of entry is unknown in most invasive GAS infections but presumably is skin or mucous membranes. Such infections very rarely follow symptomatic GAS pharyngitis. An association between nonsteroidal anti-inflammatory drugs and invasive GAS infections in children with varicella has been suggested, but a causal relationship has not been established.

STSS can occur at any age. Fewer than 5% of invasive streptococcal infections in children are associated with STSS. Childhood STSS has been reported with focal lesions (eg, varicella, cellulitis, trauma, osteomyelitis, pneumonia), and with bacteremia without a defined focus. Mortality rates are substantially lower for children than for adults with STSS.

During GAS epidemics on military bases in the 1950s, ARF developed in up to 3% of untreated acute GAS pharyngitis; rare cases have occurred in treated patients. The current incidence in the United States is not precisely known but is believed to be <0.5%, with higher rates reported among people of Samoan ancestry living in Hawaii or residents of American Samoa. Focal outbreaks of ARF in school-aged children occurred in several areas in the 1990s, and small clusters continue to be reported periodically, most likely related to circulation of particularly rheumatogenic strains.

The **incubation period** for streptococcal pharyngitis is 2 to 5 days. For impetigo, a 7- to 10-day period between GAS acquisition on healthy skin and development of lesions has been demonstrated. The **incubation period** for STSS is not known but is as short as 14 hours when associated with subcutaneous inoculation of organisms (eg, puerperal sepsis, penetrating trauma).

DIAGNOSTIC TESTS[1]:

Testing for Group A Streptococci in Pharyngitis. Children with acute onset of sore throat and clinical signs and symptoms such as pharyngeal exudate, pain on swallowing, fever, and enlarged tender anterior cervical nodes are more likely to have GAS infection and should be tested. Children with pharyngitis and obvious viral symptoms (eg, rhinorrhea, cough, hoarseness, oral ulcers) should not be tested or treated for GAS infection; testing also generally is not recommended for children younger than 3 years. Laboratory confirmation before initiation of antimicrobial treatment is required for children with pharyngitis without viral symptoms, because many will not have GAS pharyngitis. A specimen should be obtained by vigorously swabbing both tonsils and the posterior pharynx for rapid antigen testing or other diagnostic test, as discussed below. A second swab specimen from a child with a negative rapid antigen test should be submitted for culture. Culture on sheep blood agar can confirm GAS infection, with latex agglutination differentiating group A streptococci from other beta-hemolytic streptococci (eg, group C or G). False-negative culture results occur in <10% of symptomatic patients when an adequate throat swab specimen is obtained and cultured by trained personnel. Recovery of GAS organisms from the pharynx, including the number of colonies on a culture plate, does not distinguish patients with true acute streptococcal infection from chronic streptococcal carriers with intercurrent viral pharyngitis. Cultures negative for GAS organisms after 18 to 24 hours incubation should be reincubated for a second day to optimize recovery from GAS infection.

Several rapid tests for GAS pharyngitis are available. The specificity of these tests generally is high (very few false-positive results), but reported sensitivities vary considerably and generally are 80% to 85% (ie, false-negatives occur). As with throat cultures, the sensitivity of these tests is highly dependent on the quality of the throat swab specimen, experience of the test performer, and the rigor of the culture method used for comparison.

Because of very high specificity of rapid antigen-based tests, a positive result does not require culture confirmation, but negative results require a confirmatory test in children. Other diagnostic tests using techniques such as polymerase chain reaction (PCR), chemiluminescent DNA probes, and isothermal nucleic acid amplification tests have

---

[1]Shulman ST, Bisno AL, Clegg HW, et al. Clinical practice guideline for the diagnosis and management of group a streptococcal pharyngitis: 2012 update by the Infectious Diseases Society of America. *Clin Infect Dis.* 2012;55(10):e86-e102

been developed. The US Food and Drug Administration has cleared some nucleic acid amplification tests for detection of group A streptococci from throat swab specimens as stand-alone tests that, because of high sensitivity, do not require routine culture confirmation of negative test results. Some studies suggest that in addition to providing more timely results, these tests may be more sensitive than standard throat swab cultures on sheep blood agar, although the device labeling states that culture is still required if the test result is negative and the patient's symptoms persist or in the event of an outbreak of rheumatic fever. Additional studies are ongoing to establish the benefits and limitations of these tests.

Testing Contacts for GAS Infection. Indications for testing contacts for GAS infection are few. Testing asymptomatic household contacts is not recommended, except when the contacts are at increased risk for sequelae of GAS infection, such as ARF or AGN; if test results are positive, the contacts should be treated.

In schools, child care centers, or other environments where many people are in close contact, the prevalence of GAS pharyngeal carriage in healthy children can reach 25% in the absence of an outbreak of streptococcal disease. Therefore, classroom or more widespread culturing generally is not indicated.

Follow-up Throat Cultures. Post-treatment throat cultures are indicated only for those at particularly high risk of ARF (eg, with previous history of ARF).

Patients with repeated episodes of pharyngitis at short intervals in whom GAS infection is documented by culture or rapid antigen or nucleic acid amplification test present a special problem. Most often, they are chronic GAS carriers experiencing frequent viral illnesses for whom repeated testing and antimicrobials are unnecessary. In assessing these patients, inadequate adherence to oral treatment also should be considered. Testing asymptomatic household contacts usually is not helpful. However, if multiple household members have pharyngitis or other GAS infections, simultaneous cultures of all household members and treatment of all positive test results may be of value.

Testing for Group A Streptococci in Nonpharyngitis Infections. Cultures of impetigo lesions often yield both streptococci and staphylococci, and determination of the primary pathogen is generally difficult. Culture is useful to determine *S aureus* susceptibility. In suspected invasive GAS infections, cultures of blood and focal sites of possible infection are indicated. In necrotizing fasciitis, imaging studies may delay, rather than facilitate, establishing the diagnosis. Clinical suspicion of necrotizing fasciitis should prompt urgent surgical evaluation with possible urgent debridement of affected tissues, with Gram stain and culture of surgical specimens. STSS is diagnosed on the basis of clinical and laboratory findings and isolation of GAS organisms (Table 3.55); more than 50% of patients with STSS have blood cultures positive for group A streptococci. Cultures of focal sites of infection are also usually positive and can remain positive for several days after initiation of an appropriate antimicrobial agents.

TREATMENT[1]:

S pyogenes is uniformly susceptible to all beta-lactam antibiotics (penicillins and cephalosporins); thus, susceptibility testing is needed only for non–beta-lactam agents, such as a macrolide or clindamycin, to which *S pyogenes* can be resistant.

---

[1]Shulman ST, Bisno AL, Clegg HW, et al. Clinical practice guideline for the diagnosis and management of group a streptococcal pharyngitis: 2012 update by the Infectious Diseases Society of America. *Clin Infect Dis.* 2012;55(10):e86-e102

Table 3.55. Streptococcal Toxic Shock Syndrome: Clinical Case Definition[a]

I. Isolation of group A *Streptococcus (Streptococcus pyogenes)*

  A. From a normally sterile site (eg, blood, cerebrospinal fluid, peritoneal, joint, pleural, or pericardial fluid)

  B. From a nonsterile site (eg, throat, sputum, vagina, open surgical wound, or superficial skin lesion)

II. Clinical signs of severity

  A. Hypotension: systolic pressure 90 mm Hg or less in adults or lower than the fifth percentile for age in children <16 years of age

AND

  B. Two or more of the following signs of multi-organ involvement:

- Renal impairment: creatinine concentration 177 μmol/L (2 mg/dL) or greater for adults or at least 2 times the upper limit of normal for age[b]
- Coagulopathy: platelet count 100 000/mm^3 or less and/or disseminated intravascular coagulation defined by prolonged clotting times, low fibrinogen, and presence of fibrin degradation products
- Hepatic involvement: elevated alanine aminotransferase, aspartate aminotransferase, or total bilirubin concentrations at least 2 times the upper limit of normal for age[b]
- Acute respiratory distress syndrome defined by acute onset of diffuse pulmonary infiltrates and hypoxemia in absence of cardiac failure or by evidence of diffuse capillary leak
- A generalized erythematous macular rash that may desquamate
- Soft tissue necrosis, including necrotizing fasciitis or myositis, or gangrene

Adapted from: The Working Group on Severe Streptococcal Infections. Defining the group A streptococcal toxic shock syndrome: rationale and consensus definition. *JAMA.* 1993;269(3):390–391

[a] An illness fulfilling criteria IA and IIA and IIB can be defined as a *confirmed* case. An illness fulfilling criteria IB and IIA and IIB can be defined as a *probable* case if no other cause for the illness is identified. Manifestations need not be detected within the first 48 hours of illness or hospitalization.

[b] In patients with preexisting renal or hepatic disease, concentrations twofold or greater over patient's baseline.

Pharyngitis.

- Penicillin V is the drug of choice for GAS pharyngitis. Prompt administration of penicillin shortens the clinical course, decreases risk of transmission and suppurative sequelae, and prevents ARF, even when administered up to 9 days after illness onset. All patients with ARF should receive a complete course of penicillin or another appropriate antimicrobial agent for GAS pharyngitis, even if group A streptococci are not recovered from the throat.
- Amoxicillin, orally as a single daily dose (50 mg/kg; maximum, 1000–1200 mg) for 10 days, is as effective as penicillin V or amoxicillin administered orally multiple times per day for 10 days and is a more palatable suspension than penicillin V. This regimen is endorsed by the American Heart Association and the Infectious Disease Society of America in its guidelines for the treatment of GAS pharyngitis and the prevention of ARF.[1] Adherence is particularly important for once-daily dosing regimens.

[1] Gerber MA, Baltimore RS, Eaton CB, et al. Prevention of rheumatic fever and diagnosis and treatment of acute streptococcal pharyngitis. A scientific statement from the American Heart Association, Rheumatic Fever, Endocarditis, and Kawasaki Disease Committee, Council on Cardiovascular Disease in the Young, and the Quality of Care and Outcomes Research Interdisciplinary Working Group and endorsed by the American Academy of Pediatrics. *Circulation.* 2009;119(11):1541-1551

- The dose of oral penicillin V is 400 000 U (250 mg), 2 to 3 times per day, for 10 days for children weighing <27 kg and 800 000 U (500 mg), 2 to 3 times per day, for those weighing ≥27 kg, including adolescents and adults. To prevent ARF, oral penicillin or amoxicillin should be taken for 10 full days, regardless of promptness of clinical recovery. Treatment failures occur more often with oral penicillin than with intramuscular penicillin G benzathine because of inadequate adherence. Notably, short-course treatment (<10 days) for GAS pharyngitis, particularly with penicillin V, is associated with inferior bacteriologic eradication rates.
- Intramuscular penicillin G benzathine is appropriate therapy, ensuring adequate blood concentrations and avoiding adherence issues, but administration may be painful. See Tables of Antibacterial Drug Dosages (p 876) for dosing. Discomfort is decreased if the preparation of penicillin G benzathine is brought to room temperature before intramuscular injection. Mixtures containing shorter-acting penicillins (eg, penicillin G procaine) in addition to penicillin G benzathine are not more effective than penicillin G benzathine alone but are less painful. Although supporting data are limited, the combination of 900 000 U (562.5 mg) of penicillin G benzathine and 300 000 U (187.5 mg) of penicillin G procaine is satisfactory for most children; however, the efficacy of this combination for heavier patients has not been documented.
- For patients who have a history of nonanaphylactic allergy to penicillin, a 10-day course of a narrow-spectrum (first-generation) oral cephalosporin (eg, cephalexin) is indicated. Patients with immediate (anaphylactic) or type I hypersensitivity to penicillin should receive oral clindamycin (20 mg/kg per day in 3 divided doses; maximum, 900 mg/day for 10 days) rather than a cephalosporin.
- An oral macrolide (eg, erythromycin, azithromycin, or clarithromycin) also is acceptable for penicillin–allergic patients. This should not be used in patients who can take a beta-lactam agent. Therapy for 10 days is indicated, except for azithromycin, which is given for 5 days. GAS strains resistant to macrolides have been highly prevalent in some countries and have resulted in treatment failures. In some areas in the United States, macrolide resistance rates of more than 20% have been reported. Testing for macrolide resistance may help to decide the best antimicrobial agent for specific penicillin-allergic patients.
- Tetracyclines, sulfonamides, and fluoroquinolones should not be used for treating GAS pharyngitis.

Children with recurrent GAS pharyngitis shortly after a full course of a recommended oral agent can be retreated with the same antimicrobial agent (if it is a beta-lactam), an alternative beta-lactam oral drug (such as cephalexin or amoxicillin-clavulanate), or an intramuscular dose of penicillin G benzathine. Susceptibility testing should be performed when considering a macrolide or clindamycin.

Frequent Acute Pharyngitis With Positive GAS Testing. Management of a patient with frequently repeated episodes of acute pharyngitis and repeatedly positive test results for group A streptococci is complex. To determine whether the patient is a long-term streptococcal pharyngeal carrier who is experiencing repeated episodes of intercurrent viral pharyngitis (the most common situation), it should be determined: (1) whether clinical findings are more suggestive of GAS or viral infection; (2) whether household or community epidemiologic factors support group A streptococci or a virus as the cause; (3) the nature of the clinical response to antimicrobial therapy (in bonafide GAS pharyngitis, response to therapy usually is <24 hours); and (4) whether test results are positive for group A streptococci between episodes of acute pharyngitis (suggesting the patient is a carrier). Measurement of serologic response to GAS extracellular antigens (eg, antistreptolysin O) is discouraged, because interpretation can be very difficult. Typing (M or *emm* typing) of GAS isolates generally is available only in research laboratories, but if performed, repeated isolation of the same type suggests carriage; isolation of differing types indicates repeated infections.

Pharyngeal Carriers. Antimicrobial therapy is not indicated for most GAS pharyngeal carriers. The few specific situations in which eradication of carriage may be indicated include the following: (1) a local outbreak of ARF or poststreptococcal glomerulonephritis; (2) an outbreak of GAS pharyngitis in a closed or semiclosed community; (3) a family history of ARF; (4) multiple ("ping-pong") episodes of documented symptomatic GAS pharyngitis occurring within a family for many weeks despite appropriate therapy; or (5) when a patient is being seriously considered for tonsillectomy solely because of frequent GAS isolations.

GAS carriage is difficult to eradicate with conventional antimicrobial therapy. Several agents, including clindamycin, cephalosporins, amoxicillin-clavulanate, azithromycin, or a combination that includes either 10 days of penicillin V or IM penicillin G benzathine with rifampin for the last 4 days of treatment are more effective than penicillin alone in terminating chronic streptococcal carriage. Of these drugs, oral clindamycin, 20 to 30 mg/kg per day in 3 doses (maximum, 900 mg/day) for 10 days, has been reported to be most effective. Documented eradication of carriage is helpful in evaluation of subsequent episodes of acute pharyngitis; however, carriage can recur after reacquisition of GAS infection, as some individuals are "carrier prone."

Nonbullous Impetigo. Topical mupirocin or retapamulin ointment may be useful for limiting person-to-person spread of nonbullous impetigo and for eradicating localized disease. With multiple lesions or nonbullous impetigo in multiple family members, child care groups, or athletic teams, treatment should include oral agents active against both group A streptococci and *S aureus*.

Toxic Shock Syndrome. As outlined in Tables 3.56 and 3.57, most aspects of management are the same for TSS caused by group A streptococci or by *S aureus*. Paramount are immediate aggressive fluid resuscitation, management of respiratory and cardiac failure, if present, and prompt surgical débridement of any deep-seated infection. Because *S pyogenes* and *S aureus* TSS are difficult to distinguish clinically, initial therapy should include an antistaphylococcal agent and a protein synthesis-inhibiting agent, such as clindamycin.

Table 3.56. Management of Streptococcal Toxic Shock Syndrome Without Necrotizing Fasciitis

- Fluid management to maintain adequate venous return and cardiac filling pressures to prevent end-organ damage
- Anticipatory management of multisystem organ failure
- Parenteral antimicrobial therapy at maximum doses with the capacity to:
  - Kill organism with bactericidal cell wall inhibitor (eg, beta-lactamase–resistant antimicrobial agent)
  - Decrease enzyme, toxin, or cytokine production with protein synthesis inhibitor (eg, clindamycin)
- IGIV often is used as an adjunct, typically at 1 g/kg on day 1, followed by 0.5 g/kg on 1–2 subsequent days

IGIV indicates Immune Globulin Intravenous.

Table 3.57. Management of Streptococcal Toxic Shock Syndrome With Necrotizing Fasciitis

- Principles outlined in Table 3.56
- Immediate surgical evaluation
  - Exploration or incisional biopsy for diagnosis and culture
  - Resection of all necrotic tissue
- Repeated resection of tissue may be needed if infection persists or progresses

Addition of clindamycin to penicillin is recommended for serious GAS infections, because its antimicrobial activity is unaffected by inoculum size (does not have the eagle effect that occurs with beta-lactam antibiotics), has a long postantimicrobial effect, and inhibits bacterial protein synthesis, which results in suppression of synthesis of *S pyogenes* antiphagocytic M-protein and bacterial toxins. Clindamycin **should not be used alone** as initial antimicrobial therapy in life-threatening situations because of the potential for resistance. In 2017, 22% of invasive GAS case isolates from the Active Bacterial Core surveillance system in the United States were resistant to clindamycin (**www.cdc.gov/drugre-sistance/pdf/threats-report/2019-ar-threats-report-508.pdf**).

Once GAS infection is confirmed, antimicrobial therapy should be tailored to penicillin and clindamycin. Intravenous therapy should be continued at least until the patient is afebrile and stable hemodynamically and blood is documented to be sterile. Clindamycin may be discontinued after a few days if there is adequate source control and clinical improvement. The total duration of therapy is based on duration established for the primary site of infection.

Aggressive drainage and irrigation of accessible sites of infection should be performed as soon as possible. If necrotizing fasciitis is suspected, immediate surgical exploration or biopsy is crucial to identify and debride deep soft tissue infection.

Immune Globulin Intravenous (IGIV) should be strongly considered as adjunctive therapy for STSS or necrotizing fasciitis if the patient is moderately to severely ill, although its use is supported by limited data.

Other Infections. Parenteral antimicrobial therapy is required for severe GAS infections, such as endocarditis, pneumonia, empyema, deep abscess, septicemia, meningitis, arthritis, osteomyelitis, erysipelas, necrotizing fasciitis, and neonatal omphalitis. Treatment often is prolonged (2–6 weeks).

Acute Rheumatic Fever. Jones criteria for diagnosis of ARF were established in 1944 and revised and modified several times, most recently in 2015.[1] The 2015 Jones criteria revision (Table 3.58) differentiates major and minor criteria on the basis of whether the child is from an area at low or high risk for ARF. Laboratory evidence of antecedent GAS infection should be confirmed in suspected ARF and includes an increased or increasing antistreptolysin O or anti-DNAase B titer or a positive rapid antigen or streptococcal throat culture. Because of the long latency between GAS infection and chorea, laboratory evidence may be lacking when chorea is the major criterion. See Table 3.58 for the major and minor criteria.

---

[1]Gewitz MH, Baltimore RS, Tani LY, et al. Revision of the Jones criteria for the diagnosis of acute rheumatic fever in the era of Doppler echocardiography. *Circulation.* 2015;131(20):1806-1818

Table 3.58. Revised Jones Criteria (2015)

1. All patients require evidence of antecedent GAS infection for diagnosis of ARF (except in case of chorea, where evidence of antecedent GAS infection is not required).
2. To confirm an initial diagnosis of ARF, need 2 major OR 1 major and 2 minor criteria.
3. To confirm recurrent ARF diagnosis, need 2 major OR 1 major and 2 minor OR 3 minor criteria.
4. Criteria for diagnosis are dependent on whether patient is from a low-risk or a moderate-/high-risk population. Moderate- and high-risk populations include countries where ARF remains endemic (Africa, Asia-Pacific, indigenous population of Australia). The United States, Canada, and Europe are examples of low-risk areas.
5. Major and minor criteria are listed below, by risk categorization; differences for moderate-/high-risk populations are **bolded.**

Low-Risk Population	Moderate- and High-Risk Population
Major Criteria	**Major Criteria**
• Carditis (clinical or subclinical) • Arthritis (polyarthritis only) • Chorea • Subcutaneous nodules • Erythema marginatum	• Carditis (clinical or subclinical) • Arthritis (polyarthritis or **monoarthritis**, or **polyarthralgia**) • Chorea • Subcutaneous nodules • Erythema marginatum
Minor Criteria	**Minor Criteria**
• Polyarthralgia • Fever ≥38.5°C • ESR ≥60 mm/h and/or CRP ≥3 mg/dL • Prolonged PR interval (in absence of carditis)	• **Monoarthralgia** • **Fever ≥38°C** • **ESR ≥30 mm/h** and/or CRP ≥3 mg/dL • Prolonged PR interval (in absence of carditis)

ARF indicates acute rheumatic fever; CRP, C-reactive protein; ESR, erythrocyte sedimentation rate; GAS, group A streptococcal.

Modified from Table 7 in Gewitz MH, Baltimore RS, Tani LY, et al. Revision of the Jones criteria for the diagnosis of acute rheumatic fever in the era of Doppler echocardiography: a scientific statement from the American Heart Association. *Circulation.* 2015;131(20):1806-1818.

Treatment for ARF includes eradication of group A streptococci with a standard pharyngitis regimen, treatment of acute manifestations (eg, arthritis or valvulitis-associated heart failure), education for parents and patient, and initiation of secondary prophylaxis to prevent future GAS infection. Following initial treatment of ARF, patients with well-documented history of ARF (including cases manifested solely as Sydenham chorea) and patients with documented rheumatic heart disease (RHD) should be given continuous antimicrobial prophylaxis to prevent recurrent ARF attacks (secondary prophylaxis), because asymptomatic and symptomatic GAS infections can trigger recurrence of ARF. Continuous secondary prophylaxis should be initiated as soon as the diagnosis of ARF or rheumatic heart disease is made, and should be long-term, perhaps for life, for patients with RHD (even after prosthetic valve replacement), because they remain at risk of ARF recurrence. Risk of recurrence decreases as the interval from the most recent acute episode increases, and patients without RHD are at lower risk of recurrence than patients

Table 3.59. Duration of Prophylaxis for People Who Have Had Acute Rheumatic Fever (ARF): Recommendations of the American Heart Association[a]

Category	Duration
Rheumatic fever without carditis	5 years since last episode of ARF or until 21 years of age, whichever is longer
Rheumatic fever with carditis but without residual heart disease (no valvular disease[b])	10 years since last episode of ARF or until 21 years of age, whichever is longer
Rheumatic fever with carditis and residual heart disease (persistent valvular disease[b])	10 years since last episode of ARF or until 40 years of age, whichever is longer; consider lifelong prophylaxis for people with severe valvular disease or likelihood of ongoing exposure to group A streptococcal infection

[a]Modified from Gerber M, Baltimore R, Eaton C, et al. Prevention of rheumatic fever and diagnosis and treatment of acute streptococcal pharyngitis. A scientific statement from the American Heart Association, Rheumatic Fever, Endocarditis, and Kawasaki Disease Committee, Council on Cardiovascular Disease in the Young, and the Quality of Care and Outcomes Research Interdisciplinary Working Group. *Circulation.* 2009;119(11):1541-1551.
[b]Clinical or echocardiographic evidence.

with residual cardiac involvement. These considerations and the estimate of future exposure to GAS infection, influence the duration of secondary prophylaxis in adults but should not alter the duration of secondary prophylaxis for children and adolescents. Secondary prophylaxis for all who have had ARF should be continued for at least 5 years or until the person is 21 years of age, whichever is longer (see Table 3.59). Prophylaxis also should be continued if the risk of contact with people with GAS infection is high (eg, for parents with school-aged children, teachers, and others in frequent contact with children).

The antibiotic regimens in Table 3.60 are effective for secondary prophylaxis. The intramuscular regimen is the most reliable, because success of oral prophylaxis depends primarily on patient adherence; however, inconvenience and pain of injection may cause some patients to discontinue intramuscular prophylaxis. In non-US populations in whom risk of ARF is particularly high, administration of penicillin G benzathine every 3 weeks is justified and recommended, because serum penicillin concentrations can decrease below a protective level in the fourth week after a dose. In the United States, administration every 4 weeks is likely adequate, except for those who have developed recurrent ARF despite adherence to an every-4-week regimen. Oral sulfadiazine is as effective as oral penicillin for secondary prophylaxis but may not be as readily available in the United States. By extrapolating from sulfadiazine, sulfisoxazole has been deemed an appropriate alternative; it is available in combination with erythromycin as a generic version.

Allergic reactions to oral penicillin are less common and usually less severe than reactions to parenteral penicillin and occur much more often in adults than in children. Severe allergic reactions rarely occur with intramuscular penicillin G benzathine prophylaxis, but the incidence may be higher in patients older than 12 years with severe RHD. Most severe reactions seem to be vasovagal responses rather than anaphylaxis. A serum sickness-like reaction characterized by fever and joint pains can occur in those receiving prophylaxis and can be mistaken for recurrence of ARF.

Table 3.60. Chemoprophylaxis for Recurrences of Acute Rheumatic Fever[a]

Drug	Dose	Route
Penicillin G benzathine	1.2 million U, every 4 wk[b]; 600 000 U, every 4 wk for patients weighing less than 27 kg (60 lb)	Intramuscular
OR		
Penicillin V	250 mg, twice a day	Oral
OR		
Sulfadiazine or sulfisoxazole	0.5 g, once a day for patients weighing 27 kg (60 lb) or less	Oral
	1.0 g, once a day for patients weighing greater than 27 kg (60 lb)	
For people who are allergic to penicillin and sulfonamide drugs		
Macrolide or azalide	Variable (see text)	Oral

[a] Gerber M, Baltimore R, Eaton C, et al. Prevention of rheumatic fever and diagnosis and treatment of acute streptococcal pharyngitis. A scientific statement from the American Heart Association, Rheumatic Fever, Endocarditis, and Kawasaki Disease Committee, Council on Cardiovascular Disease in the Young, and the Quality of Care and Outcomes Research Interdisciplinary Working Group. *Circulation.* 2009;119(11):1541-1551.

[b] In particularly high-risk situations (usually non-US sites), administration every 3 weeks is recommended.

Reactions to continuous sulfadiazine or sulfisoxazole prophylaxis are rare and usually minor; evaluation of blood cell counts may be advisable after 2 weeks of prophylaxis, because leukopenia has been reported. Prophylaxis with a sulfonamide during late pregnancy is contraindicated because of interference with fetal bilirubin metabolism. Febrile mucocutaneous syndromes (erythema multiforme, Stevens-Johnson syndrome, or toxic epidermal necrolysis) rarely have been associated with penicillin and sulfonamides.

When an adverse event occurs with any prophylactic regimen, the drug should be stopped immediately and an alternative drug selected. For the rare patient allergic to both penicillins and sulfonamides, erythromycin is recommended. Other macrolides, such as azithromycin or clarithromycin, also are acceptable; they have less risk of gastrointestinal tract intolerance but increased cost.

Poststreptococcal Reactive Arthritis. After an episode of acute GAS pharyngitis, reactive arthritis may develop without sufficient clinical and laboratory findings to fulfill the Jones criteria for diagnosis of ARF. This syndrome has been termed poststreptococcal reactive arthritis (PSRA). The precise relationship of PSRA to ARF is unclear. In contrast to arthritis of ARF, PSRA does not respond dramatically to nonsteroidal anti-inflammatory agents. Because a very small proportion of patients with PSRA have been reported to develop late valvular heart disease, they should be observed carefully for 1 to 2 years for evidence of carditis, and some experts recommend secondary prophylaxis during the observation period. If carditis develops, the patient should be considered to have had ARF, and secondary prophylaxis should be initiated (see above).

ISOLATION OF THE HOSPITALIZED PATIENT: In addition to standard precautions, droplet precautions are recommended for those with GAS pharyngitis or pneumonia until

24 hours after initiation of appropriate antimicrobial therapy. For burns with secondary GAS infection and extensive or draining cutaneous infections that cannot be covered or contained adequately by dressings, contact precautions should be used until at least 24 hours after initiation of appropriate therapy.

CONTROL MEASURES: The most important means of controlling GAS disease and its sequelae is prompt identification and treatment of infections.

School and Child Care. Children with GAS pharyngitis or skin infections should not return to school or child care until well appearing and at least 12 hours after beginning appropriate antimicrobial therapy. Close contact with other children during this time should be avoided.

Care of Exposed People. Symptomatic contacts of a child with documented GAS infection with recent or current clinical evidence of a GAS infection should undergo appropriate laboratory tests and treated if test results are positive. Rates of GAS carriage are higher among sibling contacts of children with GAS pharyngitis than among parent contacts in nonepidemic settings; carriage rates as high as 50% for sibling contacts and 20% for parent contacts are reported during epidemics. Asymptomatic acquisition of GAS infection may pose some low risk of nonsuppurative complications; as many as one third of patients with ARF have no history of recent streptococcal infection and another third have minor respiratory tract symptoms not brought to medical attention. However, routine laboratory evaluation of asymptomatic household contacts is not indicated except during outbreaks or when contacts are at increased risk of developing sequelae of infection. In rare circumstances, such as a large family with documented, repeated, intrafamilial transmission resulting in frequent episodes of GAS pharyngitis over a prolonged period, physicians may elect to treat all family members identified by laboratory tests as harboring GAS organisms.

Household contacts of patients with severe invasive GAS disease, including STSS, are at some increased risk of developing severe invasive GAS disease compared with the general population. However, the risk is not sufficiently high to warrant routine testing for GAS colonization, and a clearly effective regimen has not been identified to justify routine chemoprophylaxis of all household contacts. However, because of increased risk of sporadic, invasive GAS disease among certain populations (eg, people with human immunodeficiency virus [HIV] infection) and because of increased risk of death in those 65 years and older who develop invasive GAS disease, physicians may choose to offer targeted chemoprophylaxis to household contacts 65 years and older or to members of other high-risk populations (eg, people with HIV infection, varicella, or diabetes mellitus). Because of the rarity of secondary cases and the low risk of invasive GAS infections in children, chemoprophylaxis is not recommended in schools or child care facilities.

Bacterial Endocarditis Prophylaxis.[1] The American Heart Association (AHA) has published updated recommendations regarding use of antimicrobial agents to prevent infective endocarditis (see Prevention of Bacterial Endocarditis, p 1021). The AHA no longer recommends prophylaxis for patients with RHD without a prosthetic valve. However, use of oral antiseptic solutions and maintenance of optimal oral health through daily oral

---

[1]Wilson W, Taubert KA, Gewitz M, et al. Prevention of infective endocarditis. Recommendations by the American Heart Association. A guideline from the American Heart Association Rheumatic Fever, Endocarditis, and Kawasaki Disease Committee, Council on Cardiovascular Disease in the Young, and the Council on Clinical Cardiology, Council on Cardiovascular Surgery and Anesthesia, and the Quality of Care and Outcomes Research Interdisciplinary Working Group. *Circulation.* 2007;116(15):1736–1754

hygiene and regular dental visits remain important components of an overall health care program. For individuals with a prosthetic valve, infective endocarditis prophylaxis still is recommended, and current AHA recommendations should be followed. If penicillin is being used for secondary ARF prevention, an agent other than penicillin or amoxicillin should be used for infective endocarditis prophylaxis, because penicillin-resistant alpha-hemolytic streptococci are likely to be present in the mouth.

Group B Streptococcal Infections

CLINICAL MANIFESTATIONS: Group B streptococci are a major cause of perinatal infections, including bacteremia, intra-amniotic infection (formerly called chorioamnionitis), and endometritis in pregnant and postpartum women, as well as systemic and focal infections in neonates and young infants. In newborn infants, early-onset disease (EOD) usually occurs within the first 24 hours after birth (range, 0 through 6 days), presenting with respiratory distress, apnea, shock, pneumonia, and less often, meningitis (5%–10% of cases). Late-onset disease (LOD), which typically occurs at 3 to 4 weeks of age (range, 7 through 89 days), commonly manifests as bacteremia or meningitis (approximately 30% of cases); other focal infections, such as osteomyelitis, septic arthritis, necrotizing fasciitis, pneumonia, adenitis, and cellulitis, occur less commonly. Approximately 20% of survivors of neonatal group B streptococcal meningitis have moderate to severe neurodevelopmental impairment. Cases among infants older than 90 days are reported rarely, usually in very preterm infants requiring prolonged hospitalization.

ETIOLOGY: Group B streptococci *(Streptococcus agalactiae)* are gram-positive diplococci that typically produce a narrow zone of beta hemolysis on 5% sheep blood agar. These organisms are divided into 10 types on the basis of capsular polysaccharides structures. Types Ia, Ib, II, III, IV, and V account for approximately 99% of cases in infants in the United States. Type III causes approximately 30% to 60% of EOD and LOD, respectively.

EPIDEMIOLOGY: Group B streptococci colonize the human gastrointestinal and genitourinary tracts, and less commonly the pharynx. The vaginal/rectal colonization rate in pregnant women ranges from 15% to 35% and can be persistent or intermittent. In the 1990s, recommendations were made for prevention of early-onset group B streptococcal (GBS) disease through maternal intrapartum antibiotic prophylaxis (IAP) (see Control Measures, p 709). As a result of widespread implementation of IAP, the incidence of EOD has decreased by approximately 80% to an estimated 0.25 cases per 1000 live births in 2018. The use of IAP has had no measurable effect on late-onset GBS disease incidence. In 2018, LOD incidence exceeded that of EOD at 0.28 cases per 1000 live births. The case-fatality rate for group B streptococcal disease in term infants ranges from 1% to 3% but is higher in preterm neonates (estimated to be 20% for EOD and 8% for LOD). Approximately 70% of EOD and 50% of LOD afflict term neonates.

Transmission from mother to infant generally occurs shortly before or during delivery in mothers who are colonized with GBS organisms. Less commonly, GBS infection may be transmitted in the nursery from health care professionals or visitors, or in the community via colonized family members or caregivers. The risk of EOD is increased in preterm infants, infants born 18 hours or more after membrane rupture, and infants born to women with intrapartum fever (temperature 38°C [100.4°F] or greater), intra-amniotic infection, GBS bacteriuria during the current pregnancy, or a history of a previous infant with invasive GBS disease. A higher incidence of EOD has also been associated with maternal age <20 years of age and mothers of Black race. However, the independent contribution of these factors is unclear, because both maternal age and race have also been associated with higher rates of both GBS colonization and preterm birth. Infants can remain colonized for several months despite treatment for systemic infection. Recurrent GBS disease affects an estimated 1% to 3% of appropriately treated infants.

The **incubation period** of EOD is fewer than 7 days. In LOD, the **incubation period** is unknown.

DIAGNOSTIC TESTS: Visualization of gram-positive cocci in pairs or short chains from a normally sterile body fluid provides presumptive evidence of infection, but growth of the organism in culture establishes the diagnosis. Meningitis/encephalitis multiplex panel polymerase chain reaction (PCR) assays are available in many clinical laboratories for direct testing of cerebrospinal fluid (CSF) for GBS organisms.

For prenatal GBS screening, maternal swab specimens from vaginal and rectal sites are collected (vaginal swab specimens alone underestimate GBS colonization by up to 10%–15%). Culture yield can be increased with the use of commercially available selective broth enrichment media for 18 to 24 hours of incubation before being plated on tryptic soy blood agar or other selective agars for an additional 24 to 48 hours. Alternatively, DNA probe assays, latex agglutination assays, and nucleic acid amplification tests (NAATs) are available to detect GBS organisms from enriched broth specimens. Several NAATs are approved for antepartum or intrapartum detection of GBS organisms from vaginal/rectal swab specimens collected from pregnant women. However, the sensitivity of NAATs may be significantly decreased when used for rapid intrapartum testing, because a preanalysis enrichment incubation step cannot be included in those situations. Neonatal cases of GBS disease have occurred in mothers whose screens were negative during pregnancy.

TREATMENT:

- Ampicillin plus an aminoglycoside is the initial empiric treatment of choice for a **newborn infant ≤7 days of age** with presumptive early-onset GBS infection; this reflects the need for coverage of other pathogens, such as *Escherichia coli*, which is the second-most common cause of EOD. In a critically ill neonate, particularly one with low birth weight, broader-spectrum empiric therapy should be considered when there is concern about non-GBS ampicillin-resistant infection.
- For empiric therapy of late-onset GBS disease in **infants 8 through 28 days of age** who are not critically ill and do not have evidence of meningitis, ampicillin plus either gentamicin or cefotaxime (or ceftazidime or cefepime if cefotaxime is not available) are recommended. If meningitis is suspected, ampicillin plus cefotaxime (or ceftazidime or cefepime if cefotaxime is not available) should be used; gentamicin should not be used if meningitis is suspected.
- For **infants 29 to 90 days of age**, ceftriaxone is recommended. If there is evidence of meningitis or critical illness, vancomycin should be added to expand empiric coverage.
- For a **preterm infant hospitalized beyond 72 hours**, empiric treatment for sepsis should take into account the potential for health care-associated pathogens as well as coverage for pathogens associated with neonatal sepsis, including group B streptococci.
- When GBS infection is identified definitively, penicillin G or ampicillin are recommended. See Table 4.2 (p 877) in Tables of Antibacterial Drug Dosages for dosing recommendations.

- For meningitis, especially in the neonate, some experts recommend that a second lumbar puncture be performed approximately 24 to 48 hours after initiation of therapy to assist in management and prognosis. If CSF sterility is not achieved or if increasing protein concentration is noted, a complication (eg, cerebral infarcts, cerebritis, ventriculitis, subdural empyema, ventricular obstruction) is more likely. Additional lumbar punctures and intracranial imaging may be indicated if neurologic abnormalities persist or focal neurological deficits occur. A failed hearing screen or abnormal neurologic examination at discharge mandates careful clinical follow-up.
- For infants with **bacteremia without a defined focus** or with an **isolated urinary tract infection** without bacteremia, treatment should be continued parenterally for 10 days. Shorter intravenous courses have been reported, sometimes with an oral component; however, prospective clinical studies are lacking. For infants with uncomplicated **meningitis**, 14 days of parenteral treatment is recommended, with longer courses of treatment provided for infants with prolonged or complicated courses. **Septic arthritis or osteomyelitis** requires treatment for 3 to 4 weeks. Patients who have **endocarditis or ventriculitis** require treatment for at least 4 weeks.
- Because of the reported increased risk of infection, the birth mates of a multiple-birth index case with EOD or LOD should be observed carefully and evaluated and treated empirically for suspected systemic infection if signs of illness occur; treatment should be continued for a full course for those with confirmed infection.

ISOLATION OF THE HOSPITALIZED PATIENT: Standard precautions are recommended. Routine cultures to determine whether infants are colonized with group B streptococci are not recommended.

CONTROL MEASURES:

Intrapartum Antibiotic Prophylaxis

New recommendations from the American Academy of Pediatrics[1] (**https://pediatrics.aappublications.org/content/144/2/e20191881**) and the American College of Obstetricians and Gynecology[2] (ACOG) (**www.acog.org/clinical/clinical-guidance/committee-opinion/articles/2020/02/prevention-of-group-b-streptococcal-early-onset-disease-in-newborns**) were published in 2019. Components that are directly germane to the management of neonates at risk for GBS include the following:

- All pregnant women should have culture-based screening from vaginal and rectal sites at 36 0/7 to 37 6/7 weeks' gestation, unless intrapartum antibiotic prophylaxis (IAP) for GBS infection is already planned because of predelivery maternal risk factors. For women who are at increased risk for a planned preterm delivery for medical indications, GBS screening within 5 weeks of anticipated delivery can be considered.
- For women who present with preterm labor, baseline GBS screening should be performed before intravenous GBS IAP is initiated.
- Intravenous penicillin G (5 million U initially, then 2.5 to 3.0 million U, every 4 hours, until delivery) is the preferred agent for GBS IAP because of its efficacy and narrow

[1]Puopolo KM, Lynfield R, Cummings JJ; American Academy of Pediatrics, Committee on Fetus and Newborn, Committee on Infectious Diseases. Management of infants at risk for group B streptococcal disease. *Pediatrics.* 2019;144(2):e20191881

[2]American College of Obstetricians and Gynecologists. Prevention of group B streptococcal early-onset disease in newborns: ACOG Committee Opinion Number 797. *Obstet Gynecol.* 2020;135(2):e51-e72

spectrum of antimicrobial activity. Intravenous ampicillin (2 g initially, then 1 g every 4 hours until delivery) can be used as an alternative when penicillin is unavailable. Oral or intramuscular antimicrobial agents should *not* be used as IAP. Women who report a mild or unknown penicillin allergy should receive intravenous cefazolin for IAP. Women who report penicillin allergies placing them at high risk for anaphylaxis should receive either intravenous clindamycin or vancomycin for IAP, depending on organism susceptibilities, with dosing detailed in the ACOG guidelines (**www.acog. org/clinical/clinical-guidance/committee-opinion/articles/2020/02/ prevention-of-group-b-streptococcal-early-onset-disease-in-newborns**).

- Penicillin allergy testing is safe during pregnancy and should be considered for women with a history of allergy to penicillin to optimize the antibiotic choice for GBS IAP.
- For the purpose of newborn evaluation regardless of gestational age, "adequate" GBS IAP is defined as the administration of at least 1 dose of penicillin G, ampicillin, or cefazolin 4 or more hours prior to delivery. Available evidence suggests that administration of penicillin G, ampicillin, or cefazolin for periods of time <4 hours prior to delivery confers some level of protection from GBS EOD. Of note, in the Neonatal Early-Onset Sepsis Risk calculator, "GBS specific antibiotics >2 hours prior to birth" is one of the calculator variables. The 2-hour timing is used because multiple factors in addition to GBS IAP are considered when using these multivariate models.
- The ACOG recommendations updated in 2020 detail the indications for IAP, management of mothers with penicillin allergy, use of alternative agents, and management of women with preterm prelabor rupture of membranes, taking into account gestational age, presence of labor, and availability of GBS test results. See **www.acog.org/clinical/clinical-guidance/committee-opinion/articles/2020/02/preventionof-group-b-streptococcal-early-onset-disease-in-newborns** for full discussion.

Management of Neonates at Risk for Early-Onset GBS Disease.
　　Please refer to the AAP clinical report "Management of Infants at Risk for GBS Disease"[1] for detailed discussion. Recommendations include the following:

- Routine use of antimicrobial chemoprophylaxis for neonates born to mothers who have received adequate IAP is *not* recommended. Antimicrobial therapy is appropriate only for infants with suspected systemic infection.
- Early-onset GBS disease is diagnosed by blood or CSF culture. Lumbar puncture should be performed for culture and analysis of CSF when there is a high suspicion for early onset GBS disease. All cultures should include testing for antibiotic susceptibility. Complete blood cell counts and measurement of C-reactive protein are not accurate enough to reliably identify infected infants. Chest radiography and other studies should be performed as clinically indicated.
- Infants born at ≥35 weeks' gestation can be assessed for risk of early-onset sepsis based upon one of three methods: (1) a categorical algorithm, (2) a multivariate risk assessment, or (3) enhanced clinical observation (see Fig 3.13).
  - A categorical approach (Fig 3.13A) uses threshold values to identify infants at increased risk for GBS disease. Because thresholds are used, the risk will vary greatly among newborn infants recommended to undergo laboratory evaluation and receive empiric treatment, and it will include relatively low-risk newborn infants.

[1]Puopolo KM, Lynfield R, Cummings JJ; American Academy of Pediatrics, Committee on Fetus and Newborn, Committee on Infectious Diseases. Management of infants at risk for group B streptococcal disease. *Pediatrics*. 2019;144(2):e20191881

Fig 3.13. Risk Assessment for Early-Onset Group B Streptococcal Disease Among Infants Born at ≥35 Weeks of Gestation

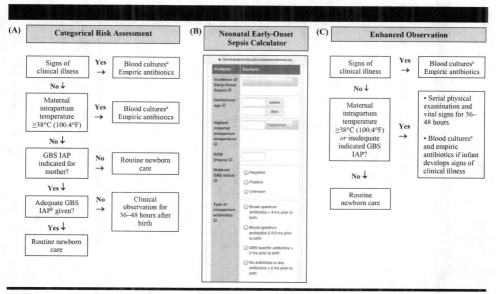

Reproduced from Puopolo KM, Lynfield R, Cummings JJ; American Academy of Pediatrics, Committee on Fetus and Newborn, Committee on Infectious Diseases. Management of infants at risk for group B streptococcal disease. *Pediatrics*. 2019;144(2):e20191881. The screenshot of the Neonatal Early-Onset Sepsis Calculator (**https://neonatalsepsiscalculator.kaiserpermanente.org/**) was used with permission from Kaiser-Permanente Division of Research.

[a]Consider lumbar puncture and CSF culture before initiation of empiric antibiotics for infants who are at the highest risk of infection, especially those with critical illness. Lumbar puncture should not be performed if the infant's clinical condition would be compromised, and antibiotics should be administered promptly and not deferred because of procedure delays.

[b]Adequate GBS IAP is defined as the administration of penicillin G, ampicillin, or cefazolin ≥4 hours before delivery.

- ◆ Multivariate risk assessment (Fig 3.13B, Neonatal Early-Onset Sepsis Calculator, and as an example: **https://neonatalsepsiscalculator.kaiserpermanente.org**) uses the individual infant's combination of risk factors for early-onset sepsis (including maternal components) and the infant's clinical status to estimate the risk of early-onset sepsis, including risk for GBS disease. It provides recommended clinical actions, such as enhanced clinical observation or laboratory evaluation and empiric antibiotics, on the basis of predicted risk estimates. This tool has been prospectively validated in large newborn cohorts.
- ◆ Enhanced clinical observation (Fig 3.13C) is a risk assessment based on newborn clinical conditions. Good clinical condition at birth in term infants is associated with an approximately 60% to 70% reduction in risk for EOD of all infections, including GBS infection. Infants who appear ill at birth and those who develop signs of illness over the first 48 hours after birth will undergo laboratory evaluation and receive empiric antibiotics. This approach can be combined with a categorical or multivariate assessment for risk factors or used on its own for infants born at ≥35 weeks' gestation. Use of this approach requires processes to ensure serial and structured physical assessments and clear criteria for additional evaluation and empiric antibiotic administration.

FIG 3.14. RISK ASSESSMENT FOR EARLY-ONSET GROUP B STREPTOCOCCAL DISEASE AMONG INFANTS BORN AT ≤34 WEEKS' GESTATION

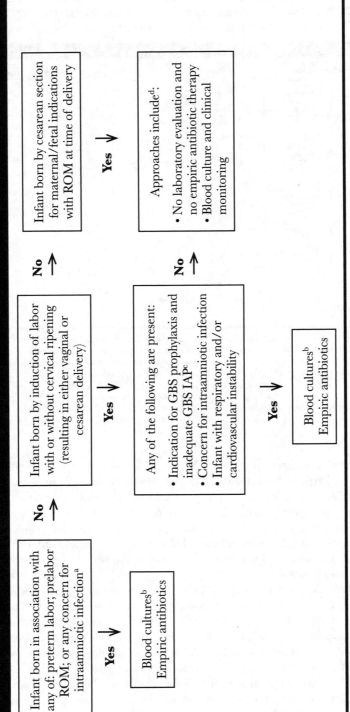

Reproduced from Puopolo KM, Lynfield R, Cummings JJ; American Academy of Pediatrics, Committee on Infectious Diseases. Management of infants at risk for group B streptococcal disease. *Pediatrics.* 2019;144(2):e20191881

[a] Intraamniotic infection should be considered when a pregnant woman presents with unexplained decreased fetal movement and/or there is sudden and unexplained poor fetal testing.

[b] Lumbar puncture and CSF culture should be performed before initiation of empiric antibiotics for infants who are at the highest risk of infection unless the procedure would compromise the infant's clinical condition. Antibiotics should be administered promptly and not deferred because of procedural delays.

[c] Adequate GBS IAP is defined as the administration of penicillin G, ampicillin, or cefazolin ≥4 hours before delivery.

[d] For infants who do not improve after initial stabilization and/or those who have severe systemic instability, the administration of empiric antibiotics may be reasonable but is not mandatory.

- Infants born at ≤34 weeks' gestation are at higher risk for early-onset sepsis, including GBS sepsis, than are full-term infants. However, the risk varies and is dependent on several maternal, peripartum, and neonatal factors. Management is outlined in Fig 3.14, with additional summary provided in the bullets below.
  - Infants born preterm because of cervical insufficiency, preterm labor, prelabor rupture of membranes, intra-amniotic infection, and/or acute and otherwise unexplained onset of concerning fetal status are at the highest risk of early-onset sepsis, including from group B streptococci. The administration of GBS IAP can decrease this risk; however, these infants remain at high risk and a laboratory evaluation should be done and empiric antibiotics for pathogens causing early-onset sepsis, including group B streptococci should be given. The most reasonable approach to these infants is to obtain a blood culture and start empiric antibiotic treatment. A lumbar puncture for culture and analysis of CSF should be considered in clinically ill infants when there is a high suspicion for GBS EOD, unless the procedure will compromise the neonate's clinical condition.
  - Some infants born at ≤34 weeks' gestation are at much lower risk for early onset sepsis, including GBS sepsis, if they have *all* of the following: (1) delivery for maternal indications (such as pre-eclampsia, other noninfectious medical illness, or placental insufficiency); (2) mothers who were not in labor; (3) mothers who did not experience efforts to induce labor; (4) mothers who did not have rupture of membranes prior to delivery, and (5) delivery by cesarean section. Acceptable initial approaches to these infants include (a) no laboratory evaluation and no empiric antibiotic therapy, or (b) blood culture and clinical monitoring. For infants who do not receive empiric antibiotics and do not improve after initial stabilization and/or those who have severe systemic instability, the administration of empiric antibiotics may be reasonable but is not mandatory; given that, infants can develop instability as a result of noninfectious factors.
  - Infants born at ≤34 weeks' gestation who are delivered for maternal indications but who are ultimately born by vaginal or cesarean delivery after efforts to induce labor and/or with rupture of membranes before delivery are subject to factors associated with the pathogenesis of GBS EOD. If the mother has an indication for GBS IAP, including a positive screen, and adequate IAP is not given or if any other concerns for infection occur during delivery, the infant should be managed as recommended for infants born at ≤34 weeks' gestation who are at highest risk for early-onset sepsis (see first bullet under "Infants born at ≤34 weeks' gestation"). If there are no concerns and these preterm infants are clinically well at birth, an acceptable approach to these infants is close observation and to conduct a laboratory evaluation and initiate empiric antibiotic therapy for infants with respiratory and/or cardiovascular instability after birth.

Non-Group A or B Streptococcal and Enterococcal Infections

CLINICAL MANIFESTATIONS: Streptococci other than Lancefield groups A or B can be associated with invasive disease in infants, children, adolescents, and adults. The principal clinical syndromes of groups C and G streptococci (most belong to the *Streptococcus dysgalactiae* group) are bacteremia, septicemia, upper and lower respiratory tract infections (eg, pharyngitis, sinusitis, and pneumonia), skin and soft tissue infections, septic arthritis, osteomyelitis, meningitis with a parameningeal focus, brain abscess, toxic shock syndrome, pericarditis, and endocarditis with various clinical manifestations. Viridans streptococci are the most common cause of bacterial endocarditis in children, especially children with congenital or valvular heart disease. Viridans streptococci are a common cause of bacteremia in neutropenic patients with cancer, especially following intensive induction chemotherapy for acute myeloid leukemia, after hematopoietic stem cell transplantation, and as a cause of central line-associated bacteremia. Among the viridans streptococci, group F streptococci (most belong to the *Streptococcus anginosus* group) are implicated in complicated sinus infections but are an infrequent cause of invasive infection. More serious *S anginosus* group infections include brain or dental abscesses or abscesses in other sites, including lymph nodes, liver, pelvis, and lung. These organisms may also cause sinusitis and other head and neck infections, meningitis, spondylodiskitis, spinal epidural abscesses, subdural empyema, peritonitis, complicated intra-abdominal infections, and cholangitis. Enterococci are associated with bacteremia in neonates and immunocompromised hosts, device-associated infections, intra-abdominal abscesses, and urinary tract infections in patients with anatomical anomalies.

ETIOLOGY: Changes in taxonomy and nomenclature of the *Streptococcus* genus have evolved with advances in molecular technology (see Table 3.61). Among gram-positive organisms that are catalase negative and display chains by Gram stain, the genera associated most often with human disease are *Streptococcus* and *Enterococcus*.

The genus *Streptococcus* has been subdivided into 6 species groups on the basis of 16S rRNA gene sequencing. Members of the genus that are beta-hemolytic on blood agar plates include *Streptococcus pyogenes* (see Group A Streptococcal Infections, p 694), *Streptococcus agalactiae* (see Group B Streptococcal Infections, p 707), and groups C and G streptococci; *S dysgalactiae* subspecies *equisimilis* is the group C subspecies most often associated with human infections. Streptococci that are non-beta–hemolytic (alpha-hemolytic or nonhemolytic) on blood agar plates include: (1) *Streptococcus pneumoniae* (see *Streptococcus pneumoniae* (Pneumococcal) Infections, p 717); (2) the *Streptococcus gallolyticus* (formerly *S bovis*) group; and (3) viridans streptococci clinically relevant in humans, which

Table 3.61. Classification of Streptococci Most Commonly Associated With Disease, by Lancefield Group and by Hemolysis

Species	Lancefield Group	Hemolysis
Streptococcus pyogenes	A	β
Streptococcus agalactiae	B	β
Streptococcus dysgalactiae subspecies *equisimillis*, *Streptococcus equi* subspecies *zooepidemicus*	C	β
Enterococcus faecalis, *Enterococcus faecium*, *Streptococcus gallolyticus*	D	γ
Streptococcus canis	G	β
Streptococcus pneumoniae, viridans streptococci	Not groupable[a]	α

[a]Occasional viridans streptococci have variable hemolysis and can possess Lancefield group A, C, F, or G antigens.

include 5 *Streptococcus* species groups (*S anginosus* group, *mitis* group, *sanguinis* group, *salivarius* group, and *mutans* group). The *anginosus* group (formerly *Streptococcus milleri* group) includes *S anginosus, Streptococcus constellatus,* and *Streptococcus intermedius.* This group can have variable hemolysis, and approximately one third possess group A, C, F, or G antigens. Nutritionally variant streptococci, once believed to be viridans streptococci, now are classified in the genera *Abiotrophia* and *Granulicatella.* Group D streptococci include *S gallolyticus, Streptococcus infantarius,* and *Streptococcus pasteurianus,* now classified under the *S gallolyticus* group.

The genus *Enterococcus* contains at least 25 species, with *Enterococcus faecalis* and *Enterococcus faecium* accounting for most human enterococcal infections. Outbreaks and health care-associated spread of vancomycin-resistant enterococcal species including *Enterococcus gallinarum, Enterococcus casseliflavus,* or *Enterococcus flavescens* have occurred.

EPIDEMIOLOGY: The habitats that non-group A and B streptococci and enterococci occupy in humans include the skin (groups C and G), oropharynx (groups C and G and the *mutans* group), gastrointestinal tract (groups C and G streptococci, *S gallolyticus* group, and *Enterococcus* species), and vagina (groups C, D, and G streptococci and *Enterococcus* species). Typical human habitats of species of viridans streptococci are the oropharynx, epithelial surfaces of the oral cavity, teeth, skin, and gastrointestinal and genitourinary tracts. Intrapartum transmission is responsible for most cases of early-onset neonatal infection caused by non-group A and B streptococci and enterococci. Environmental contamination or transmission via hands of health care professionals can lead to colonization of patients. Groups C and G streptococci can cause foodborne outbreaks of pharyngitis.

The **incubation period** and the period of communicability are unknown.

DIAGNOSTIC TESTS: Diagnosis is established by culture of usually sterile body sites or abscesses with appropriate biochemical testing and serologic analysis for definitive identification. Mass spectrometry is unreliable in differentiation of *S pneumoniae* from viridians streptococci. Genomic methods are being used increasingly, particularly for rapid identification of positive blood cultures. Antimicrobial susceptibility testing of isolates from usually sterile sites should be performed to guide treatment of infections caused by viridans streptococci or enterococci. The proportion of vancomycin-resistant enterococci (the vast majority of which are *E faecium*) among hospitalized patients can be as high as 30%. Selective agars are available for screening of vancomycin-resistant enterococcus from stool specimens. Molecular assays are available for direct detection of *vanA* and *vanB* genes (which confer vancomycin resistance) from rectal and blood specimens to identify vancomycin-resistant enterococci (VRE).

TREATMENT: Penicillin G is the drug of choice for groups C and G streptococci. Other agents with good activity include ampicillin, third- and fourth-generation cephalosporins, vancomycin, and linezolid. The combination of gentamicin (when high level resistance is not present) with a beta-lactam antimicrobial agent (eg, penicillin or ampicillin) or vancomycin may enhance bactericidal activity needed for treatment of life-threatening infections (eg, endocarditis or meningitis).

Many viridans streptococci remain susceptible to penicillin (minimum inhibitory concentration [MIC] ≤ 0.12 µg/mL). Infections caused by strains susceptible to penicillin, including endocarditis, can be treated with penicillin or ceftriaxone. Strains with an MIC >0.12 µg/mL and <0.5 µg/mL are considered relatively resistant to penicillin by criteria in the American Heart Association guidelines for treatment of infective endocarditis in childhood.[1] In this situation, penicillin, ampicillin, or ceftriaxone for 4 weeks, combined for the first 2 weeks with gentamicin, is recommended for endocarditis treatment. Strains with a penicillin MIC ≥ 0.5 µg/mL are considered resistant. Nonpenicillin antimicrobial agents with good activity against viridans streptococci include cephalosporins (especially ceftriaxone), vancomycin, linezolid, and tigecycline, although pediatric experience with tigecycline is limited. *Abiotrophia* and *Granulicatella* organisms can exhibit relative or high-level resistance to penicillin. The combination of high-dose penicillin or vancomycin and an aminoglycoside can enhance bactericidal activity.

Enterococci exhibit uniform resistance to cephalosporins (except ceftaroline and, where available, ceftobiprole), aztreonam, and antistaphylococcal penicillins. Most are intrinsically resistant to clindamycin and trimethoprim-sulfamethoxazole even if in vitro susceptibility indicates otherwise. The vast majority of *E faecalis* strains are susceptible to ampicillin (which can be extrapolated to amoxicillin, piperacillin-tazobactam, and imipenem, but not to penicillin). *E faecium* strains may be multidrug resistant. Two types of vancomycin resistance are identified: intrinsic low-level resistance that occurs with *E gallinarum* and *E casseliflavus/E flavescens* (these strains are ampicillin susceptible), and acquired resistance, which has been seen in *E faecium* and some *E faecalis* strains but also has been recognized in *Enterococcus raffinosus*, *Enterococcus avium*, and *Enterococcus durans*.

Systemic enterococcal infections, such as endocarditis or meningitis, should be treated with penicillin or ampicillin (if the isolate is susceptible) combined with ceftriaxone or gentamicin (see endocarditis guidelines[1]); vancomycin plus an aminoglycoside (with appropriate monitoring of renal function) is suggested for patients unable to tolerate penicillins and who cannot be desensitized. Gentamicin should not be used if in vitro susceptibility testing demonstrates high-level resistance. In general, children with a central line-associated bloodstream infection caused by enterococci should have the device removed promptly. Combination therapy for treating central line-associated bloodstream infections generally is not needed. Linezolid or daptomycin are options for treatment of other systemic infections caused by vancomycin-resistant *E faecium*. Linezolid is approved for use in children, including neonates. Isolates of VRE that are resistant to linezolid have been described, and resistance can develop during prolonged linezolid treatment. Most vancomycin-resistant isolates of *E faecalis* and *E faecium* are daptomycin-susceptible. Data suggest that clearance of daptomycin is more rapid in young children compared with adolescents and adults, and dosing may need to be adjusted accordingly. Daptomycin should not be used to treat pneumonia, as tissue concentrations are poor and daptomycin is inactivated by surfactants. Microbiologic and clinical cure has been reported in children infected with vancomycin-resistant *E faecium* who were treated with quinupristin-dalfopristin. This drug frequently causes phlebitis in peripheral intravenous lines, and pediatric dosing in children younger than 12 years is unclear. Tigecycline is approved for use in adults with complicated skin and skin structure infections caused by vancomycin-susceptible *E faecalis*. Tigecycline is bacteriostatic against both vancomycin-resistant *E faecalis* and vancomycin-resistant *E faecium*, but experience with this drug in children is limited. There are case reports of successful use of daptomycin plus tigecycline for endocarditis and with intraventricular daptomycin for VRE ventriculitis.

---

[1]Baltimore RS, Gewitz M, Baddour LM, et al. Infective endocarditis in childhood: 2015 update. A scientific statement from the American Heart Association. *Circulation* 2015;132(15):1487-1515

ISOLATION OF THE HOSPITALIZED PATIENT: Standard precautions are recommended. For patients with infection or colonization attributable to VRE, contact precautions in addition to standard precautions are indicated. Patients harboring vancomycin resistant strains of *E gallinarum, E casseliflavus,* or *E flavescens* may be managed using only standard precautions, because these species harbor chromosomally encoded vancomycin resistance genes (*vanC, vanT*) that are not easily exchanged between bacterial populations. Common practice is to maintain precautions until the patient no longer harbors the organism or is discharged from the health care facility. Some experts recommend discontinuation of contact precautions if screening cultures are negative; there is, however, no accepted standard regarding the frequency (1, 2, or 3 cultures), timing (weekly, daily) or preferred site selection (eg, stool, axilla, etc).

CONTROL MEASURES: Use of vancomycin and treatment with broad-spectrum antimicrobial agents are risk factors for colonization and infection with VRE. Hospitals should develop institution-specific guidelines for the proper use of vancomycin.

Patients with a prosthetic valve or prosthetic material used for cardiac valve repair, previous infective endocarditis, or congenital heart disease associated with the highest risk of adverse outcome from endocarditis should receive antimicrobial prophylaxis to prevent endocarditis at the time of certain dental procedures (see Prevention of Bacterial Endocarditis, p 1021). For these patients, early instruction in proper diet; oral health, including use of dental sealants and adequate fluoride intake; and prevention or cessation of smoking will aid in prevention of dental caries and potentially will lower their risk of recurrent endocarditis.

Streptococcus pneumoniae (Pneumococcal) Infections[1]

CLINICAL MANIFESTATIONS: *Streptococcus pneumoniae* is a common bacterial cause of acute otitis media, sinusitis, community-acquired pneumonia, and pediatric conjunctivitis; pleural empyema, mastoiditis, and periorbital cellulitis occur. It is the most common cause of bacterial meningitis in infants and children ages 2 months to 11 years in the United States. *S pneumoniae* also may cause endocarditis, pericarditis, peritonitis, pyogenic arthritis, osteomyelitis, soft tissue infection, and neonatal septicemia. Overwhelming septicemia in patients with splenic dysfunction is noted, and hemolytic-uremic syndrome can accompany pneumococcal infection.

ETIOLOGY: *S pneumoniae* organisms (pneumococci) are lancet-shaped, gram-positive, catalase-negative diplococci. More than 90 pneumococcal serotypes have been identified on the basis of unique polysaccharide capsules.

EPIDEMIOLOGY: Nasopharyngeal carriage rates in children range from 21% in industrialized settings to more than 90% in resource-limited settings. Transmission is from person to person by respiratory droplet contact. Viral upper respiratory tract infections, including influenza, can predispose to pneumococcal infection and transmission. Pneumococcal infections are most prevalent during winter months. The period of communicability is unknown and may be as long as the organism is present in respiratory tract secretions but probably is less than 24 hours after effective antimicrobial therapy is begun.

---

[1] Centers for Disease Control and Prevention. Prevention of pneumococcal disease among infants and children—use of 13-valent pneumococcal conjugate vaccine and 23-valent pneumococcal polysaccharide vaccine. *MMWR Recomm Rep.* 2010;59(RR-11):1-18

Table 3.62. Underlying Medical Conditions That Are Indications for Immunization With 23-Valent Pneumococcal Polysaccharide Vaccine (PPSV23)[a] Among Children, by Risk Group[b]

Risk group	Condition
Immunocompetent children	Chronic heart disease[c]
	Chronic lung disease[d]
	Diabetes mellitus
	Cerebrospinal fluid leaks
	Cochlear implant
Children with functional or anatomic asplenia	Sickle cell disease and other hemoglobinopathies
	Chronic or acquired asplenia, or splenic dysfunction
Children with immunocompromising conditions	HIV infection
	Chronic renal failure and nephrotic syndrome
	Diseases associated with treatment with immunosuppressive drugs or radiation therapy, including malignant neoplasms, leukemias, lymphomas, and Hodgkin disease; or solid organ transplantation
	Congenital immunodeficiency[e]

[a] PPSV23 is indicated starting at 24 months of age.
[b] Centers for Disease Control and Prevention. Licensure of a 13-valent pneumococcal conjugate vaccine (PCV13) and recommendations for use among children. Advisory Committee on Immunization Practices (ACIP). *MMWR Morb Mortal Wkly Rep.* 2010;59(9):258-261; and Centers for Disease Control and Prevention. Use of 13-valent pneumococcal conjugate vaccine and 23-valent pneumococcal polysaccharide vaccine among children aged 6-18 years with immunocompromising conditions: recommendation of the ACIP. *MMWR Morb Mortal Wkly Rep.* 2013;62(25):521-524.
[c] Particularly cyanotic congenital heart disease and cardiac failure.
[d] Including asthma if treated with prolonged high-dose oral corticosteroids.
[e] Includes B- (humoral) or T-lymphocyte deficiency; complement deficiencies, particularly C_1, C_2, C_3, and C_4 deficiency; and phagocytic disorders (excluding chronic granulomatous disease).

The incidence and severity of infections are increased in people with congenital or acquired humoral immunodeficiency, human immunodeficiency virus (HIV) infection, absent or deficient splenic function (eg, sickle cell disease, congenital, or surgical asplenia), certain complement deficiencies, diabetes mellitus, chronic liver disease, chronic renal failure or nephrotic syndrome, or abnormal innate immune responses. HIV-exposed uninfected infants are also at increased risk of severe pneumococcal infections. Children with cochlear implants, particularly those who had placement of an older model that involved a cochlear electrode, have high rates of pneumococcal meningitis, as do children with congenital or acquired cerebrospinal fluid (CSF) leaks.[1] Other categories of children at presumed high risk or at moderate risk of developing invasive pneumococcal disease are outlined in Table 3.62. Infection rates are highest in infants, young children, elderly

---

[1] American Academy of Pediatrics, Committee on Infectious Diseases. Policy statement: cochlear implants in children: surgical site infections and prevention and treatment of acute otitis media and meningitis. *Pediatrics.* 2010;126(2):381-391

people, and Black, Alaska Native, and some American Indian populations. Since introduction of the heptavalent pneumococcal conjugate vaccine (PCV7) in 2000 and the 13-valent pneumococcal conjugate vaccine (PCV13) in 2010, racial disparities have diminished; however, rates of invasive pneumococcal disease (IPD) among some American Indian (Alaska Native, Navajo, and White Mountain Apache) populations remain more than fourfold higher than the rate among children in the general US population. Recent data from Alaska and the Southwestern US indicate that the majority of IPD cases among American Indian/Alaska Native children are now caused by serotypes not contained in the PCV-13 vaccine.

By 2016, 6 years after the introduction of PCV13, the incidence of vaccine-type invasive pneumococcal infections decreased by 98% compared with incidence before introduction of PCV7, and the incidence of all IPD decreased by 95% in children younger than 5 years. In adults 65 years and older, IPD caused by PCV13 serotypes decreased 87% compared with baseline, and all IPD decreased by 61%. The reduction in cases in this latter group indicates the significant indirect (ie, herd) benefits of PCV13 immunization achieved by interruption of transmission of pneumococci from vaccinated children to adults. Although *S pneumoniae* strains that are nonsusceptible to penicillin G, ceftriaxone, and other antimicrobial agents have been identified throughout the United States and worldwide, a reduction in the proportion of isolates that are penicillin-resistant and ceftriaxone -resistant has been observed since introduction of PCV7 and PCV13.

The **incubation period** varies by type of infection but can be as short as 1 day.

DIAGNOSTIC TESTS: Recovery of *S pneumoniae* from a normally sterile site confirms the diagnosis. The finding of lancet-shaped gram-positive organisms and white blood cells in expectorated sputum (older children and adults) or pleural exudate suggests pneumococcal pneumonia. Recovery of pneumococci by culture of an upper respiratory tract swab specimen is not sufficient to assign an etiologic diagnosis of pneumococcal disease involving the middle ear, upper or lower respiratory tract, or sinus.

There are at least 2 multiplexed nucleic acid amplification tests cleared by the US Food and Drug Administration (FDA) designed to identify *S pneumoniae* and other bacterial and fungal pathogens from positive blood culture bottles. At least 1 real-time polymerase chain reaction (PCR) assay is cleared by the FDA for detection of *S pneumoniae* in CSF. The assay is a multiplexed PCR designed to detect a number of agents of bacterial, fungal, and viral meningitis or encephalitis. PCR testing should be accompanied by culture of CSF to obtain an isolate, which is needed for antimicrobial susceptibility testing.

Detection of C-polysaccharide (common to all pneumococci) in urine for diagnosis of pneumococcal pneumonia may have some utility in adults but is not useful in children, because asymptomatically colonized children may have positive test results. Similarly, commercially available antigen detection tests performed on CSF or blood are not recommended for routine use because of low sensitivity.

Susceptibility Testing. All *S pneumoniae* isolates from normally sterile body fluids should be tested for antimicrobial susceptibility to determine the minimum inhibitory concentration (MIC) of penicillin, cefotaxime or ceftriaxone, and clindamycin. CSF isolates also should be tested for susceptibility to vancomycin, meropenem, and rifampin. If the patient has a nonmeningeal infection caused by an isolate that is nonsusceptible to penicillin, cefotaxime, and ceftriaxone, susceptibility testing to other agents such as clindamycin, erythromycin, trimethoprim-sulfamethoxazole, levofloxacin, linezolid, meropenem, and vancomycin should be performed.

TREATMENT:

Bacterial Meningitis Possibly or Proven to Be Caused by S pneumoniae. For children with bacterial meningitis possibly or known to be caused by *S pneumoniae*, vancomycin should be administered in addition to cefotaxime (or ceftriaxone for patients >1 month of age) because of the possibility of *S pneumoniae* resistant to penicillin and third-generation cephalosporins. In neonates, when cefotaxime is not available, then ceftazidime or cefepime can be used in addition to vancomycin. Vancomycin should be stopped if susceptibility to third-generation cephalosporins is documented (using central nervous system [CNS] breakpoints for thresholds of resistance), if another organism not requiring vancomycin is identified, or if the CSF culture is negative. Antibiotic dosing recommendations for meningitis are included in Tables 4.2 (neonatal) and 4.3 (nonneonatal) in Tables of Antibacterial Drug Dosages, p 876. If the *S pneumoniae* isolate is nonsusceptible (intermediate or resistant) to penicillin or third-generation cephalosporins, treatment options are provided in Table 3.63. Consultation with an infectious diseases specialist should be considered for all children with bacterial meningitis.

For children with serious proven hypersensitivity reactions to third- or fourth-generation cephalosporins, a pediatric infectious diseases specialist should be consulted for consideration of use of vancomycin plus either meropenem or rifampin.

A repeat lumbar puncture should be considered after 48 hours of therapy in the following circumstances:

Table 3.63. Antimicrobial Therapy for Infants and Children With Meningitis Caused by *Streptococcus pneumoniae* on the Basis of Susceptibility Test Results

Susceptibility Test Results	Antimicrobial Management[a]
Susceptible to penicillin	Discontinue vancomycin **AND EITHER** Continue cefotaxime or ceftriaxone alone[b] **OR** Begin penicillin (and discontinue cephalosporin)
Nonsusceptible to penicillin (*intermediate* or *resistant*) **AND** *Susceptible* to cefotaxime and ceftriaxone	Discontinue vancomycin **AND** Continue cefotaxime or ceftriaxone
Nonsusceptible to penicillin (*intermediate* or *resistant*) **AND** *Nonsusceptible* to cefotaxime and ceftriaxone (*intermediate* or *resistant*) **AND** *Susceptible* to rifampin	Continue vancomycin and high-dose cefotaxime or ceftriaxone **AND** Rifampin may be added in selected circumstances (see text)

[a]Initial empiric therapy of nonallergic children older than 1 month of age with presumed bacterial meningitis should be vancomycin and cefotaxime or ceftriaxone. See Tables 4.2 (neonatal) and 4.3 (nonneonatal) in Tables of Antibacterial Drug Dosages, p 876, for dosages. Some experts recommend the maximum dosages.

[b]Some physicians may choose this alternative for convenience and cost savings but only in treatment of meningitis.

- The organism is penicillin nonsusceptible by oxacillin disk or quantitative (MIC) testing, and results from cefotaxime and ceftriaxone quantitative susceptibility testing are not yet available or the isolate is cefotaxime and ceftriaxone nonsusceptible; or
- The patient's condition has not improved or has worsened; or
- The child has received dexamethasone, which can interfere with the ability to interpret the clinical response, such as resolution of fever.

Dexamethasone. For infants and children 6 weeks and older, adjunctive therapy with dexamethasone may be considered after weighing the potential benefits and risks. Some experts recommend use of corticosteroids in pneumococcal meningitis, but this issue is controversial and data are not sufficient to make a routine recommendation for children. The Infectious Diseases Society of America recommends use of dexamethasone in adults with suspected or proven pneumococcal meningitis. If used, dexamethasone should be administered before or concurrently with the first dose of parenteral antimicrobial agents.

Nonmeningeal Invasive Pneumococcal Infections Requiring Hospitalization. For nonmeningeal invasive infections in previously healthy children who are not critically ill, antimicrobial agents currently used to treat infections with *S pneumoniae* and other potential pathogens should be initiated at the usually recommended dosages (see Tables 4.2 (neonatal) and 4.3 (nonneonatal) in Tables of Antibacterial Drug Dosages, p 876).

For critically ill infants and children with invasive infections potentially attributable to *S pneumoniae,* vancomycin, in addition to empiric antimicrobial therapy (eg, cefotaxime or ceftriaxone or others), can be considered. Such patients include those with presumed septic shock, severe pneumonia with empyema, or significant hypoxia or myopericardial involvement. If vancomycin is administered, it should be discontinued as soon as antimicrobial susceptibility test results demonstrate effective alternative agents.

If the organism has in vitro resistance to penicillin, cefotaxime, and ceftriaxone according to guidelines of the Clinical and Laboratory Standards Institute (CLSI), therapy should be modified on the basis of clinical response, susceptibility to other antimicrobial agents, and results of follow-up cultures of blood and other infected body fluids. Consultation with an infectious diseases specialist should be considered.

For children with severe hypersensitivity to beta-lactam antimicrobial agents (ie, penicillins and cephalosporins), initial management should include vancomycin or clindamycin, in addition to antimicrobial agents for other potential pathogens, as indicated. Vancomycin should not be continued if the organism is susceptible to other appropriate non–beta-lactam antimicrobial agents. Consultation with an infectious diseases specialist should be considered.

Acute Otitis Media.[1] According to clinical practice guidelines of the American Academy of Pediatrics (AAP) and the American Academy of Family Physicians (AAFP) on acute suppurative otitis media (AOM), amoxicillin (80–90 mg/kg/day) is recommended for infants younger than 6 months, for those 6 through 23 months of age with bilateral disease, and for those older than 6 months with severe signs and symptoms (see *Haemophilus influenzae* Infections, p 345, and Appropriate and Judicious Use of Antimicrobial Agents, p 868). A watch-and-wait option can be considered for older children and those with nonsevere disease. Optimal duration of therapy is uncertain. For younger children and children with severe disease at any age, a 10-day course is recommended; for children 6 years and older

[1]Lieberthal AS, Carroll AE, Chonmaitree T, et al. Clinical practice guideline: diagnosis and management of acute otitis media. *Pediatrics.* 2013;131(3):e964-e999

with mild or moderate disease, a duration of 5 to 7 days is appropriate. Otalgia should be treated symptomatically.

Patients who fail to respond to initial management should be reassessed at 48 to 72 hours to confirm the diagnosis of AOM and exclude other causes of illness. If AOM is confirmed in the patient managed initially with observation, amoxicillin should be administered. If the patient has failed initial antibacterial therapy, a change in antibacterial agent is indicated. Suitable alternative agents should be active against penicillin-nonsusceptible pneumococci as well as beta-lactamase–producing *Haemophilus influenzae* and *Moraxella catarrhalis*. Such agents include high-dose oral amoxicillin-clavulanate; oral cefdinir, cefpodoxime, or cefuroxime; or once-daily doses of intramuscular ceftriaxone for 3 consecutive days. Macrolide resistance among *S pneumoniae* is high, so clarithromycin and azithromycin are not considered appropriate alternatives for initial therapy even in patients with a type I (immediate, anaphylactic) reaction to a beta-lactam agent. In such cases, treatment with clindamycin (if susceptibility is known) or levofloxacin is preferred. For patients with a history of non-type I allergic reaction to penicillin, agents such as cefdinir, cefuroxime, or cefpodoxime can be used orally.

Myringotomy or tympanocentesis should be considered for children failing to respond to second-line therapy, for severe cases to obtain cultures to guide therapy, and for patients with invasive pneumococcal infection. For multidrug-resistant strains of *S pneumoniae,* use of levofloxacin or other agents should be considered in consultation with an infectious diseases specialist and based on the specific susceptibility profile.

Sinusitis. Antimicrobial agents effective for treatment of AOM also are likely to be effective for acute sinusitis and are recommended when a child meets clinical criteria for diagnosis.

Pneumonia.[1] Oral amoxicillin at a dose of 45 mg/kg/day in 3 equally divided doses or 90 mg/kg/day in 2 divided portions is likely to be effective in ambulatory children with pneumonia caused by susceptible and relatively resistant pneumococci, respectively. Ampicillin is recommended for intravenous therapy of community acquired pneumonia. Cefotaxime or ceftriaxone is recommended for treatment of inpatients infected with pneumococci suspected or proven to be penicillin-resistant strains, for serious infections including empyema, or in those not fully immunized with PCV13. Vancomycin should be included in those with life-threatening infection. For patients with isolates resistant to penicillin (MICs of 4.0 µg/mL or higher) or significant allergy to beta lactam antimicrobials, treatment with clindamycin (if susceptible) or levofloxacin should be considered, assuming that concurrent meningitis has been excluded.

ISOLATION OF THE HOSPITALIZED PATIENT: Standard precautions are recommended, including for patients with infections caused by drug-resistant *S pneumoniae.*

CONTROL MEASURES:

Active Immunization. Two pneumococcal vaccines are available for use in children in the United States: the 13-valent pneumococcal conjugate vaccine (PCV13) and the 23-valent pneumococcal polysaccharide vaccine (PPSV23). PCV13 is licensed for use in infants and children 6 weeks and older as well as in adults. PCV13 is composed of the 13 purified capsular polysaccharide serotypes (1, 3, 4, 5, 6A, 6B, 7F, 9V, 14, 18C, 19A, 19F, and

---

[1]Bradley JS, Byington CL, Shah SS, et al. The management of community-acquired pneumonia in infants and children older than 3 months of age: clinical practice guidelines by the Pediatric Infectious Diseases Society and the Infectious Diseases Society of America. *Clin Infect Dis.* 2011;53(7):e25–e76

23F). PCV13 is available in single-dose, prefilled syringes that do not contain latex or preservative. PPSV23 is licensed for use in children 2 years and older and adults. PPSV23 is composed of 23 capsular polysaccharides, including all of those in PCV13 except 6A. PPSV23 is available in single or multidose vials and single-dose prefilled syringes that do not contain latex. Each available vaccine is recommended in a dose of 0.5 mL to be administered intramuscularly. In contrast to immunization with PCV13, immunization with PPSV23 does not induce immunologic memory or boosting with subsequent doses, has no effects on nasopharyngeal carriage, and therefore does not interrupt transmission and indirectly protect unimmunized people.

Routine Immunization With Pneumococcal Conjugate Vaccine. PCV13 is recommended for all infants and children 2 through 59 months of age. For infants, the vaccine should be administered at 2, 4, 6, and 12 through 15 months of age; catch-up immunization is recommended for all children 59 months of age or younger (Table 3.64). Infants should begin the PCV13 immunization series in conjunction with other recommended vaccines at the time of the first regularly scheduled health maintenance visit after 6 weeks of age. Infants of very low birth weight (1500 g or less) should be immunized when they attain a chronologic age of 6 to 8 weeks, regardless of their gestational age at birth. PCV13 can be administered concurrently with all other age-appropriate childhood immunizations (except MenACWY-D [Menactra, Sanofi Pasteur], see *General Recommendations for Use of Pneumococcal Vaccines*, below) using a separate syringe and a separate injection site.

Immunization of Children Unimmunized or Incompletely Immunized With PCV13. For children 2 through 59 months of age who have not received PCV13, the dose schedule is outlined in Table 3.64. PCV13 is recommended for all children younger than 18 years who are at high risk or presumed high risk of acquiring invasive pneumococcal infection (Table 3.65), as defined in Table 3.62 (p 718).

Immunization of Children 6 Through 18 Years of Age With High-Risk Conditions[1]

PPSV23-Naïve Children. For children 6 through 18 years of age who previously have not received PCV13 or PPSV23 and who are at increased risk of IPD because of anatomic or functional asplenia (including sickle cell disease [SCD]), HIV infection, cochlear implant, CSF leak, or other immunocompromising conditions (Table 3.62, p 718), administration of a single PCV13 dose followed by a dose of PPSV23 at least 8 weeks after the PCV13 dose is recommended. A second PPSV23 dose is recommended 5 years after the first PPSV23 dose for children with anatomic or functional asplenia (including SCD), HIV infection, or other immunocompromising conditions. No more than a total of 2 PPSV23 doses should be administered before 65 years of age.

Immunization of Children 2 Through 18 Years of Age Who Are at Increased Risk of IPD With PPSV23 After PCV7 or PCV13.[2] Children 2 years or older with an underlying medical condition increasing the risk of IPD should receive PPSV23 after completing all recommended doses of PCV13. These children should receive a single dose of PPSV23 at least 8 weeks after the most recent dose of PCV13. In children who are candidates for solid organ transplantation and in cases when a splenectomy is planned for a

---

[1]Centers for Disease Control and Prevention. Use of 13-valent pneumococcal conjugate vaccine and 23-valent pneumococcal polysaccharide vaccine among children aged 6–18 years with immunocompromising conditions: recommendations of the Advisory Committee on Immunization Practices (ACIP). *MMWR Morb Mortal Wkly Rep.* 2013;62(25):521-524

[2] American Academy of Pediatrics, Committee on Infectious Diseases. Immunization for *Streptococcus pneumoniae* infections in high-risk children. *Pediatrics.* 2014;134(6):1230–1233

Table 3.64. Recommended Schedule for Doses of PCV13, Including Catch-up Immunizations in Previously Unimmunized and Partially Immunized Children 2 Through 59 Months of Age

Age at Examination	Immunization History	Recommended Regimen[a,b]
2 through 6 mo	0 doses	3 doses, 8 wk apart; fourth dose at 12 through 15 mo of age
	1 dose	2 doses, 8 wk apart; fourth dose at 12 through 15 mo of age
	2 doses	1 dose, 8 wk after the most recent dose; fourth dose at 12 through 15 mo of age
7 through 11 mo	0 doses	2 doses, 4 wk apart; third dose at 12 mo of age
	1 or 2 doses before age 7 mo	1 dose at age 7 through 11 mo, with another dose at 12 through 15 mo of age (≥2 mo later)
12 through 23 mo	0 doses	2 doses, ≥8 wk apart
	1 dose at <12 mo	2 doses, ≥8 wk apart
	1 dose at ≥12 mo	1 dose, ≥8 wk after the most recent dose
	2 or 3 doses at <12 mo	1 dose, ≥8 wk after the most recent dose
24 through 59 mo[c] Healthy children	Any incomplete schedule	1 dose, ≥8 wk after the most recent dose[c]

PCV13 indicates 13-valent pneumococcal conjugate vaccine.

[a]For children immunized at younger than 12 months, the minimum interval between doses is 4 weeks. Doses administered at 12 months or older should be at least 8 weeks apart.

[b]Centers for Disease Control and Prevention. Licensure of a 13-valent pneumococcal conjugate vaccine (PCV13) and recommendations for use among children. Advisory Committee on Immunization Practices (ACIP). *MMWR Morb Mortal Wkly Rep.* 2010;59(RR-11):1-18

[c]A single dose should be administered to all healthy children 24 through 59 months of age with any incomplete schedule.

patient older than 2 years, PPSV23 should be administered at least 2 weeks before transplant or splenectomy. In candidates for solid organ transplantation not previously vaccinated with PCV13, a dose of PCV13 should be administered, even for those older than 6 years.

If a child previously has received PPSV23, the child also should receive the recommended doses of PCV13. A second dose of PPSV23 is recommended 5 years after the first dose in children with sickle cell disease or functional or anatomic asplenia, HIV infection, or other immunocompromising conditions, but no more than a total of 2 PPSV23 doses should be administered before 65 years of age.

Table 3.65. Recommendations for Pneumococcal Immunization with PCV13 and/or PPSV23 Vaccine for Children at High Risk or Presumed High Risk of Pneumococcal Disease, as Defined in Table 3.62 (p 718)

Age	Previous Dose(s) of Any Pneumococcal Vaccine	Recommendations
23 mo or younger	None	PCV13, as in Table 3.62 (p 718).
24 through 71 mo	4 doses of PCV13	1 dose of PPSV23 vaccine at 24 mo of age, ≥8 wk after last dose of PCV13.
24 through 71 mo	3 previous doses of PCV13 before 24 mo of age	1 dose of PCV13.
		1 dose of PPSV23, ≥8 wk after the last dose of PCV13.
24 through 71 mo	<3 doses of PCV13 before 24 mo of age	2 doses of PCV13, ≥8 wk after last dose of PCV13 (if applicable).
		1 dose of PPSV23 vaccine, ≥8 wk after the last dose of PCV13.
24 through 71 mo	1 dose of PPSV23	2 doses of PCV13, 8 wk apart, beginning at 8 wk after last dose of PPSV23.
6 years through 18 years with immunocompromising conditions[a,b]	No previous doses of PCV13 or PPSV23	1 dose of PCV13 followed by 1 dose of PPSV23 at least 8 weeks later and a second dose of PPSV23 5 years after the first.[c]
	1 dose of PCV13	1 dose of PPSV23 and a second dose of PPSV23 5 years after the first
	≥1 dose of PPSV23 and no previous dose of PCV13	1 dose of PCV13 (even if PCV7 previously administered) ≥8 weeks after the last PPSV23 dose; if a second PPSV23 dose is indicated, it should be administered ≥5 years after the first PPSV23 dose

PCV13 indicates 13-valent pneumococcal conjugate vaccine; PPSV23, 23-valent pneumococcal polysaccharide vaccine.

[a]Includes anatomic or functional asplenia, human immunodeficiency virus (HIV) infection, cochlear implant, cerebrospinal fluid (CSF) leak, nephrotic syndrome, chronic renal failure, or other immunocompromising conditions.

[b]American Academy of Pediatrics, Committee on Infectious Diseases. Policy statement: Immunization for *Streptococcus pneumoniae* infections in high-risk children. *Pediatrics*. 2014;134(6):1230–1233

[c]A second dose of PPSV23 5 years after the first dose is recommended only for children who have functional or anatomic asplenia, HIV infection, or other immunocompromising conditions (Table 3.62, p 718). No more than 2 doses of PPSV23 are recommended. All other children with underlying medical conditions should receive 1 dose of PPSV23.

General Recommendations for Use of Pneumococcal Vaccines.

- Either PPSV23 or PCV13 should not be given together but can be administered concurrently with other childhood vaccines, with one exception. For children for whom quadrivalent meningococcal conjugate vaccine is indicated, MenACWY-D (Menactra [Sanofi Pasteur]) should not be administered concomitantly OR within 4 weeks of administration of PCV13 immunization to avoid potential interference with the immune response to PCV13. Because of their high risk for IPD, children with functional or anatomic asplenia should not be immunized with MenACWY-D (Menactra) before 2 years of age so that they can complete their PCV13 series; only MenACWY-CRM (Menveo [Novartis Vaccines and Diagnostics]) should be used in this age group because it has been shown to not interfere with the immune response to PCV13 and because the only other alternative, MenACWY-TT (MenQuadfi [Sanofi Pasteur]), is only approved in children ≥2 years of age (see Table 3.38, p 528).
- When elective splenectomy is performed for any reason, immunization with PCV13 should be completed at least 2 weeks before splenectomy. Immunization also should precede initiation of immune-compromising therapy or placement of a cochlear implant by at least 2 weeks. PPSV23 should be administered 8 or more weeks after PCV13 (see Immunization and Other Considerations in Immunocompromised Children, p 72).
- Generally, pneumococcal vaccines should be deferred during pregnancy. However, a pregnant woman who has an underlying medical condition that predisposes to IPD is at risk for severe disease and should receive PPSV23 if it has been >5 years since prior PPSV23 and she has not previously received 2 doses.

Case Reporting. Cases of IPD in children younger than 5 years should be reported according to state standards. The vast majority of cases of invasive disease cases are caused by non-PCV13 serotypes. Therefore, the overwhelming majority of invasive pneumococcal disease cases occurring among immunized children do not represent vaccine failures. To differentiate PCV13 failure in an immunized child from disease caused by a serotype not included in PCV13, the isolate should be serotyped. A protocol for serotyping pneumococci using PCR is available for state public health laboratories on the CDC website (**www.cdc.gov/streplab/downloads/triplex-pcr-us.pdf**). If the invasive isolate is a serotype included in the vaccine, an evaluation of the patient's HIV status and immunologic function should be considered if the child had received an age-appropriate regimen of PCV13 at least 2 weeks before the onset of the invasive infection.

Adverse Reactions to Pneumococcal Vaccines. Adverse reactions after administration of polysaccharide or conjugate vaccines generally are mild to moderate. The most commonly reported adverse reactions are local reactions of injection site, pain, redness, or swelling in addition to irritability, decreased appetite, or impaired sleep. Fever may occur within the first 1 to 2 days after injections, particularly after use of conjugate vaccine. Other systemic reactions include fatigue, headache, generalized muscle pain, decreased appetite, and chills.

Passive Immunization. Intravenous administration of Immune Globulin is recommended for preventing pneumococcal infection in patients with certain congenital or acquired immunodeficiency diseases.

Chemoprophylaxis. Daily antimicrobial prophylaxis is recommended for certain children with functional or anatomic asplenia, regardless of their immunization status, for prevention of pneumococcal disease on the basis of results of a large, multicenter study (see Asplenia and Functional Asplenia, p 85). Oral penicillin V (125 mg, twice a day, for children younger than 3 years; 250 mg, twice a day, for children 3 years and older) is recommended. The study, performed before routine use of PCV7 or PCV13 in the United States, demonstrated that oral penicillin V given to infants and young children with sickle cell disease decreased the incidence of pneumococcal bacteremia by 84% compared with the placebo control group. Although overall incidence of IPD is decreased after penicillin prophylaxis, cases of penicillin-resistant IPD and nasopharyngeal carriage of penicillin-resistant strains in patients with sickle cell disease have increased since these studies were conducted. Parents should be informed that penicillin prophylaxis may not be effective in preventing all cases of IPD. In children with suspected or proven penicillin allergy, erythromycin is an alternative agent for prophylaxis.[1]

The age at which prophylaxis is discontinued is an empiric decision. Most children with sickle cell disease who have received all recommended pneumococcal vaccines for age and who had received penicillin prophylaxis for prolonged periods, who are receiving regular medical attention, and who have not had a previous severe pneumococcal infection or a surgical splenectomy may discontinue prophylactic penicillin safely at 5 years of age. However, they must be counseled to seek medical attention promptly for all febrile events. The duration of prophylaxis for children with asplenia attributable to other causes is unknown. Some experts continue prophylaxis throughout childhood or longer.

Control of Transmission of Pneumococcal Infection and Invasive Disease Among Children Attending Out-of-Home Child Care. Antimicrobial chemoprophylaxis is not recommended for contacts of children with IPD, regardless of their immunization status.

Strongyloidiasis
(Strongyloides stercoralis)

CLINICAL MANIFESTATIONS: Most infections with *Strongyloides stercoralis* are asymptomatic. When symptoms occur, they are related most often to larval tissue migration and/or the presence of adult worms in the intestine. Infective (filariform) larvae are acquired from skin contact with contaminated soil, which may produce transient pruritic papules at the site of penetration. Larvae then migrate to the lungs, where they may cause a transient pneumonitis or Löffler-like syndrome. After ascending the tracheobronchial tree, larvae are swallowed and mature into adult forms within the gastrointestinal tract. Symptoms of intestinal infection may include nonspecific abdominal pain, malabsorption, vomiting, and diarrhea. Larval migration may produce migratory serpiginous pruritic erythematous skin lesions. These tracks are referred to as "larva currens" and are pathognomonic for *Strongyloides*. The most feared complication is *Strongyloides* hyperinfection syndrome and disseminated disease, in which larvae migrate via the systemic circulation to distant organs, including the brain, liver, kidney, heart, and skin. Hyperinfection syndrome typically occurs in immunocompromised people, most often those receiving immunosuppressive agents, particularly glucocorticoids, for underlying disease (eg, malignancy or autoimmunity), but also in recipients of solid organ or hematopoietic stem cell transplants (through either reactivation of prior asymptomatic infection in the recipient or donor-derived

---

[1] American Academy of Pediatrics, Committee on Genetics. Health supervision for children with sickle cell disease. *Pediatrics.* 2002;109(3):526-535 (Reaffirmed January 2011, February 2016)

infection), and patients with human T-lymphotropic virus 1 (HTLV-1) coinfection. *Strongyloides* hyperinfection syndrome is characterized by fever, abdominal pain, diffuse pulmonary infiltrates, and septicemia or meningitis caused by enteric gram-negative bacilli and may be fatal. For unknown reasons, it is extremely rare during childhood.

ETIOLOGY: *S stercoralis* is a nematode (roundworm).

EPIDEMIOLOGY: Strongyloidiasis is endemic in the tropics and subtropics, including the southeastern United States, wherever suitable moist soil and improper disposal of human waste coexist. Humans are the principal hosts, but dogs, cats, and other animals can serve as reservoirs. Transmission involves penetration of skin by filariform larvae from contact with contaminated soil. Infections can also be acquired via fecal-oral route with ingestion of food contaminated with human feces containing larvae or from inadvertent coprophagy. Adult females release eggs in the small intestine, where they hatch as first-stage (rhabditiform) larvae that are excreted in feces. A small percentage of larvae molt to the infective (filariform) stage during intestinal transit, at which point they can penetrate the bowel mucosa or perianal skin, thus maintaining the life cycle within a single person (autoinfection). Because of the capacity for autoinfection, people can remain infected for decades even after leaving an endemic area.

The **incubation period** in humans is unknown.

DIAGNOSTIC TESTS: Strongyloidiasis can be difficult to diagnose. Testing may be performed on stool or serologically. Visualization through direct microscopy for larvae (rhabditiform, or less often, filariform) in the stool (or from duodenal biopsy or fluid, obtained using the string test [Entero-Test] or a direct aspirate through a flexible endoscope) confirms the diagnosis. At least 3 consecutive stool specimens should be examined microscopically using a concentration method (eg, sedimentation techniques) for characteristic larvae (not eggs), but a negative test does not exclude infection because larvae excretion can be intermittent and of low intensity. Other techniques that provide greater sensitivity but are not available routinely in the United States include stool PCR, stool agar culture, or other specialized tests on stool specimens. Filariform larvae may be identified in disseminated strongyloidiasis from other specimens such as sputum or bronchoalveolar lavage fluid, spinal fluid, pleural fluid, peritoneal fluid, or in skin biopsies. Serologic tests, including enzyme-linked immunosorbent assays (ELISAs) that detect immunoglobulin (Ig) G to filariform larvae, are highly sensitive but cross reactivity may occur in patients with filariasis and other nematode infections. Serologic tests using recombinant antigens have similar high sensitivity but greater specificity for strongyloidiasis. Serologic testing has several limitations. Detection does not confirm active infection, because antibodies may remain positive for a period of time following infection resolution. False-negative results also may occur, so a negative test result does not eliminate the possibility of ongoing infection. Serologic monitoring may be useful in following treatment in immunocompetent patients, because antibody concentrations decline over time (usually within 6 months) with successful treatment. The Centers for Disease Control and Prevention performs reference serologic testing to confirm equivocal results.

Eosinophilia (blood eosinophil count greater than $500/\mu L$) generally is present during acute and chronic infection, but its absence does not eliminate infection from consideration. When eosinophilia is absent in hyperinfection syndrome, it may predict poor outcome. Gram-negative bacillary meningitis and bacteremia may occur with disseminated disease and carry a high mortality rate.

TREATMENT: Ivermectin is the treatment of choice for all forms of strongyloidiasis and is approved by the US Food and Drug Administration for the treatment of intestinal strongyloidiasis. Ivermectin is contraindicated in people with confirmed or suspected coinfection with *Loa loa*. The safety of ivermectin in children weighing less than 15 kg and in pregnant women has not been established. An alternative agent is albendazole, although it is associated with lower cure rates (see Drugs for Parasitic Infections, p 967). Studies in children as young as 1 year suggest that albendazole can be administered safely to this population. Mebendazole is not recommended. Prolonged or repeated treatment may be necessary in people with hyperinfection and disseminated strongyloidiasis, and relapse can occur.

ISOLATION OF THE HOSPITALIZED PATIENT: Standard precautions are recommended.

CONTROL MEASURES: Sanitary disposal of human waste is effective at interrupting transmission of *S stercoralis*. Any individual at risk epidemiologically for strongyloidiasis who will undergo a solid organ or hematopoietic stem cell transplant or immunosuppressant therapy, particularly with corticosteroids or TNF alpha inhibitors, either should be treated presumptively for strongyloidiasis or tested serologically and treated if the serologic test result is positive before initiation of immunosuppression. Screening for *Strongyloides* also should be considered in organ donors from areas with endemic infection, patients with hematologic malignancies, people with HTLV-1 infection, people with persistent or unexplained eosinophilia, household contacts with shared risk factors, or people who traveled recently to areas with endemic disease.

Syphilis

CLINICAL MANIFESTATIONS:

Congenital Syphilis. Intrauterine infection with *Treponema pallidum* can result in stillbirth, hydrops fetalis, or preterm birth or may be asymptomatic at birth. Infected infants can have hepatosplenomegaly; snuffles (copious nasal secretions); lymphadenopathy; mucocutaneous lesions; pneumonia; osteochondritis, periostitis, and pseudoparalysis; edema; rash (maculopapular consisting of small dark red-copper spots that is most severe on the hands and feet); hemolytic anemia; or thrombocytopenia at birth or within the first 4 to 8 weeks of age. Untreated infants, including those asymptomatic at birth, may develop late manifestations, which usually appear after 2 years of age and involve the central nervous system (CNS), bones and joints, teeth, eyes, and skin. Some findings may not become apparent until many years after birth, such as interstitial keratitis, eighth cranial nerve deafness, Hutchinson teeth (peg-shaped, notched central incisors), anterior bowing of the shins, frontal bossing, mulberry molars, saddle nose, rhagades (perioral fissures), and Clutton joints (symmetric, painless swelling of the knees). Late manifestations can be prevented by treatment of early infection.

Acquired Syphilis. Acquired disease can be divided into 3 stages. The **primary stage** (or "**primary syphilis**") appears as painless indurated ulcers (chancres) of the skin or mucous membranes at the site of inoculation. These lesions appear, on average, 3 weeks after exposure (10–90 days) and heal spontaneously in a few weeks. Adjacent lymph nodes frequently are enlarged but are nontender. The **secondary stage** (or "**secondary syphilis**"), beginning 1 to 2 months later, is characterized by fever, sore throat, muscle aches, rash, mucocutaneous lesions, hepatitis, and generalized lymphadenopathy. The polymorphic maculopapular rash is generalized and typically includes the palms and soles. In moist areas of the perineum, hypertrophic papular lesions (condyloma lata) can be confused with condyloma acuminata secondary to human papillomavirus (HPV) infection. Malaise, splenomegaly, headache, alopecia, and arthralgia can be present. This stage resolves spontaneously without treatment in approximately 3 to 12 weeks. A variable asymptomatic latent period follows but may be interrupted during the first few years by recurrences of symptoms of secondary syphilis. **Latent syphilis** is the period after infection when patients are seroreactive but demonstrate no clinical manifestations of disease. Development of latent syphilis within the preceding year is referred to as **early latent syphilis;** if >1 year in duration, it is known as **late latent syphilis.** If the duration of infection is unknown, the patient should be considered to have late latent syphilis for the purposes of management. The **tertiary stage** of syphilis occurs 15 to 30 years after the initial infection and can include gumma formation (soft, noncancerous, granulomatous growths that can destroy tissue) or cardiovascular involvement (including aortitis). Neurosyphilis infection of the central nervous system (CNS) can occur at any stage of infection, especially in people with human immunodeficiency virus (HIV) and in neonates with congenital syphilis; manifestations include meningitis, uveitis, seizures, optic atrophy, hearing loss, and (typically years after infection) dementia and posterior spinal cord degeneration (tabes dorsalis, including a characteristic high-stepping gait with the feet slapping the ground with each step because of loss of proprioception).

ETIOLOGY: *T pallidum* subspecies *pallidum (T pallidum)* is a thin, motile spirochete that is extremely fastidious, surviving only briefly outside the host. It is very closely related to 3 other organisms causing nonvenereal human disease in distinct geographic regions of the world: *T pallidum* subspecies *pertenue,* which causes yaws; *T pallidum* subspecies *endemicum,* which causes endemic syphilis; and *Treponema carateum,* which causes pinta. The genus *Treponema* is classified in the family *Spirochaetaceae.*

EPIDEMIOLOGY: During 2013–2017, the primary and secondary syphilis rate increased 72.7% nationally, and 155.6% among women, from 5.5 to 9.5 cases per 100 000 population. Syphilis rates increased by 17.6% overall from 2015 to 2016, with most primary and secondary cases occurring among men, particularly gay, bisexual, and other men who have sex with men (MSM). Also, half of MSM in whom syphilis was diagnosed also had a diagnosis of human immunodeficiency virus (HIV) infection. In 2017, among women 15 through 24 years of age, the rate of reported primary and secondary syphilis was 5.5 cases per 100 000, which was a 7.8% increase from 2016 (5.1 cases per 100 000) and an 83.3% increase from 2013 (3.0 cases per 100 000). Among men 15 through 24 years of age, the rate was 26.1 cases per 100 000, which was an 8.3% increase from 2016 (24.1 cases per 100 000) and a 50.9% increase from 2013 (17.3 cases per 100 000). During 2016–2017, the rate of reported syphilis cases increased 9.8% among people 15 through 19 years of age and 7.8% among people 20 through 24 years of age.

In 2018, the number of infants born with syphilis was the highest since 1997, increasing from 9.2 cases per 100 000 live births to 33.1 per 100 000 live births from 2013 to 2018, with an absolute increase in cases over that period from 362 to 1306 in 2018. This trend mirrors the rise in primary and secondary syphilis cases seen in women of reproductive age. From 2013 to 2018, rates of early syphilis among women of reproductive age (15–44 years) increased from 2.5 to 15.1 per 100 000 population, reflecting an increase from 3386 to 9651 per year.

Congenital syphilis may be contracted at any stage of maternal infection via transplacental transmission at any time during pregnancy, or via contact with maternal lesions at the time of delivery. Among pregnant women with untreated early syphilis, up to 40% of their pregnancies will result in spontaneous abortion, stillbirth, or perinatal death. The rate of maternal-fetal transmission is 60% to 100% in the setting of primary and secondary syphilis during pregnancy and decreases with later stages of maternal infection (approximately 40% with early latent infection and <8% with late latent infection). Among women who acquire syphilis during pregnancy, the risk of transmission to the infant increases directly with the gestational age at the time of maternal infection. HIV-infected women, in particular, have a higher prevalence of untreated or inadequately treated syphilis during pregnancy; therefore, their newborn infants may be at higher risk of congenital syphilis. In addition, syphilis coinfection during pregnancy may also increase the rate of mother-to-child transmission of HIV.

T pallidum is not transmitted through human milk, but transmission may occur if the breastfeeding mother has an infectious lesion (chancre) on her breast.

Acquired syphilis almost always is contracted through direct sexual contact with ulcerative lesions of the skin or mucous membranes of infected people. Open, moist lesions of the primary or secondary stages are highly infectious. Syphilis acquired beyond the neonatal period should be considered diagnostic of sexual abuse in infants and young children once rare vertical transmission is excluded (see Sexual Assault and Abuse in Children and Adolescents/Young Adults, p 150).

The **incubation period** for acquired primary syphilis typically is 3 weeks but ranges from 10 to 90 days.

DIAGNOSTIC TESTS: Definitive diagnosis is made when spirochetes are identified by microscopic darkfield examination of lesion exudate, nasal discharge, or tissue, such as placenta, lymph node, umbilical cord, or autopsy specimens. *T pallidum* can be detected by polymerase chain reaction (PCR) assay. Specimens from mouth lesions can contain nonpathogenic treponemes that can be difficult to distinguish from *T pallidum* by darkfield microscopy. Darkfield microscopy, however, no longer is routinely available in most clinics and laboratories because of its complexity and the availability and accuracy of newer serologic and molecular diagnostic techniques.

Presumptive diagnosis requires the use of both nontreponemal and treponemal serologic tests. Nontreponemal tests for syphilis include the Venereal Disease Research Laboratory (VDRL) slide test and the rapid plasma reagin (RPR) test. These tests are inexpensive, can be performed across a range of laboratory levels of complexity with fairly rapid turnaround times for analysis, and provide semiquantitative results that can both help define disease activity and monitor response to therapy. Nontreponemal test results may be falsely negative (ie, nonreactive) in early primary syphilis, latent acquired syphilis of long duration, and late congenital syphilis. Occasionally, a nontreponemal test performed on serum containing high concentrations of antibody will be weakly reactive or falsely negative, a reaction termed the prozone phenomenon; diluting the serum being tested will then result in a positive test result. The prozone phenomenon may be observed more often in HIV coinfected individuals. When nontreponemal tests are used serially to monitor treatment response, the same test (RPR or VDRL), ideally from the same laboratory, must be used throughout the follow-up period to ensure comparability of results.

Except for congenital infection, a reactive nontreponemal test result should be confirmed by one of the specific treponemal tests to exclude a false-positive test result. False-positive nontreponemal results can be caused by certain viral infections (eg, Epstein-Barr virus infection, hepatitis, HIV, varicella, measles), lymphoma, tuberculosis, malaria, endocarditis, connective tissue disease, pregnancy, older age, abuse of injection drugs, or laboratory or technical error. In cases in which a cord blood sample is being used to test a newborn infant's RPR status, Wharton's jelly has been shown to be a potential confounder for results, and an actual neonatal blood sample, when feasible, is a preferred specimen for testing. Treponemal tests in use include the *T pallidum* particle agglutination (TP-PA) test (which is the preferred treponemal test), *T pallidum* enzyme immunoassay (TP-EIA), *T pallidum* chemiluminescence assay (TP-CIA), and fluorescent treponemal antibody absorption (FTA-ABS) test. Most people who have reactive treponemal test results remain reactive for life, even after successful therapy. However, 15% to 25% of patients treated during primary syphilis revert to being serologically nonreactive on treponemal testing after 2 to 3 years. Treponemal test results may also be variably positive in patients with other spirochetal diseases, such as yaws, pinta, leptospirosis, rat-bite fever, relapsing fever, and Lyme disease.

In most cases, if a patient has a positive RPR or VDRL result in low titer and has a negative treponemal test result, the nontreponemal test result will be a false positive. However, because false-negative test results can occur in early syphilis, retesting in 2 to 4 weeks and again later if clinically indicated should be considered in people at increased risk for syphilis, especially in pregnant women.

The Centers for Disease Control and Prevention (CDC)[1] and the US Preventive Services Task Force[2] recommend syphilis serologic screening with a nontreponemal test; this screening is followed by confirmation using one of the several available treponemal tests ("conventional diagnostic" approach). Some clinical laboratories and blood banks, however, have begun to screen samples using treponemal tests first rather than beginning with a nontreponemal test. This "reverse-sequence screening" approach may result in false-positive results, especially in low-prevalence populations. When the reverse-sequence algorithm is used, people with a positive treponemal test result and a negative nontreponemal test result (eg, EIA positive, RPR negative) should have a second treponemal test targeting a different *T pallidum* antigen performed to confirm the results of the original test. If the second treponemal-specific test result is negative (eg, EIA-positive, RPR-negative, then TP-PA-negative) and the person is at low risk for syphilis, the original treponemal test result likely was a false positive. However, in individuals at high-risk for infection, retesting in 2 to 4 weeks and again later if clinically indicated should be considered.

Cerebrospinal Fluid Tests. Cerebrospinal fluid (CSF) abnormalities in patients with neurosyphilis can include increased protein concentration, increased white blood cell (WBC) count, and/or a reactive CSF-VDRL test result. Outside the neonatal period, the CSF-VDRL is highly specific but insensitive; therefore, a negative result does not exclude a diagnosis of neurosyphilis. Conversely, a reactive CSF-VDRL test in a neonate can be the result of nontreponemal IgG antibodies that cross the blood-brain barrier. The CSF leukocyte count usually is elevated in neurosyphilis (>5 WBCs/mm[3]). Interpretation of CSF test results requires a nontraumatic lumbar puncture (ie, a CSF sample that is not contaminated with blood). CSF test results obtained during the neonatal period can be difficult to interpret; normal values differ by gestational age and are higher in preterm infants. Studies suggest that 95% of healthy neonates have values ≤16 to 19 white blood

---

[1]Centers for Disease Control and Prevention. Sexually transmitted infections treatment guidelines, 2021. *MMWR Recomm Rep.* 2021; in press

[2]US Preventive Services Task Force. Screening for syphilis infection in non-pregnant adults and adolescents. *JAMA.* 2016;315(21):2321-2327

cells (WBCs)/mm^3 and/or protein ≤115 to 118 mg/dL on CSF examination. During the second month of life, 95% of normal infants have ≤9 to 11 WBCs/mm^3 and/or protein of ≤89 to 91 mg/dL. Lower values (ie, 5 WBCs/mm^3 and protein of 40 mg/dL) might be considered the upper limits of normal in older infants. Other causes of elevated values should be considered when an infant is being evaluated for congenital syphilis. A positive CSF FTA-ABS or TP-PA result can support the diagnosis of neurosyphilis but does not establish the diagnosis definitively. Fewer data exist for the EIA or RPR test for CSF, and these tests should not be used for CSF evaluation.

Testing During Pregnancy. Prevention of congenital syphilis requires that pregnant women be screened serologically early in pregnancy. False-negative test results are possible in recent infection, and syphilis may be acquired later in pregnancy. Therefore, in communities and populations in which the prevalence of syphilis is high and for women at high risk for infection, serologic testing also should be performed at 28 weeks' gestation and again at delivery. A nontreponemal test (RPR or VDRL) is recommended for screening, followed by a treponemal test if the screening result is positive. In most cases, if the treponemal antibody test result is negative, the nontreponemal test result is falsely positive and no further evaluation is necessary. However, retesting in 2 to 4 weeks, and again later if clinically indicated, should be considered for pregnant women who are at high risk of syphilis.

If the reverse-sequence screening algorithm is used, pregnant women with reactive treponemal screening test results should have confirmatory testing with a quantitative nontreponemal test. If the nontreponemal test result is negative (eg, EIA positive, RPR negative), a second treponemal-specific test using a different *T pallidum* antigen should be obtained to determine whether the initial treponemal test result was a false positive (TP-PA preferred). If the second treponemal test result is negative (eg, EIA positive, RPR negative, then TP-PA negative) and the person is at low risk for syphilis, the original treponemal test result likely was a false positive. However, retesting in 2 to 4 weeks and again later if clinically indicated should be considered for pregnant women who are at high risk of syphilis.

Ultrasonographic evaluation of the fetus from the second trimester onward should be performed when syphilis is diagnosed at any time during pregnancy, even if appropriate maternal treatment has been administered. Pathologic examination of the placenta and/or umbilical cord at delivery also should be performed.

Evaluation of Infants for Congenital Infection During the Newborn Period to 1 Month of Age. No newborn infant should be discharged from the hospital without determination of the mother's serologic status for syphilis. All infants born to seropositive mothers require a careful examination and nontreponemal testing. A negative maternal RPR or VDRL test result at delivery does not rule out the possibility of the infant having congenital syphilis, although such a situation is rare. The diagnostic approach to infants being evaluated for congenital syphilis is presented in Fig 3.15 (p 734).

Evaluation of Infants >1 Month of Age and Children. Infants and children identified as having reactive serologic tests for syphilis should have maternal serologic test results and records reviewed to assess whether they have congenital or acquired syphilis. Evaluation for congenital syphilis after 1 month of age includes: (1) CSF analysis for VDRL, cell count, and protein; (2) CBC, differential, and platelet count; (3) other tests as clinically indicated (eg, long-bone radiographs, chest radiograph, liver function tests, abdominal ultrasonography, ophthalmologic examination, neuroimaging, and auditory brain-stem response); and (4) testing for HIV infection.

FIG 3.15. ALGORITHM FOR DIAGNOSTIC APPROACH OF INFANTS BORN TO MOTHERS WITH REACTIVE SEROLOGIC TESTS FOR SYPHILIS.

RPR indicates rapid plasma reagin; VDRL, Venereal Disease Research Laboratory.

[a] *Treponema pallidum* particle agglutination (TP-PA) (which is the preferred treponemal test) or fluorescent treponemal antibody absorption (FTA-ABS).

[b] Test for human immunodeficiency virus (HIV) antibody. Infants of HIV-infected mothers do not require different evaluation or treatment for syphilis.

[c] A fourfold change in titer is the same as a change of 2 dilutions. For example, a titer of 1:64 is fourfold greater than a titer of 1:16, and a titer of 1:4 is fourfold lower than a titer of 1:16. When comparing titers, the same type of nontreponemal test should be used (eg, if the initial test was an RPR, the follow-up test should also be an RPR).

[d] Stable VDRL titers 1:2 or less or RPR 1:4 or less beyond 1 year after successful treatment are considered low serofast.

[e] Complete blood cell (CBC) count and platelet count; cerebrospinal fluid (CSF) examination for cell count, protein, and quantitative VDRL; other tests as clinically indicated (eg, chest radiographs, long-bone radiographs, eye examination, liver function tests, neuroimaging, and auditory brainstem response). For neonates, pathologic examination of the placenta or umbilical cord with specific fluorescent antitreponemal antibody staining, if possible.

TREATMENT[1]: Parenteral penicillin G is the preferred drug for treatment of syphilis at any stage. The type and duration of penicillin G therapy varies depending on the stage of disease and clinical manifestations. Parenteral penicillin G is the only documented effective therapy for patients who have neurosyphilis, congenital syphilis, or syphilis during pregnancy and also is recommended for people with HIV infection.

Penicillin Allergy. Infants and children with a history of penicillin allergy or who develop presumed penicillin allergy during treatment should be desensitized and then treated with penicillin whenever possible. Data to support the use of alternatives to penicillin are limited, but options for nonpregnant patients who are allergic to penicillin may include doxycycline, tetracycline, and for neurosyphilis, ceftriaxone. These therapies should be used with close clinical and laboratory follow-up to ensure expected serologic response and cure. In pregnancy, desensitization and treatment with doses of intramuscular benzathine penicillin, guided by the stage of syphilis diagnosed, is the only appropriate therapy in the setting of a maternal penicillin allergy. Erythromycin and azithromycin, which have been suggested as extended-course alternatives in nonpregnant adults with penicillin allergy, are not appropriate for treatment in pregnancy because they may suboptimally treat the mother and will not cross the placenta adequately to treat the fetus. Similarly, doxycycline is not appropriate for extended use in pregnancy, especially in the second and third trimesters.

Congenital Syphilis: Newborn Period to 1 Month of Age. The management of congenital syphilis is based on whether the infant has proven or probable congenital syphilis, has possible congenital syphilis, or is considered less likely or unlikely to have syphilis, as detailed in Figure 3.15 (p 734) and Table 3.66 (p 736). If more than 1 day of therapy is missed, the entire course should be restarted. Data supporting use of other antimicrobial agents (eg, ampicillin) for treatment of congenital syphilis are not available. When possible, a full 10-day course of penicillin is preferred, even if ampicillin initially was provided for possible sepsis. Use of agents other than penicillin requires close serologic follow-up to assess adequacy of therapy.

Congenital Syphilis: Infants ≥1 Month of Age and Children. Infants older than 1 month who possibly have congenital syphilis and children older than 2 years who have late and previously untreated congenital syphilis should be treated with intravenous aqueous crystalline penicillin (200 000–300 000 U/kg/day, intravenously, administered as 50 000 U/kg, every 4–6 hours for 10 days). Some experts suggest giving such patients a single dose of penicillin G benzathine (50 000 U/kg, intramuscularly, not to exceed 2.4 million U) after the 10-day course of intravenous aqueous crystalline penicillin. If the patient has no clinical manifestations of disease, the CSF examination is normal, and the CSF-VDRL test result is negative, some experts would treat with 3 weekly doses of penicillin G benzathine (50 000 U/kg, intramuscularly, not to exceed 2.4 million U).

Congenital Syphilis: Penicillin Shortage. During periods when the availability of aqueous crystalline penicillin G is compromised, check local sources for aqueous crystalline penicillin G (potassium or sodium).

For infants with proven or highly probably congenital syphilis, if intravenous penicillin G is limited, then substitute some or all daily doses with procaine penicillin G (50,000 U/kg/dose intramuscularly a day in a single daily dose for 10 days). If aqueous or procaine penicillin G is not available, ceftriaxone (50 to 75 mg/kg/day intravenously

---

[1]Centers for Disease Control and Prevention. Sexually transmitted infections treatment guidelines, 2021. *MMWR Recomm Rep.* 2021; in press

Table 3.66. Evaluation and Treatment of Infants *Up To 1 Month of Age* With Possible, Probable, or Confirmed Congenital Syphilis[a]

Category	Findings	Recommended Evaluation	Treatment
Proven or highly probable congenital syphilis	Abnormal physical examination consistent with congenital syphilis OR A serum quantitative nontreponemal serologic titer fourfold higher than the mother's titer OR A positive result of darkfield test or PCR assay of lesions or body fluid(s)	CSF analysis (CSF VDRL, cell count, and protein) CBC count with differential and platelet count Other tests (as clinically indicated): Long-bone radiography Chest radiography Aminotransferases Neuroimaging Ophthalmologic examination Auditory brain stem response	Aqueous crystalline penicillin G, 50 000 U/kg, IV, every 12 hours (1 wk or younger), then every 8 h for infants older than 1 wk, for a total of 10 days of therapy[b] **(preferred)** OR Procaine penicillin G, 50 000 U/kg, IM, as single daily dose for 10 days

Table 3.66. Evaluation and Treatment of Infants *Up To 1 Month of Age* With Possible, Probable, or Confirmed Congenital Syphilis,[a] continued

Category	Findings	Recommended Evaluation	Treatment
Possible congenital syphilis	Normal infant examination AND A serum quantitative nontreponemal serologic titer equal to or less than fourfold the maternal titer AND ONE OF THE FOLLOWING: Mother was not treated, was inadequately treated, or had no documentation of receiving treatment; OR Mother was treated with a regimen other than recommended in the guideline (ie, a nonpenicillin regimen) OR Mother received recommended treatment <4 wk before delivery	CSF analysis (CSF VDRL, cell count, and protein) CBC count with differential and platelet count Long-bone radiography	Aqueous crystalline penicillin G, 50 000 U/kg, IV, every 12 h (1 wk or younger), then every 8 h for infants older than 1 wk, for a total of 10 days of therapy[b] (**preferred**) OR Procaine penicillin G, 50 000 U/kg, IM, as single daily dose for 10 days OR Benzathine penicillin G, 50 000 U/kg, IM, single dose (recommended by some experts, but **only** if all components of the evaluation are obtained and are normal[c] and follow-up is certain

Table 3.66. Evaluation and Treatment of Infants *Up To 1 Month of Age With Possible, Probable, or Confirmed Congenital Syphilis*,[a] continued

Category	Findings	Recommended Evaluation	Treatment
Congenital syphilis less likely	Normal infant examination AND A serum quantitative nontreponemal serologic titer equal to or less than fourfold the maternal titer AND Mother was treated during pregnancy, treatment was appropriate for stage of infection, and treatment was administered >4 wk before delivery AND Mother has no evidence of reinfection or relapse	Not recommended	Benzathine penicillin G, 50 000 U/kg, IM, single dose (**preferred**) Alternatively, infants whose mothers' nontreponemal titers decreased at least fourfold after appropriate therapy for early syphilis or remained stable at low titer (eg, VDRL ≤1:2; RPR ≤1:4) may be followed every 2–3 mo without treatment until the nontreponemal test becomes nonreactive Nontreponemal antibody titers should decrease by 3 mo of age and should be nonreactive by 6 mo of age; patients with increasing titers or with persistent stable titers 6 to 12 mo after initial treatment should be reevaluated, including a CSF examination, and treated with a 10-day course of parenteral penicillin G, even if they were treated previously

Table 3.66. Evaluation and Treatment of Infants *Up To 1 Month of Age* With Possible, Probable, or Confirmed Congenital Syphilis,[a] continued

Category	Findings	Recommended Evaluation	Treatment
Congenital syphilis is unlikely	Normal infant examination AND A serum quantitative nontreponemal serologic titer equal to or less than fourfold the maternal titer AND Mother was treated adequately before pregnancy AND Mother's nontreponemal serologic titer remained low and stable (ie, serofast) before and during pregnancy and at delivery (eg, VDRL ≤1:2; RPR ≤1:4)	Not recommended	None, but infants with reactive nontreponemal tests should be followed serologically to ensure test result returns to negative Benzathine penicillin G, 50 000 U/kg, IM, single dose can be considered if follow-up is uncertain and infant has a reactive test (some experts) Neonates with a negative nontreponemal test result at birth and whose mothers were seroreactive at delivery should be retested at 3 mo to rule out incubating congenital syphilis

PCR indicates polymerase chain reaction; CSF, cerebrospinal fluid; CBC, complete blood cell count; VDRL, Venereal Disease Research Laboratory; IV, intravenously; IM, intramuscularly; RPR, rapid plasma reagin.

Adapted and modified from Centers for Disease Control and Prevention. Sexually transmitted diseases treatment guidelines, 2015. *MMWR Recomm Rep.* 2015;64(RR-3):45-47.

[a] For treatment of infants ≥1 month of age with congenital syphilis, see text on p 735.

[b] If 24 hours or more of therapy is missed, the entire course must be restarted.

[c] If CSF is not obtained or uninterpretable (eg, bloody tap), a 10-day course is recommended.

every 24 hours) can be considered with careful clinical and serologic follow-up and in consultation with a pediatric infectious diseases specialist, as evidence is insufficient to support the use of ceftriaxone for the treatment of congenital syphilis. In neonates ≤28 days of age, ceftriaxone is contraindicated if they are hyperbilirubinemic or if they require treatment with calcium-containing intravenous solutions because of the risk of precipitation of ceftriaxone-calcium.

For infants with possible congenital syphilis or in whom congenital syphilis is less likely, with procaine penicillin G (50 000 U/kg/dose intramuscularly a day in a single dose for 10 days) or benzathine penicillin G (50 000 U/kg intramuscularly as a single dose) should be used. If any part of the evaluation for congenital syphilis is abnormal or was not performed, CSF examination is not interpretable, or follow-up is uncertain, procaine penicillin G is recommended. A single dose of ceftriaxone is inadequate therapy. However, for preterm infants who might not tolerate intramuscularly injections because of decreased muscle mass, intravenous ceftriaxone can be considered with careful clinical and serologic follow-up and in consultation with a pediatric infectious diseases specialist; ceftriaxone dosing must be adjusted according to birth weight, and has the contraindications listed above for jaundice or if calcium-containing intravenous solutions are being administered concomitantly.

Syphilis in Pregnancy. Regardless of stage of pregnancy, women should be treated with penicillin according to the dosage schedules appropriate for the stage of syphilis as recommended for nonpregnant patients (see Table 3.67). Nonpenicillin treatment of syphilis during pregnancy cannot be considered reliable to cure infection in the mother and will not cross the placenta adequately to ensure fetal treatment.

Acquired Primary, Secondary, Early Latent Syphilis; Late Latent Syphilis; Tertiary Syphilis; and Neurosyphilis. Treatment recommendations for children and adults are detailed in Table 3.67.

Other Considerations.

- All nonneonatal patients with syphilis should be tested for other sexually transmitted infections (STIs), including *Neisseria gonorrhoeae, Chlamydia trachomatis,* HIV, hepatitis B, and hepatitis C. Patients who have syphilis should be retested for HIV infection after 3 months if the first HIV test result is negative. Immunization status for hepatitis B and HPV should be reviewed and vaccines should be administered if not up to date.

- All recent sexual contacts of people with acquired syphilis should be evaluated for other STIs as well as syphilis (see Control Measures, p 744).

- Children with acquired primary, secondary, or latent syphilis should be evaluated for possible sexual assault or abuse (see Sexual Assault and Abuse in Children and Adolescents/Young Adults, p 150).

Follow-up and Management.

Congenital Syphilis. All infants who have reactive serologic tests for syphilis or were born to mothers who were seroreactive at delivery should receive careful follow-up evaluations during well-child care visits at 2, 4, 6, and 12 months of age. Serologic nontreponemal tests should be performed every 2 to 3 months until the test becomes nonreactive. Nontreponemal antibody titers typically decrease by 3 months of age and should be nonreactive by 6 months of age, whether the infant was infected and adequately treated or was not infected and initially seropositive because of transplacentally acquired maternal antibody. The serologic response after therapy may be slower for infants treated after

Table 3.67. Recommended Treatment for Acquired Primary, Secondary, Early Latent Syphilis; Late Latent Syphilis; Tertiary Syphilis; and Neurosyphilis[a]

Status	Children	Adults
Primary, secondary, and early latent syphilis[b]	Penicillin G benzathine,[c] 50 000 U/kg, IM, up to the adult dose of 2.4 million U in a single dose *If allergic to penicillin and not pregnant,* Doxycycline, 4.4 mg/kg divided in 2 doses, max 200 mg per day, orally, twice a day for 14 days **OR** Tetracycline, 25–50 mg/kg divided in 4 doses, max 2 g per day, orally, for 14 days **(for age ≥8 years)**	Penicillin G benzathine, 2.4 million U, IM, in a single dose *If allergic to penicillin and not pregnant,* Doxycycline, 100 mg, orally, twice a day for 14 days **OR** Tetracycline, 500 mg, orally, 4 times/day for 14 days
Late latent syphilis[d]	Penicillin G benzathine, 50 000 U/kg, IM, up to the adult dose of 2.4 million U, administered as 3 single doses at 1-wk intervals (total 150 000 U/kg, up to the adult dose of 7.2 million U) *If allergic to penicillin and not pregnant,* Doxycycline, 4.4 mg/kg divided in 2 doses, max 200 mg per day, orally, twice a day for 4 wk **(for age ≥8 years)** **OR** Tetracycline, 25–50 mg/kg divided in 4 doses, max 2 g per day, orally, for 4 wk **(for age ≥8 years)**	Penicillin G benzathine, 7.2 million U total, administered as 3 doses of 2.4 million U, IM, each at 1-wk intervals; pregnant women who have delays in any dose of therapy beyond 9 days between doses should repeat the full course of therapy **OR** *If allergic to penicillin and not pregnant,* Doxycycline, 100 mg, orally, twice a day for 4 wk **OR** Tetracycline, 500 mg, orally, 4 times/day for 4 wk

Table 3.67. Recommended Treatment for Acquired Primary, Secondary, Early Latent Syphilis; Late Latent Syphilis; Tertiary Syphilis; and Neurosyphilis,[a] continued

Status	Children	Adults
Tertiary	…	Penicillin G benzathine, 7.2 million U total, administered as 3 doses of 2.4 million U, IM, at 1-wk intervals *If allergic to penicillin and not pregnant, consult an infectious diseases expert*
Neurosyphilis[e]	Aqueous crystalline penicillin G, 200 000–300 000 U/kg/day, IV, administered as 50 000 U/kg every 4–6 h for 10–14 days, in doses not to exceed the adult dose	Aqueous crystalline penicillin G, 18–24 million U per day, administered as 3–4 million U, IV, every 4 h for 10–14 days[f] **OR** Penicillin G procaine,[e] 2.4 million U, IM, once daily **PLUS** probenecid, 500 mg, orally, 4 times/day, both for 10–14 days[f]

IV indicates intravenously; IM, intramuscularly.

[a] Excludes patients with either early or late recognition of congenital syphilis

[b] Early latent syphilis is defined as being acquired within the preceding year.

[c] Penicillin G benzathine and penicillin G procaine are approved for intramuscular administration only.

[d] Late latent syphilis is defined as syphilis beyond 1 year's duration.

[e] Patients who are allergic to penicillin should be desensitized.

[f] Some experts administer penicillin G benzathine, 2.4 million U, IM, once per week for up to 3 weeks after completion of these neurosyphilis treatment regimens.

the neonatal period. Patients with increasing titers or with persistent stable titers 6 to 12 months after initial treatment should be reevaluated, including a CSF examination. Retreatment with a 10-day course of parenteral penicillin G may be indicated, even if they were treated previously. Neonates with a negative nontreponemal test at birth whose mothers were seroreactive at delivery should be retested at 3 months to rule out incubating congenital syphilis.

Treponemal tests should not be used to evaluate treatment response, because results can remain positive despite effective therapy. Passively transferred maternal treponemal antibodies can persist in an infant until 15 months of age. A reactive treponemal test after 18 months of age is diagnostic of congenital syphilis and should be followed by evaluation and, if necessary, treatment for congenital syphilis. If the treponemal test is nonreactive at this time, no further evaluation or treatment is necessary.

Neonates whose initial CSF evaluations are abnormal do not need repeat lumbar puncture unless they exhibit persistent nontreponemal serologic test titers at age 6–12 months. After 2 years of follow-up, a reactive CSF VDRL test or abnormal CSF indices that cannot be attributed to another ongoing illness at the 6-month interval are indications for retreatment.

Acquired Syphilis. People with acquired primary or secondary syphilis should have clinical and serologic evaluations at 6 and 12 months after treatment. More frequent evaluation might be necessary if adherence to follow-up or reinfection is a concern. If signs or symptoms persist or recur, or a fourfold or greater increase in nontreponemal titers occurs, treatment failure or reinfection may be responsible. CSF analysis, HIV testing, and retreatment based on CSF findings are indicated. Failure of nontreponemal titers to decline fourfold within 6 to 12 months may also indicate treatment failure.

Following treatment, people with acquired latent syphilis should have serologic evaluation at 6, 12, and 24 months after treatment; HIV-infected people should also have serologic testing at 3 and 9 months in addition to 6, 12, and 24 months. Patients should experience a fourfold or greater decline in nontreponemal titers within 12 to 24 months. If titers increase at least fourfold or initial high titers fail to fall fourfold, or symptoms of syphilis develop, reevaluation, including a CSF examination, is warranted. Additional guidance can be found in the current CDC guidelines for the management of STIs.[1]

Patients with neurosyphilis associated with acquired syphilis must have periodic serologic testing, clinical evaluation at 6-month intervals, and repeat CSF examinations. If the CSF WBC has not decreased after 6 months or if the CSF WBC count or protein concentration is not normal after 2 years, retreatment should be considered. CSF abnormalities may persist for extended periods of time in people with HIV infection with neurosyphilis.

ISOLATION OF THE HOSPITALIZED PATIENT: Standard precautions are recommended for all patients, including infants with suspected or proven congenital syphilis. Because moist open lesions, secretions, and possibly blood are contagious in all patients with syphilis, gloves should be worn when caring for patients with congenital, primary, and secondary syphilis with skin and mucous membrane lesions until 24 hours of treatment has been completed.

---

[1]Centers for Disease Control and Prevention. Sexually transmitted diseases treatment guidelines, 2021. *MMWR Recomm Rep.* 2021; in press

CONTROL MEASURES:

- All recent sexual contacts of a person with acquired syphilis should be identified, examined, serologically tested, and treated as needed. Sexual contacts of people with primary, secondary, or early latent syphilis exposed within the preceding 90 days may be infected even if seronegative and should be treated for early-acquired syphilis. People exposed >90 days previously should be treated presumptively if serologic test results are not available immediately and follow-up is uncertain. For identification of at-risk sexual partners, the periods before treatment are as follows: (1) 3 months plus duration of symptoms for primary syphilis; (2) 6 months plus duration of symptoms for secondary syphilis; and (3) 1 year for early latent syphilis.
- All people who have had close unprotected contact with a patient with early congenital syphilis before identification of the disease or during the first 24 hours of therapy should be examined clinically for the presence of lesions 2 to 3 weeks after contact. Serologic testing should be performed and repeated 3 months after contact or sooner if symptoms occur. If the degree of exposure is considered substantial, immediate treatment should be considered.
- Congenital syphilis is a nationally notifiable disease in the United States.

Tapeworm Diseases
(Taeniasis and Cysticercosis)

CLINICAL MANIFESTATIONS:

Taeniasis. Infection with adult tapeworms often is asymptomatic. The most common symptom is noting passing tapeworm segments from the anus or in feces. Other mild gastrointestinal tract symptoms, such as nausea or diarrhea, can occur.

Cysticercosis. Cysticercosis, caused by larval pork tapeworm (*Taenia solium*) infection, can have serious consequences. Manifestations depend on the location and number of pork tapeworm larval cysts (cysticerci) and on the host response. Cysticerci may be found anywhere in the body. The most common and serious clinical manifestations are caused by cysticerci in the central nervous system. Larval cysts of *T solium* in the brain (neurocysticercosis) can result in seizures, headache, obstructive hydrocephalus, and other neurologic signs and symptoms. Neurocysticercosis is the leading infectious cause of epilepsy in the developing world. Most symptoms result from the host reaction to degenerating cysticerci. Cysts in the spinal column can cause gait disturbance, pain, or transverse myelitis. Subcutaneous cysticerci produce palpable nodules, and ocular involvement can cause visual impairment.

ETIOLOGY: Taeniasis is caused by intestinal infection by the adult tapeworm, *Taenia saginata* (beef tapeworm) or *T solium* (pork tapeworm). *Taenia asiatica* causes taeniasis in Asia. Human cysticercosis is caused only by the larvae of *T solium.*

EPIDEMIOLOGY: Tapeworm diseases have worldwide distribution. Prevalence is high in areas with poor sanitation and human fecal contamination in areas where cattle graze or swine are fed. Most cases of *T solium* infection in the United States are imported from Latin America, although the disease is prevalent in parts of Asia and sub-Saharan Africa as well. *T saginata* infection occurs at high rates in East Africa and the Middle East and also is prevalent in Latin America, much of Asia, and eastern Europe. *T asiatica* is common in China, Taiwan, and Southeast Asia. Taeniasis is acquired by eating undercooked beef *(T saginata)*, pork *(T solium)*, or pig viscera *(T asiatica)* that contain encysted larvae.

Cysticercosis in humans is acquired by ingesting eggs of the pork tapeworm *(T solium)*. Transmission is fecal-oral, usually by ingestion of food contaminated by feces from a person harboring the adult tapeworm. Autoinfection, in which tapeworm carriers infect themselves, also occurs. Humans are the obligate definitive host and the only host to shed the eggs. Eggs liberate oncospheres in the intestine that migrate through the blood and lymphatics to tissues throughout the body, including the central nervous system, where the oncospheres develop into cysticerci. Although nearly all cases of cysticercosis in the United States are imported, cysticercosis can be acquired in the United States from tapeworm carriers who emigrated from an area with endemic infection and still have *T solium* intestinal-stage infection. *T saginata* and *T asiatica* do not cause cysticercosis.

The **incubation period** for taeniasis (the time from ingestion of the larvae until segments are passed in the feces) is 2 to 3 months. For cysticercosis, the time between infection and onset of symptoms is typically several years.

DIAGNOSIS[1]: Diagnosis of taeniasis (adult tapeworm infection) is based on demonstration of the proglottids or ova in feces or the perianal region, although these techniques are insensitive. Antigen detection, nucleic acid tests, and immunoblot assays for tapeworm stage-specific antibody are more sensitive but are not commercially available. Species identification of the parasite is based on the different structures of gravid proglottids and scolex or on polymerase chain reaction (PCR) assay.

Diagnosis of neurocysticercosis typically depends on clinical presentation and imaging of the central nervous system. Serologic testing also can be helpful in certain cases. Computed tomography (CT) scanning or magnetic resonance imaging (MRI) of the brain or spinal cord are used to demonstrate lesions compatible with cysticerci. CT scans are helpful in identifying calcifications. MRI is better at identifying extraparenchymal cysts (eg, in ventricles or the subarachnoid space) and the invaginated scolex within the parasite cysticercus. Antibody assays that detect specific antibodies to larval *T solium* in serum can be useful to confirm the diagnosis. Most commercially available antibody tests use crude antigen in an ELISA format. These tests have problems with sensitivity and specificity and are not reliable diagnostic techniques. In the United States, immunoblot assays (including the Enzyme-linked ImmunoTransfer Blot [EITB]) are available through the Centers for Disease Control and Prevention and a few commercial laboratories and are the antibody tests of choice. In general, immunoblot assays are more sensitive with serum specimens than with cerebrospinal fluid specimens. Even immunoblot tests can have limited sensitivity if only one cysticercus or only calcified cysticerci are present, and results often are negative in children with solitary parenchymal lesions. A negative serologic test result does not exclude the diagnosis of neurocysticercosis when clinical suspicion is high. A serologic test result could be positive in patients from areas of high endemicity who do not have neurocysticercosis. Antigen-detection assays are available commercially in Europe and available from the Centers for Disease Control and Prevention and National Institutes of Health for selected cases.

---

[1]White AC Jr, Coyle CM, Rajshekhar V, et al. Diagnosis and treatment of neurocysticercosis: 2017 clinical practice guidelines by the Infectious Diseases Society of America (IDSA) and the American Society of Tropical Medicine and Hygiene (ASTMH). *Clin Infect Dis.* 2018;66(8):1159-1163

TREATMENT[1]:

Taeniasis. Praziquantel is highly effective for eradicating infection with the adult tapeworm (see Drugs for Parasitic Infections, p 984). Praziquantel is not approved for this indication, but dosing recommendations are available for children 4 years and older. Safety is not established in children younger than 4 years, but this drug has been used successfully to treat cases of *Dipylidium caninum* infection in children as young as 6 months. Praziquantel is detected in the milk of lactating women, and women should not breastfeed on the day of treatment or during the subsequent 72 hours. Niclosamide is an alternative agent for treatment of taeniasis but is not available commercially in the United States.

Cysticercosis. Neurocysticercosis treatment should be individualized on the basis of the number, location, and viability of cysticerci as assessed by neuroimaging studies (MRI or CT scan) and clinical manifestations. Symptomatic therapy is critical and should include antiseizure medications for patients with seizures and surgery for patients with hydrocephalus. Two antiparasitic drugs—albendazole and praziquantel—are available (see Drugs for Parasitic Infections, p 984). Studies in children as young as 1 year suggest that albendazole can be administered safely to this population. Praziquantel is not approved by the US Food and Drug Administration for this indication. Both drugs are cysticercidal and hasten radiologic resolution of cysts, but symptoms result from host inflammatory response and may be exacerbated by treatment. In symptomatic patients with a single cyst within brain parenchyma, controlled studies demonstrate that clinical resolution and seizure recurrence rates are slightly improved when children are treated with albendazole along with corticosteroids. Two studies have demonstrated that in those with more than 2 lesions, the response rate was better when albendazole was coadministered with praziquantel and corticosteroids. When a single agent is used, albendazole is preferred over praziquantel, because it has fewer drug-drug interactions with anticonvulsants and steroids. Patients with calcified cysts do not benefit from antiparasitic treatment. An ophthalmic examination should be performed before antiparasitic treatment to rule out intraocular cysticerci (see below). Coadministration of corticosteroids during antiparasitic therapy decreases adverse effects during treatment and is required for some forms of the disease (eg, basilar or subarachnoid, extensive parenchymal, or spinal involvement). See footnote 66 of Drugs for Parasitic Infections, p 989, for steroid dosing. Duration of corticosteroid therapy is longer in patients with subarachnoid disease, vasculitis, or encephalitis. Arachnoiditis, vasculitis, or diffuse cerebral edema (cysticercal encephalitis) are treated with corticosteroid therapy until the cerebral edema is controlled. Corticosteroids can affect the tissue concentrations of albendazole. Patients requiring steroids may need screening for strongyloidiasis, latent tuberculosis, and vitamin D deficiency.

Medical and surgical management of cysticercosis can be highly complex and often needs to be conducted in consultation with a neurologist or neurosurgeon and an infectious diseases or other specialist with experience treating neurocysticercosis. Seizures may recur for months or years. Anticonvulsant therapy is recommended until there is neuroradiologic evidence of resolution and seizures have not occurred for 6 months (for a single lesion) or 1 to 2 years (for multiple lesions). Calcification of cysts may require prolonged or indefinite use of anticonvulsants. Subarachnoid cysticercosis does not respond well to the regimens used for parenchymal disease and generally should be treated with

---

[1]White AC Jr, Coyle CM, Rajshekhar V, et al. Diagnosis and treatment of neurocysticercosis: 2017 clinical practice guidelines by the Infectious Diseases Society of America (IDSA) and the American Society of Tropical Medicine and Hygiene (ASTMH). *Clin Infect Dis.* 2018;66(8):1159-1163

prolonged courses of antiparasitic and anti-inflammatory medications. Methotrexate and/or tumor necrosis factor inhibitors have been used as steroid-sparing agents. Intraventricular cysticerci and hydrocephalus usually should be treated surgically. Surgical removal of intraventricular cysticerci is the treatment of choice when possible and often can be accomplished by endoscopic surgery (lateral, third, and sometimes 4th ventricles) or open surgery (4th ventricle). If cysticerci cannot be removed easily, hydrocephalus should be corrected with placement of intraventricular shunts. Adjunctive chemotherapy with antiparasitic agents and corticosteroids may decrease the rate of subsequent shunt failure. Ocular cysticercosis is treated by surgical excision of the cysticerci. Ocular cysticercosis generally is not treated with anthelminthic drugs, which can exacerbate inflammation. Spinal cysticercosis may be treated with medical and/or surgical therapy. There is not adequate evidence to guide the choice of medical versus surgical therapy.

ISOLATION OF THE HOSPITALIZED PATIENT: Standard precautions are recommended.

CONTROL MEASURES: Eating raw or undercooked beef or pork should be avoided. Whole cuts of meat should be cooked to at least 145°F (63°C) and then allowed to rest for 3 minutes before consuming, and ground meat and wild game meat should be cooked to at least 160°F (71°C). Freezing pork or beef below −5°C (23°F) for more than 4 days kills cysticerci. People known to harbor the adult tapeworm of *T solium* should be treated immediately. Careful attention to hand hygiene and appropriate disposal of fecal material is important.

Adequate hand hygiene is a key preventive measure. People traveling to resource-limited countries with high endemic rates of cysticercosis should avoid eating uncooked vegetables and fruits that cannot be peeled. If someone in a household is found to have cysticercosis, household members should be screened for taeniasis (see Diagnosis, above), and people with compatible neurologic signs and symptoms should be evaluated for cysticercosis.

Other Tapeworm Infections
(Including Hydatid Disease)

Most tapeworm (cestode) infections are asymptomatic, but nausea, abdominal pain, and diarrhea have been observed in people who are heavily infected.

ETIOLOGIES, DIAGNOSIS, AND TREATMENT

Hymenolepis nana. This tapeworm, also called the dwarf tapeworm because it is the smallest of the adult human tapeworms (about 3 to 4 cm long), can complete its entire life cycle within humans. Transmission occurs by ingestion of eggs present in feces of infected people resulting in human-to-human spread via the fecal-oral route or rarely by ingestion of infected arthropods (certain species of beetles and fleas) present in food. Autoinfection, in which eggs can hatch within the intestine and reinitiate the life cycle, leads to development of new worms and increases the worm burden. Most infections are asymptomatic. Young children may develop abdominal cramps, diarrhea, and irritability with heavy infection. Anal pruritus and difficulty sleeping mimic pinworm infections. Diagnosis is by identification of the characteristic eggs in stool. Praziquantel is the treatment of choice, with nitazoxanide as an alternative drug; niclosamide is another therapeutic option but is not available commercially in the United States (see Drugs for Parasitic Infections, p 962). Praziquantel and nitazoxanide are not approved for this indication. These drugs have been used safely and effectively in children as young as 6 months (praziquantel) and 1 year (nitazoxanide) for other indications. Stools should be reexamined 1 month after treatment to document cure. If infection persists, retreatment with praziquantel is indicated.

Dipylidium caninum. This is the most common tapeworm of dogs and cats and has a wide geographic distribution. Children develop infection with *D caninum* after inadvertently swallowing a dog or cat flea (the intermediate host). Most cases are asymptomatic and come to attention when motile proglottids are passed in stool. Some children have abdominal pain, diarrhea, and anal pruritus. Diagnosis is made by finding the characteristic eggs or motile proglottids in stool. Proglottids resemble rice kernels and may be mistaken for maggots or fly larvae. Their appearance can be mistaken for recurrent pinworm infections. Infection is self-limiting in the human host and typically clears spontaneously by 6 weeks. Therapy with praziquantel is effective. Niclosamide is an alternative therapeutic option but is not available commercially in the United States (see Drugs for Parasitic Infections, p 957). Praziquantel and niclosamide are not approved for this indication. These drugs have been used safely and effectively in children as young as 6 months (praziquantel) and 2 years (niclosamide) (**www.cdc.gov/parasites/dipylidium/ health_professionals/index.html**).

Diphyllobothrium *species (and Related Species).* These are the largest tapeworms that can infect humans. Fish are intermediate hosts of the *Diphyllobothrium* tapeworm, also called fish tapeworm or broad tapeworm (based on the shape of the proglottids). Consumption of infected, raw, or undercooked freshwater (including trout and pike), saltwater (at least 17 species including one shark), or anadromous (salmon) fish leads to infection. Three to 6 weeks after ingestion, the adult tapeworm matures and begins to lay eggs. The most common symptom is noting passage of proglottids. Abdominal pain and diarrhea may occur. The worm rarely may cause mechanical obstruction of the bowel or gallbladder, diarrhea, or abdominal pain. Megaloblastic anemia secondary to vitamin B_{12} deficiency has been noted only with the species *Diphyllobothrium latum* (found in northern Europe and North America and also known as *Dibothriocephalus latus*). Diagnosis is made by recognition of the characteristic proglottids or eggs passed in stool. Therapy with praziquantel is effective; niclosamide is an alternative but is not available commercially in the United States (see Drugs for Parasitic Infections, p 957). Praziquantel and niclosamide are not approved for this indication. These drugs have been used safely and effectively in children as young as 6 months (praziquantel) and 2 years (niclosamide).

Echinococcus granulosus *and* Echinococcus multilocularis.[1] The larval forms of these tapeworms cause human echinococcosis. *Echinococcus granulosus* causes the disease cystic echinococcosis, also known as hydatid disease. The distribution of *E granulosus* is related to areas where sheep or cattle are raised and dogs, the definitive host, are used for herding. Areas of high prevalence include parts of South America, East Africa, Eastern Europe, the Middle East, the Mediterranean region, China, and Central Asia. The parasite also is endemic in Australia and New Zealand. In the United States, small foci of endemic transmission have been reported historically in Arizona, California, New Mexico, and Utah, and a strain of the parasite has adapted to wolves, moose, and caribou in Alaska and Canada. Dogs, coyotes, wolves, dingoes, and jackals can become infected by swallowing protoscolices of the parasite within hydatid cysts in the organs of slaughtered sheep

---

[1]Brunetti E, Kern P, Vuitton DA; Writing Panel for the WHO-Informal Working Group on Echinococcosis. Expert consensus for the diagnosis and treatment of cystic and alveolar echinococcosis in humans. *Acta Trop.* 2010;114(1):1-16

or other intermediate hosts. Dogs pass embryonated eggs in their feces, and humans become intermediate hosts by ingesting the viable parasite eggs. Humans then develop cysts in various organs, such as the liver, lungs, kidneys, and spleen. Cysts caused by larvae of *E granulosus* usually grow slowly (1 cm in diameter per year in the liver) and eventually can contain several liters of fluid. If a cyst ruptures, anaphylaxis and multiple secondary cysts from seeding of protoscolices can result. Clinical diagnosis often is difficult. A history of contact with dogs in an area with endemic infection is helpful. Cystic lesions can be demonstrated by radiography, ultrasonography, or computed tomography of various organs. Serologic testing is helpful, but false-negative results occur. Treatment depends on ultrasonographic staging and may include antiparasitic therapy, PAIR (**p**uncture, **a**spiration, **i**njection of protoscolicidal agents, and **r**easpiration), surgical excision, or no treatment but with watchful waiting. Optimal therapy varies with the location, size, and stage of the parasite (**www.cdc.gov/parasites/echinococcosis/health_professionals/ index.html#tx**). Small cysts in the liver may respond to antiparasitic drugs alone. For larger, uncomplicated liver cysts, treatment of choice is PAIR. Contraindications to PAIR include communication of the cyst with the biliary tract (eg, bile staining after initial aspiration), superficial cysts, and heavily septated cysts. Surgical therapy is indicated for complicated cases and requires meticulous care to prevent spillage, including preparations such as soaking of surgical drapes in hypertonic saline. In general, the cyst should be removed intact, because leakage of contents is associated with a higher rate of complications, including anaphylactic reactions to cyst contents. Treatment with albendazole generally should be initiated days to weeks before surgery or PAIR and continued for several weeks to months thereafter (see Drugs for Parasitic Infections, p 957). Studies in children as young as 1 year suggest that albendazole can be administered safely to this population. Degenerating cysts can be managed by watchful waiting with follow-up imaging studies. For lung lesions, small cysts often resolve with antiparasitic drugs alone. Larger cysts are best removed surgically. Many surgeons prefer to avoid preoperative antiparasitic drugs for lung cysts.

Echinococcus multilocularis, the causative agent for alveolar echinococcosis, has definitive hosts (foxes, coyotes, other wild canines) and intermediate hosts (rodents). Alveolar echinococcosis is characterized by invasive growth of the larvae in the liver (which may mimic neoplasm) with occasional metastatic spread, most worrisomely to the brain. Alveolar echinococcosis is limited to the Northern Hemisphere and usually is diagnosed in people 50 years or older. The disease has been reported frequently from Western China and is also endemic in central Europe. Diagnosis can be confirmed by imaging and serologic testing. The preferred treatment is surgical removal of the entire larval mass followed by treatment with albendazole. In nonresectable cases, continuous treatment with albendazole has been associated with clinical improvement (see Drugs for Parasitic Infections, p 957). Two other species, *Echinococcus vogeli* and *Echinococcus oligarthrus*, infect humans; they cause polycystic echinococcosis.

ISOLATION OF THE HOSPITALIZED PATIENT: Standard precautions are recommended.

CONTROL MEASURES: Preventive measures for *H nana* include educating the public about personal hygiene and sanitary disposal of feces.

Infection with *D caninum* is prevented by keeping dogs and cats free of fleas and worms. Children should wash their hands after playing with dogs and cats and after playing in areas soiled with pet feces.

To protect against *D latum (D latus)*, freshwater fish should be cooked thoroughly to an internal temperature of 63°C (145°F) or should be frozen per the following recommendations:

- At −4°F (−20°C) or below for 7 days (total time), or
- At −31°F (−35°C) or below until solid, and storing at −31°F (−35°C) or below for 15 hours, or
- At −31°F (−35°C) or below until solid and storing at −4°F (−20°C) or below for 24 hours.

Control measures for prevention of *E granulosus* and *E multilocularis* include educating the public about hand hygiene and avoiding exposure to dog and wild canid feces. Prevention and control of infection in dogs (preventing dogs from feeding on rodents or carcasses of sheep, treating dogs for parasitic infections) decreases the risk of subsequent human infection.

Tetanus
(Lockjaw)

CLINICAL MANIFESTATIONS: Tetanus is caused by neurotoxin produced by the anaerobic bacterium *Clostridium tetani* in a contaminated wound and can manifest in 3 overlapping clinical forms: generalized, local, and cephalic.

Generalized tetanus (lockjaw) is a neurologic disease manifesting as trismus and severe muscular spasms, including risus sardonicus, which is a facial expression characterized by raised eyebrows and grinning distortion of the face resulting from spasm of facial muscles. Onset is gradual, occurring over 1 to 7 days, and symptoms progress to severe painful generalized muscle spasms, which often are aggravated by any external stimulus. Autonomic dysfunction, manifesting as diaphoresis, tachycardia, labile blood pressure, and arrhythmias, often is present. Other potential complications include fractures associated with muscle spasms, laryngospasm, pulmonary embolism, and aspiration pneumonia. Severe spasms persist for 1 week or more and subside over several weeks in people who recover. Neonatal tetanus is a form of generalized tetanus occurring in newborn infants lacking protective passive immunity because their mothers are not immune. Early symptoms include inability to suck or breastfeed and excessive crying that then progress to findings typical of generalized tetanus.

Local tetanus manifests as local muscle spasms in areas contiguous to a wound. **Cephalic tetanus** is the rarest form of tetanus and usually causes flaccid cranial nerve palsies, although trismus can occur. It is associated with infected wounds on the head and neck including, rarely, suppurative otitis media. Local and cephalic tetanus can precede generalized tetanus.

ETIOLOGY: *C tetani* is a spore-forming, obligate anaerobic, gram-positive bacillus. This organism is a wound contaminant that causes neither tissue destruction nor an inflammatory response. The vegetative form of *C tetani* produces a potent plasmid-encoded exotoxin (tetanospasmin). The heavy chain of tetanospasmin binds to the presynaptic motor neuron and facilitates entry of the light chain, a zinc-dependent protease, into the cytosol. As a result, gamma-aminobutyric acid- and glycine-containing vesicles are not released, and inhibitory action on motor and autonomic neurons is lost.

EPIDEMIOLOGY: Tetanus occurs worldwide and is more common in warmer climates and during warmer months, in part because of higher frequency of contaminated wounds associated with those locations and seasons. The organism, a normal inhabitant of soil and animal and human intestines, is ubiquitous in the environment, especially where contamination by excreta is common. Organisms multiply in wounds, recognized or unrecognized, and elaborate toxins in the presence of anaerobic conditions. Contaminated wounds, especially wounds with devitalized tissue and deep-puncture trauma, are at greatest risk. Neonatal tetanus is common in many resource-limited countries where pregnant women are not immunized appropriately against tetanus and nonsterile umbilical cord-care practices are followed. Globally, activities are ongoing to eliminate maternal and neonatal tetanus by improving vaccination coverage among pregnant women and promoting safe delivery practices. During 2000-2018, 45 countries achieved maternal and neonatal tetanus elimination, reported cases of neonatal tetanus decreased 90%, and estimated deaths declined 85%.[1]

Widespread active immunization against tetanus has modified the epidemiology of disease in the United States, where it is now rare. Tetanus is not transmissible from person to person.

In the United States, nearly all cases of tetanus occur in individuals who have never received a tetanus vaccine or who have not received their 10-year booster vaccine. At particular risk are people with immune-compromising conditions, people with diabetes mellitus, or people who use intravenous drugs.

The **incubation period** ranges from 3 to 21 days, with most cases occurring within 8 days. In general, the farther the injury site from the central nervous system, the longer the incubation period. Shorter incubation periods have been associated with more heavily contaminated wounds, more severe disease, and a worse prognosis. In neonatal tetanus, symptoms usually appear from 4 to 14 days after birth, averaging 7 days. Cephalic tetanus may have an **incubation period** as short as 1 to 2 days.

DIAGNOSTIC TESTS: The diagnosis of tetanus is made clinically by excluding other causes of tetanic spasms, such as hypocalcemic tetany, phenothiazine reaction, strychnine poisoning, and conversion disorder. Attempts to culture *C tetani* are associated with poor yield, and a negative culture does not rule out disease. A protective serum antitoxin concentration should not be used to exclude the diagnosis of tetanus, because tetanus disease has been known to occur rarely despite adequate antibody level.

TREATMENT: Human Tetanus Immune Globulin (TIG) binds circulating unbound toxin and prevents further progression of disease, but it does not reverse the effects of already bound toxin. A single dose of human TIG is recommended for treatment. However, the optimal therapeutic dose has not been established. Most experts recommend 500 IU, which appears to be as effective as higher doses ranging from 3000 to 6000 IU and causes less discomfort. Available preparations must be administered intramuscularly. Infiltration of part of the dose locally around the wound is recommended, although the efficacy of this approach has not been proven. Results of studies on the benefit from intrathecal administration of TIG are conflicting. The TIG preparation in use in the United States is not licensed or formulated for intrathecal or intravenous use. If TIG is not available (as is the case in some countries), Immune Globulin Intravenous (IGIV) can be used at a dose of 200 to 400 mg/kg. IGIV is not approved by the US Food and Drug Administration for this use, and antitetanus antibody concentrations can vary from lot to lot. In some

[1] Njuguna HN, Yusuf N, Raza AA, Ahmed B. Tohme RA. Progress toward maternal and neonatal tetanus eliminiation—worldwide, 2000–2018. *MMWR Morb Mortal Wkly Rep.* 2020;69(17):515-520. DOI: **http://dx.doi.org/10.15585/mmwr.mm6917a2**

countries, equine tetanus antitoxin may be considered if TIG is not available and the patient is tested for sensitivity and desensitized as necessary.

- All wounds should be cleaned and débrided properly, especially if extensive necrosis is present. In neonatal tetanus, wide excision of the umbilical stump is not indicated.
- Supportive care and pharmacotherapy to control tetanic spasms and autonomic instability are of major importance.
- Oral (or intravenous) metronidazole is effective in decreasing the number of vegetative forms of *C tetani* and is the antimicrobial agent of choice. Parenteral penicillin G is an alternative treatment. Therapy for 7 to 10 days is recommended.
- Active immunization against tetanus always should be undertaken during convalescence from tetanus. Because of the extreme potency of tiny amounts of toxin, tetanus disease may not result in immunity.

ISOLATION OF THE HOSPITALIZED PATIENT: Standard precautions are recommended.

CONTROL MEASURES:

Care of Exposed People (see Table 3.68). Risk of tetanus disease depends on the type of wound and immune status of the patient. Depending on the clinical scenario, there are 3 potential interventions to prevent tetanus: wound care, active immunization, and passive immunization. Antimicrobial prophylaxis has not been shown to prevent tetanus and is not recommended.

- Wound care: Although any open wound is a potential source of tetanus, wounds contaminated with dirt, feces, soil, or saliva (eg, animal bites) are at increased risk. Punctures and wounds containing devitalized tissue, including necrotic or gangrenous wounds, frostbite, crush and avulsion injuries, and burns, are particularly conducive to *C tetani* infection. Wounds with devitalized tissue should be débrided and have dirt removed. It is not necessary or appropriate to débride puncture wounds extensively.
- Active immunization: Immunization status should be assessed for all wounds, and age-appropriate vaccine should be administered (see Immunization) if not contraindicated on the basis of clinical scenario (Table 3.68). For infants younger than 6 months, prior infant doses and maternal tetanus toxoid immunization history at time of delivery should be considered in determining need for infant immunization (and need for TIG, if clinically indicated).
- Passive immunization: Patients with tetanus-prone wounds who have not completed a primary series of tetanus vaccine should be considered nonimmune and receive passive immunization with TIG (in addition to active immunization with tetanus toxoid vaccine, as clinically appropriate). In patients with HIV or other severe immunodeficiency, TIG should be administered for tetanus-prone wounds regardless of the history of tetanus toxoid immunization. When TIG is required for wound prophylaxis, it is administered intramuscularly in a dose of 250 U (regardless of age or weight). If tetanus toxoid vaccine and TIG are administered concurrently, separate syringes and sites should be used. Administration of tetanus toxoid vaccine simultaneously with or at an interval after receipt of TIG does not impair development of protective antibody substantially. Efforts should be made to initiate active immunization and arrange for its completion.

Immunization. Antibody to tetanus toxoid is detectable 4 to 7 days after a dose of tetanus vaccine, and its concentration peaks at 2 to 4 weeks. Protective antibody is not reliably achieved following a first dose of vaccine to prevent tetanus disease. After completing a vaccination series, circulating antitoxin usually lasts at least 10 years and for a longer time after a booster dose.

Table 3.68. Guide to Tetanus Prophylaxis in Routine Wound Management

History of Adsorbed Tetanus Toxoid (Doses)	Clean, Minor Wounds		All Other Wounds[a]	
	DTaP, Tdap, or Td[b]	TIG[c]	DTaP, Tdap, or Td[b]	TIG[c,d]
Fewer than 3 or unknown	Yes	No	Yes	Yes
3 or more	No if <10 y since last tetanus-containing vaccine dose	No	No if <5 y since last tetanus-containing vaccine dose	No
	Yes if ≥10 y since last tetanus-containing vaccine dose	No	Yes if ≥5 y since last tetanus-containing vaccine dose	No

DTaP indicates diphtheria and tetanus toxoids and acellular pertussis vaccine; Td, adult-type diphtheria and tetanus toxoids vaccine; Tdap, booster tetanus toxoid, reduced diphtheria toxoid, and acellular pertussis vaccine; TIG, Tetanus Immune Globulin (human).

[a] Such as, but not limited to, wounds contaminated with dirt, feces, soil, and saliva (eg, following animal bites); puncture wounds; avulsions; and wounds resulting from missiles, crushing, burns, and frostbite.

[b] DTaP is used for children younger than 7 years. Tdap is preferred over Td for underimmunized children 7 years and older who have not received Tdap previously.

[c] Immune Globulin Intravenous should be used when TIG is not available.

[d] People with human immunodeficiency virus (HIV) infection or severe immunodeficiency who have contaminated wounds should also receive TIG regardless of their history of tetanus immunization.

Active immunization against tetanus always should be undertaken during convalescence from tetanus, because this exotoxin-mediated disease usually does not confer immunity.

Active immunization with tetanus toxoid vaccine is recommended for all people. For all appropriate indications, tetanus immunization is administered with diphtheria toxoid-containing vaccines or with diphtheria toxoid- and acellular pertussis-containing vaccines. Vaccine is administered intramuscularly and may be administered concurrently with other vaccines (see Simultaneous Administration of Multiple Vaccines, p 36). Conjugate vaccines containing tetanus toxoid (eg, *Haemophilus influenzae* type b) are not substitutes for tetanus toxoid immunization. Recommendations for use of tetanus toxoid-containing vaccines (**http://aapredbook.aappublications.org/site/resources/izschedules. xhtml**) are as follows:

- Immunization for children from 6 weeks through 6 years (up to the seventh birthday) of age:
  - Recommended schedule: should consist of 5 doses of tetanus- and diphtheria toxoid-containing vaccine. All doses are administered as DTaP (or DTaP-containing vaccines) at 2, 4, and 6 months of age, then a dose at 15 through 18 months of age, and another dose at 4 through 6 years of age (recommended before kindergarten or elementary school entry). DTaP can be administered concurrently with other vaccines (see Simultaneous Administration of Multiple Vaccines, p 36). If a dose of Tdap is administered inadvertently instead of DTaP as any one of the primary 3 dose series, then it should not be counted as valid. DTaP can be administered at any interval after the Tdap dose and remaining DTaP doses can be administered as per the recommended schedule. If Tdap is inadvertently administered as the 4th or 5th dose in the series the Tdap dose is counted as valid toward the 5-dose DTaP series.

- Catch up vaccination: the 5-dose DTaP series can be administered with a minimum of 4 weeks between each of the first 3 doses and 6 months between dose 3 and 4 as well as dose 4 and 5. If the fourth dose is administered at 4 years or older, the fifth dose is not needed.
- Pertussis vaccination contraindicated (see Pertussis, p 578): DT should be administered (can be administered concurrently with other vaccines). If the vaccine series is initiated at younger than 1 year, 5 doses are administered on a schedule similar to the DTaP schedule. If the DT series is started at or after 1 year of age, DT is administered as a 4-dose series with a minimum of 4 weeks between dose 1 and 2 and 6 months between dose 2 and 3, with a final dose administered at 4 through 6 years of age. With either regimen, the final dose can be omitted if the most recent dose was administered at 4 years or older.
- Series was started with DT, but pertussis vaccination is desired and is not contraindicated: doses of DTaP should be administered to complete the recommended pertussis immunization schedule (see Pertussis, p 578); however, the total number of doses of diphtheria and tetanus toxoid vaccines (as DT, DTaP, or DTwP) should not exceed 6 before the seventh birthday.
- Immunization for children ≥7 years (see **http://aapredbook.aappublications. org/site/resources/izschedules.xhtml** and Pertussis [Whooping Cough], p 578)[1]:
  - Adolescents 11 years and older should receive a single dose of Tdap instead of Td for booster immunization against tetanus, diphtheria, and pertussis. The preferred age for Tdap immunizations is 11 through 12 years of age.
  - Adolescents who received Td but not Tdap should receive a single dose of Tdap to provide protection against pertussis regardless of time since receipt of Td.
  - Simultaneous administration of Tdap and all other recommended vaccines is recommended when feasible.
  - Inadvertent administration of DTaP instead of Tdap in people 7 years and older is counted as a valid dose of Tdap.
  - Children 7 through 10 years of age who have not completed their immunization schedule with DTaP before 7 years of age or who have an unknown vaccine history should receive at least one dose of Tdap. If further dose(s) of tetanus and diphtheria toxoids are needed in a catch-up schedule, either Td or Tdap can be used. The preferred schedule is Tdap followed by Td or Tdap at 2 months and 6 to 12 months (if needed).
  - Children 7 through 9 years of age who receive Tdap or DTaP for any reason should receive the adolescent Tdap booster at 11 through 12 years of age.
  - A Tdap or DTaP dose received by a 10 year-old for any reason can count as the adolescent Tdap booster dose.
- If more than 5 years have elapsed since the last dose, a booster dose of a tetanus-containing vaccine should be considered for people at risk of occupational exposure in locations where tetanus boosters may not be available readily. Tdap is preferred over Td if the person has not received Tdap previously.

---

[1]Havers FP, Moro PL, Hunter P, Hariri S, Berstein H. Use of tetanus toxoid, reduced diphtheria toxoid, and acellular pertussis vaccines: updated recommendations of the Advisory Committee on Immunization Practices—United States, 2019. *MMWR Morb Mortal Wkly Rep.* 2020;69(3):77-83. DOI: **http://dx.doi. org/10.15585/mmwr.mm6903a5**

- Pregnant women should receive Tdap during each pregnancy, preferably between 27 and 36 weeks' gestation, but the vaccine may be administered at any time during the pregnancy. Pregnant women who have not completed their primary tetanus series should receive 3 vaccinations containing tetanus and reduced diphtheria toxoids, if time permits. The recommended schedule is 0, 4 weeks, and 6 months or later. The risk of neonatal tetanus is minimal if a previously unimmunized woman receives at least 2 properly spaced doses of tetanus toxoid-containing vaccines. If there is insufficient time, 2 doses of Td or Tdap should be administered at least 4 weeks apart, and the second dose should be administered at least 2 weeks before delivery. Tdap should be used for at least one of the tetanus-containing doses, preferably early in the interval between 27 and 36 weeks of gestation (see Pertussis, p 578).

Adverse Events, Precautions, and Contraindications. Severe anaphylactic reactions, Guillain-Barré syndrome (GBS), and brachial neuritis attributable to tetanus toxoid have been reported but are rare. No increased risk of GBS has been observed with use of DTaP in children. For a child with a history of GBS, the decision to administer additional doses of DTaP should be made on the basis of consideration of the benefit of further immunization versus the risk of recurrence of GBS.

An immediate anaphylactic reaction to tetanus- and diphtheria toxoid-containing vaccines (ie, DTaP, Tdap, DT, Td, or conjugate vaccine containing diphtheria or tetanus toxoid) is a contraindication to further doses unless the patient can be desensitized to these toxoids (see Pertussis, p 578). Injection site pain and erythema are common. Fever may occur, and rarely, whole limb swelling occurs (with or without pain and erythema). Repeat vaccination, as age appropriate, appears to be safe in children who had whole limb swelling. Arthus-type hypersensitivity reaction has been reported in adults who received excessive doses of Td over a short period and usually is associated with high concentrations of tetanus antitoxin. Arthus reactions are rare in children and did not occur in clinical trials of Tdap vaccines.

People who experienced an Arthus-type hypersensitivity reaction after a previous dose of a tetanus toxoid-containing preparation usually have very high serum tetanus antibody concentrations and should not receive dose(s) of tetanus toxoid-containing preparation more frequently than every 10 years, even if they have a wound that is neither clean nor minor.

Other Control Measures. Sterilization of hospital supplies will prevent the rare instances of tetanus that may occur in a hospital from contaminated sutures, instruments, or plaster casts.

For prevention of neonatal tetanus, preventive measures (in addition to maternal immunization) include community immunization programs for adolescent girls and women of childbearing age and appropriate training of midwives in recommendations for immunization and sterile technique.

Tinea Capitis
(Ringworm of the Scalp)

CLINICAL MANIFESTATIONS: Dermatophytic fungal infections of the scalp usually present with an area of localized alopecia and scaling but may include subtle findings of mild hair loss with faint scaling or a large hairless, boggy erythematous area (kerion). Other manifestations include a common "black dot" pattern reflecting stubs of broken-off hairs at the scalp surface; a less common "grey patch" pattern with prominent, well-demarcated alopecic areas of scaling and erythema; or a vesiculopustular pattern resembling bacterial folliculitis. Regional lymphadenopathy may be present.

The differential diagnosis for tinea capitis depends on the clinical presentation. In the classic scaling presentation, clinicians should consider atopic dermatitis, seborrheic dermatitis, and psoriasis. Alopecia should raise the possibility of trichotillomania and alopecia areata, although these disorders usually are not associated with scaling. When vesiculopustular in nature, lice infestation and bacterial infection should be considered. A boggy fluctuant mass likely represents a kerion, but primary (or secondary) bacterial infection can be considered. Although scalp scarring can result from tinea, particularly when a kerion suppurates, presence of scalp scarring should raise the possibility of an autoimmune disorder, such as discoid lupus.

An associated skin eruption, known as a dermatophytic or "id" reaction, can occur as a hypersensitivity reaction to the infecting fungus and can manifest as diffuse, pruritic, papular, vesicular, and/or eczematous lesions occurring at sites distant from the fungal infection. Id reactions may begin after starting therapy but do not represent a drug allergy.

Tinea capitis can occur in association with tinea corporis. Examination of the body (face, trunk, and limbs) should be performed, particularly in wrestlers and others engaged in contact sports.[1]

ETIOLOGY: Tinea capitis develops when dermatophyte fungal elements invade the scalp hair follicle and shaft. The specific pathogen varies by geographic region and mode of transmission. The primary causes are fungi of the genus *Trichophyton*, including *Trichophyton tonsurans* and *Trichophyton violaceum*, as well as *Microsporum*, including *Microsporum canis* and *Microsporum audouinii*.

EPIDEMIOLOGY: Tinea capitis primarily occurs in prepubertal children but may occur in children of all ages and in adults. In the United States, *T tonsurans* is responsible for up to 95% of tinea capitis and is most common in Black school-aged children but occurs in all racial and ethnic groups. Infection with *T tonsurans* is contracted from direct contact with an infected individual, animal, or contaminated object such as hat or brush. *T violaceum* is the dominant organism in eastern Europe and south Asia and is seen more frequently in immigrant populations in the United States.

M canis is associated with less than 5% of infections in the United States, but is distributed more evenly among racial/ethnic groups. *M canis* infection almost always results from contact with infected pets, particularly kittens or puppies. *M canis* outbreaks in schools and child care facilities have followed visits from infected animals.

The dermatophyte organism remains viable for prolonged periods on fomites (eg, brushes, combs, hats, towels), and rate of asymptomatic carriage and infected individuals among family members of index cases is high. Asymptomatic carriers almost certainly serve as a reservoir of infection within families, schools, and communities.

Immunocompromised people and those with trisomy 21 have an increased susceptibility to dermatophyte infections.

The **incubation period** is unknown but is believed to be 1 to 3 weeks. Dermatophyte infections have been reported as early as 3 days of age.

---

[1]Davies HD, Jackson MA, Rice SG; American Academy of Pediatrics, Committee on Infectious Diseases, Council on Sports Medicine and Fitness. Infectious diseases associated with organized sports and outbreak control. *Pediatrics.* 2017;140(4):e20172477

DIAGNOSTIC TESTS: The presence of alopecia, pruritus, scale, and posterior cervical lymphadenopathy makes the diagnosis of tinea capitis almost certain. Most clinicians will choose to treat empirically, but it is prudent to obtain a fungal culture first. Diagnosis can be confirmed by dermatoscopic examination of the affected area, by microscopic evaluation of a potassium hydroxide wet mount of cutaneous scrapings, or by isolation in culture. Dermatoscopic evaluation of areas of alopecia with a lighted magnifier may show comma, corkscrew, or elbow-shaped hairs. Potassium hydroxide wet mount microscopy may be used to examine hairs and scale obtained by gentle scraping of a moistened area of the scalp with a blunt scalpel, hairbrush, toothbrush, or cotton swab or by plucking with tweezers. Visualization of spores filling the interior of the hair shaft indicates an endothrix infection caused by *T tonsurans*, while coating of the outside of the hair shaft with spores indicates an ectothrix infection, such as from *M canis*. In both forms, septate hyphae may be visualized in scrapings from the scalp surface. Clinicians may use fungal culture to establish a diagnosis, in conjunction with or instead of microscopy. If fungal culture is desired, a cotton-tipped applicator can be used to swab an affected area. The sample is transported to a mycology laboratory for processing; 2 to 4 weeks of incubation on Sabouraud dextrose agar are required for results. Polymerase chain reaction is very useful but expensive and not yet widely available. Under Wood lamp, tinea lesions are not fluorescent unless the etiologic agent is of the *Microsporum* genus, in which blue-green fluorescence is noted because it is an ectothrix infection.

TREATMENT: Tinea capitis always requires systemic medication, because the fungal infection is found within the hair follicles, where topical agents do not reach. Optimal treatment of tinea capitis includes consideration of drug tolerability, availability, and cost. Current treatment options are summarized in Table 3.69.

Griseofulvin is approved by the US Food and Drug Administration (FDA) for children 2 years and older, is available in either liquid or tablet form, can be administered on a daily basis, and should be taken with fatty foods. Experts generally use higher doses of griseofulvin than have been approved by the FDA or that were used in clinical trials. Laboratory testing of serum hepatic enzymes is not required if duration of griseofulvin therapy is less than 8 weeks (but treatment of longer than 8 weeks is often required for resolution of infection). High-dose griseofulvin is considered standard of care for *M canis* infection.

Terbinafine granules are approved by the FDA for tinea capitis in children 4 years and older and can be split and mixed with foods such as pudding and peanut butter to increase palatability (although bioavailability is not dependent on food). Advantages of terbinafine for *T tonsurans* infection include possibility of shorter duration of therapy (Table 3.69) and equal or superior effectiveness compared with griseofulvin. Terbinafine clearance is higher in children than adults; pharmacokinetic data derived from studies of a granule formulation that is no longer on the market are the best information available regarding terbinafine clearance in children, and some experts extrapolate this "higher dosing" when utilizing tablets.

Two triazole agents can be considered in therapy. Fluconazole is the only oral antifungal agent approved by the FDA for children younger than 2 years, albeit not for tinea capitis. It had lower cure rates than other oral agents in a large randomized controlled trial. Accumulating evidence supports that itraconazole (currently not FDA approved for use in children or for tinea capitis) can be effective and safe for this disease. Liver function testing need not be assessed at baseline unless the child has preexisting liver disease or is

Table 3.69. Recommended Systemic Therapy for Tinea Capitis

Drug	Dosage	Duration	FDA Approved for Tinea Capitis
Griseofulvin microsize (liquid, 125 mg/5 mL)	20–25 mg/kg/day (max 1 g/day)	≥6 wk; continue until clinically clear	Yes (children ≥2 y)
Griseofulvin ultramicrosize (tablets of varying size)	10–15 mg/kg/day (max 750 mg/day)		
Terbinafine tablets (250 mg)[a]	4–6 mg/kg/day (max: 250 mg); or 10–20 kg: 62.5 mg 20–40 kg: 125 mg >40 kg: 250 mg	*T tonsurans*: 4–6 wk *M canis*: 8–12 wk	No
Terbinafine granules (125 mg and 187.5 mg)[b]	<25 kg: 125 mg 25–35 kg: 187.5 mg >35 kg: 250 mg	*T tonsurans*: 4–6 wk *M canis*: 8–12 wk	Yes (children ≥4 y)
Fluconazole (liquid, 10 mg/mL; tablet, 50 and 100 mg)	6 mg/kg/day (max 400 mg/day)	3–6 wk	No (but approved for pediatric patients ≥6 mo for other indications)
Itraconazole solution (10 mg/mL)	3 mg/kg/day (max 600 mg/day)	2–4 wk	No
Itraconazole capsule (100 mg)	5 mg/k/day (max 600 mg/day)		

[a]Some experts use "higher" dosing listed for terbinafine granules instead.
[b]Terbinafine granules have been discontinued in the United States.

on concomitant hepatotoxic medications. Monitoring while on therapy need not occur unless treatment duration is >4 weeks or if the child develops symptoms while receiving treatment.

Topical treatment, such as shampoos containing selenium sulfide, ketoconazole, or ciclopirox, may be useful as an adjunct to systemic therapy to decrease carriage of viable conidia for all forms of tinea capitis. Shampoo can be applied 2 to 3 times per week and left in place for 5 to 10 minutes. Treatments should continue for at least 2 weeks, and some experts recommend continuing topical treatments until clinical and mycologic cure occurs.

Affected patients receiving therapy should be reassessed in 1 month for clinical response. Fungal cultures may be obtained to evaluate for a mycologic response. Poor response may prompt retreatment with a different agent, if compliance with the initial drug is confirmed.

Kerion is managed by systemic antifungal treatment as outlined previously. Removal of crusts with wet compresses is thought to decrease the risk of secondary bacterial infection. Combined antifungal and corticosteroid therapy (either oral or intralesional) has not been shown to be superior to antifungal therapy alone. Nonetheless, if the condition is unresponsive to traditional therapy, most experts will add systemic prednisone, 1 mg/kg/day for 2 weeks, to decrease likelihood of scarring. Treatment with antimicrobial agents is unnecessary unless secondary bacterial infection occurs.

ISOLATION OF THE HOSPITALIZED PATIENT: Standard precautions apply.

CONTROL MEASURES: If discovered while at school, the affected student need not be sent home early. Once therapy is initiated, children should not be excluded from school. Family members and close contacts should be questioned regarding symptoms, and anyone with symptoms should be evaluated. Some experts recommend topical antifungal shampoo therapy for asymptomatic family members, but evidence is lacking regarding efficacy of this intervention. Sharing of items such as hats and combs/brushes should be avoided in households with an affected person. If pets are suspected as a source of *M canis* infection, evaluation and appropriate treatment of the affected animal should be implemented.

Tinea Corporis
(Ringworm of the Body)

CLINICAL MANIFESTATIONS: Superficial tinea infections of the nonhairy (glabrous) skin, termed tinea corporis, involve the face, trunk, or limbs. Lesions often are ring-shaped or circular (hence, the lay term "ringworm") and are sharply marginated. Involved skin is slightly erythematous and scaly, with color variations from red to brown. The classic eruption displays a scaly, vesicular, or pustular border (often serpiginous) with central clearing. Small confluent plaques or papules as well as multiple lesions can occur, particularly in wrestlers (tinea gladiatorum).[1]

The differential diagnosis for tinea corporis includes pityriasis rosea (particularly the herald patch), candidiasis, psoriasis, other dermatitides (seborrheic, atopic, irritant or allergic, generally caused by therapeutic agents applied to the area), pityriasis versicolor (tinea versicolor), nummular eczema, erythema annulare centrifugum, and erythrasma (an eruption of reddish brown patches resulting from superficial bacterial skin infection caused by *Corynebacterium minutissimum*).

The typical appearance of the lesions is altered in patients who have been treated erroneously with topical corticosteroids. Known as tinea incognito, this altered appearance includes diminished erythema and absence of typical scaling borders. Such patients also can develop Majocchi granuloma, a fungal invasion of the hair shaft and surrounding dermis, which causes a granulomatous dermal reaction that can extend into the surrounding subcutaneous fat. Majocchi granuloma also can occur without prior use of corticosteroids.

An associated dermatophytic or "id" reaction can be present as a hypersensitivity reaction to the infecting fungus, manifesting as diffuse, pruritic, papular, vesicular, or eczematous lesions, which can occur at sites distant from the fungal infection. Sometimes id reactions first appear following institution of therapy, but they do not represent a drug allergy.

---

[1]Davies HD, Jackson MA, Rice SG; American Academy of Pediatrics, Committee on Infectious Diseases, Council on Sports Medicine and Fitness. Infectious diseases associated with organized sports and outbreak control. *Pediatrics.* 2017;140(4):e20172477

Skin lesions can occur as grouped papules or pustules without erythema or scaling in patients with diminished T-lymphocyte function (eg, human immunodeficiency virus infection).

Tinea corporis can occur in association with tinea capitis. The scalp should be examined, particularly in wrestlers and others engaged in contact sports.

ETIOLOGY: Tinea corporis develops when dermatophytic fungi invade the outer skin layers at the affected body region. Primary etiologic agents are *Trichophyton* species, especially *Trichophyton tonsurans*, *Trichophyton rubrum*, and *Trichophyton mentagrophytes*; *Microsporum* species, especially *Microsporum canis*; and *Epidermophyton floccosum*.

EPIDEMIOLOGY: Causative fungi occur worldwide and are transmissible by direct contact with infected humans, animals, soil, or fomites (eg, brushes, combs, hats, towels), where organisms can remain viable for prolonged periods.

Immunocompromised people have an increased susceptibility to dermatophyte infections.

The **incubation period** is believed to be 1 to 3 weeks but can be shorter, as reported cases have occurred at 3 days of age.

DIAGNOSTIC TESTS: Tinea corporis is diagnosed by clinical manifestations and can be confirmed by microscopic examination of a potassium hydroxide wet mount of skin scrapings or fungal culture. Skin scrapings, ideally at the scaly edges of lesions for best recovery of organisms, are obtained by gentle scraping of a moistened area with a glass coverslip, blunt scalpel, toothbrush, or brush or by plucking with tweezers. If fungal culture is desired, a cotton-tipped applicator can be used to swab an affected area gently. The sample is transported to a mycology laboratory for processing; 2 to 4 weeks of incubation on Sabouraud dextrose agar are required for results. Polymerase chain reaction of specimens is available but expensive, and generally is not necessary. Under Wood lamp, tinea is not fluorescent unless the etiologic agent is of the genus *Microsporum*, in which case a blue-green fluorescence can be seen because it is an ectothrix infection.

TREATMENT: A myriad of topical antifungal options are available for treatment and should be applied on the lesions and 1 to 2 cm beyond the borders. Some topical agents are approved by the US Food and Drug Administration (FDA) only for certain lesion locations and age groups and with applications specified as once or twice daily (Table 3.70). Any of the following products (applied twice daily) are reasonable first-line therapies if appropriate for age: miconazole, clotrimazole, tolnaftate, or ciclopirox. Any of the following products also can be used (applied once daily) if appropriate for age: ketoconazole, terbinafine, econazole, naftifine, luliconazole, or butenafine. Oxiconazole and sulconazole can be used (once or twice daily) if appropriate for age (also see Topical Drugs for Superficial Fungal Infections, p 922).

Although clinical resolution may be evident within 2 weeks of therapy, continuing therapy for another 2 to 4 weeks generally is recommended. If significant clinical improvement is not observed after 2 weeks of treatment, an alternate diagnosis and/or systemic therapy should be considered. Topical preparations of antifungal medication combined with a corticosteroid should not be used because of inferior effectiveness, the possibility of leading to Majocchi granuloma, and increase in the rate of relapse, higher cost, and potential for adverse corticosteroid effects.

Table 3.70. Products for Topical Treatment of Tinea Corporis, Cruris, and Pedis

Topical Product	Age for Use	Daily Application
Miconazole (cream, 2%)	Age ≥2 y	Twice
Clotrimazole (cream or solution, 1%)	All ages	Twice
Tolnaftate (cream or solution, 1%)	All ages	Twice
Ciclopirox (cream or suspension, 0.77%)	Age ≥10 y	Twice
Ciclopirox (gel, 0.77%)	Age ≥16 y for tinea corporis or pedis	Twice
Ketoconazole (cream, 2%)[a]	All ages	Once
Terbinafine (cream, 1%)	Age ≥12 y	Once for tinea corporis and cruris
		Twice for tinea pedis
Econazole (cream, 1%)	All ages	Once
Naftifine (cream, 2%)	Age ≥12 y for tinea corporis and pedis	Once
Luliconazole (cream, 1%)	Age ≥2 y for tinea corporis	Once
	Age ≥12 y for tinea cruris and pedis	
Butenafine (cream, 1%)	Age ≥12 y	Once for tinea corporis and tinea cruris
		Twice for tinea pedis
Oxiconazole (cream, 1%)	All ages	Once or twice
Sulconazole (cream or solution, 1%)	Adults only	Once or twice
Sertaconazole (cream, 2%)	Age ≥12 y, for tinea pedis only	Twice

[a]Safety and effectiveness in children have not been established for ketoconazole 2% cream.

If lesions are extensive or unresponsive to topical therapy, griseofulvin (for children ≥2 years) or terbinafine (for children ≥4 years; oral formulation not approved for this indication but approved for tinea capitis [granules] and onychomycosis in adults [tablets]) may be administered orally for 4 to 6 weeks (see Tinea Capitis, p 755). Oral itraconazole and fluconazole do not have FDA indications for treatment of any tinea condition; oral fluconazole is approved for other indications in children 6 months and older. If a Majocchi granuloma is present, oral antifungal therapy is recommended, because topical therapy is unlikely to penetrate adequately to eradicate infection.

Dermatophyte infections in other locations, if present, should be treated concurrently.

ISOLATION OF THE HOSPITALIZED PATIENT: Standard precautions apply. Recent outbreaks of tinea infection in both acute and chronic care facilities among patients and caregivers illustrate the need for education regarding clinical manifestations of tinea and infection control procedures in the care of infected individuals.

CONTROL MEASURES[1]: Infections should be treated promptly. Direct contact with known or suspected sources of infection should be avoided. Periodic inspections of contacts for early lesions and prompt therapy are recommended. Athletic mats and equipment should be cleaned frequently, and actively infected athletes in sports with person-to-person contact must be excluded from competitions. Athletes with tinea corporis can participate in matches 72 hours after commencement of topical therapy and when the affected area can be covered. Prophylaxis of wrestling team members is controversial. Fluconazole, 100 mg per day for 3 days, given prophylactically before initiation of competitive interscholastic high school wrestling and given again 6 weeks into the season, has been reported to reduce the incidence of *T corporis* significantly, from 67.4% to 3.5%. The risk-benefit analysis of giving fluconazole prophylactically in this manner has not been determined, however, and its use should be in consultation with an infectious diseases expert. Infected pets also should receive antifungal treatment.

Tinea Cruris
(Jock Itch)

CLINICAL MANIFESTATIONS: Tinea cruris is a common superficial fungal disorder of the groin, pubic/perianal area, and upper thighs. It is more common in male adults and adolescents and uncommon in prepubertal children. The lesions often are ring-shaped or circular (hence, the lay term "ringworm"), are sharply marginated, and can be intensely pruritic (jock itch). The involved skin is slightly erythematous and scaly, with color variations from red to brown. Lesions can display a scaly, vesicular, or pustular border (often serpiginous) with central clearing. Maceration may also develop. The disorder usually spares the scrotum unless candidiasis also is present. The margins can be subtle in chronic infections, and lichenification may be present.

The differential diagnosis for tinea cruris includes intertrigo, candidiasis, psoriasis, other dermatitides (seborrheic, atopic, irritant or allergic, generally caused by therapeutic agents applied to the area), pityriasis versicolor (tinea versicolor), nummular eczema, erythema annulare centrifugum, and erythrasma (an eruption of reddish brown patches resulting from superficial bacterial skin infection caused by *Corynebacterium minutissimum*).

An altered appearance known as tinea incognito can occur in patients who have been treated erroneously with topical corticosteroids, which includes diminished erythema and absence of typical scaling borders. Such patients also can develop Majocchi granuloma when fungi invade the hair shaft and surrounding dermis, causing a granulomatous dermal reaction that can extend into the surrounding subcutaneous fat. Majocchi granuloma also can occur without prior use of topical corticosteroid.

---

[1]Davies HD, Jackson MA, Rice SG; American Academy of Pediatrics, Committee on Infectious Diseases, Council on Sports Medicine and Fitness. Infectious diseases associated with organized sports and outbreak control. *Pediatrics.* 2017;140(4):e20172477

An associated skin eruption, known as a dermatophytic or "id" reaction, can occur as a hypersensitivity reaction to the infecting fungus and manifests as diffuse, pruritic, papular, vesicular, or eczematous lesions at sites distant from the fungal infection. An id reaction can first occur following institution of therapy but does not represent a drug allergy.

Concomitant tinea pedis, tinea unguium, and tinea corporis have been reported in patients with tinea cruris.

ETIOLOGY: Tinea cruris develops when dermatophyte fungi invade the outer skin layers of the affected body region. The fungi *Epidermophyton floccosum*, *Trichophyton rubrum*, and *Trichophyton mentagrophytes* are the most common causes. *Trichophyton tonsurans*, *Trichophyton verrucosum*, and *Trichophyton interdigitale* also have been identified as causes.

EPIDEMIOLOGY: Tinea cruris occurs predominantly in adolescent and adult males and is acquired principally through indirect contact with desquamated epithelium or hair. Direct person-to-person transmission also occurs. Moisture, close-fitting garments, noncotton underwear, friction, and obesity are predisposing factors. Recurrence is common.

Immunocompromised patients have increased susceptibility to dermatophyte infections. In patients with diminished T-lymphocyte function (eg, human immunodeficiency virus infection), skin lesions can appear as grouped papules or pustules unaccompanied by scaling or erythema.

The **incubation period** is unknown but is thought to be approximately 1 to 3 weeks.

DIAGNOSTIC TESTS: Confirmatory diagnostic modalities for tinea cruris are similar to that for tinea corporis (see Tinea Corporis, p 759).

TREATMENT: Treatment is similar to that for tinea corporis (see Tinea Corporis, Table 3.70, p 761). Treatment of concurrent onychomycosis (tinea unguium) and tinea pedis may reduce recurrence. Recurrence is common, particularly if predisposing factors such as moisture and friction are not minimized. Loose-fitting clothing and use of antifungal powders, such as tolnaftate and miconazole, should aid in recovery and prevent recurrence.

Oral terbinafine, itraconazole, and fluconazole are options but do not have a US Food and Drug Administration indication for tinea cruris. Griseofulvin, administered orally for 4 to 6 weeks, may be effective if lesions are unresponsive to topical therapy (see Tinea Capitis, p 755). Oral antifungal therapy is recommended if a Majocchi granuloma (deep folliculitis) is present, because topical therapy is unlikely to penetrate adequately to eradicate infection. Dermatophyte infections in other locations, if present, should be treated concurrently, and may be an indication for oral therapy.

Topical steroids are not recommended, even in formulations coupled with anti-fungal agents, as these may exacerbate the infection.

ISOLATION OF THE HOSPITALIZED PATIENT: Standard precautions apply.

CONTROL MEASURES: Infections should be treated promptly. Involved areas should be kept dry to prevent recurrences, and antifungal powders and wearing loose fitting undergarments may be useful. Patients should be advised to dry the groin area before drying their feet to avoid inoculating dermatophytes of tinea pedis into the groin area. When infection is present, towel sharing should be avoided.

Tinea Pedis and Tinea Unguium (Onychomycosis)
(Athlete's Foot, Ringworm of the Feet)

CLINICAL MANIFESTATIONS: Tinea pedis can have a variety of clinical manifestations in children. Lesions can involve all areas of the foot but usually are patchy in distribution, with a predisposition to cause fissures, macerated areas, and scaling between toes, particularly in the third and fourth interdigital spaces. A pruritic, fine scaly, or vesiculopustular eruption is most common. "Moccasin foot" exhibits confluent, hyperkeratotic, dry scaling of the soles. Recurrence of tinea pedis is common, and it can be a chronic infection. Toenails can be infected (onychomycosis or tinea unguium) and become distorted, discolored, and thickened with accumulation of subungual debris. A superficial white form of foot and toenail fungal infection can occur in children. Toenails may be the source for recurrent tinea pedis.

Tinea pedis must be differentiated from dyshidrotic eczema, atopic dermatitis, contact dermatitis, juvenile plantar dermatosis, palmoplantar keratoderma, and erythrasma (reddish brown patches which can affect the feet and axillae resulting from superficial bacterial skin infection caused by *Corynebacterium minutissimum*).

An associated skin eruption, known as a dermatophytic or "id" reaction, can occur as a hypersensitivity reaction to the infecting fungus and manifests as diffuse, pruritic, papular, vesicular, or eczematous lesions at sites distant from the fungal infection. An id reaction can occur first following institution of therapy but does not represent a drug allergy.

Skin lesions may appear as grouped papules or pustules unaccompanied by erythema or scaling in patients with diminished T-lymphocyte function (eg, human immunodeficiency virus infection).

The differential diagnosis of tinea unguium includes trauma (particularly if only 1 nail is involved), psoriasis, twenty nail dystrophy (trachyonychia), and occasionally subungual exostosis if only 1 nail is involved.

Concomitant tinea in other body sites has been reported in patients with tinea pedis and tinea unguium.

ETIOLOGY: Tinea pedis and unguium develop when dermatophytic fungi invade the skin layers and nails of the affected body region. The fungi *Trichophyton rubrum*, *Trichophyton mentagrophytes*, and *Epidermophyton floccosum* are the most common causes of tinea pedis.

EPIDEMIOLOGY: Tinea pedis is a common infection worldwide in adolescents and adults but is less common in young children. Fungi are acquired by contact with infected skin scales or organisms present in damp areas, such as swimming pools, locker rooms, and showers. Tinea pedis may spread among family members in the household; this may represent enhanced genetic susceptibility as well as increased exposure to the organism. The incidence of onychomycosis, which is more common in toenails, increases with age, with worldwide prevalence estimated to be from 0.1% to 0.87%. The increased use of occlusive footwear earlier in childhood and exposure to high-risk areas (eg, swimming pools, gyms) earlier in life may be associated with an increase of tinea pedis in children. Childhood onychomycosis is associated with a history of tinea pedis, a history of family member infection, increased number of siblings, and male sex.

Immunocompromised people and those with trisomy 21 have increased susceptibility to dermatophyte infections.

The **incubation period** is unknown, although it is believed to be approximately 1 to 3 weeks.

DIAGNOSTIC TESTS: Confirmatory diagnostic tests for tinea pedis are similar to those for tinea corporis (see Tinea Corporis, p 759). Fungal infection of the nail (tinea unguium or onychomycosis) can be verified by direct microscopic examination with potassium hydroxide, fungal culture of desquamated subungual material, or fungal stain of a nail clippings fixed in formalin. Polymerase chain reaction is a useful tool but is expensive and not yet widely available.

TREATMENT: A myriad of topical options are available for treatment of tinea pedis (see Tinea Corporis, Table 3.70, p 761; also see Topical Drugs for Superficial Fungal Infections, p 922). Therapy duration of 2 weeks usually is sufficient for milder cases of tinea pedis in children. Acute vesicular lesions can be treated with intermittent use of open wet compresses (eg, with Burow solution, diluted 1:80). Tinea pedis that is severe, chronic, or refractory to topical treatment can be treated with oral therapy similar to that for tinea capitis (see Tinea Capitis, Table 3.69, p 758).

Recurrence of tinea pedis is prevented by proper foot hygiene, which includes keeping the feet dry and cool, cleaning gently, drying between the toes, use of absorbent antifungal foot powder, exposing affected areas to air frequently, and avoidance of occlusive footwear, nylon socks, and other fabrics that interfere with dissipation of moisture. Protective footwear should be worn in common areas such as pools, gyms, and other public facilities.

Topical antifungal lacquers and solutions that are effective for distal toenail infections that do not involve the nail matrix now are available. Despite lower cure rates, topical agents are preferred because of substantially lower adverse effects, lack of drug-drug interactions, and avoidance of need for laboratory test monitoring for toxicity. Topical ciclopirox 8% lacquer, with a US Food and Drug Administration (FDA) indication for tinea unguium for patients 12 years and older, can be applied to affected toenail(s) twice daily for up to 48 weeks, in combination with a comprehensive nail management program. Efinaconazole 10% solution and tavaborole 5% solution have an FDA indication for tinea unguium in adults; both have higher cure rates in adults than ciclopirox. Topical therapies appear to show a higher cure rate in children than in adults, possibly because of thinner nail plates and faster nail growth rate in children. Most of these agents are expensive and not usually covered by insurance.

Studies in adults have demonstrated the best cure rates for onychomycosis (tinea unguium) are with oral terbinafine or itraconazole. Although oral therapies are more likely to lead to cure, they also require laboratory monitoring and can induce drug–drug interactions. Guidelines for dosing of terbinafine for children are based on studies for treatment of tinea capitis and are weight based (see Table 3.69, p 758). The duration of therapy is the same as for adults (6 weeks for fingernail infection, 12 weeks for toenail infection). Pediatric dosing of oral itraconazole is not established for superficial mycoses, although a suggested dosing may follow that for tinea capitis (Table 3.69, p 758). Griseofulvin, although approved by the FDA for treatment of tinea unguium, is rarely used for this indication.

Factors that influence choice of therapy include severity of infection, results of fungal culture or potassium hydroxide preparation (if performed), prior treatments, concomitant drug therapy for other illnesses, patient preference, and cost. Topical and systemic therapy may be used concurrently to increase therapeutic response. Cure rates following oral or combined therapy approach 80% in children. Mechanical and chemical debridement of the nail, using 40% urea ointment daily under occlusion for 10 days to soften the nail, should be performed in refractory cases or when severe thickening of the nail is likely to decrease absorption and response to therapy.

Dermatophyte infections in other locations, if present, should be treated concurrently.

ISOLATION OF THE HOSPITALIZED PATIENT: Standard precautions apply.

CONTROL MEASURES: Treatment of patients with active infections should decrease transmission. Using public areas conducive to transmission (eg, swimming pools) is discouraged in those with active infection. Chemical foot baths can facilitate spread of infection. Because recurrence after treatment is common, proper foot hygiene is important (as described in Treatment). Patients should be advised to dry the groin area before drying the feet to avoid inoculating dermatophytes from tinea pedis into the groin area. Prevention of tinea unguium includes keeping nails short and clean, and avoid sharing of nail clippers.

Toxocariasis

CLINICAL MANIFESTATIONS: Clinical disease is caused by parasitic nematode larva migration through tissues. Signs and symptoms differ depending on the affected organ and host inflammatory response. Toxocariasis can be of following types: covert toxocariasis, visceral larva migrans, neurotoxocariasis, or ocular larva migrans. Most infected children are asymptomatic. Covert disease most often presents with simple, persistent eosinophilia and may be attributed to the continuation of the migratory phase, which may last for many years. Symptoms of visceral toxocariasis include fever, cough, wheezing, abdominal pain, and malaise and uncommonly may include myocarditis and rash. Neurotoxocariasis may manifest with an eosinophilic meningoencephalitis, space-occupying lesions, myelitis, or cerebral vasculitis and may present with seizures. Laboratory abnormalities include leukocytosis, eosinophilia, and hypergammaglobulinemia. Ocular invasion (resulting in uveitis, endophthalmitis, or retinal granulomas) most often manifests as unilateral vision loss, often without other systemic signs of infection.

ETIOLOGY: Toxocariasis is caused by *Toxocara* species, which are nematode parasites (roundworms) of dogs and cats (especially puppies or kittens), specifically *Toxocara canis* and *Toxocara cati*, respectively; most cases are caused by *T canis*.

EPIDEMIOLOGY: A nationally representative survey found 5% of the US population 6 years and older to have serologic evidence of *Toxocara* infection. Visceral toxocariasis typically occurs in children 2 to 7 years of age but can occur in older children and adults. Ocular toxocariasis usually occurs in older children and adolescents, and the majority of reported cases of ocular toxocariasis occur in patients living in southern states. Infection is more likely among people who own dogs and people living in poverty and is more prevalent in hot and humid regions where eggs remain viable in soil. Humans are infected by ingestion of soil containing infective eggs of the parasite. Eggs may be found wherever dogs and cats defecate, often in sandboxes and playgrounds. Eggs become infective after 2 to 4 weeks in the environment and may persist long-term in the soil. Direct contact with dogs or cats is not necessary, because eggs are not infectious immediately when shed in the feces.

The **incubation period** cannot be determined accurately.

DIAGNOSTIC TESTS: Laboratory findings include marked leukocytosis with eosinophilia and occasionally anemia and hypergammaglobulinemia. Patients with visceral disease frequently have increased titers of isohemagglutinin to the A and B blood group antigens. An enzyme-linked immunosorbent assay (ELISA) for *Toxocara* antibodies in serum or vitreous fluid is available through the Centers for Disease Control and Prevention and is preferred over testing by commercial laboratories. A positive antibody test result does not distinguish between past and current infection, and the test is less sensitive for diagnosis of ocular toxocariasis. For visceral disease, imaging of the liver using ultrasonography, computed tomography, or magnetic resonance imaging may reveal diffuse nodular lesions measuring less than 2 cm in diameter. Microscopic identification of larvae in a liver biopsy specimen is diagnostic, but this test is not sensitive or specific and therefore rarely indicated.

TREATMENT: Albendazole is recommended for treatment of visceral and ocular toxocariasis (see Drugs for Parasitic Infections, p 949). The drug has been approved by the US Food and Drug Administration but not for this indication. Studies in children as young as 1 year suggest that albendazole can be administered safely to this population. Mebendazole is an alternative. In severe cases with myocarditis or involvement of the central nervous system, corticosteroid therapy administered concurrently with albendazole is warranted. Control of inflammation of the eye with oral or topical corticosteroids may be warranted; surgical therapy may be helpful in complicated cases.

ISOLATION OF THE HOSPITALIZED PATIENT: Standard precautions are recommended. There is no person-to-person spread.

CONTROL MEASURES: Proper disposal of cat and dog feces is essential. Regular veterinary care and periodic deworming of dogs and cats, and especially puppies and kittens, decreases environmental contamination with *Toxocara* eggs and has public health benefit. Covering sandboxes when not in use is helpful. No specific management following exposure is recommended.

Toxoplasma gondii Infections[1]
(Toxoplasmosis)

CLINICAL MANIFESTATIONS: Up to 50% of patients with acute *Toxoplasma* infection are asymptomatic. When present, common signs and symptoms of acute *Toxoplasma* infection can include flu-like symptoms, lymphadenopathy with atypical lymphocytosis, fever, myalgia, arthralgia, sweats, chills, fatigue, headache, chorioretinitis, hepatic dysfunction, pneumonitis, meningoencephalitis, myocarditis, myositis, acute disseminated encephalomyelitis (ADEM), and myelitis. Reactivation of chronic *Toxoplasma* infection in immunocompromised patients may result in fever, pneumonia, septic shock, brain abscesses, diffuse encephalitis without brain-space occupying lesions, seizures, chorioretinitis, myocarditis, myelitis, and polymyositis.

Congenital Infection. Mothers are not screened routinely for toxoplasmosis during pregnancy in the United States. Clinically apparent signs and symptoms of congenital

---

[1]Maldonado YA, Read JS; American Academy of Pediatrics, Committee on Infectious Diseases. Diagnosis, treatment, and prevention of congenital toxoplasmosis in the United States. *Pediatrics.* 2017;139(2):e20163860

toxoplasmosis are found on routine physical examination in a minority of infected infants at birth, but more specific testing (of cerebrospinal fluid [CSF], dilated eye examination, or central nervous system [CNS] imaging) can reveal evidence of infection. Visual or hearing impairment, learning disabilities, or severe developmental delay will become apparent later in life in a large proportion of congenitally infected infants. Chorioretinitis occurs in approximately 70% of congenitally infected infants whose mothers were not treated during pregnancy and in up to 25% of those who were treated.

Clinical illness is more likely to be severe when infection occurs in the first trimester and is not treated during gestation. The classic triad of chorioretinitis, cerebral calcifications, and hydrocephalus is highly suggestive of congenital toxoplasmosis. Additional signs at birth include microcephaly, seizures, hearing loss, strabismus, petechial rash, jaundice, generalized lymphadenopathy, hepatomegaly, splenomegaly, pneumonia, thrombocytopenia, and anemia. Meningoencephalitis may be associated with CSF abnormalities including high protein concentrations, hypoglycorrhachia, and eosinophilia. Some severely affected fetuses/infants with disseminated congenital toxoplasmosis die in utero or within a few days of birth. Cerebral calcifications can be demonstrated by ultrasonography, computed tomography (CT), or magnetic resonance imaging (MRI) of the head. CT is the radiologic technique of choice, because it is the most sensitive for calcifications and can reveal brain abnormalities when ultrasonographic studies are normal.

Postnatally Acquired Primary Infection. Postnatally acquired *Toxoplasma gondii* infections in immunocompetent patients usually are asymptomatic. When symptoms develop, they may be nonspecific and can include malaise, fever, headache, sore throat, arthralgia, and myalgia. Lymphadenopathy, frequently cervical, is the most common sign. Patients occasionally have a mononucleosis-like illness associated with a maculopapular rash, hepatosplenomegaly, hepatic dysfunction, and atypical lymphocytosis. The clinical course usually is benign and self-limited.

In a subset of patients, primary infection may be severe and/or persistent disease including fever, myocarditis, pericarditis, myositis, hepatitis, pneumonia, encephalitis with and without brain abscesses, and skin lesions (maculopapular rash). These severe syndromes are especially common in patients who acquired primary *T gondii* infections with high parasite loads and/or in areas where atypical, more virulent strains are present (eg, Mexico, French Guiana, Brazil, and Colombia).

Chorioretinitis. Toxoplasmic chorioretinitis can occur: (a) with congenital infection; (b) from a postnatally acquired acute infection; and (c) from reactivation of a congenital or postnatally acquired infection. Acute onset of blurred vision, eye pain, decreased visual acuity, floaters, scotoma, photophobia, epiphora, nystagmus, or strabismus are noted. Ocular findings in toxoplasmic eye disease include white focal retinitis with overlying vitreous inflammation ("headlight in the fog"), nearby prior pigmented retinochoroidal scar, retinal vasculitis, vitreous inflammation, cataracts, iridocyclitis and stellate keratic precipitates (accompanying chorioretinitis), and elevated intraocular pressure. Complications can include retinal detachment, cystoid macular edema, optic atrophy, chronic iridocyclitis, cataract formation, secondary glaucoma, or band keratopathy.

Reactivation of Chronic Infection in Immunocompromised Patients. Reactivation of latent infection may occur in immunosuppressed patients. Reactivation can result in encephalitis, brain abscesses, seizures, pneumonia, myocarditis, hepatitis, skin lesions, posterior uveitis or panuveitis with chorioretinitis, fever of unknown origin, and disseminated disease and death. Toxoplasmic encephalitis (TE) can present as a single or multiple brain lesions on MRI or as a "diffuse form" with a rapidly progressive clinical course leading to death despite apparently normal brain imaging. MRI is superior to CT for the diagnosis of TE. In patients with acquired immunodeficiency syndrome (AIDS), TE is the most common cause of space-occupying brain lesions and typically presents with acute to subacute neurologic or psychiatric symptoms and multiple ring-enhancing brain lesions. In these patients, a clear improvement in the neurologic examination within 7 to 10 days of beginning empiric anti-*Toxoplasma* therapy is considered diagnostic of TE. Lack of radiographic response 2 weeks after initiation of anti-*Toxoplasma* therapy is an indication to consider alternative diagnoses. Non-AIDS patients with multiple brain lesions should not be treated empirically for only toxoplasmosis, and other etiologies should be entertained for diagnostic and empiric treatment purposes.

Seropositive hematopoietic stem cell transplant and solid organ transplant recipients are at risk of reactivation of latent infection in the absence of appropriate prophylaxis. Toxoplasmosis in this setting presents as pneumonia, unexplained fever or seizures, myocarditis, hepatitis, hepatosplenomegaly, lymphadenopathy, skin lesions, or brain abscesses and diffuse encephalitis. Transplant donors and recipients should be screened pretransplant for *Toxoplasma* infection, including heart, other solid organ, and hematopoietic stem cell/bone marrow donors.

ETIOLOGY: *T gondii* is a protozoan and obligate intracellular parasite. The infectious forms include tachyzoites, tissue cysts containing bradyzoites, and oocysts containing sporozoites. The tachyzoite and the corresponding host immune reaction are responsible for observed symptoms. The tissue cyst is responsible for latent infection and usually is present in brain, eye, cardiac tissue, and skeletal muscle.

EPIDEMIOLOGY: Seroprevalence of *T gondii* infection varies by geographic locale and socioeconomic strata of the population. The overall *T gondii* seropositivity rate in the United States (according to the National Health and Nutrition Examination Survey 2011–2014) in people older than 6 years is 11.1% and among women 15 to 44 years of age is 7.5%.

Congenital transmission occurs in most cases as a result of acute primary maternal infection acquired during pregnancy or within 3 months prior to conception. In utero infection rarely can occur as a result of reactivated parasitemia in a latently infected immunocompromised woman in the absence of prophylaxis. Rarely, congenital toxoplasmosis is acquired from an immunocompetent pregnant women reinfected with a different *T gondii* strain. Incidence of acute primary *T gondii* infection during pregnancy in the United States is estimated to be 0.2 to 1.1/1000 pregnant women on the basis of data from Massachusetts and New Hampshire, which are the only 2 states in the United States with universal toxoplasmosis newborn screening.

The **incubation period** of postnatally acquired infection is approximately 7 days, with a range of 4 to 21 days. Parasites can be detected in the blood for up to 2 weeks after acute infection; prolonged parasitemia also has been reported.

DIAGNOSTIC TESTS: Serologic tests are the primary means of diagnosis. *Toxoplasma* immunoglobulin (Ig) G and IgM can be performed by commercial laboratories in most situations; exceptions are testing of pregnant women with suspected acute *Toxoplasma* infections during gestation and neonates with suspected congenital toxoplasmosis, for whom testing should be performed at a reference laboratory (see below). *Toxoplasma* IgM results from commercial laboratories can be falsely positive; confirmation should be obtained from reference laboratories with special expertise such as the Palo Alto Medical Foundation Toxoplasma Serology Laboratory (PAMF-TSL; Palo Alto, CA; **www.sutterhealth.org/RemingtonLab**; telephone: (650) 853-4828; email: **RemingtonLab@sutterhealth.org**). Confirmatory testing at the reference laboratory may include IgM testing IgA, IgE, IgG avidity, and the differential agglutination (of acetone [*AC*]-fixed versus that of formalin [*HS*]-fixed tachyzoites) test (*AC/HS* test).

IgG-specific antibodies achieve a peak concentration 3 to 5 months after infection and remain positive indefinitely. IgM-specific antibodies can be detected 1 to 2 weeks after infection (IgG-specific antibodies usually are negative during this period), achieve peak concentrations in 1 month, and usually become undetectable within 6 to 9 months, but may also persist for years without apparent clinical significance. The lack of *T gondii*-specific IgM antibodies in a person with low-positive titers of IgG antibodies (eg, a dye test at PAMF-TSL ≤1:512) indicates infection of at least 6 months' duration. In contrast, detectable *T gondii*-specific IgM antibodies can indicate recent infection, chronic (latent) infection, or a false-positive reaction. If timing of infection is clinically important (eg, in a pregnant woman), sera with positive *T gondii* IgM test results can be sent to PAMF-TSL to establish acute versus chronic infection using an additional panel of tests such as IgG avidity, AC/HS, and IgA- and IgE-specific antibody tests.

Polymerase chain reaction (PCR) detection has been applied to body fluid or tissue, and *T gondii*-specific immunoperoxidase staining can be performed with any tissue, depending on the clinical scenario. A positive PCR test result in tissue must be interpreted with caution, because it may amplify tachyzoite or bradyzoite DNA and cannot distinguish between tachyzoites with acute infection or reactivation or bradyzoites with chronic latent infection. CSF PCR for *T gondii* has high specificity (96%–100%) but sensitivity is only 50%. CSF PCR results can also be negative because of anti-toxoplasma therapy.

Congenital Toxoplasmosis. During pregnancy, PCR assay of amniotic fluid is the method of choice to confirm fetal infection. Fetal ultrasonography can assess for anatomical abnormalities. Examination of the placenta by histologic testing and PCR assay may provide additional information but is not sufficiently sensitive or specific for diagnostic purposes. At birth or postnatally, serologic tests for IgG, IgM, and IgA should be performed on the neonate, and CSF, urine, and whole blood should be sent for *T gondii* PCR assay. Positive neonatal serum *Toxoplasma* IgM (after 5 days of life) and/or IgA (after 10 days of life), along with a positive IgG, is considered diagnostic of congenital toxoplasmosis. IgM immunosorbent agglutination assay (ISAGA) test results can be falsely positive after transfusion of blood products but usually becomes negative 14 days after transfusion. Occasionally, false-positive results for IgG, IgM, and IgA can be observed as a result of platelet transfusions or Immune Globulin Intravenous infusions. The diagnosis of congenital toxoplasmosis also can be made definitively in an infant who remains *Toxoplasma* IgG positive at 12 months of life.

Newborn infants being evaluated for toxoplasmosis also should have a CBC with differential, liver function tests, and cerebrospinal fluid cell count, differential, protein, and glucose performed (in addition to *T gondii* PCR, above). Ophthalmologic and audiologic assessments should be conducted, and head ultrasonography or brain MRI should be performed. Abdominal ultrasonography can be considered to evaluate for hepatospleno-megaly or intrahepatic calcifications.

Asymptomatic newborn infants with low suspicion for congenital toxoplasmosis but who were initially IgG positive but IgM and IgA negative should have follow-up sero-logic testing with IgG only at 4- to 6-week intervals until complete disappearance of IgG antibodies, usually within 6 to 12 months. In the absence of postnatal treatment, disappearance of IgG antibodies in the infant safely excludes the diagnosis of congenital toxoplasmosis.

Expert advice for evaluation and management of neonates/infants with sus-pected or confirmed congenital toxoplasmosis is available at: (a) the PAMF-TSL (**www.sutterhealth.org/RemingtonLab**; telephone [650] 853-4828; email **RemingtonLab@sutterhealth.org**) and (b) the Toxoplasmosis Center, University of Chicago, Chicago, IL (**www.toxoplasmosis.org**; telephone [773] 834-4131; email **rmcleod@bsd.uchicago.edu**).

TREATMENT: Most cases of acquired acute *T gondii* infections in immunocompetent hosts do not require specific therapy unless: (a) infection occurs during pregnancy; (b) there is ocular involvement; or (c) symptoms are severe or persistent. Treatment of acute *T gondii* infections in immunocompromised patients is always recommended.

Newborns and infants with confirmed/strongly suspected congenital toxoplasmosis should receive oral therapy with pyrimethamine, sulfadiazine, and folinic acid (P/S/FA), usually for 12 months, as outlined in Table 3.71. While receiving pyrimeth-amine, neonates/infants should be monitored for development of neutropenia weekly for 4 weeks; if the absolute neutrophil count (ANC) is stable, then CBCs should be obtained every 2 weeks for 2 to 3 months and then every 3 to 4 weeks for the remainder of treat-ment. If the ANC decreases to <750, the frequency of folinic acid administration should be increased to daily dosing and pyrimethamine therapy should be held temporarily.

Ophthalmologic evaluations should be continued at least every 3 to 6 months during the first 3 years of life for children with confirmed/probable congenital toxoplasmosis, even if the initial evaluation at or near birth was normal. Long-term neurodevelopmental evaluation also is required.

Infected neonates/infants with asymptomatic congenital toxoplasmo-sis with normal fetal ultrasonography and normal findings in all postnatal evaluations, including head ultrasonography or head MRI, abdominal ultrasonography, eye exami-nation, hearing test, CBC, and liver function tests, should be managed with the regi-men used for symptomatic infants (P/S/FA). Treatment duration may be shorter than 12 months (but should be at least 3 months) and should be discussed with a congenital toxoplasmosis expert. Ophthalmologic and neurodevelopmental follow-up should be per-formed as detailed above.

Older children with active toxoplasmic chorioretinitis represent a medi-cal emergency, and treatment should be initiated as soon as possible, as outlined in Table 3.72. Close monitoring by a retinal specialist with expertise in management of toxoplasmic eye disease and a toxoplasmosis infectious diseases expert is recommended. Treatment for eye disease usually is given for 1 to 2 weeks beyond complete resolution of all clinical signs and symptoms and usually is approximately 4 to 6 weeks total. Treatment courses up to 3 months total are required occasionally.

Table 3.71. Treatment of Neonates/Infants With Confirmed or Strongly Suspected Congenital Toxoplasmosis

Regimen	Dosing and Duration
Pyrimethamine PLUS Sulfadiazine PLUS Folinic acid[a]	Doses: Pyrimethamine[b]: 1 mg/kg every 12 hours orally for 2 days, followed by 1 mg/kg once daily for 2–6 months (6 months should be considered for symptomatic cases), followed by 1 mg/kg once per day every Monday, Wednesday, Friday to complete a total course of 12 months PLUS Sulfadiazine: 50 mg/kg every 12 hours orally for 12 months PLUS Folinic acid (leucovorin): 10 mg/dose 3 times per week orally (during and up to 1 week after completing pyrimethamine) Duration: Treatment usually is recommended for 1 year[c] Prednisone (if CSF protein ≥1 g/dL or severe chorioretinitis in vision threatening area): 0.5 mg/kg (maximum 20 mg/dose) every 12 hours orally until CSF protein <1 g/dL or resolution of severe chorioretinitis (if prednisone is used, it should be started 48–72 hours after the initiation of anti-*Toxoplasma* therapy)

CSF indicates cerebrospinal fluid.

[a] Folic acid should not be used as a substitute for folinic acid (leucovorin).

[b] In some centers in Europe, the regimen of pyrimethamine/sulfadoxine (Fansidar) every 10 days, plus folinic acid, is used for subclinical/mild forms of congenital toxoplasmosis and/or for poor compliance and/or frequent hematologic adverse effects. This regimen is used after the first 2 months of daily therapy with pyrimethamine/sulfadiazine (plus folinic acid 2 to 3 times per week). No other alternative medications have been studied adequately for treatment of congenital toxoplasmosis.

[c] For infants with delayed diagnosis of congenital toxoplasmosis (several months after birth), optimal duration of treatment should be discussed with a toxoplasmosis expert.

Immunocompetent and immunocompromised children with severe primary (acute) toxoplasmosis and *immunocompromised children with reactivation of latent (chronic) Toxoplasma infection* should receive oral therapy with P/S/FA, as outlined in Table 3.73. In patients for whom P/S/FA is not immediately available, who are allergic or unable to take P or S, or who have significant issues with absorption of oral medications, see alternative regimens listed in Table 3.73.

While children are receiving pyrimethamine, weekly monitoring with CBC and differential is recommended. If neutropenia is detected, the dose of leucovorin should be increased.

Table 3.72. Treatment of Older Children With Active Toxoplasmic Chorioretinitis

- Active toxoplasmic chorioretinitis, particularly in patients with severe eye disease in vision-threatening areas, is a medical emergency and treatment should begin as soon as possible.
- Duration: Treatment is usually given for 1 to 2 weeks beyond resolution of clinical manifestations, and usually is approximately 4–6 weeks total; prolonged treatment courses up to 3 months sometimes may be needed.
- Consultation with a retinal specialist (with experience in management of patients with toxoplasmic chorioretinitis) AND with a toxoplasmosis infectious diseases expert should be requested to assist with optimal medication dosing, duration of therapy, and necessary monitoring.

Doses:

Pyrimethamine[a,b,c]:
Loading dose: 1 mg/kg once every 12 hours orally (maximum 50 mg/day) for 2 days, followed by maintenance dose: 1 mg/kg once per day orally (maximum 25 mg/day)

PLUS

Sulfadiazine:
Loading dose: 75 mg/kg (first dose), followed (12 hours later) by maintenance dose: 50 mg/kg every 12 hours orally (maximum 4 g/day)

PLUS

Folinic acid (leucovorin)[d]:
10–20 mg/dose daily orally (during and 1 week after therapy with pyrimethamine)

Prednisone (for severe eye disease in vision-threatening areas [eg, fovea/macula]): 0.5 mg/kg every 12 hours orally (maximum 40 mg/day). If steroids are used, they should be started after 48–72 hours of anti-*Toxoplasma* therapy, with rapid taper. Use steroids at the lowest possible dose and for the shortest possible duration.

Suppressive therapy for recurrent toxoplasmic chorioretinitis:
Although there are no pediatric clinical trials for primary or secondary prophylaxis (suppressive therapy), 2 adult randomized trials in Brazil for secondary prophylaxis showed that after recurrent active toxoplasmic chorioretinitis, initiation of chronic suppressive anti-toxoplasma therapy (1 double strength TMP/SMX every 2–3 days, for 12–20 months) significantly decreased the incidence of recurrences.[e]

BID indicates twice a day.

[a]If pyrimethamine tablets cannot be obtained immediately, compounded pyrimethamine can be obtained by calling Imprimis Rx at: (844) 446-6979. Treatment should change back to pyrimethamine tablets as soon as they are acquired.

[b]Trimethoprim/sulfamethoxazole (TMP/SMX) can also be used when the first-line therapy (pyrimethamine/sulfadiazine) is not readily available, but ONLY until the first-line therapy with pyrimethamine/sulfadiazine/folinic acid becomes available.

[c]While on pyrimethamine therapy, a complete blood cell count should be performed weekly. Screening for glucose-6-phosphate dehydrogenase (G6PD) deficiency before starting sulfadiazine or TMP/SMX should be performed for patients from regions with high prevalence of severe G6PD deficiency.

[d]Folic acid should not be used as a substitute for folinic acid (leucovorin).

[e]Silveira C, Belfort R Jr, Muccioli C, et al. The effect of long-term intermittent trimethoprim/sulfamethoxazole treatment on recurrences of toxoplasmic retinochoroiditis. *Am J Ophthalmol.* 2002;134(1):41-46; and Fernandez Felix JP, Cavalcanti Lira RP, Santos Zacchia R, et al. Trimethoprim-sulfamethoxazole versus placebo to reduce the risk of recurrences of toxoplasma gondii retinochoroiditis: randomized controlled clinical trial. *Am J Ophthalmol.* 2014;157(4):762-766.e1

Table 3.73. Treatment Regimens for Children and Adolescents With Severe Primary (Acute) Toxoplasmosis[a] and Immunocompromised Children and Adolescents With Severe Toxoplasmosis Attributable to Reactivation[b]

Regimen	Dose
PREFERRED REGIMEN	
Pyrimethamine[c,d] (PO)	Loading dose: 1 mg/kg every 12 hours (maximum 100 mg/day) for 2 days; followed by 1 mg/kg once per day (up to 50 mg/day [if <60 kg] or up to 75 mg/day [if ≥60 kg] in older patients with severe disease)
PLUS	
Folinic acid[e] (PO)	10–20 mg/dose once per day (up to 50 mg/day) (during and 1 week after therapy with pyrimethamine)
PLUS	
Sulfadiazine (PO)	100–200 mg/kg/day divided every 6 hours (maximum 4–6 grams/day for severe disease)
PREFERRED ALTERNATIVE REGIMEN	
Trimethoprim-Sulfamethoxazole[d] (IV or PO)	
ALTERNATIVE REGIMENS (WITH LIMITED DATA)	
Pyrimethamine + Folinic acid + Clindamycin	
Pyrimethamine + Folinic acid + Atovaquone	
Pyrimethamine + Folinic acid + Clarithromycin	
Pyrimethamine + Folinic acid + Azithromycin	
Atovaquone + Sulfadiazine	

BID indicates twice a day; IV intravenous; PO, oral.

[a] Includes immunocompetent or immunocompromised children with severe acute *Toxoplasma gondii* infection, particularly in the setting of myocarditis, myositis, hepatitis, pneumonia, brain lesions, and lymphadenopathy accompanied by severe or persisting symptoms **(for drug dosing for ocular toxoplasmosis, see Table 3.72).** For toxoplasmic encephalitis in HIV patients, treatment should be continued for 3–6 weeks followed by suppressive therapy.

[b] Expert advice is available at the PAMF-TSL **(www.sutterhealth.org/RemingtonLab**; telephone [650] 853-4828; email **RemingtonLab@sutterhealth.org)** and the Toxoplasmosis Center, University of Chicago, Chicago, IL **(www.toxoplasmosis.org;** telephone [773] 834-4131; email **rmcleod@bsd.uchicago.edu).**

[c] If pyrimethamine tablets cannot be obtained immediately, compounded pyrimethamine can be obtained by calling Imprimis Rx at: (844) 446-6979. Treatment should change back to pyrimethamine tablets as soon as they are acquired.

[d] Trimethoprim/sulfamethoxazole (TMP/SMX) can also be used when the first-line therapy (pyrimethamine/sulfadiazine) is not readily available, and ONLY until the first-line therapy with pyrimethamine/sulfadiazine/folinic acid becomes available. In those cases, the highest doses of TMP/SMX should be used (10–15 mg/kg/day of the TMP component, divided Q8–Q12 hours).

[e] Folinic acid = leucovorin; folic acid must not be used as a substitute for folinic acid.

Primary and Secondary Prophylaxis. Current treatment recommendations and recommendations for primary and secondary toxoplasmosis prophylaxis in children and adolescents with human immunodeficiency virus (HIV) infection are available at **https://clinicalinfo. hiv.gov/sites/default/files/inline-files/oi_guidelines_pediatrics.pdf.**

ISOLATION OF THE HOSPITALIZED PATIENT: Standard precautions are recommended.

CONTROL MEASURES: Testing household or close family members of individuals diagnosed with acute *Toxoplasma* infection should be considered in settings in which there are individuals at high risk (eg, pregnant women, immunocompromised individuals, and young children in whom visual impairment associated with acute infection may be missed). HIV-infected, immunocompromised, and pregnant individuals should be counseled about avoidance of sources of *Toxoplasma* infection (see below). Pregnant women and immunocompromised patients whose serostatus for *T gondii* is negative or unknown should avoid activities that may expose them to cat feces by avoiding changing litter boxes, gardening, and landscaping, or wearing gloves while doing so and washing hands immediately thereafter. If it must be done, daily changing of cat litter decreases risk of infection, because oocysts are not infective during the first 1 to 2 days after passage. Domestic cats can be protected from infection by feeding them commercially prepared cat food and preventing them from eating undercooked meat and hunting wild rodents and birds.

Oral ingestion of viable *T gondii* can be prevented by the following:
- Avoiding consumption of raw or undercooked meat and cooking meat—particularly pork, lamb, and venison—to an internal temperature of 65.5°C to 76.6°C (150°F–170°F), whole cuts of meat (excluding poultry) to at least 145°F (63°C), ground meat (excluding poultry) to at least 160°F (71°C), and all poultry to at least 165°F (74°C) before consumption;
- Avoiding consumption of smoked meat and meat cured in brine;
- Freezing meat to −20°C for 48 hours before consumption;
- Washing fruits and vegetables;
- Washing hands and cleaning kitchen surfaces after handling fruits, vegetables, and raw meat;
- Washing hands after gardening or other contact with soil;
- Preventing contamination of food with raw or undercooked meat or soil;
- Avoiding ingestion of raw shellfish such as oysters, clams, and mussels;
- Avoiding ingestion of raw goat milk; and
- Avoiding ingestion of untreated water, particularly in resource-limited countries.

Additional resources for health care personnel can be found at **www.cdc.gov/ parasites/toxoplasmosis/health_professionals/index.html.**

Trichinellosis
(*Trichinella spiralis* and Other Species)

CLINICAL MANIFESTATIONS: The clinical spectrum of *Trichinella* infection ranges from inapparent infection to fulminant and fatal illness; most infections are asymptomatic. Severity of disease is proportional to the infective dose and varies with the causative species of *Trichinella*. During the first week after ingesting infected meat, a person may experience abdominal discomfort, nausea, vomiting, and/or diarrhea as excysted larvae penetrate the intestinal mucosa. Two to 8 weeks later, as progeny larvae migrate into tissues, fever, myalgia, periorbital edema, urticarial rash, and conjunctival and subungual hemorrhages may develop. In severe infections, myocarditis, neurologic involvement, and pneumonitis can occur in 1 or 2 months. Larvae may remain viable in tissues for years; calcification of some larvae in skeletal muscle usually occurs within 6 to 24 months and may be detected using various imaging modalities.

ETIOLOGY: Infection is caused by nematodes (roundworms) of the genus *Trichinella*. Seven species have been implicated in human disease; worldwide, *Trichinella spiralis* is the most common cause of human infection.

EPIDEMIOLOGY: Animal infections occur worldwide in carnivores and omnivores, especially scavengers. Humans acquire the infection following ingestion of raw or insufficiently cooked meat containing larvae of *Trichinella* species. Commercial and home-raised pork remain a source of human infections, but meats other than pork, such as venison, horse meat, and particularly meats from wild carnivorous or omnivorous game (especially bear, boar, seal, and walrus) now are the most common sources of infection. The disease is not transmitted from person to person.

The **incubation period** usually is less than 1 month.

DIAGNOSTIC TESTS: Eosinophilia of up to 70% in the setting of compatible symptoms and dietary history suggests the diagnosis. Increases in concentrations of muscle enzymes, such as creatinine phosphokinase and lactic dehydrogenase, may occur but are not always present. Larvae can be detected in suspect meat, but this is not often feasible. Encapsulated larvae in a skeletal muscle biopsy specimen (particularly deltoid and gastrocnemius) are visible under light microscopy beginning 2 weeks after infection by examining hematoxylin-eosin–stained slides or sediment from digested muscle tissue. Serologic testing is available through the Centers for Disease Control and Prevention, some state reference laboratories, and commercial laboratories. Serum antibodies are detectable at 3 or more weeks postinfection and may remain for years. Testing of paired acute and convalescent serum specimens showing an increase in titer is diagnostic, but a single positive test result in the appropriate clinical setting makes the diagnosis likely.

TREATMENT: Albendazole and mebendazole are each recommended for treatment of acute trichinellosis (see Drugs for Parasitic Infections, p 985), although anthelmintics typically do not kill larvae that have already encysted within muscles. Studies in children as young as 1 year suggest that albendazole can be administered safely to this population. Coadministration of corticosteroids with anthelmintics is recommended when systemic symptoms are severe. Corticosteroids can be lifesaving when the central nervous system or heart is involved.

ISOLATION OF THE HOSPITALIZED PATIENT: Standard precautions are recommended. There is no person-to-person spread.

CONTROL MEASURES: Transmission to pigs can be prevented by not feeding them garbage, by preventing cannibalism among animals, and by effective rat control. The public should be educated about the importance of cooking pork and wild game meat thoroughly. Specific recommendations include the following:

- For whole cuts of meat (excluding poultry and wild game): cook to at least 145°F (63°C) as measured with a food thermometer placed in the thickest part of the meat, then allow the meat to rest for 3 minutes before carving or consuming.

- For ground meat (including wild game, excluding poultry): cook to at least 160°F (71°C); ground meats do not require a rest time.
- For all wild game (whole cuts and ground): cook to at least 160°F (71°C).

Freezing pork less than 6 inches thick at 5°F (−15°C) for 20 days kills *T spiralis*. *Trichinella* organisms in wild animals, such as bears and raccoons, are resistant to freezing. For people who have ingested undercooked meat known to be contaminated with *Trichinella* organisms, preemptive therapy with albendazole or mebendazole may be considered; a case series suggests that this may be effective if initiated within 6 days of exposure. Case reporting to appropriate health authorities is required in many jurisdictions (see Appendix III: Nationally Notifiable Infectious Diseases in the United States, p 1033).

Trichomonas vaginalis Infections
(Trichomoniasis)

CLINICAL MANIFESTATIONS: Infection with *Trichomonas vaginalis* (TV), which has been described as the most common nonviral sexually transmitted infection (STI) affecting approximately 3.7 million people in the United States, is asymptomatic in 70% to 85% of infected individuals. Untreated infections may persist for months to years. Clinical manifestations in symptomatic pubertal or postpubertal females may include a diffuse vaginal discharge, odor, and vulvovaginal pruritus and irritation. Dysuria and, less often, lower abdominal pain can occur. Vaginal discharge may be any color but classically is yellow-green, frothy, and malodorous. The vulva and vaginal mucosa can be erythematous and edematous. The cervix can be inflamed and sometimes is covered with numerous punctate cervical hemorrhages and swollen papillae, referred to as "strawberry" cervix. This finding occurs in fewer than 5% of infected females but is highly suggestive of trichomoniasis. Clinical manifestations in symptomatic men include urethritis and, rarely, epididymitis or prostatitis. Reinfection is common, and resistance to treatment is uncommon but increasing. Rectal infections are uncommon, and oral infections have not been described.

TV infections in pregnant females have been associated with increased risks of premature rupture of the membranes and preterm delivery, although direct causation has not been clearly established. Perinatal infection may occur in up to 5% of neonates of infected mothers. TV in female newborn infants may cause vaginal discharge during the first weeks of life but usually is self-limited. Respiratory infections in newborn infants may occur as well.

ETIOLOGY: *T vaginalis* is a flagellated protozoan approximately the size of a leukocyte. It requires adherence to host cells for survival.

EPIDEMIOLOGY: The United States population-based TV prevalence is 2.1% among females and 0.5% among males, with the highest rate among Black women (9.6%) and Black men (3.6%), compared with non-Hispanic white females 0.8% and Hispanic females 1.4%. Unlike chlamydia and gonorrhea, TV prevalence rates are as high among women 24 years and older as they are for women younger than 24 years. Other risk factors for *T vaginalis* include having 2 or more sex partners in the past year, having less than a high school education, and living below the poverty level. Women with bacterial vaginosis are at higher risk for TV. Male partners of women with TV are likely to have infection, although the prevalence of trichomoniasis in men who have sex with men is low. TV commonly coexists with other infections, particularly with *Neisseria gonorrhoeae* and herpes simplex virus. Transmission results almost exclusively from sexual contact. The presence of TV in a child or preadolescent beyond the perinatal period is considered indicative of sexual abuse (see STI Evaluation of Prepubertal Victims, p 152, and Table 2.5, p 151). TV infection can increase both the acquisition and transmission of human immunodeficiency virus (HIV).

The **incubation period** averages 1 week but ranges from 5 to 28 days.

DIAGNOSTIC TESTS[1]: Wet mount microscopy of vaginal discharge traditionally has been used as the preferred diagnostic test for TV in women, but its sensitivity is low (44%–68%) compared with culture. TV culture in Diamond media or other trichomonas-specific culture systems is a specific method of diagnosis in females with a sensitivity of 75% to 96% but has lower sensitivity in males. In women, vaginal secretions are the preferred specimen type for culture, because urine culture is less sensitive. In men, culture specimens require a urethral swab, urine sediment, and/or semen specimen.

In contrast, nucleic acid amplification tests (NAATs) are highly sensitive, detecting more TV infections than wet-mount microscopy among women. Sensitivities and specificities generally are in the 95% to 100% range. Some but not all are cleared for use in both women (vaginal, endocervical, urine) and men (urine). There also are several FDA-cleared rapid tests available to detect TV with improved sensitivities and specificities compared with wet mount. These rapid tests detect TV antigen or nucleic acid (via DNA hybridization) and result within 15 to 45 minutes. Sensitivity and specificity of antigen tests generally are in the 85% to 95% and 97% to 100% range, respectively, and for the nucleic acid rapid tests they generally are 90% to 98%. These rapid tests currently are not cleared for use in men.

When highly sensitive (eg, NAAT) testing on specimens is not readily available, a testing algorithm (eg, wet mount first, followed by NAAT if the result is negative) can improve diagnostic sensitivity in people with an initial negative result by wet mount. Some commercially available molecular-based diagnostic tests are able to simultaneously detect several different pathogens that cause vaginitis, typically *Candida*, TV, and bacterial vaginosis.

TREATMENT[1]: The recommended treatment for TV infection in women is metronidazole, 500 mg, orally, twice daily for 7 days. In men, the recommended treatment is metronidazole 2 g, orally in a single dose. An alternative regimen in both women and men is tinidazole 2 g, orally, in a single dose. Tinidazole is generally more expensive, reaches higher concentrations in serum and the genitourinary tract, has a longer half-life than metronidazole (12.5 hours versus 7.3 hours), and has fewer gastrointestinal adverse effects. Metronidazole gel does not reach therapeutic concentrations in the urethra and perivaginal glands. Because it is less efficacious than oral metronidazole, it is not recommended.

If treatment failure occurs in a woman after completing a treatment course of metronidazole, 500 mg, twice daily for 7 days, and she has been reexposed to an untreated partner, a repeat course of the same regimen is recommended. If there has been no

[1]Centers for Disease Control and Prevention. Sexually transmitted infections treatment guidelines, 2021. *MMWR Recomm Rep.* 2021; in press

reexposure, she should be treated with 2 g of metronidazole or tinidazole, once daily, for 7 days. If a man is still infected with TV after a single dose of 2 g of metronidazole and has been reexposed to an untreated partner, he should be given another single dose of 2 g of metronidazole. If he has not been reexposed, he should be given a course of metronidazole, 500 mg, twice daily for 7 days. For people who are experiencing persistent infection not attributable to reexposure, clinicians should request a kit from the CDC (**www.cdc.gov/std**) to perform drug resistance testing (**www.cdc.gov/laboratory/specimen-submission/detail.html?CDCTestCode=CDC-10239**). Treatment can then be determined on the basis of the test results.

Pregnancy. TV infection in pregnant females has been associated with adverse pregnancy outcomes, particularly premature rupture of membranes, preterm delivery, and delivery of an infant with low birth weight. Although metronidazole treatment produces parasitologic cure, trials have shown no significant difference in perinatal morbidity following metronidazole treatment. In symptomatic infected pregnant females, regardless of pregnancy stage, consideration should be given to treatment with metronidazole. Metronidazole crosses the placental barrier and its effects on the human fetal organogenesis are not known, but studies in animals have not shown evidence of harm to the fetus. Metronidazole is secreted in human milk. With maternal oral therapy, breastfed infants receive metronidazole in doses that are lower than those used to treat infections in infants. Although several reported case series found no evidence of adverse effects in infants exposed to metronidazole in human milk, some clinicians advise deferring breastfeeding for 12 to 24 hours following maternal treatment with metronidazole. Data from studies involving human subjects are limited regarding use of tinidazole in pregnancy; however, animal data suggest this drug poses moderate risk. Thus, tinidazole should be avoided in pregnant women, and breastfeeding should be deferred for 72 hours following a single 2-g dose of tinidazole.

Neonatal. For newborn infants, infection with TV acquired maternally is self-limited, and treatment generally is not recommended.

ISOLATION OF THE HOSPITALIZED PATIENT: Standard precautions are recommended.

CONTROL MEASURES: Measures to prevent STIs, particularly the consistent and correct use of condoms, are indicated. Patients should be instructed to avoid sexual activity until they and their sexual partners are treated and there is resolution of symptoms. Testing for other STIs including HIV, syphilis, gonorrhea, and chlamydia should be performed in people with TV.

Follow-up. Because of the high rate of trichomoniasis reinfection among females, retesting for TV is recommended for all sexually active females within 3 months following initial treatment regardless of whether they are symptomatic or believe their sex partners were treated. If retesting at 3 months is not possible, clinicians should retest at the next presentation for medical care within 12 months following initial treatment. Data are insufficient to support retesting males.

Routine Screening Tests.[1] Although routine TV screening of asymptomatic adolescents is not recommended, screening should be considered for people receiving care in

---

[1] American Academy of Pediatrics, Committee on Adolescence; Society for Adolescent Health and Medicine. Screening for nonviral sexually transmitted infections in adolescents and young adults. *Pediatrics*. 2014;134(1):e302-e311

high-prevalence settings (eg, STI clinics and correctional facilities) and for asymptomatic people at high risk of infection. Risk factors that may put females at higher risk of TV include new or multiple partners, exchanging sex for payment, illicit drug use, or an STI history. The CDC recommends screening for TV in all women with HIV infection at least annually and at their first prenatal visit.

Management of Sexual Partners. All people with a known exposure to TV infection should be treated routinely, regardless of a diagnostic test result. Expedited partner therapy might have a role in partner management for trichomoniasis and may be used in states where this approach is permissible.

Trichuriasis
(Whipworm Infection)

CLINICAL MANIFESTATIONS: Disease caused by the whipworm *Trichuris trichiura* generally is proportional to the intensity of the infection. Most infected children are asymptomatic, but those with heavy infestations can develop a colitis that mimics inflammatory bowel disease and can lead to anemia, chronic abdominal pain and diarrhea, physical growth restriction, and clubbing. A more serious condition is *Trichuris* dysentery syndrome, which is characterized by severe abdominal pain, tenesmus, bloody diarrhea, and occasionally rectal prolapse.

ETIOLOGY: *T trichiura*, the human whipworm, is the causative agent of trichuriasis. Adult worms are 30 to 50 mm long with a large, thread-like anterior end that embeds in the mucosa of the large intestine. Adult worms typically reside in the cecum and ascending colon; with heavy infection, worms may extend further into the colon and rectum.

EPIDEMIOLOGY: *T trichiura* is the second most prevalent soil-transmitted helminth in the world, with approximately 600 to 800 million people infected worldwide, most in tropical regions that lack proper sanitation infrastructure. It is frequently coendemic with *Ascaris* and hookworm species. Humans are the natural reservoir. Eggs excreted in moist soil require a range of 10 days to 4 weeks of incubation, depending on temperature, before they are infectious. Children become infected by accidental ingestion of infective eggs in food or on hands contaminated with soil. The disease is not communicable directly from person to person.

The time between infection and appearance of eggs in the stool (**incubation period**) is approximately 12 weeks; worms may live 1 to 3 years or more.

DIAGNOSTIC TESTS: Quantitative techniques like the Kato-Katz, McMaster, and FLOTAC methods are used typically in research settings to quantify fecal egg excretion as a measure of infection intensity. Direct microscopic visualization of eggs using stool concentrating techniques is recommended in routine clinical settings and screening at-risk populations such as immigrants, refugees, and international adoptees. Adult worms may be seen on proctoscopy or colonoscopy.

TREATMENT: Mebendazole and albendazole are first-line therapies in the treatment of trichuriasis; some recommend mebendazole over albendazole given its higher early cure rate (11% vs 2%). Ivermectin is an alternative treatment (see Drugs for Parasitic Infections, p 985). Longer duration of therapy (5 to 7 days) is recommended for heavy infections. Studies in children as young as 1 year suggest that albendazole can be administered safely to this population. The safety of ivermectin in children weighing less than 15 kg and in pregnant women has not been established.

The cure rate for any single drug is low; stool specimens should be reexamined approximately 2 weeks after therapy to document cure. Those who fail therapy should be retreated. In clinical studies, combination therapy with 2 anthelmintics (eg, albendazole plus ivermectin or albendazole plus oxantel pamoate) has been associated with higher cure rates than single-drug therapy with mebendazole and should be considered in patients who persistently test positive following single-agent treatment. Iron supplements should be prescribed in patients with severe or symptomatic anemia.

ISOLATION OF THE HOSPITALIZED PATIENT: Standard precautions are recommended; there is no direct person-to-person transmission.

CONTROL MEASURES: Proper disposal of contaminated feces is the most effective means of control for whipworm and other soil-transmitted helminths. Annual (20% or more baseline prevalence) or biannual (50% or more baseline prevalence) administration of single doses of benzimidazoles (albendazole or mebendazole) in communities with endemic infection is recommended by the World Health Organization for control of soil-transmitted helminth infections. Evidence of sustained benefit attributable to preventive chemotherapy programs is mixed.

African Trypanosomiasis
(African Sleeping Sickness)

CLINICAL MANIFESTATIONS: The clinical course of human African trypanosomiasis has 2 stages: the hemolymphatic stage, in which the parasite multiplies in subcutaneous tissues, lymph, and blood, and the neurologic stage, after the parasite crosses the blood-brain barrier and infects the central nervous system (CNS). The rapidity of disease progression and clinical manifestations vary with the infecting subspecies. With *Trypanosoma brucei gambiense* infection (West African sleeping sickness), initial symptoms may be mild and include intermittent fever, headaches, muscle and joint aches, and malaise. Pruritus, rash, hepatosplenomegaly, weight loss, and lymphadenopathy (mainly posterior cervical [Winterbottom sign] but also possible in axillary, inguinal, and epitrochlear areas) can occur. CNS involvement typically develops after 1 to 2 years with development of confusion, behavioral changes, cachexia, headache, sensory disturbances, poor coordination and movement disorders, seizures, tremors, speech disorders (eg, dysarthria, logorrhea), hallucinations, delusions, and daytime somnolence followed by nighttime insomnia. Trypanosome infiltration of endocrine organs (mainly thyroid and adrenal glands) and the heart may lead to disruptions of hormonal secretions and mild perimyocarditis.

Symptoms of *Trypanosoma brucei rhodesiense* infection (East African sleeping sickness) are similar to those of *T brucei gambiense* infection. An inoculation chancre may develop at the site of the tsetse fly bite. Initial manifestations include high fever, headaches, pruritis, lymphadenopathy (more often submandibular, axillary, and inguinal), rash, and muscle and joint aches. Thyroid dysfunction, adrenal insufficiency, and hypogonadism are found more frequently in *T brucei rhodesiense* infection and myopericarditis may be more severe.

Edema is reported more frequently in *T brucei rhodesiense* infection, and liver involvement with hepatomegaly is usually moderate, sometimes with ascites.

Clinical meningoencephalitis can develop after onset of the untreated systemic illness caused by both *Trypanosoma* subspecies. As the disease progresses, severe but less frequent complications can include renal failure requiring dialysis, multiorgan failure, disseminated intravascular coagulopathy, and coma. Both forms of African trypanosomiasis have high fatality rates; without treatment, infected patients usually die within 6 months after clinical onset of disease caused by *T brucei rhodesiense* and within 2 to 3 years from disease caused by *T brucei gambiense*.

ETIOLOGY: Human African trypanosomiasis (sleeping sickness) is caused by *Trypanosoma brucei* subspecies, which are protozoan parasites transmitted by blood-feeding tsetse flies. The west and central African (Gambian) form is caused by *T brucei gambiense*, and the east and southern African (Rhodesian) form is caused by *T brucei rhodesiense*. Both are extracellular protozoan hemoflagellates that live in blood and tissue of the human host.

EPIDEMIOLOGY: The number of cases of human African trypanosomiasis is decreasing, with 977 cases reported to the World Health Organization (WHO) in 2018, a greater than 90% reduction since 2000. Most of total reported cases worldwide (>95%) are caused by *T brucei gambiense*. There are occasional reported cases of African trypanosomiasis in the United States, typically in returning travelers who became infected with *T brucei rhodesiense* while on safari in East Africa. Transmission of *T brucei* subspecies is confined to an area in Africa between the latitudes of 14° north and 29° south, corresponding precisely with the distribution of the tsetse fly vector (*Glossina* species). In West and Central Africa, humans are the main reservoir of *T brucei gambiense*, although the parasite sometimes can be found in domestic animals, such as dogs and pigs. In East Africa, wild animals, such as antelope, bush buck, and hartebeest, constitute the major reservoirs for sporadic infections with *T brucei rhodesiense*, although cattle serve as reservoir hosts in local outbreaks. *T brucei* subspecies also can be transmitted congenitally. Accidental infections in laboratories as a result of pricks with contaminated needles have occurred.

The **incubation period** for *T brucei rhodesiense* infection ranges from 3 to 21 days, and for most cases is 5 to 14 days. For *T brucei gambiense* infection, the **incubation period** usually is longer but is not well defined; it is generally <1 month for travelers from countries without endemic disease.

DIAGNOSTIC TESTS: Diagnosis is made by identification of trypanosomes in specimens of blood, cerebrospinal fluid (CSF), or fluid aspirated from a chancre or lymph node, or by inoculation of susceptible laboratory animals (mice) with heparinized blood in the case of *T brucei rhodesiense* infection. Examination of CSF is critical to management, and all patients diagnosed in the United States should undergo lumbar puncture; concentration methods (such as the double-centrifugation technique) typically should be used. Concentration and Giemsa staining of the buffy coat layer of peripheral blood is easier for *T brucei rhodesiense*, because the density of organisms in circulating blood is higher than for *T brucei gambiense*. Wet preparations of the buffy coat and of concentrated CSF sediment should be examined for motile trypanosomes. *T brucei gambiense* is more likely to be found in lymph node aspirates than in blood. The most widely used criteria for stage determination to assess CNS involvement include identification of trypanosomes in CSF or a CSF white blood cell count of 6 or higher; elevated CSF neopterin and an increase in intrathecal immunoglobulin M also may suggest second-stage disease. Serologic testing for antibodies to *T brucei gambiense* is available outside the United States and typically is used only for screening purposes to help identify suspect cases; there is no comparable serologic screening test for *T brucei rhodesiense*.

TREATMENT: The choice of drug(s) used for treatment depends on the type and stage of African trypanosomiasis (**www.cdc.gov/parasites/sleepingsickness/health_professionals/index.html#tx**). When no evidence of CNS involvement is present, the drug of choice for the acute hemolymphatic stage of infection is pentamidine for *T brucei gambiense* infection and suramin for *T brucei rhodesiense* infection. For treatment of infection with CNS involvement, the drug of choice is eflornithine alone or in combination with nifurtimox, if available, for *T brucei gambiense* infection; for *T brucei rhodesiense* infection, the drug of choice is melarsoprol (eflornithine is not effective for CNS treatment of *T brucei rhodesiense* infection). Melarsoprol encephalopathy may be reduced in severity by concomitant administration of corticosteroids. Safety of eflornithine in children has not been established, and the drug is not approved by the US Food and Drug Administration (FDA) for use in pediatric patients. Suramin, eflornithine, and melarsoprol can be obtained from the Centers for Disease Control and Prevention (phone: [404] 718-4745). For specific dosing recommendations, see Drugs for Parasitic Infections (p 949). Consultation with a specialist familiar with the disease and its treatment is recommended. Patients who have had CNS involvement should undergo repeated CSF examinations every 6 months for 2 years because of the risk of relapse. The optimal approach to treatment of relapse is uncertain. The WHO has developed interim updated guidelines for the treatment of human African trypanosomiasis caused by *T brucei gambiense*. These guidelines allow for certain patients (older children and adults without clinically apparent severe disease) to forego a lumber puncture. They also describe recommendations for the use of oral fexinidazole, a nitroimidazole, to be given under directly observed therapy in select patients (**apps.who.int/iris/bitstream/handle/10665/326178/9789241550567-eng.pdf?ua=1**). Fexinidazole is not available in the United States.

ISOLATION OF THE HOSPITALIZED PATIENT: Standard precautions are recommended.

CONTROL MEASURES: Travelers to areas with endemic infection should avoid known foci of sleeping sickness and tsetse fly infestation and should minimize fly bites by wearing long-sleeved shirts and pants of medium-weight material in neutral colors. Newborn babies of infected mothers should be examined clinically and their blood should be tested for trypanosomes; breastfeeding may continue during treatment.

American Trypanosomiasis
(Chagas Disease)

CLINICAL MANIFESTATIONS: The acute phase of *Trypanosoma cruzi* infection (Chagas disease) lasts 2 to 3 months, followed by the chronic phase that, in the absence of successful antiparasitic treatment, is lifelong. The acute phase commonly is asymptomatic or characterized by mild, nonspecific symptoms. When disease is acquired by oral transmission, patients are more likely to exhibit symptoms of febrile illness. In the minority of patients with symptomatic acute-phase infection, fever, edema, cutaneous rash, myalgia, pallor, malaise, lymphadenopathy, and hepatosplenomegaly may develop. Meningoencephalitis and/or acute myocarditis are rare manifestations. Unilateral edema of the eyelids, known as the Romaña sign, may occur if the portal of entry is the conjunctiva. The edematous skin may be violaceous and associated with conjunctivitis and enlargement of the ipsilateral preauricular lymph node. In some patients, a red, indurated nodule known as a chagoma develops at the site of the original inoculation, usually on the face or arms.

Symptoms of acute Chagas disease can resolve without treatment within 3 months, and patients pass into the chronic phase of the infection. Most people with chronic *T cruzi* infection have no signs or symptoms and are said to have the indeterminate form of chronic Chagas disease. Serious progressive sequelae affecting the heart and/or gastrointestinal tract develop in 20% to 40% of cases years to decades after the initial infection (called determinate forms of chronic Chagas disease). Chagas cardiomyopathy is characterized by conduction system abnormalities, especially right bundle branch block and ventricular arrhythmias, and may progress to dilated cardiomyopathy and congestive heart failure. Patients with Chagas cardiomyopathy may die suddenly from ventricular arrhythmias, complete heart block, or embolic phenomena; death also may occur from intractable congestive heart failure. Less commonly, patients with chronic Chagas disease may develop digestive disease with dilatation of the colon and/or esophagus with swallowing difficulties accompanied by severe weight loss.

Congenital Chagas disease occurs in 1% to 10% of infants born to infected mothers and may be characterized by low birth weight, hepatosplenomegaly, and anemia; myocarditis and/or meningoencephalitis with seizures and tremors are rare. Most infants with congenital *T cruzi* infection have no signs or symptoms of disease.

Reactivation of chronic *T cruzi* infection with parasitemia may be life threatening and may occur in immunocompromised people, including people infected with human immunodeficiency virus and those who are immunosuppressed after transplantation.

ETIOLOGY: *Trypanosoma cruzi*, a protozoan hemoflagellate, causes American trypanosomiasis (Chagas disease). Chagas disease is named after the Brazilian physician Carlos Chagas, who discovered it in 1909.

EPIDEMIOLOGY: Parasites are transmitted in feces of infected triatomine insects (sometimes called "kissing bugs," a type of reduviid; local Spanish/Portuguese names include vinchuca, chinche picuda, or barbeiro). When found indoors, they tend to be found in pet areas, under bedding, and in areas of rodent infestation. The bugs defecate during or after taking a blood meal. The bitten person is inoculated through inadvertent rubbing of insect feces containing the parasite into the site of the bite through the harmed skin or mucous membranes of the eye. The parasite also can be transmitted congenitally, during solid organ transplantation, through blood transfusion, and by ingestion of food or drink contaminated by the vector's excreta. Accidental laboratory infections can result from handling parasite cultures or blood from infected people or laboratory animals, usually through needlestick injuries. Vectorborne transmission of the disease is limited to the Western Hemisphere, predominantly Mexico and Central and South America.

In the United States, 11 species of kissing bugs have been identified, and most have been found to be infected naturally with *T cruzi*. Triatomines have been found throughout the southern half of the United States, from California to Florida and as far north as Illinois and Pennsylvania. Significant numbers of wild animals are infected, including opossums, armadillos, wood rats, and raccoons. Animals usually acquire the parasite by eating infected triatomines. Rare vectorborne cases of Chagas disease have been noted in the United States. Most *T cruzi*-infected individuals in the United States are immigrants from areas of Latin America with endemic infection.

An estimated 300 000 individuals with *T cruzi* infection live in the United States. Assuming a 1% to 5% risk of congenital transmission, based on estimates of maternal infection, approximately 63 to 315 infants are born with Chagas disease in the United States every year. Several transfusion- and transplantation-associated cases have been documented in the United States.

The disease is an important cause of morbidity and death in Latin America, where an estimated 6 million people are infected, of whom approximately 20% to 40% either have or will develop cardiomyopathy and/or gastrointestinal tract disorders.

The **incubation period** for the acute phase of disease is 1 to 2 weeks or longer. Chronic manifestations do not appear for years to decades.

DIAGNOSTIC TESTS: During the acute phase of disease, the parasite is demonstrable in blood specimens by Giemsa staining after a concentration technique or in direct wet-mount or buffy coat preparations. Molecular detection techniques (available at the Centers for Disease Control and Prevention [CDC]) also have high sensitivity in the acute phase. The chronic phase of *T cruzi* infection is characterized by low-level intermittent parasitemia. Diagnosis in the chronic phase relies on serologic tests to demonstrate immunoglobulin (Ig) G antibodies against *T cruzi*. Serologic tests include indirect immunofluorescent and enzyme immunosorbent assays; no single serologic test is sufficiently sensitive or specific to confirm a diagnosis of chronic *T cruzi* infection. The Pan American Health Organization and the World Health Organization recommend that samples be tested using 2 diagnostic assays of different formats before treatment decisions are made.

The diagnosis of congenital Chagas disease can be made during the first 3 months of life by identification of motile trypomastigotes by direct microscopy of fresh anticoagulated blood specimens or by polymerase chain reaction (PCR) testing, which is a useful tool in infants and has higher sensitivity than serologic testing. If not diagnosed earlier, serologic testing should be performed after 9 months of age, once serum IgG measurements are expected to reflect infant response rather than maternal antibody. The CDC has developed algorithms for evaluation of Chagas disease in pregnant women and infants (**www.cdc.gov/parasites/chagas/health_professionals/congenital_chagas.html**). Some countries have congenital Chagas disease screening programs, which combine maternal screening with microscopic examination of cord blood from infants of seropositive mothers.

Low sensitivity of screening tests and low rates of follow-up likely lead to underestimation of infection rates. Diagnostic testing and consultation, including after positive screens for blood donors, are available from the CDC Division of Parasitic Diseases and Malaria (phone: [404] 718-4745; email: **parasites@cdc.gov**; CDC Emergency Operator [after business hours and on weekends]: [770] 488-7100).

TREATMENT: The only drugs with proven efficacy are benznidazole and nifurtimox (see Drugs for Parasitic Infections, p 950). Benznidazole was approved in 2017 by the US Food and Drug Administration (FDA) for use in children 2 to 12 years of age for the treatment of Chagas disease. Nifurtimox was approved by the FDA on August 7, 2020, for the treatment of Chagas disease in children from birth to less than 18 years of age.

Antitrypanosomal treatment is recommended for all cases of acute and congenital Chagas disease, reactivated infection attributable to immunosuppression, and chronic *T cruzi* infection in children younger than 18 years. Treatment of chronic *T cruzi* infection in adults without advanced cardiomyopathy generally is recommended.

Trypanocidal therapy with benznidazole in patients with established Chagas cardiomyopathy significantly reduces serum parasite detection by PCR but does not significantly reduce cardiac clinical deterioration or death through 5 years of follow-up and is, therefore, not recommended. Both drugs have significant adverse event profiles. The recommended treatment courses are at least 60 days. Careful consideration of potential risks and benefits in consultation with an expert in treatment of the disease or with CDC may be necessary, especially for patients in whom chronic infection is diagnosed and/or who do not fall under a clearly recommended treatment category.

ISOLATION OF THE HOSPITALIZED PATIENT: Standard precautions should be followed.

CONTROL MEASURES: Risk to travelers is low. Travelers to areas with endemic infection should avoid contact with triatomine bugs by avoiding habitation in buildings vulnerable to infestation, particularly those constructed of mud, palm thatch, or adobe brick. The use of insecticide-impregnated bed nets, tucked under the mattress on all sides, also may be beneficial. Camping or sleeping outdoors in areas with endemic transmission is not recommended. Travelers to regions with endemic infection also should avoid ingestion of unpasteurized juices, such as sugar cane, guava, or açaí palm fruit juice, which have been linked to oral transmission of Chagas disease. Diagnostic testing should be performed on members of households with an infected patient if they have had exposure to the vector similar to that of the patient. All children of women with *T cruzi* infection should be tested for Chagas disease.

Education about the mode of spread and methods of prevention is warranted in areas with endemic infection. Homes should be examined for the presence of the vectors, and if found, measures to eliminate the vector should be taken.

People with known *T cruzi* infection should not donate blood. Most US blood collection agencies started screening for *T cruzi* infection in 2007; final guidance to all blood collection agencies for appropriate use of serologic tests to screen blood donors for *T cruzi* infection was issued by the FDA in December 2010.

Tuberculosis

CLINICAL MANIFESTATIONS: Tuberculosis (TB) disease is caused by organisms of the *Mycobacterium tuberculosis* complex. Most infections caused by *M tuberculosis* complex in children and adolescents are asymptomatic. When pulmonary TB occurs, clinical manifestations most often appear 1 month to 2 years after infection and include fever, weight loss or poor weight gain, cough, night sweats, and chills. Chest radiographic findings rarely are specific for TB and include lymphadenopathy of the hilar, subcarinal, paratracheal, or mediastinal nodes; atelectasis or infiltrate of a segment or lobe; pleural effusion that can conceal small interstitial lesions; interstitial cavities; or miliary-pattern infiltrates. In selected instances, computed tomography or magnetic resonance imaging of the chest can clarify nonspecific or subtle radiographic findings. Although cavitation is a typical presentation of reactivated TB in adults (and sometimes in adolescents) who were infected as children, cavitation is uncommon in childhood TB. Necrosis and cavitation, however, can result from a progressive primary focus in very young or immunocompromised patients and in patients with lymphobronchial disease. Extrapulmonary manifestations include meningitis and granulomatous inflammation of the lymph nodes, bones, joints, skin, and middle ear and mastoid. Gastrointestinal tract TB can mimic inflammatory bowel disease. Renal TB is unusual in younger children but can occur in adolescents. In addition, chronic abdominal pain with peritonitis and intermittent partial intestinal obstruction can be present in disease caused by *Mycobacterium bovis*. Congenital TB can mimic neonatal sepsis, or the infant may come to medical attention in the first 90 days of life with bronchopneumonia and hepatosplenomegaly. Clinical findings in patients with drug-resistant TB disease are indistinguishable from manifestations in patients with drug-susceptible disease.

ETIOLOGY: The causative agent is *M tuberculosis* complex, a group of closely related acid-fast bacilli: *M tuberculosis, M bovis, Mycobacterium africanum,* and a few additional species infrequently associated with human infection. *M africanum* is rare in the United States, so clinical laboratories do not distinguish it routinely, and treatment recommendations are the same as for *M tuberculosis. M bovis* can be distinguished from *M tuberculosis* in reference laboratories, and although the spectrum of illness caused by *M bovis* is similar to that of *M tuberculosis,* the epidemiology, treatment, and prevention are different, as detailed later in the chapter.

Definitions:

- **Bacille Calmette-Guérin (BCG)** is a live attenuated vaccine strain of *M bovis.* BCG vaccine rarely is administered to children in the United States but is one of the most widely used vaccines in the world. An isolate of BCG can be distinguished from wild-type *M bovis* only in a reference laboratory.
- **Positive tuberculin skin test (TST).** A positive TST result (see Table 3.74) indicates possible infection with *M tuberculosis* complex. Tuberculin reactivity appears 2 to 10 weeks after initial infection; the median interval is 3 to 4 weeks (see "Tuberculin Skin Test," p 791). BCG immunization can produce a positive TST result (see Diagnostic Tests, Testing for *M tuberculosis* Infection).
- **Positive interferon-gamma release assay (IGRA).** A positive IGRA result indicates probable infection with *M tuberculosis* complex. IGRAs measure ex vivo interferon-gamma production from T lymphocytes in response to stimulation with antigens specific to *M tuberculosis* complex, including *M tuberculosis* and *M bovis.* The antigens used in IGRAs are not found in BCG or most pathogenic nontuberculous mycobacteria (eg, are not found in *Mycobacterium avium* complex, but are found in *Mycobacterium kansasii, Mycobacterium szulgai,* and *Mycobacterium marinum*).
- **TB infection (TBI)** is *M tuberculosis* complex infection in a person who has no symptoms or signs of disease and chest radiograph findings that are normal or reveal evidence of healed infection (eg, calcification in the lung, lymph nodes, or both) and a positive TST or IGRA result. Note that hilar adenopathy is evidence of TB disease, not TBI. TBI is also known as latent tuberculosis infection, or LTBI, but TBI is a more accurate term, because infection is not actually "latent" prior to manifesting as TB disease.

Table 3.74. Definitions of Positive Tuberculin Skin Test (TST) Results in Infants, Children, and Adolescents[a,b]

Induration 5 mm or greater

Children in close contact with known or suspected contagious people with tuberculosis (TB) disease

Children suspected to have TB disease:
- Findings on chest radiograph consistent with active or previous TB disease
- Clinical evidence of TB disease[c]

Children receiving immunosuppressive therapy[d] or with immunosuppressive conditions, including human immunodeficiency (HIV) infection

Induration 10 mm or greater

Children at increased risk of disseminated TB disease:
- Children younger than 4 y
- Children with other medical conditions, including Hodgkin disease, lymphoma, diabetes mellitus, chronic renal failure, or malnutrition (see Table 3.75)
- Children born in high-prevalence regions of the world
- Children with significant travel to high-prevalence regions of the world[e]
- Children frequently exposed to adults who are living with HIV, experiencing homelessness, or incarcerated, or to people who inject or use drugs or have alcohol use disorder

Induration 15 mm or greater

Children without any risk factors

[a] See www.cdc.gov/tb/publications/guidelines/pdf/ciw778.pdf.
[b] These definitions apply regardless of previous bacille Calmette-Guérin (BCG) immunization (see Testing for *M tuberculosis* Infection, p 791); erythema alone at TST site does not indicate a positive test result. Tests should be read at 48 to 72 hours after placement.
[c] Evidence by physical examination or laboratory assessment that would include tuberculosis in the working differential diagnosis (eg, meningitis).
[d] Including immunosuppressive doses of corticosteroids (see Corticosteroids, p 807) or tumor necrosis factor-alpha antagonists or blockers (see Biologic Response-Modifying Drugs Used to Decrease Inflammation, p 82) or immunosuppressive drugs used in transplant recipients (see Solid Organ Transplantation p 84).
[e] Some experts define significant travel as travel or residence in a country with an elevated TB rate for at least 1 month.

- **TB disease** is illness in a person with infection in whom symptoms, signs, or radiographic manifestations caused by *M tuberculosis* complex are apparent; disease can be pulmonary, extrapulmonary, or both.
- **Multidrug-resistant TB** (MDR TB) is defined as infection or disease caused by a strain of *M tuberculosis* complex that is resistant to at least isoniazid and rifampin.
- **Extensively drug-resistant TB** (XDR TB) is defined as infection or disease caused by a strain of *M tuberculosis* complex that is resistant to isoniazid and rifampin, at least 1 fluoroquinolone, and at least 1 of the following parenteral drugs: amikacin, kanamycin, or capreomycin.
- **Drug-resistant tuberculosis** (DR TB) is infection or disease caused by a strain of *M tuberculosis* that is resistant to any drug used to treat drug-susceptible tuberculosis and includes isoniazid-resistant TB, rifampin-resistant TB, MDR TB, and XDR TB.
- **Directly observed therapy** (DOT) is an intervention by which medications are taken by the patient while a health care professional or trained third party (not a relative or friend) observes and documents that the patient ingests each dose of medication and assesses for possible adverse drug effects.

Table 3.75. Tuberculin Skin Test (TST) and IGRA Recommendations for Infants, Children, and Adolescents[a]

Children for whom immediate TST or IGRA is indicated[b]:
- Contacts of people with confirmed or suspected contagious tuberculosis (contact investigation)
- Children with radiographic or clinical findings suggesting tuberculosis disease
- Children immigrating from countries with endemic infection (eg, Asia, Middle East, Africa, Latin America, countries of the former Soviet Union), including international adoptees
- Children with history of significant[c] travel to countries with endemic infection who have substantial contact with the resident population[d]

Children who should have annual TST or IGRA:
- Children living with HIV infection

Children at increased risk of progression of TBI to TB disease: Children with other medical conditions, including diabetes mellitus, chronic renal failure, malnutrition, congenital or acquired immunodeficiencies, and children receiving tumor necrosis factor (TNF) antagonists, deserve special consideration. Underlying immune deficiencies associated with these conditions theoretically would enhance the possibility for progression to severe disease. Initial histories of potential exposure to tuberculosis should be included for all these patients. If these histories or local epidemiologic factors suggest a possibility of exposure, immediate and periodic TST or IGRA should be considered. **A TST or IGRA should be performed before initiation of immunosuppressive therapy, including prolonged systemic corticosteroid administration, organ transplantation, use of TNF-alpha antagonists or blockers, or other immunosuppressive therapy in any child requiring these treatments.**

IGRA indicates interferon-gamma release assay; HIV, human immunodeficiency virus; TBI, *M tuberculosis* infection.
[a] Bacille Calmette-Guérin (BCG) immunization is not a contraindication to a TST; IGRA is generally preferred for BCG-vaccinated children.
[b] Beginning as early as 3 months of age for TST and 2 years of age for IGRAs, for TBI and disease.
[c] Some experts define significant travel as birth, travel, or residence in a country with an elevated tuberculosis rate for at least 1 month.
[d] If the child is well and has no history of exposure, the TST or IGRA should be delayed for 8 to 10 weeks after return.

- **Exposed person** is anyone who has had recent (less than 3 months) contact with another person with suspected or confirmed contagious TB disease (ie, pulmonary, laryngeal, tracheal, or endobronchial disease) and has a negative TST or IGRA result, normal physical examination findings, and chest radiographic findings that are normal or not compatible with TB. Some exposed people are or become infected (and subsequently develop a positive TST or IGRA result), and others do not become infected after exposure; the 2 groups cannot be distinguished initially.
- **Source person** is the person who has transmitted *M tuberculosis* complex to another person who subsequently develops TB infection or disease.

EPIDEMIOLOGY: Case rates of TB in all ages in North America are higher in urban, low-income areas and in nonwhite racial and ethnic groups; more than 87% of reported cases in the United States occur in Hispanic and nonwhite people. In recent years, more than 70% of all US cases have been in people born outside the United States. Almost 80% of childhood TB disease in the United States is associated with some form of foreign contact of the child, parent, or a household member. Specific groups with greater rates of TB include immigrants, international adoptees, refugees from or travelers to high-prevalence regions (eg, Asia, Africa, Latin America, and countries of the former Soviet Union), people experiencing homelessness or those with unstable housing, people who inject or use drugs, people with alcohol use disorders, and residents of certain correctional facilities and other congregate settings. Secondhand smoke exposure increases the risk of TB disease developing in infected children.

Infants and postpubertal adolescents are at increased risk of progression from TBI to TB disease. Other predictive factors for development of disease include recent infection (within the past 2 years); immunodeficiency, especially from human immunodeficiency virus (HIV) infection; use of immunosuppressive drugs, such as prolonged or high-dose corticosteroid therapy or chemotherapy and drugs for preventing transplant organ rejection (see Solid Organ Transplantation, p 84); and certain diseases or medical conditions, including Hodgkin disease, lymphoma, diabetes mellitus, chronic renal failure, and malnutrition. Patients with TBI who are being treated with tumor necrosis factor-alpha (TNF-alpha) antagonists or blocking agents (see Biologic Response-Modifying Drugs Used to Decrease Inflammation, p 82) are at higher risk of progressing to TB disease. A positive TST or IGRA result should be accepted as indicative of infection in individuals receiving or soon to receive these medications,[1,2] and the patient should be evaluated and treated accordingly.

A diagnosis of TBI or TB disease in a young child is a public health sentinel event often representing recent transmission. Transmission of *M tuberculosis* complex is airborne, with inhalation of droplet nuclei usually produced by an adult or adolescent with contagious pulmonary, endobronchial, or laryngeal TB disease. The probability of transmission increases if the index person has a positive acid-fast sputum smear, productive cough, or pulmonary cavities or is a household contact. Although contagiousness usually lasts only a few days to weeks after initiation of effective drug therapy, it can last longer if the source patient does not adhere to medical therapy or is infected with a drug-resistant strain. If the sputum smear becomes negative for acid-fast bacilli (AFB) on 3 separate specimens at least 8 hours apart after treatment is initiated and the patient has improved clinically, the treated patient can be considered at low risk of transmitting *M tuberculosis*. Children younger than 10 years with only adenopathy in the chest or small pulmonary lesions (paucibacillary disease) and nonproductive cough are not contagious. Rare cases of pulmonary disease in young children, particularly with lung cavities or presence of AFB on sputum microscopy, and infants with congenital TB can be contagious.

M bovis is transmitted most often by unpasteurized dairy products, but airborne human-to-human transmission can occur.

The **incubation period** from infection to development of a positive TST or IGRA result is 2 to 10 weeks. The risk of developing TB disease is highest during the 12 months after infection and remains high for 2 years; however, many years can elapse between initial *M tuberculosis* infection and subsequent disease.

---

[1]Starke JR; American Academy of Pediatrics, Committee on Infectious Diseases. Technical report: Interferon-γ release assays for diagnosis of tuberculosis infection and disease in children. *Pediatrics*. 2014;134(6):e1763-e1773 (Reaffirmed July 2018)

[2]Nolt D, Starke JR, American Academy of Pediatrics Committee on Infectious Diseases. Clinical report: Tuberculosis infection in children: testing and treatment. *Pediatrics*. 2021; in press

DIAGNOSTIC TESTS:

Testing for M tuberculosis Infection

Tuberculin Skin Test. The TST is one of two indirect methods for detecting *M tuberculosis* infection, the other method being IGRA (p 792). Both methods rely on specific lymphocyte sensitization after infection. Conditions that decrease lymphocyte numbers or function, including severe TB disease, can reduce the sensitivity of these tests. Tuberculin is a purified protein derivative (PPD) from heat-inactivated *M tuberculosis*. The routine (ie, Mantoux) technique of administering the skin test consists of 5 tuberculin units of solution (PPD; 0.1 mL) injected intradermally using a 27-gauge needle and a 1.0-mL syringe into the volar aspect of the forearm. Creation of a palpable wheal 6 to 10 mm in diameter is crucial to accurate testing.

Administration of TSTs and interpretation of results should be performed by trained and experienced health care personnel, because administration and interpretation by unskilled people or family members are unreliable. The standardized time for assessing the TST result is 48 to 72 hours after administration. The diameter of **induration** is measured transversely to the long axis of the forearm, and the result should be recorded in millimeters. Positive TST results, as defined in Table 3.74 (p 788), can persist for several weeks.

Lack of reaction to a TST does not exclude TBI or TB disease. Approximately 10% to 40% of immunocompetent children with culture-documented TB disease do not react initially to a TST. Host factors, such as young age, poor nutrition, immunosuppression, viral infections (especially measles, varicella, and influenza), recent *M tuberculosis* infection, and disseminated TB disease, can decrease TST reactivity.

Classification of TST results is based on epidemiologic and clinical factors. Interpretation of the size of induration (mm) as a positive result varies with the person's epidemiologic risk of TBI and likelihood of progression to TB disease. Current guidelines from the Centers for Disease Control and Prevention (CDC), the American Thoracic Society, and the American Academy of Pediatrics (AAP) recommend interpretation of TST findings on the basis of an individual's risk stratification and are summarized in Table 3.74 (p 788). Prompt clinical and radiographic evaluation of all children and adolescents with a positive TST result is recommended (see Assessing for *M tuberculosis* Disease, p 795).

BCG immunization, because of cross-reacting antigens present in the PPD, can result in induration of a TST. Distinguishing between a positive TST result caused by *M tuberculosis* complex infection and that caused by BCG requires a qualitative assessment of several factors. Reactivity of the TST (ie, mm of induration) attributable to prior BCG immunization may be absent or variable and depends on many factors, including age at BCG immunization, quality and strain of BCG vaccine used, number of doses of BCG vaccine received, nutritional and immunologic status of the vaccine recipient, frequency of TST administration, and time between immunization and TST. Evidence that increases the probability that a positive TST result is attributable to TBI includes known contact with a person with contagious TB, a family history of TB disease, more than 2 years since neonatal BCG immunization, and a TST reaction 15 mm or greater. Generally, interpretation of TST results in BCG recipients who are known contacts of a person with TB disease or who are at high risk of developing TB disease is the same as for people who have not received BCG vaccine.

Blood-Based Testing With IGRAs.[1,2,3] IGRAs measure ex vivo interferon-gamma production from T lymphocytes in response to stimulation with proprietary polypeptide mixtures that simulate antigens specific to *M tuberculosis* complex, which includes *M tuberculosis* and *M bovis.* The IGRA antigens used are not found in BCG or most pathogenic nontuberculous mycobacteria (eg, *M avium* complex) but are found in the nontuberculous mycobacteria *M kansasii, M szulgai,* and *M marinum.* Examples of IGRAs are the QuantiFERON-TB Gold Plus assay and the T-SPOT.TB assay. As with TSTs, IGRAs cannot distinguish between TBI and TB disease, and a negative result from these tests cannot exclude TBI or the possibility of TB disease in a patient with suggestive clinical findings. The sensitivity of IGRA tests is similar to that of TSTs for detecting infection in adults and children who have untreated culture-confirmed TB. In many clinical settings, the specificity of IGRAs is higher than that for the TST, because the antigens used are not found in BCG or most pathogenic nontuberculous mycobacteria. The published experience testing children with IGRAs demonstrates that IGRAs consistently perform well in children 2 years and older, and some data support their use for even younger children. The negative predictive value of IGRAs is not clear, but in general, if the IGRA result is negative and the TST result is positive in an asymptomatic, unexposed child, the diagnosis of TBI is unlikely, especially if the child has received a BCG vaccine. A negative result for either a TST or an IGRA should be considered especially unreliable in infants younger than 3 months.

TST Versus IGRA. For children younger than 2 years, TST is the preferred method for detection of *M tuberculosis* infection. For children 2 years and older, either TST or IGRA can be used, but in people previously vaccinated with BCG, IGRA is preferred to avoid a false-positive TST result caused by a previous vaccination with BCG. Low-grade, false-positive IGRA results occur in some individuals. A negative IGRA result cannot be interpreted universally as evidence of absence of infection. Indeterminate or invalid IGRA results have several possible causes that could be related to the patient, the assay itself, or its performance; these results do not exclude *M tuberculosis* infection and may necessitate repeat testing, possibly with a different test. Indeterminate/invalid IGRA results should not be used to make clinical decisions.

Specific recommendations for TST and IGRA use are provided in Table 3.75 (p 789) and Fig 3.16 (p 793).

Use of Tests for M tuberculosis *Infection.* The most reliable strategies for identifying TBI and preventing TB disease in children are based on identification of known risk factors for TBI and thorough and expedient contact tracing associated with cases of TB disease rather than nonselective testing of large populations. Contact tracing is an intervention that should be coordinated through the local public health department. Universal testing with TST or IGRA, including programs based at schools, child care centers, and camps that include populations at low risk, is discouraged because it results in either a low yield of positive results or a large proportion of false-positive results, leading to an inefficient use of health care resources. However, using a questionnaire to determine risk

[1]Centers for Disease Control and Prevention. Updated guidelines for using interferon gamma release assays to detect *Mycobacterium tuberculosis* infection—United States. *MMWR Recomm Rep.* 2010;59(RR-5):1-26

[2]Starke JR; American Academy of Pediatrics, Committee on Infectious Diseases. Technical report: Interferon-γ release assays for diagnosis of tuberculosis infection and disease in children. *Pediatrics.* 2014;134(6):e1763-e1773 (Reaffirmed July 2018)

[3]Nolt D, Starke JR, American Academy of Pediatrics Committee on Infectious Diseases. Clinical report: Tuberculosis infection in children: testing and treatment. *Pediatrics.* 2021; in press

FIG 3.16. GUIDANCE ON STRATEGY FOR USE OF TST AND IGRA FOR DIAGNOSIS OF TBI IN CHILDREN WITH AT LEAST 1 RISK FACTOR, BY AGE AND BCG IMMUNIZATION STATUS

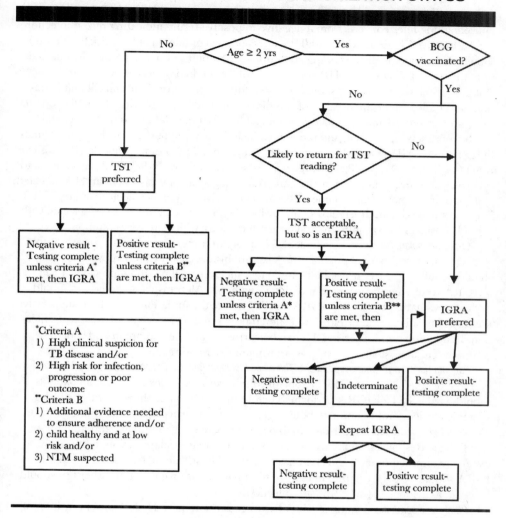

Table 3.76. Validated Questions for Determining Risk of TBI in Children in the United States

- Has a family member or contact had tuberculosis disease?
- Has a family member had a positive tuberculin skin test result?
- Was your child born in a high-risk country (countries other than the United States, Canada, Australia, New Zealand, or Western and North European countries)?
- Has your child traveled to a high-risk country? How much contact did your child have with the resident population?

TBI indicates *M tuberculosis* infection.

factors for TBI and identifying who should have a TST or IGRA performed can be useful (see Table 3.76). Risk assessment for TB should be performed at the first medical home encounter with a child and then annually if possible. Testing children for TBI and clinical evaluation for possible TB disease is indicated whenever a TST or IGRA result of a household member converts from a negative to positive result (indicating recent infection).

HIV Infection. Children living with HIV infection are considered at high risk for TB and should be tested annually beginning at 3 through 12 months of age if perinatally infected or at the time of diagnosis of HIV infection in older children or adolescents. Conversely, children who have TB disease should be tested for HIV infection. The clinical manifestations and radiographic appearance of TB disease in children living with HIV infection tend to be similar to those in immunocompetent children, but manifestations in these children can be more severe, unusual, and more often include extrapulmonary involvement of multiple organs. In HIV-infected patients, a TST induration of ≥5 mm is considered a positive result (see Table 3.74, p 788); however, a false-negative TST or IGRA result attributable to HIV-related immunosuppression also can occur. Diagnosing TB disease in an HIV-infected child with microbiological specimens is challenging, given the paucibacillary nature of TB in this population. Antituberculosis therapy in HIV-infected children must be selected with careful consideration of antiretroviral drug interactions, which are very common.

Organ Transplant Recipients. The risk of TB in organ transplant recipients is several-fold greater than in the general population. A careful history of previous exposure to TB should be taken from all transplant candidates, including details about previous TST or IGRA results and exposure to individuals with TB. All transplant candidates should undergo evaluation by TST or IGRA for TBI before the initiation of immunosuppressive therapy. A positive result of either test should be taken as evidence of *M tuberculosis* infection. In addition, donor-derived TB can be carried in an infected organ and should be considered as a possible cause of post-transplant fever and related symptoms.

Patients Receiving Immunosuppressive Therapies Including Biologic Response Modifiers. In addition to a detailed history of risk factors for *M tuberculosis* complex infection, all patients should have a TST or IGRA performed before the initiation of therapy with high-dose systemic corticosteroids, antimetabolite agents, and tumor necrosis factor antagonists or blockers (eg, adalimumab, certolizumab pegol, etanercept, golimumab, and infliximab; see Biologic Response-Modifying Drugs Used to Decrease Inflammation, p 82). Some experts recommend that if the child has at least 1 TB risk factor, both a TST and an IGRA should be performed to maximize sensitivity; a positive result of either test should be taken as evidence of *M tuberculosis* infection.

Other Considerations. Testing for TB at any age is not required before administration of live-virus vaccines. Live attenuated measles, mumps, and rubella vaccines temporarily can suppress tuberculin reactivity for at least 4 to 6 weeks, and data suggest a similar suppression with varicella and yellow fever vaccines. The effect of live attenuated influenza vaccines on TST reactivity and IGRA results is not known. If indicated, a TST can be performed or blood drawn for an IGRA at the same visit during which these vaccines are administered (ie, before substantial replication of the vaccine virus). The effects of live-virus vaccination on IGRA characteristics have not been determined; the same precautions as for TST should be followed.

Sensitivity to PPD tuberculin antigen persists for years in most instances, even after effective treatment. The durability of positive IGRA results has not been determined. Repeat testing with either TST or IGRA has no known clinical utility for assessing the effectiveness of treatment or for diagnosing newly acquired infection in patients who previously were infected with *M tuberculosis*.

Assessing for M tuberculosis Disease. Although both IGRA and TST provide evidence for infection with *M tuberculosis*, they cannot distinguish TBI from TB disease. Therefore, patients testing positive for *M tuberculosis* infection by IGRA or TST should be assessed for TB disease before initiating any therapeutic intervention. This assessment should include: (1) asking about symptoms of TB disease and exposure to TB patients; (2) physical examination for signs of TB disease; and (3) a chest radiograph. If radiographic signs of TB (eg, airspace opacities, pleural effusions, cavities, or changes on serial radiographs) are seen, then sputum or gastric aspirate sampling should then be performed, as described below. Most experts recommend that children younger than 12 months who are suspected of having pulmonary or extrapulmonary TB disease (eg, have a positive TST result <u>and</u> symptoms, physical examination signs, or chest radiograph abnormalities consistent with TB disease), with or without neurologic symptoms, should have a lumbar puncture to evaluate for tuberculous meningitis. Children 12 months and older with TB disease require a lumbar puncture only if they have neurologic signs or symptoms.

Laboratory Confirmation of M tuberculosis. Laboratory isolation of *M tuberculosis* complex by culture from a specimen of sputum, gastric aspirate, bronchial washing, pleural fluid, cerebrospinal fluid (CSF), urine, or other body fluid or a tissue biopsy specimen confirms the diagnosis of TB disease. Positive results from a rapid molecular method (eg, nucleic acid amplification tests [NAATs]) increasingly are also considered confirmatory, but culture isolation of the organism still is required after diagnosis with molecular methods for phenotypical susceptibility testing, genotyping, rapid molecular detection of drug-resistance genes, and species identification with the *M tuberculosis* complex. Children older than 2 years and adolescents frequently produce sputum spontaneously or by induction with aerosolized hypertonic saline. Studies have demonstrated successful collection of induced sputum from infants with pulmonary TB, but this requires special expertise. The best specimen for diagnosis of pulmonary TB in any child or adolescent in whom cough is absent or nonproductive and sputum cannot be induced is an early-morning gastric aspirate, which should be obtained with a nasogastric tube on awakening the child and before ambulation or feeding. Aspirates collected on 3 separate mornings should be submitted for AFB staining and culture.

Fluorescent staining methods for specimen smears are more sensitive than the traditional Kinyoun acid fast smears and are preferred. The overall diagnostic yield of microscopy of gastric aspirates and induced sputum is low in children with clinically suspected pulmonary TB, and false-positive stain results caused by the presence of nontuberculous mycobacteria occur rarely. Histologic examination for and demonstration of AFB and granulomas in biopsy specimens from lymph node, pleura, mesentery, liver, bone marrow, or other tissues can be useful, but *M tuberculosis* complex organisms cannot be distinguished reliably from other mycobacteria in stained specimens; the CDC offers molecular species identification of mycobacteria including *M tuberculosis* in fixed tissues. Regardless of results of the AFB smears, each specimen should be cultured.

Because *M tuberculosis* complex organisms are slow growing, detection of these organisms may take as long as 10 weeks using solid media; use of liquid media and continuous monitoring systems allows detection within 1 to 6 weeks and usually within 3 weeks. Even with optimal culture techniques, *M tuberculosis* complex organisms are isolated from fewer than 75% of infants and 50% of children with pulmonary TB diagnosed by clinical criteria; the culture yields for most forms of extrapulmonary TB are even lower. Current methods for species identification of isolates from culture include molecular probes, NAATs, genetic sequencing, mass spectrometry, and biochemical tests. *M bovis* usually is suspected because of isolated pyrazinamide resistance, which is characteristic of almost all *M bovis* isolates, but further biochemical or molecular testing is required to distinguish *M bovis* from *M tuberculosis*.

For a child with clinically suspected TB disease, finding the culture-positive source person supports the child's presumptive diagnosis and provides the likely drug susceptibility of the child's organism. Culture material should be collected from children with evidence of TB disease, especially when (1) an isolate from a source person is not available; (2) the presumed source person has drug-resistant TB; (3) the child is immunocompromised or ill enough to require hospital admission; or (4) the child has extrapulmonary disease. Traditional methods of determining drug susceptibility require bacterial isolation. Several new molecular methods of rapidly determining drug resistance directly from clinical samples now are available.

NAATs cleared by the FDA are available for rapid detection of *M tuberculosis* complex organisms from smear-positive and smear-negative sputum specimens, and other laboratory-developed tests for rapid molecular detection are available locally. Some tests have been validated for specimens other than sputum: expert consultation is recommended for test availability and interpretation of results. Molecular methods that find *M tuberculosis* genetic markers associated with drug resistance are supplementing the culture-based (ie, phenotypic) methods for drug susceptibility testing as they decrease the time to detection of drug resistance from weeks to hours, and in some instances the results could be more reliable for patient care decisions. Some of the methods are verified for direct testing of patient specimens. However, culture-based results are still required for confirming susceptibility to each drug when drug resistance genes are not detected, because the absence of resistance genes is not entirely predictive of susceptibility. The molecular methods are constantly evolving, and expert consultation should be sought for a testing strategy when drug resistance is suspected.

TREATMENT (SEE TABLE 3.77)[1]:

Specific Drugs. Regimen and dosage recommendations and the more commonly reported adverse reactions of first-line antituberculosis drugs are summarized in Tables 3.77, 3.78, and 3.79 (p 803). The less commonly used (eg, "second-line") antituberculosis drugs, their doses, and adverse effects are listed in Table 3.80 (p 805). Some of these drugs have less effectiveness and greater toxicity; they should be used only in consultation with a specialist familiar with treatment of childhood TB. For treatment of TB disease, drugs always must be used in recommended combination and dosage to minimize emergence of drug-resistant strains. Use of nonstandard regimens for any reason (eg, drug allergy, drug resistance) should be undertaken only by an expert in treating TB.

Occasionally, a patient cannot tolerate oral medications. Isoniazid, rifampin, amikacin and related drugs, linezolid, and fluoroquinolones can be administered parenterally.

Treatment Regimens for Tuberculosis Infection (TBI). Several regimens are recommended, depending on the circumstances for individual patients. Dosages and intervals are provided in Table 3.78.

---

[1]Nolt D, Starke JR, American Academy of Pediatrics Committee on Infectious Diseases. Clinical report: Tuberculosis infection in children: testing and treatment. *Pediatrics*. 2021; in press

Table 3.77. Recommended Usual Treatment Regimens for Drug-Susceptible TB Infection and TB Disease in Infants, Children, and Adolescents

Infection or Disease Category	Regimen	Remarks
M tuberculosis infection (positive TST or IGRA result, no disease)[a]		
• Isoniazid susceptible	12 weeks of isoniazid plus rifapentine, once a week	Most experts consider isoniazid-rifapentine to be the preferred regimen for treatment of TBI for children 2 years and older, and some experts prefer isoniazid-rifapentine therapy for TBI in children 2 years and older.
	OR	
	4 mo of rifampin, once a day	Continuous daily therapy is required. Intermittent therapy even by DOT is not recommended.
	OR	
	3 mo of isoniazid plus rifampin, once a day	To be considered if above 2 regimens are not feasible.
	OR	
	6 or 9 mo of isoniazid, once a day	If daily therapy is not possible, DOT twice a week can be used; medication doses differ with daily and twice-weekly regimens.
• Isoniazid resistant	4 mo of rifampin, once a day	Continuous daily therapy is required. Intermittent therapy even by DOT is not recommended.
• Isoniazid-rifampin resistant	Consult a tuberculosis specialist	Moxifloxacin or levofloxacin with or without ethambutol or pyrazinamide are most commonly given.

Table 3.77. Recommended Usual Treatment Regimens for Drug-Susceptible TB Infection and TB Disease in Infants, Children, and Adolescents, continued

Infection or Disease Category	Regimen	Remarks
Pulmonary and extrapulmonary disease (except meningitis)[b]	2 mo of rifampin, isoniazid, pyrazinamide, and ethambutol (RIPE) daily or 3 times per week, followed by 4 mo of isoniazid and rifampin[c] by DOT[d] for drug-susceptible *M tuberculosis*	Some experts recommend a 3-drug initial regimen (isoniazid, rifampin, and pyrazinamide) if the risk of drug resistance is low. DOT is highly desirable. If hilar adenopathy only and the risk of drug resistance is low, a 6-mo course of isoniazid and rifampin is sufficient. DOT is required for intermittent regimens. Drugs can be given daily or 3 times/wk; 2 times/wk is acceptable if DOT resources are scarce.
Meningitis	At least 9 mo of isoniazid and rifampin for *Mycobacterium bovis* susceptible to these drugs	See text for information on corticosteroids.
	2 mo of isoniazid, rifampin, pyrazinamide, and ethionamide, if possible, or an aminoglycoside[e] or capreomycin, once a day[f,g]; followed by 4–10 mo of isoniazid and rifampin, once a day or 3 times per week (9–12 mo total) for drug-susceptible *M tuberculosis*	
	At least 12 mo of therapy without pyrazinamide for *M bovis* susceptible to isoniazid and rifampin	

TST indicates tuberculin skin test; IGRA, interferon-gamma release assay; DOT, directly observed therapy.

[a] See text for comments and additional acceptable/alternative regimens.

[b] Duration of therapy may be longer for people living with HIV infection, and additional drugs and dosing intervals may be indicated (see Tuberculosis Disease and HIV Infection, p 808).

[c] Medications should be administered daily for the first 2 weeks to 2 months of treatment and then can be administered daily or 3 times per week by DOT; twice weekly is acceptable if resources for DOT are limited. Intermittent therapy is not recommended for people living with HIV infection.

[d] If initial chest radiograph shows pulmonary cavities and/or sputum culture after 2 months of therapy remains positive, the continuation phase is extended to 7 months, for a total treatment duration of 9 months.

[e] Parenteral streptomycin, kanamycin, or amikacin.

[f] Many experts add a fluoroquinolone to this initial regimen.

[g] When susceptibility to first-line drugs is established, the ethionamide, aminoglycoside (or capreomycin), and/or fluoroquinolone can be discontinued.

Table 3.78. Regimens and Dosages Used in Pediatric Patients With TB Infection (TBI)

Agent(s)	Dose and Age Group	Administration	Duration (months)	Age Restriction	Comments
INH + Rifapentine (3HP)	**Age ≥12 y** INH: 15 mg/kg, rounded up to nearest 50 or 100 mg (max 900 mg) Rifapentine (by weight): 10–14 kg: 300 mg 14.1–25 kg: 450 mg 25.1–32 kg: 600 mg 32.1–49.9 kg: 750 mg ≥50.0 kg: 900 mg **Age 2–11 y** INH: 25 mg/kg, rounded up to nearest 50 or 100 mg (max 900 mg) Rifapentine: see above	Weekly (SAT or DOT)	3	Not for children <2 y	Take with food, containing fat if possible; pyridoxine for selected patients[a]
Rifampin (4R)	**Adult:** 10 mg/kg (max 600 mg) **Child:** 15–20 mg/kg (max 600 mg)	Daily (SAT)	4	None	Drug-drug interactions

Table 3.78. Regimens and Dosages Used in Pediatric Patients With TB Infection (TBI), continued

Agent(s)	Dose and Age Group	Administration	Duration (months)	Age Restriction	Comments
INH + Rifampin	Same doses as when drugs are used individually	Daily (SAT)	3	None	Not considered unless 3HP or 4R are not feasible
INH	**Adult:** 5 mg/kg (max dose 300 mg) **Child:** 10–15 mg/kg (max 300 mg)	Daily (SAT)	6 or 9	None	Seizures with overdose; pyridoxine for selected patients[a]
	Adult: 15 mg/kg (max dose 900 mg) **Child:** 20–30 mg/kg (max 900 mg)	Twice weekly (DOT)			

Table adapted from Nolt D, Starke JR; American Academy of Pediatrics, Committee on Infectious Diseases. Clinical report: Tuberculosis infection in children: testing and treatment. *Pediatrics*. 2021; in press.

INH, isoniazid; DOT, directly observed therapy; SAT, self-administrated therapy.

[a]Exclusively breastfed infants and for children and adolescents on meat- and milk-deficient diets; children with nutritional deficiencies, including all symptomatic children living with HIV infection; and pregnant adolescents and women.

Isoniazid-Rifapentine Therapy for TBI.[1] A 12-week course, comprising a once-weekly dose of isoniazid and rifapentine, is a regimen that is safe, well tolerated, and at least as efficacious as 9 months of isoniazid taken daily. Extensive published and unpublished experience with this combination in children has demonstrated similar results. Most experts consider isoniazid-rifapentine to be the preferred regimen for treatment of TBI for children 2 years and older, although the pill burden in younger children is substantial and sometimes not well tolerated. Isoniazid-rifapentine should not be used in children younger than 2 years because of a lack of pharmacokinetic data in this age group.

Rifampin Therapy for TBI. A 4-month course of rifampin given daily also is an acceptable regimen for the treatment of TBI. It is the preferred regimen when isoniazid resistance is likely, as judged from the exposure history. The data supporting the efficacy and safety of this regimen are from randomized controlled trials and case control studies in adults and several studies that included children. The regimen has been as effective as 9 months of daily isoniazid, the rates of adverse effects have been low, and the completion rates of therapy have been much higher than for 9 months of isoniazid. There has been extensive published and unpublished experience with this regimen in children demonstrating safety, tolerability, and high rates of completion.

Isoniazid-Rifampin Therapy for TBI. An additional possible regimen for treatment of TBI is 3 months of daily isoniazid and rifampin, with no age restriction on it use. This regimen is quite similar in principle to the isoniazid-rifapentine option; however, the medications are given daily because of the relatively short half-life of rifampin compared with rifapentine. Efficacy and rates of completion of are comparable or better when compared with isoniazid monotherapy.

Isoniazid Therapy for TBI. Isoniazid monotherapy has been the most widely recommended and utilized treatment for pediatric TBI. The efficacy of isoniazid monotherapy reaches 98% against development of TB disease, but many studies have shown that the long duration of isoniazid monotherapy results in poor adherence and low completion rates. The World Health Organization (WHO) recommends a treatment duration of 6 months to provide high coverage of the population in countries with a high disease burden. A 9-month regimen gives an additional 20% to 30% increase in efficacy. The CDC and National TB Controllers Association recommend 6-month or 9-month durations of isoniazid monotherapy, if shorter-course rifamycin-based regimens cannot be used. Although isoniazid is readily available, the long duration of isoniazid monotherapy results in poor adherence and low completion rates. This option may be very unattractive to patients and families. Many TB care providers and clinics use this regimen only when a rifamycin-containing regimen cannot be used because of drug interactions.

For infants, children, and adolescents, including those living with HIV infection or other immunocompromising conditions, the recommended duration of isoniazid therapy in the United States is 9 months. The WHO recommends a 6-month course of isoniazid, but modeling studies have shown that the efficacy of 6 months of treatment is approximately 30% less than that of a 9-month course. Although there have been no formal trials of interrupted 9-month courses, many experts in North America accept 6 months of uninterrupted treatment as adequate. When adherence with daily therapy with isoniazid cannot be ensured, twice-a-week DOT on the basis of expert opinion and published

---

[1]Sterling TR, Njie G, Zenner D, et al. Guidelines for the treatment of latent tuberculosis infection: recommendations from the National Tuberculosis Controllers Association and CDC, 2020. *MMWR Recomm Rep.* 2020;69(1):1-11

experience can be considered, but each dose should be observed. Determination of serum aminotransferase concentrations before or during therapy is not indicated except in patients with underlying liver or biliary disease, during pregnancy or the first 12 weeks postpartum, with concurrent use of other potentially hepatotoxic drugs (eg, anticonvulsant or HIV agents), or if there is clinical concern of possible hepatotoxicity.

Therapy for TBI and Contacts of Patients With Isoniazid-Resistant M tuberculosis *and When Isoniazid Cannot Be Administered.* The incidence of isoniazid resistance among *M tuberculosis* complex isolates from US patients in 2017 was approximately 9%. Risk factors for drug resistance are listed in Table 3.81. If the source case is found to have isoniazid-resistant, rifampin-susceptible organisms, isoniazid should be discontinued and rifampin should be administered daily to contacts with TBI for a total course of 4 months. Optimal therapy for children with TBI caused by organisms with resistance to isoniazid and rifampin (ie, multidrug resistance) is not known. In these circumstances, a fluoroquinolone alone and multidrug regimens have been used in observational studies, but the safety and the efficacy of these empiric regimens have not been assessed in controlled clinical trials. Drugs to consider include levofloxacin or moxifloxacin, with or without the addition of pyrazinamide or ethambutol, depending on susceptibility of the isolate. Consultation with a TB specialist is indicated.

Treatment of Tuberculosis Disease. The goal of treatment is to achieve killing of replicating organisms in the tuberculous lesion in the shortest possible time. Achievement of this goal minimizes the possibility of development of resistant organisms. The major problem limiting successful treatment is poor adherence to prescribed treatment regimens. The use of DOT decreases the rates of relapse, treatment failures, and drug resistance; therefore, DOT is strongly recommended for treatment of all children and adolescents with TB disease in the United States. Intervals and dosages are provided in Tables 3.77, 3.79, and 3.80.

Therapy for Presumed or Known Drug-Susceptible Pulmonary Tuberculosis. A 6-month, 4-drug regimen consisting initially of rifampin, isoniazid, pyrazinamide, and ethambutol (RIPE) for the first 2 months and isoniazid and rifampin for the remaining 4 months is recommended for treatment of pulmonary disease, pulmonary disease with hilar adenopathy, and hilar adenopathy disease in infants, children, and adolescents when resistance to isoniazid, rifampin, or pyrazinamide is not suspected on the basis of exposure history or when favorable drug-susceptibility results are available from the patient or the likely source case. If the chest radiograph shows one or more pulmonary cavities and/or the sputum culture result remains positive after 2 months of therapy, the duration of therapy should be extended to at least 9 months. Some experts administer 3 drugs (isoniazid, rifampin, and pyrazinamide) as the initial regimen if a presumed source person has been identified with known pan-susceptible *M tuberculosis* or has no risk factors for drug-resistant *M tuberculosis*. For children with only hilar adenopathy in whom drug resistance is not a consideration, a 6-month regimen of only isoniazid and rifampin is considered adequate by some experts.

In the 6-month regimen with 4-drug RIPE therapy, drugs are administered once a day for at least the first 2 weeks by DOT at least 5 days per week. An alternative to daily dosing between 2 weeks and 2 months of treatment is to administer these drugs 3 times a week by DOT (except in people living with HIV, in whom intermittent dosing is not recommended). After the initial 2-month period, a DOT regimen of isoniazid and rifampin usually is given daily or 3 times a week, although 2 times a week is acceptable (see Table 3.79, p 803, for doses). Several alternative regimens with differing durations of daily therapy and total therapy have been used successfully in adults and children. These alternative regimens should be prescribed and managed by a specialist in pediatric TB.

Table 3.79. Drugs for Treatment of Drug-Susceptible TB Disease in Infants, Children, and Adolescents

Drugs	Dosage Forms	Daily Dosage (Range), mg/kg	Three Times per Week Dosage, mg/kg per Dose	Maximum Dose	Most Common Adverse Reactions
Ethambutol	Tablets 100 mg 400 mg	20 (15–25)	50	Daily, 1 g Twice a week, 2.5 g	Optic neuritis (usually reversible), decreased red-green color discrimination, gastrointestinal tract disturbances, hypersensitivity
Isoniazid[a]	Scored tablets 100 mg 300 mg	10 (10–15)[b]	20–30	Daily, 300 mg Twice a week, 900 mg	Mild hepatic enzyme elevation, hepatitis,[b] peripheral neuritis, hypersensitivity
Pyrazinamide[a]	Scored tablets 500 mg	35 (30–40)	50	2 g	Hepatotoxic effects, hyperuricemia, arthralgia, gastrointestinal tract upset, pruritus, rash
Rifampin[a]	Capsules 150 mg 300 mg Syrup formulated capsules	15–20[c]	15–20[c]	600 mg	Orange discoloration of secretions or urine, staining of contact lenses, vomiting, hepatitis, influenza-like reaction, thrombocytopenia, pruritus; oral contraceptives may be ineffective

[a]Rifamate is a capsule containing 150 mg of isoniazid and 300 mg of rifampin. Two capsules provide the usual adult (greater than 50 kg) daily doses of each drug. Rifater, in the United States, is a capsule containing 50 mg of isoniazid, 120 mg of rifampin, and 300 mg of pyrazinamide. Isoniazid and rifampin also are available for parenteral administration.

[b]When isoniazid in a dosage exceeding 10 mg/kg/day is used in combination with rifampin, the incidence of hepatotoxic effects may be increased.

[c]Many experts recommend using a daily rifampin dose of 20–30 mg/kg/day for infants and toddlers and for serious forms of tuberculosis, such as meningitis and disseminated disease.

Therapy for Drug-Resistant Pulmonary Tuberculosis Disease. Consultation with an expert in treating drug-resistant tuberculosis is strongly recommended when drug resistant-TB is suspected or occurs. Drug resistance is more common in certain groups (Table 3.81). When resistance to drugs other than isoniazid is likely (see Table 3.81), initial therapy should be adjusted by adding at least 2 drugs to match the presumed drug susceptibility pattern until drug susceptibility results are available. If an isolate from the pediatric case under treatment is not available, drug susceptibilities can be inferred by the drug susceptibility pattern of isolates from the presumed source person. Data for guiding drug selection may not be available for foreign-born children or in circumstances of international travel or adoption. If this information is not available, a 4- or 5-drug initial regimen should be strongly considered with close monitoring for clinical response.

Most cases of pulmonary TB in children that are caused by an isoniazid-resistant but rifampin- and pyrazinamide-susceptible strain of *M tuberculosis* complex can be treated with a 6-month regimen of rifampin, pyrazinamide, and ethambutol. If disease is extensive, many experts add a fluoroquinolone to this regimen. For cases of MDR TB disease, the treatment regimen needed for cure should include at least 4 or 5 antituberculosis drugs to which the organism is susceptible. Bedaquiline is approved by the FDA as part of combination therapy in the treatment for adults with multidrug-resistant pulmonary TB for whom an effective regimen could not be instituted; there currently are few safety, tolerability, efficacy, or pharmacokinetic data on use of bedaquiline in children, but many experts recommend its use in children 12 years and older.[1] The profile for delamanid is similar, but this drug is available under a compassionate use protocol only. Therapy for MDR TB is administered for 12 to 24 months from the time of culture conversion to negativity. An injectable drug initially administered 5 days per week, such as amikacin, kanamycin, or capreomycin, often is used for the first 4 to 6 months of treatment, as tolerated; some experts, however, are no longer recommending injectable drugs. Regimens in which drugs are administered intermittently are not recommended for drug-resistant disease (with the exception of aminoglycosides and capreomycin, which are typically intermittent to limit toxicity); daily DOT is critical to prevent emergence of additional resistance. An expert in DR TB should be consulted for all drug-resistant cases.

Extrapulmonary Tuberculosis Disease. In general, extrapulmonary TB—with the exception of meningitis—can be treated with the same regimens as used for pulmonary TB. For suspected drug-susceptible tuberculous meningitis, daily treatment with isoniazid, rifampin, pyrazinamide, and ethionamide, if possible, or an aminoglycoside (parenteral streptomycin, kanamycin, amikacin) or capreomycin should be initiated. Many experts add a fluoroquinolone to this initial regimen. When used to treat CNS TB, rifampin should be given at a dose of 20 to 30 mg/kg/day to ensure adequate CNS penetration (see Table 3.79, footnote c). When susceptibility to first-line drugs is established, the ethionamide, aminoglycoside (or capreomycin), and/or fluoroquinolone can be discontinued. Pyrazinamide is given for a total of 2 months, and isoniazid and rifampin are given for a total of 6 to 12 months. Isoniazid and rifampin can be given daily or 3 times per week after the first 2 months of treatment if the child has responded well.

Evaluation and Monitoring of Therapy in Children and Adolescents. Careful monthly monitoring of clinical and bacteriologic responses to therapy is important. With DOT, clinical

---

[1]Centers for Disease Control and Prevention. Provisional CDC guidelines for the use and safety monitoring of bedaquiline fumarate (Sirturo) for the treatment of multidrug-resistant tuberculosis. *MMWR Recomm Rep.* 2013;62(RR-9):1-11

Table 3.80. Drugs for Treatment of Drug-Resistant TB Disease in Infants, Children, and Adolescents[a]

Drugs	Dosage, Forms	Daily Dosage	Maximum Dose	Adverse Reactions
Amikacin[b,c]	Vials, 500 mg and 1 g	15–30 mg/kg (intravenous or intramuscular administration)	1 g	Auditory and vestibular toxic effects, nephrotoxic effects
Bedaquiline[d]	Tablets, 100 mg	Children ≥12 y: 400 mg daily for first 2 wk, then 200 mg 3 times/wk with 48 h between doses for wk 3–24	400 mg	Arthralgia, nausea, abdominal pain, headache; can prolong QTc interval, can elevate hepatic enzymes
Capreomycin[c]	Vials, 1 g	15–30 mg/kg (intramuscular administration)	1 g	Auditory and vestibular toxicity and nephrotoxic effects
Cycloserine	Capsules, 250 mg	10–20 mg/kg, given in 2 divided doses	1 g	Psychosis, personality changes, seizures, rash
Ethionamide	Tablets, 250 mg	15–20 mg/kg, given in 2–3 divided doses	1 g	Gastrointestinal tract disturbances, hepatotoxic effects, hypersensitivity reactions, hypothyroidism
Kanamycin[b,c]	Vials 75 mg/2 mL 500 mg/2 mL 1 g/3 mL	15–30 mg/kg (intramuscular or intravenous administration)	1 g	Auditory and vestibular toxic effects, nephrotoxic effects
Levofloxacin[b,e]	Tablets 250 mg 500 mg 750 mg Oral solution 25 mg/mL Vials 5 mg/mL 25 mg/mL	Adults: 750–1000 mg (once daily) Children: 15–20 mg/kg	1 g	Hypersensitivity reactions; theoretical effect on growing cartilage, tendonitis, gastrointestinal tract disturbances, cardiac disturbances, peripheral neuropathy, rash, headache, restlessness, confusion; can prolong QTc interval

Table 3.80. Drugs for Treatment of Drug-Resistant TB Disease in Infants, Children, and Adolescents,[a] continued

Drugs	Dosage, Forms	Daily Dosage	Maximum Dose	Adverse Reactions
Linezolid[b,f]	Tablet 400 mg Intravenous 400 mg/250 mL	Adults: 600 mg (once daily) Children <10 y: 10 mg/kg/dose, every 12 h Children ≥10 y: 10 mg/kg/dose daily	600 mg	Used for treatment of multidrug-resistant TB; adverse events include bone marrow suppression
Moxifloxacin[b,e]	Tablet 400 mg Intravenous 400 mg/250 mL	Adults: 400 mg (once daily) Children: 10 mg/kg (once daily)	400 mg	Hypersensitivity reactions; theoretical effect on growing cartilage; tendonitis, gastrointestinal tract disturbances, cardiac disturbances, peripheral neuropathy, rash, headache, restlessness, confusion; can prolong QTc interval
Para-aminosalicylic acid (PAS)	Packets, 3 g	200–300 mg/kg (2–4 times a day)	10 g	Gastrointestinal tract disturbances, hypersensitivity, hepatotoxic effects, hypothyroidism
Streptomycin[c]	Vials 1 g 4 g	20–40 mg/kg (intramuscular administration)	1 g	Auditory and vestibular toxic effects, nephrotoxic effects and rash

[a] These drugs should be used in consultation with a specialist in TB.

[b] These drugs do not have an indication from the US Food and Drug Administration (FDA) for treatment of TB.

[c] Dose adjustment in renal insufficiency; capreomycin and kanamycin are not recommended for longer individualized regimens of multidrug-resistant TB (**https://apps.who.int/iris/bitstream/handle/10665/311389/9789241550529-eng.pdf?ua=1**).

[d] Bedaquiline is not FDA-approved for use in children <18 years. It has been used for children ≥12 years and ≥30 kg together with 4 other drugs for which the patient's MDR TB isolate is likely to be susceptible; safety and efficacy have not been established in children <12 years. Use with caution in end-stage renal impairment.

[e] Levofloxacin and moxifloxacin are not approved for use in children younger than 18 years; its use in younger children necessitates assessment of the potential risks and benefits (see Antimicrobial Agents and Related Therapy, p 863).

[f] Linezolid pharmacokinetics have not been well established in children. The doses listed will yield a drug exposure approximately equal to that in adults taking 600 mg daily.

Table 3.81. People at Increased Risk of Drug-Resistant Tuberculosis Infection or Disease[a]

- People with a history of treatment for tuberculosis disease (or whose source case for the contact received such treatment)
- Contacts of a patient with drug-resistant contagious tuberculosis disease
- People from countries with high prevalence of drug-resistant tuberculosis, such as Russia and certain nations of the former Soviet Union, Asia, Africa, and Latin America
- Infected people whose source case has positive smears for acid-fast bacilli or cultures after 2 months of appropriate antituberculosis therapy and patients who do not respond to a standard treatment regimen
- Residence in geographic area with a high percentage of drug-resistant isolates

[a] See **wwwnc.cdc.gov/travel/page/yellowbook-home.**

evaluation is an integral component of each visit for drug administration. For patients with pulmonary TB, chest radiographs often are obtained after 2 months of therapy to evaluate response. After initiation of treatment, alveolar or interstitial infiltrates often start to decrease within 1 to 2 weeks but take much longer to resolve completely. Pleural effusions are slower to resolve and may require drainage for symptom relief; partial reaccumulation is common as an isolated finding but does not indicate treatment failure. Even with successful 6-month regimens, hilar adenopathy can persist for 2 to 3 years; normal radiographic findings are not necessary to discontinue therapy. Follow-up chest radiography beyond termination of successful therapy usually is not necessary unless clinical deterioration occurs.

If therapy has been interrupted, the date of completion should be extended. Although guidelines cannot be provided for every situation, factors to consider when establishing the date of completion include the following: (1) length of interruption of therapy; (2) time during therapy (early or late) when interruption occurred; and (3) the patient's clinical, radiographic, and bacteriologic status before, during, and after interruption of therapy. The total doses administered by DOT should be calculated to guide the duration of therapy. Consultation with a specialist in TB is advised.

Untoward effects of TB therapy, including severe hepatitis in otherwise healthy infants, children, and adolescents, are rare. Routine determination of serum aminotransferase concentrations is not recommended (see "Isoniazid Therapy for TBI," p 801) during treatment of TBI or in most cases of TB disease unless the child develops symptoms suggestive of hepatotoxicity. Monthly clinical evaluations to observe for signs or symptoms of hepatitis and other adverse effects of drug therapy without routine monitoring of aminotransferase concentrations is appropriate follow-up. Regular physician-patient contact to assess drug adherence, efficacy, and adverse effects is an important aspect of management. DOT visits also are opportunities for checking on well-being and treatment tolerance. Patients should be provided with written instructions and advised to call a physician immediately if symptoms of adverse events, in particular hepatotoxicity (ie, nausea, vomiting, abdominal pain, jaundice), develop.

Other Treatment Considerations

Corticosteroids. The evidence supporting adjuvant treatment with corticosteroids for children with TB disease is incomplete. Corticosteroids are definitely indicated for children with tuberculous meningitis, because corticosteroids decrease rates of mortality and long-term neurologic impairment. Corticosteroids can be considered for children with pleural and pericardial effusions (to hasten reabsorption of fluid), severe miliary disease (to mitigate alveolocapillary block), endobronchial disease (to relieve obstruction and atelectasis), and abdominal TB (to decrease the risk of strictures). Corticosteroids should be given only when accompanied by appropriate antituberculosis drug therapy. Most experts give 2 mg/kg per day of prednisone (maximum, 60 mg/day) or its equivalent for 4 to 6 weeks followed by tapering.

Tuberculosis Disease and HIV Infection.[1] Most adults living with HIV with drug-susceptible TB respond well to standard treatment regimens. However, optimal therapy for TB in children living with HIV infection has not been established. Treating TB in a child living with HIV infection is complicated by antiretroviral drug interactions with the rifamycins and overlapping toxicities. Therapy always should include at least 4 drugs initially, should be administered daily via DOT, and should be continued for at least 6 months. Rifampin, isoniazid, pyrazinamide, and ethambutol (RIPE) should be administered for at least the first 2 months. Ethambutol can be discontinued once DR TB disease is excluded. Rifampin may be contraindicated in people who are receiving antiretroviral therapy. Rifabutin is substituted for rifampin in some circumstances. Consultation with a specialist who has experience in managing patients living with HIV infection with TB is strongly advised. If TB is diagnosed in an HIV-infected individual who is not yet receiving antiretroviral therapy, even in the presence of severe immune suppression, antiretroviral therapy can be safely initiated within 2 weeks of antituberculosis therapy, despite the risk of inciting immune reconstitution syndrome.

Immunizations. Patients who are receiving treatment for TB can receive measles and other age-appropriate attenuated live-virus vaccines unless they are receiving high-dose systemic corticosteroids, are severely ill, or have other specific contraindications to immunization.

Tuberculosis During Pregnancy and Breastfeeding. Pregnant women who have a positive TST or IGRA result, are asymptomatic, have a normal chest radiograph, and had recent contact with a contagious person should be considered for therapy, which usually should begin after the first trimester. If there has been no recent contact with a contagious case, therapy can be delayed until after delivery. Pyridoxine supplementation is indicated for all pregnant and breastfeeding women receiving isoniazid.

If TB disease is diagnosed during pregnancy, a standard 6-month regimen for drug-susceptible TB is usually initiated; however, 9 months of therapy is indicated if pyrazinamide is not used initially. Prompt initiation of therapy is mandatory to protect mother and fetus.

There are no adequate and well-controlled studies evaluating the adverse effects of isoniazid, rifampin, ethambutol, and pyrazinamide on the fetus. Isoniazid, ethambutol, and rifampin are believed to be relatively safe for the fetus. The benefit of ethambutol and rifampin for therapy of TB disease in the mother outweighs the risk to the infant. Because aminoglycosides (streptomycin, kanamycin, amikacin) or capreomycin may cause ototoxic effects in the fetus, they should not be used unless administration is essential for effective treatment. Ethionamide has been demonstrated to be teratogenic, so its use

---

[1]Panel on Opportunistic Infections in HIV-Exposed and HIV-Infected Children. Guidelines for the Prevention and Treatment of Opportunistic Infections in HIV-Exposed and HIV-Infected Children. Department of Health and Human Services. Available at: **https://clinicalinfo.hiv.gov/sites/default/files/inline-files/oi_guidelines_pediatrics.pdf**

during pregnancy is contraindicated. The effects of other second-line drugs on the fetus are unknown.

Women with tuberculosis who have been treated appropriately for 2 or more weeks and who are not considered contagious (smear-negative sputum) may breastfeed. Women with tuberculosis disease suspected of being contagious should refrain from breastfeeding and from other close contact with the infant because of potential spread of *M tuberculosis* through respiratory tract droplets or airborne transmission (see Breastfeeding and Human Milk, p 107). However, expressed human milk can be fed to the infant, as long as there is no evidence of tuberculosis mastitis, which is rare. Although isoniazid is secreted in human milk, no adverse effects of isoniazid on nursing infants have been demonstrated. Breastfed infants do not require pyridoxine supplementation unless they are receiving isoniazid, but breastfeeding mothers who are taking isoniazid should take pyridoxine. The isoniazid dosage of a breastfed infant whose mother is taking isoniazid does not require adjustment for the small amount of drug in the milk.

Congenital Tuberculosis. Congenital TB is rare, but in utero infections can occur after maternal bacillemia and have been reported following in vitro fertilization of women from countries with endemic disease in whom infertility likely was related to subclinical maternal genitourinary tract TB.

None of the possible signs of congenital TB, such as fever, tachypnea, lethargy, organomegaly, or pulmonary infiltrates, distinguish it from other systemic infections of the newborn infant. The prognosis is poor without prompt treatment. If a newborn infant is suspected of having congenital TB, a TST and IGRA test, chest radiography, lumbar puncture, and appropriate cultures and radiography should be performed promptly. The TST result usually is negative in newborn infants with congenital or perinatally acquired infection; IGRA sensitivity in this context is not known but is likely to be low. Regardless of the TST or IGRA results, treatment of the infant should be initiated promptly with rifampin, isoniazid, pyrazinamide, and either ethambutol (RIPE) or an aminoglycoside (streptomycin, kanamycin, amikacin) or capreomycin. If meningitis is confirmed, corticosteroids should be added (see Corticosteroids, p 807). The placenta should be examined histologically for granulomata and AFB, and a specimen should be cultured for *M tuberculosis* complex. The mother should be evaluated for presence of pulmonary or extrapulmonary disease, including genitourinary tuberculosis. HIV testing of the mother is essential.

Management of the Newborn Infant Whose Mother Has TBI or Tuberculosis Disease. Management of the newborn infant is based on categorization of the maternal infection. Although protection of the infant from exposure and infection is of paramount importance, contact between infant and mother should be allowed when possible. Differing circumstances and resulting recommendations are as follows:

- **Mother has a positive TST or IGRA result and normal chest radiographic findings.** If the mother is asymptomatic, no separation is required. The mother usually is a candidate for treatment of TBI after the initial postpartum period. The newborn infant needs no special evaluation or therapy. Because of the young infant's exquisite susceptibility and because the mother's positive TST or IGRA result could be a marker of an unrecognized case of contagious TB within the household, other household members should be questioned about having symptoms of TB and have a TST or IGRA and further evaluation; this should not delay the infant's discharge from the hospital. These mothers can breastfeed their infants.

- **Mother has clinical signs and symptoms or abnormal findings on chest radiograph consistent with TB disease.** Cases of suspected or proven TB disease in mothers should be reported immediately to the local health department, and evaluation of all household members should be initiated as soon as possible. If the mother has TB disease, the infant should be evaluated for congenital TB (see Congenital Tuberculosis, p 809), and the mother should be tested for HIV infection. The mother and the infant should be separated until the mother has been evaluated and, if TB disease is suspected, until the mother and infant are receiving appropriate antituberculosis therapy, the mother wears a mask, and the mother understands and is willing to adhere to infection control measures. Women with tuberculosis who have been treated appropriately for 2 or more weeks and who are not considered contagious (smear-negative sputum) may breastfeed; women with tuberculosis disease suspected of being contagious should refrain from breastfeeding and from other close contact with the infant because of potential spread of *M tuberculosis* through respiratory tract droplets or airborne transmission (see Tuberculosis During Pregnancy and Breastfeeding, p 808). During separation, expressed human milk can be fed to the infant unless mother has signs of tuberculous mastitis, which is rare. Once the infant is receiving isoniazid (see next paragraph), separation is not necessary unless the mother has possible isoniazid-resistant TB disease or has poor adherence to treatment and DOT is not possible. If the mother is suspected of having isoniazid-resistant TB disease, an expert in TB disease management should be consulted.

  If congenital TB is excluded, isoniazid is administered until the infant is 3 or 4 months of age, when a TST should be performed. If the TST result is negative at 3 to 4 months of age and the mother has good adherence and response to treatment and no longer is contagious, isoniazid should be discontinued. If the TST result is positive, the infant should be reassessed for TB disease. If TB disease is excluded, isoniazid alone should be continued for a total of 9 months, or a 4-month course of rifampin can be given. The infant should be evaluated monthly during treatment for signs of illness or poor growth.

- **Mother has a positive TST or IGRA result and abnormal findings on chest radiography but no evidence of TB disease.** If the chest radiograph of the mother appears abnormal but is not suggestive of TB disease and the history, physical examination, and sputum smear indicate no evidence of TB disease, the infant can be assumed to be at low risk of *M tuberculosis* infection and need not be separated from the mother. The mother and her infant should receive follow-up care and the mother should be treated for TBI. Other household members should have a TST or IGRA and further evaluation.

TUBERCULOSIS CAUSED BY *M BOVIS*. Infections with *M bovis* account for approximately 1% to 2% of TB cases in the United States, with higher rates along the border with Mexico. Children who come from countries where *M bovis* is prevalent in cattle or whose parents come from those countries are more likely to be infected. Most infections in humans are transmitted from cattle by unpasteurized milk and its products, such as fresh cheese,[1] although human-to-human transmission by the airborne route has been documented. In children, *M bovis* more commonly causes cervical lymphadenitis,

---

[1]American Academy of Pediatrics, Committee on Infectious Diseases and Committee on Nutrition. Consumption of raw or unpasteurized milk and milk products by pregnant women and children. *Pediatrics.* 2014;133(1):175-179 (Reaffirmed November 2019)

intestinal TB disease and peritonitis, and meningitis. In adults, *M bovis* infection can progress to advanced pulmonary disease with a risk of transmission to others.

The TST result typically is positive in a person infected with *M bovis*; IGRAs have not been studied systematically for diagnosing *M bovis* infection in particular, but theoretically they should have acceptable test characteristics (see Blood-Based Testing With Interferon-Gamma Release Assays [IGRAs], p 792). The definitive diagnosis of *M bovis* infection requires an isolate. The commonly used methods for identifying a microbial isolate as *M tuberculosis* complex do not distinguish *M bovis* from *M tuberculosis, M africanum,* and BCG, which is a live attenuated vaccine strain of *M bovis*; *M bovis* is suspected in clinical laboratories by its typical resistance to pyrazinamide. This approach can be unreliable, and species confirmation at a reference laboratory should be requested when *M bovis* is suspected. Molecular genotyping through the state health department may assist in identifying *M bovis*. BCG rarely is isolated from pediatric clinical specimens in the United States; however, it should be suspected from localized BCG suppuration or draining lymphadenitis in children who recently (within several months) received BCG vaccine, or in infants with selected congenital immunodeficiency syndromes who received a BCG vaccine. Only a reference laboratory can distinguish an isolate of BCG from an isolate of *M bovis*.

Therapy for M bovis *Disease.* Controlled clinical trials for treatment of *M bovis* disease have not been conducted, and treatment recommendations for *M bovis* disease in adults and children are based on results from treatment trials for *M tuberculosis* disease. Although most strains of *M bovis* are pyrazinamide-resistant and resistance to other first-line drugs has been reported, MDR strains are rare. Initial therapy for disease caused by *M bovis* should include 3 or 4 drugs, excluding pyrazinamide, that would be used to treat disease attributable to *M tuberculosis*. For isoniazid- and rifampin-susceptible strains, a total treatment course of at least 9 months is recommended.

Parents should be counseled about the many infectious diseases transmitted by unpasteurized milk and its products,[1] and parents who might import traditional, unpasteurized dairy products from countries where *M bovis* infection is prevalent in cattle should be advised against giving those products to their children. When people are exposed to an adult who has pulmonary disease caused by *M bovis* infection, they should be evaluated by the same methods as for *M tuberculosis*.

ISOLATION OF THE HOSPITALIZED PATIENT: Most children with TB disease, especially children younger than 10 years, are not contagious. Exceptions are the following: (1) children with pulmonary cavities; (2) children with positive sputum AFB smears; (3) children with laryngeal involvement; (4) children with extensive pulmonary infection; or (5) neonates or infants with congenital TB undergoing procedures that involve the oropharyngeal airway (eg, endotracheal intubation). In these instances, airborne infection isolation precautions for TB are indicated until effective therapy has been initiated, sputum smears are negative, and coughing has abated. Additional criteria apply to suspected or known MDR TB.

Children with no cough and smear-negative sputum AFB smears can be hospitalized in an open ward. Infection prevention measures for hospital personnel and visitors exposed to contagious patients should include the use of personally "fit tested" and "sealed" N95 particulate respirators for all patient contacts (see Infection Prevention and Control for

---

[1]American Academy of Pediatrics, Committee on Infectious Diseases and Committee on Nutrition. Consumption of raw or unpasteurized milk and milk products by pregnant women and children. *Pediatrics.* 2014;133(1):175-179 (Reaffirmed November 2019)

Hospitalized Children, p 133). If they have or are suspected to have DR TB, consultation regarding infection prevention and control should be made with public health authorities.

The major concern in infection control relates to adult household members and contacts who can be the source of infection. Visitation should be limited to people who have been evaluated by symptom screening and chest radiograph and do not have TB.

CONTROL MEASURES[1,2]: Reporting of suspected and confirmed cases of TB disease is mandated by law in all states. TBI is reportable in some states. Control of TB disease in the United States requires collaboration between health care providers and health department personnel, obtaining a thorough history of exposure(s) to people with contagious TB, timely and effective contact tracing, proper interpretation of TST or IGRA results, and appropriate antituberculosis therapy, including DOT services. A plan to control and prevent XDR TB has been published.[3] Eliminating ingestion of unpasteurized dairy products will prevent most *M bovis* infection.[4]

Management of Contacts, Including Epidemiologic Investigation.[5,6] Children with a positive TST or IGRA result or TB disease ideally should be the starting point for epidemiologic investigation by the local health department. Close contacts of a TST- or IGRA-positive child, if the test was performed because the child has 1 or more risk factors, should have a TST or IGRA, and people with a positive TST or IGRA result or with symptoms consistent with TB disease should be investigated further. Because children with TB usually are not contagious unless they have an adult-type multibacillary form of pulmonary or laryngeal disease, their contacts are not likely to be infected unless they also have been in contact with an adult source person. After the presumptive adult source of the child's TB is identified, other contacts of that adult should be evaluated.

Therapy for Contacts. Children and adolescents recently exposed to a contagious case of TB disease should have a TST or IGRA test performed and should have an evaluation for TB disease (history and physical examination, as well as chest radiography if symptomatic or positive TST or IGRA results) performed. For exposed contacts with impaired immunity (eg, HIV infection) and all contacts younger than 5 years, treatment for presumptive TBI should be initiated, even if the initial TST or IGRA result is negative, once TB disease is excluded (see Treatment Regimens for TBI, p 796). Infected children can have a negative TST or IGRA result because a cellular immune response has not yet developed

[1]American Thoracic Society, Centers for Disease Control and Prevention, and Infectious Diseases Society of America. Controlling tuberculosis in the United States. Recommendations from the American Thoracic Society, CDC, and the Infectious Diseases Society of America. *MMWR Recomm Rep.* 2005;54(RR-12):1–81

[2]Starke JR; American Academy of Pediatrics, Committee on Infectious Diseases. Technical report: interferon-γ release assays for diagnosis of tuberculosis infection and disease in children. *Pediatrics.* 2014;134(6):e1763-e1773 (Reaffirmed July 2018)

[3]Centers for Disease Control and Prevention. Plan to combat extensively drug-resistant tuberculosis: recommendations of the Federal Tuberculosis Task Force. *MMWR Recomm Rep.* 2009;58(RR-3):1–43

[4]American Academy of Pediatrics, Committee on Infectious Diseases and Committee on Nutrition. Consumption of raw or unpasteurized milk and milk products by pregnant women and children. *Pediatrics.* 2014;133(1):175-179 (Reaffirmed November 2019)

[5]National Tuberculosis Controllers Association and Centers for Disease Control and Prevention. Guidelines for the investigation of contacts of persons with infectious tuberculosis. Recommendations from the National Tuberculosis Controllers Association and CDC. *MMWR Recomm Rep.* 2005;54(RR-15):1–47

[6]Starke JR; American Academy of Pediatrics, Committee on Infectious Diseases. Technical report: interferon-γ release assays for diagnosis of tuberculosis infection and disease in children. *Pediatrics.* 2014;134(6):e1763-e1773 (Reaffirmed July 2018)

or because of anergy. Children with a negative TST or IGRA result should be retested 8 to 10 weeks after the last exposure to a source of infection. If the TST or IGRA result still is negative in an immunocompetent person, treatment can be discontinued. If the contact is immunocompromised and TBI cannot be excluded, after an evaluation for TB disease, treatment should be continued to the completion of the regimen. If a TST or IGRA result of a contact becomes positive, the regimen for TBI should be completed after an evaluation for TB disease.

Child Care and Schools. Children with TB disease can attend school or child care if they are receiving therapy (see Children in Group Child Care and Schools, p 116). They can return to regular activities as soon as effective therapy has been instituted, adherence to therapy has been documented, and clinical symptoms have diminished. Children with TBI can participate in all activities whether they are receiving treatment or not.

BCG Vaccines. BCG vaccine is a live vaccine originally prepared from attenuated strains of *M bovis.* Use of BCG vaccine[1] is recommended by the Expanded Programme on Immunization of the World Health Organization for administration at birth (see Table 1.7, p 15). BCG is used in more than 100 countries to reduce the incidence of disseminated and other life-threatening manifestations of TB in infants and young children. Although BCG immunization appears to decrease the risk of serious complications of TB disease in children, the various BCG vaccines used throughout the world differ in composition and efficacy.

Two meta-analyses of published clinical trials and case-control studies concerning the efficacy of BCG vaccines concluded that BCG vaccine has relatively high protective efficacy (approximately 80%) against meningeal and miliary TB in children. The protective efficacy against pulmonary TB differed significantly among the studies, precluding a specific conclusion. Protection afforded by BCG vaccine in one meta-analysis was estimated to be 50%. Comparative evaluations of the BCG vaccine that is licensed in the United States for the prevention of TB disease versus other BCG vaccines globally have not been performed.

Indications. In the United States, administration of BCG vaccine should be considered only in limited and select circumstances, such as unavoidable risk of exposure to TB and failure or unfeasibility of other control methods. Recommendations for use of BCG vaccine for control of TB among children and health care personnel have been published by the Advisory Committee on Immunization Practices of the CDC and the Advisory Council for the Elimination of Tuberculosis.[2] For infants and children, BCG immunization should be considered only for those who have a negative TST result and who do not have contraindications in the following circumstances:

- The child is exposed continually to a person or people with contagious pulmonary TB resistant to isoniazid and rifampin and the child cannot be removed from this exposure, OR
- The child is exposed continually to a person or people with untreated or ineffectively treated contagious pulmonary TB and the child cannot be removed from such exposure or given antituberculosis therapy.

Careful assessment of the potential risks and benefits of BCG vaccine and consultation

---

[1] **www.bcgatlas.org**

[2] Centers for Disease Control and Prevention. The role of BCG vaccine in the prevention and control of tuberculosis in the United States: a joint statement by the Advisory Committee for the Elimination of Tuberculosis and the Advisory Committee on Immunization Practices. *MMWR Recomm Rep.* 1996;45(RR-4):1–18

with personnel in local TB control programs are strongly recommended before use of BCG vaccine.

Adverse Reactions. Uncommonly (1%–2% of immunizations), BCG vaccine can result in local adverse reactions, such as subcutaneous abscess and regional lymphadenopathy, which generally are not serious. One rare complication, osteitis affecting the epiphysis of long bones, can occur as long as several years after BCG immunization. Disseminated fatal infection occurs rarely (approximately 2 per 1 million people), primarily in people who are severely immunocompromised, such as children with poorly controlled HIV infection or severe combined immunodeficiency. Antituberculosis therapy is recommended to treat osteitis and disseminated disease caused by BCG vaccine. Pyrazinamide is not believed to be effective against BCG and should not be included in treatment regimens.

Children with complications caused by BCG vaccine should be referred for management, if possible, to a TB expert and also should have consideration of evaluation for an immune deficiency.

Contraindications. People with burns, skin infections, and primary or secondary immunodeficiencies should not receive BCG vaccine. The World Health Organization no longer recommends BCG in healthy children living with HIV infection, because an increasing number of cases of localized and disseminated BCG have been described in infants and children living with HIV infection. Use of BCG vaccine is contraindicated for people receiving immunosuppressive medications including high-dose corticosteroids (see Corticosteroids, p 807). Although no untoward effects of BCG vaccine on the fetus have been observed, immunization of women during pregnancy is not recommended.

Nontuberculous Mycobacteria
(Environmental Mycobacteria, Mycobacteria other than *Mycobacterium tuberculosis*)

CLINICAL MANIFESTATIONS: Several syndromes are caused by nontuberculous mycobacteria (NTM).

- In children, the most common of these syndromes is cervical lymphadenitis.
- Cutaneous infection may follow soil- or water-contaminated traumatic wounds, surgeries, or cosmetic procedures (eg, tattoos, pedicures, body piercings).
- Less common syndromes include skin and soft tissue infection, osteomyelitis, otitis media, central catheter-associated bloodstream infections, and pulmonary infections, especially in adolescents with cystic fibrosis.
- NTM, especially *Mycobacterium avium* complex (MAC [including *M avium* and *Mycobacterium avium-intracellulare*]) and *Mycobacterium abscessus,* can be recovered from sputum in 10% to 20% of adolescents and young adults with cystic fibrosis and can be associated with fever and declining clinical status.
- Disseminated infections almost always are associated with impaired cell-mediated immunity, as found in children with congenital immune defects (eg, interleukin-12 deficiency, cytokine–JAK–STAT pathways abnormalities, NF-kappa-B essential modulator [NEMO] mutation and related disorders, and interferon-gamma receptor defects), hematopoietic stem cell transplants, or advanced human immunodeficiency virus (HIV) infection. Disseminated NTM infection, most commonly MAC, is rare in children living with HIV during the first year of life. The frequency of disseminated MAC increases

with increasing age and declining CD4+ T-lymphocyte counts, typically less than 50 cells/μL, in children 6 years or older.[1] Manifestations of disseminated NTM infections depend on the species and route of infection and include fever, night sweats, weight loss, abdominal pain, fatigue, diarrhea, and anemia. These signs and symptoms also are found in advanced immunosuppressed children living with HIV infection without disseminated MAC. For children living with HIV infection who have disseminated MAC, respiratory symptoms and isolated pulmonary disease are uncommon. In patients living with HIV infection who develop immune restoration with initiation of combination antiretroviral therapy (ART), local NTM symptoms can worsen temporarily. This immune reconstitution syndrome usually occurs 2 to 4 weeks after initiation of ART. Symptoms can include worsening fever, swollen lymph nodes, local pain, and laboratory abnormalities.

ETIOLOGY: Of the close to 200 species of NTM that have been identified, only a few cause most human infections. However, gene sequencing has led to identification of new species that cause human disease infrequently. The species most commonly infecting children in the United States are MAC, *Mycobacterium fortuitum*, *M abscessus*, and *Mycobacterium marinum* (Table 3.82). Several new species, which can be detected by nucleic acid amplification testing but cannot be grown by routine culture methods, have been identified in lymph nodes of children with cervical adenitis. NTM disease in patients living with HIV infection usually is caused by MAC. *M fortuitum*, *Mycobacterium chelonae*, *Mycobacterium smegmatis*, and *M abscessus* commonly are referred to as "rapidly growing" mycobacteria, because sufficient growth and identification can be achieved in the laboratory within 3 to 7 days on solid media, whereas MAC, *M marinum*, *Mycobacterium szulgai*, and most other NTM usually require several weeks before sufficient growth occurs for identification and are referred to as "slow growing" mycobacteria. Rapidly growing mycobacteria have been implicated most often in wound, soft tissue, bone, pulmonary, central venous catheter, and middle-ear infections. Other mycobacterial species that usually are not pathogenic have caused infections in immunocompromised hosts or have been associated with the presence of a foreign body.

EPIDEMIOLOGY: Many NTM species are ubiquitous in nature, being found in soil, food, water, and animals. Tap water is the major reservoir for *Mycobacterium kansasii*, *Mycobacterium lentiflavum*, *Mycobacterium xenopi*, *Mycobacterium simiae*, and health care-associated infections attributable to *M abscessus* and *M fortuitum*. Outbreaks have been associated with contaminated water used for acupuncture and pedicures and inks used for tattooing. Health care-associated outbreaks have occurred among children undergoing pulpotomy or other dental procedures associated with improperly maintained dental unit water lines. Outbreaks of otitis media caused by *M abscessus* have been associated with polyethylene ear tubes and use of contaminated equipment or water. Health care-associated outbreaks of *M chelonae* have been associated with the use of commercial-grade misting humidifiers and nonsterile ice for invasive procedures. For *M marinum*, water in a fish tank or aquarium or an injury in a salt-water environment are the major sources of infection. A waterborne route of transmission has been implicated for MAC infection in some immunocompromised hosts.

---

[1] Panel on Opportunistic Infections in HIV-Exposed and HIV-Infected Children. Guidelines for the Prevention and Treatment of Opportunistic Infections in HIV-Exposed and HIV-Infected Children. Department of Health and Human Services. Available at: **https://clinicalinfo.hiv.gov/sites/default/files/inline-files/oi_guidelines_pediatrics.pdf**

Table 3.82. Diseases Caused by Nontuberculous *Mycobacterium* Species

Clinical Disease	Species
Cutaneous infection	*Mycobacterium marinum* *Mycobacterium chelonae* *Mycobacterium fortuitum* *Mycobacterium abscessus* *Mycobacterium ulcerans*[a]
Lymphadenitis	MAC *Mycobacterium haemophilum* *Mycobacterium lentiflavum* *Mycobacterium kansasii* *M fortuitum* *M abscessus* *Mycobacterium malmoense*[b]
Otologic infection	*M abscessus* *M fortuitum*
Pulmonary infection	MAC *M kansasii* *M abscessus* *Mycobacterium xenopi* *M malmoense*[b] *Mycobacterium szulgai* *M fortuitum* *Mycobacterium simiae*
Catheter-associated infection	*M chelonae* *M fortuitum* *M abscessus*
Prosthetic valve endocarditis	*M chelonae* *M fortuitum* *Mycobacterium chimaera*
Skeletal infection	MAC *M kansasii* *M fortuitum* *M chelonae* *M marinum* *M abscessus* *M ulcerans*[a]
Disseminated	MAC *M kansasii* *Mycobacterium genavense* *M haemophilum* *M chelonae*

MAC indicates *Mycobacterium avium* complex.
[a]Not endemic in the United States.
[b]Found primarily in Northern Europe.

An international outbreak of *Mycobacterium chimaera* infection (including prosthetic valve endocarditis, vascular graft infection, and disseminated infection) was associated with heater-cooler devices used in heart surgery requiring cardiopulmonary bypass, and was likely attributable to aerosolization of *M chimaera* from contaminated devices. Clinical presentation was indolent and included fever, myalgia, arthralgia, fatigue, and weight loss, with diagnosis in patients occurring up to several years after exposure. The US Food and Drug Administration (FDA) has determined that all heater-cooler devices have common design features that could lead to bioaerosol formation.

Although many people are exposed to NTM, it is unknown why some exposures result in acute or chronic infection. Usual portals of entry for NTM infection are believed to be abrasions in the skin, such as cutaneous lesions caused by *M marinum*; penetrating trauma, such as needles and organic material most often associated with *M abscessus* and *M fortuitum*; surgical sites, especially for cosmetic surgery and central vascular or perito-neal dialysis catheters; oropharyngeal mucosa, which is the presumed portal of entry for cervical lymphadenitis; tooth eruption, which is the presumed portal of entry for sub-mandibular lymphadenitis; gastrointestinal or respiratory tract, for disseminated MAC; and respiratory tract, including tympanostomy tubes for otitis media. Pulmonary disease and rare cases of mediastinal adenitis and endobronchial disease occur. NTM are impor-tant pathogens in patients with cystic fibrosis and are emerging pathogens in individuals receiving biologic response modifiers, such as antitumor necrosis factor-alpha agents (see Biologic Response-Modifying Drugs Used to Decrease Inflammation, p 82). Most infec-tions remain localized at the portal of entry or in regional lymph nodes. Dissemination to distal sites primarily occurs in severely immunocompromised hosts.

No definitive evidence of person-to-person transmission of NTM exists outside of reports of possible occurrence in cystic fibrosis clinics.

Buruli ulcer disease is a skin and bone infection caused by *Mycobacterium ulcerans*, an emerging disease causing significant morbidity and disability in tropical areas such as Africa, Asia, South America, Australia, and the western Pacific.

The **incubation periods** are variable.

DIAGNOSTIC TESTS: Routine screening of respiratory or gastrointestinal tract specimens for MAC microorganisms is not recommended. Definitive diagnosis of NTM disease requires isolation of the organism. Consultation with the laboratory should occur to ensure that cultures and other specimens are handled correctly. For example, isolation of *Mycobacterium haemophilum* requires that the culture be maintained at 30°C and that heme-containing medium is added for isolation. Because NTM commonly are found in the environment, contamination of cultures or transient colonization can occur. Caution must be exercised in interpretation of cultures obtained from nonsterile sites, such as gastric washing specimens, endoscopy material, a single expectorated sputum sample, or urine specimens, and when the species cultured usually is nonpathogenic (eg, *Mycobacterium terrae* complex or *Mycobacterium gordonae*). An acid-fast bacilli smear-positive sample and repeated isolation on culture media of a single species from any site are more likely to indicate dis-ease than culture contamination or transient colonization. Diagnostic criteria for NTM lung disease in adults include 2 or more separate sputum samples or 1 bronchial alveolar lavage specimen that grows NTM. These criteria have not been validated in children and apply best to MAC, *M kansasii*, and *M abscessus*. NTM isolates from draining sinus tracts or wounds almost always are significant clinically. Recovery of NTM from sites that usu-ally are sterile, such as cerebrospinal fluid, pleural fluid, bone marrow, blood, lymph node aspirates, middle ear or mastoid aspirates, or surgically excised tissue, is very likely to be significant. However, rare instances of sample or laboratory contamination leading to a false-positive culture result have been reported. With radiometric or nonradiometric broth techniques, blood cultures are highly sensitive in recovery of MAC and other bloodborne NTM species. If disseminated MAC disease is confirmed, the patient should be evaluated to identify an underlying immunodeficiency condition. Polymerase chain reaction-based assays for some NTM have been developed but are not yet widely available in commercial diagnostic laboratories.

Patients with NTM infection such as *M marinum, M kansasii,* or MAC cervical lymph-adenitis can have a positive tuberculin skin test (TST) result, because the purified protein derivative preparation, derived from *Mycobacterium tuberculosis,* shares a number of anti-gens with these NTM species. These TST reactions usually measure less than 10 mm of induration but can measure more than 15 mm (see Tuberculosis, p 786). The interferon-gamma release assays (IGRAs) use 2 or 3 antigens specific to *M tuberculosis* complex and results in less cross-reactivity from *M avium-intracellulare* and most other NTM species com-pared with TST. However, cross-reactions can occur with infection caused by *M kansasii, M marinum,* and *M szulgai* (see Tuberculosis, p 786).

TREATMENT[1,2]: Many NTM are relatively resistant in vitro to antituberculosis drugs, but this does not necessarily correlate with clinical response, especially with MAC infections. Only limited controlled trials of drug treatment have been performed in adults with NTM infections, and none have been conducted in children. The approach to initial ther-apy should be directed by the following: (1) the species causing the infection; (2) the results of drug-susceptibility testing, especially to macrolides; (3) the site(s) of infection; (4) the patient's immune status; and (5) the need to treat a patient presumptively for tuberculosis while awaiting culture reports that subsequently reveal NTM.

For NTM lymphadenitis in otherwise healthy children, especially when the disease is caused by MAC, complete surgical excision is curative and limits scar formation. Therapy with clarithromycin or azithromycin combined with ethambutol and/or rifampin or rifab-utin may be beneficial for children in whom surgical excision is not possible or is incom-plete and for children with recurrent disease (see Table 3.83), although published reports of antimicrobial therapy without surgical incision have had variable success rates. The natural history of NTM lymphadenitis without curative surgical excision is slow resolu-tion but with a high risk of spontaneous drainage through the skin and resulting scarring, even when antimicrobial management is used. Joint decision making with the parent(s) and possibly the child, depending on age, and the surgeon is important in developing the best treatment plan for each patient.

The choice of drugs, dosages, and duration should be reviewed with a consultant experienced in the management of NTM infections, but always includes 2 or more drugs (see Table 3.83). Indwelling foreign bodies must be removed, and surgical débridement for serious localized disease is optimal. Clinical isolates of MAC usually are resistant to many

[1]Daley CL, Iaccarino JM, Lange C, et al. Treatment of nontuberculous mycobacterial pulmonary dis-ease: an official ATS/ERS/ESCMID/IDSA clinical practice guideline: executive summary. *Clin Infect Dis.* 2020;71(4):e1-e36. DOI: **10.1093/cid/ciaa241**

[2]Floto RA, Olivier KN, Saiman L, et al. US Cystic Fibrosis Foundation and European Cystic Fibrosis Society consensus recommendations for the management of non-tuberculous mycobacteria in individuals with cys-tic fibrosis. *Thorax.* 2016;71:i1-i22. Available at: **https://thorax.bmj.com/content/thoraxjnl/71/Suppl_1/i1.full.pdf**

Table 3.83. Treatment of Nontuberculous Mycobacteria Infections in Children[a]

Organism	Disease	Initial Treatment
Slowly Growing Species		
Mycobacterium avium complex (MAC); Mycobacterium haemophilum; Mycobacterium lentiflavum	Lymphadenitis	Complete excision of lymph nodes; if excision incomplete or disease recurs, clarithromycin or azithromycin plus ethambutol and/or rifampin (or rifabutin).
	Pulmonary infection	Clarithromycin or azithromycin plus ethambutol with rifampin or rifabutin (pulmonary resection in some patients who fail to respond to drug therapy). For severe disease, an initial course of amikacin or streptomycin often is included. Clinical data in adults with mild to moderate disease support that 3-times-weekly therapy is as effective as daily therapy, with less toxicity. For patients with advanced or cavitary disease, drugs should be given daily.
Mycobacterium chimaera	Prosthetic valve endocarditis	Valve removal, prolonged antimicrobial therapy based on susceptibility testing.
	Disseminated	See text.
Mycobacterium kansasii	Pulmonary infection	Rifampin plus ethambutol with isoniazid daily. If rifampin resistance is detected, a 3-drug regimen based on drug susceptibility testing should be used.
	Osteomyelitis	Surgical débridement and prolonged antimicrobial therapy using rifampin plus ethambutol with isoniazid.
Mycobacterium marinum	Cutaneous infection	None, if minor; rifampin, trimethoprim-sulfamethoxazole, clarithromycin, or doxycycline[b] for moderate disease; extensive lesions may require surgical débridement. Susceptibility testing not routinely required.
Mycobacterium ulcerans	Cutaneous and bone infections	Daily intramuscular streptomycin and oral rifampin for 8 weeks; excision to remove necrotic tissue, if present; potential response to thermotherapy.

Table 3.83. Treatment of Nontuberculous Mycobacteria Infections in Children,[a] continued

Organism	Disease	Initial Treatment
Rapidly Growing Species		
Mycobacterium fortuitum group	Cutaneous infection	Initial therapy for serious disease is amikacin plus meropenem, IV, followed by clarithromycin, doxycycline[b] or trimethoprim-sulfamethoxazole, or ciprofloxacin, orally, on the basis of in vitro susceptibility testing; may require surgical excision. Up to 50% of isolates are resistant to cefoxitin.
	Catheter infection	Catheter removal and amikacin plus meropenem, IV; clarithromycin, trimethoprim-sulfamethoxazole, or ciprofloxacin, orally, on the basis of in vitro susceptibility testing.
Mycobacterium abscessus	Otitis media; cutaneous infection	There is no reliable antimicrobial regimen because of variability in drug susceptibility. Clarithromycin plus initial course of amikacin plus cefoxitin or imipenem/meropenem; may require surgical débridement on the basis of in vitro susceptibility testing (50% are amikacin resistant).
	Pulmonary infection (in cystic fibrosis)	Serious disease, clarithromycin, amikacin, and cefoxitin or imipenem/meropenem on the basis of susceptibility testing; most isolates have very low MICs to tigecycline; may require surgical resection.
Mycobacterium chelonae	Catheter infection, prosthetic valve endocarditis	Catheter removal; débridement, removal of foreign material; valve replacement; and tobramycin (initially) plus clarithromycin, meropenem, and linezolid.
	Disseminated cutaneous infection	Tobramycin and meropenem or linezolid (initially) plus clarithromycin.

IV indicates intravenously; MIC, minimum inhibitory concentration.

[a]Treatment always includes 2 or more drugs.

[b]Doxycycline can be used for short durations (ie, 21 days or less) without regard to patient age, but for longer treatment durations is not recommended for children younger than 8 years (see Tetracyclines, p 866). Only 50% of isolates of *M marinum* are susceptible to doxycycline.

of the approved antituberculosis drugs, including isoniazid, but generally are susceptible to clarithromycin and azithromycin and often are susceptible to combinations of ethambutol, rifabutin or rifampin, and amikacin or streptomycin. Secondary agents include moxifloxacin and linezolid. Susceptibility testing to these other agents has not been standardized and, thus, is not recommended routinely. Isolates of rapidly growing mycobacteria (*M fortuitum*, *M abscessus*, and *M chelonae*) should be tested in vitro against drugs to which they commonly are susceptible and that have been used with some therapeutic success (eg, amikacin, imipenem, sulfamethoxazole or trimethoprim-sulfamethoxazole, cefoxitin, ciprofloxacin, clarithromycin, linezolid, clofazimine, doxycycline, and tigecycline).

The duration of therapy for NTM infections will depend on host status, site(s) of involvement, and severity. Patients receiving therapy should be monitored. Patients receiving clarithromycin plus rifabutin or high-dose rifabutin (with another drug) should be observed for the rifabutin-related development of leukopenia, uveitis, polyarthralgia, and pseudojaundice.

Most patients who respond ultimately show substantial clinical improvement in the first 4 to 6 weeks of therapy. Elimination of the organisms from blood cultures can take longer, often up to 12 weeks. Most experts recommend a minimum treatment duration of 3 to 6 months or longer.

For patients with cystic fibrosis and isolation of MAC species, treatment is suggested only for those with clinical symptoms not attributable to other causes, worsening lung function, and chest radiographic progression. The decision to embark on therapy should take into consideration susceptibility testing results and should involve consultation with a specialist in cystic fibrosis care.

In patients with living with HIV infection and in other immunocompromised people with disseminated MAC infection, multidrug therapy is recommended. Treatment of disseminated MAC infection should be undertaken in consultation with an expert because the infections are life threatening and drug-drug interactions may occur between medications used to treat disseminated MAC and HIV infections.

The optimal time to initiate ART in a child in whom HIV infection and disseminated MAC are newly diagnosed is not established. Many experts provide treatment of disseminated MAC for 2 weeks before initiating ART in an attempt to minimize occurrence of the immune reconstitution syndrome and minimize confusion relating to the cause of drug-associated toxicity.

Chemoprophylaxis. The most effective way to prevent disseminated MAC in children living with HIV infection is to preserve their immune function through use of combination ART. Children living with HIV infection who have advanced immunosuppression should be offered prophylaxis against disseminated MAC with azithromycin or clarithromycin based on their CD4+ T-lymphocyte counts, provided disseminated MAC has been excluded by 3 negative blood cultures in AFB-specific blood culture bottles.[1] Combination therapy for prophylaxis should be avoided in children, if possible, because it has not been shown to be cost-effective and increases rates of adverse events. Children with a history of disseminated MAC and continued immunosuppression should receive lifelong prophylaxis

---

[1]Panel on Opportunistic Infections in HIV-Exposed and HIV-Infected Children. Guidelines for the Prevention and Treatment of Opportunistic Infections in HIV-Exposed and HIV-Infected Children. Department of Health and Human Services. Available at: **https://clinicalinfo.hiv.gov/sites/default/files/inline-files/oi_guidelines_pediatrics.pdf**

to prevent recurrence. Prophylaxis can be discontinued in some children living with HIV infection after immune reconstitution as detailed in the AIDS guidelines.[1]

ISOLATION OF THE HOSPITALIZED PATIENT: Standard precautions are recommended.[2]

CONTROL MEASURES: Control measures include chemoprophylaxis for high-risk patients living with HIV infection (see Treatment, p 818) and avoidance of tap water contamination of central venous catheters, dental procedures, surgical procedures and wounds, injections and injectable medications, skin, or endoscopic equipment and other medical devices.

FDA instructions are available regarding the use of filtered water (not tap water) for heater-cooler devices and for other recommendations for these devices (**www.fda.gov/ medical-devices/what-heater-cooler-device/recommendations-use-any-heater-cooler-device**). If heater-cooler devices are implicated in *M chimaera* infection or have been or are to be used in cardiac surgeries, patients should be informed (preferably before their surgery) of the risk and monitored after surgery for signs and symptoms suggestive of infection. These devices are also used for extracorporeal membrane oxygenation (ECMO), but to date, no cases related to use in this setting have been reported. If *M chimaera* infection is suspected or documented, an FDA medical device report should be filed with MedWatch (see MedWatch – the FDA Safety Information and Adverse Event-Reporting Program, p 1004).

Tularemia

CLINICAL MANIFESTATIONS: There are several common presentations of tularemia in children, with ulceroglandular disease being the most frequently identified. Characterized by a maculopapular lesion at the entry site with subsequent ulceration and slow healing, the ulceroglandular variant is associated with tender regional lymphadenopathy that can drain spontaneously. The glandular variant (regional lymphadenopathy with no ulcer) also is common. Less common disease variants include oculoglandular (severe conjunctivitis with preauricular lymphadenopathy), oropharyngeal (severe exudative stomatitis, pharyngitis, or tonsillitis with cervical lymphadenopathy), typhoidal (high fever, hepatomegaly, splenomegaly, systemic infection including septicemia; pneumonia and or meningitis may be seen as complications), and secondary eruptions that can include vesicular skin lesions, which can be mistaken for herpes simplex virus or varicella zoster virus cutaneous infections. Pneumonic tularemia, characterized by influenza-like symptoms often without chest radiograph abnormalities, presents with fever, dry cough, chest pain, and hilar adenopathy and normally is associated with farming or lawn maintenance activities that create aerosols and dust. Pneumonic tularemia would also be the anticipated variant after intentional release of aerosolized organisms.

---

[1] Panel on Opportunistic Infections in HIV-Exposed and HIV-Infected Children. Guidelines for the Prevention and Treatment of Opportunistic Infections in HIV-Exposed and HIV-Infected Children. Department of Health and Human Services. Available at: **https://clinicalinfo.hiv.gov/sites/default/files/inline-files/oi_guidelines_pediatrics.pdf**

[2] The Cystic Fibrosis Foundation has additional recommendations for infection prevention and control in patients with cystic fibrosis, regardless of respiratory tract culture results: Saiman L, Seigel JD, LiPuma JJ, et al. Infection prevention and control guideline for cystic fibrosis: 2013 update. *Infect Control Hosp Epidemiol.* 2014;35(Suppl 1): S1-S67. Available at: **www.cff.org/Care/Clinical-Care-Guidelines/Infection-Prevention-and-Control-Clinical-Care-Guidelines/Infection-Prevention-and-Control-Clinical-Care-Guidelines/**

ETIOLOGY: *Francisella tularensis* is a small, weakly staining, gram-negative pleomorphic coccobacillus. Two subspecies cause human infection in North America: *F tularensis* subspecies *tularensis* (type A), and *F tularensis* subspecies *holarctica* (type B). Type A generally is considered more virulent, although either can be lethal, especially if inhaled.

EPIDEMIOLOGY: *F tularensis* can infect more than 100 animal species; the vertebrate species considered most important in enzootic cycles are rabbits, hares, and rodents, especially muskrats, voles, beavers, and prairie dogs. Domestic cats and dogs are an additional but rare source of infection. In the United States, most human cases are attributed to tick bites but may also result from bites of other arthropod vectors, such as deer flies, or direct from contact with any of the aforementioned animal species. Infections attributable to tick and deer fly bites usually take the form of ulceroglandular or glandular tularemia. *F tularensis* bacteria can be transmitted to humans via the skin when handling infected animal tissue, as can occur when hunting or skinning infected rabbits, muskrats, prairie dogs, and other rodents. Infection has been reported in commercially traded hamsters and prairie dogs. Infection also can be acquired following ingestion of contaminated water or inadequately cooked meat, or by inhalation of contaminated aerosols generated during lawn mowing, brush cutting, or certain farming activities (eg, baling contaminated hay). At-risk people have occupational or recreational exposure to infected animals or their habitats; this includes rabbit hunters and trappers, people exposed to certain ticks or biting insects, and laboratory technicians working with *F tularensis,* which is highly infectious and may be aerosolized when grown in culture. In the United States, most cases occur during May through September. Approximately two thirds of cases occur in males, and one quarter of cases occur in children younger than 15 years.

Tularemia has been reported in all US states except Hawaii. It is most common in central and western states and parts of Massachusetts (particularly Martha's Vineyard). In 2018, a total of 229 cases in the United States were reported. Tularemia has been a nationally notifiable disease since 2000.

Organisms can be present in blood during the first 2 weeks of disease and in cutaneous lesions for as long as 1 month if untreated. Person-to-person transmission has not been reported.

The **incubation period** usually is 3 to 5 days, with a range of 1 to 21 days.

DIAGNOSTIC TESTS: Diagnosis is established most often by serologic testing. Patients do not develop antibodies until the second week of illness. A single serum antibody titer of 1:128 or greater determined by microagglutination (MA) or of 1:160 or greater determined by tube agglutination (TA) is consistent with recent or past infection and constitutes a presumptive diagnosis. For those with suspected disease and an initial nondiagnostic titer, a repeat titer should be obtained in 4 weeks. Confirmation by serologic testing requires a fourfold or greater titer change between serum samples obtained 4 weeks apart, with at least 1 of the specimens having a minimum titer of 1:128 or greater by MA or 1:160 or greater by TA. Nonspecific cross-reactions can occur with specimens containing heterophile antibodies, or antibodies to *Brucella* species, *Legionella* species, or other Gram-negative bacteria. However, cross-reactions rarely result in MA or TA titers that are diagnostic. Because of its propensity for causing laboratory-acquired infections, laboratory personnel should be alerted immediately when *F tularensis* infection is suspected.

F tularensis in ulcer exudate or aspirate material can be identified by laboratory-developed polymerase chain reaction (PCR) assay or direct fluorescent antibody assay.

Immunohistochemical staining is specific for detection of *F tularensis* in fixed tissues; however, this method is not available in most clinical laboratories. Isolation of *F tularensis* from specimens of blood, skin, ulcers, lymph node drainage, gastric washings, or respiratory tract secretions is best achieved by inoculation of cysteine-enriched media. Because *F tularensis* is a biosafety level 3 agent, if suspected on the basis of clinical and epidemiologic history or Gram stain identification of tiny, gram-negative coccobacillus, further work should only be performed in a certified Class II Biosafety Cabinet using appropriate personal protective equipment (back fastening gown, dual gloves, N95 respirator). All isolates suspected to be *F tularensis* should be forwarded for confirmation to local reference laboratories (usually the state laboratory) that are part of the Laboratory Response Network.

TREATMENT: Gentamicin (5 mg/kg/day, divided twice or 3 times/day, intravenously or intramuscularly, with the dose adjusted to maintain the desired peak serum concentrations of at least 5 µg/mL) is the drug of choice for the treatment of tularemia in children because of the limited availability of streptomycin (30–40 mg/kg/day, divided twice/day, intramuscularly; maximum 2 g/day) and the fewer adverse effects of gentamicin. Duration of therapy usually is 10 days. A 5- to 7-day course may be sufficient in mild disease, but a longer course is required for more severe illness (eg, meningitis). Ciprofloxacin is an alternative for mild disease (10- to 14-day course of oral ciprofloxacin; 20–40 mg/kg daily in 2 divided doses, maximum of 500 mg/dose) but is not approved by the US Food and Drug Administration for the treatment of tularemia. Doxycycline is associated with a higher rate of relapse compared with other therapies and is not recommended for definitive treatment. Suppuration of lymph nodes can occur despite antimicrobial therapy. *F tularensis* is not susceptible to beta-lactam drugs, including carbapenems. Because of the difficulty in achieving adequate cerebrospinal fluid concentrations of gentamicin, combination therapy with doxycycline or ciprofloxacin plus gentamicin may be considered for patients with tularemic meningitis. Because treatment delay is associated with therapeutic failure, treatment should be initiated as soon as tularemia is suspected.

ISOLATION OF THE HOSPITALIZED PATIENT: Standard precautions are recommended.

CONTROL MEASURES:

- People should protect themselves against arthropod bites by wearing protective clothing, by frequent inspection for and removal of ticks from the skin and scalp, and by using insect repellents (see Prevention of Mosquitoborne and Tickborne Infections, p 175).
- Drinking untreated surface water should be avoided.
- Gloves should be worn by those handling the carcasses of wild rabbits, muskrats, prairie dogs, and other potentially infected animals. Children should not handle sick or dead animals, including pets.
- People should avoid mowing over live or dead animals, because this may aerosolize infective material.
- Game meats should be cooked thoroughly.
- Primary clinical specimens may be handled in the laboratory using Biological Safety Level (BSL) 2 precautions. Work with suspected cultures requires BSL3 precautions. Note that F tularensis is a tier 1 select agent and must be handled as such after it has been identified. Additional information on laboratory safety can be found in the Centers for Disease Control and Prevention (CDC) Biosafety in Microbiological and Biomedical Laboratories manual (**www.cdc.gov/biosafety/publications/bmbl5/**).

- Standard precautions should be used for handling clinical materials.
- A 14-day course of doxycycline or ciprofloxacin is recommended for children and adults after exposure to an intentional release of tularemia (eg, a bioterrorism attack) and for laboratory workers with inadvertent exposure to *F tularensis*.
- A vaccine that had been available to protect laboratory workers and other high-risk personnel is under review by the US Food and Drug Administration but is not currently available in the United States except through the Special Immunization Program administered by the Department of Defense.

Louseborne Typhus
(Epidemic or Sylvatic Typhus)

CLINICAL MANIFESTATIONS: Louseborne or epidemic typhus is an uncommon disease that is spread through contact with infected human body lice. Patients develop abrupt onset of high fever, chills, and myalgia accompanied by severe headache and malaise. Rash often develops by day 4 to 7 after the start of illness but may not always be present and should not be relied on for diagnosis. When present, the rash usually begins on the trunk and axilla, spreads centrifugally to the limbs, and generally spares the face, palms, and soles. The rash typically is macular to maculopapular but in advanced stages can become petechial or hemorrhagic. The rash can be difficult to observe on patients with darkly pigmented skin and is absent in up to 40% of patients. There is no eschar, as might be present in many other rickettsial diseases. Abdominal complaints (stomach pain, nausea) and changes in mental status are common, including delirium, drowsiness, seizures, and coma. Cough and tachypnea may be present. Myocardial and renal failure can occur when disease is severe. The fatality rate in untreated people can be as high as 30%. Mortality is less common in children and increases with advancing age. Untreated patients who recover typically have an illness lasting 2 weeks.

Brill-Zinsser disease is a relapse of epidemic typhus that can occur years after the initial episode, and generally occurs when the body's immune system is weakened from illness, medications, or advanced age. The symptoms of Brill-Zinsser disease generally are milder in nature and shorter in duration than the initial infection. Factors that reactivate the rickettsiae are unknown.

Laboratory abnormalities in epidemic typhus may include thrombocytopenia, increased hepatic enzymes, hyperbilirubinemia, and elevated blood urea nitrogen.

ETIOLOGY: Epidemic typhus is caused by *Rickettsia prowazekii*, which are gram-negative obligate intracellular bacteria.

EPIDEMIOLOGY: Epidemic typhus is transmitted by the human body louse (*Pediculus humanus corporis*), which is infected through feeding on patients with acute typhus fever. Humans are the primary reservoir of the organism. Infected lice excrete the bacteria in their feces and usually defecate at the time of feeding. Disease transmission can occur when infected louse feces are rubbed into broken skin or mucous membranes or are inhaled. All ages can be affected. Poverty, crowding, and poor sanitary conditions such as those found in war, famine, drought, and other natural disasters contribute to the spread of body lice and, hence, the disease. Cases have occurred throughout the world, including the colder, mountainous areas of Asia, Africa, some parts of Europe, and Central and South America, particularly in refugee camps and jails in resource-limited countries. Epidemic typhus is most common during winter, when conditions favor person-to-person transmission of the vector. Cases of epidemic typhus are rare in the United States, but there is no formal system for epidemic typhus surveillance. The last known epidemic in the United States occurred in 1921; sporadic human cases associated with close contact with infected flying squirrels (*Glaucomys volans*), their nests, or their ectoparasites occasionally are reported in the eastern United States. Cases have been reported in people who reside or work in flying squirrel-infested dwellings, even when direct contact is not reported. Flying squirrel-associated disease, called sylvatic typhus, typically presents with a similar but generally milder illness to that observed with body louse-transmitted infection. Untreated illness can be severe, although no fatal cases of sylvatic typhus have been reported; the later development of Brill-Zinsser disease has been confirmed in at least 1 case of untreated sylvatic typhus.

People with Brill-Zinsser disease harbor active *R prowazekii* and, therefore, may pose a risk for reintroduction of the organism and new outbreaks. *Amblyomma* ticks in the Americas and in Ethiopia have been shown to carry *R prowazekii*, but their vector potential is unknown. Rickettsiae are present in the blood and tissues of patients during the early febrile phase but are not found in secretions. Direct person-to-person spread of the disease does not occur in the absence of the louse vector.

The **incubation period** is 1 to 2 weeks.

DIAGNOSTIC TESTS: Louseborne typhus may be diagnosed via indirect immunofluorescence antibody (IFA) assay; immunohistochemistry (IHC); polymerase chain reaction (PCR) assay of blood, plasma, or tissue samples; or isolation by culture. Serologic tests are the most common means of confirmation and can be used to detect either immunoglobulin (Ig) G or IgM antibodies. The specimen preferably should be obtained within the first week of symptoms and before (or within 24 hours of) doxycycline administration. The gold standard for serologic diagnosis of louseborne typhus is a fourfold increase in IgG antibody titer by the IFA test between acute sera obtained in the first week of illness and convalescent sera obtained 2 to 4 weeks later. A negative acute serologic test result does not rule out a diagnosis of louseborne typhus, because detectable levels of IgG and IgM antibodies generally do not appear until around 7 to 10 days after onset of symptoms. An elevated acute titer may represent past infection rather than acute infection. Low-level elevated antibody titers can be an incidental finding in a significant proportion of the general population in some regions. IgM antibodies may remain elevated for months and are not highly specific for acute louseborne typhus. Cross-reactivity may be observed to antibodies to *Rickettsia typhi* (the agent of endemic typhus), *Rickettsia rickettsii* (the agent of Rocky Mountain spotted fever), and other spotted fever group rickettsiae. *R prowazekii* also may be cultured and identified through submission to specific reference laboratories that are equipped to culture and identify epidemic typhus. Cell culture cultivation of the organism must be confirmed by molecular methods.

TREATMENT: Doxycycline is the drug of choice to treat louseborne typhus, regardless of patient age. The recommended dosage of doxycycline for adults is 100 mg twice per day, intravenously or orally, and for children under 45 kg (100 lb) is 2.2 mg/kg per dose, administered twice a day (maximum 100 mg/dose [see Tetracyclines, p 866]). Treatment should be continued for at least 3 days after defervescence and evidence of clinical improvement is documented, and the total treatment course is usually 7 to 10 days. Some patients may relapse if not treated for the full 7 to 10 days. Other broad-spectrum antimicrobial agents, including ciprofloxacin, are not recommended and may be more likely to result in fatal outcome. Chloramphenicol, where available, may be used in cases of absolute contraindication of doxycycline (life-threatening allergy) but also carries significant risks (ie, aplastic anemia). In epidemic situations in which antimicrobial agents may be limited (eg, refugee camps), a single 200-mg dose of doxycycline in adults (or 4.4 mg/kg, maximum dose 200 mg as a single dose for children) may provide effective treatment and facilitate outbreak control when combined with delousing efforts.

ISOLATION OF THE HOSPITALIZED PATIENT: Standard precautions are recommended. Precautions should be taken to delouse hospitalized patients using pediculicide when louse infestations are present.

CONTROL MEASURES: Thorough delousing in epidemic situations, particularly among exposed contacts of cases, is recommended. Several applications of pediculicides may be needed, because lice eggs are resistant to most insecticides. Washing clothes in hot water kills lice and eggs. During epidemics, insecticides dusted onto clothes of louse-infested populations are effective. In situations involving outbreaks of epidemic typhus in prisons and refugee settings, active surveillance for fever is important to assess efficacy of control measures and to ensure rapid and effective treatment. To halt the spread of disease to other people, louse-infested patients should be treated with cream or gel pediculicides containing pyrethrins or permethrin; malathion is prescribed most often when pyrethroids fail. Prevention and control of flying squirrel-associated typhus requires application of insecticides and precautions to prevent contact with these animals and their ectoparasites and to exclude them from nesting in, or entering into, human dwellings. No prophylaxis is recommended for people exposed to flying squirrels. Cases should be reported to local, state, regional, or national public health departments.

Murine Typhus
(Endemic or Fleaborne Typhus)

CLINICAL MANIFESTATIONS: Murine typhus, also known as endemic typhus or fleaborne typhus, resembles epidemic (louseborne) typhus but usually has a less abrupt onset with less severe systemic symptoms. The disease can be mild in young children. Fever, present in almost all patients, can be accompanied by myalgia and a persistent, usually severe, headache. Nausea, vomiting, anorexia, and abdominal pain and tenderness also develop in approximately half of patients. A macular or maculopapular rash appears by day 4 to 7 of illness in approximately 50% of patients, and lasts 4 to 8 days. The rash often is distributed on the patient's trunk, although extremities also can be involved. Illness seldom lasts longer than 2 weeks. The clinical course is usually uncomplicated, but severe manifestations, such as central nervous system abnormalities, are possible. Laboratory findings include thrombocytopenia, elevated liver aminotransferases, hypoalbuminemia, hypocalcemia, and hyponatremia. Fatal outcome is rare but has been reported in up to 4% of hospitalized patients.

ETIOLOGY: Murine typhus is caused by *Rickettsia typhi*, which are gram-negative obligate intracellular bacteria.

EPIDEMIOLOGY: Rats, in which infection is inapparent, are the natural reservoirs for *R typhi*. The disease is worldwide in distribution and tends to occur most commonly in male adults; in children, males and females are affected equally. Outside the United States, the primary vector for transmission among rats and transmission to humans is the rat flea, *Xenopsylla cheopis*, although other fleas and mites have been implicated. A suburban cycle involving cat fleas (*Ctenocephalides felis*) and opossums (*Didelphis virginiana*) or feral cats has emerged as an important cause of murine typhus in the United States. Infection occurs when infected flea feces are rubbed into broken skin or mucous membranes or are inhaled. Murine typhus is rare in most of the United States, although it is likely underdiagnosed. Most diagnosed cases occur during the months of April to October and in southern California, southern Texas, the southeastern Gulf Coast, and Hawaii.

The **incubation period** is 6 to 14 days.

DIAGNOSTIC TESTS: Antibody titers determined with *R typhi* antigen by an indirect fluorescent antibody (IFA) assay are measured most commonly. Enzyme immunoassay or latex agglutination tests also are available. Antibody concentrations peak at around 4 weeks after infection, but results of antibody tests may be negative early in the course of illness. A fourfold increase in immunoglobulin (Ig) G titer between acute and convalescent serum specimens obtained 2 to 4 weeks apart is confirmatory for laboratory diagnosis. Although more prone to false-positive results, immunoassays demonstrating increases in specific IgM antibody can aid in distinguishing clinical illness from previous exposure if interpreted with a concurrent IgG test result; use of IgM assays alone is not recommended. Because of cross-reactivity, standard serologic tests might not differentiate murine typhus caused by *R typhi* from epidemic (louseborne) typhus (*Rickettsia prowazekii*) or from infection with spotted fever rickettsiae, such as *Rickettsia rickettsii*. More specific testing with antibody cross-absorption for immunofluorescence antibody (IFA) assay or western blot analyses is not available routinely. Isolation of the organism in cell culture potentially is hazardous and is performed best by specialized laboratories, such as those at the Centers for Disease Control and Prevention (CDC). Routine hospital blood cultures are not suitable for culture of *R typhi*. Molecular diagnostic assays on infected whole blood and skin biopsies can distinguish murine and epidemic typhus and other rickettsioses and are performed at the CDC. Immunohistochemical procedures on formalin-fixed skin biopsy tissues also can be performed at the CDC.

TREATMENT: Doxycycline is the treatment of choice for murine typhus, regardless of patient age. The recommended dosage of doxycycline is 4.4 mg/kg per day, divided every 12 hours, intravenously or orally (maximum 100 mg/dose [see Tetracyclines, p 866]). Early diagnosis should be based on clinical suspicion and epidemiology. In a patient with disease that is clinically compatible with murine typhus, treatment should not be withheld because of a negative laboratory result or while awaiting laboratory confirmation, because severe or fatal infection can develop when treatment is delayed. Treatment should be continued for at least 3 days after defervescence and evidence of clinical improvement is documented. The total treatment course usually is 7 to 14 days. Fluoroquinolones or chloramphenicol are alternative medications but may not be as effective; fluoroquinolones are not approved for this use in children younger than 18 years (see Fluoroquinolones, p 864).

ISOLATION OF THE HOSPITALIZED PATIENT: Standard precautions are recommended.

CONTROL MEASURES: Fleas should be controlled by appropriate insecticides before use of rodenticides, because fleas will seek alternative hosts, including humans. Suspected animal populations should be controlled by species-appropriate means. No prophylaxis is recommended for exposed people. The disease should be reported to local or state public health departments.

Ureaplasma urealyticum and *Ureaplasma parvum* Infections

CLINICAL MANIFESTATIONS: The role of *Ureaplasma* species in human disease is controversial. There has been an inconsistent association between presence of *Ureaplasma urealyticum* and nongonococcal urethritis (NGU). Without treatment, the urethritis usually resolves within 1 to 6 months. There also has been an inconsistent relationship of infection by *Ureaplasma* species with prostatitis and epididymitis in men and upper genital tract syndromes in women, including salpingitis, endometritis, and pelvic inflammatory disease. *Ureaplasma* organisms commonly are detected in placentas with histologic chorioamnionitis (now known as intra-amniotic infection), and studies suggest that there is an association of upper genital tract infection by *Ureaplasma* species and adverse pregnancy outcomes. Some reports also describe an association between the presence of *Ureaplasma* in the vaginal flora and preterm birth.

U urealyticum and *Ureaplasma parvum* are frequently isolated from the lower respiratory tract and from lung biopsy specimens of preterm infants, and studies have demonstrated an association of *Ureaplasma* species with the development of bronchopulmonary dysplasia in preterm infants. These organisms also have been recovered from respiratory tract secretions of infants 3 months or younger with pneumonia, but their role in development of lower respiratory tract disease in otherwise healthy young infants is unclear. *Ureaplasma* species have been isolated from the bloodstream of newborn infants and from cerebrospinal fluid of infants with meningitis, intraventricular hemorrhage, and hydrocephalus. The contribution of *U urealyticum* to the outcome of infants with infections of the central nervous system is unclear given the confounding effects of preterm birth and intraventricular hemorrhage.

Cases of *U urealyticum* or *U parvum* arthritis, osteomyelitis, pneumonia, pericarditis, meningitis, and progressive sinopulmonary disease have been reported, almost exclusively in immunocompromised patients. Patients with solid organ transplants appear to be the major risk group. A recently described syndrome of *Ureaplasma* sepsis with hyperammonemia (attributable to rapid hydrolysis of host urea by the organism) in lung transplant patients appears to be attributable to the introduction of the organism in the transplanted lung into naïve recipients who are immunosuppressed.

ETIOLOGY: *Ureaplasma* organisms are small pleomorphic bacteria that lack a cell wall. The genus contains 2 species capable of causing human infection, *U urealyticum* and *U parvum*. At least 14 serotypes have been described, 4 for *U parvum* and 10 for *U urealyticum*.

EPIDEMIOLOGY: The principal reservoir of human *Ureaplasma* species is the genital tract of sexually active adults. Colonization occurs in approximately half of sexually active women; the incidence in sexually active men is lower. Colonization is uncommon in prepubertal children and adolescents who are not sexually active, but a positive genital tract culture is not clearly definitive of sexual abuse. *Ureaplasma* species may colonize the throat, eyes, umbilicus, and perineum of newborn infants and may persist for several months after birth. *U parvum* generally is more common than *U urealyticum* as a colonizer in pregnant women and their offspring.

Because *Ureaplasma* species commonly are isolated from the female lower genital tract and neonatal respiratory tract in the absence of disease, a positive culture does not establish its causative role in acute infection. However, recovery of these organisms from an upper genital tract or lower respiratory tract specimen in the appropriate host who has evidence of clinical disease is much more indicative of true infection.

The **incubation period** after sexual transmission is 10 to 20 days.

DIAGNOSTIC TESTS: Specimens for culture require *Ureaplasma* compatible transport media, with refrigeration at 4°C (39°F). If the specimen cannot be transported to the reference laboratory within 24 hours, the sample should be frozen at $-70°$ C (not $-20°$ C). If a vaginal or urethral swab is used for collection, Dacron or calcium alginate swabs should be used to collect and inoculate transport media; cotton swabs should be avoided. Several rapid, sensitive real-time polymerase chain reaction assays for detection of *U urealyticum* and *U parvum* have been developed. Many of these assays have greater sensitivity than culture, but they are not widely available outside of reference laboratories. Transport medium is not necessary for urine to be tested only by polymerase chain reaction (PCR) assay. Such specimens can be concentrated 10-fold and frozen at $-70°$ C immediately after collection and shipped on dry ice. *Ureaplasma* species can be cultured in urea-containing broth and agar in 2 to 4 days. Serologic testing is of limited value for diagnostic purposes and is not available commercially.

TREATMENT: A positive *Ureaplasma* culture or PCR assay does not indicate need for therapy if the patient is asymptomatic. *Ureaplasma* species generally are susceptible to macrolides, tetracyclines, and quinolones, but because they lack a cell wall they are not susceptible to penicillins or cephalosporins. They also are not susceptible to trimethoprim-sulfamethoxazole or clindamycin. For symptomatic children, adolescents, and adults, doxycycline can be used for treatment. Doxycycline can be used for short durations (ie, 21 days or less) without regard to patient age (see Tetracyclines, p 866); azithromycin is the preferred antimicrobial agent for children younger than 8 years or people who are allergic to tetracyclines. Persistent urethritis after doxycycline treatment may be attributable to doxycycline-resistant *U urealyticum* or *Mycoplasma genitalium*. Recurrences are common, and tetracycline resistance may occur in up to 50% of *Ureaplasma* isolates in some patient populations. If tetracycline resistance is likely, azithromycin is indicated; a quinolone is an option if azithromycin resistance also is possible. On the basis of very limited data, quinolone and macrolide coresistance remains uncommon, at less than 5% in the United States, but up to 10% elsewhere including Australia and Southeast Asia. Such infections are difficult to treat, and pristinamycin (not approved by the US Food and Drug Administration) has proven effective.

In neonates, antimicrobial treatment with erythromycin has generally failed to prevent chronic pulmonary disease in small randomized trials, possibly because erythromycin does not eliminate *Ureaplasma* organisms from the airways in a large proportion of infants. One small randomized trial suggests that bronchopulmonary dysplasia or death may be reduced by azithromycin (10 mg/kg/day for 7 days followed by 5 mg/kg/day for a maximum of 6 weeks). Pharmacokinetic studies suggest that a 3-day course of 20 mg/kg/day of intravenous azithromycin may be more effective in clearance of *Ureaplasma* organisms from preterm infants, although efficacy in improving clinical outcomes needs to be demonstrated. Definitive evidence of efficacy of antimicrobial agents in the treatment of central nervous system infections caused by *Ureaplasma* species in infants and children also is lacking. There are reports of preterm infants with *Ureaplasma* species identified in cerebrospinal fluid who have or have not received antimicrobial therapy and who have had documentation of sterilization of cerebrospinal fluid.

ISOLATION OF THE HOSPITALIZED PATIENT: Standard precautions are recommended.

CONTROL MEASURES: None recommended.

Varicella-Zoster Virus Infections

CLINICAL MANIFESTATIONS: Primary infection results in varicella (chickenpox), manifesting in unvaccinated people as a generalized, pruritic, erythematous vesicular rash typically consisting of 250 to 500 lesions in varying stages of development (papules, vesicles) and resolution (crusting), low-grade fever, and other systemic symptoms. Complications include bacterial superinfection of skin lesions with or without bacterial sepsis, pneumonia, central nervous system involvement (acute cerebellar ataxia, encephalitis, stroke/vasculopathy), thrombocytopenia, and rarer complications such as glomerulonephritis, arthritis, and hepatitis. Primary viral pneumonia is uncommon among immunocompetent children but is the most common complication in adults. Varicella tends to be more severe in adults, infants, and adolescents than in other children. Despite widespread use of varicella vaccine, breakthrough cases can occur in immunized children, as described in Active Immunization (p 13), but usually are mild and rash presentation is modified. Reye syndrome may follow varicella, although this outcome has become very rare with the recommendation not to use salicylate-containing compounds (eg, aspirin, bismuth-subsalicylate) for children with chickenpox. In immunocompromised children, progressive, severe varicella may occur with continuing eruption of lesions (sometimes including hemorrhagic skin lesions) along with high fever persisting into the second week of illness and visceral dissemination (ie, encephalitis, hepatitis, and pneumonia). Severe and even fatal varicella has been reported in otherwise healthy children on high-dose corticosteroids (greater than 2 mg/kg/day of prednisone or equivalent) for treatment of asthma and other illnesses.

Varicella-zoster virus (VZV) establishes latency in sensory (dorsal root, cranial nerve, and autonomic including enteric) ganglia during primary VZV infection. This latency occurs with both wild-type VZV and the vaccine strain. Reactivation results in herpes zoster (shingles), typically characterized by grouped vesicular skin lesions on an erythematous base in the unilateral distribution of 1 to 3 contiguous sensory dermatomes, most commonly in the thoracic and lumbar regions, frequently accompanied by localized pain and/or itching. Zoster may also result in cranial neuropathy, particularly in the fifth, seventh, and eighth cranial nerve distributions. Postherpetic neuralgia (PHN), pain that persists after resolution of the zoster rash, may last for weeks to months but is unusual in children. Zoster occasionally becomes disseminated in immunocompromised patients, with lesions appearing outside the primary dermatomes and/or visceral complications. VZV reactivation less frequently occurs in the absence of skin rash (zoster sine herpete); these patients may present with aseptic meningitis, encephalitis, stroke, acute retinal necrosis, or gastrointestinal tract involvement (visceral zoster). Recurrent zoster is rare and should prompt a consideration for an evaluation for immunodeficiency. A vesicular rash, especially in the distribution of the trigeminal ganglion or sacral sensory roots, may represent herpes simplex virus infection (so-called zosteriform HSV) and should be assessed virologically (eg, by polymerase chain reaction testing of swabbed material from the base of an unroofed vesicle) to distinguish this from zoster attributable to VZV.

Fetal infection after maternal varicella during the first or early second trimester of pregnancy occasionally results in fetal death or varicella embryopathy, characterized by limb hypoplasia, cutaneous scarring, eye abnormalities, and damage to the central nervous system (congenital varicella syndrome). The incidence of the congenital varicella syndrome among infants born to mothers who experience gestational varicella is approximately 2% when infection occurs between 8 and 20 weeks of gestation. Rarely, cases of congenital varicella syndrome have been reported in infants of women infected after 20 weeks of pregnancy, the latest occurring at 28 weeks' gestation. Children infected with VZV in utero may develop zoster early in life without having had extrauterine varicella.

Varicella infection has a higher case-fatality rate in infants when the mother develops varicella from 5 days before to 2 days after delivery, because there is little opportunity for development and transfer of maternal antibody across the placenta prior to delivery and the infant's cellular immune system is immature.

ETIOLOGY: VZV (also known as human herpesvirus 3) is a member of the *Herpesviridae* family, the subfamily *Alphaherpesvirinae*, and the genus *Varicellovirus*.

EPIDEMIOLOGY: Humans are the only source of infection for this highly contagious virus. Infection occurs when the virus comes in contact with the mucosa of the upper respiratory tract or the conjunctiva of a susceptible person. Person-to-person transmission occurs either from direct contact with VZV lesions from varicella or herpes zoster or from airborne spread. Varicella is more contagious than herpes zoster. There is no evidence of VZV spread from fomites; the virus is extremely labile and is unable to survive for long in the environment. Varicella infection in a household member usually results in infection of almost all susceptible people in that household. Children who acquire their infection at home (secondary family cases) often have more skin lesions than the index case. Health care-associated transmission is well documented.

In temperate climates in the prevaccine era, varicella was a disease with a marked seasonal distribution, with peak incidence during winter and spring mainly among children younger than 10 years. In tropical climates, acquisition of varicella often occurs later, resulting in a significant proportion of susceptible adults. High rates of vaccine coverage in the United States have eliminated discernible seasonality of varicella. Following implementation of universal immunization in the United States in 1995, varicella incidence declined by approximately 98% in all age groups as a result of personal and herd immunity.

The age of peak varicella incidence has shifted from children younger than 10 years to children 10 through 14 years of age. Immunity to wild type varicella generally is lifelong. Symptomatic reinfection is uncommon in immunocompetent people. Asymptomatic primary infection is unusual.

Immunocompromised people with primary (varicella) or reactivated (herpes zoster) infection are at increased risk of severe disease. Severe varicella and disseminated zoster are more likely to develop in children with congenital T-lymphocyte defects or acquired immunodeficiency syndrome than in people with B-lymphocyte abnormalities. Other groups of pediatric patients who may experience more severe or complicated varicella include infants, adolescents, patients with chronic cutaneous or pulmonary disorders, and patients receiving systemic corticosteroids or other immunosuppressive therapy or long-term salicylate therapy.

Patients are considered contagious from 1 to 2 days before onset of the rash until all lesions have dried/crusted.

The **incubation period** usually is 14 to 16 days, with a range of 10 to 21 days after exposure to rash. The **incubation period** may be prolonged for as long as 28 days after receipt of Varicella-Zoster Immune Globulin or Immune Globulin Intravenous (IGIV), and may be shortened in immunocompromised patients. Varicella can develop after birth in infants born to mothers with active varicella around the time of delivery; the usual interval from onset of rash in a mother to onset in her neonate is 9 to 15 days.

Table 3.84. Diagnostic Tests for Varicella-Zoster Virus (VZV) Infection

Test	Specimen	Comments
PCR	Vesicular swabs or scrapings, scabs from crusted lesions, biopsy tissue, CSF	Very sensitive method. Specific for VZV. Methods have been designed that distinguish vaccine strain from wild-type (see text).
DFA	Vesicle scraping, swab of lesion base (must include cells)	Specific for VZV. More rapid and more sensitive than culture, less sensitive than PCR.
Viral culture	Vesicular fluid, CSF, biopsy tissue	Distinguishes VZV from HSV. High cost, limited availability, requires up to a week for result. Least sensitive.
Serology (IgG)	Acute and convalescent serum specimens for IgG	Specific for VZV. Commercial assays generally have low sensitivity to reliably detect vaccine-induced immunity.
Serology (IgM)	Acute serum specimens for IgM	IgM serology is less specific than IgG serology. IgM inconsistently detected. Not reliable method for routine confirmation.

CSF indicates cerebrospinal fluid; DFA, direct fluorescent antibody; HSV, herpes simplex virus; IgG, immunoglobulin G; IgM, immunoglobulin M; PCR, polymerase chain reaction.

DIAGNOSTIC TESTS: Diagnostic tests for VZV are summarized in Table 3.84. Vesicular fluid or a scab can be used to identify VZV using a polymerase chain reaction (PCR) test, which currently is the diagnostic method of choice. During the acute phase of illness, VZV also can be identified by polymerase chain reaction (PCR) assay of saliva or buccal swab specimens, although VZV is more likely to be detected in vesicular fluid or scabs. VZV can be demonstrated by direct fluorescent antibody (DFA) assay, using scrapings of a vesicle base early in the eruption or by viral isolation in cell culture from vesicular fluid. Viral culture and DFA assay both are much less sensitive than PCR assay. PCR testing that discriminates between vaccine and wild type VZV is available free of charge through the specialized reference laboratory at the Centers for Disease Control and Prevention (CDC [404-639-0066]), through a safety research program sponsored by Merck & Co (1-800-672-6372), and from 4 state public health laboratories serving as vaccine-preventable disease reference centers (Wisconsin, Minnesota, California, and New York).

A significant increase (4-fold increase in titer) in serum varicella immunoglobulin (Ig) G antibody between acute and convalescent samples by any standard serologic assay can confirm a diagnosis retrospectively, but this may not reliably occur in immunocompromised people (see Care of Exposed People, p 836). However, diagnosis of varicella by serologic testing seldom is indicated. Commercially available enzyme immunoassay (EIA) tests usually are not sufficiently sensitive to demonstrate reliably a vaccine-induced antibody response, and therefore, routine postvaccination serologic testing is not recommended. Commercial IgM tests are not reliable for routine confirmation or ruling out of acute infection because of potential false-negative and false-positive results.

TREATMENT: Nonspecific therapies for varicella include keeping fingernails short to prevent trauma and secondary bacterial infection from scratching, frequent bathing, application of lotion to reduce pruritus, and acetaminophen for fever. Children with varicella should not receive salicylates or salicylate-containing products (eg, aspirin, bismuth-subsalicylate) because these products increase the risk of Reye syndrome. Salicylate therapy should be stopped if possible in an unimmunized child who is exposed to varicella. Treatment with ibuprofen is controversial, because some data suggest an association with life-threatening streptococcal skin infections, perhaps because of delays in recognition, and should be avoided if possible.

The decision to use antiviral therapy and the route and duration of therapy should be determined by host factors and extent of infection. Antiviral drugs have a limited window of opportunity to affect the outcome of VZV infection. In immunocompetent hosts, most virus replication has stopped by 72 hours after onset of rash; the duration of replication may be extended in immunocompromised hosts. Oral acyclovir and valacyclovir are not recommended for routine use in otherwise healthy younger children with varicella, because their use results in only a modest decrease in symptoms. Antiviral therapy should be considered for otherwise healthy people at increased risk of moderate to severe varicella, such as unvaccinated people older than 12 years, those with chronic cutaneous or pulmonary disorders, those receiving long-term salicylate therapy, or those receiving short or intermittent courses of corticosteroids. Some experts also recommend use of oral acyclovir or valacyclovir for secondary household cases in which the disease usually is more severe than in the primary case or in children who have immunocompromised household contacts. Acyclovir therapy should also be considered for children with zoster and the continuing development of new lesions. For recommendations on dosage and duration of therapy, see Non-HIV Antiviral Drugs (p 930).

The American College of Obstetricians and Gynecology recommends that pregnant women with varicella should be considered for treatment to minimize maternal morbidity. No controlled data are available that treatment will impact the likelihood or severity of congenital varicella syndrome. Intravenous acyclovir is recommended for pregnant patients with serious complications of varicella.

Intravenous acyclovir therapy is recommended for immunocompromised patients, including patients being treated with high-dose corticosteroid therapy for more than 14 days. Therapy initiated early in the course of the illness, especially within 24 hours of rash onset, maximizes benefit. Oral acyclovir should not be used to treat immunocompromised children with varicella because of poor oral bioavailability. In the event of national shortages of intravenous acyclovir (as occurred in 2011–2012 and 2019), intravenous ganciclovir or foscarnet may be reasonable alternatives. Valacyclovir (20 mg/kg per dose, with a maximum dose of 1000 mg, administered orally 3 times daily for 5 days) is licensed for treatment of varicella in children 2 through 17 years of age. Some experts have used valacyclovir, with its improved bioavailability compared with oral acyclovir, in selected immunocompromised patients perceived to be at low to moderate risk of developing severe varicella, such as human immunodeficiency virus (HIV)-infected patients with relatively normal concentrations of CD4+ T-lymphocytes and children with leukemia in whom careful follow-up is ensured. Famciclovir is available for treatment of VZV infections in adults, but its efficacy and safety have not been established for children. Although Varicella Zoster Immune Globulin or IGIV, administered shortly after exposure, can prevent or modify the course of disease, immune globulin preparations are not effective treatment once disease is established (see Care of Exposed People, p 836).

Antiviral susceptibility testing is not validated but can be considered in cases of poor response to standard therapy; susceptibility testing requires growth of the virus in cell culture, however, which is challenging with VZV. Infections caused by acyclovir-resistant VZV strains, which generally are rare and limited to immunocompromised hosts with prior prolonged exposure to antiviral therapy or prophylaxis have been successfully treated with parenteral foscarnet.

CONTROL MEASURES:

Evidence of Immunity to Varicella. Evidence of immunity to varicella includes any of the following:
1. Documentation of age-appropriate immunization
   - Preschool-aged children (ie, ≥12 months of age): 1 dose
   - School-aged children, adolescents, and adults: 2 doses
2. Laboratory evidence of immunity or laboratory confirmation of disease
3. Varicella diagnosed by a clinician or verification of history of varicella disease
4. History of herpes zoster diagnosed by a clinician

Isolation and Exclusions

Child Care and School. Children with uncomplicated varicella who have been excluded from school or child care may return when the rash has crusted or, in immunized people without crusts, until no new lesions appear within a 24-hour period. Exclusion of children with zoster whose lesions cannot be covered is based on similar criteria. Zoster lesions that are covered pose little risk to susceptible people, although transmission has been reported.

Hospitalized Patients.

VARICELLA. In addition to standard precautions, airborne and contact precautions are recommended for patients with varicella until all lesions are dry and crusted, typically at least 5 days after onset of rash but a week or longer in immunocompromised patients. In patients with varicella pneumonia, precautions are maintained for the duration of illness. For previously immunized patients with breakthrough varicella with only maculopapular lesions, isolation is recommended until no new such lesions appear within a 24-hour period, even if lesions have not resolved completely. For exposed patients without evidence of immunity (see Evidence of Immunity to Varicella), airborne and contact precautions from 8 until 21 days after exposure to the index patient also are indicated; these precautions should be maintained until 28 days after exposure for those who received Varicella Zoster Immune Globulin or IGIV.

ZOSTER. Airborne and contact precautions are recommended for both immunocompetent and immunocompromised patients with disseminated zoster for the duration of illness. Immunocompromised patients with localized disease require airborne and contact precautions until disseminated infection is ruled out. For immunocompetent patients with localized zoster, standard precautions and complete covering of the lesions (if possible) are indicated until all lesions are crusted.

NEWBORN INFANTS. For neonates born to mothers with varicella or disseminated zoster or to mothers with localized zoster in whom the lesions cannot be covered, airborne and contact precautions are recommended until 21 days of age or until 28 days of age if Varicella Zoster Immune Globulin or IGIV was administered. To minimize risk of transmission to the infant, the mother and the infant should be isolated separately until the mother's vesicles have dried, even if the infant has received Varicella Zoster Immune Globulin. Neither wild-type VZV nor Oka vaccine strain virus has been shown to be transmitted by human milk; expressed/pumped milk from a mother with varicella or zoster can be fed to the infant, provided no lesions are evident on the breast. If the infant develops clinical varicella, the mother may care for the infant. If the neonate is born with varicella, the mother and her newborn infant should be isolated together and discharged home when clinically stable. Infants born to mothers with localized zoster may be in contact with the mother as long as the lesions can be covered. The mother should be advised to practice good hand hygiene before holding her infant.

If an infant is clinically stable for discharge during the potential incubation period and has not yet developed varicella, isolation to complete the 21- or 28-day period may continue at home after ensuring that all relatives and contacts have evidence of immunity to varicella. If the infant needs to see the health care provider during that period, the office should be notified of the need for airborne and contact precautions.

Infants with varicella embryopathy do not require isolation if they do not have active skin lesions.

Care of Exposed People. Potential interventions for people without evidence of immunity exposed to a person with varicella or herpes zoster include: (1) varicella vaccine, administered ideally within 3 days but up to 5 days after exposure; (2) when indicated, Varicella Zoster Immune Globulin; or (3) if the child cannot be immunized and Varicella Zoster Immune Globulin is not indicated, preemptive oral acyclovir or valacyclovir starting day 7 after exposure. These options and their use in different settings are discussed in detail below.

Postexposure Immunization. Varicella vaccine should be administered to healthy people without evidence of immunity who are 12 months or older, including adults, as soon as possible, preferably within 3 days and up to 5 days after exposure. This approach may prevent or modify disease. Patients should be counseled that not all close exposures result in infection, so vaccination even after 3 to 5 days following exposure is still warranted.

Passive Immunoprophylaxis. The decision to administer Varicella Zoster Immune Globulin depends on 3 factors: (1) the likelihood that the exposed person is susceptible to varicella; (2) the probability that a given exposure to varicella or zoster will result in infection; (3) the likelihood that complications of varicella will develop if the person is infected. Fig 3.17 identifies what constitutes a significant exposure and people without evidence of immunity who should receive Varicella Zoster Immune Globulin if exposed, including immunocompromised people, pregnant women, and certain newborn infants. Varicella Zoster Immune Globulin is commercially available in the United States from a broad network of specialty distributors (list available at **www.varizig.com**).

Data are not available regarding the sensitivity and specificity of serologic tests in immunocompromised patients. Detection of VZV IgG after 1 dose of varicella vaccine might not correspond to adequate protection in immunocompromised people, and false-positive results can occur. Therefore, regardless of serologic test results, careful questioning of the child and parents about potential past disease or exposure to disease can be helpful in determining immunity. Administration of Varicella Zoster Immune Globulin is recommended as soon as possible within 10 days to immunocompromised children without evidence of immunity (see Figure 3.17 for dosing). However, the degree and type of

FIG 3.17. MANAGEMENT OF EXPOSURES TO VARICELLA-ZOSTER VIRUS

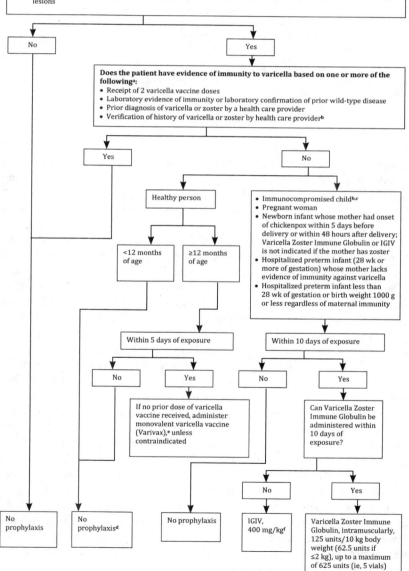

Significant exposure:
- Household: residing in the same household
- Playmate: face-to-face indoor play ≥5 minutes (some experts use >1 hour)
- Newborn infant
- Hospital:
  - Varicella: In same 2- to 4-bed room or adjacent beds in a large ward, face-to-face contact with an infectious staff member or patient, or visit by a person deemed contagious
  - Zoster: Contact (eg, touching or hugging) with a person with disseminated zoster or with uncovered uncrusted lesions

No

Yes

Does the patient have evidence of immunity to varicella based on one or more of the following[a]:
- Receipt of 2 varicella vaccine doses
- Laboratory evidence of immunity or laboratory confirmation of prior wild-type disease
- Prior diagnosis of varicella or zoster by a health care provider
- Verification of history of varicella or zoster by health care provider[b]

Yes

No

Healthy person

- Immunocompromised child[b,c]
- Pregnant woman
- Newborn infant whose mother had onset of chickenpox within 5 days before delivery or within 48 hours after delivery; Varicella Zoster Immune Globulin or IGIV is not indicated if the mother has zoster
- Hospitalized preterm infant (28 wk or more of gestation) whose mother lacks evidence of immunity against varicella
- Hospitalized preterm infant less than 28 wk of gestation or birth weight 1000 g or less regardless of maternal immunity

<12 months of age

≥12 months of age

Within 5 days of exposure

Within 10 days of exposure

No

Yes

No

Yes

If no prior dose of varicella vaccine received, administer monovalent varicella vaccine (Varivax),[e] unless contraindicated

Can Varicella Zoster Immune Globulin be administered within 10 days of exposure?

No

Yes

No prophylaxis

No prophylaxis[d]

No prophylaxis

IGIV, 400 mg/kg[f]

Varicella Zoster Immune Globulin, intramuscularly, 125 units/10 kg body weight (62.5 units if ≤2 kg), up to a maximum of 625 units (ie, 5 vials)

IGIV indicates Immune Globulin Intravenous.

[a] People who receive hematopoietic stem cell transplants should be considered nonimmune regardless of previous history of varicella disease or varicella vaccination in themselves or in their donors.

[b] To verify a history of varicella in an immunocompromised child, health care providers should inquire about an epidemiologic link to another typical varicella case or to a laboratory confirmed case, or evidence of laboratory confirmation. Immunocompromised children who have neither an epidemiologic link nor laboratory confirmation of varicella should not be considered as having a valid history of disease.

[c] Immunocompromised children include those with congenital or acquired T-lymphocyte immunodeficiency, including leukemia, lymphoma, and other malignant neoplasms affecting the bone marrow or lymphatic system; children receiving immunosuppressive therapy, including ≥2 mg/kg/day of systemic prednisone (or its equivalent) for ≥14 days, and certain biologic response modifiers; all children with human immunodeficiency virus (HIV) infection regardless of CD4+ T-lymphocyte percentage; and all hematopoietic stem cell transplant patients regardless of pretransplant immunity status.

[d] If the exposed person is an adolescent or adult, has chronic illness, or there are other compelling reasons to try to avert varicella, some experts recommend preemptive therapy with oral acyclovir (see p 000 for dosing). For exposed people ≥12 months of age, vaccination is recommended for protection against subsequent exposures.

[e] If 1 prior dose of varicella vaccine has been received, a second dose should be administered at ≥4 years of age. If the exposure occurred during an outbreak, a second dose is recommended for preschool-aged children younger than 4 years for outbreak control if at least 3 months have passed after the first dose.

[f] If Varicella Zoster Immune Globulin and IGIV are not available, some experts recommend preemptive therapy with oral valacyclovir or oral acyclovir; see p 838 for dosing.

immunosuppression should be considered in making this decision, and consultation with pediatric infectious diseases or immunology specialists can assist in decision making.

Patients receiving monthly high-dose IGIV (400 mg/kg or greater) at regular intervals are likely to be protected if the last dose of IGIV was administered 3 weeks or less before exposure.

Any patient to whom Varicella Zoster Immune Globulin is administered to prevent varicella subsequently should receive age-appropriate varicella vaccine, provided that receipt of live vaccines is not contraindicated. Administration of varicella; measles, mumps, and rubella (MMR); and measles, mumps, rubella, and varicella (MMRV) vaccines should be delayed until 5 months after Varicella Zoster Immune Globulin administration. Varicella vaccine is not needed if the patient develops varicella despite receipt of Varicella Zoster Immune Globulin.

Chemoprophylaxis. Some experts recommend preemptive antiviral therapy in select circumstances for mildly immunocompromised patients without evidence of immunity or for immunocompetent patients for whom varicella prevention is desired (eg, healthy older adolescent or adult contacts for whom vaccination is not possible) who have been exposed to varicella or herpes zoster (Fig 3.17). Acyclovir (20 mg/kg per dose, administered orally 4 times per day, with a maximum daily dose of 3200 mg) or valacyclovir (20 mg/kg per dose, administered orally 3 times per day, with a maximum daily dose of 3000 mg) beginning 7 days after exposure and continuing for 7 days can be used. Limited data on acyclovir as postexposure prophylaxis are available for healthy children, and no studies have been performed for adults or immunocompromised people. VZV seropositive patients receiving intensive and/or myeloablative chemotherapy routinely receive antiviral prophylaxis; children receiving cytomegalovirus prophylaxis or treatment with valganciclovir, ganciclovir, or foscarnet do not require additional antiviral prophylaxis against VZV.

Hospital Exposures. The CDC recommends health care institutions evaluate employees proactively for evidence of immunity to varicella and establish protocols and recommendations for vaccinating and managing health care personnel following workplace exposures. If an exposure occurs in the hospital to an infected person by a patient, health care professional, or visitor, the following control measures are recommended:

- Health care professionals, patients, and visitors who have been exposed (see Fig 3.17, p 837) and who lack evidence of immunity to varicella should be identified.
- Varicella immunization is recommended for people without evidence of immunity, provided there are no contraindications to vaccine use.
- Varicella Zoster Immune Globulin should be administered to appropriate candidates (see Fig 3.17, p 837) up to day 10 after exposure.
- If vaccine cannot be administered and Varicella Zoster Immune Globulin is not indicated, preemptive oral acyclovir or valaciclovir can be considered.
- All exposed patients without evidence of immunity should be discharged as soon as possible. Patients who remain hospitalized should be isolated from day 8 through 21 after exposure or through day 28 if they received Varicella Zoster Immune Globulin.
- Health care professionals who have received 2 doses of vaccine and who are exposed to VZV should self-monitor or be monitored daily during days 8 through 21 after exposure through the employee health program or by infection-control staff to determine clinical status. They should be restricted from work immediately if symptoms such as fever, headache, other constitutional symptoms, or any suspicious skin lesions occur.
- Health care professionals who have received only 1 dose of vaccine and who are exposed to VZV should receive the second dose with a single-antigen live attenuated varicella vaccine (ie, not given in combination as in MMRV vaccine), preferably within 3 to 5 days of exposure, provided at least 4 weeks have elapsed after the first dose. After immunization, management is similar to that of 2-dose vaccine recipients.
- Health care professionals who lack evidence of immunity should receive varicella vaccine as soon as possible and be restricted from work from day 8 through 21 after exposure or through day 28 if they received Varicella Zoster Immune Globulin.

Previously immunized health care professionals who develop breakthrough infection should be considered infectious until vesicular lesions have crusted or, if they had maculopapular lesions, until no new lesions appear within a 24-hour period.

Exposure of Newborn Infants

Infant Exposure to Varicella or Zoster. Preterm infants and term infants whose mothers had varicella in the immediate peripartum period may need Varicella Zoster Immune Globulin (see Figure 3.17, p 837). For healthy term infants exposed postnatally to mothers with varicella outside of the immediate perinatal period or who have zoster, Varicella Zoster Immune Globulin is not indicated. However, some experts advise use of Varicella Zoster Immune Globulin for exposed newborn infants within the first 2 weeks of life whose mothers do not have evidence of immunity to varicella.

Active Immunization.[1]

Vaccine. Varicella vaccine is a live attenuated vaccine licensed in 1995 by the FDA for use in healthy people 12 months or older who have not had varicella illness. Quadrivalent MMRV vaccine was licensed in September 2005 by the FDA for use in healthy children 12 months through 12 years of age.

---

[1]Centers for Disease Control and Prevention. Prevention of varicella: recommendations of the Advisory Committee on Immunization Practices (ACIP). *MMWR Recomm Rep.* 2007;56(RR-4):1–40

Dose and Administration. The recommended dose of vaccine is 0.5 mL, administered subcutaneously.

Immunogenicity. Approximately 76% to 85% of immunized healthy children older than 12 months develop a humoral immune response to VZV at levels considered associated with protection after a single dose of varicella vaccine. Seroprotection rates and cell-mediated immune responses approach 100% after 2 doses.

Effectiveness. The effectiveness of 1 dose of varicella vaccine is about 82% against any clinical varicella and 98% against severe disease. Two doses of vaccine demonstrated 92% effectiveness against any clinical varicella.

Simultaneous Administration With Other Vaccines or Antiviral Agents. Varicella-containing vaccines may be administered simultaneously with other childhood immunizations recommended for children 12 through 15 months of age and 4 through 6 years of age (**https://aapredbook.aappublications.org/site/resources/izschedules. xhtml**). If not administered at the same visit or as MMRV vaccine, the interval between administration of a varicella-containing vaccine and MMR vaccine should be at least 28 days (see Table 1.9, p 33). The minimal interval between MMRV vaccine doses is 3 months. Because of susceptibility of vaccine virus to acyclovir, valacyclovir, or famciclovir, these antiviral agents may interfere with immunogenicity and, thus, should be avoided from 1 day before to 21 days (the outer limit of likely viral replication) after receipt of a varicella-containing vaccine.

Adverse Events. Varicella vaccine is safe; reactions generally are mild and occur with an overall frequency of approximately 5% to 35%. Approximately 20% to 25% of immunized children will experience minor injection site reactions (eg, pain, redness, swelling). In approximately 1% to 3% of immunized children, a localized rash develops, and in an additional 3% to 5%, a generalized varicella-like rash develops. These rashes typically consist of 2 to 5 lesions and may be maculopapular rather than vesicular; lesions usually appear 5 to 26 days after immunization, usually at or near the injection site when localized. After MMRV or monovalent varicella vaccine plus MMR, a measles-like rash was reported in 2% to 3% of recipients. Fever was reported in a higher proportion after the first dose of MMRV than after the first dose of monovalent varicella vaccine plus MMR (22% vs 15%) in young children. Both fever and measles-like rash usually occurred within 5 to 12 days of immunization, were of short duration, and resolved without sequelae.

A slightly increased risk of febrile seizures is associated with the higher likelihood of fever following the first dose of MMRV compared with MMR and monovalent varicella vaccine. One additional febrile seizure is expected to occur per approximately 2300 to 2600 young children immunized with a first dose of MMRV compared with a first dose of MMR and monovalent varicella vaccine. After the second vaccine dose administered in older children (4 to 6 years of age), there were no differences in incidence of fever, rash, or febrile seizures among recipients of MMRV vaccine compared with recipients of simultaneous MMR and varicella vaccines.[1]

Breakthrough Disease. Breakthrough disease is defined as a case of infection with wild-type VZV occurring more than 42 days after immunization. Varicella in vaccine recipients usually is very mild, with rash frequently atypical (predominantly maculopapular) with a median of fewer than 50 lesions), a lower rate of fever, and faster recovery than

---

[1]Centers for Disease Control and Prevention. Use of combination measles, mumps, rubella, and varicella vaccine: recommendations of the Advisory Committee on Immunization Practices (ACIP). *MMWR Recomm Rep.* 2010;59(RR-3):1-12

disease in unimmunized children. It may be mistaken for other conditions, such as insect bites or poison ivy.

Herpes Zoster After Immunization. Vaccine-strain VZV can cause herpes zoster in immunocompetent and immunocompromised people. However, data from postlicensure surveillance indicate that the age-specific risk of herpes zoster is much lower among immunocompetent children immunized with varicella vaccine than among children who have had natural varicella infection.

Transmission of Vaccine-Strain VZV. Vaccine-strain VZV transmission to contacts is rare. In all cases in which transmission has occurred, the immunized person had a rash following vaccine. Some experts believe that immunocompromised people with skin lesions that are presumed to be attributable to vaccine virus should receive acyclovir or valacyclovir treatment.

Recommendations for Immunization.

Children 12 Months Through 12 Years of Age. Both monovalent varicella vaccine and MMRV have been licensed for use for healthy children 12 months through 12 years of age.[1] Children in this age group should receive two 0.5-mL doses of monovalent varicella vaccine or MMRV administered subcutaneously, separated by at least 3 months. However, provided the second dose is administered a minimum 28 days after the first dose, it does not need to be repeated.

All healthy children should receive the first dose of varicella-containing vaccine at 12 through 15 months of age. The second dose of vaccine is recommended routinely when children are 4 through 6 years of age (ie, before a child enters kindergarten or first grade) but can be administered at an earlier age. The American Academy of Pediatrics expresses no preference between MMR plus monovalent varicella vaccine or MMRV for toddlers receiving their first immunization of this kind. Parents should be counseled about the rare possibility of their child developing a febrile seizure 1 to 2 weeks after immunization with MMRV for the first immunizing dose. For the second dose at 4 through 6 years of age, MMRV generally is preferred over MMR plus monovalent varicella to minimize the number of injections. A catch-up second dose of varicella vaccine should be offered to all children 7 years and older who have received only 1 dose.

People 13 Years or Older. Immunocompetent individuals 13 years or older without evidence of immunity should receive two 0.5-mL doses of monovalent varicella vaccine, separated by at least 28 days. For people who previously received only 1 dose of varicella vaccine, a second dose is necessary. Only monovalent varicella vaccine is licensed for use in this age group.

Contraindications and Precautions.

Allergy to Vaccine Components. Varicella vaccine should not be administered to people who have had an anaphylactic or severe allergic reaction to any component of the vaccine, including gelatin and neomycin, or to a previous dose of a varicella-containing vaccine.

Immunization of Immunocompromised Patients.

GENERAL RECOMMENDATIONS.[2] Varicella vaccine (as a 2-dose regimen if there is sufficient time) should be administered to immunocompetent patients without

---

[1]Centers for Disease Control and Prevention. Use of combination measles, mumps, rubella, and varicella vaccine: recommendations of the Advisory Committee on Immunization Practices (ACIP). *MMWR Recomm Rep.* 2010;59(RR-3):1-12

[2]Rubin LG, Levin MJ, Ljungman P, et al. 2013 IDSA clinical practice guideline for vaccination of the immunocompromised host. *Clin Infect Dis.* 2014;58(3):e44-e100

evidence of varicella immunity, if it can be administered ≥4 weeks before initiating immunosuppressive therapy. Varicella vaccine should not be administered to highly immunocompromised patients. Certain categories of patients (eg, patients with HIV infection without severe immunosuppression or with a primary immune deficiency disorder without defective T-lymphocyte–mediated immunity, such as primary complement component deficiency disorder, isolated impairment of humoral immunity, or chronic granulomatous disease [CGD]) should receive varicella vaccine. Immunodeficiency should be excluded before immunization in children with a family history of hereditary immunodeficiency.

In people with possible altered immunity, only monovalent varicella vaccine (not MMRV) should be used for immunization against varicella. The Oka vaccine strain remains susceptible to acyclovir, and if a high-risk patient develops vaccine-related rash, then acyclovir or valacyclovir may be used as treatment.

MALIGNANCY.[1] The interval until immune reconstruction varies with the intensity and type of immunosuppressive therapy, radiation therapy, underlying disease, and other factors, complicating the ability to make a broadly applicable recommendation for an interval after cessation of immunosuppressive therapy when live-virus vaccines can be administered safely and effectively. Current recommendations are for patients to be vaccinated with varicella vaccine when in remission and at least 3 months after cancer chemotherapy, with evidence of restored immunocompetence. In regimens that included anti–B-lymphocyte antibodies, vaccinations should be delayed at least 6 months.

TRANSPLANT RECIPIENTS.[1] A 2-dose series of varicella vaccine should be administered a minimum of 24 months after hematopoietic stem cell transplant to varicella-seronegative patients who do not have graft-versus-host disease, are considered immunocompetent, and whose last dose of IGIV was 8 to 11 months previously. Varicella immunization generally is not recommended for solid organ transplant recipients after transplantation, although this is an evolving area, especially for certain organs.[2]

HIV INFECTION.[3] The live-virus MMR vaccine and monovalent varicella vaccine can be administered to asymptomatic HIV-infected children and adolescents without severe immunosuppression (that is, can be administered to children 1 through 13 years of age with a CD4+ T-lymphocyte percentage ≥15% and to adolescents ≥14 years with a CD4+ T-lymphocyte count ≥200 lymphocytes/mm^3). Eligible children should receive 2 doses of single-antigen varicella vaccine at the appropriate intervals. The quadrivalent MMRV vaccine should not be administered to any HIV-infected patient, regardless of degree of immunosuppression, because of lack of safety data in this population.

---

[1]Rubin LG, Levin MJ, Ljungman P, et al. 2013 IDSA clinical practice guideline for vaccination of the immunocompromised host. *Clin Infect Dis.* 2014;58(3):e44-e100

[2]Danziger-Isakov L, Kumar D, AST ID Community of Practice. Vaccination of solid organ transplant candidates and recipients: Guidelines from the American society of transplantation infectious diseases community of practice. *Clin Transplant.* 2019;33(9):e13563

[3]Panel on Opportunistic Infections in HIV-Exposed and HIV-Infected Children. Guidelines for the Prevention and Treatment of Opportunistic Infections in HIV-Exposed and HIV-Infected Children. Department of Health and Human Services. Available at: **https://clinicalinfo.hiv.gov/sites/default/files/inline-files/oi_guidelines_pediatrics.pdf**

CHILDREN RECEIVING CORTICOSTEROIDS. Varicella vaccine should not be administered to people who are receiving high doses of systemic corticosteroids (2 mg/kg per day or more of prednisone or its equivalent or 20 mg/day of prednisone or its equivalent) for 14 days or more. The recommended interval between discontinuation of high-dose corticosteroid therapy and immunization with varicella vaccine is at least 1 month. Varicella vaccine may be administered to individuals receiving only inhaled, nasal, or topical steroids.

HOUSEHOLDS WITH POTENTIAL CONTACT WITH IMMUNOCOMPROMISED PEOPLE. Household contacts of immunocompromised people should be immunized if they have no evidence of immunity to decrease the likelihood that wild-type VZV will be introduced into the household. No precautions are needed following immunization of healthy people who do not develop a rash. Immunized people in whom a postimmunization rash develops should avoid direct contact with an immunocompromised host who lacks evidence of immunity for the duration of the rash.

Pregnancy and Lactation. Varicella vaccine should not be administered to pregnant women, because the possible effects on fetal development are unknown, although no cases of congenital varicella syndrome or patterns of malformation have been identified after inadvertent immunization of pregnant women. Pregnancy should be avoided for at least 1 month after immunization. A pregnant mother or other household member is not a contraindication for immunization of a child in the household. Breastfeeding is not a contraindication to immunization.

Immune Globulin. Whether Immune Globulin (IG) can interfere with varicella vaccine-induced immunity is unknown, although IG can interfere with immunity induction by measles vaccine. Pending additional data, varicella vaccine should be withheld for the same intervals after receipt of any form of IG or other blood product as for measles vaccine (see Measles, p 503; and Table 1.11, p 40). Conversely, IG should be withheld for at least 2 weeks after receipt of varicella vaccine.

Salicylates. No cases of Reye syndrome have been reported following varicella vaccination with >140 million doses distributed in the United States. However, because use of salicylates during varicella infection is associated with Reye syndrome, the vaccine manufacturer recommends that salicylates be avoided for 6 weeks after administration of varicella vaccine.

VIBRIO INFECTIONS

Cholera
(Vibrio cholerae)

CLINICAL MANIFESTATIONS: Cholera is characterized by voluminous watery diarrhea and rapid onset of life-threatening dehydration. Hypovolemic shock may occur within hours of the onset of diarrhea. Stools have a characteristic rice-water appearance, are white-tinged with small flecks of mucus, and contain high concentrations of sodium, potassium, chloride, and bicarbonate. Vomiting is a common feature of cholera. Fever and abdominal cramps usually are absent. In addition to dehydration and hypovolemia, common complications of cholera include hypokalemia, metabolic acidosis, and hypoglycemia, particularly in children. Although severe cholera is a distinctive illness characterized by profuse diarrhea and rapid dehydration, people infected with toxigenic *Vibrio cholerae* O1 may have either no symptoms or mild to moderate diarrhea lasting 3 to 7 days.

ETIOLOGY: *V cholerae* is a curved or comma-shaped motile gram-negative rod. There are more than 200 *V cholerae* serogroups, some of which carry the cholera toxin (CT) gene. Although those serogroups with the CT gene and others without the CT gene can cause acute watery diarrhea, only toxin-producing serogroups O1 and O139 have caused epidemic cholera, with O1 causing the vast majority of cases of cholera. *V cholerae* O1 is classified into 2 biotypes, classical and El Tor, and 2 major serotypes, Ogawa and Inaba. Since 1992, toxigenic *V cholerae* serogroup O139 has been recognized as a cause of epidemic cholera in Asia. Aside from the substitution of the O139 for the O1 antigen, the organism is almost identical to *V cholerae* O1 El Tor. All other serogroups of *V cholerae* are known collectively as *V cholerae* non-O1/non-O139. Toxin-producing strains of *V cholerae* non-O1/non-O139 can cause sporadic cases of severe dehydrating diarrheal illness but have not caused large outbreaks of cholera. Non–toxin-producing strains of *V cholerae* non-O1/non-O139 are associated with sporadic cases of gastroenteritis, sepsis, and rare cases of wound infection (discussed in Other Vibrio Infections, p 847).

EPIDEMIOLOGY: Since the early 1800s, there have been 7 cholera pandemics. The current pandemic began in 1961 and is caused by *V cholerae* O1 El Tor. Molecular epidemiology shows that this pandemic has occurred in 3 successive waves, with each one spreading from South Asia to other regions in Asia, Africa, and the Western Pacific Islands (Oceania). In 1991, epidemic cholera caused by toxigenic *V cholerae* O1 El Tor appeared in Peru and spread to most countries in South, Central, and North America, causing more than 1 million cases of cholera before subsiding. In 2010, *V cholerae* O1 El Tor was introduced into Haiti, on the island of Hispaniola, initiating a massive epidemic of cholera with more than 650 000 cases and 8000 deaths. In the United States, sporadic cases resulting from travel to or ingestion of contaminated food transported from regions with endemic cholera are reported, including at least 40 cases imported from Hispaniola since 2010. Domestically acquired cases in the United States have been reported from eating Gulf coast seafood.

Humans are the only documented natural host, but free-living *V cholerae* organisms can persist in the aquatic environment. Infection primarily is acquired by ingestion of large numbers of organisms from contaminated water or food (particularly raw or undercooked shellfish, raw or partially dried fish, or moist grains or vegetables held at ambient temperature). People with low gastric acidity and with blood group O are at increased risk of severe cholera infection.

The median **incubation period** usually is 1 to 2 days, with a range of a few hours to 5 days.

DIAGNOSTIC TESTS: *V cholerae* can be cultured from fecal specimens (preferred) or vomitus plated on thiosulfate citrate bile salts sucrose agar. Because most laboratories in the United States do not culture routinely for *V cholerae* or other *Vibrio* organisms, clinicians should request appropriate cultures for clinically suspected cases. Isolates of *V cholerae* should be sent to a state health department laboratory for confirmation and then forwarded to the Centers for Disease Control and Prevention (CDC) for confirmation, serogrouping, and detection of the cholera toxin gene (**www.cdc.gov/laboratory/**

specimen-submission/detail.html?CDCTestCode=CDC-10119). Tests to detect serum antibodies to *V cholerae,* such as the vibriocidal assay and an anticholera toxin enzyme-linked immunoassay, are available at the CDC, subject to preapproval. Both assays require submission of acute and convalescent serum specimens and, thus, provide a retrospective diagnosis. A fourfold increase in vibriocidal antibody titers between acute and convalescent sera suggests the diagnosis of cholera. Several commercial tests for rapid antigen detection of *V cholerae* O1 and O139 in stool specimens have been developed. These *V cholerae* O1 and O139 rapid diagnostic tests (RDTs) have sensitivities ranging from approximately 80% to 97% and specificities of approximately 70% to 90% compared with culture on thiosulfate citrate bile salts sucrose agar. RDTs are not a substitute for stool culture but potentially provide a rapid presumptive indication of a suspect cholera outbreak in regions where stool culture is not immediately available. Multiplex polymerase chain reaction (PCR) panels have been cleared by the US Food and Drug Administration for detection of various bacteria, parasites, and viruses associated with gastrointestinal tract infections, and some can specifically detect *V cholerae* from unpreserved stool specimens and/or stool specimens preserved in Cary Blair media.

TREATMENT: Timely and appropriate rehydration therapy is the cornerstone of management of cholera and reduces the mortality of severe cholera from more than 10% to less than 0.5%. Rehydration therapy should be based on World Health Organization (WHO) standards, with the goal of replacing the estimated fluid deficit within 3 to 4 hours of initial presentation. In patients with severe dehydration, isotonic intravenous fluids should be used, and lactated Ringer solution is the preferred commercially available option.[1] For patients without severe dehydration, oral rehydration therapy using the WHO's reduced-osmolality oral rehydration solution (ORS) has been the standard, but data suggest that rice-based ORS or amylase-resistant starch ORS are more effective.

Antimicrobial therapy decreases the duration and volume of diarrhea and decreases the shedding of viable bacteria. Antimicrobial therapy should be considered for people who are moderately to severely ill. The choice of antimicrobial therapy should be made on the basis of the age of the patient (Table 3.85) as well as prevailing patterns of antimicrobial resistance. In cases in which prevailing patterns of resistance are unknown, antimicrobial susceptibility testing should be performed and monitored. Zinc supplementation should be considered as an adjunct to rehydration in children (**www.cdc.gov/cholera/treatment/zinc-treatment.html**).

ISOLATION OF THE HOSPITALIZED PATIENT: In addition to standard precautions, contact precautions are indicated for diapered children or incontinent people for the duration of illness.

CONTROL MEASURES:

Hygiene. Disinfection of drinking water through chlorination or boiling prevents waterborne transmission of V cholerae. Thoroughly cooking crabs, oysters, and other shellfish from the Gulf Coast before eating is recommended to decrease the likelihood of transmission. Foods such as fish, rice, or grain gruels should be refrigerated promptly and thoroughly reheated before eating, and fruits and vegetables should be peeled before eating. The use of latrines or burying feces is recommended, and defecation should be avoided

---

[1]World Health Organization. *The Treatment of Diarrhoea, a Manual for Physicians and Other Senior Health Workers.* 4th Rev. WHO/FCH/CAH/05.1. Geneva, Switzerland: World Health Organization; 2005

Table 3.85. Antibiotics for Suspected Cholera

Antibiotic	Pediatric Dose[a]	Adult Dose	Comment(s)
Doxycycline	4.4 mg/kg, single dose	300 mg, single dose	Use should be in epidemics caused by susceptible isolates. Not recommended for pregnant women.
Ciprofloxacin[b]	15 mg/kg, twice daily for 3 days (single dose 20 mg/kg has been used)	500 mg, twice daily for 3 days	Decreased susceptibility to fluoroquinolones is associated with treatment failure. Ciprofloxacin is not recommended in children and pregnant women.
Azithromycin	20 mg/kg, single dose	1 g, single dose	
Erythromycin	12.5 mg/kg, 4 times/day for 3 days	250 mg, 4 times/day for 3 days	
Tetracycline[c]	12.5 mg/kg, 4 times/day for 3 days	500 mg, 4 times/day for 3 days	

[a] Not to exceed adult dose.
[b] Fluoroquinolones are not approved for children for children younger than 18 years for this indication.
[c] For use in children ≥8 y.

near any body of water. Appropriate hand hygiene after defecating and before preparing or eating food is important for preventing transmission.

Treatment of Contacts. Although administration of appropriate antimicrobial agents within 24 hours of identification of the index case may prevent additional cases of cholera among household contacts, chemoprophylaxis of contacts currently is not recommended.

Vaccine. A single-dose, live attenuated monovalent oral vaccine (Vaxchora) has been approved by the US Food and Drug Administration and is available in the United States for use for travelers 2 through 64 years of age who are traveling to areas where cholera is a risk. In addition to following safe food and water precautions, the Advisory Committee on Immunization Practices of the CDC recommends cholera vaccine for adult travelers (18 through 64 years old) to an area of active cholera transmission[1] and, as of February 2021, is considering decreasing this recommendation down to 2 years of age. An area of active cholera transmission is defined as a province, state, or other administrative subdivision within a country with endemic or epidemic cholera caused by toxigenic *V cholerae* O1 and includes areas with cholera activity within the past year that are prone to recurrence of cholera epidemics; it does not include areas where rare sporadic cases only have been reported. Information about destinations with active cholera transmission is available at **wwwnc.cdc.gov/travel/.** Note that in December 2020, the manufacturer of Vaxchora temporarily stopped making and selling it; this vaccine may be in limited supply or unavailable.

Three inactivated oral vaccines are approved by the WHO and available outside the United States. Dukoral is a monovalent inactivated vaccine based on heat-killed whole

[1] Wong KK, Burdette E, Mahon BE, Mintz ED, Ryan ET, Reingold AL. Recommendations of the Advisory Committee on Immunization Practices for use of cholera vaccine. *MMWR Morb Mortal Wkly Rep.* 2017;66:482–485. Available at: **http://dx.doi.org/10.15585/mmwr.mm6618a6**

cells of serogroup O1 plus recombinant cholera toxin B subunit. The vaccine also may provide some protection against heat-labile enterotoxigenic *Escherichia coli* infection and is primarily used by travelers to areas with endemic cholera. Children between 2 and 6 years of age require 3 doses, and adults and children 6 years and older require 2 doses at least 1 week apart. Two bivalent (O1 and O139) vaccines, ShanChol and Euvichol, provide durable protection in older children and adults but do not provide significant protection in young children. In 2011, the WHO initiated a global oral cholera vaccine stockpile, comprised of bivalent vaccine, to allow for its rapid deployment during cholera epidemics and other emergencies. Instructions regarding access to the stockpile are available at **www.who.int/cholera/vaccines/ocv_stockpile_2013/en/.**

Cholera immunization is not required for travelers entering the United States from cholera-affected areas, and the WHO no longer recommends immunization for travel to or from areas with cholera infection. No country requires cholera vaccine for entry.

Public Health Reporting. Confirmed cases of cholera must be reported to health authorities in any country in which they occur and were contracted. Local and state health departments should be notified immediately of presumed or known cases of cholera.

Other *Vibrio* Infections

CLINICAL MANIFESTATIONS: Illness attributable to the following (mostly nontoxigenic) species of the *Vibrionaceae* family is known as vibriosis: (1) *Vibrio parahaemolyticus, Vibrio vulnificus,* and other *Vibrio* species; (2) nontoxigenic *Vibrio cholerae*; (3) toxigenic *Vibrio cholerae* O75 and O141; and (4) members of the *Vibrionaceae* family that are not in the genus *Vibrio* (eg, *Grimontia hollisae*). Associated clinical syndromes include gastroenteritis, wound infection, and septicemia. Gastroenteritis is the most common syndrome and is characterized by acute onset of watery nonbloody stools and crampy abdominal pain. Approximately half of affected people will have low-grade fever, headache, and chills; approximately 30% will have vomiting. Spontaneous recovery follows in 2 to 5 days. Wound infections typically start as cellulitis with vesicles and can progress to hemorrhagic bullae, necrosis, and/or necrotizing fasciitis. Septicemia can be primary or follow gastroenteritis or wound infection and often is fulminant and accompanied by development of metastatic skin lesions within 36 hours. Risk factors for severe wound infections and for septicemia include liver disease, iron overload, hemolytic anemia, chronic renal failure, diabetes mellitus, low gastric acidity, and immunosuppression. Various otolaryngologic manifestations attributable to *Vibrio alginolyticus* have been linked to swimming in salt water.

ETIOLOGY: *Vibrio* organisms are facultatively anaerobic, motile, gram-negative bacilli that are tolerant of salt. The most commonly reported nontoxigenic *Vibrio* species associated with diarrhea are *V parahaemolyticus* and *V cholerae* non-O1/non-O139. *V vulnificus* typically causes primary septicemia and severe wound infections, but the other species also can cause these syndromes. *V alginolyticus* typically causes wound and ear infections, with ear infections more common in children.

EPIDEMIOLOGY: *Vibrio* species are natural inhabitants of marine and estuarine environments. In temperate climates, most noncholera *Vibrio* infections occur during summer and autumn months, when *Vibrio* populations in seawater are highest. Gastroenteritis usually follows ingestion of raw or undercooked seafood, especially oysters, clams, crabs, and shrimp. Wound infections usually are attributable to *V vulnificus* and can result from exposure of a preexisting wound to contaminated seawater or from punctures resulting from handling of contaminated fish or shellfish. Exposure to contaminated water during natural disasters, such as hurricanes, has resulted in wound infections. Person-to-person transmission has not been reported. Infections associated with noncholera *Vibrio* organisms became nationally notifiable since January 2007. It is estimated that 80 000 cases, 500 hospitalizations, and 100 deaths from vibriosis occur each year in the United States.

The **incubation period** for gastroenteritis is typically 24 hours (with a range of 5 to 92 hours) and is 1 to 7 days for wound infections and septicemia.

DIAGNOSTIC TESTS: Depending on the clinical syndrome, *Vibrio* organisms can be isolated from stool, wound exudates, or blood. Because identification of the organism requires special techniques, laboratory personnel should be notified when infection with *Vibrio* species is suspected. Multiplex molecular panels are available, but the specificity in some diagnostic tests is poor. Infection should be confirmed by culture, and isolates (or clinical specimens if isolates are not available on a positive nonculture diagnostic test) should be forwarded as required to the local or state public health laboratory for characterization and outbreak investigation.

TREATMENT: Diarrhea typically is mild and self-limited and requires only oral rehydration. Wound infections require prompt surgical débridement of necrotic tissue, if present. Antimicrobial therapy is indicated for severe diarrhea, wound infection, and septicemia. Septicemia with or without hemorrhagic bullae and wound infections should be treated with a third-generation cephalosporin plus either doxycycline or ciprofloxacin. Severe diarrhea should be treated with doxycycline or ciprofloxacin. Doxycycline can be used for short durations (ie, 21 days or less) without regard to patient age (see Tetracyclines, p 866). A combination of trimethoprim-sulfamethoxazole and an aminoglycoside is an alternative regimen.

ISOLATION OF THE HOSPITALIZED PATIENT: In addition to standard precautions, contact precautions are recommended for diapered or incontinent children.

CONTROL MEASURES: Seafood should be cooked fully and refrigerated if not consumed immediately. Cross-contamination of cooked seafood by contact with surfaces and containers contaminated by raw seafood should be avoided. Uncooked mollusks and crustaceans should be handled with care, and gloves can be worn during preparation. Abrasions suffered by ocean bathers should be rinsed with clean fresh water. All children, immunocompromised people, and people with chronic liver disease should avoid eating raw oysters or clams, and all individuals should be advised of risks associated with seawater exposure if a wound is present or likely to occur. Vibriosis is a nationally notifiable disease, and cases should be reported to local or state health departments.

West Nile Virus

CLINICAL MANIFESTATIONS: An estimated 70% to 80% of people infected with West Nile virus (WNV) are asymptomatic. Most symptomatic people experience an acute systemic febrile illness that often includes headache, myalgia, arthralgia, vomiting, diarrhea, or a transient maculopapular rash. Less than 1% of infected people develop neuroinvasive disease, which typically manifests as meningitis, encephalitis, or acute flaccid myelitis. WNV meningitis is indistinguishable clinically from aseptic meningitis caused by other viruses. Patients with WNV encephalitis usually present with fever, headache, seizures, mental status changes, focal neurologic deficits, or movement disorders. WNV acute flaccid myelitis often is clinically and pathologically identical to poliovirus-associated poliomyelitis, with damage of anterior horn cells, and may progress to respiratory paralysis requiring mechanical ventilation. WNV-associated Guillain-Barré syndrome also has been reported and can be distinguished from WNV acute flaccid myelitis by clinical manifestations, findings on cerebrospinal fluid analysis, and electrophysiologic testing. Cardiac dysrhythmias, myocarditis, rhabdomyolysis, optic neuritis, uveitis, chorioretinitis, orchitis, pancreatitis, and hepatitis have been described rarely after WNV infection.

Routine clinical laboratory results are nonspecific in WNV infections. In patients with neuroinvasive disease, cerebrospinal fluid (CSF) examination generally shows lymphocytic pleocytosis, but neutrophils may predominate early in the illness. Brain magnetic resonance imaging frequently is normal, but signal abnormalities may be seen in the basal ganglia, thalamus, and brainstem with WNV encephalitis and in the spinal cord with WNV acute flaccid myelitis.

Most patients with WNV nonneuroinvasive disease or meningitis recover completely, but fatigue, malaise, and weakness can linger for weeks or months. Recovery from WNV encephalitis or acute flaccid myelitis often takes weeks to months, and patients commonly have residual neurologic deficits. Among patients with neuroinvasive disease, the overall case-fatality rate is approximately 10% but is significantly higher in WNV encephalitis and acute flaccid myelitis than in WNV meningitis.

Most women known to have been infected with WNV during pregnancy have delivered infants without evidence of infection or clinical abnormalities. Rare cases of congenital infection and probable transmission via human milk (see Breastfeeding and Human Milk, p 107) have been reported. If WNV disease is diagnosed during pregnancy, a detailed examination of the fetus and of the newborn infant should be performed.[1]

ETIOLOGY: WNV is an RNA virus of the *Flaviviridae* family (genus *Flavivirus*) that is related antigenically to St. Louis encephalitis and Japanese encephalitis viruses.

EPIDEMIOLOGY: WNV is an <u>ar</u>thropod <u>borne</u> <u>virus</u> (arbovirus) that is transmitted in an enzootic cycle between mosquitoes and amplifying vertebrate hosts, primarily birds. WNV is transmitted to humans primarily through bites of infected *Culex* mosquitoes. Humans usually do not develop a level or duration of viremia sufficient to infect mosquitoes, and therefore are dead-end hosts. Person-to-person WNV transmission can occur through blood transfusion and solid organ transplantation. Intrauterine and probable breastfeeding transmission have been described rarely. Transmission through percutaneous and mucosal exposure has occurred in laboratory workers and occupational settings.

WNV transmission has been documented on every continent except Antarctica. Since the 1990s, the largest outbreaks of WNV neuroinvasive disease have occurred in the Middle East, Europe, and North America. WNV first was detected in the Western Hemisphere in New York City in 1999 and subsequently spread across the continental United States and Canada. From 1999 through 2018, there were 24 657 cases of WNV neuroinvasive disease reported in the United States, with peaks in national incidence in 2002, 2003, and 2012. WNV is the leading cause of neuroinvasive arboviral disease in the United States. In 2018, there were 1658 cases of WNV neuroinvasive disease reported, more than 11 times the number of neuroinvasive disease cases reported for all other domestic arboviruses combined (eg, Eastern equine encephalitis, Jamestown

---

[1]Centers for Disease Control and Prevention. Interim guidelines for the evaluation of infants born to mothers infected with West Nile virus during pregnancy. *MMWR Morb Mortal Wkly Rep.* 2004;53(7):154-157. Available at: **www.cdc.gov/mmwr/preview/mmwrhtml/mm5307a4.htm**

Canyon, La Crosse, Powassan, and St. Louis encephalitis viruses). Alaska and Hawaii are the only states that have not reported local transmission of WNV. A map of the distribution of WNV neuroinvasive disease across the United States can be found on the Centers for Disease Control and Prevention (CDC) website (**www.cdc.gov/westnile/ statsMaps**).

In temperate and subtropical regions, most human WNV infections occur in summer or early autumn. All age groups and both genders are susceptible to WNV infection, but incidence of severe disease (eg, encephalitis and death) is highest among older adults. Chronic renal failure, history of cancer, history of alcohol abuse, diabetes, and hypertension have been associated with developing severe WNV disease.

The **incubation period** usually is 2 to 6 days but ranges from 2 to 14 days and can be up to 21 days in immunocompromised people and up to 37 days in solid organ transplant recipients.

DIAGNOSTIC TESTS: Detection of anti-WNV immunoglobulin (Ig) M antibodies in serum or cerebrospinal fluid (CSF) is the most common way to diagnose WNV infection. The presence of anti-WNV IgM usually is good evidence of recent WNV infection but may indicate infection with another closely related flavivirus. Because anti-WNV IgM can persist in the serum of some patients for longer than 1 year, a positive test result occasionally may reflect past infection. Detection of WNV IgM in CSF generally is indicative of recent neuroinvasive infection. WNV IgM antibodies are detectable in most WNV-infected patients within 3 to 8 days of symptom onset and typically remain detectible for 30 to 90 days. For patients from whom serum collected within 8 days of illness lacks detectable IgM, testing should be repeated on a convalescent-phase sample. IgG antibody generally is detectable shortly after IgM and can persist for years. Plaque reduction neutralization tests can be performed to measure virus-specific neutralizing antibodies and to discriminate between cross-reacting antibodies from closely related flaviviruses. A fourfold or greater increase in virus-specific neutralizing antibodies between acute- and convalescent-phase serum specimens collected 2 to 3 weeks apart may be used to confirm recent WNV infection.

Viral culture and WNV nucleic acid amplification tests (including reverse transcriptase-polymerase chain reaction) can be performed on acute-phase serum, CSF, or tissue specimens. By the time most immunocompetent patients present with clinical symptoms, WNV RNA usually no longer is detectable; therefore, polymerase chain reaction assay is not recommended for diagnosis in immunocompetent hosts. Sensitivity of these tests is likely higher in immunocompromised patients. Immunohistochemical staining can detect WNV antigens in fixed tissue, but negative results are not definitive.

WNV disease should be considered in the differential diagnosis of febrile or acute neurologic illnesses associated with recent exposure to mosquitoes, blood transfusion, or solid organ transplantation and of illnesses in neonates whose mothers were infected with WNV during pregnancy or while breastfeeding. WNV and other arboviruses should be considered in the differential diagnosis of aseptic meningitis and encephalitis along with other causes such as herpes simplex virus and enteroviruses.

TREATMENT: No specific therapy is available; management of WNV disease is supportive. Although various therapies have been evaluated or used empirically for WNV disease, none has shown specific benefit thus far. A review summarizing potential treatments (including Immune Globulin Intravenous with or without a high titer of WNV antibody,

WNV recombinant humanized monoclonal antibody, interferon, corticosteroids, ribavirin) is available online at **www.cdc.gov/westnile/healthcareproviders/health-CareProviders-TreatmentPrevention.html.** Updated information about ongoing or completed clinical trials is available online (**http://clinicaltrials.gov/ct2/results?term=west+nile+virus&Search=Search**).

ISOLATION OF THE HOSPITALIZED PATIENT: Standard precautions are recommended.

CONTROL MEASURES: Candidate WNV vaccines are being evaluated, but none are licensed for use in humans. Prevention of WNV disease depends on community-level mosquito control programs to reduce vector densities, personal protective measures to decrease exposure to infected mosquitoes, and screening of blood and organ donors. Personal protective measures include use of mosquito repellents, wearing long-sleeved shirts and long pants, and limiting outdoor exposure from dusk to dawn (see Prevention of Mosquitoborne and Tickborne Infections, p 175). Using air conditioning, installing window and door screens, and reducing peridomestic mosquito breeding sites can decrease the risk of WNV exposure further. Blood donations in the United States are screened for WNV infection, but physicians should remain vigilant for the possible transmission of WNV through blood transfusion or organ transplantation. Any suspected WNV infections temporally associated with blood transfusion or organ transplantation should be reported promptly to the appropriate state health department and to the United Network for Organ Sharing in the case of suspected organ transmission.

Pregnant women should take precautions to avoid mosquito bites. Products containing N,N-diethyl-meta-toluamide (DEET) can be used in pregnancy without adverse effects. Pregnant women who develop meningitis, encephalitis, acute flaccid myelitis, or unexplained fever in areas of ongoing WNV transmission should be tested for WNV infection. Confirmed WNV infections should be reported to local or state health departments, and women should be followed to determine the outcomes of their pregnancies. Although WNV probably has been transmitted through human milk, such transmission appears rare, and no adverse effects on infants have been described. Because the benefits of breastfeeding outweigh the risk of WNV disease in breastfeeding infants, mothers should be encouraged to breastfeed even in areas with ongoing WNV transmission.

Yersinia enterocolitica and *Yersinia pseudotuberculosis* Infections
(Enteritis and Other Illnesses)

CLINICAL MANIFESTATIONS: *Yersinia enterocolitica* causes several age-specific syndromes and a variety of other less commonly reported clinical illnesses. Infection with *Y enterocolitica* typically manifests as fever, diarrhea, and abdominal pain in children younger than 5 years; stool often contains leukocytes, blood, and mucus. Diarrhea commonly persists for more than 2 weeks. Relapsing disease and, rarely, necrotizing enterocolitis also have been described. In older children and adults, a pseudoappendicitis syndrome attributable to mesenteric lymphadenitis (fever, abdominal pain, tenderness in the right lower quadrant of the abdomen, and leukocytosis) is common. Bacteremia is the major complication of *Y enterocolitica*-associated enteric infection occurring mostly in children younger than 1 year and in older children with predisposing conditions, such as excessive iron storage (eg, deferoxamine use, sickle cell disease, and beta-thalassemia) and immunosuppressive states. Extraintestinal manifestations of *Y enterocolitica* are uncommon and include pharyngitis, meningitis, osteomyelitis, pyomyositis, conjunctivitis, pneumonia, empyema, endocarditis, acute peritonitis, abscesses of the liver and spleen, urinary tract infection, and primary cutaneous infection. Postinfectious sequelae with *Y enterocolitica* infection include erythema nodosum, reactive arthritis, uveitis, and glomerulonephritis. These sequelae occur most often in older children and adults, particularly people with HLA-B27 antigen.

Major manifestations of *Yersinia pseudotuberculosis* infection include fever, scarlatiniform rash, acute gastroenteritis, and abdominal symptoms. Acute pseudoappendiceal abdominal pain is common, resulting from ileocecal mesenteric adenitis or terminal ileitis. Other uncommon findings reported have been intestinal intussusception, erythema nodosum, septicemia mainly among individuals with underlying conditions, acute renal failure with nephritis, and sterile pleural and joint effusions. Clinical features can mimic those of Kawasaki disease; in Hiroshima, Japan, nearly 10% of children with a diagnosis of Kawasaki disease have serologic or culture evidence of *Y pseudotuberculosis* infection.

ETIOLOGY: The genus *Yersinia* consists of 17 species of gram-negative bacilli belonging to the family *Enterobacteriaceae*. *Y enterocolitica*, *Y pseudotuberculosis*, and *Yersinia pestis* (see Plague, p 592) are the 3 most recognized human pathogens; however, other *Yersinia* species also have been isolated from clinical specimens. Isolates of *Y enterocolitica* involved in human infections belong to several serotypes (O:3, O:8, O:9, and O:5.27) and are divided into 3 groups according to their pathogenic potential: nonpathogenic biotype 1A, weakly pathogenic biotypes 2 through 5, and highly pathogenic biotype 1B. Strains from biotype 1A can induce infections only in immunocompromised individuals. Serotype O:8, from biotype 1B, is the most virulent and has been responsible for several food poisoning outbreaks in the United States. At present, *Y enterocolitica* serotype O:3, found primarily in pigs, is the most frequent cause of yersiniosis in Europe and North America. The 3 *Yersinia* species have in common a tropism for lymphoid tissue and share factors that promote serum resistance, coordinate gene expression, and facilitate iron acquisition. Differences in virulence gene distribution exist among *Yersinia* species; for example, *Y enterocolitica* has a chromosomal gene encoding for an enterotoxin, and *Y pseudotuberculosis* produces a superantigen toxin among other factors. Virulence can be attributed to adhesion/invasion genes (*ail*, *inv*), enterotoxins (YstA, YstB), iron-scavenging genomic islands, and secretion systems. Highly pathogenic *Yersinia* are known to carry a 70 kb pYV virulence plasmid, which encodes a type III secretion system that is activated at human body temperatures and promotes entry into lymph tissues and subsequent evasion of host defense mechanisms.

EPIDEMIOLOGY: *Yersinia* infections are reported uncommonly in the United States, and infection is not nationally notifiable but is reportable in most US states. *Y enterocolitica* and *Y pseudotuberculosis* are isolated most often during the cool months of temperate climates. The Foodborne Disease Active Surveillance Network (FoodNet) conducts active surveillance for infections caused by 9 pathogens, including *Yersinia*. During 2018, FoodNet identified 465 *Yersinia* cases of infection, with an average incidence of 0.9 per 100 000 population, which represents a 58% increase in comparison to 2015–2017.[1] This increased incidence likely resulted from increased use of culture-independent diagnostic

---

[1]Tack DM, Marder MP, Griffen PM, et al. Preliminary incidence and trends of infections with pathogens transmitted commonly through food—Foodborne Diseases Active Surveillance Network, 10 U.S Sites, 2015-2018. *Morb Mortal Wkly Rep.* 2019;68(16):369-373

tests that detect bacterial antigens and genes for *Y enterocolitica*. *Yersinia* incidence is highest in children younger than 5 years and in Black people; however, in recent years, a significant declining incidence among Black children has been observed. Based on the FoodNet data from 1996–2007, compared with *Y enterocolitica* infection, *Y pseudotuberculosis* infection average annual incidence is much lower (0.04 cases per 1 million population), occurs in older people (median age was 47 years), and is more severe and invasive (72% were hospitalized, 11% died, and two thirds of isolates were recovered from blood).

The principal reservoir of *Y enterocolitica* is swine, although it can be isolated from a variety of domestic and wildlife animals; *Y pseudotuberculosis* has been isolated from ungulates (deer, elk, goats, sheep, cattle), rodents (rats, squirrels, beaver), rabbits, and many bird species. Infection with *Y enterocolitica* is believed to be transmitted by ingestion of contaminated food (raw or incompletely cooked pork products, tofu, and unpasteurized or inadequately pasteurized milk[1]), by contaminated surface or well water, by direct or indirect contact with animals, and rarely by transfusion with contaminated packed red blood cells and by person-to-person transmission. Cross-contamination has been documented to lead to infection in infants if their caregivers handle raw pork intestines (ie, chitterlings) and do not clean their hands or food preparation surfaces adequately before handling the infant or the infant's toys, bottles, or pacifiers. *Y pseudotuberculosis* can follow exposure to well and mountain waters contaminated with animal feces. Household pets can be source of infection for children. Infections in Finland have been associated with eating fresh produce, presumably contaminated by wild animals carrying the organism.

The **incubation period** typically is 4 to 6 days, with a range of 1 to 14 days. Organisms typically are excreted for 2 to 3 weeks and up to 2 to 3 months in untreated cases. Prolonged asymptomatic carriage is possible.

DIAGNOSTIC TESTS: *Y enterocolitica* and *Y pseudotuberculosis* can be recovered from stool, throat swab specimens, mesenteric lymph nodes, peritoneal fluid, and blood. *Y enterocolitica* also has been isolated from synovial fluid, bile, urine, cerebrospinal fluid, sputum, pleural fluid, and wounds. Stool cultures generally yield bacteria during the first 2 weeks of illness, regardless of the nature of gastrointestinal tract manifestations. *Yersinia* organisms are not sought routinely in stool specimens by most laboratories in the United States. Laboratory personnel should be notified when *Yersinia* infection is suspected so that stool can be cultured on suitable media (eg, CIN agar); however, strains of *Y enterocolitica* 3/O:3 and *Y pseudotuberculosis* may be inhibited on CIN agar, and MacConkey is preferred. DNA-based gastrointestinal syndrome panels that can reliably detect *Yersinia* are commercially available; these tests typically target only *Y enterocolitica* but may cross-react with other *Yersinia* species. Biotyping and serotyping for further identification of pathogenic strains are available through public health reference laboratories. Infection also can be confirmed by demonstrating increases in serum antibody titer after infection, but these tests generally are available only in reference or research laboratories. Cross-reactions of these antibodies with *Brucella, Vibrio, Salmonella, Rickettsia* organisms, and *Escherichia coli* can lead to false-positive *Y enterocolitica* and *Y pseudotuberculosis* titers. In patients with thyroid disease, persistently increased *Y enterocolitica* antibody titers can result from antigenic similarity of the organism with antigens of the thyroid epithelial cell membrane. Characteristic ultrasonographic features demonstrating edema of the wall of the terminal ileum and cecum

[1]American Academy of Pediatrics, Committee on Infectious Diseases and Committee on Nutrition. Consumption of raw or unpasteurized milk and milk products by pregnant women and children. *Pediatrics.* 2014;133(1):175-179 (Reaffirmed November 2019)

with normal appendix help to distinguish pseudoappendicitis from appendicitis and can help avoid exploratory surgery. Several DNA-based methods have been developed for both *Y enterocolitica* and *Y pseudotuberculosis* for use in clinical, food, and environmental samples.

TREATMENT: Neonates, immunocompromised hosts, and all patients with septicemia or extraintestinal disease require treatment for *Yersinia* infection. Parenteral therapy with a third-generation cephalosporin is appropriate, and evaluation of cerebrospinal fluid should be performed for infected neonates. Otherwise healthy nonneonates with enterocolitis can be treated symptomatically. Although a clinical benefit of antimicrobial therapy for immunocompetent patients with enterocolitis, pseudoappendicitis syndrome, or mesenteric adenitis has not been established, some clinicians consider treatment because of its favorable effect on decreasing the duration of shedding of *Y enterocolitica* and *Y pseudotuberculosis*. In addition to third-generation cephalosporins, *Y enterocolitica* and *Y pseudotuberculosis* usually are susceptible to trimethoprim-sulfamethoxazole, aminoglycosides, fluoroquinolones, chloramphenicol, tetracycline, and doxycycline. *Y enterocolitica* isolates usually are resistant to first-generation cephalosporins and most penicillins.

ISOLATION OF THE HOSPITALIZED PATIENT: In addition to standard precautions, contact precautions are indicated for diapered or incontinent children for the duration of diarrheal illness.

CONTROL MEASURES: Ingestion of uncooked or undercooked meat (especially pork), unpasteurized milk,[1] or contaminated water should be avoided. People who handle raw meat products should minimize contact with young children and their possessions while handling raw products. Meticulous hand hygiene and proper sanitization of food preparation surfaces should be practiced before and after handling and preparation of uncooked products.

Zika

CLINICAL MANIFESTATIONS: Most Zika virus infections are asymptomatic. In situations in which infection is symptomatic, the clinical disease usually is mild, and symptoms last for a few days to a week. Commonly reported signs and symptoms include fever, pruritic maculopapular rash, arthralgia, and conjunctival hyperemia. Other findings include myalgia, headache, edema of the extremities, vomiting, retro-orbital pain, and lymphadenopathy. Clinical laboratory abnormalities are observed uncommonly in symptomatic patients but can include thrombocytopenia, leukopenia, and increased liver aminotransferase concentrations. Severe disease requiring hospitalization and deaths are rare. However, Guillain-Barré syndrome and rare reports of other neurologic complications (eg, meningoencephalitis, myelitis, and uveitis) have been associated with Zika virus infection.

Congenital Zika virus infection can cause fetal loss as well as microcephaly and other serious neurologic anomalies. Clinical findings reported in infants with confirmed congenital Zika virus infection include brain anomalies (eg, subcortical calcifications, ventriculomegaly, abnormal gyral patterns, corpus callosum agenesis, and cerebellar hypoplasia),

---

[1]American Academy of Pediatrics, Committee on Infectious Diseases and Committee on Nutrition. Consumption of raw or unpasteurized milk and milk products by pregnant women and children. *Pediatrics.* 2014;133(1):175-179 (Reaffirmed November 2019)

ocular anomalies (eg, microphthalmia, cataracts, chorioretinal atrophy, and optic nerve hypoplasia), congenital contractures (eg, clubfoot and arthrogryposis), and neurologic sequelae (eg, hypertonia, hypotonia, irritability, tremors, swallowing dysfunction, hearing loss, and visual impairment).

Rare cases of perinatal transmission from mothers who were viremic at delivery have been reported. These generally result in asymptomatic or mildly symptomatic illness in the neonate.

ETIOLOGY: Zika virus is a single-stranded, RNA virus in the genus *Flavivirus* that is related antigenically to dengue, yellow fever, West Nile, St. Louis encephalitis, and Japanese encephalitis viruses. Two major lineages, African and Asian, have been identified through phylogenetic analyses.

EPIDEMIOLOGY: Zika virus is transmitted to humans primarily by *Aedes aegypti* mosquitoes and less commonly by *Aedes albopictus* and possibly other *Aedes* (*Stegomyia*) species (eg, *Aedes polynesiensis* and *Aedes hensilli*). In the United States, *Ae aegypti* mosquitoes are found primarily in southern states. *Ae albopictus* mosquitoes have a wider distribution (see map at **www.cdc.gov/zika/vector/range.html**). Both *Aedes* species bite humans during the day and night. These are the same vectors that transmit dengue, chikungunya, and yellow fever viruses. Human and nonhuman primates are the main reservoirs of the virus, with humans acting as the primary host in which the virus multiplies, allowing spread to additional mosquitoes and then other humans. Additional modes of transmission have been identified, including perinatal, in utero, sexual, blood transfusion, and laboratory exposure. Although Zika virus has been detected in human milk, and a few probable cases of transmission of Zika virus by breastfeeding have been reported, to date there is no consistent evidence that infants acquire Zika virus through breastfeeding.

Zika virus first was identified in the Zika forest of Uganda in 1947. Prior to 2007, only sporadic human disease cases were reported from countries in Africa and Asia. In 2007, the first documented Zika virus disease outbreak was reported in the Federated States of Micronesia. In subsequent years, outbreaks of Zika virus disease were identified in countries in Southeast Asia and the Western Pacific. In 2015, Zika virus was identified for the first time in the Western hemisphere, with large outbreaks reported in Brazil. Since then, the virus has spread throughout much of the Americas, with 48 countries and territories in the Americas reporting local transmission. During 2016 in the United States, large outbreaks occurred in Puerto Rico and the US Virgin Islands, and limited local transmission was identified in parts of Florida and Texas. Current information on Zika virus transmission and travel guidance can be found at **www.cdc.gov/zika/geo/index.html** and **wwwnc.cdc.gov/travel/page/zika-travel-information,** respectively.

The **incubation period** is 3 to 14 days after the bite of an infected mosquito, with 50% of symptomatic cases developing symptoms 1 week after exposure.

DIAGNOSTIC TESTS: Zika virus infection should be considered in patients with acute onset of fever, maculopapular rash, arthralgia, or conjunctivitis who live in or have traveled to an area with ongoing transmission in the 2 weeks preceding illness onset. Because dengue and chikungunya virus infections share a similar geographic distribution and symptomology with Zika virus infection, patients with suspected Zika virus infection also should be evaluated and managed for possible dengue or chikungunya virus infection. Other considerations in the differential diagnosis include malaria, rubella, measles, parvovirus, adenovirus, enterovirus, leptospirosis, rickettsiosis, and group A streptococcal infections.

Laboratory testing for Zika virus has a number of limitations. Zika virus RNA is only transiently present in body fluids; thus, a negative real-time reverse transcriptase-polymerase chain reaction (RT-PCR) result does not rule out infection. Likewise, a negative immunoglobulin (Ig) M serologic test result does not rule out infection, because the serum specimen might have been collected before the development or after waning of IgM antibodies. Alternatively, IgM antibodies might be detectable for months after the initial infection, making it difficult to distinguish the timing of Zika acquisition. Cross-reactivity of the Zika virus IgM antibody tests with other flaviviruses can result in a false-positive test result. Recent epidemiologic data indicate a declining prevalence of Zika virus infection in the Americas; this lower prevalence will result in a lower pretest probability of infection and a higher probability of false-positive test results.

Zika Laboratory Testing in Nonpregnant Symptomatic Individuals. For people with suspected Zika virus disease, Zika virus RT-PCR assay should be performed on serum and urine specimens collected <14 days after onset of symptoms. Serum IgM antibody testing should be performed if the RT-PCR result is negative or when ≥14 days have passed since illness onset.

Zika Laboratory Testing in Pregnant Women. Current recommendations from the Centers for Disease Control and Prevention (CDC) take into account the decreasing prevalence of Zika virus disease cases in the Americas that occurred in 2017.[1] Zika virus testing is not routinely recommended for asymptomatic pregnant women who have possible recent but not ongoing Zika virus exposure. Zika virus RT-PCR testing should be offered as part of routine obstetric care to asymptomatic pregnant women with ongoing possible Zika virus exposure (at first prenatal visit and if negative, at 2 other times during pregnancy). Because of the potential for persistence of IgM antibodies over several months, serologic testing is no longer routinely recommended to screen asymptomatic women.

Zika Laboratory Testing for Congenital Infection. Zika virus testing is recommended for infants with clinical findings consistent with congenital Zika syndrome and possible maternal Zika virus exposure during pregnancy, regardless of maternal testing results, and for infants without clinical findings consistent with congenital Zika syndrome who are born to women with laboratory evidence of possible infection during pregnancy. Recommended laboratory testing for possible congenital Zika virus infection includes evaluation for Zika virus RNA in infant serum and urine and Zika virus IgM antibodies in serum. In addition, if cerebrospinal fluid (CSF) is obtained for other reasons, RT-PCR and IgM antibody testing should be performed on CSF, because CSF was the only sample that tested positive in a limited number of infants with congenital Zika virus infection.

Laboratory testing of infants should be performed as soon as possible after birth (within the first few days of life), although testing specimens within the first few weeks to months after birth might still be useful. If CSF was not collected for other reasons, testing CSF for Zika virus RNA and Zika virus IgM should be considered to improve the likelihood of diagnosis, especially if serum and urine testing are negative and another etiology has not been identified. Diagnosis of congenital Zika virus infection is confirmed by a positive Zika virus RT-PCR or by a positive Zika virus IgM and neutralizing antibody

[1]Oduyebo T, Polen KD, Walke HT, et al. Update: Interim guidance for health care providers caring for pregnant women with possible zika virus exposure—United States (including U.S. territories), July 2017. *MMWR Morb Mortal Wkly Rep.* 2017;66(29):781-793

result. If neither Zika virus RNA nor Zika IgM antibodies are detected on the appropriate specimens obtained within the first few days after birth, congenital Zika virus infection is unlikely.

The plaque reduction neutralization test (PRNT), which measures virus-specific neutralizing antibodies, can be used to help identify false-positive results. If the infant's initial sample is IgM nonnegative (nonnegative serology terminology varies by assay and might include "positive," "equivocal," "presumptive positive," or "possible positive") and RT-PCR negative, and PRNT was not performed on the mother's sample, PRNT for Zika and dengue viruses should be performed on the infant's initial sample. If the Zika virus PRNT result is negative, this suggests that the infant's Zika virus IgM test result is a false positive. For infants with clinical findings consistent with congenital Zika syndrome or maternal evidence of possible Zika virus infection during pregnancy who were not tested near birth, PRNT at age ≥18 months (after maternal antibodies have dissipated from the infant's system) might help confirm or rule out congenital Zika virus infection. If the PRNT result is negative at age ≥18 months, congenital Zika virus infection is unlikely.

TREATMENT: No specific antiviral treatment currently is available for Zika virus disease. Only supportive care is indicated, including rest, fluids, and symptomatic treatment (acetaminophen to relieve fever and antihistamines to treat pruritus). Aspirin and nonsteroidal anti-inflammatory drugs (NSAIDs) should be avoided until dengue can be ruled out to reduce the risk of hemorrhagic complications.

Guidance is updated as new information is obtained; for the most recent guidance, visit: **www.cdc.gov/Zika.** Fig 3.18 (p 858) outlines the current recommended evaluation of infants with possible maternal and congenital Zika virus exposure during pregnancy.[1]

Clinical Management of Infants With Clinical Findings Consistent With Congenital Zika Infection. Zika virus testing is recommended (see Zika Laboratory Testing for Congenital Infection, p 856), ultrasonography of the head should be performed, and a comprehensive ophthalmologic examination should be performed by age 1 month by an ophthalmologist experienced in assessment of infants. Referrals to a developmental specialist and early intervention are recommended. Additional consultation should be considered by infectious disease (for evaluation of other congenital infections and assistance with Zika virus diagnosis and testing), clinical genetics (for evaluation for other causes of microcephaly or congenital anomalies), and neurology by age 1 month (for comprehensive neurologic examination and consideration for other evaluations, such as advanced neuroimaging and electroencephalography [EEG]). The initial clinical evaluation, including subspecialty consultations, can be performed before hospital discharge or as an outpatient. Ophthalmologic follow-up after the initial examination should be based on ophthalmology recommendations. Infants should be referred for automated brainstem response (ABR) testing by age 1 month if the newborn hearing screen was passed using only otoacoustic emissions (OAE) methodology.

Clinical Management of Infants Without Clinical Findings Consistent With Congenital Zika Infection but Maternal Laboratory Evidence of Possible Zika Virus Infection During Pregnancy. Zika virus testing is recommended (see Zika Laboratory Testing for Congenital Infection, p 856),

---

[1] Adebanjo T, Godfred-Cato S, Viens L, et al. Update: interim guidance for the diagnosis, evaluation, and management of infants with possible congenital Zika virus infection—United States, October 2017. *MMWR Morb Mortal Wkly Rep.* 2017;66(41):1089–1099

FIG 3.18. RECOMMENDATIONS FOR THE EVALUATION OF INFANTS WITH POSSIBLE CONGENITAL ZIKA VIRUS INFECTION BASED ON INFANT CLINICAL FINDINGS,[a,b] MATERNAL TESTING RESULTS,[c,d] AND INFANT TESTING RESULTS[e,f]—UNITED STATES[1]

[1]Adebanjo T, Godfred-Cato S, Viens L, et al. Update: interim guidance for the diagnosis, evaluation, and management of infants with possible congenital Zika virus infection—United States, October 2017. *MMWR Morb Mortal Wkly Rep.* 2017;66(41):1089–1099

Fig 3.18. Recommendations for the Evaluation of Infants with Possible Congenital Zika Virus Infection Based on Infant Clinical Findings,[a,b] Maternal Testing Results,[c,d] and Infant Testing Results[e,f]—United States,[1] Continued

ABR indicates auditory brainstem response; CSF, cerebrospinal fluid; CZS, congenital Zika syndrome; IgM, immunoglobulin M; NAAT, nucleic acid amplification test; PRNT, plaque reduction neutralization test.

[a]All infants should receive a standard evaluation at birth and at each subsequent well-child visit by their health care providers, including (1) comprehensive physical examination, including growth parameters; and 2) age-appropriate vision screening and developmental monitoring and screening using validated tools. Infants should receive a standard newborn hearing screen at birth, preferably using auditory brainstem response.

[b]Automated ABR by age 1 month if newborn hearing screen passed but performed with otoacoustic emission methodology.

[c]Laboratory evidence of possible Zika virus infection during pregnancy is defined as (1) Zika virus infection detected by a Zika virus RNA NAAT on any maternal, placental, or fetal specimen (referred to as NAAT-confirmed), or (2) diagnosis of Zika virus infection, timing of infection cannot be determined or unspecified *Flavivirus* infection, timing of infection cannot be determined by serologic tests on a maternal specimen (ie, positive/equivocal Zika virus IgM and Zika virus PRNT titer ≥10, regardless of dengue virus PRNT value; or negative Zika virus IgM, and positive or equivocal dengue virus IgM, and Zika virus PRNT titer ≥10, regardless of dengue virus PRNT titer). The use of PRNT for confirmation of Zika virus infection, including in pregnant women, is not routinely recommended in Puerto Rico (**www.cdc.gov/zika/laboratories/lab-guidance.html**).

[d]This group includes women who were never tested during pregnancy as well as those whose test result was negative because of issues related to timing or sensitivity and specificity of the test. Because the latter issues are not easily discerned, all mothers with possible exposure to Zika virus during pregnancy who do not have laboratory evidence of possible Zika virus infection, including those who tested negative with currently available technology, should be considered in this group.

[e]Laboratory testing of infants for Zika virus should be performed as early as possible, preferably within the first few days after birth, and includes concurrent Zika virus NAAT in infant serum and urine, and Zika virus IgM testing in serum. If CSF is obtained for other purposes, Zika virus NAAT and Zika virus IgM testing should be performed on CSF.

[f]Laboratory evidence of congenital Zika virus infection includes a positive Zika virus NAAT or a nonnegative Zika virus IgM with confirmatory neutralizing antibody testing, if PRNT confirmation is performed.

and ultrasonography of the head should be performed by age 1 month to detect subclinical brain findings. All infants should have a comprehensive ophthalmologic examination by age 1 month to detect subclinical eye findings; further follow-up visits with an ophthalmologist after the initial examination should be based on ophthalmology recommendations. Infants should be referred for automated ABR testing by 1 month of age if newborn screen was passed using only OAE methodology. Infants should be monitored for findings consistent with congenital Zika syndrome that could develop over time (eg, impaired visual acuity/function, hearing problems, developmental delay, delay in head growth).

Clinical Management of Infants Without Clinical Findings Consistent with Congenital Zika Infection Born to Mothers With Possible Zika Virus Infection During Pregnancy but Without Laboratory Evidence of Zika Virus During Pregnancy. Zika virus testing is not routinely recommended, and specialized clinical evaluation or follow-up is not routinely indicated. Health care providers can consider additional evaluation in consultation with families. If findings suggestive of congenital Zika syndrome are identified at any time, referrals to the appropriate specialists should be made.

---

[1]Adebanjo T, Godfred-Cato S, Viens L, et al. Update: interim guidance for the diagnosis, evaluation, and management of infants with possible congenital Zika virus infection—United States, October 2017. *MMWR Morb Mortal Wkly Rep.* 2017;66(41):1089–1099

ISOLATION OF THE HOSPITALIZED PATIENT: Standard precautions are recommended, with attention to the potential for bloodborne transmission. People infected with Zika virus, as well as other arboviruses, should be protected from further mosquito exposure, especially during the first week of illness, to reduce the risk of local transmission to others.

CONTROL MEASURES: Vaccines to prevent Zika virus infection currently are not available. Prevention and control measures rely on personal prevention measures to avoid mosquito bites, and community-level programs to reduce vector densities in areas with endemic infection. Personal measures include using insect repellent; wearing long pants, socks, and long-sleeved shirts while outdoors; and staying in air-conditioned buildings or buildings with window and door screens. Permethrin-treated clothing and gear can repel mosquitoes. Travelers returning to the United States from an area with risk of Zika, even if asymptomatic, should take steps to prevent mosquito bites for 3 weeks to minimize spread to local mosquito populations (**www.cdc.gov/zika/prevention/prevent-mosquito-bites.html**).

Insect repellents registered by the US Environmental Protection Agency (EPA) can be used according to directions on the product labels. Products containing N,N-diethyl-meta-toluamide (DEET), picaridin, oil of lemon eucalyptus, IR3535, para-menthane-diol (PMD), and 2-undecanone provide protection from mosquito bites (see Prevention of Mosquitoborne and Tickborne Infections, p 175). All travelers should take precautions to avoid mosquito bites to prevent Zika virus infection and other mosquitoborne diseases.

Sexual Transmission. Zika virus can be transmitted sexually. Couples in whom the man or woman has had possible Zika virus exposure who want to maximally reduce their risk for sexually transmitting Zika virus to the uninfected partner should use condoms or abstain from sex for at least 3 months for men or 8 weeks for women after symptom onset (if symptomatic) or last possible Zika virus exposure (if asymptomatic) (**www.cdc.gov/zika/prevention/sexual-transmission-prevention.html**). Men should not donate sperm for at least 3 months from infection or last exposure.

Women Who Are Pregnant or Seeking to Become Pregnant. Pregnant women should postpone travel to any area where local Zika virus transmission is ongoing. Pregnant women who do travel to one of these areas should talk to their health care provider before traveling and should strictly follow steps to avoid mosquito bites during travel. There is no restriction on the use of insect repellents by pregnant women if used in accordance with the instructions on the product label. Male partners of pregnant women who have traveled to areas with local transmission of Zika virus should abstain from sex or use condoms for the duration of the pregnancy to avoid sexual transmission to their pregnant partners (**www.cdc.gov/zika/prevention/sexual-transmission-prevention.html**).

For couples who have possible Zika virus exposure and who are considering pregnancy, the CDC recommends postponing pregnancy for 3 months following potential exposure or diagnosis of Zika infection (**www.cdc.gov/zika/prevention/sexual-transmission-prevention.html**).

Pregnant women who develop a clinically compatible illness during or within 2 weeks of returning from an area with Zika virus transmission should be tested for Zika virus infection. Fetuses and infants of women with possible Zika virus exposure or known Zika virus infection during pregnancy should be evaluated for possible congenital infection (Fig 3.18).

Blood and Tissue Donation. The US Food and Drug Administration (FDA) recommends temporary deferral of blood donors who recently were infected with Zika virus infection as well as testing of all blood donations collected in the United States and its territories to reduce the risk for transfusion-associated transmission of Zika virus. Because of universal Zika virus testing of blood donors, people who traveled to areas with local Zika virus transmission and who did not exhibit any evidence of infection may donate blood.

The CDC also has developed guidance to reduce potential Zika virus transmission from human cells, tissues, and cellular and tissue-based products (HCT/Ps). The guidance addresses donation of HCT/Ps from both living and deceased donors, including donors of umbilical cord blood, placenta tissue, or other gestational tissues. The guidance recognizes the potential risk of transmission of Zika virus from HCT/Ps. Living donors should be considered ineligible to donate HCT/Ps if they had a diagnosis of Zika virus infection, were in an area with Zika virus transmission, or had sex with a male with either of these risk factors, within the past 6 months. Donors of umbilical cord blood, placenta tissue, or other gestational tissues should be considered ineligible if any of the aforementioned risk factors occurred at any point during pregnancy. This guidance may change as more evidence becomes available about persistence of Zika virus in human tissues and fluids.

Breastfeeding. The World Health Organization and Centers for Disease Control and Prevention (CDC) recommend infants born to women with suspected, probable, or confirmed Zika virus infection, or to women who live in or have traveled to areas with Zika virus, should be fed according to local infant feeding guidelines. Because of the benefits of breastfeeding, mothers are encouraged to breastfeed even in areas where Zika virus is found.

REPORTING: Health care professionals should report suspected Zika virus infection to their state or local health departments to facilitate diagnosis and mitigate the risk of local transmission. Zika virus disease and congenital infections were added to the list of nationally notifiable diseases in 2016 (see Appendix III: Nationally Notifiable Infectious Diseases in the United States, p 1033). State health departments should then report cases to the CDC through ArboNET, the national surveillance system for arboviral diseases.

Antimicrobial Agents and Related Therapy

······························
INTRODUCTION

The product label (package insert) approved by the US Food and Drug Administration (FDA) for a given antimicrobial drug provides information on indications (the clinical infections that require antimicrobial treatment, such as "complicated urinary tract infection") based on clinical trial data reviewed by the FDA. Virtually all current antimicrobial product labels are available at **https://dailymed.nlm.nih.gov/dailymed/.** The FDA also maintains a general website (**www.accessdata.fda.gov/scripts/cder/daf/**) of approved drug products with therapeutic equivalence evaluations that can be searched by active ingredient or proprietary names as well as an online repository of labels for approved drugs (**https://labels.fda.gov/**).

An FDA-approved indication usually means that adequate and well-controlled studies were conducted (usually by the drug's manufacturer), presented to, and reviewed by the FDA and, if appropriate, approved for use in the populations in which the drug was investigated. However, accepted medical practice (ie, when to use which antimicrobial agent for a specific infection or "indication") often includes use of drugs that are not reflected in approved indications found in the drug label. These additional uses of antimicrobial agents usually are based on studies that may or may not have been supported by the drug's original manufacturer, particularly for generic drugs. Clinical investigators may not always present clinical studies formally to the FDA for review because of the substantial cost of conducting the clinical trials, collecting and analyzing the data, and presenting the data for that specific indication. For this reason, lack of FDA approval may not necessarily mean lack of effectiveness, because it is possible either that FDA-required studies have not been performed or that studies have not been submitted for FDA approval for that specific indication. Therefore, unapproved use does not imply improper use, provided that reasonable supporting medical evidence exists and that use of the drug is deemed to be in the best interest of the patient. Conversely, some vaccines or drugs are not recommended for use by the American Academy of Pediatrics (AAP) or Centers for Disease Control and Prevention (CDC), despite licensed indications noted in the package label. The decision to prescribe a drug is the responsibility of the medical provider, who must weigh the risks and benefits of using the drug for a specific situation.

Manufacturing of drugs is the responsibility of the pharmaceutical industry, which is regulated by the FDA. On occasion, drug shortages can occur. The pharmaceutical company may share information about the shortage with the FDA (**www.accessdata.fda.gov/scripts/drugshortages/default.cfm**). When drug shortages occur, alternative, nonstandard therapy may be required.

Some antimicrobial agents with proven therapeutic benefit in adults are not approved by the FDA for use in pediatric patients or, rarely, are considered contraindicated in children because of possible toxicity. The following information delineates general principles for use of fluoroquinolones, tetracyclines, and other approved agents.

Fluoroquinolones

Fluoroquinolones (eg, ciprofloxacin, levofloxacin, gemifloxacin, moxifloxacin, delafloxacin) should not be used routinely as first-line agents in children younger than 18 years except when specific indications exist or in specific conditions for which there are no alternative agents (including oral agents) and the drug is known to be effective for the specific situation. Use of fluoroquinolones in adults and children is a driver of fluoroquinolone resistance, and therefore, using fluoroquinolones judiciously is an important strategy to combat antibiotic resistance and improve patient safety. Information on the safety of fluoroquinolones for children was reviewed and published by the AAP.[1]

Although generally well tolerated, transient arthralgia has been reported in patients treated with fluoroquinolones; however, this reported symptom has not been confirmed by clinical examination. Arthralgia also has been noted in some children in the control groups in these studies, making it difficult to assess whether the fluoroquinolone caused this adverse effect. For some fluoroquinolones, cartilage damage in animal models occurs at doses that approximate therapeutic doses in humans. The mechanism of damage remains speculative, but there are emerging in vitro data to suggest direct collagen effects. In some pediatric studies, an increased incidence of reversible adverse events involving joints or surrounding tissues has been observed with fluoroquinolones compared with other agents. Long-term safety data have been reported for both levofloxacin and moxifloxacin. To date, there is no compelling evidence of long-term sequelae related to fluoroquinolone bone or joint toxicity in children.

Risks related to fluoroquinolones are summarized as follows:
- *Clostridioides difficile* (formerly called *Clostridium difficile*) disease: Fluoroquinolones are one of the most common antimicrobials to be associated with *Clostridioides difficile* disease.
- Tendinopathy: Fluoroquinolones are associated in adults with an increased risk of tendon rupture (with a predilection for the Achilles tendon) and tendonitis, with further increased risk in people older than 60 years; in those who have received renal, heart, kidney, or lung transplants; and in those with concurrent use of corticosteroids. To date, there have been no reports of Achilles tendon rupture in children in association with quinolone use.
- QT interval prolongation: Certain fluoroquinolones (moxifloxacin, levofloxacin, ciprofloxacin) can prolong the QT interval and should be avoided in patients with long QT syndrome, those with hypokalemia or hypomagnesemia, those with organic heart disease including congestive heart failure, those receiving an antiarrhythmic agent from class Ia (particularly quinidine) or class III, those who are receiving a concurrent drug that prolongs the QTc interval independently, and those with hepatic insufficiency-related metabolic derangements that may promote QT prolongation.

---

[1] Jackson MA, Schutze GE, American Academy of Pediatrics Committee on Infectious Diseases. The use of systemic and topical fluoroquinolones. *Pediatrics*. 2016;138(5):e20162706

- Aortic aneurysms: In population-based studies, fluoroquinolones have been associated in adults with an small but increased risk of aortic aneurysms and dissection and should not be given to patients with aortic aneurysms or at risk for aortic aneurysms (eg, Marfan and Ehlers-Danlos syndromes).
- Central nervous system toxicity: Neurologic complications associated with fluoroquinolone use, although very uncommon in children, include peripheral neuropathy, seizures, lightheadedness, sleep disorders, hallucinations, dizziness, headaches, disturbances in attention, disorientation, agitation, nervousness, memory impairment, delirium, and pseudotumor cerebri.
- Myasthenia gravis: Fluoroquinolones also may unmask or worsen muscle weakness in people with myasthenia gravis.
- Thrombocytopenia, hepatic dysfunction, renal dysfunctions (interstitial nephritis and crystal nephropathy), hyperglycemia/hypoglycemia, hypersensitivity, and photosensitivity reactions have also been reported.

The FDA has issued a Drug Safety Communication for the fluoroquinolone class, advising that health care providers should not prescribe systemic fluoroquinolones to patients who have other treatment options for acute bacterial sinusitis, acute bacterial exacerbation of chronic bronchitis, and uncomplicated urinary tract infections because the risks outweigh the benefits in these patients.[1]

Although ciprofloxacin is approved for complicated urinary tract infection or pyelonephritis in children, it should not be a first-line agent, and other agents should be used preferentially if the pathogens are susceptible. The significant exceptions in which ciprofloxacin may be used as a first-line agent in children are for postexposure prophylaxis for inhalation anthrax (ciprofloxacin primarily, with levofloxacin and moxifloxacin considered equivalent alternatives) and treatment of plague (ciprofloxacin, levofloxacin, or moxifloxacin). Circumstances in which use of systemic fluoroquinolones may be justified in children include the following: (1) parenteral therapy is not practical and no other safe and effective oral agent is available; and (2) infection is caused by a multidrug-resistant pathogen for which there is no other effective intravenous or oral agent available. These clinical situations may include the following:

- Urinary tract, bone, or other invasive infections, including chronic suppurative otitis media or malignant otitis externa caused by *Pseudomonas aeruginosa* or other multidrug-resistant, gram-negative bacteria resistant to beta-lactams and other classes of antimicrobial agents;
- Multidrug-resistant (beta-lactam–, carbapenem–, macrolide–, and trimethoprim-sulfamethoxazole–resistant) pneumococcal infections;
- Gastrointestinal tract infection or bacteremia caused by suspected or documented multidrug-resistant *Shigella* species, *Salmonella* species, *Vibrio cholerae*, *Campylobacter jejuni*, or *Campylobacter coli*;
- Mycobacterial infections that are multidrug resistant for which no other oral drug is available or appropriate;
- Serious infections attributable to fluoroquinolone-susceptible pathogen(s) in children with severe allergy to alternative agents.

---

[1] US Food and Drug Administration. FDA Drug Safety Communication: FDA advises restricting fluoroquinolone antibiotic use for certain uncomplicated infections; warns about disabling side effects that can occur together. Available at: **www.fda.gov/Drugs/DrugSafety/ucm500143.htm**

- Otorrhea associated with tympanic membrane perforation as well as tympanostomy tube otorrhea, for which topical fluoroquinolone-containing agents are considered as safer alternatives to aminoglycoside-containing agents.

Tetracyclines

Use of tetracyclines as a class of drugs in pediatric patients historically has been limited because of reports that this class could cause permanent dental discoloration in children younger than 8 years, because their degradation products are incorporated in tooth enamel. After 8 years of age, it was believed that tetracyclines can be given without concern for dental staining because enamel formation in permanent teeth is complete. The period of odontogenesis to completion of formation of enamel in permanent teeth appears to be the critical time for effects of these drugs, and it is now known that the calcification stage of tooth development actually starts at the sixth week of development in utero and is usually completed at 3 to 4 months of life. The degree of staining appears to depend on dosage, duration of therapy, and which drug in the tetracycline class is used.

Doxycycline binds less readily to calcium compared with other members of the tetracycline class, but because of concern for a drug class effect with tetracyclines, its use previously has been limited largely to patients 8 years and older, and these older children have been studied more thoroughly than younger children. More recent data from the United States and Europe in younger children, however, suggest that doxycycline is not likely to cause visible teeth staining or enamel hypoplasia in children younger than 8 years. These reassuring data support the recommendation by the AAP that doxycycline can be administered for short durations (ie, 21 days or less) without regard to the patient's age. When used, patients should be careful to avoid excess sun exposure because of photosensitivity associated with doxycycline.

Antimicrobial Agents Approved for Use in Adults but Not Children

Antimicrobial agents in a variety of classes have been studied and approved by the FDA for use in adults for certain indications but still are under investigation for pharmacokinetics, safety, and efficacy in children. These agents include but are not limited to dalbavancin, oritavancin, telavancin, tedizolid, ceftolozane/tazobactam, plazomicin, eravacycline, omadacycline, and tigecycline. These drugs should be used in children only when no other safe and effective agents that are FDA approved for use in children are available and when benefits are expected to exceed risks for that patient. For these agents with relatively undefined or emerging safety and efficacy in pediatrics, consultation with an expert in pediatric infectious diseases should be considered.

Cephalosporin Cross-Reactivity With Other Beta Lactam Antibiotics

Patients with cephalosporin allergy appear to be at a higher risk for a reaction to other beta-lactam antibiotics because of shared chemical structures (beta-lactam ring, R group side chains). Cephalosporin-allergic subjects most often tolerate other cephalosporins with different R1 group side chains. A cephalosporin cross-reactivity matrix has been published (Fig 4.1) that quantifies the likelihood of cross-reactivity. This figure indicates side-chain cross-reactivity only; when considering cross-reactivity between penicillins and cephalosporins, cross-reactivity is also possible with the core beta-lactam ring.

FIG 4.1. CEPHALOSPORIN CROSS-REACTIVITY MATRIX.

	Cefazolin (1st)	Cefaclor (2nd)	Cefadroxil (1st)	Cefamandole (2nd)	Cefdinir (3rd)	Cefepime (4th)	Cefixime (3rd)	Cefoperazone (3rd)	Cefotaxime (3rd)	Cefotetan (2nd)	Cefoxitin (2nd)	Cefpirome (4th)	Cefpodoxime (3rd)	Cefprozil (2nd)	Ceftazidime (3rd)	Ceftolozane (2nd)	Ceftibuten (3rd)	Ceftizoxime (3rd)	Ceftriaxone (3rd)	Cefuroxime (2nd)	Cephalexin (1st)	Cephaloridine (1st)	Cephradine (1st)	Cefditoren (3rd)	Ceftaroline (5th)	Amoxicillin	Ampicillin	Penicillin G	Aztreonam
Cefazolin (1st)	-																												
Cefaclor (2nd)		-	X	X										X							X		X			X	X		
Cefadroxil (1st)		X	-	X										X							X		X			X	X		
Cefamandole (2nd)		X	X	-				X		X																			
Cefdinir (3rd)					-		X																						
Cefepime (4th)						-	X		X			X	X		X	X		X	X	X				X					X
Cefixime (3rd)					X	X	-		X			X	X		X	X		X	X	X				X					X
Cefoperazone (3rd)				X				-		X																			
Cefotaxime (3rd)						X	X		-			X	X					X	X	X				X					X
Cefotetan (2nd)				X				X		-																			
Cefoxitin (2nd)											-														X			X	
Cefpirome (4th)						X	X		X			-	X		X	X		X	X	X				X					X
Cefpodoxime (3rd)						X	X		X			X	-		X	X		X	X	X				X					X
Cefprozil (2nd)		X	X											-							X		X			X	X		
Ceftazidime (3rd)						X	X		X			X	X		-	X		X	X	X									X
Ceftolozane (2nd)						X	X		X			X	X		X	-		X	X	X									X
Ceftibuten (3rd)																	-												
Ceftizoxime (3rd)						X	X		X			X	X		X	X		-	X	X				X					X
Ceftriaxone (3rd)						X	X		X			X	X		X	X		X	-	X				X					X
Cefuroxime (2nd)						X	X		X			X	X		X	X		X	X	-				X					X
Cephalexin (1st)		X	X											X							-		X			X	X		
Cephaloridine (1st)																						-					X		
Cephradine (1st)		X	X											X							X		-			X	X		
Cefditoren (3rd)						X	X		X			X	X					X	X	X				-					X
Ceftaroline (5th)											X														-				
Amoxicillin		X	X											X							X		X			-	X		
Ampicillin		X	X											X							X	X	X			X	-		
Penicillin G											X																	-	
Aztreonam						X	X		X			X	X		X	X		X	X					X					-

This matrix describes the risk of cross-reactivity between 2 beta-lactam antibiotics. Boxes with a symbol indicate either a similar (light gray) or an identical (dark gray) side chain and, therefore, higher risk for an allergic reaction. Empty boxes indicate a lack of side-chain similarity and decreased risk of allergic reaction. Reproduced with permission from Blumenthal KG, Shenoy ES, Wolfson AR, et al. Addressing inpatient beta-lactam allergies: a multihospital implementation. *J Allergy Clin Immunol Pract.* 2017;5(3):616-625.

··
ANTIMICROBIAL RESISTANCE AND ANTIMICROBIAL STEWARDSHIP: APPROPRIATE AND JUDICIOUS USE OF ANTIMICROBIAL AGENTS

Antimicrobial Resistance

The Centers for Disease Control and Prevention (CDC), World Health Organization (WHO), and other international agencies have identified antimicrobial resistance as one of the world's most pressing public health threats. In the United States, it is estimated that more than 2.8 million people are infected with antimicrobial-resistant bacteria, and at least 35 000 people die annually as a direct result of these infections. Highly resistant gram-negative pathogens (carbapenemase-producing *Enterobacteriaceae* and *Acinetobacter* species, multidrug resistant *Pseudomonas aeruginosa,* and extended-spectrum beta-lactamase–producing *Enterobacteriaceae*), gram-positive pathogens (methicillin-resistant *Staphylococcus aureus* and *Enterococcus* species resistant to ampicillin and vancomycin), and drug-resistant *Candida* species are increasingly associated with invasive infections. *Clostridioides difficile* disease is the most common cause of diarrhea acquired in a health care facility and an infection that usually results from antimicrobial exposure. *C difficile* causes approximately 223 900 infections and at least 12 800 deaths annually. The CDC has ranked the antimicrobial-resistant bacteria and fungi that have the most impact on human health in categories of urgent, serious, and concerning threats (Table 4.1).

The presence of resistant pathogens complicates patient management, increases morbidity and mortality, and increases medical expenses for patients and the health care system. Studies have estimated that antimicrobial resistance in the United States adds as much as $20 billion in excess costs to the health care system each year, and the costs to society as a result of lost productivity are as high as $35 billion.

Factors Contributing to Resistance

The use of antimicrobial agents is a key driver of antimicrobial resistance. Antimicrobial agents are among the most commonly prescribed drugs used in human medicine. Many studies have measured the extent of inappropriate or unnecessary antibiotic use; results have been remarkably consistent at 30% to 50% in both inpatient and outpatient studies.

The number of antibiotic-resistant bacteria and the diversity of molecular mechanisms of resistance continue to increase, but the development of newer, effective antimicrobial agents has not kept pace. The loss of effective antimicrobial agents will hamper clinicians' efforts to treat potentially life-threatening infections. At the same time, many advances in medical treatment involve immunosuppression, and these patients' ability to control infections depends even more on the receipt of effective antimicrobial agents. When first- and second-line treatment options are limited by resistance or are unavailable, health care providers are forced to use antimicrobial agents that may be more toxic, more expensive, and/or less effective.

The overuse of antimicrobial agents in animal agriculture also contributes substantially to the problem of antimicrobial resistance. The CDC has determined

Table 4.1. Antimicrobial-Resistant Bacteria and Fungi Posing Health Threats

Urgent Threats	Serious Threats	Concerning Threats	Watch List
Carbapenem-resistant *Acinetobacter*	Drug-resistant *Campylobacter*	Erythromycin-resistant group A *Streptococcus*	Azole-resistant *Aspergillus fumigatus*
Candida auris	Drug-resistant *Candida*	Clindamycin-resistant group B *Streptococcus*	Drug-resistant *Mycoplasma genitalium*
Clostridioides difficile	ESBL-producing *Enterobacteriaceae*		Drug-resistant *Bordetella pertussis*
Carbapenem-resistant *Enterobacteriaceae*	Vancomycin-resistant enterococci (VRE)		
Drug-resistant *Neisseria gonorrhoeae*	Multidrug-resistant *Pseudomonas aeruginosa*		
	Drug-resistant nontyphoidal *Salmonella*		
	Drug-resistant *Salmonella* serotype Typhi		
	Drug-resistant *Shigella*		
	Methicillin-resistant *Staphylococcus aureus* (MRSA)		
	Drug-resistant *Streptococcus pneumoniae*		
	Drug-resistant tuberculosis		

Adapted from **www.cdc.gov/drugresistance/biggest-threats.html.**

that antimicrobial use in animals is linked to resistance in humans. The US Food and Drug Administration has described a pathway toward reducing inappropriate antimicrobial use in animals, and many major medical and public health organizations, including the American Academy of Pediatrics (AAP), have called for stronger action.

Actions to Prevent or Slow Antimicrobial Resistance

Antimicrobial resistance can only be addressed through concerted and collaborative efforts. The CDC's Antibiotic Resistance Solutions initiative invests in US infrastructure to detect, respond to, contain, and prevent antimicrobial resistant infections (**www.cdc.gov/drugresistance/solutions-initiative/index.html**). Actions to combat antimicrobial resistance include:

1. **Prevent infections and prevent the spread of resistance.** Antimicrobial-resistant infections can be prevented by immunization, infection prevention in health care settings, safe food preparation and handling, and handwashing. The CDC has

also provided guidance on the containment of highly resistant pathogens of public health concern (**www.cdc.gov/hai/containment/**).

2. **Track antimicrobial resistant infections.** The CDC, in collaboration with health care facilities and state and local health departments, gathers data on antimicrobial-resistant infections to help inform strategies and interventions for prevention. The CDC Antibiotic Resistance Laboratory Network (**www.cdc.gov/drugresistance/solutions-initiative/ar-lab-network.html**) provides regional capacity to detect and characterize resistant pathogens.

3. **Improve antimicrobial use and promote antimicrobial stewardship.** It is critical to modify the way antimicrobial agents are used in humans and animals. Unnecessary and inappropriate use of antimicrobial agents is common across the continuum of care. Inappropriate use of antimicrobial agents often is a result of errors in antimicrobial selection, dosing, or duration of therapy. Unnecessary exposure to antimicrobial agents results in adverse drug reactions, subsequent treatment challenges related to the development of antimicrobial resistance, and complications including *C difficile* disease. Every health care facility should have a formal antimicrobial stewardship program (ASP) built on the CDC's Core Elements of Antimicrobial Stewardship (see next section). Outpatient antimicrobial stewardship also is important to combat inappropriate antibiotic prescribing and antibiotic resistance.

4. **Develop drugs and improved diagnostic tests.** Discovery of new antimicrobial agents is needed to keep pace with the emergence of pathogen resistance. Unfortunately, the number of antimicrobial agents in late-phase clinical development is low; in particular, few agents are being developed with a new mechanism of action to treat resistant gram-negative infections. In addition, new diagnostic tests are needed to guide antimicrobial therapy and to track the development of resistance.

Antimicrobial Stewardship

The primary goal of antimicrobial stewardship is to optimize antimicrobial use with the aim of decreasing inappropriate use that leads to unwarranted toxicity and spread of resistant organisms. The CDC's Core Elements of Antibiotic Stewardship provide a framework for implementing stewardship across the spectrum of health care and include guidance for hospitals, including small and critical access hospitals; nursing homes; outpatient settings; and resource-limited settings outside the United States (**www.cdc.gov/antibiotic-use/core-elements/index.html**).

For **inpatient facilities**, the CDC describes 7 core elements needed for a successful ASP (**www.cdc.gov/antibiotic-use/healthcare/implementation/core-elements.html**):

- *Hospital leadership commitment.* Hospital administration should support and provide dedicated time to a stewardship program leader and a pharmacist coleader as well as financial and technologic resources needed to accomplish the programmatic goals.
- *Accountability.* A program leader (often a physician) should work collaboratively with a pharmacy leader and other core members of the ASP team (infectious diseases specialists, clinical pharmacists, clinical microbiologists, hospital epidemiologists, infection prevention professionals, and information systems specialists). This leader should ensure that other core elements of a successful program are implemented.

- *Pharmacy expertise.* A pharmacy leader should work collaboratively with the physician leader to implement the key actions and other core elements to have a successful ASP.
- *Action.* Numerous actions have been described to successfully improve the use of antibiotics. Key interventions that have had significant success include prospective audit with feedback including "handshake" stewardship, preauthorization, and implementation of guidelines. Additional actions include education, conversion from intravenous to oral agents, and dose optimization.
- *Tracking.* Antibiotic use data should be monitored and reported as days of therapy per 1000 patient days or days present. The CDC has developed the Antimicrobial Use and Resistance (AUR) module within the National Healthcare Safety Network (NHSN) that can provide the standardized antimicrobial administration ratio (SAAR) for a specific institution. This is a benchmarked measure similar to the standardized infection ratio (**www.cdc.gov/nhsn/pdfs/ pscmanual/11pscaurcurrent.pdf**). Other data to be monitored may include hospital-onset *C difficile* disease rates, length of stay, adverse drug events, and rates of concerning antibiotic-resistant pathogens (eg, carbapenem-resistant *Enterobacteriaceae*, methicillin-resistant *S aureus*), and hospital costs.
- *Reporting.* Regular updates on process and outcome measures regarding antibiotic resistance and other related issues should be given to prescribers, pharmacists, nurses, and senior administrators.
- *Education.* All health care workers should receive annual education regarding current antimicrobial stewardship practices and additional methods to improve use. Furthermore, efforts are needed to educate patients, families, and caregivers about antimicrobial stewardship and the impact of inappropriate antibiotic use.

As part of the Choosing Wisely campaign, the AAP and the Pediatric Infectious Diseases Society (**www.pids.org**) have published "Five Things Physicians and Patients Should Question" about antimicrobial therapy: (**www.choosingwisely. org/societies/american-academy-of-pediatrics-committee-on-infectious- diseases-and-the-pediatric-infectious-diseases-society/**).

- Don't initiate empiric antibiotic therapy in the patient with suspected invasive bacterial infection without first confirming that blood, urine, or other appropriate cultures have been obtained, excluding exceptional cases.
- Don't use a broad-spectrum antimicrobial agent for perioperative prophylaxis or continue prophylaxis after the incision is closed for uncomplicated clean and clean-contaminated procedures.
- Don't treat uncomplicated community-acquired pneumonia in otherwise healthy, immunized, hospitalized patients with antibiotic therapy broader than ampicillin.
- Don't use vancomycin or carbapenems empirically for neonatal intensive care patients unless an infant is known to have a specific risk for pathogens resistant to narrower-spectrum agents.
- Don't place peripherally inserted central catheters (PICC) and/or use prolonged intravenous antibiotics in otherwise healthy children with infections that can be transitioned to an appropriate oral agent.

Although inpatients are frequently exposed to broad-spectrum and potentially toxic antimicrobial agents, the vast majority of antibiotic exposure occurs in the **outpatient setting.** The CDC has developed the Core Elements of Outpatient Antibiotic

Stewardship to help improve the use of antibiotics in this setting (**www.cdc.gov/ antibiotic-use/core-elements/outpatient.html**). These core elements include: commitment, action for policy and practice, tracking and reporting, and education and expertise. Actions that have been successful in the outpatient setting include provider audit and feedback with peer comparisons, "nudge" posters, communications training, clinical decision support, patient education, and provider education. Interventions that incorporate a combination of approaches tend to be most effective. In addition, pediatricians should seek understanding of parents' expectations for antibiotic agents, because prescribing significantly increases when clinicians believe a parent is expecting an antibiotic agent.

The AAP, along with the Pediatric Infectious Diseases Society (**www.pids.org**), has developed pediatric antibiotic safety toolkits for use in the inpatient and outpatient settings (**www.aap.org/en-us/advocacy-and-policy/aap-health-initiatives/ Pages/antibiotic-safety.aspx**).

Role of the Medical Provider

Medical providers can integrate key recommendations that focus on antibiotic prescribing for common infections in children. These include the following:

1. Confirm the diagnosis of urinary tract infection by documenting that the patient is symptomatic and has a properly obtained urinalysis and positive quantitative culture. When the infection is confirmed and susceptibility tests are completed, choose an appropriate agent with the narrowest spectrum of activity to target the isolated organism.

2. Before treating a patient for bacterial pneumonia, ensure that there is not an alternate diagnosis. The vast majority of respiratory syncytial virus infections in infants are not complicated by bacterial infection, but migratory atelectasis is common. For infants with bronchiolitis, antimicrobial agents are not indicated, unless a concomitant bacterial infection is present.[1]

3. Standardize processes to ensure that appropriate cultures and other diagnostic tests are obtained before antimicrobial agents are administered.

4. Know how to access local antibiograms and be aware of antimicrobial resistance patterns.

5. Initiate antimicrobial therapy promptly for suspected or proven infection, and document indication, dose, timing, and anticipated duration.

6. Perform an "antibiotic timeout" in hospitalized patients. Reassess response to therapy within 48 hours, considering new clinical and laboratory data. Focus definitive therapy to use the most appropriate agent with the narrowest spectrum and to discontinue antibiotic therapy when a treatable bacterial infection is excluded.

7. Collaborate with the local antimicrobial stewardship team and request formal infectious diseases consultation for cases in which the patient has comorbidities, a severe illness, difficult to treat organism, or if the diagnosis is uncertain.

Additional information for health care professionals and parents on judicious use of antimicrobial agents and antimicrobial resistance is available on the CDC website (**www.cdc.gov/antibiotic-use/community/materials-references/index. html** and **www.cdc.gov/drugresistance**).

---

[1] Ralston SL, Lieberthal AS, Meissner HC, et al. Clinical practice guideline: the diagnosis, management, and prevention of bronchiolitis. *Pediatrics*. 2015;136(4):2015-2862

Principles of Appropriate Use of Antimicrobial Therapy for Upper Respiratory Tract Infections

More than half of all outpatient prescriptions for antimicrobial agents for children are given for 5 conditions: otitis media, sinusitis, cough illness/bronchitis, pharyngitis, and nonspecific upper respiratory tract infection (the common cold). Antimicrobial agents often are prescribed, even though many of these illnesses are caused by viruses, which are unresponsive to antibiotic therapy. Children treated with an antimicrobial agent for respiratory tract infections are at increased risk of becoming colonized with resistant respiratory tract flora, including *Streptococcus pneumoniae* and *Haemophilus influenzae*. These same children, who may experience future respiratory tract infections, are more likely to experience failure of subsequent antimicrobial therapy and are likely to spread resistant bacteria to close contacts. The following principles can assist pediatricians in using antibiotic agents appropriately and only when needed for these common pediatric conditions.

OTITIS MEDIA

- The decision to initiate antimicrobial therapy versus observation for children diagnosed with acute otitis media (AOM) should incorporate information about illness severity, laterality of infection, age of patient, and assurance of follow-up. Children <6 months of age, children 6 months and older with otorrhea or severe signs and symptoms (temperature ≥39°F [102.2°F], ear pain for ≥48 hours, or moderate to severe ear pain), and children 6 through 23 months of age with bilateral AOM (regardless of severity) should receive immediate antibiotic treatment. Children 6 through 23 months of age without severe symptoms and unilateral AOM and children 24 months and older without severe symptoms (with unilateral or bilateral AOM) can be offered observation and pain management for 48 to 72 hours with close follow-up, on the basis of shared decision making with the parent or caregiver.
- When antimicrobial agents are used for AOM, a narrow-spectrum antimicrobial agent (eg, amoxicillin, 80–90 mg/kg per day in 2 divided doses) should be used for most children. For children younger than 24 months or with severe symptoms at any age, a 10-day course should be used. For children 2 through 5 years of age without severe symptoms, a 7-day course may be used. For children 6 years and older without severe symptoms, a 5- to 7-day course may be used. Microbiologic and clinical failure with high-dose amoxicillin has been associated with highly penicillin-resistant pneumococci (uncommon currently with widespread use of the 13-valent pneumococcal conjugate vaccine [PCV13]) and with beta-lactamase–producing *Haemophilus* species and *Moraxella* species (an increasing problem as the proportion of cases of AOM caused by pneumococci decreases). Including β-lactamase coverage (by using amoxicillin-clavulanate) when treating a child for AOM is indicated if the child has received amoxicillin in the last 30 days, has concurrent purulent conjunctivitis, or has a history of recurrent AOM unresponsive to amoxicillin.
- Children with underlying medical conditions, craniofacial abnormalities, chronic or recurrent otitis media, or perforation of the tympanic membrane represent a more complicated and diverse population. Initial therapy with a 10-day course of an antimicrobial agent is likely to be more effective than shorter courses for many of these children.

- Persistent middle ear effusion (MEE) is common and can be detected by pneumatic otoscopy (with or without verification by tympanometry) after resolution of acute symptoms. Two weeks after successful antibiotic treatment of AOM, 60% to 70% of children have MEE, decreasing to 40% at 1 month and 10% to 25% at 3 months after successful antibiotic treatment. The presence of MEE without clinical symptoms is defined as otitis media with effusion (OME). OME must be differentiated clinically from AOM and requires infrequent additional monitoring and no antibiotic therapy. Assuring families that OME resolves is particularly important for children with cognitive or developmental delay that may be affected adversely by transient hearing loss associated with MEE.

ACUTE SINUSITIS

- Clinical practice guidelines from the AAP[1] and the Infectious Diseases Society of America[2] delineate evidence-based criteria for the diagnosis and treatment of acute bacterial sinusitis. A clinical diagnosis of acute bacterial sinusitis requires the presence of one of the following criteria: (1) persistent nasal discharge (of any quality) or daytime cough (which may be worse at night) without evidence of clinical improvement for ≥10 days; (2) a worsening course (worsening or new onset of nasal discharge, daytime cough, or fever after initial improvement); or (3) body temperature of ≥39°C (≥102.2°F) with either purulent nasal discharge and/or facial pain concurrently for at least 3 consecutive days in a child who appears ill. Most diagnoses are made by criteria 1 and 2. Findings on sinus imaging correlate poorly with disease and should not be used for acute uncomplicated bacterial sinusitis or to distinguish acute bacterial sinusitis from viral upper respiratory infection. Computed tomography and/or magnetic resonance imaging of sinuses is indicated when complications (eg, orbital or central nervous system complications) are suspected.
- Antimicrobial therapy is indicated for children with severe onset or a worsening course. For children with nonsevere, persistent illness with ≥10 days of symptoms, either observation for an additional 3 days or antimicrobial therapy is indicated.
- When antibiotic therapy is initiated, amoxicillin alone or with clavulanate is preferred. Amoxicillin may be used in standard dose (45 mg/kg/day in 2 divided doses); in areas with high prevalence (>10%) of nonsusceptible *S pneumoniae*, a high dose (80–90 mg/kg/day in 2 divided doses) should be used. Amoxicillin-clavulanate (80–90 mg/kg/day of amoxicillin with 6.4 mg/kg/day of clavulanate [14:1 formulation] in 2 divided doses) may be indicated for children with moderate-to-severe illness, children younger than 2 years, or children attending child care or when antimicrobial resistance is likely (eg, recent treatment with antibiotic agents). Treatment duration typically is 10 days, although the optimal duration of therapy is unclear and clinical trials are underway to evaluate a shorter versus longer course of therapy.

[1]Wald ER, Applegate KE, Bordley C, et al; American Academy of Pediatrics. Clinical practice guideline for the diagnosis and management of acute bacterial sinusitis in children aged 1 to 18 years. *Pediatrics.* 2013;132(1):e262-e280

[2]Chow AW, Benninger MS, Brook I, et al; Infectious Disease Society of America. IDSA clinical practice guideline for acute bacterial rhinosinusitis in children and adults. *Clin Infect Dis.* 2012;54(8):e72-e112

- As noted in the guidelines from the AAP[1] and Infectious Diseases Society of America,[2] existing clinical criteria are limited in their ability to differentiate bacterial from viral acute rhinosinusitis. The guidelines also highlight the changing prevalence and antimicrobial susceptibility profiles of bacterial isolates associated with sinusitis and the impact of pneumococcal conjugate vaccines on the microbiology of sinusitis.

COUGH ILLNESS/BRONCHITIS

- Nonspecific cough illness/bronchitis in children does not warrant antimicrobial treatment.
- Prolonged cough may be caused by *Bordetella pertussis*, *Bordetella parapertussis*, *Mycoplasma pneumoniae* and other *Mycoplasma* species, or *Chlamydia pneumoniae*. When infection caused by one of these organisms is suspected clinically or is confirmed, appropriate antimicrobial therapy is indicated (see Pertussis, p 578, *Mycoplasma pneumoniae* Infections, p 543, and Chlamydial Infections, p 256).

PHARYNGITIS

(See Group A Streptococcal Infections, p 694.)
- Diagnosis of group A streptococcal pharyngitis should be made on the basis of results of appropriate laboratory tests in conjunction with clinical and epidemiologic findings.
- Group A streptococcal testing should only be performed in patients with signs and symptoms of pharyngitis without evidence of a viral upper respiratory infection.
- Most cases of pharyngitis are viral in origin. Antimicrobial therapy should not be given to a child with pharyngitis in the absence of positive group A streptococcal testing. Rarely, other bacteria may cause pharyngitis (eg, *Arcanobacterium haemolyticum*, *Corynebacterium diphtheriae*, *Francisella tularensis*, groups G and C hemolytic streptococci, *Neisseria gonorrhoeae*), and treatment should be provided according to recommendations in disease-specific chapters in Section 3.
- Penicillin remains the drug of choice for treating group A streptococcal pharyngitis. Amoxicillin suspension may be more acceptable to children in taste than penicillin and is equally as effective.

THE COMMON COLD

- Antimicrobial agents should not be given for the common cold.
- Mucopurulent rhinitis (thick, opaque, or discolored nasal discharge that begins a few days into a viral upper respiratory tract infection) commonly accompanies the common cold and is not an indication for antimicrobial treatment.

---

[1] Wald ER, Applegate KE, Bordley C, et al; American Academy of Pediatrics. Clinical practice guideline for the diagnosis and management of acute bacterial sinusitis in children aged 1 to 18 years. *Pediatrics*. 2013;132(1):e262-e280

[2] Chow AW, Benninger MS, Brook I, et al; Infectious Disease Society of America. IDSA clinical practice guideline for acute bacterial rhinosinusitis in children and adults. *Clin Infect Dis*. 2012;54(8):e72-e112

DRUG INTERACTIONS

Use of multiple drugs for treatment increases the probability of adverse drug-drug interactions. Complete drug interaction software programs are used by most hospital and health care system pharmacies and can be consulted for advice. Mobile device-based software applications are available for health care providers to check drug-drug interactions. Labels for individual drugs often include information about clinically significant drug interactions. Individual drug labels can be found online through 2 websites: the DailyMed (**https://dailymed.nlm.nih.gov/dailymed/**) or Drugs@ FDA (**www.accessdata.fda.gov/scripts/cder/daf/**).

TABLES OF ANTIBACTERIAL DRUG DOSAGES

Recommended dosages for antibacterial agents commonly used for neonates (see Table 4.2, p 877) and for infants and children (see Table 4.3, p 882) are provided separately because of the pharmacokinetic and dosing differences between these 2 groups.

Table 4.2 is organized by variables such as gestational age (GA), postnatal age (PNA), and postmenstrual age (PMA) that best guide neonatal dosing for a given group of agents. Aminoglycosides and vancomycin are listed in separate tables to highlight their target serum concentration. For agents used to treat *Bacillus anthracis*, see Fluoroquinolones (p 864) and Anthrax (p 196).

Recommended dosages are not absolute and are intended only as a guide. When a dosage range is provided, the high dose generally is intended for severe infections. Clinical judgment about the disease, predicted drug concentration at the site of infection, alterations in renal or hepatic function, drug interactions, patient response, and laboratory results may dictate modifications of these recommendations in an individual patient. In some cases, monitoring of serum drug concentrations is recommended to avoid toxicity and to achieve concentrations associated with therapeutic efficacy. For vancomycin, this includes a recent consensus recommendation to utilize AUC guided therapeutic monitoring, preferably with Bayesian estimation, for all pediatric age groups, as explained in the tables' footnotes.

Product label information or a pediatric pharmacist should be consulted for details such as the appropriate methods of preparation and administration, measures to be taken to avoid drug interactions, and other precautions. US Food and Drug Administration (FDA)-approved drug labels can be found online at DailyMed (**https://dailymed.nlm.nih.gov/dailymed/**), on the FDA website (**https:// labels.fda.gov/**), and at Drugs@FDA (**www.accessdata.fda.gov/scripts/ cder/daf/**).

For antimicrobial agents not yet approved for children by the FDA but under study, the infections and dosages used for investigational treatments may be found at **http://clinicaltrials.gov**.

Table 4.2. Antibacterial Drugs for Neonates (≤28 Postnatal Days of Age)

Penicillins

Drug	Route	GA ≤34 wk		GA >34 wk	
		PNA ≤7 d	PNA >7 d	PNA ≤7 d	PNA >7 d
Bacteremia					
Ampicillin	IV, IM	50 mg/kg every 12 h	75 mg/kg every 12 h	50 mg/kg every 8 h	50 mg/kg every 8 h
Penicillin G aqueous	IV, IM	50 000 U/kg every 12 h	50 000 U/kg every 8 h	50 000 U/kg every 12 h	50 000 U/kg every 8 h
Meningitis					
Ampicillin	IV, IM	100 mg/kg every 8 h	75 mg/kg every 6 h	100 mg/kg every 8 h	75 mg/kg every 6 h
Penicillin G aqueous	IV, IM	150 000 U/kg every 8 h	125 000 U/kg every 6 h	150 000 U/kg every 8 h	125 000 U/kg every 6 h

Drug	Route	GA ≤34 wk		GA >34 wk	
		PNA ≤7 days	PNA >7 days	PNA ≤7 days	PNA >7 days
Nafcillin, oxacillin[a]	IV, IM	25 mg/kg every 12 h	25 mg/kg every 8 h	25 mg/kg every 8 h	25 mg/kg every 6 h

Drug	Route	PNA ≤7 days	PNA >7 days
Penicillin G procaine	IM only	50 000 U/kg every 24 h	50 000 U/kg every 24 h
Amoxicillin	PO	15 mg/kg every 12 h	15 mg/kg every 12 h

Drug	Route	PMA ≤30 wk	PMA >30 wk
Piperacillin-tazobactam	IV	100 mg/kg every 8 h	80 mg/kg every 6 h

Table 4.2. Antibacterial Drugs for Neonates (≤28 Postnatal Days of Age), continued

Cephalosporins

Drug	Route	GA <32 wk		GA ≥32 wk	
		PNA <7 days	PNA ≥7 days	PNA ≤7 days	PNA >7 days
Cefazolin	IV, IM	25 mg/kg every 12 h	25 mg/kg every 8 h	50 mg/kg every 12 h	50 mg/kg every 8 h
Cefotaxime[b]	IV, IM	50 mg/kg every 12 h	50 mg/kg every 8 h	50 mg/kg every 12 h	50 mg/kg every 8 h
Ceftazidime[c]	IV, IM	50 mg/kg every 12 h	50 mg/kg every 8 h	50 mg/kg every 12 h	50 mg/kg every 8 h
Cefuroxime	IV, IM	50 mg/kg every 12 h	50 mg/kg every 8 h	50 mg/kg every 12 h	50 mg/kg every 8 h

Drug	Route	GA <32 wk		GA ≥32 wk
		PNA ≤7 days	PNA >7 days	
Cefoxitin	IV, IM	35 mg/kg every 12 h	35 mg/kg every 8 h	35 mg/kg every 8 h

Drug	Route	All neonates
Ceftriaxone[c]	IV, IM	50 mg/kg every 24 h

Drug	Route	GA <36 wk	GA ≥36 wk
Cefepime[c]	IV	30 mg/kg every 12 h	50 mg/kg every 12 h[d]

Carbapenems

Drug	Route	GA <32 wk		GA ≥32 wk	
		PNA <14 days	PNA ≥14 days	PNA <14 days	PNA ≥14 days
Meropenem[a]	IV	20 mg/kg every 12 h	20 mg/kg every 8 h	20 mg/kg every 8 h	30 mg/kg every 8 h

Table 4.2. Antibacterial Drugs for Neonates (≤28 Postnatal Days of Age), continued

Drug	Route	PNA ≤7 days	PNA >7 days
Imipenem-cilastatin	IV	25 mg/kg every 12 h	25 mg/kg every 8 h

Other agents

Drug	Route	All neonates
Azithromycin[e]	IV, PO	10 mg/kg every 24 h[f]
Erythromycin[e]	IV, PO	10 mg/kg every 6 h
Rifampin[g]	IV, PO	10 mg/kg every 24 h

Drug	Route	GA <34 wk		GA ≥34 wk	
		PNA ≤7 days	PNA >7 days	PNA ≤7 days	PNA >7 days
Aztreonam[a]	IV	30 mg/kg every 12 h	30 mg/kg every 8 h	30 mg/kg every 8 h	30 mg/kg every 6 h

Drug	Route	PMA ≤32 wk	PMA 33–40 wk	PMA >40 wk
Clindamycin	IV, PO	5 mg/kg every 8h	7 mg/kg every 8 h	9 mg/kg every 8 h

Drug	Route	GA <34 wk		GA ≥34 wk	
		PNA ≤7 days	PNA >7 days	PNA ≤7 days	PNA >7 days
Linezolid	IV, PO	10 mg/kg every 12 h	10 mg/kg every 8 h	10 mg/kg every 8 h	10 mg/kg every 8 h

Table 4.2. Antibacterial Drugs for Neonates (≤28 Postnatal Days of Age), continued

Drug	Route	PMA ≤34 wk	PMA 35–40 wk	PMA >40 wk
Metronidazole[h]	IV	7.5 mg/kg every 12 h	7.5 mg/kg every 8 h	10 mg/kg every 8 h

Aminoglycosides

Drug	Route	GA <30 wk		GA 30–34 wk		GA ≥35 wk	
		PNA ≤14 days	>14 days	≤10 days	>10 days	≤7 days	>7 days
Amikacin[i]	IV, IM	15 mg/kg every 48 h	15 mg/kg every 24 h	15 mg/kg every 36 h	15 mg/kg every 24 h	15 mg/kg every 24 h	18 mg/kg every 24 h
Gentamicin[j]	IV, IM	5 mg/kg every 48 h	5 mg/kg every 36 h	5 mg/kg every 36 h	5 mg/kg every 24 h	4 mg/kg every 24 h	5 mg/kg every 24 h
Tobramycin[j]	IV, IM	5 mg/kg every 48 h	5 mg/kg every 36 h	5 mg/kg every 36 h	5 mg/kg every 24 h	4 mg/kg every 24 h	5 mg/kg every 24 h

Vancomycin

Begin with a 20-mg/kg loading dose followed by a maintenance dose, according to the table

GA ≤28 wk		GA >28 wk	
Serum Creatinine (mg/dL)	Dosage[k]	Serum Creatinine (mg/dL)	Dosage[k]
<0.5	15 mg/kg every 12 h	<0.7	15 mg/kg every 12 h
0.5–0.7	20 mg/kg every 24 h	0.7–0.9	20 mg/kg every 24 h
0.8–1	15 mg/kg every 24 h	1–1.2	15 mg/kg every 24 h
1.1–1.4	10 mg/kg every 24 h	1.3–1.6	10 mg/kg every 24 h
>1.4	15 mg/kg every 48 h	>1.6	15 mg/kg every 48 h

CNS indicates central nervous system; GA, gestational age; GBS, Guillain-Barré syndrome; IM, intramuscular; IV, intravenous; MIC, minimum inhibitory concentration; PNA, postnatal age; PO, oral.

[a] Higher doses than those listed may be required for meningitis, although safety and efficacy data for dosing of neonates with CNS infection are lacking for these agents.

[b] Cefotaxime is available by importation from Canada. See www.fda.gov/media/130296/download for details.

[c] This dose is appropriate for all degrees of neonatal infection, including meningitis. Neonates should not receive IV cefriaxone if they also are receiving IV calcium in any form, including parenteral nutrition. Use in hyperbilirubinemic neonates should be undertaken thoughtfully, especially for those who were born preterm. In vitro studies have shown that ceftriaxone can displace bilirubin from its binding to serum albumin.

[d] May give 30 mg/kg, every 12 h, if target pathogen MIC is ≤4 mg/L.

[e] An association between orally administered erythromycin and azithromycin and infantile hypertrophic pyloric stenosis (IHPS) has been reported in infants younger than 6 weeks. Infants treated with either of these antimicrobials should be followed for signs and symptoms of IHPS.

[f] 20 mg/kg, every 24 hours, is recommended for infants with pneumonia due to *Chlamydia pneumoniae*.

[g] See *Haemophilus influenzae* Infections, p 345, and Meningococcal Infections, p 519, for alternate dosing in special situations.

[h] Begin with a 15-mg/kg loading dose.

[i] Desired serum concentrations: 20–40 mg/L or 10 x MIC (peak), <7 mg/L (trough).

[j] Desired serum concentrations: 6–12 mg/L or 10 x MIC (peak), <2 mg/L (trough).

[k] The maintenance dose should begin at the same number of hours after the loading dose as the maintenance interval. Serum creatinine concentrations normally fluctuate and are partly influenced by transplacental maternal creatinine in the first week of postnatal age. Cautious use of creatinine-based dosing strategy with frequent reassessment of renal function and vancomycin serum concentrations is recommended in neonates ≤7 days of age. The area-under-the-curve to minimum inhibitory concentration (AUC/MIC) has been identified as the most appropriate pharmacokinetic/pharmacodynamic (PK/PD) target vancomycin in adult patients with MRSA. Although there are limitations in prospective outcomes data in pediatric patients with serious MRSA infections, the most recent consensus guideline from the American Society of Health-System Pharmacists, the Infectious Diseases Society of America, the Pediatric Infectious Diseases Society, and the Society of Infectious Diseases Pharmacists recommend AUC-guided therapeutic monitoring, preferably with Bayesian estimation, for all pediatric age groups receiving vancomycin.[1] This estimation accounts for developmental changes of vancomycin clearance from newborn to adolescent. Dosing in children should be designed to achieve an AUC of 400–600 µg-hr/L (assuming MIC of 1) and/or trough levels <15 µg/mL to minimize AKI risks. Bayesian estimation can be completed with 2 levels, with 1 level being recommended 1–2 hours after end of vancomycin infusion, and the second level being drawn 4–6 hours after end of infusion. Levels can be obtained as early as after the second dose. Software to assist with these calculations is available online and for purchase. It is recommended to avoid AUC >800 and troughs >15. In situations in which AUC calculation is not feasible, a trough concentration 10–15 mg/L is very highly likely (>90%) to achieve the AUC target in neonates and children when the MIC is 1 mg/L.

[l] Rybak MJ, Le J, Lodise TP, et al. Therapeutic monitoring of vancomycin for serious methicillin-resistant *Staphylococcus aureus* infections: a revised consensus guideline and review by the American Society of Health-System Pharmacists, the Infectious Diseases Society of America, the Pediatric Infectious Diseases Society, and the Society of Infectious Diseases Pharmacists. *Am J Health Syst Pharm.* 2020;77(11):835–864. DOI: https://doi.org/10.1093/ajhp/zxaa036; Rybak MJ, Le J, Lodise TP, et al. Executive summary: Therapeutic monitoring of vancomycin for serious methicillin-resistant *Staphylococcus aureus* infections: A revised consensus guideline and review by the American Society of Health-System Pharmacists, the Infectious Diseases Society of America, the Pediatric Infectious Diseases Society, and the Society of Infectious Diseases Pharmacists. *J Pediatric Infect Dis Soc.* 2020;9(3):281–284. DOI: https://doi.org/10.1093/jpids/piaa057; and Heil EL, Claeys KC, Mynatt RP, et al. Making the change to area under the curve-based vancomycin dosing. *Am J Health Syst Pharm.* 2018;75(24):1986–1995. DOI: https://doi.org/10.2146/ajhp180034

Adapted from *2021 Nelson's Pediatric Antimicrobial Therapy.* 27th ed. Itasca, IL: American Academy of Pediatrics; 2021.

Table 4.3. Antibacterial Drugs for Pediatric Patients Beyond the Newborn Period[a]

Drug Generic (Trade Name)	Generic Available	Route	Dosage per kg per Day (absolute maximum dosage provided if known)	Comments[b]
Aminoglycosides[c]				See Table 4.2 footnotes for serum concentration targets. Not ideal for CNS infections. Once-daily dosing preferred for parenteral agents except for some endocarditis treatment regimens. Higher doses than those given may be needed to achieve concentration targets in children with cancer or cystic fibrosis.
Amikacin	Y	IV, IM	15–22.5 mg, divided in 2–3 doses or once daily	
Gentamicin	Y	IV, IM	6–7.5 mg, divided in 3 doses, or 5–7.5 mg once daily	
Neomycin	Y	PO	100 mg, divided in 4 doses, max 12 g per day	For some enteric infections.
Tobramycin	Y	IV, IM	6–7.5 mg, divided in 3–4 doses, or 5–7.5 mg once daily	
		Inhaled	300 mg solution or 112 mg powder, inhaled every 12 h	
Aztreonam (Azactam)	Y	IV, IM	90–120 mg, divided in 3 or 4 doses, max 8 g per day	A monobactam antibiotic. Can be used for CNS infections.
Carbapenems[d]				
Imipenem/cilastatin (Primaxin)	Y	IV	60–100 mg, divided in 4 doses, max 4 g per day	Caution when treating CNS infections because of increased risk of seizures. Higher dose should be used for *Pseudomonas aeruginosa* infections.

Table 4.3. Antibacterial Drugs for Pediatric Patients Beyond the Newborn Period,[a] continued

Drug Generic (Trade Name)	Generic Available	Route	Dosage per kg per Day (absolute maximum dosage provided if known)	Comments[b]
Meropenem (Merrem)	Y	IV	30 mg, divided in 3 doses for complicated skin and skin structure infections, max 3 g per day 60 mg, divided in 3 doses for complicated intra-abdominal or *Pseudomonas aeruginosa* skin infections, max 3 g per day 120 mg, divided in 3 doses for meningitis, max 6 g per day	Extended infusion may be needed for susceptible dose-dependent infections.
Ertapenem (Invanz)	N	IV/IM	30 mg, divided in 2 doses, max 1 g per day ≥13 y and adults, 1 g, once daily	Poor activity against *Pseudomonas* and *Acinetobacter* species. Should not be used for CNS infections.
Cephalosporins[d]				The generation of each agent is listed as a guide to antimicrobial spectrum.
Cefaclor (Ceclor)	Y	PO	20–40 mg, divided in 2 or 3 doses, max 1 g per day	Second generation.
Cefadroxil (Duricef)	Y	PO	30 mg, divided in 2 doses, max 2 g per day	First generation.
Cefazolin (Ancef)	Y	IV, IM	25–75 mg, divided in 3 doses, max 6 g per day Up to 150 mg, divided in 3–4 doses for bone/joint infections, max 12 g per day	First generation. Limited data on dosages above 100 mg/kg/day. Should not be used for CNS infections.
Cefdinir (Omnicef)	Y	PO	14 mg, divided in 1 or 2 doses, max 600 mg/day	Third generation. Inadequate activity against penicillin-resistant pneumococci.
Cefepime (Maxipime)	Y	IV, IM	100 mg, divided in 2 doses, max 4 g per day 150 mg, divided in 3 doses for *Pseudomonas* infections, susceptible-dose-dependent *Enterobacterales* infections, febrile neutropenia, or meningitis, max 6 g per day	Fourth generation. Extended infusion may be needed for susceptible dose-dependent infections. Can be used for CNS infections.

Table 4.3. Antibacterial Drugs for Pediatric Patients Beyond the Newborn Period,[a] continued

Drug Generic (Trade Name)	Generic Available	Route	Dosage per kg per Day (absolute maximum dosage provided if known)	Comments[b]
Cefixime (Suprax)	Y	PO	8 mg, divided in 1 or 2 doses, max 400 mg per day	Third generation. Inadequate activity against penicillin-resistant pneumococci.
Cefotaxime (Claforan)[e]	Y	IV, IM	150–180 mg, divided in 3 doses, max 8 g per day 200–225 mg, divided in 4 doses for meningitis, max 12 g per day	Third generation. Up to 300 mg, divided in 4 or 6 doses, may be used for meningitis.
Cefotetan (Cefotan)	Y	IV, IM	60–100 mg, divided in 2 doses, max 6 g per day	Second generation. A cephamycin, active against anaerobes. Should not be used for CNS infections.
Cefoxitin (Mefoxin)	Y	IV, IM	80–160 mg, divided in 3–4 doses, max 12 g per day	Second generation. A cephamycin, active against anaerobes. Should not be used for CNS infections.
Cefpodoxime (Vantin)	Y	PO	10 mg, divided in 2 doses, max 400 mg per day 400 mg/dose, twice daily, effective in adults with severe non-MRSA SSTI.	Third generation.
Cefprozil (Cefzil)	Y	PO	15–30 mg, divided in 2 doses, max 1 g per day	Second generation.
Ceftaroline (Teflaro)	N	IV	2 mo to <2 y: 24 mg, divided in 3 doses >2 y: ≤33 kg: 36 mg, divided in 3 doses >33 kg: 1200 mg (not per kg), divided in 2–3 doses	Fifth generation with anti-MRSA activity. No activity against *Pseudomonas* species. Adult dose: 400 mg/dose, every 8 h, or 600 mg/dose, every 12 h (max 1200 mg/day). Potentially useful for CNS infections, based on limited data.

Table 4.3. Antibacterial Drugs for Pediatric Patients Beyond the Newborn Period,[a] continued

Drug Generic (Trade Name)	Generic Available	Route	Dosage per kg per Day (absolute maximum dosage provided if known)	Comments[b]
Ceftazidime (Fortaz)	Y	IV, IM	90–150 mg, divided in 3 doses 200–300 mg, divided in 3 doses for serious *Pseudomonas* infections	Third generation. Can be used for CNS infections. Max 6 g per day (12 g per day for serious *Pseudomonas* infections in children with cystic fibrosis).
Ceftazidime/avibactam (Avycaz)	N	IV	For 6 mo–18 y: 150 mg ceftazidime/37.5 mg avibactam, divided in 3 doses, max 6 g per day ceftazidime component For 3 mo–<6 mo: 120 mg ceftazidime/30 mg avibactam, divided in 3 doses	For complicated UTI including pyelonephritis and complicated intra-abdominal infections. Dosage adjustments recommended for patients 2 years and older with eGFR <50 mL/min/1.73 m²; insufficient information to recommend a dosing regimen for patients <2 y with renal impairment.
Ceftibuten (Cedax)	Y	PO	9 mg, once daily, max 400 mg per day	Third generation. Inadequate activity against penicillin-resistant pneumococci.
Ceftriaxone (Rocephin)	Y	IV, IM	50–75 mg, once daily, max 1 g per day (for non-CNS, nonendocarditis infections) 100 mg, divided in 1 or 2 doses, max 4 g per day (for CNS or endocarditis infections) 50 mg/kg, IM, once daily for 1–3 days for AOM, max 1 g per day	Third generation.

Table 4.3. Antibacterial Drugs for Pediatric Patients Beyond the Newborn Period,[a] continued

Drug Generic (Trade Name)	Generic Available	Route	Dosage per kg per Day (absolute maximum dosage provided if known)	Comments[b]
Cefuroxime (Zinacef)	Y	IV, IM	100–150 mg, divided in 3 doses, max 6 g per day	Second-generation. Limited activity against penicillin-resistant pneumococcus. Other agents preferred for CNS infections.
Cefuroxime axetil (Ceftin)	Y	PO	20–30 mg, divided in 2 doses, max 1 g per day Up to 100 mg, divided in 3 doses for bone or joint infections, max 3 g per day	Second-generation. Limited activity against penicillin-resistant pneumococcus.
Cephalexin (Keflex)	Y	PO	25–50 mg divided in 2 doses 75–100 mg divided in 3–4 doses for bone or joint infections, max 4 g per day	First-generation.
Chloramphenicol	Y	IV	50–100 mg, divided in 4 doses Adjust based on target serum concentrations (15–25 mg/L)	Reserved for serious infections because of rare risk of aplastic anemia. Can be used for CNS infections.
Clindamycin (Cleocin)	Y	IM, IV	20–40 mg, divided in 3–4 doses, max 2.7 g per day	Active against pneumococci, CA-MRSA, anaerobes. Can be used for CNS infections.
	Y	PO	10–25 mg, divided in 3 doses 30–40 mg, divided in 3–4 doses for AOM or CA-MRSA, max 1.8 g per day	

Table 4.3. Antibacterial Drugs for Pediatric Patients Beyond the Newborn Period,[a] continued

Drug Generic (Trade Name)	Generic Available	Route	Dosage per kg per Day (absolute maximum dosage provided if known)	Comments[b]
Daptomycin (Cubicin)	N	IV	For *Staphylococcus aureus* bacteremia: 1–6 y: 12 mg, once daily 7–11 y: 9 mg, once daily 12–17 y: 7 mg, once daily For skin and skin structure infections: 1–2 y: 10 mg, once daily 2–6 y: 9 mg, once daily 7–11 y: 7 mg, once daily 12–17 y: 5 mg, once daily	Neuromuscular toxicity in neonatal and juvenile canine model. FDA warns to avoid use in infants <12 mo. Not used for CNS infections.
Fluoroquinolones (see also p 864)				
Ciprofloxacin (Cipro)	Y	PO	20–40 mg, divided in 2 doses, max 1.5 g per day	Can be used to treat CNS infections.
		IV	20–30 mg, divided in 2 or 3 doses, max 0.8–1.2 g per day	
Levofloxacin (Levaquin)	Y	IV, PO	≥6 mo and <50 kg: 16 mg, divided in 2 doses, max 500 mg per day for *Bacillus anthracis* exposure >50 kg: 500 mg total daily dose (not per kg) once daily	

Table 4.3. Antibacterial Drugs for Pediatric Patients Beyond the Newborn Period,[a] continued

Drug Generic (Trade Name)	Generic Available	Route	Dosage per kg per Day (absolute maximum dosage provided if known)	Comments[b]
Macrolides				
Azithromycin (Zithromax, Zmax)	Y	PO	5–10 mg, once daily for the immediate-release products 60 mg as a single dose for the extended-release (ER) formulation Respiratory tract infection dosages (per kg, interval is once daily): AOM: 10 mg for 3 days; or 30 mg for 1 day; or 10 mg for 1 day then 5 mg for 4 days Pharyngitis: 12 mg for 1 day, then 6 mg for 4 days Sinusitis: 10 mg for 3 days CAP: 10 mg for 1 day, then 5 mg for 4 days	Per dose max 250 mg for 6 mg/kg, 500 mg for 10–12 mg/kg, 1.5 g for 30 mg/kg. Normal adult total course is 1.5–2 g. Total course max 2.5 g. Multiple additional indications. See relevant chapters in Section 3.
	Y	IV	10 mg, once daily, max 500 mg per day	See *Legionella pneumophila* Infections, p 465. Can be used for some CNS infections,
Clarithromycin (Biaxin)	Y	PO	15 mg, divided in 2 doses, max 1 g per day	Similar activity to erythromycin; more activity against *Mycobacterium avium* and *Helicobacter pylori*.

Table 4.3. Antibacterial Drugs for Pediatric Patients Beyond the Newborn Period,[a] continued

Drug Generic (Trade Name)	Generic Available	Route	Dosage per kg per Day (absolute maximum dosage provided if known)	Comments[b]
Erythromycin (numerous)	Y	PO	40–50 mg, divided in 3–4 doses, max 4 g per day	Available in base, stearate, and ethylsuccinate preparations.
	N	IV	20 mg, divided in 4 doses, max 4 g per day	Administer over at least 60 minutes to potentially prevent cardiac arrhythmias. Not used for CNS infections.
Fidaxomicin (Dificid)	N	PO	Children ≥6 mo: 4 kg to <7 kg: 160 mg total daily dose (not per kg), divided in 2 doses 7 kg to <9 kg: 240 mg total daily dose (not per kg), divided in 2 doses 9 kg to <12.5 kg: 320 mg total daily dose (not per kg), divided in 2 doses ≥12.5 kg: 400 mg total daily dose (not per kg) divided in 2 doses Adults: 400 mg total daily dose (not per kg) divided in 2 doses	For treatment of *Clostridioides difficile* disease.

Table 4.3. Antibacterial Drugs for Pediatric Patients Beyond the Newborn Period,[a] continued

Drug Generic (Trade Name)	Generic Available	Route	Dosage per kg per Day (absolute maximum dosage provided if known)	Comments[b]
Metronidazole (Flagyl)	Y	PO	Range: 15–50 mg, divided in 3 doses, max 2.25 g per day	Can be used for CNS infections.
			30 mg, divided in 3 doses for anaerobic bacterial infections including *Clostridioides difficile* (maximum 500 mg per dose)	
			For bacterial vaginosis, see Table 4.4 (p 898) and Table 4.5 (p 903)	
			For *Trichomonas vaginalis*, see Table 4.4 (p 898) and Table 4.5 (p 903)	
			For Amebiasis, see Table 4.11 (p 958)	
	Y	IV	22.5–40 mg, divided in 3 or 4 doses, max 4 g per day	Can be used for CNS infections.
Nitrofurantoin (Furadantin, Macrodantin)	Y	PO	<12 y: 5–7 mg divided in 4 doses, max 200 mg per day	For treatment of cystitis; not appropriate for pyelonephritis.
			≥12 y: 200 mg total daily dosage, divided in 2 doses	Increased risk of hemolysis in G6PD deficiency.
			UTI prophylaxis: 1–2 mg, once daily	
Oxazolidinones				

Table 4.3. Antibacterial Drugs for Pediatric Patients Beyond the Newborn Period,[a] continued

Drug Generic (Trade Name)	Generic Available	Route	Dosage per kg per Day (absolute maximum dosage provided if known)	Comments[b]
Linezolid (Zyvox)	Y	PO, IV	≤11 y: 30 mg divided in 3 doses (maximum total daily dose: 1200 mg) >11 y: 1200 mg (not per kg) divided in 2 doses	5–11 y: 20 mg divided in 2 doses for SSTI. Myelosuppression increases with duration of therapy over 10 days. Can be used for CNS infections IV or PO.
Tedizolid (Sivextro)	N	PO, IV	6 mg, divided in 2 doses, max 200 mg (not per kg) per day Adults: 200 mg (not per kg), once daily	Not known if effective for CNS infections.
Penicillins[d]				
Amoxicillin (Amoxil)	Y	PO	Standard dose: 40–45 mg, divided in 3 doses High dose: 80–90 mg, divided in 2 doses ≥12 y of age: 775 mg (not per kg), once daily of ER formulation	90 mg/kg/day divided in 2 doses for AOM. 50 mg/kg once daily for streptococcal pharyngitis (see Group A Streptococcal Infections, p 694).
Amoxicillin–clavulanic acid (Augmentin)	Y	PO	14:1 Formulation: 90 mg, divided in 2 doses 7:1 Formulation: 25–45 mg, divided in 2 doses, max 1750 mg per day 4:1 Formulation: 20–40 mg, divided in 3 doses, max 1500 mg per day	Dosed on amoxicillin component. 14:1 Formulation – Augmentin ES-600 7:1 Formulation – Augmentin 875/125 4:1 Formulation – Augmentin 500/125
Ampicillin	Y	IV, IM	50–200 mg, divided in 4 doses, max 8 g per day 300–400 mg, divided in 6 doses for meningitis, endocarditis, max 12 g per day	Can be used for CNS infections.
	Y	PO	50–100 mg, divided in 4 doses, max 2 g per day	

Table 4.3. Antibacterial Drugs for Pediatric Patients Beyond the Newborn Period,[a] continued

Drug Generic (Trade Name)	Generic Available	Route	Dosage per kg per Day (absolute maximum dosage provided if known)	Comments[b]
Ampicillin–sulbactam (Unasyn)	Y	IV	100–200 mg, divided in 4 doses, max 8 g per day 200–400 mg, divided in 4 doses for meningitis or severe infections attributable to resistant *Streptococcus pneumoniae*	Dosed on ampicillin component. Can be used for CNS infections.
Dicloxacillin (Dynapen)	Y	PO	12–25 mg, divided in 4 doses, max 1 g per day 100 mg, divided in 4 doses for bone or joint infections, max 2 g per day	Oral suspension not commercially available.
Nafcillin (Nallpen)	Y	IV, IM	100–200 mg, divided in 4–6 doses, max 12 g per day	Can be used for CNS infection.
Oxacillin (Bactocill)	Y	IV, IM	100–200 mg, divided in 4–6 doses, max 12 g per day	Can be used for CNS infection.
Penicillin G, crystalline potassium or sodium	Y	IV, IM	100 000–300 000 U, divided in 4–6 doses, 300 000–400 000 U, divided in 6 doses for CNS infection	Max 24 million U per day.
Penicillin G procaine	Y	IM	50 000 U, divided in 1–2 doses, max 1.2 million U	Not safe for IV administration. Should not be used for CNS infection.
Penicillin G benzathine (Bicillin LA)	N	IM	Group A streptococcal pharyngitis (see p 694): <27 kg (60 lb): 600 000 U (not per kg), one time >27 kg (60 lb): 1.2 million U (not per kg), one time	Not safe for IV administration. See Group A Streptococcal Infections, p 694. Should not be used for acute CNS infection (see Syphilis, p 729).

Table 4.3. Antibacterial Drugs for Pediatric Patients Beyond the Newborn Period,[a] continued

Drug Generic (Trade Name)	Generic Available	Route	Dosage per kg per Day (absolute maximum dosage provided if known)	Comments[b]
Penicillin G benzathine/procaine (Bicillin CR)	N	IM	<14 kg (30 lb): 600 000 U (not per kg), one time 14–27 kg (30–60 lb): 1.2 million U (not per kg), one time ≥27 kg (60 lb): 2.4 million U (not per kg), one time	Not safe for IV administration. Major use is treatment of group A streptococcal infections (see p 694).
Penicillin V	Y	PO	25–50 mg, divided in 4 doses, max 2 g per day	50–75 mg, divided in 4 doses for group A streptococcal pneumonia.
Piperacillin-tazobactam (Zosyn)	Y	IV	240–300 mg, divided in 3–4 doses, max 16 g per day	Dosed on piperacillin component. Extended infusion may be needed for susceptible-dose dependent infections. 400–600 mg, divided in 6 doses, max 24 g per day, may be appropriate in some patients with cystic fibrosis. Other agents preferred for CNS infections.
Polymyxins				
Colistimethate (Colymycin M)	Y	IV, IM	2.5–5 mg base, divided in 2–4 doses	Not ideal for CNS infections, local (intraventricular) administration required to achieve therapeutic concentrations. Up to 7 mg base/kg/day may be required. 1 mg base = 2.7 mg colistimethate.
Polymyxin B	Y	IV	2.5 mg, divided in 2 doses	>3 mg/kg/day not well studied. 1 mg = 10 000 U.

Table 4.3. Antibacterial Drugs for Pediatric Patients Beyond the Newborn Period,[a] continued

Drug Generic (Trade Name)	Generic Available	Route	Dosage per kg per Day (absolute maximum dosage provided if known)	Comments[b]
Quinupristin + Dalfopristin (Synercid)	N	IV	15 mg, divided in 2 doses	Moderate activity against *Staphylococcus aureus*. Limited experience in children. Not ideal for CNS infections; local (intraventricular) administration required to achieve therapeutic concentrations.
Rifamycins				
Rifampin (Rifadin)	Y	IV, PO	15–20 mg, divided in 1–2 doses, max 600 mg per day. See p 799 and 803 for *Mycobacterium tuberculosis* dosing	Should not be used routinely as monotherapy because of rapid emergence of resistance. Many experts recommend using a daily rifampin dose of at least 20 mg/kg/day for infants and toddlers, and for serious forms of tuberculosis such as meningitis and disseminated disease. Can be used for CNS infections IV or PO.
Rifaximin (Xifaxan)	N	PO	≥12 y: 600 mg/day (not per kg), divided in 3 doses. Used off-label for primary gastrointestinal tract indications (eg, SBBO, IBD) in younger children at similar dosages; consult pediatric gastroenterologist	Treatment of travelers' diarrhea caused by noninvasive *Escherichia coli*.

Table 4.3. Antibacterial Drugs for Pediatric Patients Beyond the Newborn Period,[a] continued

Drug Generic (Trade Name)	Generic Available	Route	Dosage per kg per Day (absolute maximum dosage provided if known)	Comments[b]
Sulfonamides				
Sulfadiazine	Y	PO	120–150 mg, divided in 4 doses, max 6 g per day. Rheumatic fever secondary prevention: 500 mg (not per kg), once daily in children <30 kg; 1 g, once daily in bigger children and adults	Increased risk of hemolysis in G6PD deficiency.
Trimethoprim-Sulfamethoxazole (TMP-SMX) (Bactrim, Septra)	Y	PO, IV	8–10 mg, divided in 2 doses, max 160 mg per dose 2 mg, once daily for UTI prophylaxis 15–20 mg, divided in 3–4 doses for *Pneumocystis jirovecii* treatment, no max 5 mg, divided in 2 doses 3 times/wk for prophylaxis, max 160 mg per dose	Dosed on TMP component. See also *Pneumocystis jirovecii* Infections (p 595). Can be used for CNS infections. Increased risk of hemolysis in G6PD deficiency.
Tetracyclines see also p 866				
Doxycycline (Vibramycin)	Y	PO, IV	2.2–4.4 mg, divided in 2 doses, max 200 mg per day	Can be used for CNS infections IV or PO. Higher doses reported (max 400 mg per day) in adults.
Minocycline (Minocin)	Y	PO, IV	4 mg, divided in 2 doses, max 200 mg per day	Other agents preferred for CNS infections.
Tetracycline	Y	PO	25–50 mg, divided in 4 doses, max 2 g per day	Tetracycline limited to ≥8 y of age. See p 866 for exceptions.

Table 4.3. Antibacterial Drugs for Pediatric Patients Beyond the Newborn Period,[a] continued

Drug Generic (Trade Name)	Generic Available	Route	Dosage per kg per Day (absolute maximum dosage provided if known)	Comments[b]
Vancomycin and other glycopeptides				
Vancomycin (Vancocin)	Y	IV	45–60 mg, divided in 3–4 doses	Measured serum concentrations should guide ongoing therapy.[f]
			60–70 mg, divided in 4 doses, may be necessary in some patients to achieve target serum concentrations for invasive MRSA infections	Can be used for CNS infections.
		PO	40 mg, divided in 4 doses, up to 500 mg per day	For CDI. Up to 2 g per day divided in 4 doses for severe, complicated CDI.
Dalbavancin (Dalvance)	N	IV	3 m–<6 y: 22.5 mg, one time 6 y–<18y: 18 mg, one time, max 1500 mg (not per kg)	Should not be used for CNS infections.

AOM indicates acute otitis media; CAP, community-acquired pneumonia; CA-MRSA, community associated methicillin-resistant *Staphylococcus aureus*; CDI, *Clostridioides difficile* infection; CNS, central nervous system; eGFR, estimated glomerular filtration rate; ER, extended-release; FDA, US Food and Drug Administration; G6PD, glucose-6-phosphate dehydrogenase; IBD, inflammatory bowel disease; IM, intramuscular; IV, intravenous; MRSA, methicillin-resistant *Staphylococcus aureus*; PO, oral; SBBO, small bowel bacterial overgrowth; SSTI, skin and soft tissue infection; UTI, urinary tract infection.

[a] Adapted from American Academy of Pediatrics. *2021 Nelson's Pediatric Antimicrobial Therapy.* 27th ed. Itasca, IL: American Academy of Pediatrics; 2021.

[b] Comments regarding CNS infections are based on FDA-approved indication or evidence from clinical studies in children or adults and apply to administration by the intravenous route unless otherwise specified.

[c] Extended interval ("once daily") dosing may provide equal efficacy with reduced toxicity.

[d] Children with a history of an IgE-mediated, immediate hypersensitivity reaction to penicillins (urticaria, angioedema, bronchospasm, anaphylaxis) who require treatment with an alternate β-lactam should be considered for skin testing (if available) to confirm the allergy, and/or undergo supervised graded clinical challenge or desensitization with the alternate β-lactam agent under the supervision of an expert in drug allergy and desensitization.

[e] Cefotaxime is available by importation from Canada. See www.fda.gov/media/130296/download for details.

[f] The area-under-the-curve to minimum inhibitory concentration (AUC/MIC) has been identified as the most appropriate pharmacokinetic/pharmacodynamic (PK/PD) target vancomycin in adult patients with MRSA. Although there are limitations in prospective outcomes data in pediatric patients with serious MRSA infections, the most recent consensus guideline from ASHP, IDSA, PIDS, and SIDP recommend AUC-guided therapeutic monitoring, preferably with Bayesian estimation, for all pediatric age groups receiving vancomycin.[g] This estimation accounts for developmental changes of vancomycin clearance from newborn to adolescent. Dosing in children should be designed to achieve an AUC of 400–600 µg-hr/L (assuming MIC of 1) and/or trough levels <15 µg/mL to minimize AKI risks. Bayesian estimation can be completed with 2 levels, with 1 level being recommended 1–2 hours after end of vancomycin infusion, and the second level being drawn 4–6 hours after end of infusion. Levels can be obtained as early as after the second dose. Software to assist with these calculations is available online and for purchase. It is recommended to avoid AUC >800 and troughs >15. Most children younger than 12 years will require higher doses to achieve optimal AUC/MIC compared with older children.

[g] Rybak MJ, Le J, Lodise TP, et al. Therapeutic monitoring of vancomycin for serious methicillin-resistant *Staphylococcus aureus* infections: a revised consensus guideline and review by the American Society of Health-System Pharmacists, the Infectious Diseases Society of America, the Pediatric Infectious Diseases Society, and the Society of Infectious Diseases Pharmacists. *Am J Health Syst Pharm.* 2020;77(11):835-864. DOI: **https://doi.org/10.1093/ajhp/zxaa036**; Rybak MJ, Le J, Lodise TP, et al. Executive summary: Therapeutic monitoring of vancomycin for serious methicillin-resistant *Staphylococcus aureus* infections: A revised consensus guideline and review by the American Society of Health-System Pharmacists, the Infectious Diseases Society of America, the Pediatric Infectious Diseases Society, and the Society of Infectious Diseases Pharmacists. *J Pediatric Infect Dis Soc.* 2020;9(3):281-284. DOI: **https://doi.org/10.1093/jpids/piaa057**; and Heil EL, Claeys KC, Mynatt RP, et al. Making the change to area under the curve-based vancomycin dosing. *Am J Health Syst Pharm.* 2018;75(24):1986-1995. DOI: **https://doi.org/10.2146/ajhp180034**

SEXUALLY TRANSMITTED INFECTIONS

Table 4.4. Guidelines for Treatment of Sexually Transmitted Infections in Children ≥45 kg, Adolescents, and Young Adults According to Syndrome

Preferred regimens are listed. For further information concerning other acceptable regimens and diseases not included, see recommendations in disease-specific chapters in Section 3. In addition, recommendations on treatment of sexually transmitted infections have been issued by the Centers for Disease Control and Prevention at **www. cdc.gov/std/treatment.**[a]

Syndrome	Organisms/ Diagnoses	Treatment of Children Weighing ≥45 kg, Adolescents, and Young Adults[a]
Urethritis and Cervicitis: Inflammation of urethra and/or cervix with erythema and/or mucoid, mucopurulent, or purulent discharge	*Neisseria gonorrhoeae*	45–150 kg: Ceftriaxone, 500 mg, IM, in a single dose[b] >150 kg: Ceftriaxone, 1 g, IM, in a single dose[b] If chlamydial infection has not been excluded, also treat for *Chlamydia trachomatis* (see next row)
	Chlamydia trachomatis	Doxycycline, 100 mg, orally, twice a day for 7 days (recommended) **OR** Azithromycin, 1 g, orally, in a single dose (alternative) **OR** Levofloxacin, 500 mg, orally, once daily for 7 days (alternative)
	Nongonoccal urethritis[e] or cervicitis	Doxycycline, 100 mg, orally, twice a day for 7 days (recommended) **OR** Azithromycin, 1 g, orally, in a single dose (alternative)
Persistent and Recurrent Nongonococcal Urethritis: Persistent symptoms after treatment with objective signs of urethral inflammation	The most common cause of persistent or recurrent NGU is *Mycoplasma genitalium*, especially following doxycycline therapy	*Initial regimen doxycycline:* Azithromycin, 1 g, orally, as a single dose **OR** Azithromycin, 500 mg, orally, as a single dose, followed by 250 mg, orally, daily for 4 additional days *Initial regimen azithromycin:* Moxifloxacin, 400mg, orally, daily for 7 days to 10 days (recommended) **OR** Doxycycline, 100 mg, orally, twice daily for 7 days, followed by moxifloxacin, 400 mg, orally, once daily for 7 days (alternative)

Table 4.4. Guidelines for Treatment of Sexually Transmitted Infections in Children ≥45 kg, Adolescents, and Young Adults According to Syndrome, continued

Syndrome	Organisms/ Diagnoses	Treatment of Children Weighing ≥45 kg, Adolescents, and Young Adults[a]
	T vaginalis (in males who only have sex with females)	Metronidazole, 2 g, orally, in a single dose[d,e] **OR** Tinidazole, 2 g, orally, in a single dose[d,e]
Vulvovaginitis	*T vaginalis*	Metronidazole, 500 mg, orally, twice daily for 7 days[d,e] **OR** Tinidazole, 2 g, orally, in a single dose[d,e]
	Bacterial vaginosis	Metronidazole, 500 mg, orally, twice daily for 7 days[d,e] **OR** Metronidazole gel 0.75%, 1 full applicator (5 g), intravaginally, once a day for 5 days[d,e] **OR** Clindamycin cream 2%, 1 full applicator (5 g), intravaginally at bedtime, for 7 days
	Candida albicans (and occasionally other *Candida* species or yeasts)	See Table 4.6, Recommended Regimens for Vulvovaginal Candidiasis (p 904)
Pelvic inflammatory disease (PID)[f]		**Recommended Parenteral Regimens:** Ceftriaxone, 1 g, IV, every 24 h **PLUS** Doxycycline, 100 mg, orally or IV, every 12 h **PLUS** Metronidazole, 500 mg, orally or IV, every 12 h **OR** Cefotetan, 2 g, IV, every 12 h **OR** Cefoxitin, 2 g, IV, every 6 h **PLUS** Doxycycline, 100 mg, orally or IV, every 12 h **Recommended Intramuscular/Oral Regimens[g,h]:** One of the following: Ceftriaxone, 500 mg, IM, once **OR** Cefoxitin, 2 g, IM, **and** Probenecid, 1 g, orally, in a single dose concurrently **OR** Other parenteral third-generation Cephalosporin (eg, Ceftizoxime, Cefotaxime) **PLUS**

Table 4.4. Guidelines for Treatment of Sexually Transmitted Infections in Children ≥45 kg, Adolescents, and Young Adults According to Syndrome, continued

Syndrome	Organisms/ Diagnoses	Treatment of Children Weighing ≥45 kg, Adolescents, and Young Adults[a]
		Doxycycline, 100 mg, orally, twice a day for 14 days **WITH** Metronidazole, 500 mg, orally, twice a day for 14 days[d]
Genital ulcer disease	*Treponema pallidum* (primary or secondary syphilis)	Penicillin G benzathine, 2.4 million U, IM, in a single dose
	Genital HSV—1st clinical episode[i]	Acyclovir, 400 mg, orally, 3 times/day for 7–10 days **OR** Valacyclovir, 1 g, orally, twice daily for 10 days **OR** Famciclovir, 250 mg, orally, 3 times/day for 7–10 days
	Genital HSV – episodic treatment of recurrences	Acyclovir, 800 mg, orally, twice daily for 5 days **OR** Acyclovir, 800 mg, orally, 3 times daily for 2 days **OR** Famciclovir, 1 g, orally, 2 times daily for 1 day **OR** Famciclovir, 500 mg, orally, once, followed by 250 mg, orally, twice daily for 2 days **OR** Famciclovir, 125 mg, orally, twice daily for 5 days **OR** Valacyclovir, 500 mg, orally twice daily for 3 days **OR** Valacyclovir, 1 g, orally, once daily for 5 days
	Genital HSV – suppressive therapy	Acyclovir, 400 mg, orally, twice daily **OR** Valacyclovir, 500 mg, orally, once daily **OR** Valacyclovir, 1 g, orally, once daily **OR** Famciclovir, 250 mg, orally, twice daily

Table 4.4. Guidelines for Treatment of Sexually Transmitted Infections in Children ≥45 kg, Adolescents, and Young Adults According to Syndrome, continued

Syndrome	Organisms/ Diagnoses	Treatment of Children Weighing ≥45 kg, Adolescents, and Young Adults[a]
	Haemophilus ducreyi (chancroid)	Azithromycin, 1 g, orally, in a single dose **OR** Ceftriaxone, 250 mg, IM, in a single dose **OR** Ciprofloxacin, 500 mg, orally, twice daily for 3 days[j] **OR** Erythromycin base, 500 mg, orally, 3 times/day for 7 days
	Klebsiella granulomatis (granuloma inguinale [donovanosis])	Azithromycin, 1 g, orally, once/wk or 500 mg, orally, daily, for at least 3 wk and until all lesions have healed completely
	C trachomatis serovars L1, L2, or L3 (lymphogranuloma venereum [LGV])	Doxycycline, 100 mg, orally, twice a day for 21 days
Epididymitis	*C trachomatis, N gonorrhoeae*	Ceftriaxone, 500 mg, IM, in a single dose **PLUS** Doxycycline, 100 mg, orally, twice daily for 10 days
	Enteric organisms (eg, *Escherichia coli*), *C trachomatis, N gonorrhoeae* among males who practice insertive anal sex	Ceftriaxone, 500 mg, IM, in a single dose **PLUS** Levofloxacin, 500 mg, orally, once a day for 10 days
Proctitis	*C trachomatis, N gonorrhoeae*, HSV	Ceftriaxone, 500 mg, IM, in a single dose **PLUS** Doxycycline, 100 mg, orally, twice daily for 7 days; extend to 21 days for presence of bloody discharge, perianal or mucosal ulcers, or tenesmus and a positive rectal *C trachomatis* test **PLUS** in the presence of rectal ulcers Valacyclovir, 1 g, orally, twice daily **OR** acyclovir, 400 mg, orally, three times daily **OR** famciclovir, 250 mg, orally, 3 times daily for 7–10 days

Table 4.4. Guidelines for Treatment of Sexually Transmitted Infections in Children ≥45 kg, Adolescents, and Young Adults According to Syndrome, continued

Syndrome	Organisms/ Diagnoses	Treatment of Children Weighing ≥45 kg, Adolescents, and Young Adults[a]
External anogenital warts (ie, penis, groin, scrotum, vulva, perineum, external anus, and perianus)	Human papillomavirus	*Patient-applied:* Imiquimod 3.75% or 5% cream[j,k] **OR** Podofilox 0.5% solution or gel[j] **OR** Sinecatechins 15% ointment[j] *Provider-administered:* Cryotherapy with liquid nitrogen or cryoprobe **OR** Surgical removal either by tangential scissor excision, tangential shave excision, curettage, laser, or electrosurgery **OR** Trichloroacetic acid or bichloroacetic acid 80%–90% solution

IM indicates intramuscularly; STI, sexually transmitted infection.

[a] For additional information and recommendations, see Centers for Disease Control and Prevention. Sexually transmitted infections treatment guidelines, 2021. *MMWR Recomm Rep.* 2021; in press. Available at: **www.cdc.gov/std/treatment**

[b] If ceftriaxone is not feasible, may substitute cefixime, 800 mg, orally, in a single dose.

[c] Nongonococcal urethritis (NGU) is diagnosed when microscopy indicates inflammation without gram-negative intracellular diplococci (on Gram stain) or purple intracellular diplococci (on methylene blue or gentian violet staining) on urethral smear.

[d] In areas where *T vaginalis* is prevalent, males who have sex with females and have persistent or recurrent urethritis should be presumptively treated for *T vaginalis.*

[e] Alcohol consumption should be avoided during treatment with metronidazole or tinidazole; breastfeeding should be deferred for 72 hours after mother has received a 2-g dose of tinidazole.

[f] Hospitalization and parenteral treatment is recommended if patient has severe illness such as tubo-ovarian abscess, is pregnant, or is unable to tolerate or follow ambulatory regimens.

[g] Patients with inadequate response to outpatient therapy after 72 hours should be reevaluated for possible misdiagnosis and may require parenteral therapy.

[h] The recommended third-generation cephalosporins are limited in the coverage of anaerobes. Therefore, the addition of metronidazole to treatment regimens with third-generation cephalosporins should be considered.

[i] Treatment can be extended if healing is incomplete after 10 days of therapy.

[j] Avoid in pregnancy.

[k] Wash treatment area with soap and water 6–10 hours after application.

Adapted from Centers for Disease Control and Prevention. Sexually transmitted infections treatment guidelines, 2021. *MMWR Recomm Rep.* 2021; in press

Table 4.5. Guidelines for Treatment of Sexually Transmitted Infections in Infants and Children <45 kg According to Syndrome

Preferred regimens are listed. For further information concerning other acceptable regimens and diseases not included, see recommendations in disease-specific chapters in Section 3. In addition, recommendations on treatment of sexually transmitted infections have been issued by the Centers for Disease Control and Prevention in 2021[a] (**www.cdc.gov/std/treatment**).

Syndrome	Organisms/ Diagnoses	Treatment of Infants and Children <45 kg[a,b]
Urethritis: Inflammation of urethra with erythema and/or mucoid, mucopurulent, or purulent discharge Note: Cervicitis occurs rarely in prepubertal females	*Neisseria gonorrhoeae, Chlamydia trachomatis* Other causes include *Mycoplasma genitalium,* possibly *Ureaplasma urealyticum,* and sometimes *Trichomonas vaginalis* and herpes simplex virus (HSV)	Ceftriaxone, 25–50 mg/kg, IV or IM, in a single dose, not to exceed 250 mg IM[c] **PLUS** Erythromycin base or ethylsuccinate, 50 mg/kg per day, orally, in 4 divided doses for 14 days
Prepubertal vaginitis (STI related):	*N gonorrhoeae*	Ceftriaxone, 25–50 mg/kg, IV or IM, in a single dose, not to exceed 250 mg, IM, in a single dose[c]
	C trachomatis	Erythromycin base or ethylsuccinate, 50 mg/kg per day, orally, in 4 divided doses for 14 days
	T vaginalis	Metronidazole, 45 mg/kg per day, orally, in 3 divided doses (maximum 2 g/day) for 7 days
	Bacterial vaginosis	Metronidazole, 15–25 mg/kg per day, orally, in 3 divided doses (maximum 2 g/day) for 7 days
Genital ulcer disease	*T pallidum* (primary syphilis)[d]	Benzathine penicillin G, 50 000 U/kg IM, up to the adult dose of 2.4 million U in a single dose
	HSV—1st clinical episode	Acyclovir, 80 mg/kg per day, orally, in 4 divided doses (maximum 3.2 g/day) for 7–10 days **OR** Valacyclovir, 40 mg/kg per day (maximum 2 g/day), orally, in 2 divided doses for 7–10 days

Table 4.5. Guidelines for Treatment of Sexually Transmitted Infections in Infants and Children <45 kg According to Syndrome, continued

Syndrome	Organisms/ Diagnoses	Treatment of Infants and Children <45 kg[a,b]
	Haemophilus ducreyi (chancroid)	Ceftriaxone, 50 mg/kg, IM, in a single dose (maximum 250 mg) OR Azithromycin, 20 mg/kg, orally, in a single dose (maximum 1 g)
Anogenital warts	Human papillomavirus	Same as for adolescents. See Table 4.4.

IM indicates intramuscularly; STI, sexually transmitted infection.

[a] For additional information and recommendations, see Centers for Disease Control and Prevention. Sexually transmitted infections treatment guidelines, 2021. *MMWR Recomm Rep.* 2021; in press. Available at: **www.cdc.gov/std/treatment**

[b] Infants and children aged ≥1 month with a sexually transmitted infection should be evaluated for sexual abuse (eg, through consultation with child-protection services). See Table 2.5, p 151.

[c] Providers treating patients with a severe cephalosporin allergy should consult an infectious disease specialist.

[d] Infants and children >1 mo of age who receive a diagnosis of syphilis should have birth and maternal medical records reviewed to assess whether they have congenital or acquired syphilis. Infants and children ≥1 mo of age with primary syphilis should be managed by a pediatric infectious disease specialist.

Table 4.6. Recommended Treatment Regimens for Vulvovaginal Candidiasis[a]

Over-the-Counter Intravaginal Agents[b]

Clotrimazole 1% cream, 5 g, intravaginally, for 7–14 days

OR

Clotrimazole 2% cream, 5 g, intravaginally, for 3 days

OR

Miconazole 2% cream, 5 g, intravaginally, for 7 days

OR

Miconazole 4% cream, 5 g, intravaginally, for 3 days

OR

Miconazole, 100-mg vaginal suppository, 1 suppository for 7 days

OR

Miconazole, 200-mg vaginal suppository, 1 suppository for 3 days

OR

Miconazole, 1200-mg vaginal suppository, 1 suppository for 1 day

OR

Tioconazole, 6.5% ointment, 5 g, intravaginally, in a single application

Table 4.6. Recommended Treatment Regimens for Vulvovaginal Candidiasis,[a] continued

Prescription Intravaginal Agents[b]

Butoconazole 2% cream (single-dose bioadhesive product), 5 g intravaginally in a single application

OR

Terconazole 0.4% cream, 5 g, intravaginally, daily for 7 days

OR

Terconazole 0.8% cream, 5 g, intravaginally, for 3 days

OR

Terconazole, 80-mg vaginal suppository, 1 suppository for 3 days

Oral Agent

Fluconazole, 150-mg oral tablet, 1 tablet in single dose

[a] Adapted from Centers for Disease Control and Prevention. Sexually transmitted infections treatment guidelines, 2021. *MMWR Recomm Rep.* 2021; in press.
[b] These creams and suppositories are oil-based and might weaken latex condoms and diaphragms.

ANTIFUNGAL DRUGS FOR SYSTEMIC FUNGAL INFECTIONS

Polyenes

Amphotericin B is a fungicidal agent that is effective against a broad array of fungal species. Amphotericin B, especially the "conventional" deoxycholate formulation, is associated with multiple adverse reactions, particularly acute and chronic renal toxicity, so its use is limited in certain patients. Lipid-associated formulations of amphotericin B, especially liposomal amphotericin B, limit renal toxicity but also are associated with multiple other adverse effects and do not achieve optimal concentrations in some sites of infection (eg, kidneys).

Amphotericin B deoxycholate is the preferred formulation for treatment of neonates with systemic candidiasis because of better penetration into the central nervous system, urinary tract, and eye, which often are involved in neonatal *Candida* infections; lipid-associated formulations do not penetrate as well into these body sites. Amphotericin B deoxycholate is generally administered intravenously in a single daily dose of 1 mg/kg in 5% dextrose in water at a concentration of 0.1 mg/mL and delivered through a central or peripheral venous catheter. Infusion times of 1 to 2 hours have been shown to be well tolerated in adults and older children and theoretically increase the blood-to-tissue gradient, thereby improving drug delivery. Total duration of therapy depends on the type and extent of the specific fungal infection.

Amphotericin B deoxycholate is eliminated by a renal mechanism for approximately 2 weeks after therapy is discontinued. No adjustment in dose is required for neonates or for children with impaired renal function, because serum concentrations are not increased significantly in these patients. Because of concentration-dependent killing, if renal toxicity occurs, it is recommended to maintain the dose but switch to alternate-day dosing. Neither hemodialysis nor peritoneal dialysis significantly decreases serum concentrations of the drug.

Infusion-related reactions to amphotericin B deoxycholate include fever, chills, and sometimes nausea, vomiting, headache, generalized malaise, hypotension, and arrhythmias; these reactions are rare in neonates. Onset usually is within 1 to 3 hours after starting the infusion; duration typically is less than an hour. Hypotension and arrhythmias are idiosyncratic reactions that are unlikely to occur if not observed after the initial dose but also can occur in association with rapid infusion. Multiple regimens have been used to prevent infusion-related reactions, but few have been studied in controlled clinical trials. Pretreatment with acetaminophen, alone or combined with diphenhydramine, may alleviate febrile reactions; these reactions appear to be less common in children than in adults. Hydrocortisone (25–50 mg in adults and older children) also can be added to the infusion to decrease febrile and other systemic reactions. Tolerance to febrile reactions develops with time, allowing tapering and eventual discontinuation of the hydrocortisone and often diphenhydramine and antipyretic agents. Meperidine and ibuprofen have been effective in preventing or treating fever and chills in some patients who are refractory to the conventional premedication regimen.

Toxicity from amphotericin B deoxycholate can include nephrotoxicity, hepatotoxicity, anemia, or neurotoxicity. Nephrotoxicity is caused by decreased renal blood flow and can be prevented or ameliorated by hydration, saline solution loading (0.9% saline solution over 30 minutes) before infusion of amphotericin B, and avoidance of diuretic drugs. Hypokalemia is common and can be exacerbated by sodium loading. Renal tubular acidosis can occur but usually is mild. Permanent nephrotoxicity is related to cumulative dose. Nephrotoxicity is increased by concomitant administration of amphotericin B and aminoglycosides, cyclosporine, tacrolimus, cisplatin, nitrogen mustard compounds, or acetazolamide. Anemia is secondary to inhibition of erythropoietin production. Neurotoxicity occurs rarely and can manifest as confusion, delirium, obtundation, psychotic behavior, seizures, blurred vision, or hearing loss.

Lipid preparations of amphotericin B, such as amphotericin B lipid complex (ABLC, Abelcet) and liposomal amphotericin B (L-AmB, AmBisome), are the preferred formulation in all patient populations except neonates. Acute infusion-related reactions occur with both formulations but are less frequent with AmBisome. Nephrotoxicity is less common with lipid-associated products than with amphotericin B deoxycholate. Liver toxicity, which generally is not associated with amphotericin B deoxycholate, has been reported with the lipid formulations.

Pyrimidines

Among pyrimidine antifungal agents, only flucytosine (5-fluorocytosine) is approved by the US Food and Drug Administration (FDA) for use in children. Flucytosine has a limited spectrum of activity against fungi (*Cryptococcus* and *Candida* species) and has potential for toxicity and should be avoided in the setting of renal dysfunction. When flucytosine is used as a single agent, resistance often emerges rapidly. Flucytosine should be used in combination with amphotericin B for cryptococcal meningitis. It is important to monitor serum concentrations of flucytosine to avoid bone marrow toxicity. Flucytosine is only available in oral formulation in the United States.

Azoles

Six oral azoles are available in the United States: ketoconazole, fluconazole, itraconazole, voriconazole, posaconazole, and isavuconazonium sulfate (the prodrug for isavuconazole). All have relatively broad activity against common fungi but differ in their in vitro activity (see Table 4.7, p 909), bioavailability, adverse effects, and potential for drug interactions. Fewer data are available regarding safety and efficacy of azoles in pediatric than in adult patients. Azoles are easy to administer and have little toxicity, but their use can be limited by the frequency of their interactions with coadministered drugs. These drug interactions can result in decreased serum concentrations of the azole (ie, poor therapeutic activity) or unexpected toxicity from the coadministered drug (caused by increased serum concentrations of the coadministered drug). When considering use of azoles, the patient's concurrent medications should be reviewed to avoid potential adverse clinical outcomes. The FDA reaffirmed in 2016 that it strongly discourages use of systemic ketoconazole for uncomplicated skin and nail infections because of significant risks of liver toxicity, adrenal insufficiency, and interactions with multiple medications that have resulted in at least 1 fatality.

Another potential limitation of azoles is emergence of resistant fungi, especially *Candida* species resistant to fluconazole. *Candida krusei* intrinsically are resistant to fluconazole, and strains of *Candida glabrata* increasingly are resistant to both fluconazole and voriconazole. Itraconazole is approved by the FDA for treatment of blastomycosis and histoplasmosis (nonmeningeal) and for empiric therapy of febrile neutropenic patients with suspected fungal infection. Efficacy and safety have not been established in pediatric patients. Itraconazole does not cross the blood-brain barrier and should not be used for infections of the central nervous system. Voriconazole has been approved by the FDA for individuals 2 years of age and older for primary treatment of invasive *Aspergillus* species, for candidemia in nonneutropenic patients, for esophageal candidiasis, and for refractory infection with *Fusarium* species and some *Scedosporium* species, such as *Scedosporium apiospermum*. Intravenous and oral formulations are available. Posaconazole is approved for use in adults (all formulations) and children ≥13 years of age and older (delayed release tablets and oral suspension) for prophylaxis of invasive aspergillosis and candidiasis in patients who are high risk of developing these infections, and the oral suspension is approved for treatment of oropharyngeal candidiasis. Strategies to enhance absorption are necessary (eg, administration with high-fat meal, avoidance of proton pump inhibitors) when using the oral suspension. Isavuconazole, available in oral and intravenous forms, has been approved by the FDA for patients 18 years or older for invasive aspergillosis and invasive mucormycosis. Therapeutic monitoring of azole drugs, especially itraconazole, voriconazole, and posaconazole, with measurement of serum trough concentrations is critical in patients with serious infections.

Echinocandins

Caspofungin, micafungin, and anidulafungin are the only echinocandins approved by the FDA. Caspofungin is approved for treatment of pediatric patients 3 months of age and older with invasive candidiasis and esophageal candidiasis; for empiric therapy for presumed fungal infections in febrile neutropenic patients; and for treatment of aspergillosis in patients who are refractory to or intolerant of other antifungal drugs. Clinical trials have demonstrated safety and efficacy in pediatric patients as young as 3 months of age; noncomparative anecdotal experience in neonatal infections also is reported. Micafungin is approved by the FDA for intravenous treatment of pediatric patients 4 months and older with candidemia, acute disseminated candidiasis, *Candida* peritonitis and abscesses, and esophageal candidiasis, and for prophylaxis of invasive *Candida* infections in patients undergoing hematopoietic stem cell transplantation. Although micafungin is not FDA approved for aspergillosis, data are available to support its use in the treatment of refractory disease, preferably in combination with other antifungal agent.[1] Anidulafungin is not approved by the FDA for use in children but is FDA approved for the treatment of candidemia, *Candida* infections, and esophageal candidiasis in adults. Table 4.7 provides data on the relative in vitro susceptibilities of specific fungal species with amphotericin B, azoles, echinocandins, and flucytosine.

[1]Patterson TF, Thompson GR, Denning DW, et al. Practice guidelines for the diagnosis and management of aspergillosis: 2016 update by the Infectious Diseases Society of America. *Clin Infect Dis.* 2016;63(4):e1-e60. DOI: **https://doi.org/10.1093/cid/ciw326**

Table 4.7. Fungal Species, Antifungal Drugs, Activity, Route, Clearance, CSF Penetration, Drug Monitoring Targets, and Adverse Events

Fungal Species	Amphotericin B Formulations	Fluconazole	Itraconazole	Voriconazole	Posaconazole	Isavuconazole	Flucytosine	Echinocandins[a]
Candida albicans	+	++	+	++	+	+	+	++
Candida tropicalis	+	++	+	++	+	+	+	++
Candida parapsilosis	++	++	+	++	+	+	+	+
Candida glabrata	+	−	−	−	+/−	+/−	+	+/−
Candida krusei	+	−	−	+	+	+	+	++
Candida lusitaniae	−	++	+	++	+	+	+	+
Candida guilliermondii	+	+	+	+	+	+	+	+/−
Candida auris	+/−	−	+/−	+/−	+	+	+/−	++
Cryptococcus species	++	++	+	+	+	+	++	−
Trichosporon species	+	+	+	++	+	+	−	−
Aspergillus fumigatus[b]	+	−	+	++	+	++	−	+
Aspergillus terreus[b]	−	−	+	++	+	++	−	+
Aspergillus calidoustus[b]	++	−	−	−	−	−	−	++
Fusarium species[b]	+	−	−	++	+	+	−	−

Table 4.7. Fungal Species, Antifungal Drugs, Activity, Route, Clearance, CSF Penetration, Drug Monitoring Targets, and Adverse Events, continued

Fungal Species	Amphotericin B Formulations	Flucona-zole	Itraconazole	Voriconazole	Posacona-zole	Isavucona-zole	Flucytosine	Echi-nocandins[a]
Mucor species[b]	++	–	+/-	–	+	++	–	–
Rhizopus species[b]	++	–	–	–	+	++	–	–
Scedosporium apiospermum[b]	–		+	++	+	+	–	–
Scedosporium prolificans[b]	–		+/-	+/-	+/-	+/-		–
Penicillium (Talaromyces) species[b]	+/-	–	++	+	+	+		–
Histoplasma capsulatum[c]	++	+	++	+	+	+	–	–
Coccidioides immitis[c]	++	++	++	+	+	+	–	–
Blastomyces dermatitidis[c]	++	+	++	+	+	+		–
Paracoccidioides species[c]	+	+	++	+	+	+		–
Sporothrix species[c]	+	+	++	+	+	+	–	–
IV/PO	IV only	IV and PO	PO only	IV and PO	IV and PO	IV and PO	PO only	IV only

Table 4.7. Fungal Species, Antifungal Drugs, Activity, Route, Clearance, CSF Penetration, Drug Monitoring Targets, and Adverse Events, continued

Fungal Species	Amphotericin B Formulations	Fluconazole	Itraconazole	Voriconazole	Posaconazole	Isavuconazole	Flucytosine	Echinocandins[a]
Clearance	Renal	Renal/hepatic	Hepatic	Hepatic	Hepatic	Hepatic	Renal	Hepatic (micafungin)
CSF penetration	Good	Good	Limited	Good	Minimal	Good	Good	Minimal
Therapeutic drug monitoring (treatment)	No	No	Trough 1–2 µg/mL (when measured by high-pressure liquid chromatography, both itraconazole and its bioactive hydroxy-itraconazole metabolite are reported, the sum of which should be considered in assessing drug levels)	Trough 2–6 µg/mL	Trough >1.0 µg/mL; higher rate of adverse effects when trough levels exceed 1 µg/mL	Unknown	Peak 40–80 µg/mL	No

Table 4.7. Fungal Species, Antifungal Drugs, Activity, Route, Clearance, CSF Penetration, Drug Monitoring Targets, and Adverse Events, continued

Fungal Species	Amphotericin B Formulations	Fluconazole	Itraconazole	Voriconazole	Posaconazole	Isavuconazole	Flucytosine	Echinocandins[a]
Common adverse reactions	Infusion reaction, nephrotoxicity (watch potassium, magnesium); liposomal: hepatoxicity	Hepatotoxicity, increased QTc, headache, gastrointestinal tract effects	Hepatotoxicity, increased QTc; negative inotrope (avoid in congestive heart failure)	Hepatotoxicity, increased QTc, central nervous system effects, vision changes, phototoxicity	Hepatotoxicity, increased QTc, headache, gastrointestinal tract effects	Headache, hypokalemia, Abdominal pain, nausea, diarrhea, conjunctivitis, flu-like illness, hepatotoxicity, cough	Neutropenia, hepatotoxicity (avoid in decreased renal function), gastrointestinal	Usually well tolerated; gastrointestinal tract effects, headache, hepatotoxicity

CSF indicates cerebrospinal fluid; IV, intravenous; PO, oral.

NOTE: **++**, more active, scenario dependent; **+**, usually active; **+/–**, variably active; **–**, usually not active.

[a] Caspofungin, anidulafungin, and micafungin.

[b] Mold.

[c] Endemic fungi where mold/yeast phase is temperature dependent.

RECOMMENDED DOSES OF PARENTERAL AND ORAL ANTIFUNGAL DRUGS

Table 4.8. Recommended Doses of Parenteral and Oral Antifungal Drugs

Drug	Route	Dose (per day)	Adverse Reactions[a,b]
Amphotericin B deoxycholate (see Antifungal Drugs for Systemic Fungal Infections, p 905, for detailed information)	IV	1.0 mg/kg per day (or 1.5 mg/kg every other day) (max 1.5 mg/kg/day); infuse as a single dose over 2–4 h.	Fever, chills, phlebitis, gastrointestinal tract symptoms, headache, hypotension, renal dysfunction, hypokalemia, anemia, cardiac arrhythmias, neurotoxicity, anaphylaxis.
	IT	0.01–0.025 mg, slow increase to 0.5 mg, twice/wk.	Headache, gastrointestinal tract symptoms, arachnoiditis/radiculitis.
Amphotericin B lipid complex (Abelcet)[c]	IV	3–5 mg/kg per day, infused over 2 h.	Fever, chills, other reactions associated with amphotericin B deoxycholate, but less nephrotoxicity; hepatotoxicity has been reported with lipid complex.
Liposomal amphotericin B (AmBisome)[c]	IV	3–5 mg/kg, infused over 1–2 h. IFI prophylaxis[d]: 1 mg/kg/dose every other day or 2.5 mg/kg/dose twice/wk. Doses up to 10 mg/kg have been used in patients with mucormycosis.	Fever, chills, fewer infusion reactions and less nephrotoxicity than associated with amphotericin B deoxycholate; hepatotoxicity has been reported.
Anidulafungin[c,e]	IV	For adults and adolescents 12 y and older: Candidemia and other forms of *Candida* infections: 200 mg on day 1, followed by 100-mg daily dose thereafter for at least 14 days after the last positive culture. Esophageal candidiasis: 100 mg on day 1, followed by 50-mg daily dose thereafter for a minimum of 14 days and for at least 7 days following resolution of symptoms. The rate of infusion should not exceed 1.1 mg/minute.	Fever, headache, nausea, vomiting, diarrhea, leukopenia, hypokalemia, hepatitis, hepatic enzyme elevations, hypersensitivity, and phlebitis. Because of high alcohol content of solution, the rate of infusion should not exceed 1.1 mg/minute.

Table 4.8. Recommended Doses of Parenteral and Oral Antifungal Drugs, continued

Drug	Route	Dose (per day)	Adverse Reactions[a,b]
		Dosage in pediatric patients (2 years through 11 years): Candidemia and other forms of *Candida* infections: 3-mg/kg loading dose on day 1, followed by 1.5 mg/kg once daily thereafter. Maximum loading dose and daily dose should not exceed 100 mg/day. Esophageal candidiasis: 1.5-mg/kg loading dose on day 1, followed by 0.75 mg/kg once daily thereafter. Maximum loading dose and daily dose should not exceed 50 mg.	
Caspofungin[e]	IV	Dosage in adults (18 y and older): 70-mg loading dose on day 1, followed by 50 mg once daily for all indications except esophageal candidiasis. Dosage in pediatric patients (3 months through 17 y of age): For all indications, 70-mg/m² loading dose on day 1, followed by 50 mg/m² once daily thereafter. Maximum dose should not exceed 70 mg, regardless of the patient's weight and calculated dose. Dosage in neonates: 25 mg/m² daily.	Adults: Diarrhea, pyrexia, hepatic enzymes elevations, and hypokalemia. Pediatric: diarrhea, rash, hepatic enzymes elevations, hypokalemia, infusion-related reactions. Isolated cases of hepatic dysfunction, hepatitis, or hepatic failure have been reported.
Clotrimazole	PO	10-mg lozenge, 5 times per day (dissolved slowly in mouth).	Gastrointestinal tract symptoms, hepatotoxicity.

Table 4.8. Recommended Doses of Parenteral and Oral Antifungal Drugs, continued

Drug	Route	Dose (per day)	Adverse Reactions[a,b]
Fluconazole[f]	IV, PO	Oropharyngeal and esophageal candidiasis: 6 mg/kg (adult dose: 200 mg) on the first day, followed by 3–6 mg/kg (adult dose: 100 mg) once daily. Treatment should be given for at least 2–3 wk to decrease the likelihood of relapse, and at least 2 weeks following resolution of symptoms. Doses up to 12 mg/kg/day have been used based on clinical judgment. Systemic *Candida* infections: 12 mg/kg/day. Prophylaxis in children (when indicated)[d]: 6 mg/kg once daily (max 400 mg/day) Cryptococcal meningitis (children): Following induction therapy with amphotericin B plus flucytosine, fluconazole 10–12 mg/kg/day (maximum 800 mg day) in 2 divided doses for a minimum of 8 weeks after the CSF becomes culture negative; for suppression of relapse in children with AIDS, use 6 mg/kg once daily. Cryptococcal meningitis (adults): Following induction therapy with amphotericin B plus flucytosine, fluconazole 400 mg once daily. The recommended duration of fluconazole consolidation treatment is a minimum of 8 wk after the CSF fluid becomes culture negative; 200 mg once daily is used for suppression of relapse of cryptococcal meningitis in patients with AIDS.	Rash, gastrointestinal tract symptoms, hepatotoxicity, Stevens-Johnson syndrome, anaphylaxis.

Table 4.8. Recommended Doses of Parenteral and Oral Antifungal Drugs, continued

Drug	Route	Dose (per day)	Adverse Reactions[a,b]
Flucytosine	PO	100 mg/kg/day, divided dosing every 6 h (adjust dose for renal dysfunction and neonatal age); follow 2-h post peak levels closely (therapeutic range ≤100 µg/mL).	Bone marrow suppression, hepatotoxicity, renal dysfunction, gastrointestinal tract symptoms, rash, neuropathy, confusion, hallucinations. Cytosine arabinoside, a cytostatic agent, has been reported to inactivate the antifungal activity of flucytosine by competitive inhibition; drugs that impair glomerular filtration may prolong the biological half-life of flucytosine. The hematologic parameters should be monitored frequently; liver and kidney function should be carefully monitored during therapy. Flucytosine should be used in combination with amphotericin B for the treatment of cryptococcosis because of the emergence of resistance to flucytosine.
Griseofulvin	PO	Ultramicrosize: 10–15 mg/kg, once daily; maximum dose per day, 750 mg. Microsize: 20–25 mg/kg per day divided in 2 doses; maximum dose per day, 1000 mg.	Rash, paresthesias, leukopenia, gastrointestinal tract symptoms, proteinuria, hepatotoxicity, mental confusion, headache.

Table 4.8. Recommended Doses of Parenteral and Oral Antifungal Drugs, continued

Drug	Route	Dose (per day)	Adverse Reactions[a,b]
Isavuconazole (prodrug is isavuconazonium sulfate)[g]	IV, PO	Adults: 200 mg, every 8 h for 6 doses, then 200 mg, once daily (corresponding to 372 mg of the sulfate compound every 8 h for 6 doses, then 372 mg daily), starting 12 to 24 h after the last loading dose. Pediatrics: No data or dosage regimen available.	Most frequent adverse reactions are nausea, vomiting, diarrhea, headache, elevated aminotransferases, hypokalemia, constipation, dyspnea, cough, peripheral edema, and back pain. CYP3A4 inhibitors or inducers may alter the plasma concentrations of isavuconazole. Appropriate therapeutic drug monitoring and dose adjustment of immunosuppressants (ie, tacrolimus, sirolimus, and cyclosporine) may be necessary when coadministered with isavuconazole. Drugs with a narrow therapeutic window that are P-gp substrates, such as digoxin, may require dose adjustment coadministered concomitantly with isavuconazole.
Itraconazole[c]	PO	Children: 10 mg/kg per day divided into 2 doses; acidic pH for better absorption; oral solution supplies more reliable bioavailability; confirm therapeutic trough level after several days of therapy to ensure adequate drug exposure (1–2 µg/mL; when measured by high-pressure liquid chromatography; both itraconazole and its bioactive hydroxy-itraconazole metabolite are reported, the sum of which should be considered in assessing drug levels); IFI prophylaxis[d]: 2.5 mg/kg twice a day, with minimum therapeutic level of 0.5 µg/mL. Adults: 200–400 mg/day once or twice a day for treatment of blastomycosis, histoplasmosis, and aspergillosis; 100–200 mg once daily for oropharyngeal and esophageal candidiasis.	Gastrointestinal tract symptoms, rash, edema, headache, hypokalemia, hepatotoxicity, tremor, thrombocytopenia, leukopenia; strong P450 CYP3A4 inhibitor, can heighten risk of QT prolongation via metabolism interference with drugs having that adverse effect.

Table 4.8. Recommended Doses of Parenteral and Oral Antifungal Drugs, continued

Drug	Route	Dose (per day)	Adverse Reactions[a,b]
Micafungin[h]	IV	Adults: 100 mg daily for treatment of candidemia, acute disseminated candidiasis, *Candida* peritonitis and abscesses; 150 mg daily for esophageal candidiasis; and 50 mg daily for prophylaxis of candida infections in HSCT recipients. Pediatric: 2 mg/kg/day (maximum 100 mg daily) for candidemia and acute disseminated candidiasis, *Candida* peritonitis and abscesses; 1 mg/kg/day (maximum 50 mg daily) for prophylaxis of *Candida* infections; for treatment of esophageal candidiasis, 3 mg/kg/day is used for children ≤30 kg and 2.5 mg/kg/day with a maximum 150 mg daily is used for children ≥30 kg; neonatal dosing is 10 mg/kg/day. Doses up to 7 mg/kg/day have been used for disseminated candidiasis.	Fever; headache, nausea, vomiting, diarrhea, rash, thrombocytopenia, hepatic enzyme elevations, histamine-mediated symptoms including rash, pruritus, facial swelling, and vasodilatation can occur during infusion.
Nystatin	PO	Infants: 200 000 U, 4 times a day, after meals. Children and adults: 400 000–600 000 U, 3 times a day, after meals.	Gastrointestinal tract symptoms, rash.

Table 4.8. Recommended Doses of Parenteral and Oral Antifungal Drugs, continued

Drug	Route	Dose (per day)	Adverse Reactions[a,b]
Posaconazole[c]	PO, IV[i]	Adults and adolescents[j]: for prophylaxis of invasive *Aspergillus* and *Candida* infections[d]: IV formulation is approved only for use in patients 18 y or older. 300 mg, IV, twice a day on first day, followed by 300 mg, IV, once daily starting on second day. Oral suspension and delayed-release tablets can be used in the age group 13 y and older; 300 mg delayed-release tablets twice a day on the first day followed by 300 mg once daily, starting on second day; or 200 mg (5-mL) oral solution 3 times a day; duration of therapy for both IV and oral is based on recovery from neutropenia or immunosuppression; tablet and liquid forms are not interchangeable given bioavailability and dosing differences. For oropharyngeal candidiasis: oral suspension 100 mg (2.5 mL) twice a day on first day followed by 100 mg once daily for 13 days. For oropharyngeal candidiasis refractory to itraconazole and/or fluconazole: oral suspension 400 mg (10 mL) twice a day; duration of therapy is based on the severity of the patient's underlying disease and clinical response.	Diarrhea, nausea, fever, vomiting, headache, coughing, hypokalemia, rash, edema, headache, anemia, neutropenia, thrombocytopenia, fatigue, thrombophlebitis, arthralgia, myalgia, fever; interactions with P450 CYP3A4 substrate drugs and can potentiate QT prolongation; posaconazole injection should be avoided in patients with moderate or severe renal impairment (creatinine clearance <50 mL/min), higher rate of adverse effects when trough levels exceed 1 μg/mL.

Table 4.8. Recommended Doses of Parenteral and Oral Antifungal Drugs, continued

Drug	Route	Dose (per day)	Adverse Reactions[a,b]
		Children: Non–FDA-approved dosing used by St. Jude's Children's Research Hospital suggested treatment dose range in those weighing <34 kg is 18–24 mg/kg/day and in those weighing ≥34 kg is 800 mg/day, all divided into 4 doses; minimum target trough concentrations for efficacy of 0.7 µg/mL, progressing to ≥1.25 µg/mL if poor response; IFI prophylaxis[d]: 4 mg/kg/dose (max 200 mg) 3 times daily with target trough ≥0.7 µg/mL (patients with GVHD may achieve lower levels); large variability in resultant trough levels particularly in children <12 y of age.	
Terbinafine	PO	Children: once daily dosing. Onychomycosis: 10–20 kg: 62.5 mg/day; 21–40 kg: 125 mg/day; >40 kg: 250 mg/day; treatment course of 12 wk for toenails, 6 wk for fingernails. Tinea capitis: <25 kg: 125 mg/day, 25–35 kg: 187.5 mg/day; >35 kg: 250 mg once daily; treatment course of 6 wk. Adults: 250 mg, once daily.	Common adverse events include headache, diarrhea, rash, dyspepsia, liver enzyme abnormalities, pruritus, taste disturbance, nausea, abdominal pain, and flatulence; liver failure, sometimes leading to liver transplant or death, has been reported with the use of oral terbinafine. Terbinafine is an inhibitor of CYP450 2D6 isozyme and has an effect on metabolism of desipramine. Drug interactions with cimetidine, fluconazole, cyclosporine, rifampin, and caffeine have also been reported.

Table 4.8. Recommended Doses of Parenteral and Oral Antifungal Drugs, continued

Drug	Route	Dose (per day)	Adverse Reactions[a,b]
Voriconazole[e]	IV	Treatment or IFI prophylaxis[d] in children: if 2–<12 y of age or 12–14 y of age and weight <50 kg: 9 mg/kg, IV, twice daily on day 1 of treatment; thereafter 8 mg/kg, IV, twice daily or 9 mg/kg, PO, twice daily; if ≥15 y of age or 12–14 y of age and weight ≥50 kg: 6 mg/kg, IV, on day 1 of treatment; thereafter 4 mg/kg, IV, twice daily or 200 mg, PO, twice daily; therapeutic drug monitoring is needed to ensure trough levels 2–6 µg/mL. A simpler proposed oral regimen for IFI prophylaxis[d]: 200 mg, PO, twice daily if weight is ≥40 kg and 100 mg, PO, twice daily if weight is <40 kg; if IV needed, then 4 mg/kg every 12 h is administered.	Concentration- or dose-related toxicities: hepatic toxicity, arrhythmias/QT prolongation, dermatologic reactions, visual disturbance, hallucinations, increased liver enzymes and bilirubin, encephalopathy; phototoxicity, rash; CNS related toxicities are more associated with trough levels above 6 µg/mL; there have been postmarketing reports of pancreatitis in pediatric patients; drug interactions or genetic polymorphisms involving P450 CYP2C19 can alter voriconazole pharmacokinetics markedly and enhance toxicity risk; has now been identified as an independent risk factor for development of cutaneous malignancies in lung transplant patients; pharmacogenetic testing may lead to optimized dosing earlier in the treatment course. Voriconazole is not approved for a prophylaxis indication.

CYP indicates cytochrome P; GVDH, graft versus host disease; IFI, Invasive fungal infection; IT, intrathecal; IV, intravenous; PO, oral.

[a] See package insert or listing in current edition of the *Physicians' Desk Reference* or **www.pdr.net** (for registered users only).

[b] Interactions with other drugs are common. Consult **www.fda.gov/drugs/drug-interactions-labeling/drug-development-and-drug-interactions** and the *Physicians' Desk Reference* (a drug interaction reference or database) or a pharmacist before prescribing these medications.

[c] Efficacy and safety have not been established for pediatric patients. Limited or no information about use in newborn infants is available.

[d] Invasive fungal infection prophylaxis in at-risk pediatric patients with immunosuppression attributable to cancer or hematopoietic stem cell transplant.

[e] Safety and effectiveness of anidulafungin in patients ≤16 years of age has not been established.

[f] Experience with fluconazole in neonates is limited to pharmacokinetic studies in preterm newborn infants. Based on the prolonged half-life seen in preterm newborn infants (gestational age 26 to 29 weeks), these children, in the first 2 weeks of life, should receive the same dosage (mg/kg) as in older children, but administered every 72 hours. After the first 2 weeks, these children should be dosed once daily.

[g] Safety and effectiveness of isavuconazole in patients younger than 18 years have not been established.

[h] Efficacy and safety in pediatric patients younger than 4 months of age have not been established.

[i] IV formulation of posaconazole is recommended only for 18 years or older. For systemic *Candida* infections including candidemia, disseminated candidiasis, and pneumonia, optimal therapeutic dosage and duration of therapy have not been established. In open, noncomparative studies of small numbers of patients, doses of up to 400 mg daily have been used.

[j] Safety and effectiveness of posaconazole have been established in the age groups 13 years and older.

....

TOPICAL DRUGS FOR SUPERFICIAL FUNGAL INFECTIONS

Table 4.9. Topical Drugs for Superficial Fungal Infections

Drug	Strength	Formulation	Trade Name Examples	Application(s) per Day	Adverse Reactions/Notes
Basic fuchsin, phenol, resorcinol, and acetone (Rx)		S	Castellani Paint Modified	1	Excellent for intertriginous areas. Stains everything. Also available as a colorless solution with alcohol and without basic fuchsin. This is an alternative if the patient cannot tolerate other topical antifungals. Not FDA approved. Must be compounded.
Butenafine HCl (Rx and OTC)	1%	C	Mentax; Lotrimin Ultra	1–2, typically for 2 wk; Lotrimin Ultra may be used 2/day for 1 wk or 1/day for 4 wk	Safety and efficacy in patients younger than 12 y of age have not been established. Do not occlude. Sensitivity to allylamines. Not to be used on scalp or nails.
Ciclopirox olamine (Rx)	0.77%	C, L, S, P, G, NL	Loprox; Penlac nail lacquer; Ciclodan	2 for up to 4 weeks	Irritant dermatitis, hair discoloration; shake lotion vigorously before application; safety and efficacy in children younger than 10 y of age have not been established. Precautions: diabetes mellitus; immune compromise; seizures. Do not occlude.

Table 4.9. Topical Drugs for Superficial Fungal Infections, continued

Drug	Strength	Formulation	Trade Name Examples	Application(s) per Day	Adverse Reactions/Notes
Clotrimazole (Rx and OTC)	1%	C, O, S, Com; check with pharmacist	Topical solution (more than 10 preparations); Lotrimin, Mycelex, Desenex, Cruex, FungiCURE, Fungoid, Pedesil, Trivagizole, Femcare, Alevazol	1 (Rx) 2 (OTC) for 2–4 wk	Irritant dermatitis. Avoid topical steroid combinations. [a]
Clotrimazole and betamethasone dipropionate (Rx)	1%/0.05%	C, L	Lotrim and Fungizid spray; Lotrisone	2[a] for up to 2 weeks for tinea corporis/cruris, 4 weeks for pedis	Irritant dermatitis: Not FDA approved for patients younger than 17 y and not intended for diaper dermatitis. In 2 studies in pediatric subjects, 39.5% of tinea pedis patients and 47.1% of tinea cruris patients demonstrated adrenal suppression as determined by cosyntropin testing. If used in the groin area, patients should use medication for 2 wk only and use sparingly. Do not occlude. Safety and efficacy not established in children. Contraindication: avoid steroid in varicella.
Econazole nitrate (Rx)	1%	C, F	Spectazole, Ecoza	1 (dermatophyte) 2 (candidiasis)	Irritant dermatitis; foam approved for tinea pedis in children 12 y and older.

Table 4.9. Topical Drugs for Superficial Fungal Infections, continued

Drug	Strength	Formulation	Trade Name Examples	Application(s) per Day	Adverse Reactions/Notes
Efinaconazole (Rx)	10%	S	Jublia	1, for 48 wk (*Trichophyton rubrum* and *Trichophyton mentagrophytes*)	Application site dermatitis; application site vesicles; application site pain. Safety and efficacy have not been established in children.
Iodoquinol and 2% hydrocortisone acetate (Rx)	1%	G, C	Alcortin A, Dermazene, Vytone	3–4	Burning/itching sensation. Local allergic reaction. Can stain skin and clothes. Can interfere with results of thyroid function tests. Not to be used under occlusion in the diaper area. Not intended for use on infants. Not FDA approved. Safety and efficacy in children have not been established.
Iodoquinol and 1% aloe polysaccharides (Rx)	1.25%	G	Quinja	3–4	Can interfere with thyroid function tests. False-positive ferric chloride test (used for PKU) if present in the diaper or urine. Discoloration of skin, hair, and fabric, which can be removed with normal cleansing. Not intended for use on infants, under occlusions or in the diaper area. Safety and efficacy in pediatric patients younger than 12 y not established. Not FDA approved. High risk of potential toxicity compared with other available agents (neuropathy, optic neuritis).

Table 4.9. Topical Drugs for Superficial Fungal Infections, continued

Drug	Strength	Formulation	Trade Name Examples	Application(s) per Day	Adverse Reactions/Notes
Ketoconazole (Rx and OTC)	1%, 2%	C, Sh, G, F	Nizoral, Nizoral AD, Sebizol, Xolegel, Extina, Ketodan, Kuric, Ketoderm	1 (tinea dermatophyte) for 2–6 wk 2 (candidiasis) Once to treat (Rx S) Every 3–4 days (OTC S)	Potential sulfite reaction with anaphylactic or asthmatic reaction; shampoo can cause dry or oily hair and increase hair loss; irritant dermatitis. May interfere with permanent waving or changes in hair texture. Intended for patients 12 y and older; safety and efficacy not established for younger than 12 y. Foam must not be applied directly to hands, but onto a cool surface and applied using fingertips. OTC shampoo may be used for up to 8 wk to treat, and then used as needed to control dandruff.
Luliconazole (Rx)	1%	C	Luzu	1 (x 2 weeks for tinea pedis; x 1 week for tinea cruris and tinea corporis)	Application site reactions in <1% during Phase 3 clinical trials. Safety and efficacy have been established in children 12 to <18 y with tinea pedis and tinea cruris and for children 2 to <18 y with tinea corporis.
Miconazole nitrate (Rx and OTC)	2%	O, C, P, S, SpP; check with pharmacist[b]	More than 10 preparations; Monistat-Derm, Zeasorb AF, Micatin, Daktarin tincture	2 (seborrhea), apply 2–3 times/day for several months 2 (C, L) 2 (P, L) 1 (pityriasis versicolor)	Irritant and allergic contact dermatitis. Generally not recommended for children younger than 2 y. Also available as vaginal suppository intended only for patients 12 y and older.

Table 4.9. Topical Drugs for Superficial Fungal Infections, continued

Drug	Strength	Formulation	Trade Name Examples	Application(s) per Day	Adverse Reactions/Notes
Miconazole nitrate and 15% Zinc oxide (Rx)	0.25%	O	Vusion	Every diaper change for 1 wk	Skin irritation. Can be used in children 4 wk and older. Do not routinely use for more than 7 days. Do not use in infants or children who do not have a normal immune system.
Naftifine HCl (Rx)	1%, 2% gel	C, G	Naftin	1 (C) 1–2 (Gel) for 2 wk	Burning/stinging, irritant dermatitis. Safety and efficacy in children have not been established. Do not occlude.
Nystatin (Rx and OTC	100 000 U/mL or 100 000 U/g	C, P, O, Com	Nystatin, Nystop powder; Pedi-Dri powder, Mycostatin, Nyamyc	2–4 (C) 2–3 (P)	Nontoxic except with topical steroid combinations.[c]
Nystatin and triamcinolone acetonide (Rx)	100 000 USP nystatin and 1 mg triamcinolone acetonide (0.1%)	C, O	Mytrex cream, Mytrex ointment, Mycolog-II, Mycogen II	2[a]	Pediatric patients may demonstrate greater susceptibility to topical corticosteroid-induced hypothalamic-pituitary-adrenal (HPA) axis suppression and Cushing syndrome than mature patients because of a larger ratio of skin surface area to body weight. Contraindications: Hypersensitivity to component drug. Avoid steroid use in varicella or vaccinia. Do not occlude. Use lowest effective dose. Do not routinely use for more than 2 wk.

Table 4.9. Topical Drugs for Superficial Fungal Infections, continued

Drug	Strength	Formulation	Trade Name Examples	Application(s) per Day	Adverse Reactions/Notes
Oxiconazole (Rx)	1%	C, L	Oxistat	1–2 (tinea dermatophyte)	Pruritus, burning, irritant dermatitis. Do not occlude. Intended for patients 12 y and older; safety and efficacy not established for younger than 12 y
Sertaconazole nitrate (Rx)	2%	C	Ertaczo	2 for 4 wk (pedis), 2 weeks for corporis or candida	Dry skin, skin tenderness, contact dermatitis, local hypersensitivity. Safety and efficacy in children younger than 2 y have not been established.
Sulconazole (Rx)	1%	C, S	Exelderm	1–2 (pityriasis versicolor) for 3 weeks 2 (tinea pedis) for 4 weeks	Irritant dermatitis. Safety and efficacy in children have not been established.
Tavaborole (Rx)	5%	S	Kerydin	1, for 48 wk (*Trichophyton rubrum* and *Trichophyton mentagrophytes*)	Application site exfoliation; application site erythema; application site dermatitis. Safety and efficacy have been established in children 6 y and older.
Terbinafine (Rx and OTC)	1%	C, Sp	Lamisil, Lamisil AT	1–2, tinea pedis can use up to 2 weeks	Irritant dermatitis. Avoid use of occlusive clothing or dressings. Do not apply spray to face. Safety and efficacy in children younger than 12 y have not been established.

Table 4.9. Topical Drugs for Superficial Fungal Infections, continued

Drug	Strength	Formulation	Trade Name Examples	Application(s) per Day	Adverse Reactions/Notes
Tolnaftate (OTC)	1%	C, P, S, SpP, SpL; check with pharmacist[b]	>10 preparations; Tinactin, Fungicure	2	Irritant and allergic contact dermatitis. Not recommended if younger than 2 y.
Undecylenic acid and derivatives (OTC)	8%–25%	NL, O, S, SpP, P, (dee pharmacist for formulations and applications[b])	BioRx Sponix, Elon Dual Defense, Gordochom, Hongo Cura, Myco Nail A	2 for 4 weeks	Irritant dermatitis. Generally not recommended for children younger than 2 y.
Other Remedies					
Benzoic acid and salicylic acid (OTC)	12%	O	Whitfields Ointment, Bensal HP	2	Warm, burning sensation. Avoid eyes, mouth, and nose. Keep out of the reach of children. Safety and efficacy in children not established. Not FDA approved.
Gentian violet (OTC)	1%	S	…	1–3 for 3 days	Staining. Oral mucosal ulceration reported in young children in as little as 4 days, only use as a last resort. Keep out of the reach of children. Safety and efficacy in children not established. OTC monograph not final.

Table 4.9. Topical Drugs for Superficial Fungal Infections, continued

Drug	Strength	Formulation	Trade Name Examples	Application(s) per Day	Adverse Reactions/Notes
Selenium sulfide (Rx and OTC)	1%, 2.3%, 2.5%	Sh, L	SelRx 2.3%	Use twice weekly for 2 wk (Sh) 1 for 7 days (L)	Irritant dermatitis and ulceration. For tinea capitis, to decrease spore formation and to decrease the potential spread of the dermatophyte. Hair loss, discoloration of hair, oiliness or dryness of scalp. Safety and efficacy in children not established. May damage jewelry. Not to be used when inflammation or exudation is present.
	1%	Sh, L	Head & Shoulders, Selsun Blue	Use twice weekly for at least 2 wk	For tinea capitis, to decrease spore formation and to decrease the potential spread of the dermatophyte.

C indicates cream; Com, combinations; F, foam; FDA, US Food and Drug Administration; G, gel; L, lotion; NL, nail lacquer; O, ointment; OTC, over the counter; P, powder; PKU, phenylketonuria; Rx, prescription; S, solution; Sh, shampoo; Sp, spray; SpL, spray lotion; SpP, spray powder.

[a] Topical steroids must be used with caution in young children and in areas of thin skin (eg, diaper area). In these circumstances, high systemic exposure may occur, resulting in endogenous synthesis suppression with the potential for serious adverse effects. Potential adverse effects include irritant dermatitis, folliculitis, hypertrichosis, acneiform eruptions, hypopigmentation, perioral dermatitis, allergic contact dermatitis, maceration, secondary infection, skin atrophy, striae, and miliaria.

[b] Pharmacists are an excellent resource to verify formulations that are available and new (they use *Facts and Comparisons* reference products).

[c] Any topical preparation has the potential to irritate the skin and cause itching, burning, stinging, erythema, edema, vesicles, and blister formation. For more information on individual drugs, see *Physician's Desk Reference* or **www.pdr.net** (for registered users only).

NON-HIV ANTIVIRAL DRUGS

Table 4.10. Non-HIV Antiviral Drugs[a]

Generic (Trade Name)	Indication	Route	Age	Usually Recommended Dosage
Acyclovir[b,c,d,e] (Zovirax)	Neonatal herpes simplex virus (HSV) infection	IV	Birth to ≤4 mo	Treatment dosing: 60 mg/kg per day, in 3 divided doses for 14 days (SEM disease) or 21 days (CNS or Disseminated disease) (durations >21 days are necessary if CSF PCR remains positive near end of treatment course)[g]
		Oral	2 wk to 8 mo	Oral suppressive dosing following completion of IV treatment; dosing: 300 mg/m², 3 times per day for 6 mo
	HSV encephalitis	IV	>4 mo to 12 y	30–45 mg/kg per day, in 3 divided doses for 14–21 days; FDA-approved dose of 60 mg/kg per day for this age range and indication is not recommended, as risk of acute kidney injury may increase at incremental doses exceeding 500 mg/m² or 15 mg/kg; dosing per m² causes excessive weight-based dosing in younger children[f]; concomitant ceftriaxone may enhance nephrotoxicity risk; neurotoxicity (agitation, myoclonus, delirium, altered consciousness, etc) can occur with accumulated high acyclovir levels, often a result of renal dysfunction and unadjusted dosage
		IV	≥12 y	30 mg/kg per day, in 3 divided doses for 14–21 days[g]
	Varicella in immunocompetent host[h]	Oral	≥2 y	≤40 kg: 80 mg/kg per day, in 4 divided doses for 5 days; maximum daily dose of 3200 mg/day >40 kg: 3200 mg, in 4 divided doses for 5 days (Adult dose: 4000 g per day, in 5 divided doses for 5–7 days)

Table 4.10. Non-HIV Antiviral Drugs,[a] continued

Generic (Trade Name)	Indication	Route	Age	Usually Recommended Dosage
	Varicella in immunocompetent host requiring hospitalization	IV	≥2 y	30 mg/kg per day, in 3 divided doses for 7–10 days; or 1500 mg/m^2 per day, in 3 divided doses for 7–10 days[g]
	Varicella in immunocompromised host	IV	<2 y	30 mg/kg per day, in 3 divided doses for 7–10 days
		IV	≥2 y	1500 mg/m^2 per day, in 3 divided doses for 7–10 days[g]; some experts recommend the 30 mg/kg per day, in 3 divided doses for 7–10 days
	Zoster in immunocompetent host	IV (if requiring hospitalization)	All ages	Same as for varicella in immunocompromised host
		Oral	≥12 y	4000 mg/day, in 5 divided doses for 5–7 days
	Zoster in immunocompromised host	IV	All ages	30 mg/kg per day, in 3 divided doses, for 7–10 days
	HSV infection in immunocompromised host (localized, progressive, or disseminated)	IV	All ages	30 mg/kg per day, in 3 divided doses for 7–14 days
		Oral	≥2 y	1000 mg/day, in 3–5 divided doses for 7–14 days

Table 4.10. Non-HIV Antiviral Drugs,[a] continued

Generic (Trade Name)	Indication	Route	Age	Usually Recommended Dosage
	Prophylaxis of HSV in immunocompromised hosts who are HSV seropositive	Oral	≥2 y	80 mg/kg/day, in 2–3 divided doses (maximum dose: 800 mg) during period of risk; or 600–1000 mg/day, in 3–5 divided doses during period of risk
		IV	All ages	15 mg/kg, in 3 divided doses during period of risk
	Genital HSV infection: first episode	Oral	≥12 y	1000–1200 mg/day, in 3–5 divided doses for 7–10 days. Oral pediatric dose: 40–80 mg/kg per day, divided in 3–4 doses (maximum 1000 mg/day)
		IV	≥12 y	15 mg/kg per day, in 3 divided doses for 5–7 days
	Genital HSV infection: recurrence	Oral	≥12 y	1000 mg in 5 divided doses for 5 days, or 1600 mg in 2 divided doses for 5 days, or 2400 mg in 3 divided doses for 2 days
	Chronic suppressive therapy for recurrent genital and cutaneous (ocular) HSV episodes	Oral	≥12 y	800 mg/day, in 2 divided doses for as long as 12 continuous months; decisions to continue suppressive therapy should be revisited annually
	Recurrent herpes labialis	Oral	All ages	80 mg/kg per day, in 4 divided doses, for 5 to 7 days (maximum 3200 mg/day)
Adefovir[b,i] (Hepsera)	Chronic hepatitis B	Oral	≥12 y	10 mg, once daily, in patients with CrCL ≥50 mL/min (every 48 hours for CrCL = 30–49 mL/min; every 72 for CrCL = 10–29 mL/min); optimal duration of therapy unknown, although minimum of 1 y + additional 12 mo after HBeAg seroconversion has been suggested; monitor for liver function exacerbation and renal dysfunction); monitor for viral resistance of treatment >1 y duration
		Oral	2–12 y	≥7 y–12 y: 0.25 mg/kg, 2 y–<7 y: 0.3 mg/kg once daily (both to a maximum of 10 mg) gives similar systemic exposure as in adults

Table 4.10. Non-HIV Antiviral Drugs,[a] continued

Generic (Trade Name)	Indication	Route	Age	Usually Recommended Dosage
Baloxavir (Xofluza)	Influenza A and B	Oral	≥12 y	≥80 kg: 80 mg as single dose 40–79 kg: 40 mg as single dose Avoid concomitant antacids, dairy products
Cidofovir (Vistide)	Cytomegalovirus (CMV) retinitis	IV	Adult dose[J] and adolescents	Induction: 5 mg/kg, once weekly, × 2 doses with probenecid 25–40 mg/kg (maximum 2 g) and appropriate hydration mandatory with each dose; seek alternative therapy if CrCL <55 mL/min or if ≥2+ proteinuria Maintenance: 5 mg/kg, once every 2 wk, with probenecid and hydration with each dose; duration dependent on CD4+ T-lymphocyte response to ARV therapy and regular ophthalmologic monitoring
Daclatasvir (Daklinza)	Chronic hepatitis C (genotype 1 and 3)	Oral	Adult	60 mg, once daily, together with sofosbuvir for 12 wk, with or without ribavirin; mainly used in alternative regimens Need for ribavirin is based on HCV genotype, cirrhosis status, and liver transplant status Dosages increase to 90 mg daily and decrease to 30 mg daily when concomitant use of CYP3A4 inducers and inhibitors, respectively
Elbasvir and Grazoprevir (Zepatier)	Chronic hepatitis C (genotype 1 and 4)	Oral	≥18 y	50 mg elbasvir and 100 mg grazoprevir, once daily, for 12–16 wk, with or without ribavirin Need for ribavirin is based on HCV genotype, baseline NS5A polymorphisms, and prior treatment status

Table 4.10. Non-HIV Antiviral Drugs,[a] continued

Generic (Trade Name)	Indication	Route	Age	Usually Recommended Dosage
Entecavir[b] (Baraclude)	Chronic hepatitis B	Oral	≥16 y[j]	0.5 mg, once daily, in nucleoside-therapy-naïve patients; 1 mg once daily in patients who were previously treated with a nucleoside (not first choice in this setting); optimum duration of therapy unknown but similar recommendations for minimum of 1 y + additional 12 mo after HBeAg seroconversion; full doses if in patients with CrCL ≥50 mL/min (otherwise, every 48 hours for CrCL = 30–49 mL/min; every 72 for CrCL = 10–29 mL/min)
		Oral	2 to <16 y, naïve to treatment (normal renal function)	10–11 kg: 0.15 mg oral solution once daily >11–14 kg: 0.2 mg oral solution once daily >14–17 kg: 0.25 mg oral solution once daily >17–20 kg: 0.3 mg oral solution once daily >20–23 kg: 0.35 mg oral solution once daily >23–26 kg: 0.4 mg oral solution once daily >26–30 kg: 0.45 mg oral solution once daily >30 kg: 0.5 mg oral solution or tablet once daily
			Lamivudine-treated/-refractory OR with known lamivudine or telbivudine resistance mutations	Double the dosage in each above weight bracket, up to 1 mg daily for ≥16 y

Table 4.10. Non-HIV Antiviral Drugs,[a] continued

Generic (Trade Name)	Indication	Route	Age	Usually Recommended Dosage
Famciclovir[b]	Genital HSV infection, recurrent episodes	Oral	Adult dose,[h] adolescents	Immunocompetent: 2000 mg/day, in 2 divided doses for 1 day; CDC regimens featuring smaller incremental doses and greater number of treatment days are available. HIV-infected patients: 1000 mg, in 2 divided doses for 7 days (CDC and NIH guidelines provide range of 5–14 days)
	Daily suppressive therapy	Oral	Adult dose,[j] adolescents and children	Immunocompetent: 500 mg/day, in 2 divided doses for 1 y, then reassess for recurrence of HSV infection; HIV: 1000 mg/day, in 2 divided doses for minimum of 1 y; same dosage for children and adolescents old enough to receive adult doses
	Recurrent herpes labialis	Oral	Adult dose,[j] adolescents	Immunocompetent: 1500 mg as a single dose HIV-infected patients: 1000 mg/day, in 2 divided doses for 7 days (CDC and NIH guidelines provide range of 5–10 days); comparatively slower resolution seen in adolescent patients
	Herpes zoster	Oral	Adult dose,[j] adolescents	1500 mg/day, in 3 divided doses for 7 days (7–10 days in HIV patients with localized lesions, longer if lesions resolving slowly; or to complete 10–14 days total course with initial IV acyclovir if more severe skin or visceral infection)
Foscarnet[b] (Foscavir)	CMV retinitis in HIV infected patients (drug of choice in ganciclovir-resistant disease)	IV	Adult dose[j] and infants, children, and adolescents	180 mg/kg per day, in 2–3 divided doses for 14–21 days, then 90–120 mg/kg once a day for maintenance therapy and for secondary prophylaxis; may be added to ganciclovir as induction therapy, or as follow-up to failed ganciclovir monotherapy; if sight-threatening disease; IV infused no faster than 1 mg/kg/min

Table 4.10. Non-HIV Antiviral Drugs,[a] continued

Generic (Trade Name)	Indication	Route	Age	Usually Recommended Dosage
	HSV infection resistant to acyclovir in immunocompromised host	IV	Adult dose[j] and adolescents	90–120 mg/kg per day, in 2–3 divided doses for 3 wk or until infection resolves
	VZV infection resistant to acyclovir	IV	Adult dose[j] and adolescents	Patients with HIV: 90 mg/kg per dose every 12 h
			Infants and children	40–60 mg/kg per dose, every 8 h for 7–10 days or until no new lesions have appeared for 48 h
Ganciclovir[b] (Cytovene)	Symptomatic congenital CMV disease	IV	Birth to 2 mo	12 mg/kg per day, divided every 12 h; duration of treatment is 6 mo, but most or all of the treatment should be accomplished with oral valganciclovir, as detailed below (there is no benefit to using ganciclovir instead of valganciclovir) for improved long-term developmental and hearing outcomes; dosage adjustment if neutropenia develops
	Acquired CMV retinitis in immunocompromised host[k]	IV	Adult dose[j]	Treatment: 10 mg/kg per day, in 2 divided doses for 14–21 days; long-term suppression 5 mg/kg per day for 7 days/wk or 6 mg/kg per day for 5 days/wk; HIV: duration of maintenance treatment is for at least 3–6 mo, with no active lesions, and with CD4+ T-lymphocyte count >100 cells/mm^3 for 3 to 6 mo in response to ART

Table 4.10. Non-HIV Antiviral Drugs,[a] continued

Generic (Trade Name)	Indication	Route	Age	Usually Recommended Dosage
	Disseminated CMV and retinitis	IV	Infants, children, and adolescents	10 mg/kg per day, in 2 divided doses for 14–21 days; increase to 15 mg/kg/day in 2 divided doses if needed, then 5 mg/kg body weight once daily for 5–7 days per wk for chronic suppression; discontinuation after 6 mo may be considered in children 1–5 y if CD4+ T-lymphocyte count >500/m^3 (or CD4+ T-lymphocyte percentage ≥15%); stated doses presume CrCL >50 mL/min/1.73 m^2; may add foscarnet (180 mg/kg per day divided into 2 or 3 doses) if vision at risk, or ganciclovir intravitreal injection in children 9–12 y and adolescents
	Prophylaxis of CMV in high-risk host (eg, post-transplant)	IV	All ages	10 mg/kg per day, in 2 divided doses for 5–7 days, then 5 mg/kg once daily for 100–120 days, or 6 mg/kg per day for 5 days/wk for 100 days
	Preemptive therapy of CMV in high-risk host (eg, <100 days post HSCT)	IV	All ages	10 mg/kg per day, in 2 divided doses for 7–14 days, then 5 mg/kg once daily until CMV is not detectable (antigenemia, DNA PCR, or mRNA detection methods)
	>100 days post-HSCT, OR receiving steroids for GVHD, OR if positive antigenemia or viremia/PCR x 2			10 mg/kg per day in 2 divided doses for 1–2 weeks or until CMV undetectable

Table 4.10. Non-HIV Antiviral Drugs,[a] continued

Generic (Trade Name)	Indication	Route	Age	Usually Recommended Dosage
Glecaprevir/ Pibrentasvir (Mavyret)	Chronic hepatitis C (genotypes 1–6)	Oral	≥12 y, or weighing ≥45 kg	3 tablets (total daily dose: glecaprevir 300 mg and pibrentasvir 120 mg) once daily with food Duration: 8, 12, or 16 weeks dependent on Rx-naïve vs Rx-experienced, genotype, prior vs concurrent therapy with NS3/4A protease inhibitor vs NS5A inhibitor, or other anti-hepatitis C drugs, and no cirrhosis vs compensated cirrhosis; refer to package insert for table of recommended lengths of treatment; numerous drug interactions complicates management
Interferon alfa-2b (Intron A)	Chronic hepatitis B	SC	1–18 y	Initial dosing of 3 million IU/m², SC, 3 times/wk during first wk, then 6 million IU/m², SC (maximum dose 10 million IU), 3 times/wk for 16–24 wk; 50% dose reduction if severe adverse reactions
			>18 y	5 million IU/day; or 10 million IU, IM or SC, 3 times/wk, for 16 wk; reduce dose by 50% if white blood cell count <1500/mm³ or granulocyte count <750/mm³ or platelet count <50 000/mm³ and by 75% if these counts are <1000/mm³, <500/mm³, <25 000/mm³, respectively

Table 4.10. Non-HIV Antiviral Drugs,[a] continued

Generic (Trade Name)	Indication	Route	Age	Usually Recommended Dosage
Lamivudine[b,i] (Epivir-HBV)	Chronic hepatitis B	Oral	Infants and children (HIV/HBV coinfected)	Children coinfected with HIV and hepatitis B should use the approved dose for HIV Dosing is weight based Refer to the package insert for details Tablets (150 mg scored tablets) are the preferred formulation 14 to <20 kg: 150 mg QD or 75 mg BID ≥20 to <25 kg: 225 mg QD or 75 mg AM dose + 150 mg PM dose ≥25 kg: 300 mg QD or 150 mg BID Oral solution dosing: 5 mg/kg/dose (maximum 150 mg/dose) twice daily; or 10 mg/kg/dose once daily; standard dosing for patients with CrCL >50 mL/min/1.73 m²; monitor for lamivudine-resistance
		Oral	Adolescents (HIV/HBV coinfected)	Children coinfected with HIV and hepatitis B should use the approved dose for HIV 300 mg, once daily; or 150 mg, twice daily; standard dosing for patients with CrCL >50 mL/min
		Oral	Infants and children (HIV negative)	3 mg/kg/dose, once daily (maximum of 100 mg per day); use oral solution for doses <100 mg
		Oral	Adolescents (HIV negative)	100 mg, once daily

Table 4.10. Non-HIV Antiviral Drugs,ª continued

Generic (Trade Name)	Indication	Route	Age	Usually Recommended Dosage
Ledipasvir (Harvoni as combination with sofosbuvir)	Chronic hepatitis C (genotypes 1, 4, 5, 6)	Oral	Children ≥3 y and adults	Harvoni dosing: <17 kg: 33.75 mg ledipasvir/150 mg sofosbuvir 17 kg to less than 35 kg: 45 mg ledipasvir/200 mg sofosbuvir ≥35 kg: 90 mg ledipasvir/400 mg sofosbuvir (adult dose: 90 mg ledipasvir/400 mg sofosbuvir) Ribavirin also may be added, based on genotype, cirrhosis, and liver transplant status; when used, ribavirin dosing is as follows: Children: <47 kg: oral solution at 15 mg/kg/day, in 2 divided doses 47–49 kg: 200 mg in AM and 400 mg in PM 50–65 kg: 400 mg in AM and PM 66–80 kg: 400 mg in AM and 600 mg in PM >80 kg: 600 mg in AM and PM Adults: <75 kg: 400 mg in AM and 600 mg in PM ≥75 kg: 600 mg in AM and PM Dosage modification of ribavirin based on treatment-emergent anemia (after interferon adjustment) and severe renal impairment; discontinue if severe blood dyscrasias or creatinine >2 g/dL Duration 12–24 weeks dependent on genotype and prior treatment experience
Letermovir (Prevymis)	CMV prophylaxis in seropositive patients after HSCT	IV, Oral	Adults	480 mg daily IV or oral (240 mg per day in patients taking cyclosporine) starting 0–28 between days post-transplantation and continued through day 100 post-transplantation

Table 4.10. Non-HIV Antiviral Drugs,[a] continued

Generic (Trade Name)	Indication	Route	Age	Usually Recommended Dosage
Ombitasvir, paritaprevir, and ritonavir tablets; dasabuvir tablets, copackaged for oral use (Viekira Pak)	Chronic hepatitis C (genotype 1)	Oral	≥18 y	Two ombitasvir, paritaprevir, ritonavir 12.5/75/50-mg tablets, once daily (in the morning), and one dasabuvir 250-mg tablet, twice daily (morning and evening), in additions to ribavirin (500 mg orally twice daily of <75 kg; 600 mg twice daily if ≥75 kg) for 12 wk (24 wk if liver transplant with normal hepatic function and mild fibrosis)
Oseltamivir[b,l] (Tamiflu)	Influenza A and B: treatment (see Influenza, p 447)	Oral (suspension)	Birth to <9 mo[m]	3 mg/kg twice daily for 5 days[m]; longer treatment can be considered for patients still severely ill after 5 treatment days
		Oral (suspension)	9–11 mo	3.5 mg/kg twice daily for 5 days; longer treatment can be considered for patients still severely ill after 5 treatment days
		Oral (suspension and tablets)	1–12 y	≤15 kg: 30 mg, twice daily; 15.1–23 kg: 45 mg, twice daily; 23.1–40 kg: 60 mg, twice daily; >40 kg: 75 mg, twice daily Treatment duration is for 5 days; longer treatment can be considered for patients still severely ill after 5 treatment days; half-dose given after dialysis session
		Oral (tablets)	≥13 y	75 mg, twice daily for 5 days; longer treatment can be considered for patients still severely ill after 5 treatment days; 30 mg given after dialysis session

Table 4.10. Non-HIV Antiviral Drugs,[a] continued

Generic (Trade Name)	Indication	Route	Age	Usually Recommended Dosage
	Influenza A and B: prophylaxis	Oral	3 mo–12 y	Same as the above treatment doses for patients 3 mo–12 y of age, except dose given once rather than twice daily, and given for 10 days rather than 5 (following known household exposure; 7 days for others) or for up to 6 wk (preexposure during community outbreak); not routinely recommended for infants <3 mo given lack of efficacy data
		Oral	≥13 y	75 mg, once daily for 10 days (following known household exposure; 7 days for others) or for up to 6 wk (pre-exposure during community outbreak); dosage adjustments for moderate to severe renal insufficiency in adults
Pegylated interferon alfa-2a (Pegasys)	Chronic hepatitis B	SC	>18 y[j]	180 µg, once weekly for 48 wk
Peramivir[b] (Rapivab)	Influenza A and B	IV	≥2 y	2–12 y: 12 mg/kg, once (maximum dose: 600 mg); ≥13 y: 600 mg, once; full dose for CrCL of ≥50 mL/min/1.73 m^2 Note: Not approved for neonates, but has been studied in this population at 6 mg/kg/dose once daily for 5 to 10 days
Sofosbuvir (Sovaldi)	Chronic hepatitis C (genotype 1, 2, 3, 4, depending on adult [all four genotypes] or pediatric [genotypes 2 or 3])	Oral	Children ≥3 y and adults	Sofosbuvir dosing: <17 kg: 150 mg 17 kg to less than 35 kg: 200 mg ≥35 kg: 400 mg (adult dose: 400 mg) Take once daily with or without food, as a component of combination therapy with other direct-acting antivirals (eg, daclatasvir), ribavirin, or with ribavirin plus pegylated interferon; length of treatment depending on HCV genotype and concomitant therapy used

Table 4.10. Non-HIV Antiviral Dr... ...inued

Generic (Trade Name)	Indication	Route	Age	Recommended Dosage
				Ribaviri... Children:
				<47 kg: o... in 2 divided doses
				47-49 kg: ... 5 mg/kg/day, ... 400 mg in PM
				50-65 kg: 4...5 ...and 400 mg in PM
				66-80 kg: 400 ...nd PM ...nd 600 mg in PM
				>80 kg: 600 mg ...d 600 mg in PM
				Adults: ...PM
				<75 kg: 400 mg in ...
				≥75 kg: 600 mg in ...00 mg in PM
				Dosage modification of rib... Dosage modification of rib... anemia (after interferon ad)ed on treatment-emergent discontinue if severe blood ...g) and severe renal impairment; Sofosbuvir available in a fixed-do...as or creatinine >2 g/dL ledipasvir (marketed as Harvon)...nbination tablet with 90 mg Sofosbuvir available in a fixed-do...fi)sc in children ≥3 y and adults mg velpatasvir (marketed as Ep)usa) for use in adults (includes ribavirin when decompensate(cir)hosis present) Sofosbuvir has potential for reduced efficacy when combined with to P-glycoprotein inducers
Tecovirimat (TPOXX)	Smallpox	Oral	Children ≥13 kg and adults	13 kg to less than 25 kg: 200 mg, 2 times daily for 14 days 25 kg to less than 40 kg: 400 mg, 2 times daily for 14 days ≥40 kg: 600 mg, 2 times daily for 14 days

Table 4.10. Non-HIV Antiviral Drugs, continued

Generic (Trade Name)	Indication	Route	Age	Usually Recommended Dosage
Tenofovir disoproxil fumarate (Viread)	Chronic hepatitis B	Oral	Adolescents ≥12 y and weighing ≥35 kg, with or without HIV coinfection, adults	300 mg, once daily; adjustment of dosing interval recommended for CrCL <50 mL/min; monitor liver function and bone density
			≥2 y and at least 10 kg, with or without HIV coinfection	Weight band dosing of reduced-strength tablets and oral powder formulations. Refer to the package insert for details (www.accessdata.fda.gov/drugsatfda_docs/label/2019/021356s058,022577s014lbl.pdf)
Tenofovir alafenamide fumarate (Vemlidy)	Chronic hepatitis B	Oral	Adult or ≥18 y	25 mg once daily with food; no renal dose adjustment but not recommended for CrCL <... /min); monitor for bone loss, ...osis and lactic acidosis) with severe disease exacerbation ... stoppage of treatment; int... with p-glycoprotein inhibitors and inducers
Valacyclovir (Valtrex)	Varicella	Oral	2 to <18 y	20 mg/kg, 3 times daily for up to 6 wk... not to exceed 1 g per dose, long... if lesions unresolved; ...al necrosis; HIV, same dose for acyclovir treatment ... 4-6 wk
	Genital HSV infection, first episode	Oral	Adult and adolescent dose	2 g/day, in 2 divided ...days (5-14 days in HIV infected patients); longe... incompletely healed
			Children	<45 kg: 40 mg... ≥45 kg: 2 g/... 7-10 days o...

Table 4.10. Non-HIV Antiviral Drugs,[a] continued

Generic (Trade Name)	Indication	Route	Age	Usually Recommended Dosage
	Episodic recurrent genital HSV infection	Oral	Adult and adolescent dose	1 g/day, in 2 divided doses for 3 days; HIV-infected patients should receive 2 g/day for 5–14 days
	Daily suppressive therapy for recurrent genital HSV infection	Oral	Adult dose[j]	Immunocompetent patients: 1000 mg, once daily for 1 y starting within 24 hours of symptom onset or assess history of recurrences (eg, 500 mg, once daily, in patients with ≤9 recurrences per y to reduce transmission) HIV-infected patients (CD4+ T-lymphocyte count ≥100 cells/mm³): 500 mg, twice daily for at least 6 mo
			Adolescent	500 mg or 1 g, once daily (the lower dose is less effective if frequent recurrences (eg, ≥10/y); HIV: 500 mg twice daily for indefinite duration; acyclovir for young children
	Recurrent herpes labialis	Oral	≥12 y	4 g/day, in 2 divided doses for 1 day
	Herpes zoster	Oral	Adult and adolescent dose[j]	3 g/day; in 3 divided doses for 7 days
Valganciclovir[b] (Valcyte)	Symptomatic congenital CMV disease	Oral	Birth through 6 mo	32 mg/kg per day, in 2 divided doses, started within the first mo of life and continued for a total of 6 mo of treatment; for improved long-term developmental and hearing outcomes; dosage adjustment if neutropenia or renal impairment develops
	Acquired CMV retinitis in immunocompromised host	Oral	Adult and adolescent dose[j]	Induction treatment: 900 mg, twice daily for 2–3 wk Long-term suppression: 900 mg, once daily; HIV: duration of maintenance treatment is for at least 3–6 mo, with lesions inactive, and with CD4+ T-lymphocyte count >100 cells/mm³ for 3 mo to 6 mo in response to ART

Table 4.10. Non-HIV Antiviral Drugs,ᵃ continued

Generic (Trade Name)	Indication	Route	Age	Usually Recommended Dosage
	Prevention of CMV disease in kidney, liver, or heart transplant patients	Oral	4 mo–16 y	Dose once a day within 10 days of transplantation according to dosage algorithm based on body surface area and creatinine clearance: Dose (mg) = 7 x body surface area x CrCL (calculated using the Schwartz equation with maximum value set at 150 mL/min/1.73 m²); see drug package insert; maximum 900 mg/day; round dose to the nearest 10-mg increment with solution; duration depends on type of transplant and risk status: 200 days after renal transplant, 100 days after heart or liver transplant
		Oral	Adolescents ≥17 y	900 mg, once daily, for post-transplant patients; duration in children depends on type of transplant and risk status: 200 days after renal transplant, 100 days after heart or liver transplant
	Prevention of CMV disease in HIV-infected patients (CMV-seropositive children ≥6 y with CD4+ T-lymphocyte counts <50 cells/mm³ or <6 years who are CMV-seropositive and have a CD4+ T-lymphocyte percentage <5%)	Oral	4 mo–16 y	Same calculated dose regimen as above; duration: stopping primary prophylaxis can be considered when the CD4+ T-lymphocyte count is >100 cells/mm³ for children ≥6 y, or CD4+ T-lymphocyte percentage is >10% in children <6 y

Table 4.10. Non-HIV Antiviral Drugs,[a] continued

Generic (Trade Name)	Indication	Route	Age	Usually Recommended Dosage
Velpatasvir (Epclusa as combination with sofosbuvir)	Chronic hepatitis C (genotypes 1–6)	Oral	Children ≥6 y and Adults	17 kg to less than 30 kg: 50 mg with 200 mg sofosbuvir ≥30 kg: 100 mg with 400 mg sofosbuvir Duration 12–24 wk dependent on prior treatment experience, concurrent ribavirin use
Voxilaprevir (Vosevi as combination with sofosbuvir and velpatasvir)	Chronic hepatitis C (genotypes 1–6)	Oral	Adults	100 mg combined with 400 mg sofosbuvir and 100 mg velpatasvir; taken with food; duration: 12 wk for all genotypes and treatment-experienced patient regimens
Zanamivir (Relenza)	Influenza A and B: treatment (see Influenza, p 447)	Inhalation	≥7 y (treatment)	10 mg (one 5-mg powder blister per inhalation), twice daily for 5 days; first 2 doses can be separated by as little as 2 hours; only use Diskhaler device; longer treatment can be considered for patients still severely ill after 5 treatment days
	Influenza A and B: prophylaxis	Inhalation	≥5 y (prophylaxis)	10 mg, once daily for as long as 28 days (community outbreaks) or 14 days (household setting); CDC recommends an additional 7-day course after last known exposure

ART indicates combination antiretroviral therapy; BID, twice a day; CDC, Centers for Disease Control and Prevention; CrCL, creatinine clearance; CNS, central nervous system; CSF, cerebrospinal fluid; FDA, US Food and Drug Administration; GVHD, graft-versus-host disease; HBeAg, hepatitis B e antigen; HBV, hepatitis B virus; HCV, hepatitis C virus; HIV, human immunodeficiency virus; HSCT, hematopoietic stem cell transplant; HSV, herpes simplex virus; IM, intramuscular; IV, intravenous; NIH, National Institutes of Health; PCR, polymerase chain reaction; QD, once a day; SC, subcutaneous; SEM, skin, eyes, and/or mouth; VZV, varicella-zoster virus.

[a] Drugs for human immunodeficiency virus infection are not included. See **http://aidsinfo.nih.gov** for current information on HIV drugs and treatment recommendations.

[b] Dose should be decreased in patients with impaired renal function.

[c] Oral dosage of acyclovir in children should not exceed 80 mg/kg per day (3200 mg/day).

[d] Acyclovir doses listed in this table are based on clinical trials and clinical experience and may not be identical to doses approved by the FDA.

[e] In times of shortage of intravenous acyclovir, the American Academy of Pediatrics Committee on Infectious Diseases recommends that existing supplies of intravenous acyclovir be conserved to improve availability for neonatal HSV infections, herpes simplex encephalitis, or HSV and varicella-zoster virus infections in immunocompromised patients, including more ill pregnant women with visceral dissemination of either virus. If acyclovir is not available, intravenous ganciclovir should be substituted. Alternative regimens to the use of intravenous acyclovir and other options for priority and nonpriority conditions are outlined in an exclusive Red Book Online Intravenous Acyclovir Shortage Table (**http://redbook.solutions.aap.org/selfserve/ssPage.aspx?SelfServeConte ntId=acyclovir-shortage**).

[f] Monitor for nephrotoxicity and neurologic irritation. Consider involving an infectious diseases or pharmacology specialist if weight-based dosing exceeds 800 mg per dose or if being administered with other nephrotoxic medications.

[g] Use estimate of ideal body weight in severely obese children and adolescents.

[h] Selective indications; see Varicella-Zoster Infections (p 831).

[i] "Nonpreferred" for treatment of chronic hepatitis B in the American Association for the Study of Liver Diseases 2018 Hepatitis B Guidance document (**www.aasld.org/sites/default/ files/2019-06/HBVGuidance_Terrault_et_al-2018-Hepatology.pdf**).

[j] There are not sufficient clinical data to identify the appropriate dose for use in children.

[k] Some experts use ganciclovir in immunocompromised hosts with CMV gastrointestinal tract disease and CMV pneumonitis (with or without CMV Immune Globulin Intravenous).

[l] See Influenza (p 447) and **www.cdc.gov/flu/professionals/antivirals/index.htm** for specific recommendations, which may vary on the basis of most recent influenza virus susceptibility patterns.

[m] Preterm, <38 weeks' postmenstrual age; oseltamivir, 1.0 mg/kg/dose, orally, twice daily; preterm, 38 through 40 weeks' postmenstrual age, 1.5 mg/kg/dose, orally, twice daily; preterm >40 weeks' postmenstrual age through 8 months' chronologic age, 3.0 mg/kg/dose, orally, twice daily.

For more information on individual drugs, see *Physician's Desk Reference* or **www.pdr.net** (for registered users only).

DRUGS FOR PARASITIC INFECTIONS

Table 4.11. Drugs for Parasitic Infections[1]

Disease	Drug	Adult Dosage	Pediatric Dosage	Links to CDC Web Site[2] and professional society guidelines
African trypanosomiasis (African sleeping sickness)				www.cdc.gov/ parasites/ sleepingsickness/ health_ professionals/ index.html
Trypanosoma brucei rhodesiense, hemolymphatic stage	Suramin[3]	After test dose of 100 mg,[4] 20 mg/ kg/day (max 1 g), IV, on days 1, 3, 7, 14, and 21	After test dose of 2 mg/kg (max 100 mg),[5] 20 mg/kg/day (max 1 g), IV, on days 1, 3, 7, 14, and 21	
T brucei rhodesiense, CNS involvement	Melarsoprol[6]	2–3.6 mg/kg/day IV once daily for 3 days (2 mg/kg/dose on day 1, titrating up to 3.6 mg/kg/dose on day 3) then 3.6 mg/kg/day on days 11, 12, 13, and days 21, 22, and 23	2–3.6 mg/kg/day IV once daily for 3 days (2 mg/kg/dose on day 1, titrating up to 3.6 mg/kg/dose on day 3) then 3.6 mg/kg/day on days 11, 12, 13, and days 21, 22, and 23	CDC Drug Service: www.cdc.gov/ laboratory/ drugservice/index/ html
T brucei gambiense, hemolymphatic stage	Pentamidine[7]	4 mg/kg/dose once daily, IV or IM, for 7–10 days	4 mg/kg/dose once daily, IV or IM, for 7–10 days	
T brucei gambiense, CNS involvement	Eflornithine[8]	400 mg/kg/day, IV in 4 divided doses OR 400 mg/kg/day, IV, in 2 divided doses for 14 days OR 400 mg/kg/d IV in 2 doses for 7 days when given with nifurtimox 15 mg/kg orally in 3 divided doses for 10 days	400 mg/kg/day, IV in 4 divided doses OR 400 mg/kg/day, IV, in 2 divided doses for 14 days OR 400 mg/kg/d IV in 2 doses for 7 days when given with nifurtimox 15 mg/kg orally in 3 divided doses for 10 days	

Table 4.11. Drugs for Parasitic Infections,[1] continued

Disease	Drug	Adult Dosage	Pediatric Dosage	Links to CDC Web Site[2] and professional society guidelines
American trypanosomiasis (Chagas disease; *Trypanosoma cruzi* infection)	Benznidazole[9]	5–7 mg/kg/day, orally, in 2 divided doses for 60 days	Age <12 y: 5–8 mg/kg/day, orally, in 2 divided doses for 60 days Age ≥12 y: 5–7 mg/kg/day, orally, in 2 divided doses for 60 days	www.cdc.gov/parasites/chagas/health_professionals/index.html
	OR			
	Nifurtimox[9]	8–10 mg/kg/day, orally, in 3 or 4 divided doses for 60 days	2.5 kg to 40 kg: 10–20 mg/kg/day, orally, in 3 divided doses for 60 days ≥40 kg: 8–10 mg/kg/day, orally, in 3 divided doses for 60 days	

Table 4.11. Drugs for Parasitic Infections,[1] continued

Disease	Drug	Adult Dosage	Pediatric Dosage	Links to CDC Web Site[2] and professional society guidelines
Ascariasis (*Ascaris lumbricoides*; intestinal roundworm)	Albendazole[10]	400 mg, orally, once (take with food)		www.cdc.gov/parasites/ascariasis/health_professionals/index.html
	OR			
	Mebendazole[11]	100 mg, orally, twice daily for 3 days OR 500 mg, orally, once		
	OR			
	Ivermectin[12]	150–200 µg/kg, orally, once		
	OR			
	Pyrantel pamoate[13]	11 mg/kg (up to a maximum of 1 g), orally, daily for 3 days (may be given as a single dose for adults)		
	OR			
	Nitazoxanide	500 mg, orally, twice daily for 3 days	Age 1–3 y: 100 mg, orally, twice daily for 3 days; Age 4–11 y: 200 mg, orally, twice daily for 3 days; Age ≥12 y: 500 mg, orally, twice daily for 3 days	

Table 4.11. Drugs for Parasitic Infections,¹ continued

Disease	Drug	Adult Dosage	Pediatric Dosage	Links to CDC Web Site² and professional society guidelines
Babesiosis¹⁴	Atovaquone¹⁵	750 mg, orally, twice daily (mild to moderate disease OR severe disease) for at least 7–10 days	20 mg/kg (up to 750 mg), orally, twice daily (mild to moderate disease OR severe disease) for at least 7–10 days	www.cdc.gov/parasites/babesiosis/health_professionals/index.html
	PLUS			
	Azithromycin¹⁶	500 mg, orally, on day 1, then 250 mg, orally once daily on subsequent days (mild to moderate disease); OR 500–1000 mg, IV, once daily (severe disease) until symptoms abate, then convert to all oral therapy	10 mg/kg (up to 500 mg), orally, on day 1; then 5 mg/kg/day (max 250 mg/dose), orally, on subsequent days (mild to moderate disease) OR 10 mg/kg (up to 500 mg), IV, daily (severe disease) until symptoms abate, then convert to all oral therapy	
	OR			
	Clindamycin	600 mg, orally, 3 times daily, OR 600 mg, IV, 4 times daily, for at least 7–10 days	7–10 mg/kg (up to 600 mg), orally 3 times daily (mild to moderate disease) OR IV 3 to 4 times daily (severe disease), for at least 7–10 days	
	PLUS			
	Quinine¹⁷	542 mg base (which equals 650 mg salt), orally, 3 to 4 times daily, for at least 7–10 days	6 mg base/kg (which equals 8 mg salt/kg) (up to 542 mg base or 650 mg salt/dose), orally, 3 to 4 times daily, for at least 7–10 days	

Table 4.11. Drugs for Parasitic Infections,[1] continued

Disease	Drug	Adult Dosage	Pediatric Dosage	Links to CDC Web Site[2] and professional society guidelines
Balantidiasis (*Balantidium coli*)	Tetracycline[18]	500 mg, orally, 4 times daily for 10 days	Age ≥8 y: 40 mg/kg/day (max 2 g per day), orally, in 4 doses for 10 days	www.cdc.gov/parasites/ balantidium/health_professionals/ index.html
	OR			
	Metronidazole	500–750 mg, orally, 3 times daily for 5 days	35–50 mg/kg/day, orally, in 3 doses for 5 days (max 500–750 mg/dose)	
	OR			
	Iodoquinol[19]	650 mg, orally, 3 times daily for 20 days	30–40 mg/kg/day (max 650 mg per dose), orally, in 3 doses for 20 days	
	OR			
	Nitazoxanide	500 mg, orally, twice daily for 3 days	Age 1–3 y: 100 mg, orally, twice daily for 3 days Age 4–11 y: 200 mg, orally, twice daily for 3 days Age ≥12 y: 500 mg, orally, twice daily for 3 days	
Baylisascariasis (raccoon roundworm infection)	Albendazole[10]	25–50 mg/kg/day, orally, for 10–20 days[20] (take with food)		www.cdc.gov/parasites/ baylisascaris/health_ professionals/index.html

Table 4.11. Drugs for Parasitic Infections,[1] continued

Disease	Drug	Adult Dosage	Pediatric Dosage	Links to CDC Web Site[2] and professional society guidelines
Blastocystis species infection[21]	Metronidazole	250 mg to 750 mg, orally, 3 times daily for 10 days OR 1500 mg, orally, once daily for 10 days	35–50 mg/kg/day, orally, in 3 doses for 10 days (max 500–750 mg/dose)	www.cdc.gov/parasites/ blastocystis/health_professionals/ index.html
	OR			
	Trimethoprim (TMP)/ sulfamethoxazole (SMX)	160 mg TMP, 800 mg SMX, orally, twice daily for 7 days	Age >2 mo: 8 mg/kg TMP and 40 mg/kg SMX per day, orally, in 2 divided doses for 7 days	
	OR			
	Nitazoxanide	500 mg, orally, twice daily for 3 days	Age 1–3 y: 100 mg, orally, twice daily for 3 days Age 4–11 y: 200 mg, orally, twice daily for 3 days Age ≥12 y: 500 mg, orally, twice daily for 3 days	
	OR			
	Tinidazole	2 g, orally, once	Age ≥3 y: 50 mg/kg (max 2 g) once	
Capillariasis	Mebendazole[11]	200 mg, orally, twice daily for 20 days		www.cdc.gov/parasites/capillaria/ health_professionals/index.html
	OR			
	Albendazole[10]	400 mg, orally, once daily for 10 days (take with food)		

Table 4.11. Drugs for Parasitic Infections,[1] continued

Disease	Drug	Adult Dosage	Pediatric Dosage	Links to CDC Web Site[2] and professional society guidelines
Chilomastix mesnili	No treatment is necessary; this protozoan is considered nonpathogenic but may be an indicator of ingestion of fecally contaminated food or water			**www.cdc.gov/parasites/ nonpathprotozoa/health_ professionals/index.html**
Clonorchiasis	Praziquantel[22]	75 mg/kg/day, orally, in 3 doses for 2 days		**www.cdc.gov/parasites/ clonorchis/health_professionals/ index.html**
	OR			
	Albendazole[10]	10 mg/kg/day, orally, for 7 days (take with food)		
Cryptosporidiosis	Nitazoxanide[23]	500 mg, orally, twice a day for 3 days	Age 1–3 y: 100 mg, orally, twice a day for 3 days Age 4 to 11 y: 200 mg, orally, twice a day for 3 days Age ≥12 y: 500 mg, orally, twice a day for 3 days	**www.cdc.gov/parasites/crypto/ treatment.html**
Cutaneous larva migrans (zoonotic hookworm)	Albendazole[10]	400 mg/day, orally, once daily for 3–7 days (take with food)	Age >2 y: 15 mg/kg/day (max 400 mg/day), orally, for 3 days (take with food)	**www.cdc.gov/parasites/ zoonotichookworm/health_ professionals/index.html**
	OR			
	Ivermectin[12]	200 µg/kg, orally, once daily for 1 day	Weight ≥15 kg: 200 µg/kg, orally, once daily for 1 day	
Cyclosporiasis	Trimethoprim (TMP)/ sulfamethoxazole (SMX)	160 mg TMP/800 mg SMX, orally, 2 times/day for 7–10 days[24]	Age >2 mo: 8–10 mg/kg TMP and 40–50 mg/ kg SMX per day, orally, in 2 divided doses for 7–10 days[24]	**www.cdc.gov/parasites/ cyclosporiasis/health_ professionals/index.html**

Table 4.11. Drugs for Parasitic Infections,[1] continued

Disease	Drug	Adult Dosage	Pediatric Dosage	Links to CDC Web Site[2] and professional society guidelines
Cystoisosporiasis (*Cystoisospora* infection; formerly isosporiasis)[25]	Trimethoprim (TMP)/ sulfamethoxazole (SMX)	160 mg TMP/800 mg SMX, IV or orally, 2 times/day for 7–10 days	Age >2 mo: 8–10 mg/kg TMP and 40–50 mg/kg SMX per day, IV or orally, in 2 divided doses for 7–10 days	**www.cdc.gov/parasites/ cystoisospora/health_ professionals/index.html**
	OR			
	Pyrimethamine	50–75 mg per day of pyrimethamine, either once daily or divided into 2 separate doses	--	
	PLUS			
	Leucovorin (folinic acid)	10–25 mg per day of leucovorin (folinic acid)		
	OR			
	Ciprofloxacin	500 mg, orally, 2 times/day for 7 days	--	
Dientamoeba fragilis infection[26, 27]	Iodoquinol[19]	650 mg, orally, 3 times/day for 20 days	30–40 mg/kg/day (max 650 mg/dose), orally, divided 3 times/day for 20 days	**www.cdc.gov/parasites/ dientamoeba/health_ professionals/index.html**
	OR			
	Paromomycin	25–35 mg/kg/day, orally, in 3 divided doses, for 7 days		
	OR			
	Metronidazole	500–750 mg, orally, 3 times/day for 10 days	35–50 mg/kg/day, orally, in 3 divided doses (max 500–750 mg/dose) for 10 days	

Table 4.11. Drugs for Parasitic Infections,[1] continued

Disease	Drug	Adult Dosage	Pediatric Dosage	Links to CDC Web Site[2] and professional society guidelines
Diphyllobothrium infection	Praziquantel[22]	5–10 mg/kg, orally, in a single dose taken with liquids during a meal		www.cdc.gov/parasites/diphyllobothrium/health_professionals/index.html
	OR			
	Niclosamide[28]	2 g, orally, once	50 mg/kg (max 2 g), orally, once	
Dipylidium caninum infection (dog or cat flea tapeworm)	Praziquantel[22]	5–10 mg/kg, orally, in a single dose (take with liquids during a meal)		www.cdc.gov/parasites/dipylidium/health_professionals/index.html
	OR			
	Niclosamide[28]	2 g, orally, once	50 mg/kg (max 2 g), orally, once	
Echinococcosis[29]	Albendazole[10]	400 mg, orally, twice daily for 1–6 mo (take with food)	10–15 mg/kg/day (max 800 mg/day), orally, in 2 doses for 1–6 mo (take with food)	www.cdc.gov/parasites/echinococcosis/health_professionals/index.html
Endolimax nana	No treatment is necessary; this protozoan is harmless			www.cdc.gov/parasites/nonpathprotozoa/
Entamoeba coli	No treatment is necessary; this protozoan is harmless			www.cdc.gov/parasites/nonpathprotozoa/
Entamoeba dispar	No treatment is necessary; this protozoan is harmless			www.cdc.gov/parasites/nonpathprotozoa/
Entamoeba hartmanni	No treatment is necessary; this protozoan is harmless			www.cdc.gov/parasites/nonpathprotozoa/

Table 4.11. Drugs for Parasitic Infections,[1] continued

Disease	Drug	Adult Dosage	Pediatric Dosage	Links to CDC Web Site[2] and professional society guidelines
Entamoeba histolytica (amebiasis)[30] Asymptomatic intestinal colonization	Iodoquinol[19]	650 mg, orally, 3 times/day for 20 days	30–40 mg/kg/day (max 650 mg/dose), orally, divided 3 times/day for 20 days	www.cdc.gov/parasites/amebiasis/index.html
	OR			
	Paromomycin	25–35 mg/kg/day, orally, divided 3 times/day for 7 days		
	OR			
	Diloxanide furoate[31]	500 mg, orally, 3 times/day for 10 days	20 mg/kg/day (max 500 mg/dose), orally, divided 3 times a day for 10 days	
Entamoeba histolytica (amebiasis)[30] Mild to moderate intestinal disease	Metronidazole	500 to 750 mg, orally, 3 times/day for 7–10 days	35–50 mg/kg/day, orally, divided 3 times/day for 7–10 days	www.cdc.gov/parasites/amebiasis/index.html
	OR			
	Tinidazole	2 g, orally, once daily for 3 days	Age ≥3 y: 50 mg/kg (max 2 g), orally, once daily for 3 days	
	FOLLOWED EITHER BY:			
	Iodoquinol[19]	650 mg, orally, 3 times/day for 20 days	30–40 mg/kg/day (max 650 mg/dose), orally, divided 3 times/day for 20 days	
	OR BY			
	Paromomycin	25–35 mg/kg/day, orally, divided 3 times/day for 7 days		

Table 4.11. Drugs for Parasitic Infections,[1] continued

Disease	Drug	Adult Dosage	Pediatric Dosage	Links to CDC Web Site[2] and professional society guidelines
Entamoeba histolytica (amebiasis)[30] Severe intestinal and extraintestinal disease	Metronidazole	500 to 750 mg, IV (switch to orally when tolerated), 3 times/day for 7–10 days	35–50 mg/kg/day, IV (switch to orally when tolerated), divided 3 times/day for 7–10 days (max 500–750 mg/dose)	www.cdc.gov/parasites/amebiasis/index.html
	OR			
	Tinidazole	2 g, orally, once daily for 5 days	Age ≥3 y: 50 mg/kg (max 2 g), orally, once daily for 5 days	
	FOLLOWED EITHER BY:			
	Iodoquinol[19]	650 mg, orally, 3 times/day for 20 days	30–40 mg/kg/day (max 650 mg/dose), orally, divided 3 times/day for 20 days	
	OR BY			
	Paromomycin	25–35 mg/kg/day, orally, divided 3 times/day for 7 days		
Entamoeba polecki	No treatment is necessary; this protozoan is harmless			www.cdc.gov/parasites/nonpathprotozoa/health_professionals/index.html

Table 4.11. Drugs for Parasitic Infections,[1] continued

Disease	Drug	Adult Dosage	Pediatric Dosage	Links to CDC Web Site[2] and professional society guidelines
Enterobiasis (pinworm)	Mebendazole[11]	100 mg, orally, once; repeat in 2 wk		www.cdc.gov/parasites/pinworm/health_professionals/index.html
	OR			
	Pyrantel pamoate[13]	11 mg/kg base, orally, once (max 1 g); repeat in 2 wk		
	OR			
	Albendazole[10]	400 mg orally once; repeat in 2 wk (take with food)	Age ≥2 y: 400 mg orally once; repeat in 2 wk; age <2 y 200 mg orally once; repeat in 2 wk (take with food)	
Fascioliasis (*Fasciola hepatica*; sheep liver fluke)	Triclabendazole[32]	10 mg/kg, orally, once or twice (doses separated by 12–24 hours) in patients ≥6 y (take with food)		www.cdc.gov/parasites/fasciola/health_professionals/index.html
	OR			
	Nitazoxanide	500 mg, orally, 2 times/day for 7 days (take with food)	Age 1–3 y: 100 mg, orally, 2 times/day for 7 days Age 4–11 y: 200 mg, orally, 2 times/day for 7 days Age ≥12 y: 500 mg, orally, 2 times/day for 7 days (take with food)	
Fasciolopsiasis (*Fasciolopsis buski*; intestinal fluke)	Praziquantel[22]	75 mg/kg/day, orally, in 3 divided doses for 1 day		www.cdc.gov/parasites/fasciolopsis/health_professionals/index.html

Table 4.11. Drugs for Parasitic Infections,[1] continued

Disease	Drug	Adult Dosage	Pediatric Dosage	Links to CDC Web Site[2] and professional society guidelines
Giardiasis[33]	Tinidazole	2 g, orally, once	Age ≥3 y: 50 mg/kg (max 2 g), orally, once	www.cdc.gov/parasites/giardia/audience-health-professionals.html
	OR			
	Metronidazole	250 mg, orally, 3 times/day for 5–7 days	15 mg/kg/day (max 250 mg/dose), orally, divided 3 times/day for 5–7 days	
	OR			
	Nitazoxanide	500 mg, orally, 2 times/day for 3 days	Age 1–3 y: 100 mg, orally, 2 times/day for 3 days Age 4–11 y: 200 mg, orally, 2 times/day for 3 days Age ≥12 y: 500 mg, orally, 2 times/day for 3 days	
Gnathostomiasis (cutaneous)	Albendazole[10]	400 mg, orally, 2 times/day for 21 days (take with food)		www.cdc.gov/parasites/gnathostoma/health_professionals/index.html
	OR			
	Ivermectin[12]	200 µg/kg, orally, once daily for 2 days		
Heterophyiasis	Praziquantel[22]	75 mg/kg/day, orally, divided 3 times/day for 1 day		www.cdc.gov/dpdx/heterophyiasis/index.html

Table 4.11. Drugs for Parasitic Infections,[1] continued

Disease	Drug	Adult Dosage	Pediatric Dosage	Links to CDC Web Site[2] and professional society guidelines
Hymenolepiasis (*Hymenolepis nana*; dwarf tapeworm)	Praziquantel[22]	25 mg/kg in a single-dose therapy, orally; some experts recommend a second dose 10 days later		www.cdc.gov/parasites/hymenolepis/health_professionals/index.html
	OR			
	Niclosamide[28]	2 g in a single dose for 7 days, orally	Weight 11–34 kg: 1 g in a single dose on day 1; then 500 mg per day, orally, for 6 days Weight >34 kg: 1.5 g in a single dose on day 1; then 1 g per day, orally, for 6 days	
	OR			
	Nitazoxanide	500 mg, orally, 2 times/day for 3 days	Age 1–3 y: 100 mg, orally, 2 times/day for 3 days Age 4–11 y: 200 mg, orally, 2 times/day for 3 days Age ≥12 y: 500 mg, orally, 2 times/day for 3 days	

Table 4.11. Drugs for Parasitic Infections,[1] continued

Disease	Drug	Adult Dosage	Pediatric Dosage	Links to CDC Web Site[2] and professional society guidelines
Hookworm (Human; *Ancylostoma duodenale, Necator americanus*)	Albendazole[10]	400 mg, orally once (take with food)	≥2 y: 400 mg, orally, once (take with food)	www.cdc.gov/parasites/hookworm/health_professionals/index.html
	OR			
	Mebendazole[11]	100 mg, orally, twice daily for 3 days; OR 500 mg, orally, once		
	OR			
	Pyrantel pamoate[13]	11 mg/kg (max 1 g), orally, daily for 3 days		
Iodamoeba buetschlii	No treatment is necessary; this protozoan is harmless			www.cdc.gov/parasites/nonpathprotozoa/health_professionals/index.html
Leishmaniasis[34]				
Visceral (kala-azar)	Liposomal amphotericin B	3 mg/kg/day, IV, on days 1–5, 14, and 21 (total dose 21 mg/kg) If immunocompromised, 4 mg/kg/day, IV, on days 1–5, 10, 17, 24, 31, and 38 (total dose 40 mg/kg)		www.cdc.gov/parasites/leishmaniasis/health_professionals/index.html www.idsociety.org/practice-guideline/leishmaniasis/ www.cdc.gov/laboratory/drugservice/index.html
	OR			
	Sodium stibogluconate[34]	20 mg pentavalent antimony (Sb)/kg/day, IV or IM, for 28 days		

Table 4.11. Drugs for Parasitic Infections,[1] continued

Disease	Drug	Adult Dosage	Pediatric Dosage	Links to CDC Web Site[2] and professional society guidelines
	OR			
	Miltefosine	30 through 44 kg: 50 mg, orally, twice daily, for 28 consecutive days ≥45 kg: 50 mg, orally, 3 times daily, for 28 consecutive days (contraindicated in pregnant or breastfeeding women)		
	OR			
	Amphotericin B deoxycholate	1 mg/kg, IV, daily or every second day (cumulative total usually ~15–20 mg/kg)		
	Sodium stibogluconate[34]	20 mg Sb/kg/day, IV or IM, for 20 days		
	OR			
	Miltefosine	30 through 44 kg: 50 mg, orally, twice daily, for 28 consecutive days ≥45 kg: 50 mg, orally, 3 times daily, for 28 consecutive days (contraindicated in pregnant or breastfeeding women)		
Complicated Cutaneous	OR			
	Pentamidine isethionate	2–4 mg/kg/day IV or IM, every other day, for 4–7 doses (limitations include toxicity and variable effectiveness)		
	OR			
	Amphotericin	Various regimens		
	OR			

Table 4.11. Drugs for Parasitic Infections,[1] continued

Disease	Drug	Adult Dosage	Pediatric Dosage	Links to CDC Web Site[2] and professional society guidelines
	Azoles	Fluconazole 200 mg daily for 6 weeks; or ketoconazole or itraconazole		
	OR			
	Intralesional or topical alternatives	See guidelines		
Mucosal	Sodium stibogluconate	20 mg Sb/kg/day, IV or IM, for 28 days		
	OR			
	Amphotericin B deoxycholate	0.5–1 mg/kg, IV, daily or every second day for a cumulative total of ~20–45 mg/kg		
	OR			
	Miltefosine	30–44 kg: 50 mg, PO, twice daily for 28 consecutive days ≥45 kg: 50 mg, PO, 3 times daily for 28 consecutive days (contraindicated in pregnant or breastfeeding women)		
Lice infestation (*Pediculus humanus*, *P capitis*, *P pubis*)[35]	Pyrethrins with piperonyl butoxide[36]	Topically, twice, 9–10 days apart	Topically, twice, 9–10 days apart	www.cdc.gov/parasites/lice/pubic/health_professionals/index.html
	OR			
	0.5% Ivermectin lotion[37]	Topically, once	Topically, once	www.cdc.gov/std/treatment/default.htm
	OR			
	0.9% Spinosad suspension[38]	Topically, twice (if crawling lice present), 7 days apart	Topically, twice (if crawling lice present), 7 days apart	
	OR			

Table 4.11. Drugs for Parasitic Infections,[1] continued

Disease	Drug	Adult Dosage	Pediatric Dosage	Links to CDC Web Site[2] and professional society guidelines
	1% Permethrin[36]	Topically, twice, 9–10 days apart	Topically, twice, 9–10 days apart	
	OR			
	5% Benzyl alcohol lotion[39]	Topically, twice, 7 days apart	Topically, twice, 7 days apart	
	OR			
	0.5% Malathion[40]	Topically, twice (if needed), 7–9 days apart	Topically, twice (if needed), 7–9 days apart	
	OR			
	0.74% Abametapir[41]	Topically, once	Topically, once	
	OR			
	Ivermectin[12,42]	200 µg/kg, orally, twice, 9–10 days apart OR 400 µg/kg, orally, twice, 9–10 days apart	≥15 kg: 200 µg/kg, orally, twice, 9–10 days apart OR ≥15 kg: 400 µg/kg, orally, twice, 9–10 days apart	

Table 4.11. Drugs for Parasitic Infections,[1] continued

Disease	Drug	Adult Dosage	Pediatric Dosage	Links to CDC Web Site[2] and professional society guidelines
Loiasis (*Loa loa*)	Diethylcarbamazine (DEC)[43]	Symptomatic loiasis with microfilariae of *L loa* (MF)/mL <8000: 8–10 mg/kg/day, orally, in 3 divided doses for 21 days		www.cdc.gov/parasites/loiasis/health_professionals/index.html www.cdc.gov/laboratory/drugservice/index.html
	Albendazole[10]	Symptomatic loiasis, with MF/mL <8000 and failed 2 rounds of DEC OR Symptomatic loiasis, with MF/mL ≥8000 to reduce level to <8000 prior to treatment with DEC: 200 mg, orally, twice daily for 21 days (take with food)		
	Apheresis followed by DEC[44]	Symptomatic loiasis, with MF/mL ≥8000		
Lymphatic filariasis (elephantiasis; *Wuchereria bancrofti*, *Brugia malayi*, *Brugia timori*)	Diethylcarbamazine (DEC)[43]	Treatment of lymphatic filariasis[45]: Adults and children ≥18 mo: 6 mg/kg/day, orally, in 3 divided doses for 12 consecutive days; OR 6 mg/kg as a single oral dose Treatment of tropical pulmonary eosinophilia (TPE): Adults and children ≥18 mo: 6 mg/kg/day, orally, in 3 divided doses for 14–21 days		www.cdc.gov/parasites/lymphaticfilariasis/health_professionals/index.html www.cdc.gov/laboratory/drugservice/index.html

Table 4.11. Drugs for Parasitic Infections,[1] continued

Disease	Drug	Adult Dosage	Pediatric Dosage	Links to CDC Web Site[2] and professional society guidelines
Malaria (*Plasmodium* species)	Region infection acquired			
Uncomplicated malaria *P falciparum* or species not identified If "species not identified" subsequently diagnosed as *P vivax* or *P ovale*, see below regarding radical cure with primaquine or tafenoquine	Chloroquine-resistant or unknown resistance[46,47] (All malarious regions except those specified as chloroquine-sensitive listed below.)			
	Atovaquone-proguanil[48] Adult tablet: 250 mg atovaquone/100 mg proguanil Pediatric tablet: 62.5 mg atovaquone/25 mg proguanil	1000 mg atovaquone/400 mg proguanil, orally, once daily for 3 days	Weight 5–<8 kg: 2 pediatric tablets, orally, once daily for 3 days Weight 8–<10 kg: 3 pediatric tablets, orally, once daily for 3 days Weight 10–<20 kg: 1 adult tab, orally, once daily for 3 days Weight 20–<30 kg: 2 adult tablets, orally, once daily for 3 days Weight 30–<40 kg: 3 adult tablets, orally, once daily for 3 days Weight ≥40 kg: 4 adult tablets, orally, once daily for 3 days	**www.cdc.gov/malaria/resources/pdf/Malaria_Treatment_Table_120419.pdf** Updated guidance about treatment of severe malaria: **www.cdc.gov/malaria/new_info/2019/artesunate_2019.html** CDC Malaria Hotline: (770) 488-7788 or (855) 856-4713 toll-free Monday–Friday 9 AM to 5 PM EST; (770) 488-7100 after hours, weekends, and holidays

Table 4.11. Drugs for Parasitic Infections,[1] continued

Disease	Drug	Adult Dosage	Pediatric Dosage	Links to CDC Web Site[2] and professional society guidelines
	OR			
	Artemether-lumefantrine[48] 1 tablet = 20 mg artemether and 120 mg lumefantrine	A 3-day treatment schedule with a total of 6 oral doses is recommended for both adult and pediatric patients based on weight. The patient should receive the initial dose, followed by the second dose 8 hours later, then 1 dose, orally, 2 times/day, for the following 2 days. Weight 5 to <15 kg: 1 tablet per dose Weight 15 to <25 kg: 2 tablets per dose Weight 25 to <35 kg: 3 tablets per dose Weight ≥35 kg: 4 tablets per dose		
	OR			
	Quinine sulfate[49,50] plus one of the following: Doxycycline,[51] Tetracycline,[51] or Clindamycin	Quinine sulfate: 542 mg base (=650 mg salt), orally, 3 times/day for 3 or 7 days[50] Doxycycline: 100 mg, orally, 2 times/day for 7 days Tetracycline: 250 mg, orally, 4 times/day for 7 days Clindamycin: 20 mg base/kg/day, orally, divided 3 times/day for 7 days	Quinine sulfate: 8.3 mg base/kg (=10 mg salt/kg), orally, 3 times/day for 3 or 7 days Doxycycline: 2.2 mg/kg, orally, every 12 h for 7 days (max 200 mg/day) Tetracycline: 25 mg/kg/day, orally, divided 4 times/day for 7 days Clindamycin: 20 mg base/kg/day, orally, divided 3 times/day for 7 days	

Table 4.11. Drugs for Parasitic Infections,[1] continued

Disease	Drug	Adult Dosage	Pediatric Dosage	Links to CDC Web Site[2] and professional society guidelines
	OR			
	Mefloquine[52]	684 mg base (=750 mg salt), orally, as initial dose, followed by 456 mg base (=500 mg salt), orally, given 6–12 h after initial dose Total dose = 1250 mg salt	13.7 mg base/kg (=15 mg salt/kg), orally, as initial dose, followed by 9.1 mg base/kg (=10 mg salt/kg), orally, given 6–12 h after initial dose Total dose = 25 mg salt/kg	
Uncomplicated malaria *P. falciparum* or species not identified	Chloroquine-sensitive (Central America west of Panama Canal, Haiti, and the Dominican Republic)			
	Chloroquine phosphate[53]	600 mg base (=1000 mg salt), orally, immediately; followed by 300 mg base (=500 mg salt), orally, at 6, 24, and 48 h Total dose: 1500 mg base (=2500 mg salt)	10 mg base/kg, orally, immediately; followed by 5 mg base/kg, orally, at 6, 24, and 48 h Total dose: 25 mg base/kg	
	OR			
	Hydroxychloroquine	620 mg base (=800 mg salt), orally, immediately; followed by 310 mg base (=400 mg salt), orally, at 6, 24, and 48 h Total dose: 1550 mg base (=2000 mg salt)	10 mg base/kg, orally, immediately; followed by 5 mg base/kg, orally, at 6, 24, and 48 h Total dose: 25 mg base/kg	

Table 4.11. Drugs for Parasitic Infections,[1] continued

Disease	Drug	Adult Dosage	Pediatric Dosage	Links to CDC Web Site[2] and professional society guidelines
	All regions			
Uncomplicated malaria *P malariae* or *P knowlesi*	Chloroquine phosphate[53]	600 mg base (=1000 mg salt), orally, immediately, followed by 300 mg base (=500 mg salt), orally, at 6, 24, and 48 h Total dose: 1500 mg base (=2500 mg salt)	10 mg base/kg, orally, immediately, followed by 5 mg base/kg, orally, at 6, 24, and 48 h Total dose: 25 mg base/kg	
	OR			
	Hydroxychloroquine	620 mg base (=800 mg salt), orally, immediately, followed by 310 mg base (=400 mg salt), orally, at 6, 24, and 48 h Total dose: 1550 mg base (=2000 mg salt)	10 mg base/kg, orally, immediately, followed by 5 mg base/kg, orally, at 6, 24, and 48 h Total dose: 25 mg base/kg	

Table 4.11. Drugs for Parasitic Infections,[1] continued

Disease	Drug	Adult Dosage	Pediatric Dosage	Links to CDC Web Site[2] and professional society guidelines
	All regions Note: for suspected chloroquine-resistant *P. vivax*, see row below			
	Chloroquine phosphate[53]	600 mg base (=1000 mg salt), orally, immediately, followed by 300 mg base (=500 mg salt), orally, at 6, 24, and 48 h Total dose: 1500 mg base (=2500 mg salt)	10 mg base/kg, orally, immediately, followed by 5 mg base/kg, orally, at 6, 24, and 48 h Total dose: 25 mg base/kg	
Uncomplicated malaria *P. vivax* or *P. ovale*	PLUS EITHER			
	Primaquine phosphate[54]	30 mg base, orally, once daily for 14 days	0.5 mg base/kg, orally, once daily for 14 days	
	OR			
	Tafenoquine[54]	300 mg orally on the first or second day of appropriate therapy for acute malaria	≥16 years 300 mg orally on the first or second day of appropriate therapy for acute malaria	

Table 4.11. Drugs for Parasitic Infections,[1] continued

Disease	Drug	Adult Dosage	Pediatric Dosage	Links to CDC Web Site[2] and professional society guidelines
	OR			
	Hydroxychloroquine	620 mg base (=800 mg salt), orally, immediately; followed by 310 mg base (=400 mg salt), orally, at 6, 24, and 48 h Total dose: 1550 mg base (=2000 mg salt)	10 mg base/kg, orally, immediately; followed by 5 mg base/kg, orally, at 6, 24, and 48 h Total dose: 25 mg base/kg	
	PLUS EITHER			
	Primaquine phosphate[54]	30 mg base, orally, once daily for 14 days	0.5 mg base/kg, orally, once daily for 14 days	
	OR			
	Tafenoquine[54]	300 mg orally on the first or second day of appropriate therapy for acute malaria	≥16 years 300 mg orally on the first or second day of appropriate therapy for acute malaria	

Table 4.11. Drugs for Parasitic Infections,[1] continued

Disease	Drug	Adult Dosage	Pediatric Dosage	Links to CDC Web Site[2] and professional society guidelines
	Chloroquine-resistant[55] (Papua New Guinea and Indonesia)			
	Quinine sulfate[49]	Quinine sulfate: 542 mg base (=650 mg salt),[50] orally, 3 times/day for 3 or 7 days[50]	Quinine sulfate: 8.3 mg base/kg (=10 mg salt/kg), orally, 3 times/day for 3 or 7 days[50]	
	PLUS EITHER			
	Doxycycline	Doxycycline: 100 mg, orally, 2 times/day for 7 days	Doxycycline: 2.2 mg/kg, orally, every 12 h for 7 days (max 200 mg/day)	
	OR			
Uncomplicated malaria *P vivax*	Tetracycline[51]	Tetracycline: 250 mg, orally, 4 times/day for 7 days	Tetracycline: 25 mg/kg/day, orally, divided 4 times/day for 7 days	
	PLUS EITHER			
	Primaquine phosphate[54]	Primaquine phosphate: 30 mg base, orally, once daily for 14 days	Primaquine phosphate: 0.5 mg base/kg, orally, once daily for 14 days	
	OR			
	Tafenoquine[54]	300 mg orally on the first or second day of appropriate therapy for acute malaria	≥16 years 300 mg orally on the first or second day of appropriate therapy for acute malaria	

Table 4.11. Drugs for Parasitic Infections,[1] continued

Disease	Drug	Adult Dosage	Pediatric Dosage	Links to CDC Web Site[2] and professional society guidelines
	OR			
	Atovaquone-proguanil Adult tablet: 250 mg atovaquone/100 mg proguanil Pediatric tablet: 62.5 mg atovaquone/25 mg proguanil	Atovaquone-proguanil: 1000 mg atovaquone/400 mg proguanil, orally, once daily for 3 days	Atovaquone-proguanil: 5–<8 kg: 2 pediatric tablets, orally, once daily for 3 days 8–<10 kg: 3 pediatric tablets, orally, once daily for 3 days 10–<20 kg: 1 adult tablet, orally, once daily for 3 days 20–<30 kg: 2 adult tablets, orally, once daily for 3 days 30–<40 kg: 3 adult tablets, orally, once daily for 3 days ≥40 kg: 4 adult tablets, orally, once daily for 3 days	
	PLUS EITHER			
	Primaquine phosphate[54] OR	Primaquine phosphate: 30 mg base, orally, once daily for 14 days	Primaquine phosphate: 0.5 mg base/kg, orally, once daily for 14 days	
	Tafenoquine[54]	300 mg orally on the first or second day of chloroquine or hydroxychloroquine for acute malaria	≥16 years: 300 mg orally on the first or second day of chloroquine or hydroxychloroquine for acute malaria	

Table 4.11. Drugs for Parasitic Infections,[1] continued

Disease	Drug	Adult Dosage	Pediatric Dosage	Links to CDC Web Site[2] and professional society guidelines
	OR			
	Mefloquine	Mefloquine: 684 mg base (=750 mg salt), orally, as initial dose, followed by 456 mg base (=500 mg salt), orally, given 6–12 h after initial dose Total dose= 1250 mg salt	Mefloquine: 13.7 mg base/kg (=15 mg salt/kg), orally, as initial dose, followed by 9.1 mg base/kg (=10 mg salt/kg), orally, given 6–12 h after initial dose Total dose = 25 mg salt/kg	
	PLUS EITHER			
	Primaquine phosphate[54]	Primaquine phosphate: 30 mg base, orally, once daily for 14 days	Primaquine phosphate: 0.5 mg base/kg, orally, once daily for 14 days	
	OR			
	Tafenoquine[54]	300 mg orally on the first or second day of chloroquine or hydroxychloroquine for acute malaria	≥16 years: 300 mg orally on the first or second day of chloroquine or hydroxychloroquine for acute malaria	

Table 4.11. Drugs for Parasitic Infections,[1] continued

Disease	Drug	Adult Dosage	Pediatric Dosage	Links to CDC Web Site[2] and professional society guidelines
Uncomplicated malaria: alternatives for pregnant women[56,57,58]	Chloroquine-sensitive (see uncomplicated malaria sections above for chloroquine-sensitive species by region)			
	Chloroquine phosphate[53]	600 mg base (=1000 mg salt), orally, immediately; followed by 300 mg base (=500 mg salt), orally, at 6, 24, and 48 h Total dose: 1500 mg base (=2500 mg salt)	Not applicable	
	OR			
	Hydroxychloroquine	620 mg base (=800 mg salt), orally, immediately; followed by 310 mg base (=400 mg salt), orally, at 6, 24, and 48 h Total dose: 1550 mg base (=2000 mg salt)	Not applicable	

Table 4.11. Drugs for Parasitic Infections,[1] continued

Disease	Drug	Adult Dosage	Pediatric Dosage	Links to CDC Web Site[2] and professional society guidelines
Chloroquine-resistant (see sections above for regions with chloroquine-resistant *P. falciparum* and *P. vivax*)				
	Quinine sulfate[49]	Quinine sulfate: 542 mg base (=650 mg salt),[50] orally, 3 times/day for 3 or 7 days[50]	Not applicable	
	PLUS			
	Clindamycin	Clindamycin: 20 mg base/kg/day, orally, divided 3 times/day for 7 days		
	OR			
	Artemether-lumefantrine	1 tablet = 20 mg artemether and 120 mg lumefantrine. For 2nd or 3rd trimester of pregnancy and, if no other options or benefits outweigh risks, 1st trimester. A 3-day treatment schedule with a total of 6 oral doses (4 tablets per dose) is recommended; dose 1 followed by dose 2 8 hours later, then 1 dose twice daily for the following 2 days.	Not applicable	

Table 4.11. Drugs for Parasitic Infections,[1] continued

Disease	Drug	Adult Dosage	Pediatric Dosage	Links to CDC Web Site[2] and professional society guidelines
	OR			
	Mefloquine	684 mg base (=750 mg salt), orally, as initial dose, followed by 456 mg base (=500 mg salt), orally, given 6–12 h after initial dose Total dose= 1250 mg salt	Not applicable	
Severe malaria[59,60,61]	All regions	Artesunate, IV, 2.4 mg/kg/dose at hours 0, 12, and 24, and can be continued daily for up to a total of 7 days, if needed; see CDC recommendations for further management and switch to oral regimens based on parasitemia May begin treatment with an oral regimen while awaiting arrival of IV artesunate	Artesunate, IV, 2.4 mg/kg/dose at hours 0, 12, and 24, and can be continued daily for up to a total of 7 days, if needed; see CDC recommendations for further management and switch to oral regimens based on parasitemia May begin treatment with an oral regimen while awaiting arrival of IV artesunate	

Table 4.11. Drugs for Parasitic Infections,[1] continued

Disease	Drug	Adult Dosage	Pediatric Dosage	Links to CDC Web Site[2] and professional society guidelines
Microsporidiosis				
Ocular				
Encephalitozoon hellem, E cuniculi, Vittaforma [Nosema] corneae	Fumagillin[62]	Fumagillin in saline equivalent to fumagillin 70 µg/mL eye drops 2 drops every 2 h for 4 days, then 2 drops 4 times per day		www.cdc.gov/dpdx/ microsporidiosis/index.html https://aidsinfo.nih.gov/ guidelines/html/4/adult- and-adolescent-opportunistic- infection/324/microsporidia
	PLUS for management of systemic infection:			
	Albendazole[10]	400 mg, orally, twice a day (take with food)	15 mg/kg/day, orally, divided 2 times/day (max 400 mg/dose; take with food)	

Table 4.11. Drugs for Parasitic Infections,[1] continued

Disease	Drug	Adult Dosage	Pediatric Dosage	Links to CDC Web Site[2] and professional society guidelines
Intestinal				
E bieneusi	Fumagillin[63]	20 mg, orally, 3 times/day for 14 days		
E intestinalis	Albendazole[10]	400 mg, orally, on empty stomach,[64] twice a day for 21 days	15 mg/kg/day orally, on empty stomach,[64] in 2 doses (max 400 mg/dose)	
Disseminated[65]				
E hellem, E cuniculi, E intestinalis, Pleistophora species, Trachipleistophora species, and Anncaliia [Brachiola] vesicularum	Albendazole[10]	Immunocompromised: 400 mg, orally, twice per day for 14 to 28 days (take with food). Continue treatment until CD4+ T-lymphocyte count >200 cells/µL for >6 mo after initiation of antiretroviral therapy

Immunocompetent: 400 mg, orally, twice a day for 7 to 14 days (take with food) | 15 mg/kg/day (max 400 mg/dose), orally, divided 2 times/day (take with food) | |

Table 4.11. Drugs for Parasitic Infections,[1] continued

Disease	Drug	Adult Dosage	Pediatric Dosage	Links to CDC Web Site[2] and professional society guidelines
Neurocysticercosis (*T solium*)[66]	Albendazole[10]	≥60 kg: 400 mg, orally, 2 times/day for 10–14 days (take with food) <60 kg: 15 mg/kg/day (max 1200 mg/day), orally, divided 2 times/day for 10–14 days (take with food)	15 mg/kg/day (max 1200 mg/day), orally, in 2 divided doses for 8–30 days (take with food)	**www.cdc.gov/parasites/ cysticercosis/health_professionals/ index.html** ASTMH/IDSA Guidelines: **www.idsociety.org/practice-guideline/neurocysticercosis/**
	PLUS (when > 2 intraparenchymal lesions)			
	Praziquantel[22]	50 mg/kg/day, orally, for 10–14 days		
Onchocerciasis (*Onchocerca volvulus*; River Blindness)[67]	To kill microflariae: Ivermectin[12]	150 µg/kg, orally, in 1 dose every 6–12 mo until asymptomatic		**www.cdc.gov/parasites/ onchocerciasis/health_professionals/index.html**
	To kill microfilariae: Moxidectin[68]	8 mg, orally, once (≥12 years)		
	To kill macrofilariae: Doxycycline[69]	100–200 mg, orally, daily, for 6 wk		
Opisthorchis Infection (Southeast Asian liver fluke)	Praziquantel[22]	75 mg/kg/day, orally, divided 3 times/day for 2 days (take with liquids during meals)	75 mg/kg/day, orally, divided 3 times/day for 2 days	**www.cdc.gov/parasites/ opisthorchis/health_professionals/ index.html**
	OR			
	Albendazole[10]	10 mg/kg/day, orally, for 7 days (take with food)		
Paragonimiasis (lung fluke)	Praziquantel[22]	75 mg/kg/day, orally, divided into 3 doses, for 2 days	75 mg/kg/day, orally, divided into 3 doses, for 2 days	**www.cdc.gov/parasites/ paragonimus/health_professionals/index.html**
	OR			
	Triclabendazole[32]	10 mg/kg, orally, once or twice		

Table 4.11. Drugs for Parasitic Infections,[1] continued

Disease	Drug	Adult Dosage	Pediatric Dosage	Links to CDC Web Site[2] and professional society guidelines
Scabies (Mite Infestation)	Permethrin cream 5%	Topically, twice, at least 7 days apart (≥2 months)		www.cdc.gov/parasites/scabies/ health_professionals/meds.html
	OR			
	Crotamiton lotion 10% and Crotamiton cream 10%	Topically, overnight, on days 1, 2, 3, and 8 (not FDA-approved for use in children)		
	OR			
	Sulfur (5%–10%) ointment	Apply overnight for 3 consecutive days		
	OR			
	Ivermectin[12]	200 µg/kg, orally, twice, at least 7 days apart (take with food)		
Schistosomiasis (Bilharzia)	For *Schistosoma mansoni, S haematobium, S intercalatum:*			www.cdc.gov/parasites/ schistosomiasis/health_ professionals/index.html
	Praziquantel[22]	40 mg/kg/day, orally, in 2 divided doses for 1 day		
	For *S japonicum, S mekongi:*			
	Praziquantel[22]	60 mg/kg/day, orally, in 3 divided doses for 1 day		

Table 4.11. Drugs for Parasitic Infections,[1] continued

Disease	Drug	Adult Dosage	Pediatric Dosage	Links to CDC Web Site[2] and professional society guidelines
Strongyloidiasis (*Strongyloides stercoralis*)	Ivermectin[12]	200 µg/kg, orally, daily for 1–2 days; The veterinary subcutaneous formulation of ivermectin has been used in patients who are severely ill with hyperinfection and are unable to take or reliably absorb oral medications. The subcutaneous formulation may be used under a single-patient IND protocol request to the FDA.		www.cdc.gov/parasites/ strongyloides/health_ professionals/index.html
	OR			
	Albendazole[10]	400 mg, orally, 2 times/day for 7 days (take with food)		
Taeniasis [*Taenia saginata* (beef tapeworm), *Taenia solium* (pork tapeworm), and *Taenia asiatica* (Asian tapeworm)]	Praziquantel[22]	5–10 mg/kg, orally, once		www.cdc.gov/parasites/taeniasis/ health_professionals/index.html
	OR			
	Niclosamide[28]	2 g, orally, once	50 mg/kg (max 2 g), orally, once	
Toxocariasis (Ocular Larva Migrans, Visceral Larva Migrans)	Albendazole[10]	400 mg, orally, 2 times/day for 5 days (take with food)		www.cdc.gov/parasites/ toxocariasis/health_professionals/ index.html
	OR			
	Mebendazole[11]	100–200 mg, orally, 2 times/day for 5 days		

Table 4.11. Drugs for Parasitic Infections,[1] continued

Disease	Drug	Adult Dosage	Pediatric Dosage	Links to CDC Web Site[2] and professional society guidelines
Toxoplasmosis (*Toxoplasma gondii*)[70]	See Tables in *Toxoplasma gondii* Infections (p 767)			www.cdc.gov/parasites/ toxoplasmosis/health_ professionals/index.html
Trichinellosis (trichinosis; *Trichinella* species)[71]	Albendazole[10]	400 mg, orally, twice daily for 8 to 14 days (take with food)		www.cdc.gov/parasites/ trichinellosis/health_ professionals/index.html
	OR			
	Mebendazole[11]	200–400 mg, orally, 3 times daily for 3 days; then 400–500 mg, orally, 3 times daily for 10 days		
Trichuriasis (whipworm infection; *Trichuris trichiura*)	Albendazole[10]	400 mg, orally, for 3 days		www.cdc.gov/parasites/ whipworm/health_professionals/ index.html
	OR			
	Mebendazole[11]	100 mg, orally, twice daily for 3 days		
	OR			
	Ivermectin[12]	200 μg/kg/day, orally, for 3 days		

CDC indicates Centers for Disease Control and Prevention; IV, intravenous; CNS, central nervous system; IM, intramuscular; FDA, US Food and Drug Administration.

[1] The contents of this table are provided to assist in decision making for patient management, but are not a substitute for clinical judgment or expert consultation. The table may not address drug toxicities, drug-drug interactions and issues pertinent to some special populations (eg, patients with HIV/AIDS). Recommendations in the table may not represent all potential treatment or dosage options.

[2] See CDC website for additional information on each disease and the treatment thereof. Not all recommended therapies and dosages included in this table match the recommendations on the pathogen-specific CDC web pages. Inclusion of the links to the CDC website does not suggest endorsement of the content of this table by CDC.

[3] Pentamidine is also effective against *T b rhodesiense* in the hemolymphatic stage, but suramin may have higher efficacy. Suramin is not approved by the FDA but is available through the CDC Drug Service under an investigational new drug (IND) protocol. Questions should be directed to Parasitic Diseases Inquiries (404-718-4745; e-mail **parasites@cdc.gov**).

[4] A suramin test dose of 100 mg should be given before the first dose, and the patient should be monitored for hemodynamic stability.

[5] A suramin test dose of 2 mg/kg (max 100 mg) should be given before the first dose, and the patient should be monitored for hemodynamic stability.

[6] Corticosteroids have been used to prevent melarsoprol encephalopathy (1 mg/kg/day prednisolone, up to 40 mg/day) beginning one to two days before therapy and continuing until therapy is completed). Melarsoprol is not approved by the FDA but is available through the CDC Drug Service under an IND protocol. Questions should be directed to Parasitic Diseases Inquiries (404-718-4745; e-mail **parasites@cdc.gov**).

[7] Suramin also is effective against *T b gambiense* in the hemolymphatic stage but should be used only in patients in whom onchocerciasis has been excluded. Suramin is not approved by the FDA but is available through the CDC Drug Service under an IND protocol. Questions should be directed to Parasitic Diseases Inquiries (404-718-4745; e-mail **parasites@cdc.gov**).

[8] Eflornithine is available through the CDC Drug Service; questions should be directed to Parasitic Diseases Inquiries (404-718-4745; e-mail **parasites@cdc.gov**). Nifurtimox is not FDA approved, nor is this use covered by CDC's IND protocol for nifurtimox, which solely covers treatment of Chagas disease; permission for other uses would need to be obtained.

[9] The 2 drugs used to treat infection with *Trypanosoma cruzi* are benznidazole and nifurtimox. Benznidazole was approved in 2017 by the US Food and Drug Administration (FDA) for use in children 2–12 years of age for the treatment of Chagas disease. Nifurtimox was approved in 2020 by the FDA for use in children from birth to less than 18 years of age and weighing at least 2.5 kg. For both drugs, adverse effects are common and are more frequent and more severe with increasing age.

[10] Safety of albendazole in children younger than 6 years is not certain. Studies of the use of albendazole in children as young as 1 year suggest that its use is safe. Albendazole should be taken with food.

[11] Cases of mebendazole in children has not been established. There are limited data in children 2 years and younger.

[12] Safety of ivermectin in treating pregnant women and children who weigh less than 15 kg has not been established. Ivermectin should be taken on an empty stomach with water.

[13] Safety of pyrantel pamoate in children has not been established. According to WHO guidance on preventive chemotherapy, pyrantel may be used in children age 1 year and older during mass treatment programs without diagnosis.

[14] The combination of clindamycin plus quinine, or the combination of IV azithromycin plus oral atovaquone, are options for treatment of babesiosis in patients who are severely ill.

[15] Cases of cholestatic hepatitis, elevated liver enzymes, and fatal liver failure have been reported in patients treated with atovaquone.

[16] Some immunocompromised adults with babesiosis have been treated with doses of azithromycin in the range of 600–1000 mg/day, in combination with atovaquone (750 mg twice per day).

[17] Quinine treatment is associated with thrombocytopenia, QT prolongation, ventricular arrhythmias, hypoglycemia and serious hypersensitivity reactions. Neuromuscular blocking agents should be avoided in patients receiving quinine sulfate. Use with caution in patients with atrial fibrillation or atrial flutter

[18] Tetracycline should be taken 1 hour before or 2 hours after meals containing dairy.

[19] Iodoquinol should be taken after meals.

[20] In cases in which suspicion of exposure is high, immediate treatment with albendazole (25–50 mg/kg/day, orally, for 10–20 days) may be appropriate. Treatment is successful when administered soon after exposure to abort the migration of larvae. Treatment should be initiated as soon as possible after ingestion of infectious material, ideally within 3 days. For clinical baylisascariasis, treatment with albendazole with concurrent corticosteroids to help reduce the inflammatory reaction is indicated to attempt to control the disease.

[21] Clinical significance of *Blastocystis* species is controversial.

[22] Praziquantel is not approved for treatment of children younger than 4 years, but this drug has been used successfully to treat cases of *D caninum* infection in children as young as 6 months. Take with water during meals.

[23] There are no drug regimens with proven efficacy for the treatment of cryptosporidiosis in immunosuppressed patients.

[24]HIV-infected patients may need longer courses of therapy for cyclosporiasis.

[25]Expert consultation for treatment of cystoisosporiasis is recommended if the patient is immunosuppressed.

[26]Asymptomatic infections generally do not require treatment; when *D fragilis* is the sole organism found in a patient with abdominal pain or diarrhea for a week or more treatment is appropriate.

[27]Tetracycline or doxycycline also have been used for treatment.

[28]Niclosamide is unavailable in the United States. Chew thoroughly or crush and mix with a small amount of water.

[29]See text in Other Tapeworm Infections (Including Hydatid Disease), p 747. Management depends on type and location of cysts, may involve surgery, and collaboration with specialists with experience treating this infection is advised. Albendazole is not appropriate for all forms of infection.

[30]Mild-to-moderate intestinal disease as well as severe intestinal and extraintestinal disease require different treatment regimens.

[31]Diloxanide furoate is not commercially available in the United States.

[32]Triclabendazole is approved by the FDA for treatment of fascioliasis in children 6 years of age and older. Safety and effectiveness of triclabendazole in children under age 6 have not been established.

[33]Alternative treatments for giardiasis include albendazole, mebendazole, paromomycin, quinacrine, and furazolidone.

[34]Sodium stibogluconate is not approved by the FDA but is available through the CDC Drug Service under an IND protocol; questions should be directed to Parasitic Diseases Inquiries (404-718-4745; e-mail **parasites@cdc.gov**). Only selected antileishmanial agents and regimens are listed in the table. Expert consultation about these and other potential treatment options for leishmaniasis is encouraged. For some cases of cutaneous leishmaniasis, no therapy may be needed or local (vs systemic) therapy may suffice or other systemic treatments may be considered. Miltefosine (IMPAVIDO) was approved in March 2014 by the FDA—for treatment of visceral leishmaniasis caused by *L donovani*; mucosal leishmaniasis caused by *L (Viannia) braziliensis*; and cutaneous leishmaniasis caused by *L (V) braziliensis, L (V) guyanensis,* and *L (V) panamensis* (ie, some New World cutaneous leishmaniasis species but no Old World cutaneous leishmaniasis species)—for patients who are at least 12 years of age, weigh at least 30 kg, and are not pregnant or breastfeeding during or for 5 months after the treatment course.

[35]Pediculicides should not be used for infestations of the eyelashes. Such infestations are treated with petrolatum ointment applied 2 to 4 times/day for 10 days. For pubic lice, treat with 1% permethrin, pyrethrins with piperonyl butoxide, or ivermectin.

[36]Permethrin and pyrethrin are pediculicidal; retreatment in 9–10 days is needed to eradicate the infestation. Some lice are resistant to pyrethrins and permethrin. Pyrethrins with piperonyl butoxide are recommended for use in children ≥2 years of age; permethrin for children ≥2 months of age.

[37]Ivermectin is not ovicidal, but lice that hatch from treated eggs die within 48 hours after hatching. Recommended for use in children ≥6 months of age.

[38]Spinosad causes neuronal excitation in insects leading to paralysis and death. The formulation also includes benzyl alcohol, which is pediculicidal. Two applications 7 days apart are needed. Recommended for children ≥6 months of age.

[39]Benzyl alcohol prevents lice from closing their respiratory spiracles and the lotion vehicle then obstructs their airway causing them to asphyxiate. It is not ovicidal. Two applications 9–10 days apart are needed. Recommended for use in children ≥6 months of age. Resistance, which is a problem with other drugs, is unlikely to develop.

[40]Malathion is both ovicidal and pediculicidal; 2 applications 7-9 days apart are generally necessary to kill all lice and nits. Recommended for children ≥6 years of age, and contraindicated in children <24 months of age.

[41]Abametapir is ovicidal. Contains benzyl alcohol. Use is not recommended in pediatric patients under 6 months of age because of the potential for increased systemic absorption.

[42]Ivermectin is pediculicidal but not ovicidal; more than 1 dose is generally necessary to eradicate the infestation. The number of doses and the interval between doses have not been established; animal studies have shown adverse effects on the fetus. A single oral dose of 200 μg/kg, repeated in 9–10 days, has been shown to be effective against head lice. Most recently, a single oral dose of 400 μg/kg, repeated in 9–10 days, has been shown to be more effective than 0.5% malathion lotion.

[43]Diethylcarbamazine (DEC) is not approved by the FDA but is available through the CDC Drug Service under an IND protocol; questions should be directed to Parasitic Diseases Inquiries (404-718-4745; e-mail **parasites@cdc.gov**). DEC is contraindicated in patients who may also have onchocerciasis. Before DEC therapy for lymphatic filariasis or loiasis, onchocerciasis should be excluded in all patients with a consistent exposure history because of the possibility of severe exacerbations of skin and eye involvement (Mazzotti reaction). People coinfected with *L loa* and *O volvulus* should not be treated with DEC until the onchocerciasis is treated; their onchocerciasis should not be treated with ivermectin if it is unsafe to treat their loiasis.

[44]Apheresis should be performed at an institution with experience in using this therapeutic modality for loiasis.

[45]Doxycycline is not standard treatment for lymphatic filariasis but some studies have shown adult-worm killing with doxycycline therapy (200 mg/day for 4–6 weeks).

[46] If a person develops malaria despite taking chemoprophylaxis, that particular medicine should not be used as a part of his or her treatment regimen. Use one of the other options instead.

[47] There are 4 options available for treatment of uncomplicated malaria caused by chloroquine-resistant *P falciparum*. The first 3 options are equally recommended. Because of a higher rate of severe neuropsychiatric reactions seen at treatment doses, mefloquine is not recommended unless the other options cannot be used. Because there are more data on the efficacy of quinine in combination with doxycycline or tetracycline, these treatment combinations generally are preferred to quinine in combination with clindamycin.

[48] Atovaquone-proguanil or artemether-lumefantrine should be taken with food or whole milk. If patient vomits within 30 minutes of taking a dose, the dose should be repeated. Adult tablet = 250 mg atovaquone/100 mg proguanil. Pediatric tablet = 62.5 mg atovaquone/25 mg proguanil.

[49] US-manufactured quinine sulfate capsule is in a 324-mg dosage; therefore, 2 capsules should be sufficient for adult dosing. Pediatric dosing may be difficult because of unavailability of noncapsule forms of quinine.

[50] For infections acquired in Southeast Asia, quinine treatment should continue for 7 days. For infections acquired elsewhere, quinine treatment should continue for 3 days.

[51] Tetracycline is not indicated for use in children younger than 8 years. Doxycycline can be administered for short durations (ie, 21 days or less) without regard to the patient's age (see Tetracyclines, p 866). For children younger than 8 years and > 5 kg with chloroquine-resistant *P falciparum*, atovaquone-proguanil and artemether-lumefantrine are recommended treatment options; mefloquine can be considered if no other options are available. For children younger than 8 years with chloroquine-resistant *P vivax*, mefloquine, or in those > 5 kg, atovaquone-proguanil or artemether-lumefantrine are treatment options.

[52] Treatment with mefloquine is not recommended in people who have acquired infections from Southeast Asia because of drug resistance.

[53] When treating chloroquine-sensitive infections, chloroquine and hydroxychloroquine are recommended options. Regimens used to treat chloroquine-resistant infections may also be used if available, more convenient, or preferred.

[54] Primaquine and tafenoquine are used to eradicate any hypnozoites that may remain dormant in the liver and, thus, prevent relapses in *P vivax* and *P ovale* infections. Because both drugs can cause hemolytic anemia in glucose-6-phosphate dehydrogenase (G6PD)-deficient people, G6PD screening must occur prior to starting treatment with primaquine or tafenoquine. For people with borderline G6PD deficiency or as an alternate to the above regimen, primaquine, 45 mg, orally, once per week for 8 weeks may be given; consultation with an expert in infectious disease and/or tropical medicine is advised if this alternative regimen is considered in G6PD-deficient people. Primaquine and tafenoquine must not be used during pregnancy.

[55] Three options are available for treatment of uncomplicated malaria caused by chloroquine-resistant *P vivax*. High treatment failure rates attributable to chloroquine-resistant *P vivax* have been well documented in Papua New Guinea and Indonesia. Rare case reports of chloroquine-resistant *P vivax* also have been documented in Burma (Myanmar), India, and Central and South America. People acquiring *P vivax* infections outside of Papua New Guinea or Indonesia should be started on chloroquine. If the patient does not respond, treatment should be changed to a chloroquine-resistant *P vivax* regimen and the CDC should be notified (Malaria Hotline number listed previously). For treatment of chloroquine-resistant *P vivax* infection, treatment with doxycycline or tetracycline generally

[56] For pregnant women diagnosed with uncomplicated malaria caused by chloroquine-resistant *P falciparum* or chloroquine-resistant *P vivax* infection (as recommended for nonpregnant adults) if other treatment options are not available or are not being tolerated, is not indicated. Doxycycline or tetracycline may be used in combination with quinine (as recommended for nonpregnant adults) if other treatment options are not available or are not being tolerated, and the benefit is judged to outweigh the risks.

[57] Atovaquone-proguanil generally is not recommended during pregnancy; artemether-lumefantrine is recommended in the second and third trimester and may be used in the first trimester when benefits outweigh risks

[58] For *P vivax* and *P ovale* infections, primaquine phosphate or tafenoquine for radical treatment of hypnozoites should not be given during pregnancy. Pregnant patients with *P vivax* and *P ovale* infections should be maintained on chloroquine prophylaxis for the duration of their pregnancy. The chemoprophylactic dose of chloroquine phosphate is 300 mg base (=500 mg salt), orally, once per week.

After delivery, these patients may be treated with primaquine or tafenoquine if they and their infants do not have G6PD deficiency.

[59] People with a positive blood smear OR history of recent possible exposure and no other recognized pathologic abnormality who have 1 or more of the following clinical criteria (impaired consciousness/coma, severe normocytic anemia, renal failure, pulmonary edema, acute respiratory distress syndrome, circulatory shock, disseminated intravascular coagulation, spontaneous bleeding, acidosis, hemoglobinuria, jaundice, repeated generalized convulsions, and/or parasitemia of >5%) are considered to have manifestations of more severe disease. Severe malaria is most often caused by *P falciparum*.

[60] Patients with a diagnosis of severe malaria should be treated aggressively with parenteral antimalarial therapy. IV artesunate is commercially available beginning in March 2021. If commercial IV artesunate is not available within 24 hours, clinicians can contact the CDC to acquire IV artesunate under an IND protocol. The CDC Malaria Hotline (770-488-7788) is available Monday–Friday, 9am–5pm, Eastern time. Outside these hours, providers should call 770-488-7100 and ask to speak with a CDC malaria expert.

[61] Pregnant women diagnosed with severe malaria should be treated aggressively with parenteral antimalarial therapy.

[62] An investigational agent (non–FDA approved) in the United States. Fumagillin is not FDA approved for any human indications; however fumagillin (Flisint) can be obtained through single patient investigational new drug application to the Agency after contacting Sanofi-Aventis (med.info@sanofi.com). For lesions attributable to *V corneae*, topical therapy is generally not effective and kerato-plasty may be required (RM Davis, Font RL, Keisler MS, Shadduck JA. Corneal microsporidiosis. A case report including ultrastructural observations. *Ophthalmology*. 1990;97[7]:953-957). Data are insufficient to make recommendations on the use of fumagillin in children (see "Guidelines for the Prevention and Treatment of Opportunistic Infection in HIV-Exposed and HIV-Infected Children," https://aidsinfo.nih.gov/guidelines/html/5/pediatric-opportunistic-infection/434/whats-new

[63] For gastrointestinal infections caused by *Enterocytozoon bieneusi*, fumagillin, 20 mg, orally 3 times daily, is the only drug with proven efficacy. Its use is associated with severe thrombocytopenia in 30% to 50% of patients, which is reversible on discontinuation of treatment. The drug is not currently available in the United States.

[64] For intestinal infection without systemic involvement, albendazole should be taken on an empty stomach (for systemic infections it should be taken with a fatty meal).

[65] There is no established treatment for *Pleistophora*. For disseminated disease attributable to *Trachipleistophora* or *Anncaliia*, itraconazole, 400 mg, orally, once per day, plus albendazole may also be tried.

[66] Although not all symptomatic patients with a single viable cyst of neurocysticercosis within brain parenchyma require antiparasitic medication, controlled studies demonstrate that clinical resolution and seizure recurrence rates are improved with albendazole. Two studies have demonstrated that in those with more than 2 viable intraparenchymal lesions, the response rate was better when albenda-zole was coadministered with praziquantel and corticosteroids. When a single agent is used, albendazole is preferred over praziquantel because it has fewer drug-drug interactions with anticonvulsants and steroids. Longer courses may be needed for subarachnoid disease. Anti-inflammatory therapy is recommended when anti-parasitic treatment is used though the optimal dose has not been estab-lished. Regimens such as déxamethasone 6 mg/kg/day for 10 days, beginning before starting anti-parasitic therapy; and prednisone 1–1.5 mg/kg/day during therapy have been used. Consultation with a specialist familiar with treatment of neurocysticercosis is advised.

[67] People coinfected with *O volvulus* and *L loa* should not be treated with diethylcarbamazine (DEC) until the onchocerciasis is treated; their onchocerciasis should not be treated with ivermectin if it is unsafe to treat their loiasis. Patients should only be treated with doxycycline if they no longer live in areas with endemic infection unless there is a contraindication for ivermectin.

[68] Moxidectin approved in 2018 for children 12 years of age and older; not yet available commercially in the US. Screening for loiasis recommended before use. Safety and efficacy of repeat doses have not been studied. Safety and efficacy in children under age 12 have not been established.

[69] Doxycycline is not standard therapy, but several studies support its use and safety. Treatment with a single oral dose of ivermectin (150 μg/kg) should be given 1 week before treatment with doxycycline to provide symptom relief to the patient. If the patient cannot tolerate the dosage of 200 mg, orally, daily of doxycycline, 100 mg, orally, daily is sufficient to sterilize female *Onchocerca organisms*. The safety of ivermectin in children weighing less than 15 kg and in pregnant women has not been established.

[70] For treatment and chronic suppression of toxoplasmosis in human immunodeficiency virus (HIV) infected children, see Guidelines for the Prevention and Treatment of Opportunistic Infections Among HIV-Exposed and HIV-Infected Children, at **https://aidsinfo.nih.gov/guidelines/html/5/pediatric-opportunistic-infection/434/whats-new**

[71] In addition to antiparasitic medication, treatment with corticosteroids sometimes is required in more severe cases of trichinellosis.

Table 4.12. Systems-based Treatment Table

SYSTEMS-BASED TREATMENT TABLE

System	Condition	Common Pathogens	Empiric Antibiotic Therapy	Antibiotic Duration	Notes	Key Resources
Skin and Soft Tissue Infections	Cellulitis	**Streptococcus pyogenes** (nonpurulent) **Staphylococcus aureus** (purulent)	Mild-moderate: Cefazolin OR Oxacillin/nafcillin OR Cephalexin Consider MRSA based on local prevalence (Allergy: clindamycin) Severe: Vancomycin OR Linezolid Necrotizing fasciitis: Surgical débridement ß-lactam *plus* Clindamycin (+/- Vancomycin)	5–7 days Tailor duration based on resolution of signs and symptoms	For bite wounds, see chapter p 169 Necrotizing fasciitis may require gram-negative or anaerobic coverage in the correct clinical scenario	*Bacteroides, Prevotella,* and Other Anaerobic Gram-Negative Bacilli Infections, p 224 *Staphylococcus aureus,* p 678 Group A Streptococcal Infections, p 694 Stevens et al[1]

Table 4.12. Systems-based Treatment Table, continued

System	Condition	Common Pathogens	Empiric Antibiotic Therapy	Antibiotic Duration	Notes	Key Resources
Skin and Soft Tissue Infections	Abscess	*S aureus*	Surgical drainage Mild-moderate: Cefazolin/cephalexin OR TMP/SMX OR Clindamycin OR Doxycycline Consider MRSA based on local prevalence Severe: Vancomycin OR Linezolid OR Ceftaroline OR Daptomycin	5–7 days Tailor duration based on resolution of signs and symptoms	Conversion to oral antibiotic therapy after transient[a] *S aureus* bacteremia with source control is appropriate but might warrant more prolonged therapy Surgical drainage alone may be adequate for small, completely drained abscesses	*Staphylococcus aureus*, p 678 Stevens et al[1]

Table 4.12. Systems-based Treatment Table, continued

System	Condition	Common Pathogens	Empiric Antibiotic Therapy	Antibiotic Duration	Notes	Key Resources
Skin and Soft Tissue Infections	Lymphadenitis	**Acute/unilateral:** **S pyogenes** **S aureus** **Subacute/chronic:** *Bartonella* species NTM	For acute/unilateral lymphadenitis: Consider surgical drainage Cefazolin/Cephalexin (Allergy: Clindamycin) Consider MRSA based on local prevalence	5–7 days Tailor duration based on resolution of signs and symptoms	For management of NTM or *Bartonella* infection, please see those chapters (p 814 and p 226) Bacterial adenitis is typically unilateral; bilateral disease is typically viral in etiology	*Bartonella henselae* (Cat-Scratch Disease), p 226 *Staphylococcus aureus*, p 678 Group A Streptococcal Infections, p 694 Nontuberculous Mycobacteria, p 814
Ear, Nose, and Throat/ Ophthalmologic	Mastoiditis	***Streptococcus pneumoniae*** **S pyogenes** **S aureus** *Haemophilus influenzae* **Also consider for chronic:** Microaerophilic streptococci *Fusobacterium* *Pseudomonas aeruginosa*	Consider surgical drainage/excision Ampicillin-sulbactam OR Ceftriaxone (Allergy: Clindamycin) If follows chronic AOM: Cefepime OR Levofloxacin Consider MRSA based on local prevalence	2–4 wk depending on adequate débridement, intracranial extension, extent of osteomyelitis, associated thrombosis	Transition to oral with clinical improvement Ampicillin-sulbactam may not be optimal for intracranial infections	*Haemophilus influenzae* Infections, p 345 *Fusobacterium* Infections, p 333 *Pseudomonas aeruginosa* Infections, p 614 *Staphylococcus aureus*, p 678 Group A Streptococcal Infections, p 694 Non-Group A or B Streptococcal and Enterococcal Infections, p 713 *Streptococcus pneumoniae* (Pneumococcal) Infections, p 717

Table 4.12. Systems-based Treatment Table, continued

System	Condition	Common Pathogens	Empiric Antibiotic Therapy	Antibiotic Duration	Notes	Key Resources
Ear, Nose, and Throat/ Ophthalmologic	Acute sinusitis	**S pneumoniae** *H influenzae* *Moraxella catarrhalis*	Amoxicillin OR Amoxicillin-clavulanate (Allergy: Clindamycin OR Levofloxacin)	5–7 days	Diagnosis of acute bacterial sinusitis requires the presence of one of the following criteria: (1) persistent nasal discharge or daytime cough without <u>evidence of clinical improvement</u> for ≥10 days; consider watchful waiting in this scenario (2) worsening or new onset of nasal discharge, daytime cough, or fever after initial improvement (3) temperature ≥39°C with either purulent nasal discharge and/or facial pain for at least 3 consecutive days	*Haemophilus influenzae* Infections, p 345 *Moraxella catarrhalis* Infections, p 537 *Streptococcus pneumoniae* (Pneumococcal) Infections, p 717 Chow et al[2] Wald et al[3]

Table 4.12. Systems-based Treatment Table, continued

System	Condition	Common Pathogens	Empiric Antibiotic Therapy	Antibiotic Duration	Notes	Key Resources
Ear, Nose, and Throat/ Ophthalmologic	Acute otitis media	*S pneumoniae* *H influenzae* *M catarrhalis*	Amoxicillin OR Amoxicillin-clavulanate[b] (Allergy: Cefdinir OR Cefpodoxime OR Ceftriaxone for 1–3 days, OR Cefuroxime)	>6 y: 5 days 2–5 y: 7 days <2 y or severe symptoms: 10 days	Consider observation without antibiotics for 48–72 hours for children 24 months or older without severe symptoms; if symptoms persist or worsen, use same antibiotic recommendations as for those receiving immediate therapy Consider *S aureus* and *Pseudomonas* infection for chronic otitis media	*Haemophilus influenzae* Infections, p 345 *Moraxella catarrhalis* Infections, p 537 *Streptococcus pneumoniae* (Pneumococcal) Infections, p 717 Lieberthal et al[4]

Table 4.12. Systems-based Treatment Table, continued

System	Condition	Common Pathogens	Empiric Antibiotic Therapy	Antibiotic Duration	Notes	Key Resources
Ear, Nose, and Throat/ Ophthalmologic	Streptococcal pharyngitis	*S pyogenes*	First line: Penicillin OR Amoxicillin (Allergy: Cephalexin OR Clindamycin OR Azithromycin)	10 days	Children with rhinorrhea, cough, hoarseness, or oral ulcers should not be tested or treated for GAS infection; testing also generally is not recommended for children <3 y	Group A Streptococcal Infections, p 694 Shulman et al[5]
					Management of recurrent GAS pharyngitis and pharyngeal carriers is detailed in Group A Streptococcal Infections (p 694)	
					Tetracyclines, TMP-SMX, and fluoroquinolones should not be used for treating GAS pharyngitis.	
					Return to school after ≥12 h	

Table 4.12. Systems-based Treatment Table, continued

System	Condition	Common Pathogens	Empiric Antibiotic Therapy	Antibiotic Duration	Notes	Key Resources
Ear, Nose, and Throat/ Ophthalmologic	Retropharyngeal abscess	*S aureus* *S pyogenes* *Anaerobes* *Streptococcus anginosus* *H influenzae* (often polymicrobial)	Mild-moderate: Ampicillin/sulbactam OR Clindamycin Severe: Ampicillin/sulbactam PLUS EITHER Vancomycin OR Linezolid	14 days	Longer duration of therapy may be required for complex infections with insufficient source control	
	Periorbital cellulitis (ie, non-sinus origin)	*S pyogenes* *S aureus*	Mild-moderate: Cefazolin OR Cephalexin (Allergy: Clindamycin) Severe: Vancomycin OR Linezolid	5–7 days	Switch to oral with 24 hours improvement in fever, swelling, and erythema Consider empiric MRSA coverage if high local MRSA rates	
	Orbital cellulitis	*S aureus* *S pneumoniae* *Anaerobes* *S anginosus* *H influenzae* *M catarrhalis* *S pyogenes*	Surgical drainage (if abscess): Ampicillin/ sulbactam (Allergy: Clindamycin) Severe: Add Vancomycin OR Linezolid	10–14 days May extend to 3–4 wk with extensive bone involvement	May need longer duration if insufficient source control Consider empiric MRSA coverage if high local MRSA rates	

Table 4.12. Systems-based Treatment Table, continued

System	Condition	Common Pathogens	Empiric Antibiotic Therapy	Antibiotic Duration	Notes	Key Resources
Respiratory	Community-acquired pneumonia (CAP)	*S pneumoniae* *Mycoplasma pneumoniae*	Amoxicillin OR Ampicillin OR Penicillin for fully immunized patients in regions without high prevalence of PCN-resistant pneumococcus	5 days from uncomplicated CAP improving during that time	Respiratory viruses cause the majority of CAP, especially in young children; thus, antibiotic therapy may not be indicated for all patients	Bradley et al[6]
		S pyogenes *S aureus* *H influenzae* *M catarrhalis*	(Allergy: Clindamycin OR Levofloxacin)	May extend duration when complicated by empyema, necrotizing pneumonia, or pulmonary abscess	Early switch to oral route encouraged when tolerated	
			Cefriaxone for hospitalized patients in regions with high levels PCN-resistant pneumococcus		Transient *S pneumoniae* bacteremia in otherwise uncomplicated pneumonia does not warrant prolonged or IV antibiotic therapy	
			Add macrolide if atypical pathogen (eg, *Mycoplasma* or *Chlamydia* species) suspected		Consider *S aureus* superinfection in patients with influenza	
			Add Vancomycin OR Clindamycin OR Linezolid if MRSA suspected			

Table 4.12. Systems-based Treatment Table, continued

System	Condition	Common Pathogens	Empiric Antibiotic Therapy	Antibiotic Duration	Notes	Key Resources
Genitourinary	UTI - pyelonephritis	*Escherichia coli* Klebsiella species Proteus species Enterobacter species Citrobacter species Enterococcus species Staphylococcus saprophyticus	Cephalexin OR TMP-SMX OR Ampicillin PLUS Gentamicin OR Ceftriaxone OR Ciprofloxacin	7–10 days 3–5 days (simple cystitis in adolescents) Longer durations may be required for complicated cases such as renal abscess without drainage	Drug selection should be based on local antibiogram or patient's prior urine isolates Initial short course of IV therapy (2–4 days) is as effective as longer courses of IV therapy Avoid nitrofurantoin for upper urinary tract infection or bacteremia	Roberts et al[7] Gupta et al[8]
Bone/Joint	Osteomyelitis (acute, hematogenous)	*S aureus* S pyogenes Kingella kingae	Cefazolin OR Oxacillin OR Nafcillin OR Clindamycin Severe infection: Vancomycin PLUS EITHER Cefazolin OR Oxacillin OR Nafcillin	3–4 wk Chronic osteomyelitis typically requires more prolonged antibiotic treatment and may require consideration of alternate antibiotic choice	*Kingella* infection not affected by clindamycin and not reliably susceptible to oxacillin/nafcillin Early switch to oral route encouraged with clinical improvement, even for patients with transient bacteremia	Woods et al[9]

Table 4.12. Systems-based Treatment Table, continued

System	Condition	Common Pathogens	Empiric Antibiotic Therapy	Antibiotic Duration	Notes	Key Resources
Bone/Joint	Septic arthritis	**S aureus** S pyogenes K kingae	Cefazolin OR Oxacillin OR Nafcillin OR Clindamycin Severe infection: Vancomycin PLUS EITHER Cefazolin OR Oxacillin OR Nafcillin	2–3 wk	*Kingella* not affected by clindamycin and not reliably susceptible to oxacillin/nafcillin Early switch to oral route encouraged with clinical improvement, even for patients with transient bacteremia	Woods et al[9]
Intra-abdominal	Intra-abdominal infection	**E coli** **Anaerobes** Klebsiella species (often polymicrobial)	Surgical drainage Mild-moderate: Ceftriaxone PLUS Metronidazole Severe or hospital onset: Piperacillin-tazobactam OR Ciprofloxacin PLUS Metronidazole	4–7 days	May need longer duration if insufficient source control Mild-moderate infection includes complicated appendicitis with rupture, absent sepsis	Solomkin et al[10]

Table 4.12. Systems-based Treatment Table, continued

System	Condition	Common Pathogens	Empiric Antibiotic Therapy	Antibiotic Duration	Notes	Key Resources
Neonatal Fever (Term Neonates)	Suspected UTI	*E coli* *Enterococcus* species GBS	Ampicillin PLUS Gentamicin	These are empiric recommendations; specific choice and duration of antibiotic therapy should be guided by culture results		
	Unclear source	**GBS** *E coli* HSV	Neonates 0–7 days of age: Ampicillin PLUS Gentamicin Neonates 8–28 days of age: Ampicillin PLUS Gentamicin OR Ampicillin PLUS Cefotaxime (Ceftazidime or Cefepime if Cefotaxime not available)	These are empiric recommendations; specific choice and duration of antibiotic therapy should be guided by culture results	Consider adding empiric Acyclovir with surface, blood, and CSF HSV sampling for infants at increased risk of HSV, including the presence of skin vesicles, seizures, CSF pleocytosis with a negative Gram stain, leukopenia, hepatitis, thrombocytopenia, hypothermia, mucous membrane ulcers, or maternal history of genital HSV lesions or fever from 48 hours before to 48 hours after delivery. For further discussion of HSV, see Herpes Simplex (p 407).	

Table 4.12. Systems-based Treatment Table, continued

System	Condition	Common Pathogens	Empiric Antibiotic Therapy	Antibiotic Duration	Notes	Key Resources
Neonatal Fever (Term Neonates)	Suspected meningitis	**GBS** *E coli* HSV	Neonates 0–7 days of age: Ampicillin PLUS Gentamicin (some experts will add a third or fourth generation cephalosporin if the cerebrospinal fluid gram stain shows gram negative organisms) Neonates 8–28 days of age: Ampicillin PLUS Cefotaxime (Ceftazidime or Cefepime if Cefotaxime not available) (some experts will add an aminoglycoside if the cerebrospinal fluid Gram stain shows gram-negative organisms)	These are empiric recommendations; specific choice and duration of antibiotic therapy should be guided by culture results GBS: 14 days penicillin G *E coli:* 21 days of non aminoglycoside antibiotic to which isolate is susceptible	Some experts suggest repeat lumbar puncture to document CSF sterility Consider adding empiric acyclovir with surface, blood, and CSF HSV sampling for infants at increased risk of HSV, including the presence of skin vesicles, seizures, CSF pleocytosis with a negative Gram stain, leukopenia, hepatitis, thrombocytopenia, hypothermia, mucous membrane ulcers, or maternal history of genital HSV lesions or fever from 48 hours before to 48 hours after delivery. For further discussion of HSV, see Herpes Simplex (p 407).	AAP[11,12]

Table 4.12. Systems-based Treatment Table, continued

System	Condition	Common Pathogens	Empiric Antibiotic Therapy	Antibiotic Duration	Notes	Key Resources
Central Nervous System	Meningitis (non-neonates)	S pneumoniae N meningitidis H influenzae	Ceftriaxone PLUS Vancomycin	These are empiric recommendations; specific choice and duration of antibiotic therapy should be guided by culture and susceptibility results S pneumoniae: 10–14 days H influenzae: 7–10 days N meningitidis: 5–7 days	Longer courses are necessary for patients with parenchymal brain infection (cerebritis, rhombencephalitis, brain abscess) Dexamethasone is beneficial for treatment of infants and children with Hib meningitis to diminish the risk of hearing loss, if administered before or concurrently with the first dose of antimicrobial agent(s) For all children with bacterial meningitis presumed to be caused by S pneumoniae, vancomycin should be administered in addition to ceftriaxone because of the possibility of resistant S pneumoniae Consider adding acyclovir for patients with concurrent encephalitis	

AOM indicates acute otitis media; CAP, community-acquired pneumonia; CSF, cerebrospinal fluid; GAS, group A *Streptococcus*; GBS, group B *Streptococcus*; HSV, herpes simplex virus; IV, intravenous; MRSA, methicillin-resistant *Staphylococcus aureus*; NTM, nontuberculous mycobacteria; PCN, penicillin; TMP-SMX, trimethoprim-sulfamethoxazole; UTI, urinary tract infection.

Boldface indicates primary pathogen(s) targeted by empiric antibiotic therapy.

[a]Oral antibiotics may be considered for bacteremia if bacteremia clears within 72 hours of source control and initiation of effective antibiotic therapy.

[b]Amoxicillin treatment in last 30 days, concurrent purulent conjunctivitis, or history of recurrent AOM unresponsive to amoxicillin.

[1]Stevens DL, Bisno AL, Chambers HF, et al. Practice guidelines for the diagnosis and management of skin and soft tissue infections: 2014 update by the Infectious Diseases Society of America. *Clin Infect Dis.* 2014;59(2):e10–e52. DOI: **https://doi.org/10.1093/cid/ciu296**

[2]Chow AW, Benninger MS, Brook I, et al. IDSA clinical practice guideline for acute bacterial rhinosinusitis in children and adults. *Clin Infect Dis.* 2012;54(8):e72-e112. DOI: **https://doi.org/10.1093/cid/cis370**

[3]Wald ER, Applegate KE, Bordley C, et al. Clinical practice guideline for the diagnosis and management of acute bacterial sinusitis in children aged 1 to 18 years. *Pediatrics.* 2013;132(1):e262-e280. DOI: **https://doi.org/10.1542/peds.2013-1071**

[4]Lieberthal AS, Carroll AE, Chonmaitree T, et al. Clinical practice guideline: diagnosis and management of acute otitis media. *Pediatrics.* 2013;131(3):e964-e999. DOI: DOI: **https://doi.org/10.1542/peds.2013-3791**

[5]Shulman ST, Bisno AL, Clegg HW, et al. Clinical practice guideline for the diagnosis and management of group a streptococcal pharyngitis: 2012 update by the Infectious Diseases Society of America. *Clin Infect Dis.* 2012;55(10):e86-e102. DOI: **https://doi.org/10.1093/cid/cis629**

[6]Bradley JS, Byington CL, Shah SS, et al. The management of community-acquired pneumonia in infants and children older than 3 months of age: clinical practice guidelines by the Pediatric Infectious Diseases Society and the Infectious Diseases Society of America. *Clin Infect Dis.* 2011;53(7):e25–e76. DOI: **https://doi.org/10.1093/cid/cir531**

[7]Roberts KB; Subcommittee on Urinary Tract Infection, Steering Committee on Quality Improvement and Management. Urinary tract infection: clinical practice guideline for the diagnosis and management of the initial UTI in febrile infants and children 2 to 24 months. *Pediatrics.* 2011;128(3):595–610. DOI: **https://doi.org/10.1542/peds.2011-1330** (Reaffirmed December 2016)

[8]Gupta K, Hooton TM, Naber KG, et al. International Clinical Practice Guidelines for the Treatment of Acute Uncomplicated Cystitis and Pyelonephritis in Women: A 2010 Update by the Infectious Diseases Society of America and the European Society for Microbiology and Infectious Diseases. *Clin Infect Dis.* 2011;52(5):e103-e120. DOI: **https://doi.org/10.1093/cid/ciq257**

[9]Woods CR, Bradley JS, Chatterjee A, et al. Clinical practice guideline by the Pediatric Infectious Diseases Society (PIDS) and Infectious Diseases Society of America (IDSA): 2020 Guideline on diagnosis and management of acute hematogenous osteomyelitis in pediatrics. In development

[10]Solomkin JS, Mazuski JE, Bradley JS, et al. Diagnosis and Management of Complicated Intra-abdominal Infection in Adults and Children: Guidelines by the Surgical Infection Society and the Infectious Diseases Society of America. *Clin Infect Dis.* 2010;50(2):133-164. DOI: **https://doi.org/10.1086/649554**

[11]Puopolo KM, Lynfield R, Cummings JJ; American Academy of Pediatrics, Committee on Fetus and Newborn and Committee on Infectious Diseases. Management of infants at risk for group B streptococcal disease. *Pediatrics.* 2019;144(2):e20191881. DOI: **https://doi.org/10.1542/peds.2019-188**

[12]Puopolo KM, Benitz WE, Zaoutis TE; American Academy of Pediatrics, Committee on Fetus and Newborn and Committee on Infectious Diseases. Management of neonates born at ≥35 0/7 weeks' gestation with suspected or proven early onset bacterial sepsis. *Pediatrics.* 2018;142(6):e20182894. DOI: **https://doi.org/10.1542/peds.2018-2894**

MedWatch—The FDA Safety Information and Adverse Event-Reporting Program

MedWatch, the Food and Drug Administration (FDA) Safety Information and Adverse Event Reporting Program, serves as a gateway for clinically important safety information and reporting of adverse events for human medical products, including FDA-regulated prescription and over-the-counter drugs, biologics (including human cells, tissues, and cellular and tissue-based products), medical devices (including in vitro diagnostics), special nutritional products, and cosmetics. MedWatch collects reports of drug adverse effects, product use errors, product quality problems, and therapeutic failures. Although reporting to MedWatch by health care professionals and consumers is voluntary, manufacturers of prescription medical products are required to submit adverse event reports to the FDA.

Because many prelicensure clinical trials are not large enough to reveal rare adverse events, postlicensure safety surveillance is used to identify and evaluate new safety concerns with drugs and devices after they are approved and widely used in clinical practice. MedWatch reports are used by the FDA as a pharmacovigilance data source. If a potential safety concern is identified through analysis of MedWatch reports, FDA's further evaluation might include conducting studies using other databases. On the basis of information from postmarketing safety surveillance, the FDA may take regulatory actions, such as revising and strengthening warnings, precautions, contraindications, and adverse reaction descriptions in medication package inserts or issuing "Dear Health Care Professional" letters. Safety alerts are published on the agency's website, and clinicians and the public can stay informed through email, Twitter, and RSS feed updates.

Health care professionals and consumers are encouraged to report adverse events associated with medical products. The MedWatch Form FDA3500 is a 1-page, postage-paid voluntary form (see Fig 4.2). The MedWatch form can be sent by fax (800-FDA-0178) or mail. Adverse events can also be reported online at **www.fda.gov/MedWatch/report.htm**. A toll-free number (800-FDA-1088) is available to report by phone or request blank forms with instructions. In 2013, an additional consumer-friendly reporting form (FDA3500B) became available to encourage increased reporting by patients.

Vaccine-related adverse events should be reported to the Vaccine Adverse Event Reporting System (**http://vaers.hhs.gov/**) (see p 46).

Fig 4.2 MedWatch Voluntary Reporting Form

U.S. Department of Health and Human Services
Food and Drug Administration

MEDWATCH

FORM FDA 3500 (2/19)
The FDA Safety Information and
Adverse Event Reporting Program

For VOLUNTARY reporting of
adverse events, product problems
and product use/medication errors

Page 1 of 2

Form Approved: OMB No. 0910-0291, Expires: 11-30-2021
See PRA statement on reverse.

FDA USE ONLY	
Triage unit sequence #	
FDA Rec. Date	

Note: For date prompts of "dd-mmm-yyyy" please use 2-digit day, 3-letter month abbreviation, and 4-digit year; for example, 01-Jul-2018.

A. PATIENT INFORMATION

1. Patient Identifier

2. Age
   - ☐ Year(s) ☐ Month(s)
   - ☐ Week(s) ☐ Day(s)
   - or Date of Birth (e.g., 08 Feb 1925)

In Confidence

3. Gender (check one)
   - ☐ Female
   - ☐ Male
   - ☐ Intersex
   - ☐ Transgender
   - ☐ Prefer not to disclose

4. Weight
   - ☐ lb
   - ☐ kg

5. Ethnicity (check one)
   - ☐ Hispanic/Latino
   - ☐ Not Hispanic/Latino

6. Race (check all that apply)
   - ☐ Asian ☐ American Indian or Alaskan Native
   - ☐ Black or African American ☐ White
   - ☐ Native Hawaiian or Other Pacific Islander

B. ADVERSE EVENT, PRODUCT PROBLEM

1. Type of Report (check all that apply)
   - ☐ Adverse Event ☐ Product Problem (e.g., defects/malfunctions)
   - ☐ Product Use/Medication Error ☐ Problem with Different Manufacturer of Same Medicine

2. Outcome Attributed to Adverse Event (check all that apply)
   - ☐ Death   Date of death (dd-mmm-yyyy):
   - ☐ Life-threatening
   - ☐ Hospitalization (initial or prolonged)
   - ☐ Disability or Permanent Damage
   - ☐ Congenital Anomaly/Birth Defects
   - ☐ Other Serious or Important Medical Events
   - ☐ Required Intervention to Prevent Permanent Impairment/Damage

3. Date of Event (dd-mmm-yyyy)

4. Date of this Report (dd-mmm-yyyy)

5. Describe Event, Problem or Product Use/Medication Error

(Continue on page 2)

6. Relevant Tests/Laboratory Data   Date (dd-mmm-yyyy)

(Continue on page 2)

7. Other Relevant History, Including Preexisting Medical Conditions (e.g., allergies, pregnancy, smoking and alcohol use, liver/kidney problems, etc.)

(Continue on page 2)

C. PRODUCT AVAILABILITY

1. Product Available for Evaluation? (Do not send product to FDA)
   - ☐ Yes ☐ No ☐ Returned to Manufacturer on (dd-mmm-yyyy)

2. Do you have a picture of the product? (check yes if you are including a picture)   ☐ Yes

D. SUSPECT PRODUCTS

1. Name, Strength, Manufacturer/Compounder (from product label).
   Does this report involve cosmetic, dietary supplement or food/medical food? #1 ☐ Yes #2 ☐ Yes

#1 – Name and Strength	#1 – NDC # or Unique ID
#1 – Manufacturer/Compounder	#1 – Lot #
#2 – Name and Strength	#2 – NDC # or Unique ID
#2 – Manufacturer/Compounder	#2 – Lot #

2. Dose or Amount | Frequency | Route
   #1
   #2

3. Treatment Dates/Therapy Dates (give best estimate of length of treatment (start/stop) or duration.)
   #1 Start
   #1 Stop
   Is therapy still on-going? ☐ Yes ☐ No
   #2 Start
   #2 Stop
   Is therapy still on-going? ☐ Yes ☐ No

4. Diagnosis for Use (Indication)
   #1
   #2

5. Product Type (check all that apply)
   #1 ☐ OTC #2 ☐ OTC
   ☐ Compounded ☐ Compounded
   ☐ Generic ☐ Generic
   ☐ Biosimilar ☐ Biosimilar

6. Expiration Date (dd-mmm-yyyy)
   #1
   #2

7. Event Abated After Use Stopped or Dose Reduced?
   #1 ☐ Yes ☐ No ☐ Doesn't apply
   #2 ☐ Yes ☐ No ☐ Doesn't apply

8. Event Reappeared After Reintroduction?
   #1 ☐ Yes ☐ No ☐ Doesn't apply
   #2 ☐ Yes ☐ No ☐ Doesn't apply

E. SUSPECT MEDICAL DEVICE

1. Brand Name

2a. Common Device Name | 2b. Procode

3. Manufacturer Name, City and State

4. Model # | Lot #
   Catalog # | Expiration Date (dd-mmm-yyyy)
   Serial # | Unique Identifier (UDI) #

5. Operator of Device
   - ☐ Health Professional
   - ☐ Patient/Consumer
   - ☐ Other

6a. If Implanted, Give Date (dd-mmm-yyyy) | 6b. If Explanted, Give Date (dd-mmm-yyyy)

7a. Is this a single-use device that was reprocessed and reused on a patient? ☐ Yes ☐ No | 7b. If Yes to Item 7a, Enter Name and Address of Reprocessor

8. Was this device serviced by a third party servicer?
   ☐ Yes ☐ No ☐ Unknown

F. OTHER (CONCOMITANT) MEDICAL PRODUCTS

1. Product names and therapy dates (Exclude treatment of event)

(Continue on page 2)

G. REPORTER (See confidentiality section on back)

1. Name and Address

Last Name:	First Name:
Address:	
City:	State/Province/Region:
ZIP/Postal Code:	Country:
Phone #:	Email:

2. Health Professional? ☐ Yes ☐ No

3. Occupation

4. Also Reported to:
   - ☐ Manufacturer
   - ☐ Compounder
   - ☐ User Facility
   - ☐ Distributor/Importer

5. If you do NOT want your identity disclosed to the manufacturer, please mark this box: ☐

FORM FDA 3500 (2/19)   Submission of a report does not constitute an admission that medical personnel or the product caused or contributed to the event.
* Please see instructions

Available for download at **www.fda.gov/downloads/AboutFDA/ReportsManualsForms/Forms/UCM163919.pdf.**

FIG 4.2 MEDWATCH VOLUNTARY REPORTING FORM, CONTINUED

U.S. Department of Health and Human Services
Food and Drug Administration

MEDWATCH

FORM FDA 3500 (2/19) *(continued)*
The FDA Safety Information and
Adverse Event Reporting Program

(CONTINUATION PAGE)
For VOLUNTARY reporting of
adverse events, product problems
and product use/medication errors

Page 2 of 2

B.5. Describe Event or Problem *(continued)*

Back to Item B.5

B.6. Relevant Tests/Laboratory Data *(continued)* Date *(dd-mmm-yyyy)*   Relevant Tests/Laboratory Data   Date *(dd-mmm-yyyy)*

Additional comments

Back to Item B.6

B.7. Other Relevant History *(continued)*

Back to Item B.7

F.1. Concomitant Medical Products and Therapy Dates *(Exclude treatment of event) (continued)*

Back to Item F.1

Available for download at **www.fda.gov/downloads/AboutFDA/ReportsManualsForms/Forms/UCM163919.pdf.**

Antimicrobial Prophylaxis

ANTIMICROBIAL PROPHYLAXIS

Antimicrobial prophylaxis is defined as the use of antimicrobial drugs in the absence of suspected or documented infection to prevent development of infection or disease and is a common practice in pediatrics. Although the efficacy of antimicrobial prophylaxis has been demonstrated for some conditions, this is not the case for many more conditions for which it is nevertheless used. Concerns about the emergence of resistant bacterial pathogens has led to a reexamination of the role of antimicrobial prophylaxis, especially for conditions for which prolonged administration is required, such as prevention of recurrent otitis media (OM) and urinary tract infection (UTI).

Effective chemoprophylaxis should be directed at pathogens common in the infection-prone body sites (Table 5.1). When using prophylactic antimicrobial therapy, the risk of the emergence of antimicrobial-resistant organisms and the possibility of an adverse event from the drug must be weighed against potential benefits. Ideally, prophylactic agents should have a narrow spectrum of activity and should be used for a brief period of time.

Infection-Prone Body Sites

Antibiotic prophylaxis in vulnerable body sites is most successful if (1) the period of risk is defined and brief; (2) the expected pathogens have predictable antimicrobial susceptibility; and (3) the site is accessible to adequate antimicrobial concentrations.

ACUTE OTITIS MEDIA

Universal immunization of infants with pneumococcal conjugate vaccine has reduced the burden of the incidence of acute otitis media (AOM) and recurrent OM and altered the microbiology of AOM. The proportion of disease attributable to *Streptococcus pneumoniae* has declined, but the proportion attributable to nontypeable *Haemophilus influenzae* and *Moraxella catarrhalis* has increased, potentially decreasing the effectiveness of antimicrobial prophylactic regimens relying on amoxicillin. Studies performed prior to the introduction of conjugate pneumococcal vaccines demonstrated that amoxicillin prophylaxis was modestly effective in reducing the frequency of recurrent episodes of OM in otitis-prone children but failed to alter the underlying susceptibility to recurrent attacks once prophylaxis was discontinued. In addition, greater understanding of the changes in the nasopharyngeal microbiome and increased colonization with resistant organisms has led to decreased use of antibiotic prophylaxis for the purpose of preventing AOM.

An alternative for children with recurrent OM and persistent middle ear effusion is placement of tympanostomy tubes. Tympanostomy tubes have been associated with a modest benefit of reducing episodes of AOM, by an average 1.5 episodes per child in

Table 5.1. Antimicrobial Chemoprophylaxis[a]

Anatomic Site-Related Infections	Exposed Host; Time-Limited Exposure	Vulnerable Host (Pathogen); Ongoing Exposure
Urinary tract infection with vesicoureteral reflux (VUR) Endocarditis with certain underlying cardiac conditions	*Bordetella pertussis* exposure *Neisseria meningitidis* exposure Traveler's diarrhea[b] (*Escherichia coli, Shigella* species, *Salmonella* species, *Campylobacter* species) Perinatal group B *Streptococcus* (mother/infant) exposure Bite wound (human, animal, reptile) Infants born to HIV-infected mothers, to decrease the risk of HIV transmission Influenza virus, following close family exposure in those unimmunized Susceptible contacts of index cases of invasive *Haemophilus influenzae* type b disease Exposure to aerosolized spores of *Bacillus anthracis Borrelia burgdorferi*[c] Ophthalmia neonatorum prophylaxis (*Neisseria gonorrhoeae*)	Immunosuppressed patients because of treatment of conditions, eg, oncologic, rheumatologic (*Pneumocystis jirovecii*, fungi) Solid organ and stem cell transplant patients (CMV, *P jirovecii*, fungi) HIV-infected children (*P jirovecii*, polysaccharide-encapsulated bacteria) Preterm neonates (*Candida* species) Anatomic or functional asplenia (polysaccharide-encapsulated bacteria)[d] Chronic granulomatous disease (*Staphylococcus aureus* and certain other catalase-positive bacteria and fungi) Congenital immune deficiencies (various pathogens) Rheumatic fever (group A *Streptococcus*) Treatment with Eculizumab (*Neisseria meningitidis*)

HIV indicates human immunodeficiency virus; CMV, cytomegalovirus; HSV, herpes simplex virus.

[a] Antimicrobial prophylactic regimens for exposed hosts and vulnerable hosts (pathogens) are described in each pathogen or disease-specific chapter in Section 3. Immune globulin prophylaxis is not discussed in this Section but should be considered for specific bacteria (eg, *Clostridium tetani*) or viruses (eg, respiratory syncytial virus).

[b] Prophylactic antibiotics should not be recommended for most travelers.

[c] Doxycycline prophylaxis of Lyme disease following tick bites may be considered in specific circumstances (see Lyme Disease [p 482]).

[d] See Immunization and Other Considerations in Immunosuppressed Children (p 72).

the first 6 months after placement. The most recent guidelines for prevention of recurrent OM indicate that clinicians can offer tympanostomy tube insertion but should not prescribe antimicrobial prophylaxis.[1]

URINARY TRACT INFECTION[2]

The role of chemoprophylaxis for UTI remains controversial because resistance usually will develop to any agent used for prophylaxis. The decision requires a balance between the impact of modest reduction of recurrent UTI achievable versus the

[1] Lieberthal AS, Carroll AE, Chonmaitree T, et al. The Diagnosis and Management of Acute Otitis Media. *Pediatrics.* 2013;131(3): e964-99

[2] American Academy of Pediatrics, Subcommittee on Urinary Tract Infections, Steering Committee on Quality Improvement and Management. Urinary tract infection: clinical practice guideline for the diagnosis and management of the initial UTI in febrile infants and children 2 to 24 months. *Pediatrics.* 2011;128(3):595-610

emergence of resistant organisms and its value in the prevention of subsequent renal scarring. Some experts prefer prompt diagnosis and effective treatment of a febrile UTI recurrence as the management strategy. The anatomic abnormalities of the urinary tract, the consequences of recurrent infection, the risks of infection caused by a resistant pathogen, and the anticipated duration of prophylaxis need to be carefully assessed for each patient.

People at highest risk for recurrence include those with first UTI early in life, higher grades of vesicoureteral reflux (VUR), bilateral VUR, urinary stasis related to incomplete bladder emptying or anatomic conditions such as hydroureteronephrosis, and infection not caused by *Escherichia coli*. There is agreement that data do not support use of antimicrobial prophylaxis to prevent febrile recurrent UTIs in infants without VUR or conditions causing significant urinary stasis. The Randomized Intervention for Children with Vesicoureteral Reflux (RIVUR) study among children with grade I through grade IV VUR reported that chemoprophylaxis with trimethoprim-sulfamethoxazole compared with placebo decreased recurrent UTI following a first or second febrile or symptomatic UTI by 50%. However, an increase in antibiotic resistance of causative organisms from 25% to 68% was observed, and the proportion of children with renal scarring at the 2-year follow-up was not affected by prophylaxis. In contrast, a Swedish reflux study reported that chemoprophylaxis was effective in preventing new renal scars in infant girls with grade III and IV VUR. If prophylaxis is to be offered, children with high-grade reflux are most likely to benefit; low-grade reflux is believed to play little role in renal damage, and most studies show little benefit in prophylaxis with this group.

Exposure to Specific Pathogens

Prophylaxis may be indicated if an increased risk of serious infection with a specific pathogen exists and a specific antimicrobial agent has been demonstrated to decrease the risk of infection by that pathogen (eg, prophylaxis for exposure to *Neisseria meningitidis*). Pathogen-specific prophylaxis is addressed in Section 3. It is assumed that the benefit of prophylaxis is greater than the risk of adverse effects of the antimicrobial agent or the risk of subsequent infection by antimicrobial-resistant organisms. For some pathogens that colonize the upper respiratory tract, elimination of the carrier state can be difficult and may require use of a specific antimicrobial agent that achieves microbiologically effective concentrations in nasopharyngeal secretions (eg, rifampin).

Vulnerable Hosts

Attempts to prevent serious infections in specific populations of vulnerable patients with antimicrobial prophylaxis have been successful in some carefully defined populations that are known to be at risk of infection caused by defined pathogens. In some situations, such as prophylaxis of pneumococcal bacteremia/sepsis in asplenic children, resistance to beta-lactam agents may lead to decreased effectiveness of continuous prophylaxis. In other situations, such as prophylaxis of *Pneumocystis* infection in immune-compromised children with trimethoprim-sulfamethoxazole, resistance has not appeared to develop despite years of continuous prophylaxis.

ANTIMICROBIAL PROPHYLAXIS IN PEDIATRIC SURGICAL PATIENTS

Surgical site infections (SSIs) complicate approximately 2% of surgical procedures, prolong the length of hospitalization, and increase the risk of death. Prevention of SSIs should be a priority for children's hospitals and surgical centers. Active surveillance targeting high-risk, high-volume procedures should be in place and requires education of surgeons and perioperative personnel, technological infrastructure, and use of a multidisciplinary team of trained personnel who are knowledgeable regarding SSI criteria. Institutions should monitor compliance with basic process measures and provide regular feedback to surgical personnel and hospital leadership.

Prevention of postoperative wound infections through perioperative prophylaxis is recommended for procedures with moderate or high infection rates or procedures in which a postoperative wound infection would have great consequences, such as implantation of prosthetic material into the heart. In contrast, for tissue sites already inoculated/infected, such as a ruptured appendix, antibiotics are used as treatment of infection rather than in prevention of infection. Consensus recommendations for prevention of SSIs in adults and children have been developed, although high-quality evidence for many of these recommendations is lacking. Although few data exist specifically for pediatric surgical prophylaxis, the principles of antimicrobial agent selection and exposure at surgical sites in adults should apply to children. Consequences of inappropriate use of prophylactic antimicrobial agents include increased costs, adverse events from toxicity, and emergence of resistant organisms. The emergence of drug-resistant organisms poses a risk not only to the recipient but to other patients in whom a health care-associated infection could develop.

Guidelines for Appropriate Use

Guidelines for prevention of SSIs have been published.[1,2] General principles include that agents used for antimicrobial prophylaxis should prevent SSIs and related morbidity and mortality, reduce the duration and cost of care, minimize risk of adverse effects, not create SSIs from alternative pathogens, and minimize adverse consequences on the microbial flora. Published guidelines address indications, appropriate drug selection, dosing, preoperative timing and need for intraoperative redosing, and duration of prophylaxis.

Indications for Prophylaxis

Major determinants of SSIs include the number of microorganisms in the wound during the procedure, the virulence of the microorganisms, the presence of foreign material in the wound, and host risk factors, including preoperative health status. The classification of surgical procedures is based on an estimation of bacterial contamination and, thus, risk of subsequent infection. The 4 classes are: (1) clean wounds; (2) clean-contaminated wounds; (3) contaminated wounds; and (4) dirty and infected

[1]Antimicrobial prophylaxis for surgery. *Med Lett Drugs Ther.* 2016;58(1495):63-68

[2]Berríos-Torres SI, Umscheid CA, Bratzler DW, et al. and the Healthcare Infection Control Practices Advisory Committee. Centers for Disease Control and Prevention Guideline for the Prevention of Surgical Site Infection, 2017. *JAMA Surg.* 2017;152(8):784-791

wounds. Additional risk factors for SSIs include the operative site and the duration of the procedure. A patient risk index, which incorporates the preoperative physical status assessment score of the American Society of Anesthesiologists, the duration of the operation, and the aforementioned wound classification, has been demonstrated to be a good predictor of SSIs.[1] Others have summarized patients at "high risk" of surgical site infection.[2] Although a high-risk pediatric patient is not clearly defined, high-risk factors in adult patients include obesity, coexistent infections at a remote body site, altered immune response, colonization with pathogenic microorganisms, and diabetes mellitus.

CLEAN WOUNDS

Clean wounds are uninfected operative wounds in which no inflammation is encountered; the respiratory, alimentary, and genitourinary tracts or oropharyngeal cavity are not entered; and no break in aseptic technique occurred. The operative procedures usually are elective, and wounds are closed primarily and, if necessary, drained with closed drainage. Operative incisional wounds that follow nonpenetrating (blunt) trauma are included in this category, provided that the surgical procedure does not involve entry into the gastrointestinal or genitourinary tracts. The benefits of systemic antimicrobial prophylaxis do not justify the potential risks associated with antimicrobial use in most clean wound procedures, because the risk of infection is low (usually <1%). Some exceptions exist in which prophylaxis is administered because the risks or consequences of infection are high; examples include implantation of intravascular or deep tissue prosthetic material (eg, insertion of a prosthetic heart valve or a prosthetic joint), open-heart surgery for repair of structural defects, body cavity exploration in neonates, and most neurosurgical operations.

CLEAN-CONTAMINATED WOUNDS

In clean-contaminated wounds, the respiratory, alimentary, or genitourinary tracts are entered under controlled conditions without significant contamination. Operations involving the gastrointestinal tract, the biliary tract, appendix, vagina, or oropharynx, and urgent or emergency surgery in an otherwise clean procedure, are included in this category, provided that no evidence of infection is encountered and no major break in aseptic technique occurs. Prophylaxis is limited to procedures in which a substantial amount of wound contamination is expected. The overall risk of infection for these surgical sites is 3% to 15%. On the basis of data from adults, procedures for which prophylaxis is indicated for pediatric patients include: (1) all gastrointestinal tract procedures in which there is obstruction, when the patient is receiving H_2 receptor antagonists or proton pump blockers, or when the patient has a permanent foreign body; (2) selected biliary tract operations (eg, when there is obstruction from common bile duct stones); and (3) urinary tract surgery or instrumentation in the presence of bacteriuria or obstructive uropathy.

[1] Gaynes RP, Culver DH, Horan TC, Edwards JR, Richards C, Tolson JS. Surgical site infection (SSI) rates in the United States, 1992–1998: the National Nosocomial Surveillance System basic SSI risk index. *Clin Infect Dis.* 2001;33(Suppl 2):S69–S77

[2] Bratzler DW, Dellinger EP, Olsen KM, et al; American Society of Health-System Pharmacists; Infectious Disease Society of America; Surgical Infection Society; Society for Healthcare Epidemiology of America. Clinical practice guidelines for antimicrobial prophylaxis in surgery. *Am J Health Syst Pharm.* 2013;70(3):195-283. Available at: **www.ajhp.org/content/ajhp/70/3/195.full.pdf?sso-checked=true**

CONTAMINATED WOUNDS

Contaminated wounds are previously sterile tissue sites that are likely to be heavily contaminated with bacteria and include open, fresh wounds; operative wounds in the setting of major breaks in aseptic technique or gross spillage from the gastrointestinal tract; exposed viscera at birth from congenital anomalies; penetrating trauma of fewer than 4 hours' duration; and incisions in which acute nonpurulent inflammation is encountered. The estimated rate of surgical site wound infection for these surgical sites is 15%. In contaminated wound procedures, antimicrobial prophylaxis is appropriate for some patients with acute nonpurulent inflammation isolated to, and contained within, an inflamed viscus (such as acute, nonperforated appendicitis or cholecystitis). For wounds in which contaminating bacteria have had an opportunity to establish inflammation and ongoing infection, antimicrobial use should be considered as treatment rather than prophylaxis.

DIRTY AND INFECTED WOUNDS

Dirty and infected wounds include penetrating trauma of more than 4 hours' duration from time of occurrence (the prolonged period assumes that the infection is already established), wounds with retained devitalized tissue, and wounds involving existing clinical infection or perforated viscera. This definition suggests that the organisms causing postoperative infection were present in the operative field before surgery, as noted above, and that antimicrobial use should be considered as treatment rather than prophylaxis. The estimated rate of infection for these surgical sites is 40%. In dirty and infected wound procedures, such as procedures for a perforated abdominal viscus (eg, ruptured appendix), a compound fracture, a laceration attributable to an animal or human bite >12 hours after injury, or when a major break in sterile technique occurs, antimicrobial agents are given as treatment rather than prophylaxis, although they may actually prevent an infection of the surgical wound itself.

Surgical Site Infection Criteria

Specific classification criteria for SSIs have been developed by the National Healthcare Safety Network (NHSN) and are updated yearly (**www.cdc.gov/nhsn/index. html**). Reports from the NHSN are also posted periodically on the CDC website (**www.cdc.gov/nhsn/datastat/index.html**).

SUPERFICIAL INCISIONAL SSI

A superficial incisional SSI is an infection that involves only the skin and subcutaneous layers of the incision and occurs within 30 days of the operation and from which the patient presents with one of the following: (1) purulent drainage from the superficial incision; (2) an organism(s) that is (are) identified from an aseptically obtained specimen from the superficial incision or subcutaneous tissue by culture or molecular analysis; (3) surgical wound exploration (in the absence of laboratory results) when the patient presents with one of the following signs or symptoms: pain or tenderness, localized swelling, erythema, or pain; or (4) diagnosis of superficial incisional SSI by a physician, nurse practitioner, or physician assistant.

DEEP INCISIONAL SSI

A deep incisional SSI occurs within 30 or 90 days after the operative procedure, depending on the surgery; involves only the fascial or muscle layers; and results in at least 1 of the following: (1) purulent drainage from the deep incision but not from the organ/space component of the surgical site; (2) a deep incision that spontaneously dehisces or is deliberately opened by a physician, nurse practitioner, or physician assistant and at least 1 of the following signs or symptoms: fever (>38°C), localized pain, or localized tenderness; or (3) an abscess or other evidence of infection involving the deep incision that is found on direct examination, during reoperation, or by histopathologic or radiologic examination.

ORGAN/SPACE SSI

An organ or space SSI is defined by the specific site of infection that is opened and manipulated during the procedure (eg, endocarditis, mediastinitis, osteomyelitis) and excludes the superficial, subcutaneous, fascia, or muscle layers that have been manipulated during the procedure. Organ/space SSI must occur within 30 or 90 days of the surgery (as defined by the specific procedure), and the patient must have 1 or more of the following: (1) purulent drainage from a drain that is placed through a stab wound into the organ/space; (2) organisms isolated from an aseptically obtained culture of fluid or tissue in the organ/space; or (3) an abscess or other evidence of infection involving the organ/space that is found on direct examination, during reoperation, or by histopathologic or radiologic examination.

Timing of Administration of Prophylactic Antimicrobial Agents

Effective chemoprophylaxis occurs only when the appropriate antimicrobial drug is present in tissues at sufficient local concentrations at the time of intraoperative bacterial contamination. Administration of an antimicrobial agent within 1 or 2 hours before surgery has been demonstrated to decrease the risk of wound infection. Accordingly, administration of the prophylactic agent is recommended within 60 minutes before surgical incision to ensure adequate tissue concentrations at the start of the procedure. When antimicrobial agents require longer administration times, such as glycopeptides (eg, vancomycin) or fluoroquinolones, administration should begin within 120 minutes prior to surgical incision.

Dosing and Duration of Administration of Antimicrobial Agents

Weight-based dosing for pediatric patients is routine, although not prospectively studied for prophylaxis. The preoperative doses should not exceed the usual dose for adults.

Adequate antimicrobial concentrations should be maintained throughout the surgical procedure; in most instances, a single dose of an antimicrobial agent is sufficient, and the duration of prophylaxis after any procedure should not exceed 24 hours. Intraoperative dosing is required if the duration of the procedure is greater than 2 times the half-life of the antimicrobial agent or if there is excessive blood loss (eg, >1500 mL in adults). For example, cefazolin may be administered every 3 to 4 hours during a prolonged surgical procedure or one that involves large-volume blood loss. Postoperative doses after closure generally are not recommended in clean and clean-contaminated procedures, even in the presence of a drain.

Preoperative Screening and Decolonization

The use of preoperative surveillance to identify carriers of methicillin-susceptible *Staphylococcus aureus* (MSSA) or methicillin-resistant *S aureus* (MRSA) has been explored in the adult population. Use of preoperative nasal mupirocin and chlorhexidine baths for *S aureus* carriers may reduce the risk of deep SSI and is recommended as an adjunct to intravenous prophylaxis in adult cardiac and orthopedic surgery patients. Several small studies in children undergoing cardiac surgery have suggested similar benefit in using perioperative mupirocin.

Recommended Antimicrobial Agents

An antimicrobial agent is chosen on the basis of bacterial pathogens most likely to cause infectious complications during and after the specific procedure, the antimicrobial susceptibility pattern of these pathogens, and the safety and efficacy of the drug. Antimicrobial agents administered prophylactically do not have to be active in vitro against every potential organism to be effective, because it is unlikely that all potential organisms are actually contaminating the wound. Doses are determined on the basis of the need to achieve therapeutic blood and tissue concentrations throughout the procedure. Antimicrobial prophylaxis for most surgical procedures, including gastric, biliary, thoracic (noncardiac), vascular, neurosurgical, and orthopedic operations, can be achieved effectively using an agent such as a first-generation cephalosporin (eg, cefazolin) unless the risk for MRSA infection is high, in which case vancomycin may be indicated. For colorectal surgery or appendectomy, effective prophylaxis requires antimicrobial agents that are active against aerobic and anaerobic intestinal flora. Table 5.2 provides recommendations for drugs to be used in children undergoing surgical manipulation or invasive procedures. Physicians should be aware of potential interactions and adverse effects associated with prophylactic antimicrobial agents and other medications the patient may be receiving. Routine use of broad-spectrum agents (extended-spectrum cephalosporins, beta-lactam/beta-lactamase combinations, and carbapenems) for surgical prophylaxis generally is not necessary. Hospital systems should be evaluated regularly to ensure that the process for provision, delivery, and maintenance of appropriate antimicrobial prophylaxis is in place. There are no data to support the practice of continuing antibiotic prophylaxis until all invasive lines, drains, and indwelling catheters have been removed.

Routine use of vancomycin for prophylaxis is not recommended. However, vancomycin prophylaxis may be considered for patients with congenital heart disease who undergo cardiac surgery, patients who undergo certain orthopedic procedures (eg, spinal procedures, implantation of foreign materials), children known to be colonized or previously infected by MRSA, or children living in a community with a high rate of MRSA infections. Vancomycin is not as effective as cefazolin for the prevention of infection caused by many other organisms.

Misconceptions regarding penicillin allergies may result in patients receiving alternate and less-effective antibiotics for surgical prophylaxis. Efforts toward delabeling patients of reported allergies include assessing the exact nature of the previous reaction, determining the likelihood that this reaction is a true immunoglobulin E (IgE)-mediated reaction, and determining the likelihood that the purported offending agent has cross-reactivity with the recommended perioperative antibiotic. Analysis of the chemical structure of the beta-lactams indicate little cross-reactivity between the penicillins and cefazolin, given differences in chemical side chains (see Figure 4.1, p 867). Institutions should develop programs (or at a minimum an algorithm) to manage and delabel patients with reported penicillin allergies.

Table 5.2. Recommendations for Preoperative Antimicrobial Prophylaxis

Operation	Likely Pathogens	Recommended Drugs	Preoperative Dose
Neonatal (≤72 h of age)—all major procedures	Group B streptococci, enteric gram-negative bacilli,[a] enterococci, coagulase-negative staphylococci	Ampicillin **PLUS** Gentamicin	50 mg/kg 4 mg/kg
Neonatal (>72 h of age)—all major procedures	Prophylaxis targeted to colonizing organisms, nosocomial organisms, and operative site		
Cardiac (cardiac surgical procedures, prosthetic valve or pacemaker, ventricular assist devices)	*Staphylococcus epidermidis, Staphylococcus aureus,* *Corynebacterium* species, enteric gram-negative bacilli[a]	Cefazolin **OR** (if MRSA or MRSE is likely) Vancomycin	30 mg/kg (max 2 g; 3 g if ≥120 kg) 15 mg/kg
Gastrointestinal			
Esophageal and gastroduodenal	Enteric gram-negative bacilli,[a] gram-positive cocci	Cefazolin (high risk only)[b]	30 mg/kg (max 2 g; 3 g if ≥120 kg)
Biliary tract	Enteric gram-negative bacilli,[a] enterococci	Cefazolin[c]	30 mg/kg (max 2 g; 3 g of ≥120 kg)
Colorectal or appendectomy (uncomplicated, nonperforated)	Enteric gram-negative bacilli,[a] enterococci, anaerobes (*Bacteroides* species)[d]	Cefoxitin or cefotetan **OR** Metronidazole **PLUS** Gentamicin **OR** Cefazolin **PLUS** Metronidazole	40 mg/kg (max 2 g) 15 mg/kg (max 500 mg) 2.5 mg/kg 30 mg/kg (max 2 g; 3 g if ≥120 kg) 15 mg/kg (max 500 mg)

Table 5.2. Recommendations for Preoperative Antimicrobial Prophylaxis, continued

Operation	Likely Pathogens	Recommended Drugs	Preoperative Dose
Ruptured viscus (regarded as treatment, not prophylaxis)	Enteric gram-negative bacilli,[a] enterococci, anaerobes (*Bacteroides* species)[d]	Cefoxitin **WITH OR WITHOUT**	40 mg/kg (max 2 g)
		Gentamicin	2.5 mg/kg
		OR	
		Gentamicin **PLUS**	2.5 mg/kg
		Metronidazole **PLUS**	15 mg/kg (max 500 mg)
		Ampicillin	50 mg/kg (max 2 g)
		OR	
		Ertapenem	15 mg/kg (max 1 g)
		OR	
		Other regimens for complicated appendicitis[e]	
Genitourinary	Enteric gram-negative bacilli,[a] enterococci	Cefazolin	30 mg/kg (max 2 g; 3 g if ≥120 kg)
		OR	
		Trimethoprim-sulfamethoxazole	4 mg/kg trimethoprim (max 160 mg), 20 mg/kg sulfamethoxazole (max 400 mg)

Table 5.2. Recommendations for Preoperative Antimicrobial Prophylaxis, continued

Operation	Likely Pathogens	Recommended Drugs	Preoperative Dose
Head and neck surgery (incision through oral or pharyngeal mucosa)	Anaerobes, enteric gram-negative bacilli,[a] S aureus	Cefazolin **PLUS** Metronidazole	30 mg/kg (max 2 g; 3 g if ≥120 kg) 15 mg/kg (max 500 mg)
		OR	
		Clindamycin **WITH OR WITHOUT** Gentamicin	10 mg/kg (max 900 mg) 2.5 mg/kg
		OR	
Neurosurgery (craniotomy; intrathecal baclofen shunt or ventricular shunt placement)	S epidermidis, S aureus	Ampicillin-sulbactam Cefazolin	50 mg/kg (max 3g) 30 mg/kg (max 2 g; 3 g if ≥120 kg)
		OR	
		(if MRSA or MRSE is likely) Vancomycin	15 mg/kg

Table 5.2. Recommendations for Preoperative Antimicrobial Prophylaxis, continued

Operation	Likely Pathogens	Recommended Drugs	Preoperative Dose
Ophthalmic	S epidermidis, S aureus, streptococci, enteric gram-negative bacilli,[a] Pseudomonas species	Gentamicin, ciprofloxacin, ofloxacin, moxifloxacin, tobramycin	Multiple drops topically for 2–24 h before procedure
		OR	
		Neomycin-gramicidin-polymyxin B	Multiple drops topically for 2–24 h before procedure
		OR	
		Cefazolin	100 mg, subconjunctivally at the end of the procedure
Orthopedic (internal fixation of fractures, implantation of materials including prosthetic joint and spinal procedures with and without instrumentation)	S epidermidis, S aureus	Cefazolin	30 mg/kg (max 2 g; 3 g if ≥120 kg)
		OR	
		(if MRSA or MRSE is likely) Vancomycin	15 mg/kg
Thoracic (non-cardiac)	S epidermidis, S aureus, streptococci, gram-negative enteric bacilli[a]	Cefazolin	30 mg/kg (max 2 g; 3 g if ≥120 kg)
		OR	
		(if MRSA is likely) Vancomycin	15 mg/kg

Table 5.2. Recommendations for Preoperative Antimicrobial Prophylaxis, continued

Operation	Likely Pathogens	Recommended Drugs	Preoperative Dose
Traumatic wound (exceptionally varied pathogens, based on the anatomic site injured, and the instrument causing the trauma, particularly for penetrating injuries such as motor vehicle accidents or farm injuries)	Skin: *S aureus*, group A streptococci, *S epidermidis*	Cefazolin	30 mg/kg (max 2 g; 3 g if ≥120 kg)
	Perforated viscus: gram-negative enteric bacilli, *Clostridium* species	Cefoxitin	40 mg/kg (max 2g)
		WITH OR WITHOUT	
		Gentamicin	2.5 mg/kg
		OR	
		Gentamicin	2.5 mg/kg
		PLUS	
		Metronidazole	10 mg/kg (max 500 mg)
		PLUS	
		Ampicillin	50 mg/kg (max 2g)
		OR	
		Ertapenem	15 mg/kg (max 1g)
		OR	
		Other regimens for complicated appendicitis[e]	

MRSA indicates methicillin-resistant *Staphylococcus aureus*; MRSE, methicillin-resistant *Staphylococcus epidermidis*.

[a] Selection of antibiotics should take into consideration the susceptibility patterns of isolates found in the patient and at the institution.

[b]Esophageal obstruction, decreased gastric acidity, or gastrointestinal motility; see text for additional high risk factors.

[c] Acute cholecystitis, nonfunctioning gallbladder, obstructive jaundice, common duct stones.

[d]High rates of resistance to clindamycin (~30%) now reported for *Bacteroides fragilis*. Lowest rates of resistance to carbapenems, ampicillin/sulbactam, and piperacillin/tazobactam. Resistance to cefoxitin reported at 3.5% to 9.4% (Snydman DR, Jacobus NV, McDermott LA, et al. Update on resistance of *Bacteroides fragilis* group and related species with special attention to carbapenems 2006-2009. *Anaerobe.* 2011;17[4]:147-151).

[e] Solomkin JS, Mazuski JE, Bradley JS, et al. Diagnosis and management of complicated intra-abdominal infection in adults and children: guidelines by the Surgical Infection Society and the Infectious Diseases Society of America (erratum in *Clin Infect Dis.* 2010;50(12):1695; dosage error in article text). *Clin Infect Dis.* 2010;50(2):133-164.

PREVENTION OF BACTERIAL ENDOCARDITIS

The Committee on Rheumatic Fever, Endocarditis, and Kawasaki Disease of the American Heart Association periodically issues detailed recommendations on the rationale, indications, and antimicrobial regimens for prevention of bacterial endocarditis for people at increased risk. In the guidelines published in 2007,[1] there is a lack of evidence regarding the efficacy of antibiotic prophylaxis in preventing infective endocarditis after dental procedures. Bacteremia associated with most dental procedures represents only a very small fraction of bacteremia episodes that occur with events of daily living, such as brushing teeth, chewing, and other oral hygiene measures. The committee has restricted recommendations for endocarditis prophylaxis to a considerably narrower group of people who have certain cardiac abnormalities and for fewer procedures than in the past. Although previous recommendations stressed endocarditis prophylaxis for people undergoing procedures most likely to induce bacteremia, the 2007 revision stresses only those cardiac conditions in which an episode of infective endocarditis has a high risk of an adverse outcome. Furthermore, prophylaxis is recommended only for certain dental procedures. Prophylaxis no longer is recommended for procedures involving the gastrointestinal and genitourinary tracts solely to prevent endocarditis.

In 2015, the American Heart Association issued updated guidance on the epidemiology, clinical findings, pathogenesis, diagnosis, and treatment of pediatric bacterial endocarditis that includes a short section on endocarditis prevention, which reiterates the 2007 published recommendations.[2] The 2007 document is the more comprehensive discussion of bacterial endocarditis prophylaxis.

Specific prophylactic regimens are presented in Table 5.3. Physicians should consult the published recommendations for further details (**http://circ.ahajournals. org/cgi/content/full/116/15/1736**).

Cardiac conditions associated with the highest risk of an adverse outcome from endocarditis for which prophylaxis with dental procedures is reasonable include the following:

- Prosthetic cardiac valve or prosthetic material used for repair of valve.
- Previous infective endocarditis.
- Congenital heart disease (CHD):
  - Unrepaired cyanotic CHD, including palliative shunts and conduits.
  - Completely repaired congenital heart defect with prosthetic material or device, whether placed by surgery or by catheter intervention, during the first 6 months after the procedure.

---

[1] Wilson W, Taubert KA, Gewitz M, et al. Prevention of Infective Endocarditis. Guidelines from the American Heart Association. A Guideline From the American Heart Association Rheumatic Fever, Endocarditis, and Kawasaki Diseases Committee, Council on Cardiovascular Disease in the Young, and the Council on Clinical Cardiology, Council on Cardiovascular Surgery and Anesthesia, and the Quality of Care and Outcomes Research Interdisciplinary Working Group. *Circulation.* 2007;116(15):1736–1754

[2] Baltimore RS, Gewitz M, Baddour LM, et al; American Heart Association Rheumatic Fever, Endocarditis, and Kawasaki Disease Committee of the Council on Cardiovascular Disease in the Young and the Council on Cardiovascular and Stroke Nursing. Infective endocarditis in childhood: 2015 update: a scientific statement from the American Heart Association. *Circulation.* 2015;132(15):1487-1515

Table 5.3. Regimens for Antimicrobial Prophylaxis for a Dental Procedure[a]

Situation	Agent	Regimen: Single Dose 30 to 60 min Before Procedure	
		Children	Adults
Oral	Amoxicillin	50 mg/kg	2 g
Unable to take oral medication	Ampicillin	50 mg/kg, IM or IV	2 g, IM or IV
Allergic to penicillins or oral ampicillin	Cephalexin[b,c]	50 mg/kg	2 g
		OR	
	Clindamycin	20 mg/kg	600 mg
		OR	
	Azithromycin or clarithromycin	15 mg/kg	500 mg
Allergic to penicillins or ampicillin and unable to take oral medication	Cefazolin or ceftriaxone[c]	50 mg/kg, IM or IV (cefazolin); 50 mg/kg, IM or IV (ceftriaxone)	1 g, IM or IV
		OR	
	Clindamycin	20 mg/kg, IM or IV	600 mg, IM or IV

IM, indicates intramuscular; IV, intravenous.
[a] Pediatric dosage should not exceed recommended adult dosage.
[b] Or other first- or second-generation oral cephalosporin in equivalent pediatric or adult dosage.
[c] Cephalosporins should not be used in a person with a history of anaphylaxis, angioedema, or urticaria with penicillins or ampicillin.

- ◆ Repaired CHD with residual defect(s) at the site or adjacent to the site of a prosthetic patch or prosthetic device (which inhibits endothelialization).
- • Cardiac transplantation with subsequent cardiac valvulopathy.

Dental procedures for which endocarditis prophylaxis is reasonable for patients with a cardiac condition listed above include the following:
- • All dental procedures that involve manipulation of gingival tissue or the periapical region of teeth or perforation of the oral mucosa. These procedures include biopsies, suture removal, and placement of orthodontic bands.
- • The following procedures and events **do not** require prophylaxis: routine anesthetic injections through noninfected tissue, taking dental radiographs, placement of removable prosthodontic or orthodontic appliances, adjustment of orthodontic appliances, placement of orthodontic brackets, shedding of deciduous teeth, and bleeding from trauma to the lips or oral mucosa.

In addition, antibiotic prophylaxis is reasonable for the patients with cardiac conditions listed above who undergo an invasive procedure of the respiratory tract that involves incision or biopsy of the respiratory tract mucosa.

NEONATAL OPHTHALMIA

Ophthalmia neonatorum is defined as conjunctivitis occurring within the first 4 weeks after birth. Infection usually is transmitted during passage through the birth canal. The causes and clinical characteristics of ophthalmia neonatorum are presented in Table 5.4. Neonates with ophthalmia neonatorum require clinical evaluation with appropriate laboratory testing and prompt initiation of specific therapy if an infectious etiology is identified.

Primary Prevention

The current primary strategy for prevention of neonatal ophthalmia is based on ante-partum identification and treatment of maternal infection, preventing exposure of the newborn infant. The Centers for Disease Control and Prevention (CDC) recommends routine first-trimester screening for chlamydia and gonorrhea in all pregnant women aged 24 years or younger and older women at high-risk (having new or multiple sex partners, having a sex partner with other concurrent partners, having a sex partner with a sexually transmitted infection). Additional risk factors for gonorrhea screening in pregnant women include inconsistent condom use among people who are not in mutually monogamous relationships, previous or coexisting sexually transmitted infections, exchanging sex for money or drugs, or living in an area with a high prevalence of *Neisseria gonorrhoeae*. Because determining high-risk status in pregnant women (with the exception of age) may be difficult, consideration of screening all pregnant women for *Chlamydia trachomatis* and *N gonorrhoeae* at the first prenatal visit is reasonable, especially in areas of high prevalence of either pathogen (**www.cdc.gov/std/ Gonorrhea/**; **www.cdc.gov/std/chlamydia/default.htm**). In addition, the CDC advises rescreening for chlamydia and gonorrhea during the third trimester for all women at high risk as defined above, including all females younger than 25 years. Women in whom chlamydial infection is diagnosed during the first trimester should receive a test of cure to document chlamydial eradication approximately 4 weeks after treatment and should be retested 3 months after treatment. Women in whom gonorrhea is diagnosed should be treated immediately and rescreened within 3 months. If a pregnant woman has not been tested for *C trachomatis* and/or *N gonorrhoeae* before labor/delivery, she should be tested during labor/delivery or immediately postpartum. If either pathogen is identified, the infant should receive therapy as outlined in the following sections.

Secondary Prevention

POSTEXPOSURE SYSTEMIC ANTIBIOTIC PROPHYLAXIS

To block transmission of infection, healthy infants born to women with untreated or inadequately treated gonococcal infection should receive 1 dose of ceftriaxone (25–50 mg/kg, intravenously [IV] or intramuscularly [IM], not to exceed 125 mg). Ceftriaxone should be administered cautiously to hyperbilirubinemic infants, especially those born prematurely. For infants in whom ceftriaxone is contraindicated (eg, receiving continuous intravenous calcium, as in parenteral nutrition), then 1 dose of cefotaxime (100 mg/kg, IV or IM) or 1 dose of gentamicin (2.5 mg/kg, IV or IM) can

Table 5.4. Major and Minor Etiologies in Ophthalmia Neonatorum

Etiology of Ophthalmia Neonatorum	Proportion of Cases	Incubation Period (Days)	Severity of Conjunctivitis[a]	Associated Problems
Chlamydia trachomatis	2%–40%	5–12	+	Pneumonitis 3 wk–3 mo (see Chlamydial Infections, p 256)
Neisseria gonorrhoeae	Less than 1%	2–5	+++	Disseminated infection (see Gonococcal Infections, p 338)
Pseudomonas aeruginosa	Less than 1%	5–28	+++	Sepsis, meningitis
Other bacterial microbes[b]	30%–50%	5–14	+	Variable
Herpes simplex virus	Less than 1%	6–14	+	Disseminated infection, meningoencephalitis (see Herpes Simplex, p 407); keratitis and ulceration also possible
Chemical	Varies with silver nitrate use	1	+	...

[a] + indicates mild; +++, severe.
[b] Includes skin, respiratory, vaginal and gastrointestinal tract pathogens such as *Staphylococcus aureus*; *Streptococcus pneumoniae*; *Haemophilus influenzae*, nontypeable; group A and B streptococci; *Corynebacterium* species; *Moraxella catarrhalis*; *Escherichia coli*; and *Klebsiella pneumoniae*.

be substituted for postexposure prophylaxis. Other extended-spectrum cephalosporins should be effective, although studies have not been performed. Note that gentamicin should not be used as treatment of neonates with gonococcal ocular disease attributable to inadequate penetration into the globe of the eye. Topical antimicrobial therapy alone is inadequate for *N gonorrhoeae*-exposed or infected infants and is not necessary when systemic antimicrobial therapy is administered

Infants born to mothers known to have untreated chlamydial infection are at high risk of infection; however, prophylactic antimicrobial treatment is not indicated because the efficacy of such treatment is unknown. Infants should be monitored clinically to ensure appropriate treatment if infection develops. If adequate follow-up cannot be ensured, preemptive therapy should be considered.

ROUTINE TOPICAL NEONATAL OPHTHALMIC PROPHYLAXIS

If gonorrhea is prevalent in the region and prenatal treatment cannot be ensured, or where required by law, a prophylactic agent of 0.5% erythromycin ointment should be instilled into the eyes of all newborn infants (including those born by cesarean delivery)

to prevent sight-threatening gonococcal ophthalmia. Efficacy is unlikely to be influenced by delaying prophylaxis for as long as 1 hour to facilitate parent-infant bonding. Longer delays have not been studied for efficacy. Hospitals should establish processes to ensure that infants are given prophylaxis appropriately. Before administering local prophylaxis, each eyelid should be wiped gently with sterile cotton. A 1-cm ribbon of 0.5% erythromycin ointment should then be placed in each lower conjunctival sac. Ideally ointment should be applied using single-use tubes or ampules rather than multiple-use tubes. The eyelids should then be massaged gently to spread the ointment. After 1 minute, excess ointment may be wiped away with sterile cotton. The ointment should not be flushed from the eyes after instillation, because flushing can decrease efficacy.

Periodic shortages of erythromycin ointment have occurred in recent years. If erythromycin ointment is not available, azithromycin ophthalmic solution 1% is recommended as an acceptable substitute. One to two drops of this product are placed in each conjunctival sac. Because it is a solution rather than an ointment, care must be taken to ensure the drops are placed properly. The CDC recommends that 2 people provide the prophylaxis—1 to hold the lids open and the other to instill the drops. If azithromycin ophthalmic solution 1% is not available, ciprofloxacin ophthalmic ointment 0.3% can be considered as a less suitable alternative. In most cases, potential resistance of *N gonorrhoeae* to ciprofloxacin will be overcome by the high concentrations of ciprofloxacin achieved.

Legal Mandates for Topical Prophylaxis for Neonatal Ophthalmia

Because prophylaxis with topical antimicrobial agents is highly effective in preventing blindness from gonococcal neonatal ophthalmia, it has been mandated by law in many jurisdictions. These mandates have been abandoned in many countries over the last several decades but remain in force in nearly all of the United States. The necessity for mandatory eye prophylaxis in this country has been questioned, primarily because rates of intrapartum exposure to gonorrhea have been greatly reduced by prenatal screening and treatment of maternal disease. Increasing resistance of gonococcal isolates has cast doubt on the continued efficacy of erythromycin, which is not effective for prevention of ophthalmia of other etiologies, including *C trachomatis*. When neonatal ophthalmia does develop, effective therapies are readily available, and sequelae (including loss of vision) now are exceedingly rare. Countries with well-organized systems of prenatal care, including Canada, have recommended elimination of eye prophylaxis. Resurgence either of cases of gonococcal ophthalmia neonatorum or of blindness from that condition has not been reported. The American Academy of Pediatrics supports reevaluation of the continued necessity of legislative mandates in the United States for universal neonatal eye prophylaxis, and advocates for legislation that allows adoption of alternative strategies to prevent neonatal ophthalmia on the basis of the following steps:

- Diligent compliance with CDC recommendations for prenatal screening for and treatment of *N gonorrhoeae* and *C trachomatis* to prevent intrapartum exposures.
- Testing of unscreened women for *N gonorrhoeae* and *C trachomatis* infection at the time of labor or delivery, with treatment of infected women and their infants.

- Counseling of parents to bring conjunctival discharge and inflammation to immediate medical attention resulting in optimal treatment of neonatal ophthalmia.
- Education of newborn care providers to ensure awareness that purulent conjunctivitis in a newborn infant requires thorough diagnostic evaluation and prompt specific treatment.
- Continuation of mandatory reporting of cases of gonococcal ophthalmia neonatorum to identify patterns of failure of primary prevention measures.

In regions where gonorrhea remains prevalent and prenatal screening and treatment is not routinely achievable, neonatal topical prophylaxis remains appropriate.

Pseudomonal Ophthalmia

Neonatal ophthalmia attributable to *Pseudomonas aeruginosa* is infrequent but may now be at least as common as gonococcal ophthalmia. This form of neonatal ophthalmia has a predilection for preterm infants and presents with eyelid edema and erythema, purulent discharge, and pannus formation. Because superficial infection can progress rapidly to corneal perforation, endophthalmitis, blindness, serious systemic infection (sepsis, meningitis), and death, this form of bacterial neonatal ophthalmia urgently requires a combination of systemic and topical therapy, because systemic antibiotics alone have poor penetration in the anterior chamber of the eye. The diagnosis should be suspected when Gram-stained specimens of exudate contain gram-negative bacilli, and should be confirmed by culture. Until *Pseudomonas* infection is excluded, evaluation for systemic infection and topical and systemic therapy are recommended. Ophthalmology consultation is also recommended.

Other Nongonococcal, Nonchlamydial Ophthalmia

Neonatal ophthalmia can be caused by many other bacterial pathogens (see Table 5.4). In general, uncomplicated resolution can be expected with topical treatment of these infections.

Herpes simplex keratoconjunctivitis should be considered in neonates with conjunctival inflammation and discharge, particularly when tests for bacterial and chlamydial infection are negative. The diagnosis should be suspected if there are also cutaneous vesicles or oral ulcers or vesicles and can be confirmed by demonstration of dendritic keratitis (requiring ophthalmology consultation for examination with fluorescein staining), or by virologic testing (eg, polymerase chain reaction assay or culture). Specific treatment is indicated (see Herpes Simplex, p 407). Conjunctivitis caused by other viruses generally resolves without specific treatment.

....
APPENDIX I

Directory of Resources[a]

Organization	Telephone/Fax Number	Web Site
AIDSinfo	1-800-HIV-0440 (1-800-448-0440, US) 1-301-315-2816 (Outside US) TTY: 1-888-480-3739 Fax: 1-301-315-2818	www.hivinfo.nih.gov
American Academy of Pediatrics (AAP)	1-630-626-6000 1-800-433-9016 Fax: 1-847-434-8000 Publications/Customer Service: 1-866-THE AAP1 (1-866-843-2271)	www.aap.org
American Sexual Health Association	1-919-361-8400 Fax: 1-919-361-8425	www.ashasexualhealth.org
Canadian Paediatric Society (CPS)	1-613-526-9397 Fax: 1-613-526-3332	www.cps.ca
Centers for Disease Control and Prevention (CDC)	1-800-CDC-INFO (1-800-232-4636) TTY: 1-888-232-6348	www.cdc.gov www.cdc.gov/contact/ wwwn.cdc.gov/dcs/ContactUs/Form
CDC Emergency Operations Center (24-Hour Service)	1-770-488-7100	
Advisory Committee on Immunization Practices		www.cdc.gov/vaccines/acip

Directory of Resources[a], continued

Organization	Telephone/Fax Number	Web Site
Botulism case consultation and antitoxin	1-770-488-7100	www.cdc.gov/botulism/health-professional.html
Division of Foodborne, Waterborne, and Environmental Diseases		www.cdc.gov/ncezid/dfwed
Division of Healthcare Quality Promotion	1-404-639-4000	www.cdc.gov/ncezid/dhqp/index.html
Division of High-Consequence Pathogens and Pathology	1-404-639-3574	www.cdc.gov/ncezid/dhcpp
Division of Tuberculosis Elimination	1-404-639-8120	www.cdc.gov/tb
Division of Vector-Borne Diseases	1-970-221-6400	www.cdc.gov/ncezid/dvbd
Division of Viral Hepatitis		www.cdc.gov/hepatitis/index.htm
Drug Service	1-404-639-3670 (business hours) 1-770-488-7100 (after hours) Fax: 404-639-3717	www.cdc.gov/laboratory/drugservice
Influenza		www.cdc.gov/flu
Malaria Hotline	1-770-488-7788 1-855-856-4713 (toll free) 1-770-488-7100 (after hours)	www.cdc.gov/malaria
National Prevention Information Network	1-800-458-5231	https://npin.cdc.gov
Parasitic Diseases Branch	1-404-718-4745	www.cdc.gov/parasites
Travelers' Health	1-877-394-8747	wwwnc.cdc.gov/travel
Vaccines and Immunizations		www.cdc.gov/vaccines

Directory of Resources,[a] continued

Organization	Telephone/Fax Number	Web Site
Vaccine Information Statements		www.cdc.gov/vaccines/hcp/vis/index.html
Vaccines for Children Program		www.cdc.gov/vaccines/programs/vfc/index.html
Vaccine Safety		www.cdc.gov/vaccinesafety/index.html
Food and Drug Administration (FDA)	1-888-INFO-FDA (1-888-463-6332)	www.fda.gov
Drugs	1-855-543-3784 1-301-796-3400	www.fda.gov/drugs
Pediatrics		www.fda.gov/science-research/science-and-research-special-topics/pediatrics
Vaccines, Blood, and Biologics	1-800-835-4709 1-240-402-8010	www.fda.gov/BiologicsBloodVaccines/default.htm
MedWatch	1-800-FDA-1088 (1-800-332-1088)	www.fda.gov/safety/medwatch-fda-safety-information-and-adverse-event-reporting-program
Vaccine Adverse Event Reporting System (VAERS)	1-800-822-7967 Fax: 1-877-721-0366	https://vaers.hhs.gov/index.html

Directory of Resources,[a] continued

Organization	Telephone/Fax Number	Web Site
FDA-Approved Vaccine Package Inserts		www.fda.gov/vaccines-blood-biologics/vaccines/vaccines-licensed-use-united-states
Immunization Action Coalition (IAC)	1-651-647-9009 Fax: 1-651-647-9131	www.immunize.org
Infectious Diseases Society of America (IDSA)	1-703-299-0200 Fax: 1-703-299-0204	www.idsociety.org
Institute for Vaccine Safety		www.vaccinesafety.edu
National Academy of Medicine (formerly the Institute of Medicine)	1-202-334-2000	https://nam.edu
National Institutes of Health (NIH)	1-301-496-4000 TTY: 1-301-402-9612	www.nih.gov
Eunice Kennedy Shriver National Institute of Child Health and Human Development	1-800-370-2943 Fax: 1-866-760-5947	www.nichd.nih.gov
National Institute of Allergy and Infectious Diseases (NIAID)	1-301-496-5717 1-866-284-4107 TDD: 1-800-877-8339 Fax: 1-301-402-3573	www.niaid.nih.gov
National Library of Medicine	1-888-346-3656	www.nlm.nih.gov
National Resource Center for Health and Safety in Child Care and Early Education	888-227-5125	nrckids.org

Directory of Resources,[a] continued

Organization	Telephone/Fax Number	Web Site
National Vaccine Injury Compensation Program	1-800-338-2382	www.hrsa.gov/vaccinecompensation/index.html
National Vaccine Program Office (NVPO)	1-202-690-5566	www.hhs.gov/nvpo
Parents of Kids with Infectious Diseases (PKIDS)		www.pkids.org
Pediatric Oncology Branch, Center for Cancer Research, National Cancer Institute	1-240-760-6560	https://ccr.cancer.gov/Pediatric-Oncology-Branch
Pediatric Infectious Diseases Society	1-703-299-6764 Fax: 1-703-299-0473	www.pids.org
Sociedad Latinoamericana de Infectologia Pediátrica (SLIPE)		www.slipe.org
Vaccine Education Center of the Children's Hospital of Pennsylvania		www.chop.edu/centers-programs/vaccine-education-center
Voices for Vaccines	1-678-870-5877	www.voicesforvaccines.org
World Health Organization (WHO)	(+41 22) 791 21 11 Regional Office for the Americas: 1-202-974-3000 Fax: 1-202-974-3663	www.who.int

[a] Internet addresses and telephone/fax numbers are current at the time of publication.

....

APPENDIX II

Codes for Commonly Administered Pediatric Vaccines/ Toxoids and Immune Globulins

Vaccine, toxoid, and Immune Globulin codes use a specific vaccine *Current Procedural Terminology* (CPT) code to indicate which immunization product was administered to the patient. A regularly updated listing of CPT product codes for commonly administered pediatric vaccines can be found at **www.aap.org/en-us/Documents/coding_vaccine_coding_table.pdf.**

CPT codes for vaccine administrations are reported in addition to the CPT codes for specific vaccines and toxoid products. Codes 90460 and 90461 are only reported when the physician or other qualified health care professional provides face-to-face counseling during the encounter when a vaccine is administered to a patient through 18 years of age. The 90460 code should be used for each vaccine administered. For vaccines with multiple components, code 90460 should be reported in conjunction with code 90461 for each additional component in a given vaccine (eg, DTaP administration would include 90460 x 1 and 90461 x 2). Multivalent antigens or multiple serotypes of antigens against a single organism are considered a single component of vaccines (eg, PCV-13 administration should use only one 90460). Without counseling by the physician or qualified healthcare professional, the administration codes 90471– 90474 are used, depending on the number of vaccines administered and the route of administration.

ICD-10-CM has only a single diagnosis code for reporting vaccines, Z23. When reporting vaccines administered, ICD-10 requires use of code Z23 regardless of the reason for the encounter. For example, if vaccines are given as part of a childhood preventive care visit, code Z23 should be reported in addition to code Z00.121 (encounter for routine child health examination).

Immune Globulin products are not considered vaccines, and the administration code 96372, therapeutic injection given intramuscularly or subcutaneously, should be used. For Rabies Immune Globulin and rabies vaccine administration, code Z20.3 (contact with and [suspected] exposure to rabies) should be reported as well as the ICD-10-CM codes describing the nature of the injuries and circumstances surrounding the injury, including type of animal involved (ie, codes found in the V-Y categories). The ICD-10 code Z29.14, encounter for prophylactic rabies immunoglobulin, can also be used. For RSV Immune Globulin, palivizumab, the appropriate ICD-10-CM diagnoses of gestational age and/or other medical condition(s) that support the need to administer palivizumab, should be reported.

······················
APPENDIX III

Nationally Notifiable Infectious Diseases in the United States

Nationally notifiable infectious diseases are those that public health officials from local, state, and territorial public health departments voluntarily report to the Centers for Disease Control and Prevention (CDC). Surveillance for nationally notifiable infectious diseases helps public health agencies monitor the occurrence and spread of disease across the nation and evaluate prevention and control measures, among other purposes. To ensure consistency in how the data are classified and enumerated, national surveillance case definitions are established and used for each disease. The Council of State and Territorial Epidemiologists (CSTE), with advice from the CDC, reviews the list of nationally notifiable infectious diseases on an annual basis and may recommend that a disease be added or deleted from the list or that a case definition be revised. Provisional nationally notifiable infectious disease data are published in weekly tables and finalized data are published in annual tables, available from the "Data and Statistics" section of the National Notifiable Diseases Surveillance System website (**wwwn.cdc.gov/nndss/data-and-statistics.html**). Data on approximately 120 nationally notifiable diseases, most of which are infectious diseases, are reported to the CDC from all states, Washington DC, New York City, and five US territories on either a daily or weekly basis. A subset of cases that meet the criteria for being a potential public health emergency of international concern, as per the 2015 revised International Health Regulations (**www.who.int/ihr/9789241596664/en/**), are notified by the CDC's Emergency Operations Center to the Department of Health and Human Services Secretaries Operations Center, which in turn notifies the World Health Organization. The World Health Organization makes the final determination about whether a public health emergency of international concern exists. The 2019 list of nationally notifiable infectious diseases is included in Table 1. Should a more current list of such diseases be needed, visit **wwwn.cdc.gov/nndss/conditions/.**

Nationally notifiable infectious disease reports are based on data collected at the local, state, and territorial levels as a result of legislation and regulations in those jurisdictions that require health care providers, clinical laboratories, hospitals, and other entities to submit health-related data on reportable diseases to public health departments. Case reporting to local, state, or territorial public health officials provides them the information needed to investigate these diseases and to implement prevention and control strategies, among other purposes. Because the list of reportable infectious diseases is determined by local, state, and territorial law and varies by jurisdiction, health care providers, clinical laboratories, hospitals, and other required reporters are strongly encouraged to obtain specific reporting requirements from the appropriate public health department, including the timeliness required for case reporting.

If a reportable disease meets the criteria for a nationally notifiable infectious disease, the local, state, or territorial public health department will submit a case notification to the CDC. The timeliness of such case notifications to the CDC varies by disease, with some requiring notification within 4 hours of a case meeting the notification criteria.

Table 1. Infectious Diseases and Conditions Designated as Notifiable at the National Level—United States, 2020[1,2]

- Anthrax
- Arboviral diseases, neuroinvasive, and nonneuroinvasive
  - California serogroup virus diseases
  - Chikungunya virus disease
  - Eastern equine encephalitis virus disease
  - Powassan virus disease
  - St. Louis encephalitis virus disease
  - West Nile virus disease
  - Western equine encephalitis virus disease
- Babesiosis
- Botulism
  - Botulism, foodborne
  - Botulism, infant
  - Botulism, wound
  - Botulism, other
- Brucellosis
- Campylobacteriosis
- *Candida auris*, clinical
- Carbapenemase-producing carbapenem-resistant *Enterobacteriaceae* (CP-CRE)
  - CP-CRE, *Enterobacter* species
  - CP-CRE, *Escherichia coli* (*E coli*)
  - CP-CRE, *Klebsiella* species
- Chancroid
- *Chlamydia trachomatis* infection
- Cholera
- Coccidioidomycosis
- Congenital syphilis
  - Syphilitic stillbirth
- Coronavirus disease 2019 (COVID-19)
- Cryptosporidiosis
- Cyclosporiasis

- Dengue virus infections
  - Dengue
  - Dengue-like illness
  - Severe dengue
- Diphtheria
- Ehrlichiosis and Anaplasmosis
  - *Anaplasma phagocytophilum* infection
  - *Ehrlichia chaffeensis* infection
  - *Ehrlichia ewingii* infection
  - Undetermined human ehrlichiosis/anaplasmosis
- Giardiasis
- Gonorrhea
- *Haemophilus influenzae*, invasive disease
- Hansen's disease
- Hantavirus infection, non-Hantavirus pulmonary syndrome
- Hantavirus pulmonary syndrome
- Hemolytic uremic syndrome, postdiarrheal
- Hepatitis A, acute
- Hepatitis B, acute
- Hepatitis B, chronic
- Hepatitis B, perinatal virus infection
- Hepatitis C, acute
- Hepatitis C, chronic
- Hepatitis C, perinatal infection
- HIV infection (AIDS has been reclassified as HIV Stage III)
- Influenza-associated pediatric mortality
- Invasive pneumococcal disease
- Legionellosis
- Leptospirosis

- Listeriosis
- Lyme disease
- Malaria
- Measles
- Meningococcal disease
- Mumps
- Novel influenza A virus infections
- Pertussis
- Plague
- Poliomyelitis, paralytic
- Poliovirus infection, nonparalytic
- Psittacosis
- Q fever
  - Q fever, acute
  - Q fever, chronic
- Rabies, animal
- Rabies, human
- Rubella
- Rubella, congenital syndrome
- *Salmonella* Paratyphi infection (*Salmonella enterica* serotypes Paratyphi A, B [tartrate negative], and C [*S* Paratyphi])
- *Salmonella* Typhi infection (*Salmonella enterica* serotype Typhi)
- Salmonellosis
- Severe acute respiratory syndrome-associated coronavirus disease
- Shiga toxin-producing *Escherichia coli*
- Shigellosis
- Smallpox
- Spotted fever rickettsiosis
- Streptococcal toxic shock syndrome
- Syphilis
  - Syphilis, primary
  - Syphilis, secondary

[1]wwwn.cdc.gov/nndss/conditions/notifiable/2020/infectious-diseases/

[2]wwwn.cdc.gov/nndss/data-and-statistics.html

- Syphilis, early non-primary non-secondary
- Syphilis, unknown duration or late
- Tetanus
- Toxic shock syndrome (other than streptococcal)
- Trichinellosis
- Tuberculosis
- Tularemia
- Vancomycin-intermediate *Staphylococcus aureus* and vancomycin-resistant *Staphylococcus aureus*

- Varicella
- Varicella deaths
- Vibriosis
- Viral hemorrhagic fever
  - Crimean-Congo hemorrhagic fever virus
  - Ebola virus
  - Lassa virus
  - Lujo virus
  - Marburg virus
  - New World arenavirus – Guanarito virus
  - New World arenavirus – Junin virus

- New World arenavirus – Machupo virus
- New World arenavirus – Sabia virus
- Yellow fever
- Zika virus disease and Zika virus infection
  - Zika virus disease, congenital
  - Zika virus disease, noncongenital
  - Zika virus infection, congenital
  - Zika virus infection, noncongenital

....
APPENDIX IV

Guide to Contraindications and Precautions to Immunizations

A **contraindication** to vaccination is a condition in a patient that increases the risk of a serious adverse reaction and for whom this increased risk of an adverse reaction outweighs the benefit of the vaccine. A vaccine should not be administered when a contraindication is present. The only contraindication applicable to all vaccines is a history of anaphylaxis to a previous dose or to a vaccine component, unless the patient has undergone desensitization. Refer to the Description section of manufacturer's package inserts for components of each vaccine; package inserts for vaccines that are licensed for use in the United States are available at **www.fda.gov/ BiologicsBloodVaccines/Vaccines/ApprovedProducts/ucm093833.htm.** The Centers for Disease Control and Prevention Pink Book (*Epidemiology and Prevention of Vaccine-Preventable Diseases* **www.cdc.gov/vaccines/pubs/pinkbook/genrec. html#contraindications**) also is a helpful resource.

A **precaution** is a condition in a recipient that might increase the risk or seriousness of an adverse reaction, might interfere with vaccine effectiveness, or might complicate making another diagnosis because of a possible vaccine-related reaction. People who administer vaccines should screen recipients for contraindications and precautions before administering vaccines, and this screening should be documented (eg, in the electronic health record). This information is based on recommendations of the Committee on Infectious Diseases of the American Academy of Pediatrics (AAP) and of the Advisory Committee on Immunization Practices (ACIP) of the Centers for Disease Control and Prevention (CDC). Sometimes, these recommendations differ from information in the manufacturers' package inserts.

A table that lists contraindications and precautions for commonly used vaccines can be found at **www.cdc.gov/vaccines/hcp/acip-recs/general-recs/contraindications.pdf** and **www.cdc.gov/vaccines/hcp/admin/ contraindications.html.**

APPENDIX V

Prevention of Infectious Disease From Contaminated Food Products[1]

Foodborne diseases are associated with significant morbidity and mortality in people of all ages. In 2017, the Centers for Disease Control and Prevention (CDC) reported 841 foodborne outbreaks, resulting in roughly 15 000 illnesses, 800 hospitalizations, 20 deaths, and 14 food product recalls (**www.cdc.gov/fdoss/pdf/2017_ foodborneoutbreaks_508.pdf**). Young children, pregnant women, the elderly, and immunocompromised people are especially susceptible to illnesses and complications caused by many of the organisms associated with foodborne illness. Norovirus is the most common cause of outbreaks of foodborne illness in the United States. The system for surveillance and reporting for norovirus outbreaks is known as CaliciNet (**www.cdc.gov/norovirus/reporting/calicinet/index.html**).

The Foodborne Diseases Active Surveillance Network (FoodNet) of the CDC Emerging Infections Program conducts active, population-based surveillance at 10 sites in the United States, for all laboratory-diagnosed infections with select enteric pathogens transmitted commonly through food. The FoodNet program conducts surveillance for illnesses attributable to *Campylobacter* species, *Cyclospora cayetanensis*, *Listeria monocytogenes*, *Salmonella* species, Shiga toxin-producing *Escherichia coli* (STEC) O157 and non-O157 STEC, *Shigella* species, *Vibrio* species, and *Yersinia enterocolitica*. FoodNet also conducts surveillance for hemolytic-uremic syndrome (HUS), a complication of STEC infection. In 2019, compared with the previous 3 years, the incidence of infections caused by pathogens transmitted commonly through food increased (for *Campylobacter*, *Cyclospora*, STEC, *Vibrio*, *Yersinia*) or remained unchanged (for *Listeria*, *Salmonella*, *Shigella*).[2] Additional information about FoodNet can be found at **www.cdc. gov/foodnet/index.html**.

Outbreak surveillance provides insights into the causes of foodborne illness, types of implicated foods, and settings where transmission occurs. The CDC collects data on foodborne disease outbreaks submitted from all states and territories (**www.cdc. gov/foodsafety/fdoss/index.html**). Public health, regulatory, and agricultural professionals can use this information when creating targeted control strategies and to support efforts to promote safe food preparation practices among food industry employees and the public. Data on foodborne disease outbreaks are available online through the National Outbreak Reporting System Dashboard (**wwwn.cdc.gov/ norsdashboard**).

Four general rules should be followed for food safety:

1. **Clean:** Wash hands and surfaces thoroughly and often.
2. **Separate:** Do not cross-contaminate.

---

[1]Centers for Disease Control and Prevention. Diagnosis and management of foodborne illnesses: a primer for physicians. *MMWR Recomm Rep.* 2004;53(RR-4):1–33

[2]Tack DM, Ray L, Griffin PM, et al. Preliminary incidence and trends of infections with pathogens transmitted commonly through food—Foodborne Diseases Active Surveillance Network, 10 U.S. Sites, 2016–2019. *MMWR Morb Mortal Wkly Rep.* 2020;69(17):509-514. DOI: **http://dx.doi.org/10.15585/ mmwr.mm6917a1**

3. **Chill:** Refrigerate foods promptly.
4. **Cook:** Prepare and heat food to the proper temperature.

The following preventive measures can be implemented to decrease the risk of infection from specific foods.

UNPASTEURIZED MILK AND MILK PRODUCTS

The American Academy of Pediatrics (AAP) endorses the use of pasteurized milk and recommends that parents be fully informed of the important risks associated with consumption of unpasteurized milk.[1] Interstate sale of unpasteurized (raw) milk and products made from unpasteurized milk (with the exception of certain hard cheeses) is banned by the US Food and Drug Administration (FDA). The most vulnerable populations, such as children, pregnant women, elderly people, and immunocompromised people, should not consume unpasteurized milk or products made from unpasteurized milk, including cheese, butter, yogurt, pudding, or ice cream, from any species, including cows, sheep, and goats. Serious infections attributable to *Salmonella* species, *Campylobacter* species, *Mycobacterium bovis*, *L monocytogenes*, *Brucella* species, STEC O157, *Y enterocolitica*, and *Cryptosporidium parvum* have been linked to consumption of unpasteurized milk. Although some states allow the sale of raw milk that meets state-designated arbitrary standard (certified milk), "certified" raw milk has also been linked to outbreaks. A number of outbreaks of *Campylobacter* infection among children have been associated with school field trips to farms during which children consumed raw milk. School officials should take precautions to prevent raw milk from being served to children during educational trips. Cheeses made from unpasteurized milk also have been associated with illnesses attributable to *Brucella* species, *L monocytogenes*, *Salmonella* species, *Campylobacter* species, *Shigella* species, *M bovis*, and STEC.

RAW AND UNDERCOOKED EGGS

Children and other groups at high risk of severe foodborne disease should not eat raw or undercooked eggs, unpasteurized powdered eggs, or foods that may contain raw or undercooked eggs. Ingestion of raw or improperly cooked eggs can result in severe illness attributable to *Salmonella* species. Examples of foods that may contain raw or undercooked eggs include some homemade frostings and mayonnaise, homemade ice cream, tiramisu, eggs prepared "sunny-side up," Caesar salad dressing, Hollandaise sauce, cookie dough, and cake batter.

RAW DOUGH

Children should not eat raw dough, including unbaked goods such as cookies, tortillas, pizza, biscuits, or pancakes. Children should not play with raw dough, such as at home for crafts or at restaurants. Several regional outbreaks have been linked to STEC present in raw flour. Cookie dough in ice cream sold commercially has been treated to prevent transmission of pathogens.

---

[1] American Academy of Pediatrics, Committee on Infectious Diseases and Committee on Nutrition. Consumption of raw or unpasteurized milk and milk products by pregnant women and children. *Pediatrics.* 2014;133(1):175-179

RAW AND UNDERCOOKED MEAT

Children should not eat raw or undercooked meat or meat products. Various raw or undercooked meat products can commonly harbor harmful bacteria, including STEC, *Salmonella* species, and *Campylobacter* species. Specific meat products have been linked with certain infections (pathogen-commodity pair): ground beef with STEC and *Salmonella* species; hot dogs with *L monocytogenes*; pork with *Trichinella* species; and wild game with *Brucella* species, *Francisella tularensis*, STEC, *Trichinella* species, and *Toxoplasma gondii*. Ground meats should be cooked to an internal temperature of 160°F; roasts and steaks should be cooked to an internal temperature of 145°F; and poultry should be cooked to an internal temperature of 165°F. Use of a food thermometer is the only accurate means of knowing that meat has reached a high enough temperature to destroy pathogens. Color is not a reliable indicator that ground beef patties have been cooked to a temperature high enough to kill harmful pathogens. Knives, cutting boards, plates, and other utensils used for raw meats should not be used for preparation of fresh fruits or vegetables until they have been cleaned properly (see websites at end of this Appendix for details).

UNPASTEURIZED JUICES

Children should drink only fruit or vegetable juice that has been pasteurized or that has been freshly squeezed from washed fruit or vegetables. Consumption of packaged fruit juices that have not undergone pasteurization or a comparable treatment has been associated with foodborne illness attributable to STEC O157, non-O157 STEC, *Salmonella* species, and *Cryptosporidium parvum*. To identify a packaged juice that has not undergone pasteurization or a comparable treatment, consumers should look for a warning statement that the product has not been pasteurized.

RAW SEED SPROUTS

The CDC has reaffirmed health advisories that people who are at high risk of severe foodborne disease, including children, people with compromised immune systems, pregnant women, and the elderly, should avoid eating raw seed sprouts (including alfalfa sprouts). Raw seed sprouts have been associated with outbreaks of illness attributable to *Salmonella* species, STEC, and *L monocytogenes*, as seed sprouts are grown in warm and humid environments which favor these pathogens.

FRESH FRUITS AND VEGETABLES AND RAW NUTS

Many fresh fruits and vegetables have been associated with disease attributable to *Cryptosporidium* species, *Cyclospora cayetanensis*, norovirus, hepatitis A virus, *Giardia duodenalis*, STEC, *Salmonella* species, *L monocytogenes*, and *Shigella* species. Raw nuts, commercially processed vegetable snacks, spinach, lettuce, tomatoes, cucumbers, melons, basil, and cilantro have been associated with outbreaks of salmonellosis. Nuts that have been roasted or otherwise treated can minimize the risk of foodborne illness. Washing can decrease bacterial contamination of fresh fruits and vegetables. Knives, cutting boards, utensils, and plates used for raw meats should not be used for preparation of fresh fruits or vegetables until the utensils have been cleaned properly (see websites at end of this Appendix for details).

RAW SHELLFISH AND FISH

Children should not eat raw shellfish. Raw shellfish, including mussels, clams, oysters, scallops, and other mollusks, can carry many pathogens, including norovirus, *Vibrio* species, and hepatitis A virus as well as foodborne toxins (see Appendix VI, p 1041). *Vibrio* species contaminating raw shellfish may cause severe disease in people with liver disease or other conditions associated with decreased immune function. *Vibrio* species abundance appears to be increasing because of sea surface warming, thus posing increasing concern for these infections. Some experts caution against children ingesting raw fish, which has been associated with transmission of helminths (eg, *Anisakis simplex, Diphyllobothrium latum*).

HONEY

Children younger than 1 year should not be given honey. Honey has been shown to contain spores of *Clostridium botulinum*, the agent of botulism.

POWDERED INFANT FORMULA

For many reasons, infants should be fed human milk rather than infant formula whenever possible. Powdered infant formula is not a sterile product and has been associated with severe illnesses attributable to *Cronobacter sakazakii* and *Salmonella* species. If infant formula must be used, caregivers can reduce the risk of infection by choosing sterile, liquid formula products rather than powdered products. This may be particularly important for those at greatest risk of severe infection, such as neonates and infants with immunocompromising conditions. Otherwise, water used for mixing infant formula must be from a safe water source, as defined by the state or local health department. If there are concerns or uncertainty about the safety of tap water, bottled water or cold tap water that has been brought to a rolling boil for 1 minute, then cooled to room temperature for no more than 30 minutes, may be used.

Prepared formula (including ready-to-feed products) must be discarded within 1 hour after serving to an infant. Prepared formula made from powder that has not been given to an infant may be stored in the refrigerator for 24 hours.

FOOD IRRADIATION[1]

Irradiation of food can be an effective tool to control foodborne pathogens. Irradiation involves exposing food briefly to ionizing radiation (eg, gamma rays, x-rays, or high-voltage electrons). More than 40 countries worldwide, including the United States, have approved the use of irradiation for various types of foods. Every governmental and professional organization that has reviewed the efficacy and safety of food irradiation has endorsed its use. Meat, spices, shell eggs, seeds for sprouting, and some produce items may be irradiated for sale in the United States. The risk of foodborne illness could be decreased significantly with the routine consumption of irradiated meat, poultry, and produce.

In addition to the websites previously cited in this section, detailed information on food safety issues and practices, including steps which consumers can take to protect themselves, is available on the following web sites:

- **www.foodsafety.gov**
- **www.cdc.gov/foodsafety**
- **www.fightbac.org**
- **www.fda.gov/food/resources-you-food**

---

[1]**www.fsis.usda.gov/wps/portal/fsis/topics/food-safety-education/get-answers/
food-safety-fact-sheets/production-and-inspection/irradiation-resources/
irradiation-resources**

·····················

APPENDIX VI

Clinical Syndromes Associated With Foodborne Diseases[1,2]

Foodborne disease results from consumption of contaminated foods or beverages and causes morbidity and mortality in children and adults. The epidemiology of foodborne disease is complex and dynamic because of numerous possible pathogens, the variety of disease manifestations, the increasing prevalence of immunocompromised children and adults, dietary habit changes, and trends toward centralized food production and widespread distribution. The cultural diversity of foods and food practices and international travel are also likely impacting the epidemiology of foodborne disease. Widespread availability of multiplex molecular diagnostic tests for gastrointestinal illness may lead to co-identification of multiple potential pathogens, complicating evaluation and treatment of diarrhea.

Consideration of a foodborne etiology is important in any patient with a gastrointestinal tract illness, as well as those with certain acute neurologic findings. Obtaining a detailed history is essential to assess time of onset and duration of symptoms, history of recent travel or antimicrobial use, food and water exposures, and presence of blood or mucus in stool. To aid in diagnosis, foodborne disease syndromes have been categorized by incubation period, predominant symptoms (other symptoms also occur), causative agent, and foods commonly associated with specific etiologic agents (food vehicles) (see Table 1; also **www.cdc.gov/foodsafety/outbreaks/investi-gating-outbreaks/confirming_diagnosis.html**). Diagnosis can be confirmed by laboratory testing of stool, vomitus, or blood, depending on the causative agent. Infectious Diseases Society of America Clinical Practice Guidelines for the Diagnosis and Management of Infectious Diarrhea can be found at **https://academic.oup.com/cid/article/65/12/e45/4557073.**

Sporadic (ie, non–outbreak-associated) cases account for the majority of foodborne illnesses. In localized outbreaks that affect individuals who shared a common meal, the incubation period can be estimated. In more widely dispersed outbreaks and in sporadic cases, the incubation period typically is unknown.

An outbreak should be considered when 2 or more people who have ingested the same food develop an acute illness characterized by nausea, vomiting, diarrhea, or neurologic signs or symptoms. If an outbreak is suspected, public health officials should be notified immediately to initiate an epidemiologic investigation, including diagnostic and management interventions, to curtail the outbreak.

---

[1]Centers for Disease Control and Prevention. Surveillance for foodborne-disease outbreaks—United States, 2008. *MMWR Morb Mortal Wkly Rep.* 2011;60(35):1197-1202. Additional information can be found at **www.cdc.gov/foodsafety** and **www.fsis.usda.gov/wps/portal/fsis/home**

[2]Centers for Disease Control and Prevention. Surveillance for foodborne disease outbreaks—United States, 1998–2008. *MMWR Morb Mortal Wkly Rep.* 2013;62(SS-2):1-34

Table 1. Clinical Syndromes Associated With Foodborne Diseases

Clinical Syndrome	Incubation Period	Causative Agents	Commonly Associated Vehicles[a]
Nausea and vomiting	2–4 h	*Staphylococcus aureus* (preformed enterotoxins, A through V but excluding F)	Food contaminated by infected food handler that is not cooked or is improperly cooked and stored, including ham, poultry, beef, cream-filled pastries, potato and egg salads, mushrooms, unpasteurized cheese
	<1–6 h	Preformed *Bacillus cereus* (emetic toxin cereulide)	Contaminated food that is improperly stored after cooking, including rice
	<1 h	Heavy metals (copper, tin, cadmium, iron, zinc)	Acidic beverages, metallic container
	1 h	Vomitoxin (deoxynivalenol)	Foods made from grains such as wheat, corn, barley
	12–48 h	Astrovirus	Bivalve mollusks grown in polluted waters, fresh produce (greens, berries) irrigated with contaminated water, food contaminated by infected food handler that is not cooked or is improperly cooked and stored (ready-to-eat salads/sandwiches)
Flushing, dizziness, burning of mouth and throat, headache, gastrointestinal tract symptoms, urticaria and generalized pruritis	<1 h	Histamine (scombroid toxin)	Fish (bluefish, bonita, mackerel, mahi-mahi, marlin, tuna, skipjack, and many other fish types)
Usually gastrointestinal symptoms followed by neurologic symptoms (including facial and extremity paresthesias) and reversal of hot and cold temperature sensation (characteristic of ciguatera toxin)	2–8 h[b] (can be up to 48 h)	Ciguatera toxin	Large reef-dwelling carnivorous fish (eg, amberjack, barracuda, grouper, snapper)
	Up to 18 h[c]	Neurotoxic shellfish toxin (brevetoxin)	Shellfish (eg, mussels, oysters, clams)

Table 1. Clinical Syndromes Associated With Foodborne Diseases, continued

Clinical Syndrome	Incubation Period	Causative Agents	Commonly Associated Vehicles[a]
Symptoms similar to ciguatera and neurotoxic shellfish toxin, plus short-term memory loss	1 day[b]	Domoic acid (amnesic shellfish toxin)	Mussels, clams
Neurologic, including confusion, salivation, hallucinations; gastrointestinal tract manifestations	0–2 h	Mushroom toxins (short-acting)	Mushrooms
Neuromuscular weakness, symmetric descending paralysis, respiratory weakness, neurologic symptoms may be preceded by gastrointestinal tract manifestations	12–48 h	Clostridium botulinum (preformed toxin)	Home-canned vegetables, fruits and fish, salted fish, meats, bottled garlic, potatoes baked in aluminum foil, cheese sauce
Neurologic, constipation in infant younger than 1 y	3–30 days	Clostridium botulinum (ingestion of spores with production of toxin in the intestine)	Honey
Neurologic, gastrointestinal tract[b]	10–45 min	Tetrodotoxin (ascending paralysis)	Puffer fish
	0.5–3 h	Paralytic shellfish toxins (saxitoxins, etc)	Shellfish (clams, mussels, oysters, scallops, other mollusks)
Abdominal cramps and watery diarrhea, vomiting	6–24 h	Bacillus cereus (diarrheal enterotoxin)	Meats, stews, gravies, vanilla sauce
	6–24 h	Clostridium perfringens	Meat, poultry, gravy, dried or precooked foods
	12–48 h	Norovirus	Feces-contaminated shellfish, salads, ice, cookies, water, sandwiches, fruit, leafy vegetables, ready-to-eat foods handled by infected food worker
	1–3 days	Rotavirus	Feces-contaminated salads, fruits, ready-to-eat foods handled by infected food worker

Table 1. Clinical Syndromes Associated With Foodborne Diseases, continued

Clinical Syndrome	Incubation Period	Causative Agents	Commonly Associated Vehicles[a]
Abdominal cramps, watery diarrhea	6–48 h	Enterotoxigenic *Escherichia coli*	Feces-contaminated seafood, herbs, fruits, vegetables, water, often acquired abroad—"travelers' diarrhea"
	Unknown	*Listeria monocytogenes*	Soft cheeses, raw milk, hot dogs, cole slaw, ready-to-eat delicatessen meats, produce (eg, sprouts, cantaloupe)
	4–30 h	*Vibrio parahaemolyticus*	Shellfish, especially oysters
	12–72 h	*Vibrio vulnificus*	Shellfish, especially oysters
	1–5 days	*Vibrio cholerae* O1 and O139	Shellfish (including crabs and shrimp), fish, water
	1–5 days	*V cholerae* non-O1	Shellfish, especially oysters
	1–14 days	*Cyclospora* species	Raspberries, vegetables, fresh herbs, water
	2–28 days	*Cryptosporidium* species	Vegetables, fruits, milk, water, in particular recreational water exposures
	1–3 weeks	*Giardia duodenalis*	Water, ready-to-eat foods handled by infected food worker
Diarrhea, fever, abdominal cramps, blood and mucus in stools, bacteremia	6–48 h	*Salmonella* species (nontyphoidal)	Poultry; pork; beef; eggs; dairy products, including ice cream; raw vegetables, alfalfa sprouts; fruit, including unpasteurized juices; peanut butter
	2–4 days	*Shigella* species	Feces-contaminated lettuce-based salads, potato and egg salads, salsas, dips, and oysters, ready-to-eat foods handled by infected food worker
	7–14 days	*Salmonella* Typhi	Food contaminated by infected food handler (acutely ill or chronic carrier
	2–4 wk	Amebiasis (*Entameba histolytica*)	Feces-contaminated food or water

Table 1. Clinical Syndromes Associated With Foodborne Diseases, continued

Clinical Syndrome	Incubation Period	Causative Agents	Commonly Associated Vehicles[a]
Bloody diarrhea, abdominal cramps, hemolytic-uremic syndrome (HUS)	1–10 days	Shiga toxin-producing *E coli* (STEC)	Undercooked beef (hamburger); raw milk; roast beef; salami; salad dressings; lettuce and other leafy greens; game meats, unpasteurized juices, including apple cider; sprouts; water
Febrile diarrhea or; especially in older children, abdominal pain resembling that of appendicitis	4–6 days	*Yersinia enterocolitica*	Pork chitterlings, tofu, milk
Hepatorenal failure, watery diarrhea	6–24 h	Mushroom toxins (long-acting)	Mushrooms (especially *Amanita* species)
Other extraintestinal manifestations (fever, myalgias, arthralgias, fatigue)	Varied, up to months (usually >30 days)	*Brucella* species	Goat cheese, queso fresco, raw milk, meats
Fever, chills, headache, pharyngitis, arthralgia	1–4 days	Group A *Streptococcus*	Egg and potato salad, pasta
Fever, malaise, anorexia, jaundice	15–50 days	Hepatitis A virus	Shellfish, raw produce (eg, strawberries, lettuce, green onions)
Meningoencephalitis, sepsis, fetal loss	2–6 wk	*Listeria monocytogenes*	Soft cheeses, raw milk, hot dogs, coleslaw, ready-to eat delicatessen meats, produce (eg, sprouts, cantaloupe)
Muscle soreness and pain	Varied, up to 4 wk	*Trichinella spiralis*	Wild game, pork, meat

Table 1. Clinical Syndromes Associated With Foodborne Diseases, continued

Clinical Syndrome	Incubation Period	Causative Agents	Commonly Associated Vehicles[a]
Fever, lymphadenopathy, encephalitis, retinitis (may be reactivation disease for the latter two)	5–23 days	Toxoplasma gondii	Undercooked meat (especially pork, lamb, and game meat), fruits, vegetables, raw shellfish
Sepsis, meningitis among infants	Unknown	Cronobacter sakazakii	Powdered infant formula
	Unknown	Salmonella species	Powdered infant formula
Seizures, behavioral disturbances, and other neurologic signs and symptoms	Months	Taenia solium (neurocysticercosis)	Food contaminated with feces from a human carrier of adult pork tapeworm
Epigastric discomfort, abdominal pain, cholangitis, obstructive jaundice, pancreatitis	Varied (several days to months)	Clonorchis sinensis (liver fluke); Opisthorchis species (liver fluke)	Eating raw or undercooked infected freshwater fish, crabs, crayfish
Guillain-Barré syndrome (ascending paralysis)	2–10 days	Campylobacter species Shigella Enteroinvasive E coli Yersinia enterocolitica Vibrio parahaemolyticus	Poultry, raw milk, water Feces-contaminated food or water Vegetables, hamburger, raw milk Pork chitterlings, tofu, raw milk Fish, shellfish

Table 1. Clinical Syndromes Associated With Foodborne Diseases, continued

Clinical Syndrome	Incubation Period	Causative Agents	Commonly Associated Vehicles[a]
Postdiarrheal HUS (acute renal failure, hemolytic anemia, thrombocytopenia)	7 days–2 wk after onset of diarrhea	Shiga toxin-producing *E coli* (especially serotype O157:H7), or shiga-toxin 2-producing strains of non-O157 *E coli*	Beef (hamburger); raw milk; roast beef; salami; salad dressings; lettuce and other leafy greens; unpasteurized juices, including apple cider; alfalfa and radish sprouts; water
	1–5 days after onset of diarrhea	*Shigella dysenteriae* type 1	Water, milk, other contaminated food, rare in the United States
Reactive arthritis	Varies	*Campylobacter* species	Poultry, raw milk, water
	Varies	*Salmonella* species	Poultry, pork, beef, eggs, dairy products, including ice cream; vegetables (alfalfa sprouts and fresh produce); fruit, including unpasteurized juices; peanut butter
	Varies	*Shigella* species	Feces-contaminated food or water
	Varies	*Yersinia enterocolitica*	Pork chitterlings, tofu, raw milk

[a] List of vehicles in several categories is not exhaustive, because any number of foods can be contaminated; current online literature may be helpful to sort through commonly associated vehicles.

[b] See **www.cdc.gov/habs/illness-symptoms-marine.html**

[c] See **https://emergency.cdc.gov/agent/brevetoxin/casedef.asp**

APPENDIX VII

Diseases Transmitted by Animals (Zoonoses)

Morbidity resulting from selected zoonotic diseases in the United States is reported annually by the Centers for Disease Control and Prevention (see "Summary of Notifiable Diseases" at **www.cdc.gov/mmwr/mmwr_nd/**). Information also can be obtained via the website of the National Center for Emerging and Zoonotic Infectious Diseases (**www.cdc.gov/ncezid/about-ncezid.html**) or through the main Centers for Disease Control and Prevention website (**www.cdc.gov**).

Table. Diseases Transmitted by Animals

Disease and/or Organism	Animal Sources/Reservoirs	Vector or Modes of Transmission
Bacterial Diseases		
Aeromonas species	Aquatic animals, especially shellfish, medical leeches; has also been isolated from feces of horses, pigs, sheep, and cows	Wound infection, ingestion of contaminated food or water, direct contact with infected animal or their environment
Anthrax (*Bacillus anthracis*)	Herbivores (cattle, goats, horses, sheep) Outbreaks associated with heavy rainfall, flooding, or drought; spores remain viable in soil or animal products, such as wool or hides, for decades	Direct contact with infected animals or their carcasses, or contact with products from infected animals (eg, meat, hides, hair, or wool) contaminated with *B anthracis*; ingestion of contaminated meat, inhalation of contaminated dust
Bartonellosis (*Bartonella quintana; Bartonella baciliformis*)	Cats, dogs, ruminants, rodents, human body louse	Bites from human body louse, sand flies
Brucellosis (*Brucella* species)	Cattle, coyotes, hares, chickens, goats, sheep, pigs, dogs, elk, bison, deer, camels, desert rats and other rodents, marine mammals	Direct or indirect contact with aborted fetuses, tissues, or fluids of infected animals; inoculation through mucous membranes or cuts or abrasions of the skin; inhalation of contaminated aerosols; ingestion of unpasteurized dairy products
Campylobacteriosis (*Campylobacter jejuni*)	Poultry, dogs (especially puppies), kittens, ferrets, pigs, nonhuman primates, pet rodents, cattle, sheep, birds	Ingestion of contaminated food or water, direct contact (particularly with animals with diarrhea), person-to-person (fecal-oral), fomites
Capnocytophaga canimorsus	Dogs, rarely cats	Bites, scratches, and prolonged contact with dogs
Cat-scratch disease (*Bartonella henselae*)	Cats and other felids, infrequently other animals (less than 10%)	Scratches, bites; fleas play a role in cat-to-cat transmission (evidence for transmission from cat fleas to humans is lacking)

Table. Diseases Transmitted by Animals, continued

Disease and/or Organism	Animal Sources/Reservoirs	Vector or Modes of Transmission
Erysipeloid (*Erysipelothrix rhusiopathiae*)	Pigs, horses, dogs, cats, rats, sheep, cattle, wild and domestic birds (including poultry), fresh and saltwater fish, shellfish	Direct contact with animal or contaminated animal product, or water
Hemolytic-uremic syndrome (eg, Shiga toxin-producing *Escherichia coli*) (STEC)	Cattle, sheep, goats, deer, dogs, pigs, and poultry	Ingestion of undercooked contaminated ground beef, unpasteurized milk, or other contaminated foods (eg, alfalfa sprouts and other vegetable products, mayonnaise, apple cider, and cheddar) or water; contact with infected animals or their environments (eg, farms and ranches); contact with animals in public settings including petting zoos and agricultural fairs (fecal-oral)
Leptospirosis (*Leptospira* species)	Cattle, sheep, goats, pigs, horses, dogs, rodents, and all other mammals, but rare in cats	Contact with or ingestion of water, food, or soil contaminated with urine or fluids from rodents or other infected animals, or direct contact with infected animals or their organs
Lyme disease (*Borrelia burgdorferi, Borrelia mayonii*)	White-footed mice, squirrels, shrews, and other small rodents; opossums, raccoons, birds; white-tailed deer	Tick bite (blacklegged/deer tick [*Ixodes scapularis* or *Ixodes pacificus*] in United States, castor bean tick [*Ixodes ricinus*] in Europe)
Mycobacterium marinum	Found in brackish water, fresh water, and saltwater; fish (and cleaning aquaria)	Contaminated water sources; skin injury or contamination of existing wound
Mycobacterium bovis and *Mycobacterium tuberculosis*	Cattle, elephants, giraffes, rhinoceroses, bison, deer, elk, feral pigs, badgers, possums, nonhuman primates	*M tuberculosis* is uncommon in nonhuman species, although when it is identified it is typically found in nonhuman primates and elephants Sporadic cases of *M tuberculosis* have been reported in other species, including cattle Transmission is by the airborne route

Table. Diseases Transmitted by Animals, continued

Disease and/or Organism	Animal Sources/Reservoirs	Vector or Modes of Transmission
Pasteurellosis (*Pasteurella multocida*)	Cats, dogs, rabbits, pigs, other animals, birds	Bites, scratches, licks, saliva, respiratory droplets from animals (primarily cats and dogs), and contaminated meat
Plague (*Yersinia pestis*)	Rodents, (eg, prairie dogs, chipmunks, squirrels, mice, voles, rats) cats, dogs, rabbits, wild carnivores (eg, bobcats, coyotes)	Bite of infected rodent fleas (especially Oriental rat fleas-*Xenopsylla cheopis*); in United States, most common vector is *Oropsylla montana*, a flea found on rodents including prairie dogs and squirrels; direct contact with infected animal tissues, airborne from other human or animal (eg, cat) with pneumonic plague
Q fever (*Coxiella burnetii*)	Sheep, goats, cows, cats, dogs, rabbits, rodents, horses, pigs, buffalo, camels, pigeons, geese, other wild fowl, ticks	Contact with excreta (birth products, urine, feces, milk) of infected animals, inhalation of pathogen-contaminated dust, ingestion of unpasteurized milk, and fomite transmission; (possible role of ticks not well defined); rarely by blood transfusions, sexual contact in humans, or from a pregnant woman to her fetus
Rat-bite fever (*Streptobacillus moniliformis*, *Spirillum minus*)	Rodents (especially rats, occasionally squirrels), gerbils	Bites, scratched, contact with secretions, aerosol spread, direct contact with rodent; contaminated food or water; unpasteurized, contaminated milk
Relapsing fever (tickborne) (*Borrelia* species)	Wild rodents	Soft tick bites (*Ornithodoros* species); bites from blacklegged ticks (*I scapularis* and *I pacificus*) transmit *B miyamotoi*
Salmonellosis (*Salmonella* species)	Cattle, poultry, turtles, frogs, lizards, snakes, salamanders, geckos, iguanas, fish, invertebrates, dogs, cats, pigs, sheep, horses, hedgehogs, hamsters, guinea pigs, mice, rats and other rodents, ferrets, other wild and domestic animals	Fecal-oral transmission most common; ingestion of contaminated food (eg, meat, poultry, dairy, eggs, produce, processed foods), unpasteurized milk and other raw dairy products, or contaminated water; contact with infected animals or their environments (including healthy reptiles); contaminated animal products including dry dog and cat food and pet treats

Table. Diseases Transmitted by Animals, continued

Disease and/or Organism	Animal Sources/Reservoirs	Vector or Modes of Transmission
Streptococcus iniae	Fish from many regions of the world	Skin wound during handling and preparation of infected fish
Tetanus (*Clostridium tetani*)	Any animal indirectly via soil containing animal feces	Wound infection, skin injury or soft tissue injury with inoculation of bacteria (as from soil or a contaminated object)
Tularemia (*Francisella tularensis*)	Sheep, dogs, cats, pigs, horses, wild rabbits, hares, voles, squirrels, beaver, lemmings, muskrats, moles, hamsters, birds, reptiles, and fish	Tick bites (wood tick [*Dermacentor andersoni*], dog tick [*D variabilis*], Lone-star tick bites [*Amblyomma americanum*]), deerfly bites; direct contact with infected animal, ingestion of contaminated water or meat, mechanical transmission from claws or teeth (cats/dogs), aerosolization of tissues or excreta
Vibrio species	Shellfish	Ingestion of contaminated food or water; skin injury or contamination of existing wound
Yersiniosis (*Yersinia enterocolitica, Yersinia pseudotuberculosis*)	Pigs, deer, elk, horses, goats, sheep, cattle, rodents, birds, rabbits	Ingestion of contaminated food (particularly raw or undercooked pork products), raw or unpasteurized milk or other dairy products, contaminated water; rarely direct contact
Fungal Diseases		
Cryptococcosis (*Cryptococcus neoformans*)	Excreta of birds, including pigeons, canaries, parakeets, and chickens	Inhalation of aerosols from accumulations of bird feces; can also be isolated from fruit and vegetables, house dust, air conditioners; air; and sawdust; can enter body through skin as well as inhalation
Histoplasmosis (*Histoplasma capsulatum*)	Excreta of bats, birds such as pigeons and starlings	Inhalation of aerosolized spores from accumulations of bat or bird feces, spores can also be ingested
Ringworm/tinea corporis (*Microsporum* and *Trichophyton* species)	Cats, dogs, chickens, pigs, mice, moles, horses, rodents, cattle, monkeys, goats	Direct contact; pathogenic fungi found worldwide; hot and humid climates generally increase incidence

Table. Diseases Transmitted by Animals, continued

Disease and/or Organism	Animal Sources/Reservoirs	Vector or Modes of Transmission
Parasitic Diseases		
Angiostrongylus cantonensis (rat lungworm)	Rodents and mollusks (eg, slugs and snails)	Ingestion of larvae in raw or undercooked snails or slugs, freshwater shrimp, land crabs, frogs or on contaminated raw produce
Anisakiasis (*Anisakis* species) (herring worm disease)	Crustaceans eat infective larvae from marine mammal feces; fish or squid eat the infected crustaceans.	Ingestion of larvae in raw or undercooked fish or squid (eg, sushi)
Babesiosis (several *Babesia* species)	Mice and various other rodents and small mammals; wildlife	Tick bite (in the United States, *Babesia microti* is transmitted mainly by *I scapularis*; in Europe, *Babesia divergens* is mainly transmitted by *Ixodes* tick bites)
Balantidiasis (*Balantidium coli*)	Pigs	Ingestion of contaminated food or water
Baylisascariasis (*Baylisascaris procyonis*)	Raccoons	Ingestion of eggs shed in raccoon feces found in dirt or animal waste
Clonorchiasis/Opisthorchiasis (*Clonorchis/Opisthorchis* species)	Fish, crabs, crayfish, snails, cats, dogs	Ingestion of metacercariae in raw or undercooked fish, crabs, or crayfish
Cryptosporidiosis (*Cryptosporidium* species)	*Cryptosporidium parvum* can infect all mammals; common in calves and other young ruminants; seen in pigs, rarely occurs in cats, dogs, and horses; other cryptosporidium species can infect birds and reptiles	Fecal-oral route; ingestion of contaminated water (especially groundwater) or foods; infection by inhaling aerosols can also occur
Cutaneous larva migrans [primarily *Ancylostoma* species hookworms]]	Dogs, cats	Penetration of skin by larvae, which develop in soil contaminated with animal feces

Table. Diseases Transmitted by Animals, continued

Disease and/or Organism	Animal Sources/Reservoirs	Vector or Modes of Transmission
Dog tapeworm (*Dipylidium caninum*)	Dogs are definitive hosts; cats and other animals (eg, foxes) can also be hosts	Ingestion of fleas infected with cysticercoid stage
Dwarf tapeworm (*Hymenolepis nana*) and rat tapeworm (*Hymenolepis diminuta*)	Rodents (humans are more important reservoirs than rodents for *H nana*; for *H diminuta*, rodents are primary and human infection is infrequent); arthropods including beetles and fleas can serve as intermediate hosts	Ingestion of eggs in contaminated food or water; animal-to-person (fecal-oral); person-to-person (fecal-oral); infection can occur after ingestion of cysticercoid-infected arthropods. Autoinfection may also occur in humans if eggs remain in intestine (*H nana*)
Echinococcosis, hydatid disease (*Echinococcus* species)	Definitive hosts are canids including dogs, coyotes, foxes, dingoes, jackals, hyenas, and wolves. Intermediate hosts encompass many domestic and wild animals, including herbivores such as sheep, goats, cattle, and deer	Ingestion of eggs shed in animal feces
Fascioliasis (*Fasciola* species)	Sheep, cattle	Ingestion of larvae in contaminated water, in raw watercress and other contaminated water plants, or eating raw or undercooked sheep or goat liver
Fish tapeworm (*Diphyllobothrium latum*)	Saltwater and freshwater fish	Ingestion of larvae in raw or undercooked fish (eg, sushi)
Giardiasis (*Giardia duodenalis*)	Wild and domestic animals, including dogs, cats, cattle, pigs, beavers, muskrats, rats, pet rodents, rabbits, nonhuman primates	Ingestion of contaminated water or foods, and animal-to-person (fecal-oral)

Table. Diseases Transmitted by Animals, continued

Disease and/or Organism	Animal Sources/Reservoirs	Vector or Modes of Transmission
Myiasis (*Dermatobia, Cochliomyia, Chrysomya, Cuterebra,* and *Wohlfahrtia* species)	Flies	Exposure of flies to broken or wounded skin; with *Chrysomya* screwworm flies, exposure of flies to unbroken soft skin
Taeniasis/beef tapeworm (*Taenia saginata*)	Cattle (intermediate host)	Ingestion of larvae in raw or undercooked beef; cysticercosis in cattle is caused by ingestion of embryonated eggs excreted by humans with *Taenia* infection
Taeniasis and cysticercosis/pork tapeworm (*Taenia solium; Taenia asiatica* less common)	Pigs (intermediate host)	Ingestion of larvae in raw or undercooked pork resulting in intestinal infection in humans with adult tapeworms (taeniasis); porcine cysticercosis (infection in pigs) is caused by ingestion of embryonated eggs excreted by humans with *Taenia* infection, human cysticercosis is caused by ingestion of eggs through fecal contamination of food or water, or by autoinfection
Toxoplasmosis (*Toxoplasma gondii*)	Members of the Felidae family (including domestic cats) are definitive hosts; many mammals (eg, sheep, goats, and swine) and birds can serve as intermediate hosts	Transmission can be foodborne, zoonotic, congenital, or in rare instances through organ transplantation. Zoonotic transmission can occur through ingestion of infective oocysts from hands after cleaning litter boxes or gardening (soil), or ingestion of vegetables/low growing fruits, or ingestion of anything that has become contaminated with cat feces; consumption of cysts in raw or undercooked meat (such as lamb, pork, venison) or shellfish (clams, mussels, oysters) Drinking unpasteurized goat milk; drinking contaminated water
Trichinellosis (*Trichinella spiralis* and other *Trichinella* species)	Pigs, bears, seals, walruses, rodents, horses, foxes, wolves	Ingestion of larvae in raw or undercooked meat, particularly pork or wild game meat

Table. Diseases Transmitted by Animals, continued

Disease and/or Organism	Animal Sources/Reservoirs	Vector or Modes of Transmission
Ocular or visceral toxocariasis/larva migrans (*Toxocara canis* and *Toxocara cati*)	Dogs, cats; puppies are a major source of environmental contamination	Ingestion of infected, larvated eggs, usually from soil, dirty hands, or food contaminated by animal feces
Chlamydial and Rickettsial Diseases		
Human ehrlichiosis (*Ehrlichia chaffeensis, Ehrlichia ewingii,* and *Ehrlichia muris eauclairensis*)	Dogs, red foxes, deer, coyotes, goats, and lemurs (*E chaffeensis*); dogs may be reservoir hosts along with wolves and jackals (*Ehrlichia canis* and *E ewingii*)	Tick bites (Lone star tick [*Amblyomma americanum*] for *E chaffensis, E ewingii*; blacklegged tick [*I scapularis*] for *E muris eauclairensis*); in rare cases *Ehrlichia* species have been spread through blood transfusion and organ transplantation
Human anaplasmosis (*Anaplasma phagocytophilum*)	Small mammals including wood rats and deer mice; deer may also be involved.	Tick bites (*I scapularis* and *I pacificus*)
Psittacosis (*Chlamydia psittaci*)	Most birds (especially psittacine birds such as parakeets, parrots, macaws, and cockatoos) and poultry	Inhalation of aerosols from feces of infected birds as well as fecal-oral transmission.
Rickettsialpox (*Rickettsia akari*)	House mice	Mite bites (house mouse mite, *Liponyssoides sanguineus*)
Rocky Mountain spotted fever (*Rickettsia rickettsii*)	Dogs, wild rodents, rabbits	Tick bites (American dog tick, *Dermacentor variabilis*; Rocky Mountain wood tick, *D andersoni*; and brown dog tick, *Rhipicephalus sanguineus*)
Rickettsia parkeri infection (maculatum disease, American boutonneuse fever)	Unknown; perhaps cattle, dogs, small wild rodents	Tick bites (Gulf coast tick [*Amblyomma maculatum*])
Typhus, fleaborne endemic typhus, Murine typhus (*Rickettsia typhi*)	Rats, opossums, cats, dogs	Infected flea feces scratched into abrasions; oriental rat fleas (*Xenopsylla cheopis*) and cat fleas (*Ctenocephalides felis*) are vectors.

Table. Diseases Transmitted by Animals, continued

Disease and/or Organism	Animal Sources/Reservoirs	Vector or Modes of Transmission
Typhus, louseborne epidemic typhus (*Rickettsia prowazekii*)	Flying squirrels (sylvatic typhus)	Person-to-person via infected body louse, contact with flying squirrels, their nests, or ectoparasites (role and species of ectoparasites undefined)
Viral Diseases		
B virus (formerly herpes B, monkey B virus, herpesvirus simiae, or herpesvirus B)	Macaque monkeys	Bite or exposure to secretions or tissues
Colorado tick fever virus	Rodents (eg, squirrels, chipmunks)	Tick bites (Rocky Mountain wood tick [*Dermacentor andersoni*])
Crimean Congo hemorrhagic fever (nairovirus)	Many wild and domestic animals including cattle, hares, goats, sheep	Infectious blood and body fluids from animal slaughter; Ixodid (hard) ticks, genus *Hyalomma*, are reservoir and vector; person-to-person via contact (droplet, contact) with infectious blood or body fluids; improperly sterilized medical equipment
Eastern equine encephalitis virus	Birds	Mosquito bites (*Coquillettidia* species, *Aedes* species, *Culex* species, *Ochlerotatus* species), rarely through organ transplantation
Ebola virus	Fruit bats; nonhuman primates may become infected	Direct contact through broken skin or mucous membranes (eyes, nose, mouth) with blood or body fluids, contaminated needles, prolonged presence in semen of infected individuals (possible sexual transmission), infected fruit bats or nonhuman primates
Hantaviruses	Wild and peridomestic rodents	Inhalation of aerosols of infected secreta and excreta; contact with infected rodents or infected droppings and urine
Hendra virus	Flying foxes (*Pteropus* genus) are the natural reservoir; horses can become infected	Contact with body fluids of infected horses, close contact with fruit bats

Table. Diseases Transmitted by Animals, continued

Disease and/or Organism	Animal Sources/Reservoirs	Vector or Modes of Transmission
Novel influenza (eg, H5N1, H7N9, H9N2, H3N2 variant)	Chickens, birds, pigs	Contact with infected animals or aerosols (markets, slaughterhouse)
Jamestown Canyon virus	Deer	Mosquito bites (*Aedes* species, *Anopheles* species, and *Culiseta* species)
Japanese encephalitis virus	Pigs, birds	Mosquito bites (*Culex tritaeniorhynchus*)
Kyasanur forest disease/Alkhurma hemorrhagic fever	Monkeys, rodents, and shrews are common hosts after being bitten by infected ticks	Primarily tick bites (*Haemaphysalis spinigera*), contact with infected animal
La Crosse virus	Rodents (eg, chipmunks and squirrels)	Mosquito bites (*Aedes triseriatus*)
Lassa fever	Multimammate rat (*Mastomys natalensis*)	Inhalation of aerosols or direct contact with infected secreta or excreta; consumption of food contaminated by rodents
Lymphocytic choriomeningitis virus	Rodents, particularly house mice and pet hamsters (includes feeder rodents used as reptile food), guinea pigs	Direct contact, inhalation of aerosols, ingestion of food contaminated with rodent excreta
Marburg hemorrhagic fever	African fruit bat (*Rousettus aegyptiacus*), infected nonhuman primates	Contact with fruit bats or their excreta (eg, entering caves or mines inhabited by bats); contact with infectious blood or tissue of infected monkeys
Middle East Respiratory Syndrome (MERS coronavirus)	Uncertain, virus found in camels in several countries	Respiratory droplets from infected individuals (possible airborne transmission in some cases), direct contact
Monkeypox	Natural reservoir unknown; African rodent species play a role in transmission	Animal-to-human direct contact, bite, or scratch; contact with infected body fluids or contaminated bedding

Table. Diseases Transmitted by Animals, continued

Disease and/or Organism	Animal Sources/Reservoirs	Vector or Modes of Transmission
Nipah virus	Fruit bats; pigs can become infected	Close contact with bats, consumption of bat contaminated fruit/sap; direct contact with infected pigs
Omsk hemorrhagic fever	Infected rodents including muskrats and voles	Handling infected muskrats (eg, hunting, trapping, skinning), and bites from infected ticks (*Dermacentor reticulatus*, *Ixodes persulcatus*, *Dermacentor marginatus*)
Orf (pox virus of sheep)	Sheep, goats and occasionally other ruminants	Contact with infected saliva, infected fomites
Powassan virus	Small to medium-sized rodents (eg, groundhogs, squirrels, mice)	Tick bites (*Ixodes cookei*, *Ixodes marxi*, *I scapularis*) and rarely blood transfusion
Rabies (Lyssavirus)	In the United States, primarily mammalian wildlife (bats, raccoons, skunks, foxes, coyotes, mongooses) or, less frequently, domestic animals (dogs, cats, cattle, horses, sheep, goats, ferrets)	Bites; rarely contact of open wounds, abrasions (including scratches), or mucous membranes with saliva or other infectious materials (eg, neural tissue), corneal and organ transplantation
Rift Valley fever	Domesticated livestock (eg, cattle, sheep, goats, buffalo, and camels)	Contact with blood, body fluids or tissues of infected animals. Bites from infected mosquitoes; rarely bites from other insects with virus on their mouthparts
Severe acute respiratory virus-1 (SARS-CoV-1)	Bats, civet cats, potentially other animal species	Respiratory droplets (airborne transmission believed to occur in some cases), direct contact
Severe acute respiratory virus-2 (SARS-CoV-2)	Unknown	Respiratory droplets and aerosols

Table. Diseases Transmitted by Animals, continued

Disease and/or Organism	Animal Sources/Reservoirs	Vector or Modes of Transmission
South American arenaviruses (Junin, Machupo, Guanarito, Sabia, Chapare, Lujo)	Rodents	Inhalation of aerosols of infected secretions or excreta, consumption of food or water contaminated with infected secretions or excreta, direct contact of abraded or broken skin with rodent excrement
St Louis encephalitis virus	Birds	Mosquito bites (*Culex* species) and rarely blood transfusion
Tickborne encephalitis virus	Small rodents are primary reservoirs; large animals such as cows, goats and sheep become infected but do not play a role in virus maintenance	Tick bites (*Ixodes* species); consumption of infected raw milk products, and rarely blood transfusion or organ transplantation
Venezuelan equine encephalitis virus	Sylvatic rodents, possibly birds; horses are dead-end hosts	Mosquito bites (*Aedes* species, *Anopheles* species, *Culex* species, *Deinocerites* species, *Mansonia* species, and *Psorophora* species)
West Nile virus	Birds	Mosquito bites (*Culex* species) and rarely, blood transfusion, organ transplantation
Western equine encephalitis virus	Birds	Mosquito bites (*Culex tarsalis*)
Yellow fever virus	Nonhuman primates	Mosquito bites (*Haemagogus* species, *Sabethes* species, *Aedes* [*Stegomyia*] species)

Index

Page numbers followed by "t" indicate a table. Page numbers followed by "f" indicate a figure.

Fungal diseases, 328, 329–332t. *See also*
   antifungal drugs
   ear infections, 184
   zoonotic, 1052t
Fungi-Fluor test, 535
Fusarium, 329t, 907, 909t
Fusobacterium infections, 333–335
   clinical manifestations, 333
   control measures, 335
   diagnostic tests, 334
   epidemiology, 334
   etiology, 333–334
   isolation precautions, 335
   treatment, 334–335

G

GAE. *See* granulomatous amebic encephalitis
   (GAE)
Galactomannan test, 213–214
Ganciclovir, 936–937t
   cytomegalovirus (CMV), 298
   human herpesvirus 6 and 7, 425
   human herpesvirus 8 (HHV-8), 427
Gangrene, *Haemophilus influenzae* type b (Hib), 345
Gardnerella vaginalis, 575
GAS. *See* group A streptococcal (GAS) infections
Gas gangrene, 269–271
Gastritis, *Helicobacter pylori* infections, 357
Gastrointestinal plague, 592
Gastrointestinal system
   clinical syndromes associated with foodborne
      diseases, 1041, 1042–1047t
   Listeria monocytogenes infections, 478
   preoperative antimicrobial prophylaxis for,
      1015–1016t
GBS. *See* group B streptococcal (GBS) infections;
      Guillain-Barré syndrome (GBS)
Gelatin, allergic reactions to, 53
Generalized febrile illness, arboviruses, 202
Generalized tetanus, 750
Genital herpes, 408
Genital ulcer disease, 900–901t, 903–904t
Genital warts, 902t, 904t
Genitourinary system
   manifestations of *Chlamydia trachomatis,* 260
   preoperative antimicrobial prophylaxis for,
      1016t
   treatment table, 998t
Gentamicin
   brucellosis, 239–240
   dosing for neonates, 880t
   dosing for pediatric patients beyond the
      newborn period, 882t
   Listeria monocytogenes infections, 479
   tularemia, 824

Gentian violet, topical, 928t
Gianotti-Crosti syndrome, 381
Giardia duodenalis, 335–338
   clinical manifestations, 335
   control measures, 337–338
   diagnostic tests, 336
   epidemiology, 336
   etiology, 336
   incubation period, 336
   isolation precautions, 337
Giardiasis, 1054t
   in internationally adopted, refugee, and
      immigrant children, 162
Gingivitis, *Fusobacterium* infections, 333
Gingivostomatitis, 408
Glomerulonephritis
   hepatitis B virus (HBV), 381
   mumps, 538
Gloves, 137
Glucocorticoid therapy, respiratory syncytial virus
      (RSV), 631
Gonococcal infections, 338–344
   clinical manifestations, 338–339
   control measures, 342–344
   diagnostic tests, 340–341
   epidemiology, 339–340
   etiology, 339
   incubation period, 340
   isolation precautions, 342
Gram-negative bacilli, *Enterobacteriaceae* infections,
      312
Granuloma inguinale, 344–345, 901t
   clinical manifestations, 344
   control measures, 345
   diagnostic tests, 345
   epidemiology, 345
   etiology, 345
   incubation period, 345
   isolation precautions, 345
   treatment, 345
Granulomatous amebic encephalitis (GAE), 194,
      196
Grazoprevir, 933t
Griseofulvin
   recommended doses, 916t
   tinea capitis, 757
   tinea corporis, 761
   tinea cruris, 763
Group A Coxsackieviruses, 315–318
Group A streptococcal (GAS) infections, 694–707
   acute rheumatic fever (ARF), 702–705,
      703–705t
   antimicrobial stewardship for, 875
   in child care and school settings, 121
   clinical manifestations, 694–695
   control measures, 706–707

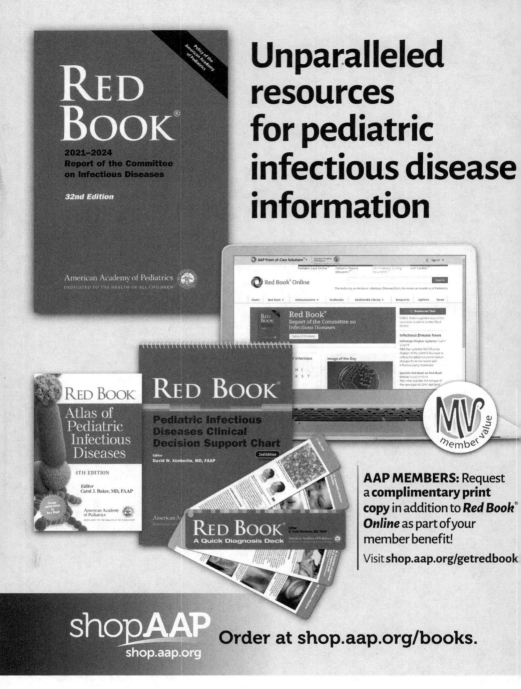